Clinics in Developmental Medicine No. 191–192

CEREBELLAR DISORDERS IN CHILDREN

Clinical in Developmental Medicine No. 191–192

Cerebellar Disorders in Children

Edited by

EUGEN BOLTSHAUSER MD
Professor of Pediatric Neurology, Department of Pediatric Neurology, University Children's Hospital, Zurich, Switzerland

and

JEREMY D. SCHMAHMANN MD
Professor of Neurology, Harvard Medical School; Ataxia Unit, Cognitive and Behavioral Neurology Unit, and Laboratory for Neuroanatomy and Cerebellar Neurobiology, Department of Neurology, Massachusetts General Hospital, Boston, MA, USA

2012
Mac Keith Press

6 Market Road, London N7 9PW

Editor: Hilary M Hart
Managing Director: Caroline Black
Production Manager: Udoka Ohuonu
Project Manager: Mirjana Misuina

First published 2012

British Library Cataloguing-in-Publication data
A catalogue record for this book is available from the British Library

Cover Illustration: Drawing of a flower by an 8-year-old girl with progressive cerebellar atrophy of unknown cause. The diagram is executed with inaccuracy, overshoot, and intention tremor, a consequence of the cerebellar motor syndrome. The figure is overly simplified, more in keeping with the drawing of a much younger child, and represents an excellent effort by a child with deficits in visual-spatial conceptualization and planning, as occurs in the cerebellar cognitive affective syndrome. The panel of magnetic resonance images at bottom in four patients reflects the characteristic features of, from left to right, prenatal Dandy-Walker malformation, cerebellar atrophy, molar tooth sign in Joubert syndrome, and cerebellar agenesis.

ISBN: 978-1-907655-01-2

Printed by TJ International, Padstow, Cornwall, UK
Mac Keith Press is supported by Scope

CONTENTS

Colour plates appear after the index.

AUTHORS' APPOINTMENTS

Annah N. Abrams	Assistant Professor of Psychiatry, Harvard Medical School; Associate Director, Child Psychiatry Consultation Liason Service; Child Psychiatrist, Division of Pediatric Hematology Oncology, Massachusetts General Hospital, Boston MA, USA
Peter G. Barth	Emeritus Professor in Pediatric Neurology, Emma Children's Hospital; Academic Medical Centre, University of Amsterdam, The Netherlands
Peter Baxter	Consultant Paediatric Neurologist, Sheffield Childrens Hospital; Honorary Senior Lecturer, University of Sheffield, Sheffield, UK
Enrico Bertini	Head, Unit of Neuromuscular and Neurodegenerative Disorders, Laboratory of Molecular Medicine, Department of Neurosciences, Bambino Gesu' Children's Research Hospital, Rome, Italy
Eugen Boltshauser	Professor of Pediatric Neurology Department of Pediatric Neurology, University Children's Hospital, Zurich, Switzerland
Francesco Brancati	Research Associate, Medical Genetics Unit, University of Rome Tor Vergata, and CSS Mendel Institute, Rome, Italy
Bruno Dallapiccola	Scientific Director, IRCCS Bambino Gesù Pediatric Hospital, Rome, Italy
Daniel A. Doherty	Associate Professor of Pediatrics, Divisions of Developmental Medicine; Genetic Medicine, University of Washington, Seattle Children's Hospital, Seattle, WA, USA
Tracey D. Graves	Specialist Registrar in Neurology, MRC Centre for Neuromuscular Disease, National Hospital for Neurology and Neurosurgery, London, UK
Michael A. Grotzer	Co-Head Oncology, Head Neuro-Oncology, University Children's Hospital, Zurich, Switzerland
Michael G. Hanna	Professor of Clinicial Neurology, MRC Centre for Neuromuscular Disease, National Hospital for Neurology and Neurosurgery, London, UK
Thierry A.G.M. Huisman	Professor of Radiology and Radiological Science; Director of Pediatric Radiology, Russell H. Morgan Department of Radiology and Radiological Science, Johns Hopkins Hospital, Baltimore, MD, USA
Andrea Klein	Consultant Paediatric Neurologist, Department of Pediatric Neurology, University Children's Hospital, Zurich, Switzerland
Deborah Levine	Professor of Radiology, Department of Radiology, Beth Israel Deaconess Medical Center; Harvard Medical School, Boston MA, USA
Catherine Limperopoulos	Associate Professor of Pediatrics, George Washington University, Division of Diagnostic Imaging and Radiology, Children's National Medical Center, Washington DC, USA
Daune L. Macgregor	Professor of Paediatrics (Neurology), Interim Head, Clinical and Metabolic Genetics, University of Toronto, The Hospital for Sick Children, Toronto, Canada
Kathleen J. Millen	Associate Professor, Seattle Children's Research Institute Center for Integrative Brain Research and The University of Washington Department of Pediatrics, Seattle WA, USA
Patricia L. Musolino	Clinical Fellow in Neurology, Partners Neurology Program; Harvard Medical School, Boston, MA, USA

Andrea H. Nemeth	Consultant in Clinical Genetics, Department of Clinical Genetics, Churchill Hospital; Senior Clinical Research Fellow, Nuffield Laboratory of Ophthalmology, University of Oxford, Oxford, UK
Michael Pike	Consultant Paediatric Neurologist, Children's Hospital, Oxford, UK
Andrea Poretti	Clinical and Research Fellow, Department of Pediatric Neurology, University Children's Hospital, Zurich, Switzerland
Samin A. Sajan	Research Scientist, Seattle Children's Research Institute Center for Integrative Brain Research, Seattle, WA, USA
Michael S. Salman	Paediatric Neurologist, Section of Paediatric Neurology, Children's Hospital; Associate Professor, Faculty of Medicine, University of Manitoba, Winnipeg, Manitoba, Canada
Ianina Scheer	Consultant Paediatric Neuroradiologist, Department of Diagnostic Imaging, University Children's Hospital, Zurich, Switzerland
Jeremy D. Schmahmann	Professor of Neurology, Harvard Medical School; Ataxia Unit, Cognitive and Behavioral Neurology Unit and Laboratory for Neuroanatomy and Cerebellar Neurobiology, Department of Neurology, Massachusetts General Hospital, Boston, MA, USA
Janet C. Sherman	Assistant Professor of Psychology, Harvard Medical School; Director, MGH Psychology Assessment Center; Chief of Neuropsychology, Massachusetts General Hospital; Co-Director, Harvard Consortium Fellowship in Neuropsychology, Massachusetts General Hospital Psychology Assessment Center, Boston, MA, USA
Katherine B. Sims	Associate Professor of Neurology, Harvard Medical School; Director, Neurogenetics DNA Diagnostic Laboratory; Director, Developmental Neurogenetics & Mitochondrial Clinics; Director, Pediatric Neurology Residency Program, Department of Neurology, Massachusetts General Hospital, Boston, MA, USA
Maja Steinlin	Head of Paediatric Neurology, Development and Rehabilitation, Division of Neuropaediatrics, Development and Rehabilitation, University Children's Hospital, Bern, Switzerland
Catherine J. Stoodley	Assistant Professor, Department of Psychology, American University, Washington DC, USA
Marc Tardieu	Professor of Paediatrics (Neurology), University Paris-Sud, Hôpitaux Universitaires Paris Sud, France
Alessandra Terracciano	Post-doctoral Fellow, Unit of Molecular Medicine for Neuromuscular and Neurodegenerative Disorders, Department of Neurosciences, Bambino Gesu' Children's Research Hospital, Rome, Italy
Peter Tsai	Fellow in Behavioural Neurology, Department of Neurology, Children's Hospital Boston; Harvard Medical School, Boston, MA, USA
Enza Maria Valente	Associate Professor of Medical Genetics, University of Messina, Messina; Head of Neurogenetics Unit, CSS-Mendel Institute, Rome, Italy
Kathryn E. Waimey	Program Director, Oncofertility Consortium, Department of Obstetrics and Gynecology, Northwestern University, Chicago, IL, USA
Nicole I. Wolf	Assistant Professor, Department of Child Neurology, VU University Medical Center, Amsterdam, The Netherlands
Ginevra Zanni	Research Scientist in Medical and Molecular Genetics, Unit of Molecular Medicine for Neuromuscular and Neurodegenerative Disorders, Department of Neurosciences, Bambino Gesu' Children's Research Hospital, Rome, Italy

FOREWORD

Many advances have taken place over the past few years in elucidating cerebellar disease in children, from clinical, genetic, neuroimaging and pathological perspectives. Nevertheless, these new data often have been overshadowed by parallel advances in disorders of the cerebral cortex, especially focal dysplasias, because of the increasingly frequent treatment of intractable epilepsy by surgical resection of epileptogenic foci. It is well documented that the cerebellum is much more than a programmed sequencer of coordinated movements with reciprocal contraction or relaxation of antagonistic muscle groups. For example, the cerebellum is not only essential to the rhythm and articulation of speech, but also participates in fluency and structure of language. The cerebellum is a strong suppressor of epileptic foci of the cerebral cortex via intermediate thalamic relay and in the 1970s implanted cerebellar stimulators were used as an early surgical treatment of refractory epilepsy, though later this treatment had to be abandoned because the stimulators caused chronic irreversible focal cerebellar degeneration. These are examples, among many, of the effects of the cerebellum on numerous higher cerebral functions unrelated to motor coordination.

This present reference book fulfills a need for a comprehensive and current update of cerebellar disorders in children. Not only is it comprehensive in scope in terms of the range of disorders that can affect the immature cerebellum, but also in terms of the various integrating disciplines, clinical, neuroimaging, genetic, and pathological. The disorders addressed include genetically-determined and acquired developmental malformations of the cerebellum; acquired lesions of fetal life from vascular, ischaemic and toxic causes, including maternal abuse of alcohol and other drugs; tumors and autoimmune paraneoplastic syndromes; effects of systemic metabolic diseases on the cerebellum; inflammatory lesions, and acute idiopathic ataxias. The hereditary ataxias are conveniently divided into chapters corresponding to Mendelian traits, but incorporate much recent molecular genetic data on specific mutations and deletions. The detailed tables, called 'Checklists' that are provided as an Appendix is a unique feature of great value in summarizing the disorders, including known genetic defects, and provide key references at a glance. The multi-authorship of the various chapters is very impressive as leading contemporary authorities from around the world have been recruited to contribute their expertise.

With the continued intensive research in cerebellar disorders that is currently underway, one can only hope that this book will be republished in a few years as a second edition to include new data not yet available. A larger array of specific genetic mutations will surely be known and perhaps the complex interactions of the many genes that programme the differentiation of granule cells will be elucidated to increase understanding of the rare 'granuloprival' form of cerebellar hypoplasia. New data on recent generations of neuroimaging equipment and functional MRI and PET studies promise to provide greater precision in early diagnosis and help explain pathogenetic mechanisms. Examples of topics to be addressed by neuropathological studies, for which present data are incomplete, include the sequence of synaptogenesis in the cerebellar system, including the Guillain-Mollaret triangle, in normal development as well as in cerebellar dysplasias; the nature of 'cell rests' and dysplastic nodules in the roof of the 4th ventricle of otherwise normal fetuses and preterm infants; the role of posterior fossa leptomeninges in influencing normal and abnormal cerebellar development, perhaps explaining the difference in selective vermal hypoplasia between fusion of the medial cerebellar hemispheres (rhombencephalosynapsis) and a subarachnoid space between them, as in Dandy-Walker malformation and Joubert syndrome; in this regard the high incidence of Dandy-Walker malformation with neurocutaneous melanosis still remains unexplained. The role of resident stem cells in the external granular layer that are capable of regenerating neurons after injury, whether traumatic or metabolic, is another topic of considerable interest with therapeutic implications. These examples of current unresolved issues in paediatric cerebellar disease are not a criticism of this very current update on cerebellar disease; they are presented, rather, to argue why I consider this book is such an excellent candidate for multiple editions in years to come, when new answers become available, balanced always by new queries to be posed for yet further editions. Such is the nature of science and medicine.

Nevertheless, despite the many exciting hypotheses to be proved and new data to discover, for the present this book brings together in a comprehensive manner the current state of knowledge on the topic. The editors are to be commended not only on the scientific quality of the contents, but for the good organization and thorough selection of topics. It is obvious that a great deal of thought has gone into the conceptualization of this outstanding work. This book is an excellent primary reference source for neurologists, paediatricians and resident physicians in treating children with cerebellar disorders.

Harvey B. Sarnat, MS, MD, FRCPC
Professor of Paediatrics, Pathology (Neuropathology) and Clinical Neurosciences
University of Calgary Faculty of Medicine and Alberta Children's Hospital, Calgary, CANADA
September 2011

PREFACE

Hidden under the tentorium and overshadowed by the large mass of the cerebral hemispheres, the cerebellum has long been neglected, regarded as something of an afterthought in clinical neurology. There have been recent advances in structural and functional neuroimaging of the cerebellum, however, and progress has been achieved in prenatal imaging, as well as in molecular genetics, and in the understanding of the neuroanatomy and clinical neurology of cerebellar non-motor functions. All these have contributed greatly to an increased interest in the cerebellum, and a quest for knowledge regarding its clinical phenomenology and underlying neurobiology. As a result, textbooks have been published over the last decade devoted to cerebellar disorders, but focusing principally on disorders of the cerebellum in adults. Many conditions that affect the cerebellum in childhood are distinct from those encountered in the adult population; cerebellar disorders that occur across the age spectrum may have clinical manifestations in children that differ substantially from the expected course in adults; and the approach to the examination of the cerebellar system in the young child has its own particular challenges and principles.

At a symposium on Revising Cerebellum, held in Montreal, Canada in 2006, and again at the annual meeting at the 10th International Child Neurology Congress of the (German-Austrian-Swiss) Society of Neonatology and Paediatric Intensive Care which took place in Zurich, Switzerland in 2008, it became apparent to us that the field of cerebellar neurobiology was ripe for a treatise devoted to an examination of this topic in children.

The distinguishing details of the many childhood cerebellar conditions are complex, and knowledge of their manifestations and long-term outcomes is evolving rapidly. It would be appropriate, we thought, to engage the paediatric neurology community in a discussion of these disorders. Our aim was to share new findings and ideas about the cerebellum in childhood in the hope of contributing to their treatment and encouraging further investigation into their etiology and pathophysiology.

We were therefore pleased to accept the proposal by Dr. Hilary Hart and Dr Peter Baxter, of Mac Keith Press, to edit a volume devoted to cerebellar disorders in the paediatric age group. The result is this first comprehensive textbook on cerebellar disorders in children, covering a wide range of topics including embryology, anatomy, motor and non-motor functions, imaging, and a broad spectrum of genetic as well as acquired disorders.

Part 1 of the book presents an overview of cerebellar development. This is followed in Part 2 by an exposition of cerebellar anatomy and functions, the neurological examination of children with cerebellar disorders, and an approach to the recognition, evaluation and management of clinically relevant cerebellar non-motor functions. Imaging of the cerebellum in health and disease, prenatally as well as in early childhood, is discussed in Part 3. The next sixteen chapters in Part 4 are devoted to cerebellar malformations, including conditions with a malformed cerebellum, some of which have a genetically identified basis, using what is essentially a neuroimaging pattern-recognition approach. We included the heterogeneous group of non-progressive congenital cerebellar ataxias (NPCA) with the malformations even though neuroimaging is often normal, and we did so because of the relationship of NPCA to the cerebellar hypoplasias. The pontocerebellar hypoplasias represent progressive disorders with prenatal onset; these are included in Part 5 that deals with the better known genetic/metabolic disorders involving the cerebellum. We readily acknowledged that the labelling of some disorders as malformative, genetic, or metabolic is sometimes arbitrary, and occasionally based on historical precedent. Part 6 deals with cerebellar disruptions, that is, prenatally acquired destructive lesions. Vascular disorders, tumors and paraneoplastic syndromes are discussed in the four chapters in Part 7. Acute ataxias are discussed in Part 8, and extrinsic insults to the cerebellum, including trauma, toxins and gluten ataxia, are discussed in Part 9. Checklists are presented in the final section, which we hope will be helpful for the clinician faced with the challenge of diagnosing cerebellar disorders in childhood. The reader is referred to the index to assist in locating a specific condition within the book.

This volume would not have been possible without the willing collaboration of many outstanding and internationally renowned clinicians and investigators. We are grateful for their enthusiastic support, and their excellent contributions. We hope this book advances our goal of enhancing interest in the paediatric cerebellum, promotes understanding of, and optimal clinical care for this and patient population. We anticipate that it will also stimulate the next generation of clinicians and investigators to address the unresolved questions that abound in this field.

We gratefully acknowledge the skilful and professional support of the editorial staff at Mac Keith Press – Caroline Black, Udoka Ohuonu, Alessy Beaver, Heather Addison, and

Mirjana Misina; as well as Susanne Staubli for the book cover design. Our research and clinical personnel have provided valuable assistance throughout this project. We are most appreciative of the dedicated efforts of Andrea Poretti, Jason MacMore and Marygrace Neal. This work of JDS in this book was supported in part by grants from the National Institutes of Mental Health, the National Organization for Rare Disorders, the Sidney R. Jr. Baer Foundation, the Massachusetts General Hospital Fund for Medical Discovery, and the ongoing commitment to research in cerebellar neurobiology by the Birmingham Foundation and the MINDlink Foundation.

We are deeply indebted to our wives, to whom this volume is dedicated, Susannne Boltshauser and Jinny Sagorin Schmahmann, for their love, patience and unswerving support for our endeavours on sunny weekends and long nights over the years.

Eugen Boltshauser, Zurich, Switzerland
Jeremy Schmahmann, Boston, Massachusetts, USA
August 2011

About the Editors

Eugen Boltshauser, Professor of Paediatric Neurology at the University of Zurich and the Kinderspital Zurich, is a paediatric neurologist with special interest in cerebellar malformations, prenatal disruptions (i.e., prenatal destructive acquired lesions) and paediatric neuroimaging. He considers the pattern recognition approach an important diagnostic signpost. His interest in the cerebellum was prompted initially by studying patients with Joubert syndrome, a designation he suggested. Over the past three decades he has contributed to the clinical, neuroimaging, and genetic aspects of this syndrome which is at present the best studied hindbrain malformation. Dr. Boltshauser was awarded the Peter-Emil Becker prize of the Society for Neuropaediatrics.

Jeremy D. Schmahmann, Professor of Neurology at Massachusetts General Hospital and Harvard Medical School, is a neurologist and neuroanatomist with a long-standing interest in the care of patients with ataxia and with cognitive disorders, the interactions between cerebellum and cerebral hemispheres, and the role of cerebellum in cognition and emotion. At the Massachusetts General Hospital he is the director of the Ataxia Unit, the Laboratory for Neuroanatomy and Cerebellar Neurobiology, and neurology clerkship, and a member of the Cognitive and the Behavioral Neurology Unit. He serves on the Medical Advisory Board and the Cooperative Ataxia Group of the National Ataxia Foundation. He is a recipient of the Norman Geschwind Prize for research in behavioral neurology, Distinguished Neurology Teacher Award of the American Neurological Association, and he is a Fellow of the American Academy of Neurology and the American Neuropsychiatric Association. Dr. Schmahmann has been recognized for excellence in teaching at Harvard Medical School. Previous books include *The Cerebellum and Cognition* (Academic Press), *MRI Atlas of the Human Cerebellum* (Academic press), and *Fiber Pathways of the Brain* (Oxford University Press).

Part 1
Cerebellar Development

1
Cerebellar Development

Kathryn E. Waimey, Samin A. Sajan,* and Kathleen J. Millen*

Introduction

The mature cerebellum coordinates movement and has additional essential roles in other central nervous system functions including learning, attention, and memory formation (Schmahmann 2004). Since normal cerebellar development is required to achieve normal function, an appreciation of cerebellar development is essential to understand dysfunction. Several features of the cerebellum make it particularly amenable to experimental manipulation in model organisms and these have led to our current understanding of cerebellar development. Importantly, loss of cerebellar function significantly impacts on motor coordination, resulting in abnormal posture (ataxia), but does not cause a complete paralysis. Mice with cerebellar dysfunction are therefore viable and mutants are often easily identifiable based on their motor phenotypes. As a result, there are over 100 ataxic spontaneous mutant strains, and more than 350 transgenic or engineered ataxic mutants (www.informatics.jax.org). Additionally, the cerebellum exhibits a fairly simple architecture in contrast to the cerebral cortex. The cerebellum is comprised of seven to nine primary neuronal subtypes each displaying a unique morphology and arranged in stereotypical laminae and circuits. This architecture facilitates analysis of cerebellar mutants since developmental disruptions of lamination and neuronal morphology are relatively easy to identify.

In this chapter, we will discuss four major, overlapping stages of cerebellar development. We will first describe how the cerebellar territory of the neural tube is defined and patterned by the expression of a series of transcription factors and signaling molecules. Then we will define the three germinal zones which arise within this territory and undergo extensive proliferation to give rise to all the neurons of the adult cerebellum. Extensive migration follows as the developing cerebellar neurons acquire their final positions within the cerebellum. Finally, we will review several developmental aspects of neuronal connectivity as the differentiating cerebellar neurons form synaptic contacts to produce the mature circuitry of the cerebellum.

Defects in one or more of these developmental processes can result in significant neurologic dysfunction and congenital human cerebellar malformations. For example, Dandy-Walker malformation (DWM), the most common congenital malformation of the cerebellum, is caused by a disconnection in signaling between the developing cerebellum and adjacent posterior fossa mesenchyme (Parisi and Dobyns 2003; Aldinger et al. 2009). Disruption of neuronal cilia causes the granule cell progenitor proliferation defects of Joubert syndrome and related disorders (JSRD). Additionally, disruption of GABAergic neuron production culminates in cerebellar agenesis (Sellick et al. 2004; Hoshino et al. 2005). Defects in neuronal migration can cause cerebellar hypoplasia accompanied by lissencephaly (Hong et al. 2000). Degenerative processes during development can cause pontocerebellar hypoplasia (Edvardson et al. 2007; Budde et al. 2008). Even spinocerebellar ataxias (SCAs), usually considered to be degenerative disorders of the mature cerebellum, appear to be developmentally based (Serra et al. 2006). Other neurodevelopmental disorders such as autism are increasingly linked with subtle cerebellar developmental abnormalities (Courchesne et al. 1994; Belmonte et al. 2004). Thus, not only are the mechanisms driving cerebellar development relevant to basic science, they are also of significant clinical interest.

Developmental origins of the cerebellum

The cerebellum arises from dorsal rhombomere 1

During early development the neural tube forms three primary vesicles at its anterior end. From anterior to posterior these vesicles give rise to the forebrain, midbrain, and hindbrain (Fig. 1.1a). The hindbrain, which will be the focus of this chapter, is divided into seven segments along the anterior posterior axis, referred to as rhombomeres (rh) 1 through 7, that express various combinations of genes. These segments are units of cell lineage restriction (Fraser et al. 1990) such that cells from one rhombomere are unable to enter neighboring rhombomeres and are destined for predefined fates based on the localized information present within that rhombomere. Along the dorsoventral axis the hindbrain is characterized by a dorsalmost single-cell layer called the roof plate, a ventrally located cell population called the floor plate, and alar (dorsal) and basal (ventral) plates or neurepithelia that lie between (Fig. 1.1b). Fate mapping studies in chick and mouse embryos indicate that the cerebellum is a direct derivative of dorsal rh1 (Martinez and Alvarado-Mallart 1989a, 1989b; Hallonet and Le Douarin 1993).

* These authors contributed equally to this work.

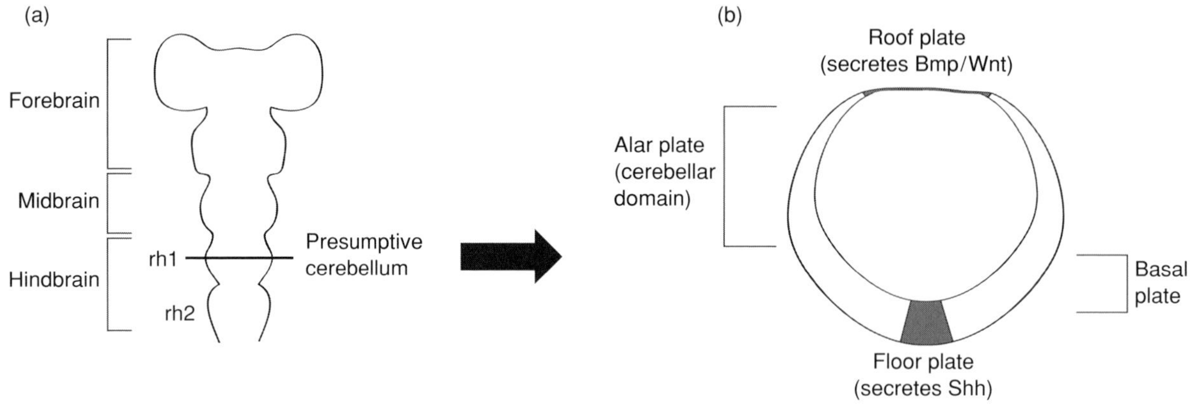

Fig. 1.1. Early neural tube development. **(a)** The early neural tube forms three primary vesicles that will form the forebrain, midbrain, and hindbrain, respectively, from anterior to posterior. The hindbrain is further subdivided into seven rhombomeres. The first two rhombomeres are illustrated (rh1 and rh2). The cerebellum is derived from rhombomere 1. **(b)** In cross-section at the level of rhombomere 1 [red line in (a)] the roof, alar, basal, and floor plates are evident. The cerebellum arises from the alar plate of rhombomere 1. The roof plate is a source of Bmp and Wnt signaling molecules, while the floor plate is a source of Shh. (See color plate 1).

Overview of major events during cerebellum development

Dorsal rh1 undergoes a series of events between mouse embryonic days (E) 9 to E12.5 during early development that rotate its rostral-caudal axis by 90 degrees and convert it into mediolateral axis of the bilateral cerebellar wings (Sgaier et al. 2005). Prolific cell division and subsequent fusion of the medial edges of the previously independent wings results in a contiguous structure that will become the medial cerebellar vermis and lateral hemispheres (Fig. 1.2a,b,c).

Two primary germinal zones, the cerebellar rhombic lip and the cerebellar ventricular zone (VZ), are established within the cerebellar anlage that give rise to all cerebellar neurons (Fig. 1.2d). The cerebellar rhombic lip arises adjacent to the roof plate and gives rise to all of the glutamatergic neurons of the cerebellum, including granule neurons, glutamatergic cerebellar nuclei, and unipolar brush cells. The ventricular zone which forms ventral to the rhombic lip, produces all cerebellar GABAergic cells, including Purkinje cells, interneurons, and inhibitory glial cells. Later, granule neuronal progenitors (GNPs) migrate from the rhombic lip to continue their proliferation in a secondary germinal zone on the surface of the developing cerebellar anlage. This secondary germinal zone is called the external granule cell layer (EGL) where they will produce differentiating granule neurons that will migrate inwards to form the internal granule layer (IGL) beneath the Purkinje cells layer (Fig. 1.2e).

During late embryogenesis and into postnatal development as the EGL proliferates, the smooth surface of the cerebellum is subdivided by four cardinal fissures that initially divide it into five lobes along the anterior-posterior axis. Postnatally, these lobes are further subdivided resulting in a basic cerebellar foliation pattern that is conserved across all mammals (Larsell and Jenson 1970). Concurrently, extensive migration of differentiating neurons results in the well-known and characteristic laminar pattern of the mature cerebellum, while extensive neuronal synaptic connections are generated to establish the well-characterized mature cerebellar circuitry.

Molecules involved in anterior-posterior axis patterning of the hindbrain and midbrain

Signals from the isthmic organizer define the cerebellar territory

The isthmic organizer (IsO) is an essential, transient embryonic signaling center that forms at the midbrain-hindbrain boundary (MHB) of the early neural tube. It secretes growth factors that pattern the adjacent nervous tissue. Loss of the IsO results in loss of both midbrain and cerebellar structures from early stages of neural tube development. The IsO forms at the boundaries of expression of two transcription factors that repress each other – *Otx2* on the anterior side/midbrain and *Gbx2* on the posterior side/hindbrain (Fig. 1.3a-b) (Simeone et al. 1992; Millet et al. 1996; Wassarman et al. 1997). Expression of *Fgf8* is the crucial signal emanating from the organizer, and is induced at the interface of *Otx2* and *Gbx2* domains at the mid-hindbrain boundary (Fig. 1.3c). Fgf8 protein induces the formation of the cerebellum by activating the Ras-ERK signaling pathway which in turn activates *Irx2* (Sato and Nakamura 2004). Coexpression of *Fgf8* and *Irx2*, but not expression of either gene alone, can induce a cerebellum in the midbrain region (Matsumoto et al. 2004). Alterations in the expression domains of *Gbx2* and *Otx2* are known to affect the location of the MHB. For example, either diminishing *Otx2* expression or extending the *Gbx2* expression domain more anteriorly results in a more anterior MHB. Conversely, either decreasing *Gbx2* expression or extending the expression domain of *Otx2* more posteriorly results in producing a more posterior MHB

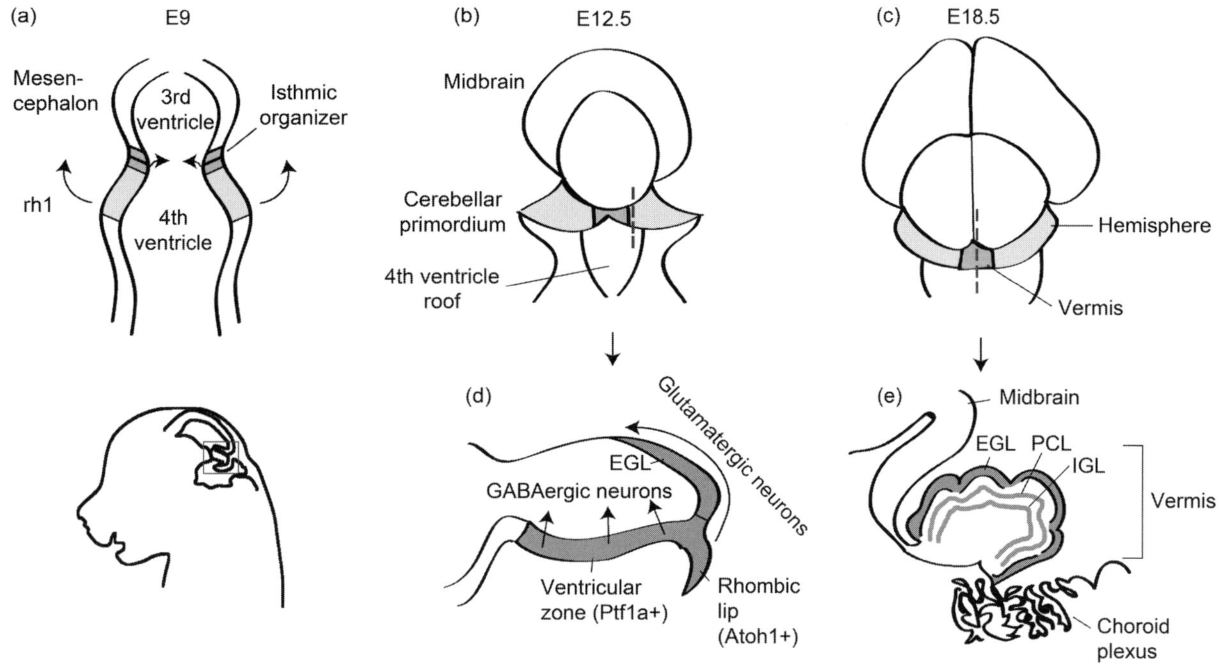

Fig. 1.2. The developing morphology of the embryonic mouse cerebellum at three stages of development. **(a–c)** Schematic dorsal views of the developing cerebellum from embryonic day 9 (E9) through E18.5. **(a)** At E9, the cerebellar territory is defined with anterior regions of rhombomere 1 (rh1) fated to become the cerebellar vermis and more posterior regions fated to become hemispheres, **(b)** after medial/lateral rotation of the bilateral cerebellar anlage wings by E12.5 **(c)** which eventually fuse on the midline to form a contiguous cerebellar anlage by E18.5. **(d)** At E12.5, the ventricular zone and rhombic lip regions of neurogenesis are evident in parasagittal view [indicated by red dotted line in (b)]. The ventricular zone gives rise to all GABAergic cerebellar neurons and the rhombic lip gives rise to glutamatergic neurons. The nascent EGL is also indicated. **(e)** At E18.5, following cell division and migration, a parasagittal schematic section reveals the locations of EGL, PCL (Purkinje cell layer), and IGL (internal granule cell layer). The fourth ventricle roof plate has also differentiated into the choroid plexus epithelium. The lower left panel shows the position of the developing cerebellum (inside red square) relative to the rest of the brain and is relevant to panels (d) and (e). (See color plate 2).

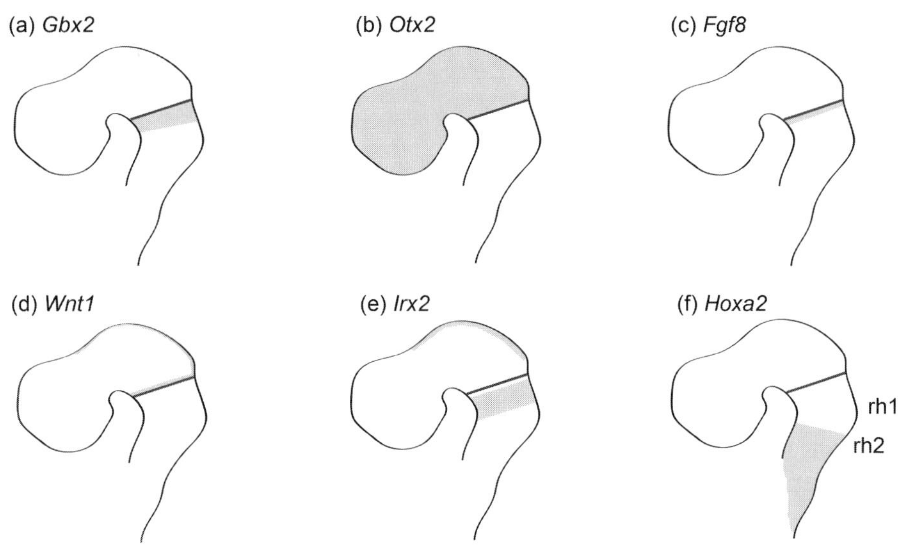

Fig. 1.3. Schematic side views of E9.5 mouse embryos illustrating the expression patterns of multiple genes (blue shading) around the mid-hindbrain boundary (red line). Each gene has been shown to be essential in establishment of the cerebellar territory along the anterior/posterior axis of the neural tube and influence positioning of the isthmic organizer. **(a, b)** The interface of *Gbx2* and *Otx2* transcription factor encoding genes at the mid-hindbrain boundary determines the expression of the secreted factor **(c)** Fgf8, a critical effector of isthmic organizer function, which in turn regulates the expression domain of **(d)** Wnt1, another essential isthmic organizer secreted factor. **(e)** The transcription factor Irx2 is required for Fgf8 function to define the cerebellar territory and **(f)** Hoxa2, yet another transcription factor, is expressed posteriorly from the rhombomere (rh) 1/2 boundary and defines the posterior limit of the cerebellar territory. (See color plate 3).

(Nakamura and Watanabe 2005). Several other genes, such as *Wnt1*, *En1*, *En2*, *Pax2*, *Pax5*, *Irx2*, and *Isl2* are also expressed around the IsO and their importance is evident by the fact that loss of function of these genes in mice also causes midbrain and hindbrain, including cerebellar developmental abnormalities (McMahon and Bradley 1990; Wurst et al. 1994; Acampora et al. 1995; Ang et al. 1996; Favor et al. 1996; Kikuchi et al. 1997; Urbanek et al. 1997; Wassarman et al. 1997; Meyers et al. 1998).

Hox genes are known to play a critical role in establishing neural tube identity along the anterior-posterior axis of the neural tube during early development, including the developing hindbrain (Tumpel et al. 2009). However, no *Hox* genes are expressed within rh1. The only known *Hox* gene expressed close to rh1 is *Hoxa2*, whose anterior-most boundary of expression lies between rh1 and 2 (Fig. 1.3f) (Gavalas et al. 1997). Loss of function of this gene in mice causes an enlargement of the cerebellum whereas its overexpression causes the opposite phenotype (Gavalas et al. 1997; Eddison et al. 2004). The lack of *Hox* gene expression in rh1, at least in part, appears to be due to Fgf8. Specifically, ectopic delivery of Fgf8 (using Fgf8-soaked beads) to chick embryos within rh1 causes the anterior boundary of *Hoxa2* to become more posterior. When Fgf8 function is inhibited, the opposite effect is observed such that the *Hoxa2* anterior boundary shifts anteriorly (Irving and Mason 2000). Thus, *Fgf8* is thought to determine the anterior-most boundary of *Hox* gene expression in the hindbrain, thereby keeping rh1 *Hox*-free. This establishes the posterior limit of the cerebellar territory at the rh1/2 boundary.

Retinoic acid gradient along the anterior-posterior axis contributes to rhombomere identity

Retinoic acid is a well-known signaling molecule important during both embryonic development and adulthood. It is derived from retinol/vitamin A. The concentration of retinoic acid diminishes from posterior to anterior regions of the developing neural tube (Horton and Maden 1995; Maden et al. 1998). The synthesis of retinoic acid occurs in the adjacent somites, facilitated by the enzyme *Raldh2*, and considerable evidence indicates that this gradient of retinoic acid influences the expression of specific *Hox* genes in the hindbrain which subsequently establish rh identity (Marshall et al. 1992). Exogenous retinoic acid during embryogenesis perturbs the anterior-posterior axis of the hindbrain so that the posterior hindbrain expands at the expense of the anterior hindbrain. When retinoic acid levels are reduced, the converse effect is seen such that the anterior hindbrain expands at the expense of the posterior hindbrain (Dupe and Lumsden 2001). It is therefore not surprising that retinoic acid exposure during human embryogenesis primarily affects anterior hindbrain-derived structures. Specifically, exposure to the acne medication, isotretinoin (Accutane), during early pregnancy is associated with cerebellar vermis hypoplasia, small cerebellar hemispheres, cystic dilation of the fourth ventricle, and malformations of the olivary and pontine nuclei (Lammer and Armstrong 1992).

Molecules involved in dorsal-ventral axis patterning of the cerebellar territory

Signals from the roof plate are dorsalizing factors

The IsO is not the only signaling center required for normal cerebellar development. The roof plate is another essential signaling center. During early neural tube development, the roof plate secretes several Bmp and Wnt proteins. In vitro, application of Bmp protein to naïve anterior hindbrain tissue is sufficient to induce formation of the cerebellar rhombic lip (Alder et al. 1999). Genetic manipulation of the roof plate in vivo in mouse embryos confirms this finding (Chizhikov et al. 2006, Mishima et al. 2009). Exposure to a balance of Bmp and Notch1 signaling molecules define the extent of the rhombic lip within the dorsoventral axis of rh1. Notch1 expression in the cerebellar ventricular zone limits the responsiveness of cerebellar ventricular zone progenitors to Bmps, such that, in the absence of Notch1, cerebellar progenitors are more responsive to BMP signalling, resulting in ectopic expression of rhombic lip markers in the ventricular zone (Machold et al. 2007). However, the correct specification of germinal zones along the dorsoventral axis is not the only function of the roof plate. Wnt signaling from the roof plate is essential to drive proliferation throughout the entire cerebellar ventricular zone (Chizhikov et al. 2006; Mishima et al. 2009).

Retinoic acid is produced by the embryonic roof plate as well as the meninges which overlies the dorsal cerebellar surface (Wilson and Maden 2005). Although during early embryonic development retinoic acid is involved in patterning the hindbrain along the anterior-posterior axis to form rhombomeres, it is later involved in the normal development of dorsal cerebellar structures. Perturbations of retinoic acid levels after hindbrain rhombomere formation appear to specifically result in malformations of structures derived from the dorsal hindbrain including cerebellar granule cells and the precerebellar olive and pontine nuclei (Yamamoto et al. 1999, 2003, 2005). The exact nature of this developmental disruption has not been elucidated.

Sonic hedgehog is a critical ventralizing signal

Sonic hedgehog (Shh) is a secreted factor which is expressed in the floor plate on the ventral midline along the entire anterior-posterior extent of the developing neural tube. The ventralizing effects of Shh signaling during early neural tube development have been studied most extensively in the spinal cord. Shh protein forms a gradient that opposes the Bmp gradient that originates from the roof plate. The graded expression of Shh and Bmps, in combination with other genes including *Hox* genes, determines the identities of the neuronal types that will form in the various regions along the dorsoventral axis of the spinal cord (Briscoe et al. 2000; Jessell 2000; Wilson and Maden 2005). In mice, Shh is required to activate its downstream transcriptional activator Gli2 to induce ventral hindbrain neuronal identities before E11.5. On the other hand, the Gli3 protein, which is a transcriptional repressor in the presence of

Shh, acts to pattern the dorsal region of the cerebellar territory by regulating *Fgf8* expression in the IsO (Blaess et al. 2006, 2008). As discussed below, however, Shh exhibits multiple functions at different stages in addition to its dorsoventral axis patterning activity at early embryonic stages.

Neurogenesis in the developing cerebellum

Once the cerebellar territory is defined by appropriate transcription factors and secreted molecules, neurogenesis in cerebellar germinal zones produces all the constituent cerebellar neurons.

Cerebellar rhombic lip neurogenesis produces glutamatergic derivatives

The rhombic lip that forms adjacent to the roof plate in rh1 is called the cerebellar rhombic lip, often also referred to as the upper rhombic lip. The cerebellar rhombic lip gives rise to all of the glutamatergic neurons of the cerebellum. Notably, the other, more posterior rhombomeres of the hindbrain also form rhombic lip structures adjacent to the roof plate. These caudal rhombic lips of the remaining hindbrain are often collectively referred to as the lower, or hindbrain, rhombic lip. Both the cerebellar rhombic lip and lower rhombic lip produce a number of glutamatergic precerebellar brainstem neurons, including those of the pontine nuclei (Machold and Fishell 2005; Wang et al. 2005; Yamada et al. 2007). The exact rhombomeric origins of these brainstem derivatives, however, are not well characterized. Thus, for this review we will primarily limit our discussion to the current understanding of cerebellar rhombic lip formation and cell fate specification of its derivatives.

The cerebellar rhombic lip produces diverse derivatives in overlapping waves of neurogenesis (Fig. 1.4a,b). In fact, the first populations of cells born from this region eventually become several hindbrain (extracerebellar) nuclei, rather than cerebellar neurons (Machold and Fishell 2005, Wang et al. 2005). These first neurons exit the rhombic lip at E10 in mice and migrate up and over the cerebellar anlage and into the rostral brainstem. Between E10 and E12, glutamatergic deep cerebellar nuclei (DCN) neurons are next produced in mice. These derivatives migrate over the cerebellar anlage, rest in an anterior nuclear transitory zone (NTZ) near the dorsal IsO, and then migrate into the cerebellar anlage. At E13.5, GNPs are generated and migrate over the surface of the cerebellar anlage to form the EGL of the anterior cerebellum. GNPs that localize to the more posterior EGL are produced later in embryonic development and during the first few postnatal days (Machold and Fishell 2005; Wang et al. 2005). Simultaneously,

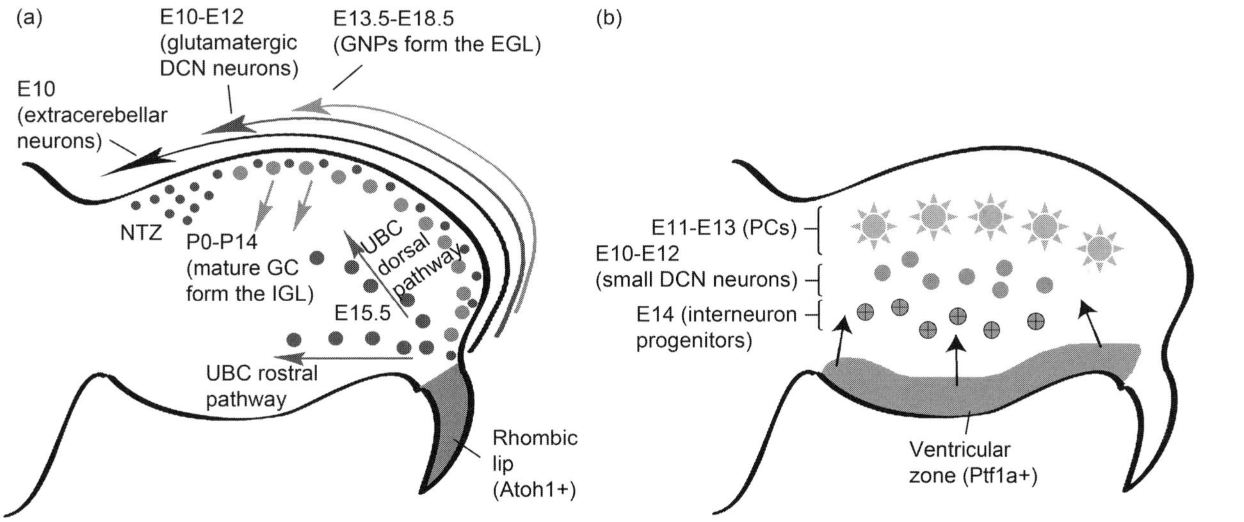

Fig. 1.4. Sagittal sections through the E16.5 cerebellum showing the migratory paths followed by various cerebellar neurons superimposed from a variety of developmental stages. **(a)** The rhombic lip produces glutamatergic neurons and traditionally has been defined by expression of the transcription factor Atoh1. Granule neuron progenitors (GNPs, orange), unipolar brush cells (UBCs, pink), and interneurons of deep cerebellar nuclei (DCN, purple) exit the rhombic lip in overlapping waves of neurogenesis, while the earliest neurons to exit the rhombic lip end up contributing to extracerebellar nuclei. Approximate exit times are indicated with arrows showing the direction of migration for these cells. The GNPs travel along a subpial tangential route to form the external granule layer (EGL) where they proliferate extensively, and eventually migrate inwards as mature granule cells along the Bergmann glial fibers (not shown in figure) through a radial route to form the internal granule layer (IGL) (see text). The UBCs migrate along two pathways – the dorsal pathway leading into the cerebellar white matter and a rostral pathway leading towards the ventricular zone and eventually the brainstem (Englund et al. 2006). The glutamatergic interneurons of the DCN follow a rostral subpial migratory path beginning from the rhombic lip and migrating to a transitory region called the nuclear transitory zone (NTZ) (Fink et al. 2006) from where they then migrate through the white matter via a poorly understood migration patter to settle deep inside the cerebellar base. **(b)** The ventricular zone, defined by expression of the transcription factor Ptf1a, gives rise to all GABAergic neurons of the cerebellum, also in overlapping waves of neurogenesis with timing indicated. The Purkinje cells (green stars) travel radially from the ventricular zone towards the surface along the fibers of radial glial cells and settle just underneath the IGL (see text). The interneuron progenitors (green with black outlines and crosses) and small neurons of the DCN (green) also travel radially away from the ventricular zone towards the prospective white matter remaining in the prospective white matter for several days before migrating to their final destinations in the cerebellar cortex and becoming committed to their final fates. (See color plate 4).

unipolar brush cells (UBCs) begin to exit the rhombic lip around E15.5 and migrate along two pathways – the dorsal pathway leading into the cerebellar white matter and a rostral pathway leading towards the ventricular zone and eventually the brainstem (Englund et al. 2006). The post-mitotic UBCs exit the rhombic lip and migrate through the developing white matter of the posterior anlage to their final positions in the posterior vermis (Wang et al. 2005, Fink et al. 2006).

Very little is known regarding the mechanisms that distinguish the fates of cerebellar rhombic lip derivatives. The basic helix-loop-helix (bHLH) transcription factor Atoh1 is used as a marker for the rhombic lip since mouse genetic fate mapping experiments demonstrated that all rhombic lip derivatives originate from Atoh1-positive progenitors (Machold and Fishell 2005; Wang et al. 2005). In mutant mice lacking *Atoh1*, the rhombic lip still forms but few if, any, derivatives are generated (Ben-Arie et al. 1997). Thus, Atoh1 is required for rhombic lip neurogenesis. However, initiation of *Atoh1* expression is itself not sufficient for normal neurogenesis. Rather, Atoh1 expression must be maintained. This finding comes from analysis of *Foxc1* mutant mice (Aldinger et al. 2009). The forkhead box transcription factor Foxc1 is expressed in the mesenchyme of the posterior fossa overlying the cerebellum where it is required to direct the expression of downstream molecules including transforming growth factor beta (TGFβ) and several Bmps. In turn, these secreted molecules are necessary for the maintenance of *Atoh1* expression. Loss of *Foxc1*, whose expression normally begins at E12.5, causes loss of these growth factors and loss of Atoh1 by E14.5. As a result, although early brainstem and DCN rhombic lip derivatives are generated, all remaining later derivatives are almost entirely absent.

Surprisingly, inducible genetic fate mapping experiments have demonstrated that Atoh1 does not actually identify rhombic lip 'stem cells'. Rather, once dividing rhombic lip cells initiate expression of Atoh1, they immediately migrate from the rhombic lip, leaving a population of Atoh1-negative proliferating progenitors behind (Machold and Fishell 2005). The nature of these rhombic lip stem cells is largely uncharacterized. However, there is evidence that the rhombic lip stem cell population is heterogeneous. In particular, a subpopulation of dividing rhombic lip cells expressing the transcription factor Lmx1a can be identified as soon as the rhombic lip forms at E12.5 in mice. Most of these cells are Atoh1 negative and Lmx1a rhombic lip expression is not dependent on Atoh1. Additional fate mapping experiments demonstrate that these Lmx1a+ progenitors give rise to just a subset of the full Atoh1+ rhombic lip lineage. Specifically Lmx1a-positive progenitors give rise to posterior GNPs (Chizhikov et al. 2010). Loss of Lmx1a function in the rhombic lip causes this population to exit the rhombic lip too early, switching their fate to anterior GNPs. Since Lmx1a is not expressed in GNPs outside of the rhombic lip, it must confer fate to its progenitor population within the rhombic lip. Together, these results suggest that the rhombic lip contains several subpopulations of progenitors whose identity is already encoded within the rhombic lip. The molecules and processes underlying these fate restrictions remain to be identified.

The cerebellar ventricular zone and mechanisms that specify cell fates of its derivatives

Once established, the cerebellar ventricular zone produces all of the GABAergic neurons of the cerebellum, including Purkinje cells, GABAergic cells of the DCN, and all the inhibitory interneurons of the cerebellum, such as basket and stellate cells. All ventricular zone cells migrate away from the germinal zone in a radial fashion into the developing cerebellum.

Expression of the bHLH transcription factor Ptf1a defines the cerebellar ventricular zone and fate mapping studies have confirmed that all GABAergic cerebellar neurons are derived from the Ptf1a-expressing domain of dorsal rh1. Ptf1a is also required for the generation of these inhibitory cells in the cerebellum since mice lacking the *Ptf1a* gene fail to produce GABAergic cerebellar neurons (Hoshino et al. 2005; Yamada et al. 2007). Interestingly, fate mapping studies show that, in the absence of Ptf1a, ventricular zone-derived cells can still proliferate and migrate into the cerebellum although they do not acquire their normal identity. Instead, they express markers of other cells such as granule neurons (Pascual et al. 2007). This suggests that Ptf1a normally prevents ventricular zone-derived cells from responding to factors such as Bmps that induce rhombic lip fates.

The roof plate is not required for the specification of the cerebellar ventricular zone. However, global proliferation within the cerebellar ventricular zone is initially driven by Wnt signaling from the roof plate (Chizhikov et al. 2006; Mishima et al. 2009). By E14.5, the mouse roof plate differentiates into the choroid plexus which secretes Shh into the fourth ventricle and appears to drive later ventricular zone proliferation (Huang et al. 2009, 2010).

Some cell fate specification decisions occur within the ventricular zone neuroepithelium, For example, the E12.5 mouse Ptf1a-positive cerebellar ventricular zone is divided into two broad domains based on levels of E-cadherin expression. Fate mapping and cell sorting experiments reveal that the dorsal E-cadherin-high domain of the cerebellar ventricular zone predominantly produces Purkinje cells, while progenitors located in the more ventral E-cadherin-low domain predominantly produce Pax2+ neurons, which include GABAergic small neurons of the DCN and all remaining cerebellar GABAergic interneurons (Mizuhara et al. 2010).

Expression of the neurogenic factor Mash1 marks all cerebellar ventricular zone lineages. However, the patchy, salt and pepper-like expression patterns of Mash1 and other neurogenic transcription factors such as Ngn1 and Ngn2 suggest that cell fate determination is not all spatially determined within the cerebellar ventricular zone (Zordan et al. 2008). In addition, significant evidence demonstrates that differentiating GABAergic interneuron precursors (e.g., basket and stellate cells) maintain a considerable level of plasticity as they exit the ventricular zone and migrate through white matter. Interestingly, the developmental potential of these differentiating GABAergic interneuron populations is not progressively restricted over time. Rather, as post-mitotic neurons, they retain a surprising plasticity, and their exact fate is only determined by local cues in their eventual location (Leto et al. 2006; Carletti et al. 2008; Leto et al. 2008; Schilling et al. 2008; Grimaldi et al. 2009; Leto et al. 2009). The nature of these external cues and the molecules which are required for this unusual model of neurogenesis remain undefined.

The external granule layer is a secondary region of neurogenesis

Regulation of external granule layer proliferation and differentiation

After GNPs leave the rhombic lip, they first migrate rostrally over the surface of the cerebellar anlage to form the EGL. The EGL is composed of two multicellular layers. The outer layer is highly proliferative, while the inner layer is composed of newly differentiating granule neurons preparing to exit the EGL and migrate radially inwards to form the inner granule cell layer.

In the outer EGL, GNP proliferation is induced by signals from ventricular zone-derived Purkinje cells that form a multicellular layer under the EGL, called the Purkinje cell layer (Fig. 1.2e). Purkinje cells secrete Shh, which acts as a mitogen and activates downstream effector genes in GNPs such as N-myc and cyclin D1 (Dahmane and Ruiz i Altaba 1999; Wallace 1999; Wechsler-Reya and Scott 1999; Kenney et al. 2003). Notch2 expression in GNPs is also important to drive their proliferation (Solecki et al. 2001).

The switch from proliferative to differentiating granule neurons is not completely understood. Tight control of this switch is essential, since unregulated proliferation of GNPs via abnormal regulation of the Shh and other signaling pathways is likely to be central to the pathogenesis of medulloblastoma, the most common malignant childhood brain tumor in humans (Eberhart 2008). Signaling pathways such as Fgf and Bmps oppose Shh-driven GNP proliferation in vitro (Rios et al. 2004; Fogarty et al. 2007). Further, cyclin-dependent kinase inhibitors, such as p27(Kip1) and p18(Ink4), are expressed in differentiating granule cells and limit expansion of this lineage in vivo (Miyazawa et al. 2000; Uziel et al. 2006). Since cell-cell contact is important to maintain GNP proliferation (Gao et al. 1991), mechanisms that alter the balance between symmetric versus asymmetric division may be central to this differentiation switch (Solecki et al. 2001, 2006). Interactions of GNPs with the overlying meninges may also regulate proliferation. For example, the ligand Cxcl12 is expressed in the meninges and its receptor Cxcr4 is expressed in the proliferating GNPs. Loss of either gene results in ectopic EGL cells within the cortex of the cerebellum (Reiss et al. 2002). Thus, the meninges appear to act as an attractant for GNPs, keeping them within their proliferative compartment.

Increased cerebellar size and foliation complexity as a consequence of external granule layer proliferation

Granule neuron progenitor proliferation is extensive, resulting in the generation of approximately 80 billion granule neurons in humans. These account for approximately 80% of the total number of all neurons within the entire brain (Azevedo et al. 2009). This increase in neuronal number directly leads to a large increase in the size of the cerebellum over the course of development. Notably, posterior fossa skull development is already nearing completion during late embryogenesis and postnatal life when EGL proliferation and granule cell differentiation are occurring. Thus, the increased cerebellar size is accommodated by the foliation of the developing cerebellum to pack it into the restricted available space, rather than an expansion of the back of the skull. The mechanisms that pattern the initial four cardinal fissures that segment the developing cerebellum into five lobules remain unclear (Sudarov and Joyner 2007). Genetic experiments do make it clear, however, that the extent of GNP proliferation directly correlates with the complexity of subsequent foliation. Increased Shh signaling results in increased GNP proliferation which in turn results in increased subdivisions of the initial lobules with additional sulci (Corrales et al. 2006). In mice there is an estimated ratio of one Purkinje cell to 200 granule neurons (Wetts and Herrup 1982). In humans, it is estimated that there are 4000 granule neurons per Purkinje cell in the mature cerebellum (Lange 1975). This substantial increase in neuron number across evolutionary distance is achieved by an extended period of EGL proliferation which continues into the first two postnatal years in humans and is accommodated by a significant increase in the complexity of human cerebellar foliation compared to rodents (Abraham et al. 2001).

Migration of cerebellar neurons

All cerebellar neurons undergo extensive migration from their origins in germinal zones to their final destinations in the mature cerebellum (Fig. 1.4a,b). Most rhombic lip-derived neurons (with the exception of UBC) initially migrate tangentially over surface of the developing cerebellar anlage. UBCs migrate directly from the rhombic lip into the white matter of the cerebellar anlage via an unknown mechanism. Tangentially migrating glutamatergic neurons of the DCN pause in the NTZ near the isthmus before initiating a complex and incompletely described migration through the anlage itself to settle with ventricular zone-derived GABAergic neurons of the DCN at the base of the mature cerebellum. Precerebellar brainstem neurons migrate tangentially over the cerebellar anlage, but exit the anlage to migrate either tangentially under the pia of the brainstem, or through the brainstem tegmentum to their final positions. GNPs also migrate tangentially over the anlage, but remain on the surface to form the EGL. As GNPs exit the EGL, they adopt a radial, glial-guided mode of migration, perpendicular to the pial surface, to settle under the Purkinje cell layer. This glial-guided aspect of granule cell migration is the best studied of all neuronal migrations in the central nervous system (CNS), due to the abundance of developing GNPs and the ease with which they can be isolated to homogeneity for in vitro and biochemical manipulations. Insights from these studies are relevant to the radial migration of the majority of neurons exiting the cerebellar ventricular zone, including Purkinje cells. They are also very broadly applicable outside the cerebellum, since glial-guided radial neuronal migration occurs ubiquitously throughout the CNS (Hatten 1999, 2002). In this section, we will overview current paradigms of granule cell migration (both tangential and radial) and Purkinje cell migration.

Granule cell migration

From rhombic lip to the external granule layer

GNPs destined for the EGL migrate over the anlage, but under the pia, occupying anterior positions first, then 'filling up' the posterior domain. Little is known about the control of this migration, although a cadherin-2 chain migration mechanism has been identified in zebrafish (Rieger et al. 2009). Signals from the pia are also important, since in hamster, removal of the pia disrupts EGL formation (von Knebel Doeberitz et al. 1986) and the Cxcr4/Cxcl12 receptor-ligand interactions between the EGL and pia described earlier in this chapter may provide some of these signals (Reiss et al. 2002). The anterior limit of GNP migration at the mid-hindbrain boundary is set by a different set of receptor-ligand interactions, this time between the GNPs of the forming EGL and the neuroepithelium. In mice mutant for the *Unc5h3* gene encoding a Netrin1 receptor, GNPs overmigrate to ectopically populate the surface of the caudal midbrain. The ligand Netrin is expressed in regions surrounding the embryonic cerebellar territory (Przyborski et al. 1998) and it is hypothesized that the Unc5h3/Netrin1 interaction is a repulsive interaction, keeping EGL cells confined to the presumptive cerebellum. *Pax6*-/- mouse mutants also express ectopic midbrain GNPs. Pax6-/- granule cells fail to express Unc5h3. This suggests that Pax6 activity, at least in part, is mediated by Unc5h3 (Engelkamp et al. 1999).

From the external granule layer to the internal granule layer

Once within the EGL and having completed their final mitosis, the granule cells alter their direction of migration from tangential to radial. In fact, these cells are known to alter the mode, tempo, and direction of migration as they pass through the different layers of the cerebellum in order to form the IGL (Komuro and Yacubova 2003). At the top of the EGL, the cells undergo extensive proliferation and remain there for 24–48 hours after their final mitosis and before initiating radial migration inwards (Komuro et al. 2001). During this window, differentiating granule cells undergo tangential migration at varying speeds within the deeper regions of the EGL and eventually extend a single vertical process into the molecular layer and initiate radial migration. The stromal-derived factor 1 and Ephrin-B reverse signaling is required for migration into deeper EGL (Lu et al. 2001), whereas interactions between Unc51.1 (a serine-threonine kinase), SynGAP (a negative regulator of Ras), and syntenin (a PDZ domain-containing scaffolding protein) are essential for the elongation of radial granule cell axons (Tomoda et al. 2004).

There is evidence to suggest that the transition from tangential to radial migration is in part due to the cessation of expression of *Sema6A*, a transmembrane semaphorin-encoding gene (Kerjan et al. 2005). Mice lacking this gene contain ectopic differentiated granule cells in the molecular layer that are synapsed with mossy fibers. Once within the molecular layer, granule cells acquire elongated cell bodies and radially migrate along the processes of Bergmann glial cells (also known as Golgi epithelial cells) (Kumuro and Rackic 1998; Hatten 1999; Sotelo 2004). The migrating granule cells secrete Fgf9 that controls the formation of Bergmann fiber scaffold, thereby guiding their own inward translocation (Lin et al. 2009). When they reach the Purkinje cell layer (PCL), the granule cells detach themselves from Bergmann glial fibers and their cell bodies become more rounded. After a stationary period within the PCL, granule cells send out motile filopodia at the distal ends of their leading processes and eventually pass the Purkinje cells and migrate into the IGL. In mouse, this entire migration from the EGL to the IGL takes approximately 2 days (Komuro and Rakic 1995, 1998; Komuro et al. 2001).

The cellular and molecular mechanisms of glial-guided (radial) migration are well studied in cerebellar granule cells. Live imaging of granule neurons migrating along glial fibers in vitro demonstrates that the migration involves multiple steps including attachment of the neuron to the glial fiber, the establishment of a leading process which wraps around the glial fiber in the direction of migration, followed by saltatory movements of the soma towards the leading process. This process is known as nucleokinesis. Soma translocation occurs in two phases, with the forward movement of a proximally located centrosome and Golgi apparatus into a swelling of the perinuclear segment of the leading process, followed by forward migration of the nucleus. The saltatory movement is in part regulated by the release and reformation of an adhesion junction complex beneath the cell soma (Edmondson and Hatten 1987). Extensive neuronal cytoskeletal remodeling is required for migration. The nucleus is surrounded by an extensive microtubule cage tethered to the centrosome, with additional microtubules extending into the leading process. This network is involved in pulling the nucleus forward (Rivas and Hatten 1995; Solecki et al. 2004). Regulation of this microtubule network is orchestrated by specialized cell polarity machinery, including the mPar6a polarity complex which is located in the centrosome and is required for its forward movement (Solecki et al. 2004). Not surprisingly, a number of microtubule and microtubule-associated proteins are essential for radial migration and, in particular, centrosome/nuclear translocation (Kawauchi and Hoshino 2008). The actin cytoskeleton is also highly regulated in radially migrating granule cells. Rapid turnover of F-actin together with myosin II motors located in the leading process power acto-myosin contractility in the leading process which is also required to organize the coordinated movement of the centrosome and nucleus (Solecki et al. 2009). Finally, highly coordinated vesicle endocytosis and exocytosis ensure that numerous surface receptors are correctly positioned throughout the migration cycle (Letinic et al. 2009; Wilson et al. 2010). These receptors include neuregulins and NMDA receptors which are likely to be involved in coupling environmental signals to cytoskeletal remodeling and neuronal-glial adhesion receptors such as astrotactin 1 (Fishell and Hatten 1991; Komuro and Rakic 1993; Rio et al. 1997; Borghesani et al. 2002).

PURKINJE CELL MIGRATION

Originating from the cerebellar ventricular zone, Purkinje cells embark on a radial migratory route, travelling dorsally towards the cortical surface. In mouse this occurs between E11 and E13, much earlier than granule cell migration from the EGL into the developing cerebellum (Morales and Hatten 2006). During this period radial glial cells of the ventricular zone (which are the progenitors of all cells from this zone) send out long smooth fibers to the pia in order to form the radial glial end feet. It is along these fibers that Purkinje cells migrate towards their final destination just beneath the EGL. There is a concurrent differentiation of some radial glial cells into Bergmann glial cell, a specialized type of astrocytic cell. The cell bodies of the differentiating Bergmann glial cells migrate in synchrony with the cell bodies of Purkinje cells towards the newly forming PCL. This process results in the shortening of the smooth Bergmann glial fibers and retention of a small descending process which disappears after maturity (Yuasa et al. 1991; Bellamy 2006). Thus, whereas granule cells migrate along the smooth fibers of Bergmann glia postnatally, Purkinje cells migrate along radial glial fibers in close association with the differentiating Bergmann glial cells during embryonic development.

While the actual cell biology of Purkinje glial-guided migration is not well studied, it is assumed that many of the features of granule cell glial-guided migration are relevant, including saltatory movements and cell polarity control. Several molecules have been identified that regulate Purkinje cell glial-guided migration, including those of the Reelin signaling pathway. Reelin is a secreted extracellular matrix protease whereas Dab1 is a cytoplasmic adapter protein. Mutations in the mouse *Reelin* or *Dab1* genes result in small cerebella with no foliation and ectopic clusters of Purkinje cells beneath the granule cell layer (Mariani et al. 1977; Sweet et al. 1996). *Reelin* is expressed by cells in the external granule layer and *Dab1* by Purkinje cell precursors from the ventricular zone of the cerebellum. During wild-type cerebellar development, differentiating Purkinje cells complete their migration just below the cells producing Reelin. However, in *Reelin* and *Dab1*-mutant animals these cells fail to respond to this 'stop' signal and become ectopically located (Goffinet et al. 1984; Goldowitz et al. 1997). As expected, mice mutant for the Reelin receptors, the lipoprotein receptors Vldlr and ApoER2, have similar

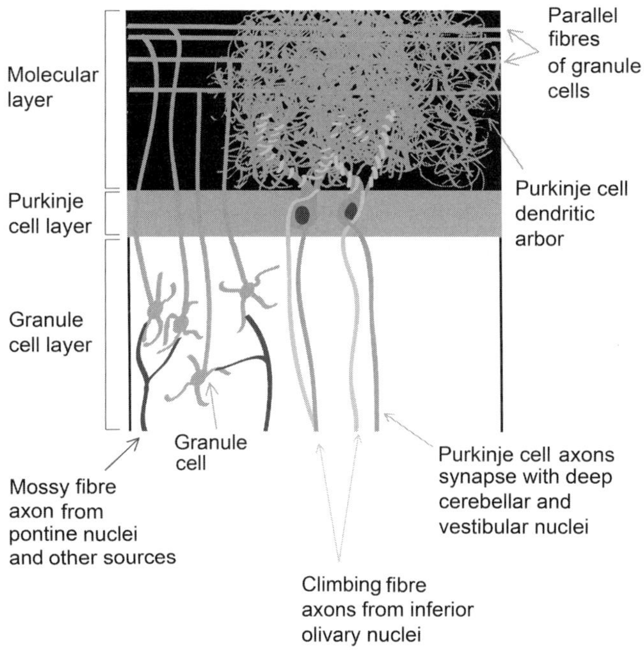

Fig. 1.5. Mature circuitry of the cerebellar cortex. Afferent input to the cerebellum is from two sources: mossy fibers (purple) and climbing fibers (blue). Granule cells (orange) receive mossy fiber (purple) inputs from multiple sources and project their extensive T-shaped axons (parallel fibers, yellow) to synapse onto the branches of dendritic arbor of Purkinje cells (green) within the upper segment of the molecular layer. Purkinje cell dendrites also receive inputs from the climbing fibers of the inferior olive (blue) within the lower segment of the molecular layer. All afferent output of the cerebellar cortex is from the axons of the Purkinje cells (green) which project to either the deep cerebellar nuclei within the base of the cerebellar cortex or the vestibular nuclei adjacent to the cerebellum. (See color plate 5).

phenotypes (D'Arcangelo et al. 1999; Trommsdorff et al. 1999). Reelin secreted from the EGL cells into the extracellular matrix binds receptors present on the surface of migrating neurons, thereby inducing receptor-mediated phosphorylation of Dab1 in the cytoplasm of Purkinje cells (Howell et al. 1999). This activates downstream genes that eventually alter the cytoskeleton of migrating neurons such as to make them post-migratory (Huang 2009). While initial studies identified the EGL as the source of Reelin that influences Purkinje cell migration, it was later shown using *Atoh1* null mice where the EGL fails to form, that Reelin is also produced from the ventricular zone as well as from the NTZ and that this expression also impinges on the migration of these neurons (Jensen et al. 2002). Notably, although first described in the developing cerebellum, the Reelin pathway is essential for glial-guided migration throughout the entire CNS (D'Arcangelo 2005).

Formation of cerebellar circuitry

The nature of the mature cerebellar circuit has long been described (Fig. 1.5). The adult cerebellar cortex receives inputs from the pontine nuclei which convey information from the cerebral cortex. In addition, the precerebellar nuclei relay sensory information from the vestibular and other nuclei. Many of the precerebellar nuclei convey information through mossy fiber axons which project to granule cells in the granule cell layer of the mature cerebellum. Granule cell parallel fiber axons then make synaptic contacts with the dendrites of Purkinje cells. In contrast to the other precerebellar nuclei, the inferior olivary nuclei directly project their climbing fiber axons to Purkinje cells, without first contacting granule cells. Purkinje cells then send inhibitory signals to the DCN which, with additional inputs from the inferior olive and other precerebellar nuclei, integrate the activity in the cerebellum and act as the sole output of the cerebellar cortex. Thus, Purkinje cells integrate the activity of parallel fibers, climbing fibers, and interneurons to project to the DCN (or vestibular nuclei) via inhibitory connections. Such projections are made in a topographic fashion such that Purkinje cells in the lateral hemispheres project to ipsilateral lateral dentate nuclei while Purkinje cells of the cerebellar vermis project to the medial fastigial nuclei. Posterior vermis Purkinje cells directly synapse with vestibular nuclei. Since Purkinje cells are so integral to cerebellar information processing, they have been the focus of much study of the development and maturation of cerebellar circuitry. Here we will overview multiple aspects of Purkinje cell differentiation, synapse formation, and maturation to demonstrate several key features of cerebellar circuit formation.

Purkinje cell dendrite formation

Mature Purkinje cells possess an elaborate dendritic tree that is completely planar in orientation yet stereotypically branched as it reaches across the molecular layer of the cerebellum. In the molecular layer, Purkinje cell dendrites intersect the parallel fibers of the granule cells which traverse through the Purkinje cell dendrites at right angles. Each parallel fiber forms weakly excitatory glutamatergic synapses with an estimated 1000 Purkinje cells and each Purkinje cell synapses with over 175 000 parallel fibers in rat (Ito 1984; Napper and Harvey 1988). In the mature cerebellum, parallel fiber synapses are segregated to the distal domain of the dendritic tree and climbing fibers from the inferior olivary nucleus neurons form strong GABAergic synapses with the proximal domain of the Purkinje cell dendritic tree. In contrast to the extensive interactions between multiple parallel fibers and Purkinje cells, each Purkinje cell receives synaptic input from a single climbing fiber terminal arbor, while each inferior olivary neuron contacts only seven Purkinje cells (Schild 1970).

Development of Purkinje cell dendrites occurs during the first 4 postnatal weeks in mice and is initially largely dependent on intrinsic cellular programs (Kapfhammer 2004, Sotelo and Dusart 2009) since early postnatal Purkinje cells grown in isolation in vitro undergo the initial stages of dendritogenesis (Baptista et al. 1994). This finding confirms in vivo analysis of mice lacking granule cells, where Purkinje cells develop a dendritic tree resembling the shape of a normal tree, but lacking higher-order dendritic branches and branchlets where parallel fibers normally synapse (Kapfhammer 2004). One major intrinsic determinant is the RORα transcription factor which is expressed in developing Purkinje cells. Purkinje cells in mice with mutations in the *RORα* gene retain an embryonic fusiform morphology. However, overexpression of RORα restores normal dendrite formation. Extrinsic influences, in particular interactions with granule cells and their parallel fibers, are required to refine the ultimate mature Purkinje cell dendritic architecture, including its exquisite planarity. These extrinsic factors include trophic factors (Mount et al. 1995; Hirai and Launey 2000; Swinny et al. 2004), hormones, such as estrogens, CRF and thyroid hormones (Heuer and Mason 2003; Shikimi et al. 2004; Swinny et al. 2004) and electrical activity (Schilling et al. 1991). Protein kinase C (PKC)-regulated signaling events within Purkinje cells are a major determinant for normal dendritic development (Kapfhammer 2004) and may represent a common downstream pathway within Purkinje cells for integration of the multiple external signals.

Integrating Purkinje cells into the cerebellar circuit

The normal function of Purkinje cells is dependent on a series of developmental processes which ensure each Purkinje cell is correctly integrated into the entire cerebellar circuit. Two particular developmental aspects of this circuit integration have been the focus of extensive study – the monoinnervation of each Purkinje cell with a single climbing fiber and the segregation of climbing and parallel fiber domains within the Purkinje cell dendritic tree.

Multiple climbing fiber elimination

During Purkinje cell dendritogenesis in late prenatal mouse stages, multiple climbing fibers innervate the proximal axon and soma of each Purkinje cell (Mason et al. 1990). Simultaneous with Purkinje cell dendritic differentiation over the first postnatal week in mice, the multiple climbing fiber connections resolve into a 1:1 climbing fiber to Purkinje cell ratio. During this maturation, climbing fibers translocate their distal axons up the proximal branch of Purkinje cell dendrites and establish hundreds of synapses along the dendrites of the proximal dendritic tree (Kano et al. 1995, 1997; Hashimoto and Kano 2005). Failure to eliminate multiple climbing fiber innervations and translocate the synaptic contacts results in significant Purkinje cell dysfunction, often leading to ataxia.

Activity between presynaptic climbing fibers and postsynaptic Purkinje cells is critical for supernumerary climbing fiber elimination. Persistent multi-climbing fiber innervation occurs in mice with impaired calcium influx caused by deficient P/Q-type voltage-dependent Ca^{2+} channel (VDCC) function (Miyazaki et al. 2004). In addition, the remaining climbing fibers fail to translocate from the Purkinje cell soma to the proximal dendrite. Activation of pre- and postsynaptic contacts leads to alterations in the strength of climbing fiber connections. A recent analysis surprisingly demonstrated that selective strengthening of one fiber's connection over the others occurs much earlier than previously believed, while the climbing fibers are still associated with the soma and prior to dendritic translocation (Hashimoto et al. 2009). Further, interaxonal competition on the cell soma causes elimination of weak synapses and axons so that the winning axon eventually occupies the majority of the synapses at that soma long before synaptic translocation.

Interestingly, the maturation of climbing fiber to Purkinje cell synapses requires intact inputs from granule cell parallel fibers, which also synapse onto Purkinje cell dendrites. When granule cell numbers or synapses are decreased, multiple climbing fibers continue to innervate Purkinje cells. Proper activity of the parallel fiber to Purkinje cell synapse is also necessary for climbing fiber synaptic maturation. This evidence comes from analysis of mice with null mutations of the glutamate receptor d2 subunit (GluRd2), which interrupt synapse formation between parallel fibers and Purkinje cell synapses, and results in a secondary failure of synaptic elimination of excess climbing fibers (Kurihara et al. 1997). This phenomenon also occurs in the *weaver*, *staggerer*, and *reeler* mutant mice which all lose granule cells via different mechanisms (Crepel and Mariani 1976; Mariani et al. 1977; Crepel et al. 1980; Steinmayr et al. 1998). Signaling through a variety of downstream molecules is specifically important for the elimination of excess climbing fiber connections later in development, as is evident from studies of MGluR1 (Kano et al. 1995, 1997), the GLAST glutamate transporter (Watase et al. 1998), and others (Miyazaki et al. 2006; Takagishi et al. 2007). Finally, the inhibitory interneurons of the molecular layer which also synapse with Purkinje cells play a role in climbing fiber elimination. For example, in TrkB neurotrophin receptor-deficient mice, parallel fiber development is unperturbed but the inhibitory GABAergic synaptic connections to Purkinje cells from basket and stellate cells is delayed, and Purkinje cells remain multiply innervated (Bosman et al. 2006; Johnson et al. 2007). Thus, synaptic elimination is a precisely conducted event requiring the functional workings of the entire circuitry of the cerebellum.

Climbing fiber/parallel fiber competition establishes distinct functional domains within the Purkinje cell dendritic tree

During development, there is progressive segregation of Purkinje cell afferents such that climbing fiber inputs to the Purkinje cell dendritic tree become restricted to the proximal branches and do not invade the upper branches where parallel fiber connections are located. Data from a number of studies demonstrate that an ongoing axonal competition between climbing fibers and parallel fibers is essential to maintain these proximal and distal domains. Ataxia can result when segregation of these domains is lost.

Two genes critical for the differential distribution of parallel and climbing fibers are GluR2d2 (mentioned in the previous section) and its ligand Clbn1 (Kashiwabuchi et al. 1995; Hirai et al. 2005; Matsuda and Yuzaki 2010). Cbln1 is secreted from granule cells and GluRd2 is expressed in Purkinje cell dendrites. Loss of either gene results in an identical phenotype – a specific and dramatic reduction of parallel fiber to Purkinje cell synapses. As a result, climbing fibers invade the distal domain of the Purkinje cell dendritic tree. A reciprocal disruption of domains can be induced when inferior olive afferents are cut or climbing fibers are chemically disrupted, causing parallel fibers to invade the de-afferented climbing fibers domain (Cesa and Strata 2009). This remarkable plasticity is important not only for response to lesions, but also for fine-tuning activity dependent learning, and is maintained throughout adulthood.

Examples of human cerebellar developmental disruptions

Advances in neuroimaging, model organism developmental biology, and molecular genetics have synergistically increased our understanding of human disorders affecting the cerebellum. As a result, significant disruptions of the major cerebellar developmental mechanisms discussed in this chapter are now known to cause a number of human congenital cerebellar malformations (also reviewed extensively in Barkovich et al. (2009)). Although a complete discussion of these malformations is beyond the scope of this chapter, here we aim to highlight several human disorders and put them in context of their associated developmental disruptions.

Human cerebellar malformations resulting from defects in neurogenesis

Defects in cerebellar neurogenesis of any of the three cerebellar germinal zones result in a variety of human cerebellar malformations.

Cerebellar agenesis can be caused by abnormal cerebellar ventricular zone neurogenesis. Specifically, mutations in *PTF1A*, a gene discussed earlier as an essential regulator of the cerebellar ventricular zone, cause a defect in cerebellar GABAergic neuron specification. Since cerebellar GABAergic neurons provide trophic support for rhombic lip-derived neurons, all glutamatergic neurons die, resulting in the very rare phenotype of cerebellar agenesis (Sellick et al. 2004; Hoshino et al. 2005).

Abnormalities of rhombic lip neurogenesis have been implicated in DWM. DWM entails hypoplasia and upward rotation of the cerebellar vermis, cystic dilatation of the fourth ventricle, and an enlarged posterior fossa, also called mega cisterna magna (MCM). Patients with mutations in *FOXC1* exhibit a spectrum of anomalies that range from isolated cerebellar vermis hypoplasia (CVH) to MCM and DWM. We recently showed that the maintenance of neurogenesis in the cerebellar rhombic lip depends on normal transcriptional regulation of growth factors and other signaling molecules by Foxc1 in the posterior fossa mesenchyme. These factors are secreted from the mesenchyme and received by the adjacent rhombic lip (Aldinger et al. 2009). Thus at least some forms of DWM are caused by a failure of normal rhombic lip neurogenesis. Notably, these data also indicate that normal posterior fossa development is essential for normal cerebellar development. The posterior fossa mesenchyme is derived from both head neural crest and head mesoderm which contribute to skull, meninges, and dermis. Defects in similar signaling pathways may underlie cerebellar malformations that also involve posterior fossa and skin disorders. These include neurocutaneous melanosis (Kadonaga et al. 1992;

Barkovich et al. 1994; Acosta et al. 2005) and PHACES syndrome (posterior fossa malformations, haemangioma, arterial anomalies, cardiac abnormalities/aortic coartation, eye abnormalities, sternal cleft defects; Frieden et al. 1996; Metry et al. 2001). Future investigations of such patient groups may identify additional genes that regulate rhombic lip maintenance.

Disruptions in EGL production of granule neurons are thought to contribute to JSRD. JRSD is characterized by hypoplasia of the cerebellar vermis and a complex brainstem phenotype including elongated cerebellar peduncles and a deep interpeduncular fissure. Recently identified JSRD genes all appear to encode for proteins involved in the structure or function of the primary cilia, a cell signaling sensor which is critical for reception of Shh (Lee and Gleeson 2010). As discussed earlier in the chapter, the Shh pathway is integral to the production of cerebellar granule cells. A loss of this signaling explains the CVH seen in JRSD (Chizhikov et al. 2007; Spassky et al. 2008) but future investigation is needed to understand additional malformations seen in JRSD. For example, the axonal defects in these disorders suggest the presence of significant axon migration abnormalities that are likely to be cilia-dependent. However, these have not yet been the focus of study in animal models of these disorders.

Abnormalities in cell proliferation and growth may cause additional malformations that can be identified based on cerebellar morphology. One syndrome, called macrocephaly-capillary malformation syndrome, consists of cerebellar (and cerebral) overgrowth (Conway et al. 2007). Abnormal growth of dysplastic cells also occurs in dysplastic gangliocytoma, or Lhermitte-Duclos disease, which results in large ganglion cells in the granule cell layer and enlarged folia of the cerebellum (Ambler et al. 1969). In addition, the cerebellar granule cells are myelinated with enlarged axons and it is postulated that an overexpression of neurofilament protein results in these morphological changes (Yachnis et al. 1988). Half of such cases result from mutations of the PTEN tumor suppressor gene, which is also found in Cowden syndrome, but the exact cause of the disease is unknown. Dysplastic cerebellar overgrowth also occurs in the cortical tubers of tuberous sclerosis caused by mutations of *TSC1* or *TSC2*. While abnormal proliferation may cause cerebellar malformations with altered size, abnormal migration may cause dislocated cell types or foliation defects of the cerebellum.

Examples of human cerebellar disorders due to defects of later developmental processes

Neuronal migration disorders

Mutations in several genes involved in neuronal migration cause cerebellar abnormalities in humans. For instance, mutations in *REELIN*, a gene essential for multiple modes of migration, including radial migration in the cerebellum, cause lissencephaly with cerebellar hypoplasia (Hong et al. 2000). Mutations in the *VLDLR* gene, a REELIN receptor, cause a very similar lissencephaly with cerebellar hypoplasia (Boycott et al. 2005). Even mutations in TUBA1A, which is a component of cytoskeletal microtubules, results in lissencephaly with cerebellar hypoplasia (Morris-Rosendahl et al. 2008; Kumar et al. 2010).

Synaptogenesis, connectivity, and degenerative disorders

As discussed in previous sections, the formation and maturation of cerebellar synapses requires the coordination of many precise events. Mutations in synaptic genes are linked to cerebellar malformations. For example, *Oliogphrenin-1* is one gene implicated in cerebellar development and X-linked mental retardation (UK: learning disability). Both mutations (Zanni et al. 2005) and deletions in the Rho-GAP *OPHN1* gene occur in families with X-linked CVH (Bergmann et al. 2003; Philip et al. 2003). Loss of this gene in mice results in immature dendritic spines (Khelfaoui et al. 2007). It remains unclear whether failure of synaptic maturation is solely responsible for the gross morphological malformation CVH in humans.

In addition to the formation of synapses, neuronal connections must also be maintained for a functional cerebellum. The calcium/calmodulin-dependent serine/threonine kinase, *CASK*, is one gene that may be required for such stabilization, as it localizes to synapses and synaptic molecules. Mutations of *CASK* are found in patients with pontocerebellar hypoplasia (PCH) (Najm et al. 2008). PCH is not a singular entity, but rather a group of rare heterogeneous conditions characterized by prenatal development of an abnormally small cerebellum and brainstem including the pontine nuclei (Barth 1993; Hevner 2007). Note that children with *CASK* mutations have a static hypoplasia. In contrast, PCH caused by mutations of the tRNA splicing pathway genes including *RARS2* (Edvardson et al. 2007), *TSEN54*, *TSEN34*, and *TSEN2* (Budde et al. 2008) is progressive in nature, with ongoing atrophy after birth. In-depth studies of animal model systems are required to determine whether tRNA splicing also regulates synaptic stabilization such that destabilization would result in cerebellar malformations and atrophy, or whether these genes are more directly required for neuronal homeostasis and survival.

Perturbation of synaptic connections in autism is also reported through functional magnetic resonance imaging (fMRI) of patients (Assaf et al. 2010; Ebisch et al. 2010). The role of the cerebellum in autism is becoming increasingly apparent since there is a significant reduction in the number of Purkinje cells in postmortem brains (Ritvo et al. 1986; Kemper and Bauman 1993; Bailey et al. 1998; Palmen et al. 2004; Amaral et al. 2008). Chimeras of wild-type and *lurcher* mice (that lose Purkinje cells postnatally) exhibit repetitive behavior and behavioral inflexibility – two of the main phenotypes of autistic patients that are negatively correlated with Purkinje cell number (Dickson et al. 2010; Martin et al. 2010). Other studies have found a 40% decrease in the transcript levels of *glutamate decarboxylase 67* (*GAD*67), a gene that codes for a GABA synthesizing enzyme, in Purkinje cells of autistic brains but an increased level in basket and stellate interneurons which form synapses with Purkinje cells (Yip et al. 2007,

2008). These observations lead to a hypothesized scenario where Purkinje cells provide reduced input to cerebellar nuclei which ultimately affects the cortex and therefore cognition.

Finally, molecular pathway analysis of combined results from many genome-wide association studies (GWAS) has revealed that the genes (in particular, *NRXN1* and *CNTNAP2*) participating in the neuronal cell adhesion pathway are significantly over-represented in schizophrenia, bipolar disorder and autism (O'Dushlaine et al. 2010). Other individual genes significantly associated with autism are *SEMA5A*, which is involved in axon guidance and whose expression was found to be lower in the brains on individuals with autism (Weiss et al. 2009), *ASTN2*, *NLGN1*, *CNTN4* (Glessner et al. 2009). These genes are involved in proper neuronal adhesion, migration, and synapse formation, further suggesting a disruption of connectivity in the brains of individuals with autism and other neurodevelopmental disorders.

Conclusion

In this chapter we discussed the major stages of cerebellar development. We have further demonstrated that an understanding of the basic processes of cerebellar development can lead to insights regarding the pathology of a wide variety of clinically important neurodevelopemental disorders.

Although we have largely discussed each developmental process in isolation, it is imperative to note that during cerebellar development, multiple processes occur simultaneously and are dependent on each other. Further, cerebellar development does not happen in isolation from the rest of the brain. Many of the developmental mechanisms driving cerebellar development also influence midbrain and hindbrain more generally. For example, anterior/posterior patterning mechanisms of the neural tube which define the cerebellar territory also define the midbrain territory. Additionally, development of the pons is dependent on normal development of the cerebellar rhombic lip, which also gives rise to cerebellar granule neurons. Thus, the pons is often hypoplastic when cerebellar hypoplasia is observed. Similarly pontine nuclear neurons undergo extensive migrations to reach their final destinations, so pontine hypoplasia is often a feature of cerebellar malformations which are caused by migration abnormalities. Finally, many of the genes that have been identified to be critical regulators of cerebellar development are expressed elsewhere in the developing CNS and examination of mouse models has clearly demonstrated roles for many of these genes in CNS development beyond the cerebellum. Thus the unraveling of the developmental pathways and molecules regulating cerebellar development in model organisms has shed considerable insight into general CNS developmental mechanisms, including those influencing cerebellar cortex development. In humans, it is likely that the cerebellar malformations and abnormalities we currently recognize represent just the 'tip of the iceberg.' The unique, stereotypical morphology and almost crystalline packing and lamination of cerebellar neurons allow structural abnormalities of the cerebellum to be visible at the relatively low resolution level of analysis possible in most MRI studies. We predict that significant abnormalities are present elsewhere in the CNS and will be revealed by detailed and comprehensive neuropathological analysis in these patients.

Acknowledgments

The authors are funded by NIH R01 grants NS050375, NS058721, R01NS072441, and NS050386.

REFERENCES

Abraham H, Tornoczky T, Kosztolanyi G, Seress L (2001) Cell formation in the cortical layers of the developing human cerebellum. Int J Dev Neurosci 19: 53–62.

Acampora D, Mazan S, Lallemand Y, Avantaggiato V, Maury M, Simeone A, Brulet P (1995) Forebrain and midbrain regions are deleted in Otx2-/- mutants due to a defective anterior neuroectoderm specification during gastrulation. Development 121: 3279–3290.

Acosta FL, Jr., Binder DK, Barkovich AJ, Frieden IJ, Gupta N (2005) Neurocutaneous melanosis presenting with hydrocephalus. Case report and review of the literature. J Neurosurg 102: 96–100.

Alder J, Lee KJ, Jessell TM, Hatten ME (1999) Generation of cerebellar granule neurons in vivo by transplantation of BMP-treated neural progenitor cells. Nat Neurosci 2: 535–540.

Aldinger KA, Lehmann OJ, Hudgins L, Chizhikov VV, Bassuk AG, Ades LC, et al. (2009) FOXC1 is required for normal cerebellar development and is a major contributor to chromosome 6p25.3 Dandy-Walker malformation. Nat Genet 41: 1037–1042.

Amaral DG, Schumann CM, Nordahl CW (2008) Neuroanatomy of autism. Trends Neurosci 31: 137–145.

Ambler M, Pogacar S, Sidman R (1969) Lhermitte-Duclos disease (granule cell hypertrophy of the cerebellum) pathological analysis of the first familial cases. J Neuropathol Exp Neurol 28: 622–647.

Ang SL, Jin O, Rhinn M, Daigle N, Stevenson L, Rossant J (1996) A targeted mouse Otx2 mutation leads to severe defects in gastrulation and formation of axial mesoderm and to deletion of rostral brain. Development 122: 243–252.

Assaf M, Jagannathan K, Calhoun VD, Miller L, Stevens MC, Sahl R, et al. (2010) Abnormal functional connectivity of default mode subnetworks in autism spectrum disorder patients. Neuroimage 53: 247–256.

Azevedo FA, Carvalho LR, Grinberg LT, Farfel JM, Ferretti RE, Leite RE, et al. (2009) Equal numbers of neuronal and nonneuronal cells make the human brain an isometrically scaled-up primate brain. J Comp Neurol 513: 532–541.

Bailey A, Luthert P, Dean A, Harding B, Janota I, Montgomery M, et al. (1998) A clinicopathological study of autism. Brain 121 (Pt 5): 889–905.

Baptista CA, Hatten ME, Blazeski R, Mason CA (1994) Cell-cell interactions influence survival and differentiation of purified Purkinje cells in vitro. Neuron 12: 243–260.

Barkovich AJ, Frieden IJ, Williams ML (1994) MR of neurocutaneous melanosis. AJNR Am J Neuroradiol 15: 859–867.

Barkovich AJ, Millen KJ, Dobyns WB (2009) A developmental and genetic classification for midbrain-hindbrain malformations. Brain 132: 3199–3230.

Barth PG (1993) Pontocerebellar hypoplasias. An overview of a group of inherited neurodegenerative disorders with fetal onset. Brain Dev 15: 411–422.

Bellamy TC (2006) Interactions between Purkinje neurones and Bergmann glia. Cerebellum 5: 116–126.

Belmonte MK, Allen G, Beckel-Mitchener A, Boulanger LM, Carper RA, Webb SJ (2004) Autism and abnormal development of brain connectivity. J Neurosci 24: 9228–9231.

Ben-Arie N, Bellen HJ, Armstrong DL, McCall AE, Gordadze PR, Guo Q, et al. (1997) Math1 is essential for genesis of cerebellar granule neurons. Nature 390: 169–172.

Bergmann C, Zerres K, Senderek J, Rudnik-Schoneborn S, Eggermann T, Hausler M, et al. (2003) Oligophrenin 1 (OPHN1) gene mutation causes syndromic X-linked mental retardation with epilepsy, rostral ventricular enlargement and cerebellar hypoplasia. Brain 126: 1537–1544.

Blaess S, Corrales JD, Joyner AL (2006) Sonic hedgehog regulates Gli activator and repressor functions with spatial and temporal precision in the mid/hindbrain region. Development 133: 1799–1809.

Blaess S, Stephen D, Joyner AL (2008) Gli3 coordinates three-dimensional patterning and growth of the tectum and cerebellum by integrating Shh and Fgf8 signaling. Development 135: 2093–2103.

Borghesani PR, Peyrin JM, Klein R, Rubin J, Carter AR, Schwartz PM, et al. (2002) BDNF stimulates migration of cerebellar granule cells. Development 129: 1435–1442.

Bosman LW, Hartmann J, Barski JJ, Lepier A, Noll-Hussong M, Reichardt LF, Konnerth A (2006) Requirement of TrkB for synapse elimination in developing cerebellar Purkinje cells. Brain Cell Biol 35: 87–101.

Boycott KM, Flavelle S, Bureau A, Glass HC, Fujiwara TM, Wirrell E, et al. (2005) Homozygous deletion of the very low density lipoprotein receptor gene causes autosomal recessive cerebellar hypoplasia with cerebral gyral simplification. Am J Hum Genet 77: 477–483.

Briscoe J, Pierani A, Jessell TM, Ericson J (2000) A homeodomain protein code specifies progenitor cell identity and neuronal fate in the ventral neural tube. Cell 101: 435–445.

Budde BS, Namavar Y, Barth PG, Poll-The BT, Nurnberg G, Becker C, van Ruissen F, et al. (2008) tRNA splicing endonuclease mutations cause pontocerebellar hypoplasia. Nat Genet 40: 1113–1118.

Carletti B, Williams IM, Leto K, Nakajima K, Magrassi L, Rossi F (2008) Time constraints and positional cues in the developing cerebellum regulate Purkinje cell placement in the cortical architecture. Dev Biol 317: 147–160.

Cesa R, Strata P (2009) Axonal competition in the synaptic wiring of the cerebellar cortex during development and in the mature cerebellum. Neuroscience 162: 624–632.

Chizhikov VV, Davenport J, Zhang Q, Shih EK, Cabello OA, Fuchs JL, et al. (2007) Cilia proteins control cerebellar morphogenesis by promoting expansion of the granule progenitor pool. J Neurosci 27: 9780–9789.

Chizhikov VV, Lindgren AG, Currle DS, Rose MF, Monuki ES, Millen KJ (2006) The roof plate regulates cerebellar cell-type specification and proliferation. Development 133: 2793–2804.

Chizhikov VV, Lindgren AG, Mishima Y, Roberts RW, Aldinger KA, Miesegaes GR, et al. (2010) Lmx1a regulates fates and location of cells originating from the cerebellar rhombic lip and telencephalic cortical hem. Proc Natl Acad Sci U S A 107: 10725–10730.

Conway RL, Pressman BD, Dobyns WB, Danielpour M, Lee J, Sanchez-Lara PA, et al. (2007) Neuroimaging findings in macrocephaly-capillary malformation: a longitudinal study of 17 patients. Am J Med Genet A 143A: 2981–3008.

Corrales JD, Blaess S, Mahoney EM, Joyner AL (2006) The level of sonic hedgehog signaling regulates the complexity of cerebellar foliation. Development 133: 1811–1821.

Courchesne E, Townsend J, Saitoh O (1994) The brain in infantile autism: posterior fossa structures are abnormal. Neurology 44: 214–223.

Crepel F, Delhaye-Bouchaud N, Guastavino JM, Sampaio I (1980) Multiple innervation of cerebellar Purkinje cells by climbing fibres in staggerer mutant mouse. Nature 283: 483–484.

Crepel F, Mariani J (1976) Multiple innervation of Purkinje cells by climbing fibers in the cerebellum of the Weaver Mutant Mouse. J Neurobiol 7: 579–582.

D'Arcangelo G (2005) The reeler mouse: anatomy of a mutant. Int Rev Neurobiol 71: 383–417.

D'Arcangelo G, Homayouni R, Keshvara L, Rice DS, Sheldon M, Curran T (1999) Reelin is a ligand for lipoprotein receptors. Neuron 24: 471–479.

Dahmane N, Ruiz i Altaba A (1999) Sonic hedgehog regulates the growth and patterning of the cerebellum. Development 126: 3089–3100.

Dickson PE, Rogers TD, Mar ND, Martin LA, Heck D, Blaha CD, et al. (2010) Behavioral flexibility in a mouse model of developmental cerebellar Purkinje cell loss. Neurobiol Learn Mem 94: 220–228.

Dupe V, Lumsden A (2001) Hindbrain patterning involves graded responses to retinoic acid signalling. Development 128: 2199–2208.

Eberhart CG (2008) Even cancers want commitment: lineage identity and medulloblastoma formation. Cancer Cell 14: 105–107.

Ebisch SJ, Gallese V, Willems RM, Mantini D, Groen WB, Romani GL, et al. (2010) Altered intrinsic functional connectivity of anterior and posterior insula regions in high-functioning participants with autism spectrum disorder. Hum Brain Mapp.

Eddison M, Toole L, Bell E, Wingate RJ (2004) Segmental identity and cerebellar granule cell induction in rhombomere 1. BMC Biol 2: 14.

Edmondson JC, Hatten ME (1987) Glial-guided granule neuron migration in vitro: a high-resolution time-lapse video microscopic study. J Neurosci 7: 1928–1934.

Edvardson S, Shaag A, Kolesnikova O, Gomori JM, Tarassov I, Einbinder T, et al. (2007) Deleterious mutation in the mitochondrial arginyl-transfer RNA synthetase gene is associated with pontocerebellar hypoplasia. Am J Hum Genet 81: 857–862.

Engelkamp D, Rashbass P, Seawright A, van Heyningen V (1999) Role of Pax6 in development of the cerebellar system. Development 126: 3585–3596.

Englund C, Kowalczyk T, Daza RA, Dagan A, Lau C, Rose MF, Hevner RF (2006) Unipolar brush cells of the cerebellum are produced in the rhombic lip and migrate through developing white matter. J Neurosci 26: 9184–9195.

Favor J, Sandulache R, Neuhauser-Klaus A, Pretsch W, Chatterjee B, Senft E, et al. (1996) The mouse Pax2(1Neu) mutation is identical to a human PAX2 mutation in a family with renal-coloboma syndrome and results in developmental defects of the brain, ear, eye, and kidney. Proc Natl Acad Sci U S A 93: 13870–13875.

Fink AJ, Englund C, Daza RA, Pham D, Lau C, Nivison M, et al. (2006) Development of the deep cerebellar nuclei: transcription factors and cell migration from the rhombic lip. J Neurosci 26: 3066–3076.

Fishell G, Hatten ME (1991) Astrotactin provides a receptor system for CNS neuronal migration. Development 113: 755–765.

Fogarty MP, Emmenegger BA, Grasfeder LL, Oliver TG, Wechsler-Reya RJ (2007) Fibroblast growth factor blocks Sonic hedgehog signaling in neuronal precursors and tumor cells. Proc Natl Acad Sci U S A 104: 2973–2978.

Fraser S, Keynes R, Lumsden A (1990) Segmentation in the chick embryo hindbrain is defined by cell lineage restrictions. Nature 344: 431–435.

Frieden IJ, Reese V, Cohen D (1996) PHACE syndrome. The association of posterior fossa brain malformations, hemangiomas, arterial anomalies, coarctation of the aorta and cardiac defects, and eye abnormalities. Arch Dermatol 132: 307–311.

Gao WO, Heintz N, Hatten ME (1991) Cerebellar granule cell neurogenesis is regulated by cell-cell interactions in vitro. Neuron 6: 705–715.

Gavalas A, Davenne M, Lumsden A, Chambon P, Rijli FM (1997) Role of Hoxa-2 in axon pathfinding and rostral hindbrain patterning. Development 124: 3693–3702.

Glessner JT, Wang K, Cai G, Korvatska O, Kim CE, Wood S, et al. (2009) Autism genome-wide copy number variation reveals ubiquitin and neuronal genes. Nature 459: 569–573.

Goffinet AM, So KF, Yamamoto M, Edwards M, Caviness VS, Jr (1984) Architectonic and hodological organization of the cerebellum in reeler mutant mice. Brain Res 318: 263–276.

Goldowitz D, Cushing RC, Laywell E, D'Arcangelo G, Sheldon M, Sweet HO, et al. (1997) Cerebellar disorganization characteristic of reeler in scrambler mutant mice despite presence of reelin. J Neurosci 17: 8767–8777.

Grimaldi P, Parras C, Guillemot F, Rossi F, Wassef M (2009) Origins and control of the differentiation of inhibitory interneurons and glia in the cerebellum. Dev Biol 328: 422–433.

Hallonet ME, Le Douarin NM (1993) Tracing neuroepithelial cells of the mesencephalic and metencephalic alar plates during cerebellar ontogeny in quail-chick chimaeras. Eur J Neurosci 5: 1145–1155.

Hashimoto K, Ichikawa R, Kitamura K, Watanabe M, Kano M (2009) Translocation of a 'winner' climbing fiber to the Purkinje cell dendrite and subsequent elimination of 'losers' from the soma in developing cerebellum. Neuron 63: 106–118.

Hashimoto K, Kano M (2005) Postnatal development and synapse elimination of climbing fiber to Purkinje cell projection in the cerebellum. Neurosci Res 53: 221–228.

Hatten ME (1999) Central nervous system neuronal migration. Annu Rev Neurosci 22: 511–539.

Hatten ME (2002) New directions in neuronal migration. Science 297: 1660–1663.

Heuer H, Mason CA (2003) Thyroid hormone induces cerebellar Purkinje cell dendritic development via the thyroid hormone receptor alpha1. J Neurosci 23: 10604–10612.

Hevner RF (2007) Progress on pontocerebellar hypoplasia. Acta Neuropathol 114: 401–402.
Hirai H, Launey T (2000) The regulatory connection between the activity of granule cell NMDA receptors and dendritic differentiation of cerebellar Purkinje cells. J Neurosci 20: 5217–5224.
Hirai H, Pang Z, Bao D, Miyazaki T, Li L, Miura E, et al. (2005) Cbln1 is essential for synaptic integrity and plasticity in the cerebellum. Nat Neurosci 8: 1534–1541.
Hong SE, Shugart YY, Huang DT, Shahwan SA, Grant PE, Hourihane JO, et al. (2000) Autosomal recessive lissencephaly with cerebellar hypoplasia is associated with human RELN mutations. Nat Genet 26: 93–96.
Horton C, Maden M (1995) Endogenous distribution of retinoids during normal development and teratogenesis in the mouse embryo. Dev Dyn 202: 312–323.
Hoshino M, Nakamura S, Mori K, Kawauchi T, Terao M, Nishimura YV, et al. (2005) Ptf1a, a bHLH transcriptional gene, defines GABAergic neuronal fates in cerebellum. Neuron 47: 201–213.
Howell BW, Herrick TM, Cooper JA (1999) Reelin-induced tyrosine [corrected] phosphorylation of disabled 1 during neuronal positioning. Genes Dev 13: 643–648.
Huang X, Ketova T, Fleming JT, Wang H, Dey SK, Litingtung Y, Chiang C (2009) Sonic hedgehog signaling regulates a novel epithelial progenitor domain of the hindbrain choroid plexus. Development 136: 2535–2543.
Huang X, Liu J, Ketova T, Fleming JT, Grover VK, Cooper MK, et al. (2010) Transventricular delivery of Sonic hedgehog is essential to cerebellar ventricular zone development. Proc Natl Acad Sci U S A 107: 8422–8427.
Huang Z (2009) Molecular regulation of neuronal migration during neocortical development. Mol Cell Neurosci 42: 11–22.
Irving C, Mason I (2000) Signalling by FGF8 from the isthmus patterns anterior hindbrain and establishes the anterior limit of Hox gene expression. Development 127: 177–186.
Ito M (1984) The cerebellum and neural control. New York: Raven Press New York.
Jensen P, Zoghbi HY, Goldowitz D (2002) Dissection of the cellular and molecular events that position cerebellar Purkinje cells: a study of the math1 null-mutant mouse. J Neurosci 22: 8110–8116.
Jessell TM (2000) Neuronal specification in the spinal cord: inductive signals and transcriptional codes. Nat Rev Genet 1: 20–29.
Johnson EM, Craig ET, Yeh HH (2007) TrkB is necessary for pruning at the climbing fibre-Purkinje cell synapse in the developing murine cerebellum. J Physiol 582: 629–646.
Kadonaga JN, Barkovich AJ, Edwards MS, Frieden IJ (1992) Neurocutaneous melanosis in association with the Dandy-Walker complex. Pediatr Dermatol 9: 37–43.
Kano M, Hashimoto K, Chen C, Abeliovich A, Aiba A, Kurihara H, et al. (1995) Impaired synapse elimination during cerebellar development in PKC gamma mutant mice. Cell 83: 1223–1231.
Kano M, Hashimoto K, Kurihara H, Watanabe M, Inoue Y, Aiba A, Tonegawa S (1997) Persistent multiple climbing fiber innervation of cerebellar Purkinje cells in mice lacking mGluR1. Neuron 18: 71–79.
Kapfhammer JP (2004) Cellular and molecular control of dendritic growth and development of cerebellar Purkinje cells. Prog Histochem Cytochem 39: 131–182.
Kashiwabuchi N, Ikeda K, Araki K, Hirano T, Shibuki K, Takayama C, et al. (1995) Impairment of motor coordination, Purkinje cell synapse formation, and cerebellar long-term depression in GluR delta 2 mutant mice. Cell 81: 245–252.
Kawauchi T, Hoshino M (2008) Molecular pathways regulating cytoskeletal organization and morphological changes in migrating neurons. Dev Neurosci 30: 36–46.
Kemper TL, Bauman ML (1993) The contribution of neuropathologic studies to the understanding of autism. Neurol Clin 11: 175–187.
Kenney AM, Cole MD, Rowitch DH (2003) Nmyc upregulation by sonic hedgehog signaling promotes proliferation in developing cerebellar granule neuron precursors. Development 130: 15–28.
Kerjan G, Dolan J, Haumaitre C, Schneider-Maunoury S, Fujisawa H, Mitchell KJ, Chedotal A (2005) The transmembrane semaphorin Sema6A controls cerebellar granule cell migration. Nat Neurosci 8: 1516–1524.
Khelfaoui M, Denis C, van Galen E, de Bock F, Schmitt A, Houbron C, et al. (2007) Loss of X-linked mental retardation gene oligophrenin1 in mice impairs spatial memory and leads to ventricular enlargement and dendritic spine immaturity. J Neurosci 27: 9439–9450.
Kikuchi Y, Segawa H, Tokumoto M, Tsubokawa T, Hotta Y, Uyemura K, Okamoto H (1997) Ocular and cerebellar defects in zebrafish induced by overexpression of the LIM domains of the islet-3 LIM/homeodomain protein. Neuron 18: 369–382.
Komuro H, Rakic P (1993) Modulation of neuronal migration by NMDA receptors. Science 260: 95–97.
Komuro H, Rakic P (1995) Dynamics of granule cell migration: a confocal microscopic study in acute cerebellar slice preparations. J Neurosci 15: 1110–1120.
Komuro H, Rakic P (1998) Distinct modes of neuronal migration in different domains of developing cerebellar cortex. J Neurosci 18: 1478–1490.
Komuro H, Yacubova E (2003) Recent advances in cerebellar granule cell migration. Cell Mol Life Sci 60: 1084–1098.
Komuro H, Yacubova E, Yacubova E, Rakic P (2001) Mode and tempo of tangential cell migration in the cerebellar external granular layer. J Neurosci 21: 527–540.
Kumar RA, Pilz DT, Babatz TD, Cushion TD, Harvey K, Topf M, et al. (2010) TUBA1A mutations cause wide spectrum lissencephaly (smooth brain) and suggest that multiple neuronal migration pathways converge on alpha tubulins. Hum Mol Genet 19: 2817–2827.
Kurihara H, Hashimoto K, Kano M, Takayama C, Sakimura K, Mishina M, et al. (1997) Impaired parallel fiber–Purkinje cell synapse stabilization during cerebellar development of mutant mice lacking the glutamate receptor delta2 subunit. J Neurosci 17: 9613–9623.
Lammer EJ, Armstrong DL (1992) Malformations of hindbrain structures among humans exposed to isotretinoin (13-cis-retinoic acid) during early embryogenesis. In: Morriss-Kay G, editor. Retinoids in Normal Development and Teratogenesis. Oxford: Oxford University Press. pp. 281–295.
Lange W (1975) Cell number and cell density in the cerebellar cortex of man and some other mammals. Cell Tissue Res 157: 115–124.
Larsell O, Jenson J (1970) The Comparative Anatomy and Histology of the Cerebellum: From Monotremes through Apes. Minnesota: University of Minnesota Press.
Lee JH, Gleeson JG (2010) The role of primary cilia in neuronal function. Neurobiol Dis 38: 167–172.
Letinic K, Sebastian R, Toomre D, Rakic P (2009) Exocyst is involved in polarized cell migration and cerebral cortical development. Proc Natl Acad Sci U S A 106: 11342–11347.
Leto K, Carletti B, Williams IM, Magrassi L, Rossi F (2006) Different types of cerebellar GABAergic interneurons originate from a common pool of multipotent progenitor cells. J Neurosci 26: 11682–11694.
Leto K, Bartolini A, Rossi F (2008) Development of cerebellar GABAergic interneurons: origin and shaping of the 'minibrain' local connections. Cerebellum 7: 523–529.
Leto K, Bartolini A, Yanagawa Y, Obata K, Magrassi L, Schilling K, Rossi F (2009) Laminar fate and phenotype specification of cerebellar GABAergic interneurons. J Neurosci 29: 7079–7091.
Lin Y, Chen L, Lin C, Luo Y, Tsai RY, Wang F (2009) Neuron-derived FGF9 is essential for scaffold formation of Bergmann radial fibers and migration of granule neurons in the cerebellum. Dev Biol 329: 44–54.
Lu Q, Sun EE, Klein RS, Flanagan JG (2001) Ephrin-B reverse signaling is mediated by a novel PDZ-RGS protein and selectively inhibits G protein-coupled chemoattraction. Cell 105: 69–79.
Machold R, Fishell G (2005) Math1 is expressed in temporally discrete pools of cerebellar rhombic-lip neural progenitors. Neuron 48: 17–24.
Machold RP, Kittell DJ, Fishell GJ (2007) Antagonism between Notch and bone morphogenetic protein receptor signaling regulates neurogenesis in the cerebellar rhombic lip. Neural Dev 2: 5.
Maden M, Sonneveld E, van der Saag PT, Gale E (1998) The distribution of endogenous retinoic acid in the chick embryo: implications for developmental mechanisms. Development 125: 4133–4144.
Mariani J, Crepel F, Mikoshiba K, Changeux JP, Sotelo C (1977) Anatomical, physiological and biochemical studies of the cerebellum from Reeler mutant mouse. Philos Trans R Soc Lond B Biol Sci 281: 1–28.
Marshall H, Nonchev S, Sham MH, Muchamore I, Lumsden A, Krumlauf R (1992) Retinoic acid alters hindbrain Hox code and induces transformation of rhombomeres 2/3 into a 4/5 identity. Nature 360: 737–741.

Martin LA, Goldowitz D, Mittleman G (2010) Repetitive behavior and increased activity in mice with Purkinje cell loss: a model for understanding the role of cerebellar pathology in autism. Eur J Neurosci 31: 544–555.

Martinez S, Alvarado-Mallart RM (1989a) Rostral Cerebellum Originates from the Caudal Portion of the So-Called 'Mesencephalic' Vesicle: A Study Using Chick/Quail Chimeras. Eur J Neurosci 1: 549–560.

Martinez S, Alvarado-Mallart RM (1989b) Transplanted mesencephalic quail cells colonize selectively all primary visual nuclei of chick diencephalon: a study using heterotopic transplants. Brain Res Dev Brain Res 47: 263–274.

Mason CA, Christakos S, Catalano SM (1990) Early climbing fiber interactions with Purkinje cells in the postnatal mouse cerebellum. J Comp Neurol 297: 77–90.

Matsuda K, Yuzaki M (2010) Cbln1 and the Delta2 Glutamate Receptor-An Orphan Ligand and an Orphan Receptor Find Their Partners. Cerebellum.

Matsumoto K, Nishihara S, Kamimura M, Shiraishi T, Otoguro T, Uehara M, et al. (2004) The prepattern transcription factor Irx2, a target of the FGF8/MAP kinase cascade, is involved in cerebellum formation. Nat Neurosci 7: 605–612.

McMahon AP, Bradley A (1990) The Wnt-1 (int-1) proto-oncogene is required for development of a large region of the mouse brain. Cell 62: 1073–1085.

Metry DW, Dowd CF, Barkovich AJ, Frieden IJ (2001) The many faces of PHACE syndrome. J Pediatr 139: 117–123.

Meyers EN, Lewandoski M, Martin GR (1998) An Fgf8 mutant allelic series generated by Cre- and Flp-mediated recombination. Nat Genet 18: 136–141.

Millet S, Bloch-Gallego E, Simeone A, Alvarado-Mallart RM (1996) The caudal limit of Otx2 gene expression as a marker of the midbrain/hindbrain boundary: a study using in situ hybridisation and chick/quail homotopic grafts. Development 122: 3785–3797.

Mishima Y, Lindgren AG, Chizhikov VV, Johnson RL, Millen KJ (2009) Overlapping function of Lmx1a and Lmx1b in anterior hindbrain roof plate formation and cerebellar growth. J Neurosci 29: 11377–11384.

Miyazaki T, Hashimoto K, Shin HS, Kano M, Watanabe M (2004) P/Q-type Ca2+ channel alpha1A regulates synaptic competition on developing cerebellar Purkinje cells. J Neurosci 24: 1734–1743.

Miyazaki T, Hashimoto K, Uda A, Sakagami H, Nakamura Y, Saito SY, et al. (2006) Disturbance of cerebellar synaptic maturation in mutant mice lacking BSRPs, a novel brain-specific receptor-like protein family. FEBS Lett 580: 4057–4064.

Miyazawa K, Himi T, Garcia V, Yamagishi H, Sato S, Ishizaki Y (2000) A role for p27/Kip1 in the control of cerebellar granule cell precursor proliferation. J Neurosci 20: 5756–5763.

Mizuhara E, Minaki Y, Nakatani T, Kumai M, Inoue T, Muguruma K, et al. (2010) Purkinje cells originate from cerebellar ventricular zone progenitors positive for Neph3 and E-cadherin. Dev Biol 338: 202–214.

Morales D, Hatten ME (2006) Molecular markers of neuronal progenitors in the embryonic cerebellar anlage. J Neurosci 26: 12226–12236.

Morris-Rosendahl DJ, Najm J, Lachmeijer AM, Sztriha L, Martins M, Kuechler A, et al. (2008) Refining the phenotype of alpha-1a Tubulin (TUBA1A) mutation in patients with classical lissencephaly. Clin Genet 74: 425–433.

Mount HT, Dean DO, Alberch J, Dreyfus CF, Black IB (1995) Glial cell line-derived neurotrophic factor promotes the survival and morphologic differentiation of Purkinje cells. Proc Natl Acad Sci U S A 92: 9092–9096.

Najm J, Horn D, Wimplinger I, Golden JA, Chizhikov VV, Sudi J, et al. (2008) Mutations of CASK cause an X-linked brain malformation phenotype with microcephaly and hypoplasia of the brainstem and cerebellum. Nat Genet 40: 1065–1067.

Nakamura H, Watanabe Y (2005) Isthmus organizer and regionalization of the mesencephalon and metencephalon. Int J Dev Biol 49: 231–235.

Napper RM, Harvey RJ (1988) Number of parallel fiber synapses on an individual Purkinje cell in the cerebellum of the rat. J Comp Neurol 274: 168–177.

O'Dushlaine C, Kenny E, Heron E, Donohoe G, Gill M, Morris D, Corvin A (2010) Molecular pathways involved in neuronal cell adhesion and membrane scaffolding contribute to schizophrenia and bipolar disorder susceptibility. Mol Psychiatry.

Palmen SJ, van Engeland H, Hof PR, Schmitz C (2004) Neuropathological findings in autism. Brain 127: 2572–2583.

Parisi MA, Dobyns WB (2003) Human malformations of the midbrain and hindbrain: review and proposed classification scheme. Mol Genet Metab 80: 36–53.

Pascual M, Abasolo I, Mingorance-Le Meur A, Martinez A, Del Rio JA, Wright CV, et al. (2007) Cerebellar GABAergic progenitors adopt an external granule cell-like phenotype in the absence of Ptf1a transcription factor expression. Proc Natl Acad Sci U S A 104: 5193–5198.

Philip N, Chabrol B, Lossi AM, Cardoso C, Guerrini R, Dobyns WB, et al. (2003) Mutations in the oligophrenin-1 gene (OPHN1) cause X-linked congenital cerebellar hypoplasia. J Med Genet 40: 441–446.

Przyborski SA, Knowles BB, Ackerman SL (1998) Embryonic phenotype of Unc5h3 mutant mice suggests chemorepulsion during the formation of the rostral cerebellar boundary. Development 125: 41–50.

Reiss K, Mentlein R, Sievers J, Hartmann D (2002) Stromal cell-derived factor 1 is secreted by meningeal cells and acts as chemotactic factor on neuronal stem cells of the cerebellar external granular layer. Neuroscience 115: 295–305.

Rieger S, Senghaas N, Walch A, Koster RW (2009) Cadherin-2 controls directional chain migration of cerebellar granule neurons. PLoS Biol 7: e1000240.

Rio C, Rieff HI, Qi P, Khurana TS, Corfas G (1997) Neuregulin and erbB receptors play a critical role in neuronal migration. Neuron 19: 39–50.

Rios I, Alvarez-Rodriguez R, Marti E, Pons S (2004) Bmp2 antagonizes sonic hedgehog-mediated proliferation of cerebellar granule neurones through Smad5 signalling. Development 131: 3159–3168.

Ritvo ER, Freeman BJ, Scheibel AB, Duong T, Robinson H, Guthrie D, Ritvo A (1986) Lower Purkinje cell counts in the cerebella of four autistic subjects: initial findings of the UCLA-NSAC Autopsy Research Report. Am J Psychiatry 143: 862–866.

Rivas RJ, Hatten ME (1995) Motility and cytoskeletal organization of migrating cerebellar granule neurons. J Neurosci 15: 981–989.

Sato T, Nakamura H (2004) The Fgf8 signal causes cerebellar differentiation by activating the Ras-ERK signaling pathway. Development 131: 4275–4285.

Schild RF (1970) On the inferior olive of the albino rat. J Comp Neurol 140: 255–260.

Schilling K, Dickinson MH, Connor JA, Morgan JI (1991) Electrical activity in cerebellar cultures determines Purkinje cell dendritic growth patterns. Neuron 7: 891–902.

Schilling K, Oberdick J, Rossi F, Baader SL (2008) Besides Purkinje cells and granule neurons: an appraisal of the cell biology of the interneurons of the cerebellar cortex. Histochem Cell Biol 130: 601–615.

Schmahmann JD (2004) Disorders of the cerebellum: ataxia, dysmetria of thought, and the cerebellar cognitive affective syndrome. J Neuropsychiatry Clin Neurosci 16: 367–378.

Sellick GS, Barker KT, Stolte-Dijkstra I, Fleischmann C, Coleman RJ, Garrett C, et al. (2004) Mutations in PTF1A cause pancreatic and cerebellar agenesis. Nat Genet 36: 1301–1305.

Serra HG, Duvick L, Zu T, Carlson K, Stevens S, Jorgensen N, et al. (2006) RORalpha-mediated Purkinje cell development determines disease severity in adult SCA1 mice. Cell 127: 697–708.

Sgaier SK, Millet S, Villanueva MP, Berenshteyn F, Song C, Joyner AL (2005) Morphogenetic and cellular movements that shape the mouse cerebellum; insights from genetic fate mapping. Neuron 45: 27–40.

Shikimi H, Sakamoto H, Mezaki Y, Ukena K, Tsutsui K (2004) Dendritic growth in response to environmental estrogens in the developing Purkinje cell in rats. Neurosci Lett 364: 114–118.

Simeone A, Acampora D, Gulisano M, Stornaiuolo A, Boncinelli E (1992) Nested expression domains of four homeobox genes in developing rostral brain. Nature 358: 687–690.

Solecki DJ, Liu XL, Tomoda T, Fang Y, Hatten ME (2001) Activated Notch2 signaling inhibits differentiation of cerebellar granule neuron precursors by maintaining proliferation. Neuron 31: 557–568.

Solecki DJ, Model L, Gaetz J, Kapoor TM, Hatten ME (2004) Par6alpha signaling controls glial-guided neuronal migration. Nat Neurosci 7: 1195–1203.

Solecki DJ, Govek EE, Tomoda T, Hatten ME (2006) Neuronal polarity in CNS development. Genes Dev 20: 2639–2647.

Solecki DJ, Trivedi N, Govek EE, Kerekes RA, Gleason SS, Hatten ME (2009) Myosin II motors and F-actin dynamics drive the coordinated movement of the centrosome and soma during CNS glial-guided neuronal migration. Neuron 63: 63–80.
Sotelo C (2004) Cellular and genetic regulation of the development of the cerebellar system. Prog Neurobiol 72: 295–339.
Sotelo C, Dusart I (2009) Intrinsic versus extrinsic determinants during the development of Purkinje cell dendrites. Neuroscience 162: 589–600.
Spassky N, Han YG, Aguilar A, Strehl L, Besse L, Laclef C, et al. (2008) Primary cilia are required for cerebellar development and Shh-dependent expansion of progenitor pool. Dev Biol 317: 246–259.
Steinmayr M, Andre E, Conquet F, Rondi-Reig L, Delhaye-Bouchaud N, Auclair N, et al. (1998) staggerer phenotype in retinoid-related orphan receptor alpha-deficient mice. Proc Natl Acad Sci U S A 95: 3960–3965.
Sudarov A, Joyner AL (2007) Cerebellum morphogenesis: the foliation pattern is orchestrated by multi-cellular anchoring centers. Neural Dev 2: 26.
Sweet HO, Bronson RT, Johnson KR, Cook SA, Davisson MT (1996) Scrambler, a new neurological mutation of the mouse with abnormalities of neuronal migration. Mamm Genome 7: 798–802.
Swinny JD, Metzger F, J IJ-P, Gounko NV, Gramsbergen A, van der Want JJ (2004) Corticotropin-releasing factor and urocortin differentially modulate rat Purkinje cell dendritic outgrowth and differentiation in vitro. Eur J Neurosci 19: 1749–1758.
Takagishi Y, Hashimoto K, Kayahara T, Watanabe M, Otsuka H, Mizoguchi A, et al. (2007) Diminished climbing fiber innervation of Purkinje cells in the cerebellum of myosin Va mutant mice and rats. Dev Neurobiol 67: 909–923.
Tomoda T, Kim JH, Zhan C, Hatten ME (2004) Role of Unc51.1 and its binding partners in CNS axon outgrowth. Genes Dev 18: 541–558.
Trommsdorff M, Gotthardt M, Hiesberger T, Shelton J, Stockinger W, Nimpf J, et al. (1999) Reeler/Disabled-like disruption of neuronal migration in knockout mice lacking the VLDL receptor and ApoE receptor 2. Cell 97: 689–701.
Tumpel S, Wiedemann LM, Krumlauf R (2009) Hox genes and segmentation of the vertebrate hindbrain. Curr Top Dev Biol 88: 103–137.
Urbanek P, Fetka I, Meisler MH, Busslinger M (1997) Cooperation of Pax2 and Pax5 in midbrain and cerebellum development. Proc Natl Acad Sci U S A 94: 5703–5708.
Uziel T, Zindy F, Sherr CJ, Roussel MF (2006) The CDK inhibitor p18Ink4c is a tumor suppressor in medulloblastoma. Cell Cycle 5: 363–365.
von Knebel Doeberitz C, Sievers J, Sadler M, Pehlemann FW, Berry M, Halliwell P (1986) Destruction of meningeal cells over the newborn hamster cerebellum with 6-hydroxydopamine prevents foliation and lamination in the rostral cerebellum. Neuroscience 17: 409–426.
Wallace VA (1999) Purkinje-cell-derived Sonic hedgehog regulates granule neuron precursor cell proliferation in the developing mouse cerebellum. Curr Biol 9: 445–448.
Wang VY, Rose MF, Zoghbi HY (2005) Math1 expression redefines the rhombic lip derivatives and reveals novel lineages within the brainstem and cerebellum. Neuron 48: 31–43.
Wassarman KM, Lewandoski M, Campbell K, Joyner AL, Rubenstein JL, Martinez S, Martin GR (1997) Specification of the anterior hindbrain and establishment of a normal mid/hindbrain organizer is dependent on Gbx2 gene function. Development 124: 2923–2934.
Watase K, Hashimoto K, Kano M, Yamada K, Watanabe M, Inoue Y, et al. (1998) Motor discoordination and increased susceptibility to cerebellar injury in GLAST mutant mice. Eur J Neurosci 10: 976–988.
Wechsler-Reya RJ, Scott MP (1999) Control of neuronal precursor proliferation in the cerebellum by Sonic Hedgehog. Neuron 22: 103–114.
Weiss LA, Arking DE, Daly MJ, Chakravarti A (2009) A genome-wide linkage and association scan reveals novel loci for autism. Nature 461: 802–808.
Wetts R, Herrup K (1982) Interaction of granule, Purkinje and inferior olivary neurons in lurcher chimaeric mice. I. Qualitative studies. J Embryol Exp Morphol 68: 87–98.
Wilson L, Maden M (2005) The mechanisms of dorsoventral patterning in the vertebrate neural tube. Dev Biol 282: 1–13.
Wilson PM, Fryer RH, Fang Y, Hatten ME (2010) Astn2, a novel member of the astrotactin gene family, regulates the trafficking of ASTN1 during glial-guided neuronal migration. J Neurosci 30: 8529–8540.
Wurst W, Auerbach AB, Joyner AL (1994) Multiple developmental defects in Engrailed-1 mutant mice: an early mid-hindbrain deletion and patterning defects in forelimbs and sternum. Development 120: 2065–2075.
Yachnis AT, Trojanowski JQ, Memmo M, Schlaepfer WW (1988) Expression of neurofilament proteins in the hypertrophic granule cells of Lhermitte-Duclos disease: an explanation for the mass effect and the myelination of parallel fibers in the disease state. J Neuropathol Exp Neurol 47: 206–216.
Yamada M, Terao M, Terashima T, Fujiyama T, Kawaguchi Y, Nabeshima Y, Hoshino M (2007) Origin of climbing fiber neurons and their developmental dependence on Ptf1a. J Neurosci 27: 10924–10934.
Yamamoto M, Ullman D, Drager UC, McCaffery P (1999) Postnatal effects of retinoic acid on cerebellar development. Neurotoxicol Teratol 21: 141–146.
Yamamoto M, Zhang J, Smith D, Hayakawa Y, McCaffery P (2003) A critical period for retinoic acid teratogenesis and loss of neurophilic migration of pontine nuclei neurons. Mech Dev 120: 701–709.
Yamamoto M, Fujinuma M, Hirano S, Hayakawa Y, Clagett-Dame M, Zhang J, McCaffery P (2005) Retinoic acid influences the development of the inferior olivary nucleus in the rodent. Dev Biol 280: 421–433.
Yip J, Soghomonian JJ, Blatt GJ (2007) Decreased GAD67 mRNA levels in cerebellar Purkinje cells in autism: pathophysiological implications. Acta Neuropathol 113: 559–568.
Yip J, Soghomonian JJ, Blatt GJ (2008) Increased GAD67 mRNA expression in cerebellar interneurons in autism: implications for Purkinje cell dysfunction. J Neurosci Res 86: 525–530.
Yuasa S, Kawamura K, Ono K, Yamakuni T, Takahashi Y (1991) Development and migration of Purkinje cells in the mouse cerebellar primordium. Anat Embryol (Berl) 184: 195–212.
Zanni G, Saillour Y, Nagara M, Billuart P, Castelnau L, Moraine C, et al. (2005) Oligophrenin 1 mutations frequently cause X-linked mental retardation with cerebellar hypoplasia. Neurology 65: 1364–1369.
Zordan P, Croci L, Hawkes R, Consalez GG (2008) Comparative analysis of proneural gene expression in the embryonic cerebellum. Dev Dyn 237: 1726–1735.

Part 2
Cerebellar Anatomy and Functions

2

Essential Anatomy of the Cerebellum and Related Structures

Patricia L. Musolino, Catherine J. Stoodley, and Jeremy D. Schmahmann

In this chapter we present an overview of the anatomic features of the cerebellum and interconnected regions essential to the understanding of the clinical manifestations of cerebellar lesions described in this volume. We emphasize organizational principles that help conceptualize the relationship of cerebellar structure to function, both in its traditional role of motor control as well as in nonmotor function.

Overview

The cerebellum (Fig. 2.1) is situated in the posterior cranial fossa, separated from the overlying occipital lobe by the tentorium cerebelli, and from the brainstem by the medullary velum that covers the roof of the fourth ventricle. It is attached to the brainstem by three bilaterally paired cerebellar peduncles, or stems. The basic internal organization of the cerebellum is a

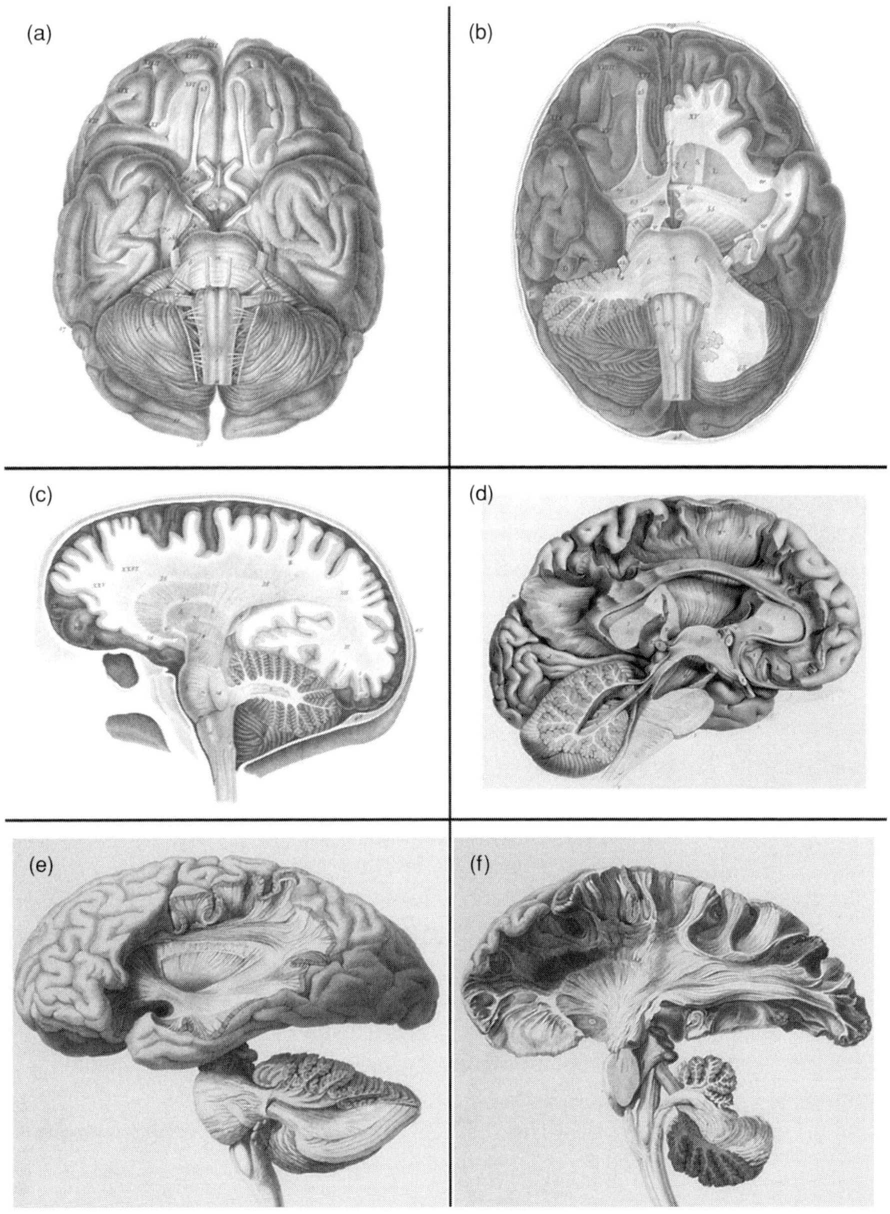

Fig. 2.1. Historic images of the human cerebellum and its relation to spinal cord, brainstem and cerebral hemispheres. **(a–c)** Depictions by Franz Joseph Gall (1758–1828) of **(a)** the ventral surface of the brain. The relations of the cerebellum to the pons and the medulla are apparent, with the pyramidal tracts and inferior olives readily identified. **(b)** Partial dissection of the cerebellum reveals the cerebellar folia and subfolia (diagram left) and part of a cerebellar nucleus (diagram right). **(c)** Sagittal dissection showing the cerebellum in the posterior fossa, a cerebellar nucleus, the pattern of cerebellar folia and subfolia, and relation to the pons, inferior olives and spinal cord. **(d)** Dissection of brain depicted by Achille-Louis Foville (1799–1878) showing the cerebellar folia and subfolia, with a tract (the superior cerebellar peduncle) emanating from the deep nuclei and traveling rostrally (to thalamus). **(e–f)** Drawing of brain dissections by Herbert Mayo (1796–1852) showing **(e)** pons and middle cerebellar peduncle entering the cerebellum, with the cerebellar folia partially displayed. The inferior olives are apparent at the lateral aspect of the medulla adjacent to the pyramidal tracts. **(f)** The superior and inferior cerebellar peduncles are clearly identified; the middle cerebellar peduncle has been dissected away. (Images from Gall and Spurzheim [1810], Foville [1844] and Mayo [1827] reproduced in Schmahmann and Pandya 2006.)

superficial cortex overlying a dense core of white matter. The cortex is multiply folded. The cerebellar fissures (equivalent to cerebral sulci) run transversely and follow the curve of the external surface. These fissures separate the folds of cerebellar tissue, or folia, that contain the trilaminate cerebellar cortex apposed on each side of a white matter lamella extending out from a central medullary core. Each folium also has multiple secondary divisions, called subfolia. Deep cerebellar nuclei (DCN) situated within the central region of the cerebellum are, from medial to lateral, the fastigial, globose, emboliform, and dentate nuclei.

Cerebellar lobules

The individual cerebellar folia group together as lobules, arising usually from a common ray of medullary white matter. Many nomenclatures for the cerebellum have been used over the years. The optimal and currently widely used approach is an updated and unified version (Schmahmann et al. 2000; Fig. 2.2) of those introduced by Lodewijk Bolk (1906) and Olaf Larsell (Larsell and Jansen 1972) that describes ten cerebellar lobules, each of which contains a vermal (midline) and hemispheric component, separated by named cerebellar fissures. The three major lobar divisions of the cerebellum are the anterior lobe (lobules I through V), the posterior lobe (lobules VI through IX), and the flocculonodular lobe (lobule X). The anterior lobe is separated from the posterior lobe by the primary fissure; and the posterior lobe is separated from the flocculonodular lobe by the posterolateral fissure. The cerebellar tonsil (important in herniation syndromes) is a gross morphological term that refers to the paired inferomedial protuberances of the cerebellum, comprising parts of lobules VIII and lobule IX.

Cerebellar peduncles

Three cerebellar peduncles carry incoming and outgoing cerebellar tracts that link the cerebellum with the spinal cord, brainstem, and cerebral hemispheres (Fig. 2.3). The peduncles also form the limiting lateral extension of the fourth ventricle. The inferior cerebellar peduncle (ICP) links the cerebellum with the medulla. It consists of a compact fiber tract situated laterally, the restiform body (a purely afferent system) and the medially situated juxtarestiform body (mainly carrying efferents from the flocculonodular lobe to the vestibular nuclei, and afferents to the same region from the vestibular nerve and nuclei). The middle cerebellar peduncle (MCP) is the largest of the three, and is composed almost entirely of afferent fibers that arise from the neurons in the contralateral basis pontis, with a small addition from nuclei in the pontine tegmentum. The superior cerebellar peduncle (SCP) links the cerebellum with the midbrain and diencephalon. It contains efferent fibers that course in the brachium conjunctivum, decussate in the midbrain, and pass via the contralateral red nucleus to terminate in the contralateral thalamus. The SCP also conveys some afferents.

Cerebellar nuclei

The fastigial nucleus is the homolog of the medial nucleus in lower primates, while the posterior and anterior interpositus nuclei are homologous with the globose and emboliform nuclei, respectively (Fig. 2.4). Among the cerebellar nuclei, the dentate, or lateral nucleus in lower vertebrates, has evolved most. Its large-celled dorsal part that has a smooth curvature is phylogenetically older. The microgyric ventral and lateral part that contains smaller neurons has expanded greatly in concert with the association cortices of the cerebral hemispheres. Each Purkinje cell contacts approximately 35 nuclear neurons, and each DCN neuron receives inhibitory GABAergic inputs from over 800 Purkinje cells. Neurons in the DCN are of three types. Large glutamatergic neurons convey excitatory output to the cerebellar cortex, thalamus, and brainstem. Small GABAergic neurons are inhibitory to the inferior olivary nucleus. Small inhibitory interneurons use both GABA and glycine as neurotransmitters. The Purkinje cell projection to the DCN is inhibitory, but the cortical interneuron influence on the Purkinje cell is inhibitory as well. The situation is further nuanced in that axo-somatic recurrent collaterals of the Purkinje cells provide inhibitory control on the Purkinje cells own output, while a further excitatory feedback to the cerebellar cortex arises from the DCN themselves. It is possible to identify the DCN on magnetic resonance images (MRI) by taking advantage of their iron content. The lateral vestibular nucleus of Deiters is located in the dorsal medulla, receives Purkinje cell axons directly from zone B of the lateral part of the anterior vermis, and may be regarded as equivalent to a DCN.

Afferent fibers

The cerebellar cortex receives excitatory inputs from two major classes of afferents – the climbing fiber and mossy fiber systems (Fig. 2.5). Climbing fibers originate exclusively from the inferior olivary nucleus, and enter the cerebellum via the ICP. The mossy fiber afferents to the cerebellar cortex arise from most of the non-olivary sources, particularly the spinocerebellar and pontocerebellar tracts, and are much more numerous than climbing fibers. The thick, heavily myelinated mossy fibers enter through the three cerebellar peduncles depending on their site of origin. Mossy fiber afferents arising in the pons terminate predominantly in the contralateral cerebellum, with a lesser projection to the ipsilateral cerebellar hemisphere after crossing the midline in the cerebellar white matter. A third contingent, monoaminergic afferent fibers, are thought to modulate the release of neurotransmitters. *Noradrenergic* innervation arises from neurons in the caudal portion of the locus coeruleus; *serotoninergic* afferents arise from the raphe nuclei; *histaminergic* fibers from neurons in the tuberomammillary nucleus of the posterior hypothalamus; and *dopaminergic* inputs from the midbrain. Diffuse *cholinergic* projections have also been observed in the cerebellum, arising particularly from the vestibular nuclei and terminating in the most rostral and caudal sectors of the vermis (Ikeda et al. 1992). The diffusible

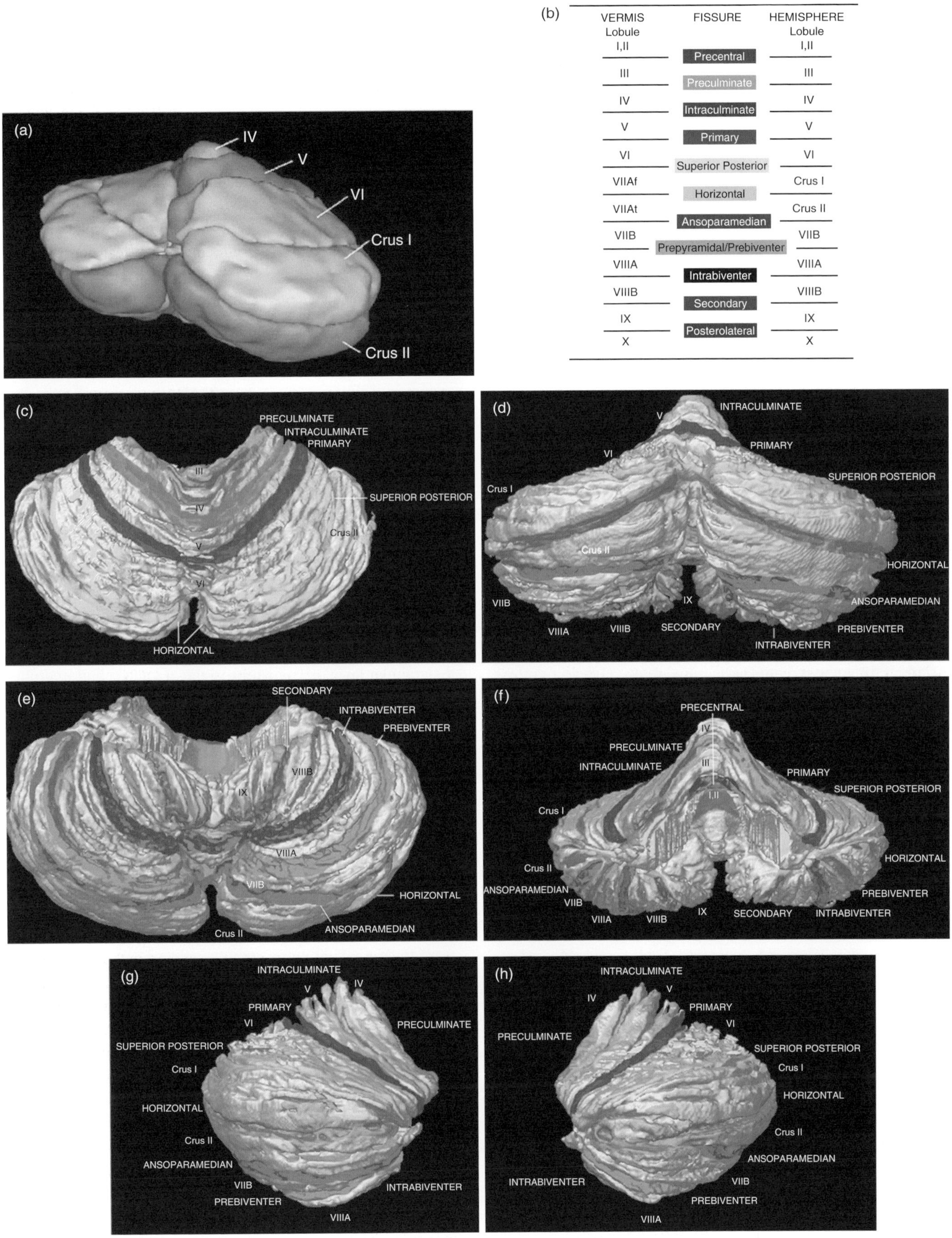

Fig. 2.2. Surface reconstructions of the human cerebellum derived from magnetic resonance images. **(a)** The cerebellum is viewed from the right posterior superior aspect, showing lobules IV through crus II as labeled. **(b)** Diagram illustrating the relationship of the named cerebellar fissures to the lobules in the vermis and hemispheres. The named fissures are demarcated in color according to the convention in (b), and the fissures and lobules are identified. The cerebellum is viewed from **(c)** superior, **(d)** posterior, **(e)** inferior, **(f)** anterior, **(g)** right lateral, and **(h)** left lateral aspects. ((a) from Makris et al. 2005; (b–h) from Schmahmann et al. 1999, 2000.) (See color plate 6).

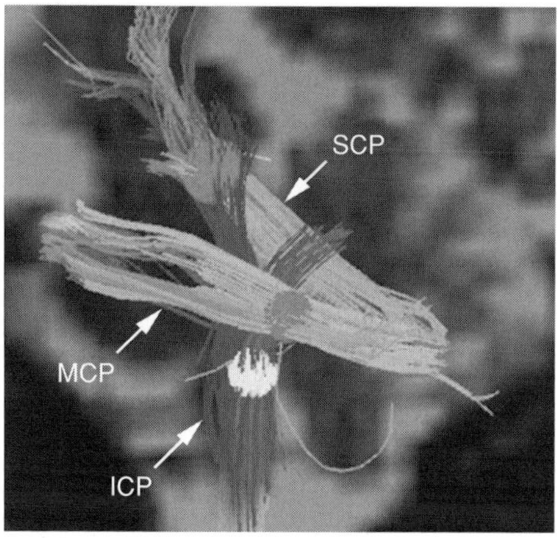

Fig. 2.3. Superior (SCP), middle (MCP) and inferior (ICP) cerebellar peduncles in human identified with diffusion spectrum magnetic resonance imaging, overlaid on a diffusion weighted image of cerebellum and brainstem. (From Granziera et al. 2009.) (See color plate 7).

messenger nitric oxide is likely to be a neurotransmitter in the cerebellar cortex as well, as the nitric oxide-producing enzyme nitric oxide synthase is present in granule cells, and soluble guanylyl cyclase through which nitric oxide acts is present in Purkinje cells, granule cells, and interneurons.

Components and circuits of the cerebellar cortex

Unlike the cerebral cortex with its multiple cortical cytoarchitectonic areas, the cerebellar cortical histology is essentially invariant throughout, with the neurons of the cerebellar cortex and nuclei linked together in multiple repeating anatomic microcircuits termed corticonuclear microcomplexes (Eccles et al. 1967; Ito 1984; Llinás 1985). The three layers of the cerebellar cortex identifiable on light microscopy (Fig. 2.6) are the molecular layer, the granule cell layer, and the Purkinje cell layer (see Cajal 1909; Fox et al. 1967; Palay and Chan-Palay 1974; Oertel 1993; Voogd 2004).

The **molecular layer** is the most superficial of the three cortical layers, is 300μm thick, and consists predominantly of axons of the granule cells that have branched to form the parallel fibers that travel along the long axis of the folium. The molecular layer also contains GABAergic inhibitory interneurons – the basket and stellate cells; dendritic arborizations of the Purkinje cells; climbing fibers; dendritic trees of the Golgi cell interneuron; and the processes of the supporting glial cells. The *basket cell* has a pyramidal or oval shape, and lies in the lower third of the molecular layer just above the Purkinje cells. Its dendrites extend up throughout the molecular layer in a parasagittal plane in a fan-shaped field of 30μm. The axon has a horizontal course in the parasagittal plane perpendicular to the long axis of the folium (that is, perpendicular to the orientation of the parallel fibers and in the same plane as the flattened plate of the Purkinje cell dendritic tree). It courses along among the lower dendrites of the Purkinje cell dendritic tree, enlarges and emits a succession of descending branches that envelope the cell bodies of 9 to 10 Purkinje cells in an axonal sheath with numerous synaptic contacts over its entire surface, hence the derivation of the basket cell's name (Fig. 2.6C). The terminal axonal branches descend to surround the initial segment of the Purkinje cell axon in a dense plexus of convoluted and branching fibers measuring 15–20μm across, that has the appearance of an old paintbrush or 'pinceau'. *Stellate cells* have small cell bodies 5–10μm in diameter. Their dendrites are contacted by parallel fibers and their axons terminate on the Purkinje cell dendrites.

The **granule cell layer** is the innermost of the three layers of the cortex. The *granule cells* are among the smallest neurons in the brain (6–8μm in diameter) and the most numerous single neuronal element in the nervous system. The granule cell contains minimal cytoplasm, and has three to five claw-like branched dendrites that participate in the granule cell glomerulus (see below). The single granule cell axon that provides excitatory (glutamatergic) input to the Purkinje cells ascends through the Purkinje cell layer into the molecular layer where it divides into two branches (like a 'T') to form the parallel fiber, one of the thinnest known vertebrate axons. The *Golgi cells* are irregularly shaped, large, rounded or polygonal, inhibitory interneurons that utilize GABA and glycine as their neurotransmitters. They number approximately 1 per 1.5 Purkinje cells in humans. The Golgi dendritic tree has a three-dimensional configuration. There are one to three distinctive Golgi axons that after a short course divide repeatedly, resulting in a multitude of fine branches that form an elaborate and dense plexus that extends throughout the entire thickness of the granular layer, participating in the granule cell glomerulus. The *Lugaro cell*, also an inhibitory interneuron, is a fusiform cell lying in the outermost third of the granular layer. It connects with an infraganglionic plexus formed by recurrent axon collaterals of the Purkinje cells and granule cells, and, via its axons, with the stellate, basket, and Golgi cells. The *unipolar brush cell* is the only excitatory (glutamatergic) cerebellar cortical interneuron, situated in the vestibulocerebellum and the vermis. It has a cell body 9–12μm in diameter and a single dendrite ending in a tight brush-like tip of dendrioles that have extensive synaptic contact with the mossy fiber rosette. The unipolar brush cell likely amplifies vestibular signals, providing feedforward excitation to granule cells.

The **Purkinje cell layer** is a 100μm monolayer, situated between the molecular and granule cell layers, consists of the elegant Purkinje cell, one of the largest cells in the nervous system, and the single most important neuronal element in the cerebellum. The proximal dendrite of the Purkinje cell arises from the apical pole of the pear-shape cell body, and divides usually into two major dendrites that then branch multiple times to form a flattened plate oriented perpendicular to the long axis of the folium with a fan-like appearance. The Purkinje cell axon arises from the pole opposite to the dendrites, descends through a constricted region surrounded by the pinceau of the basket cell axon terminals, acquires a myelin sheath about 50μm beneath the Purkinje cell soma, and descends through the granule cell layer to the DCN and (in the case of lobule X)

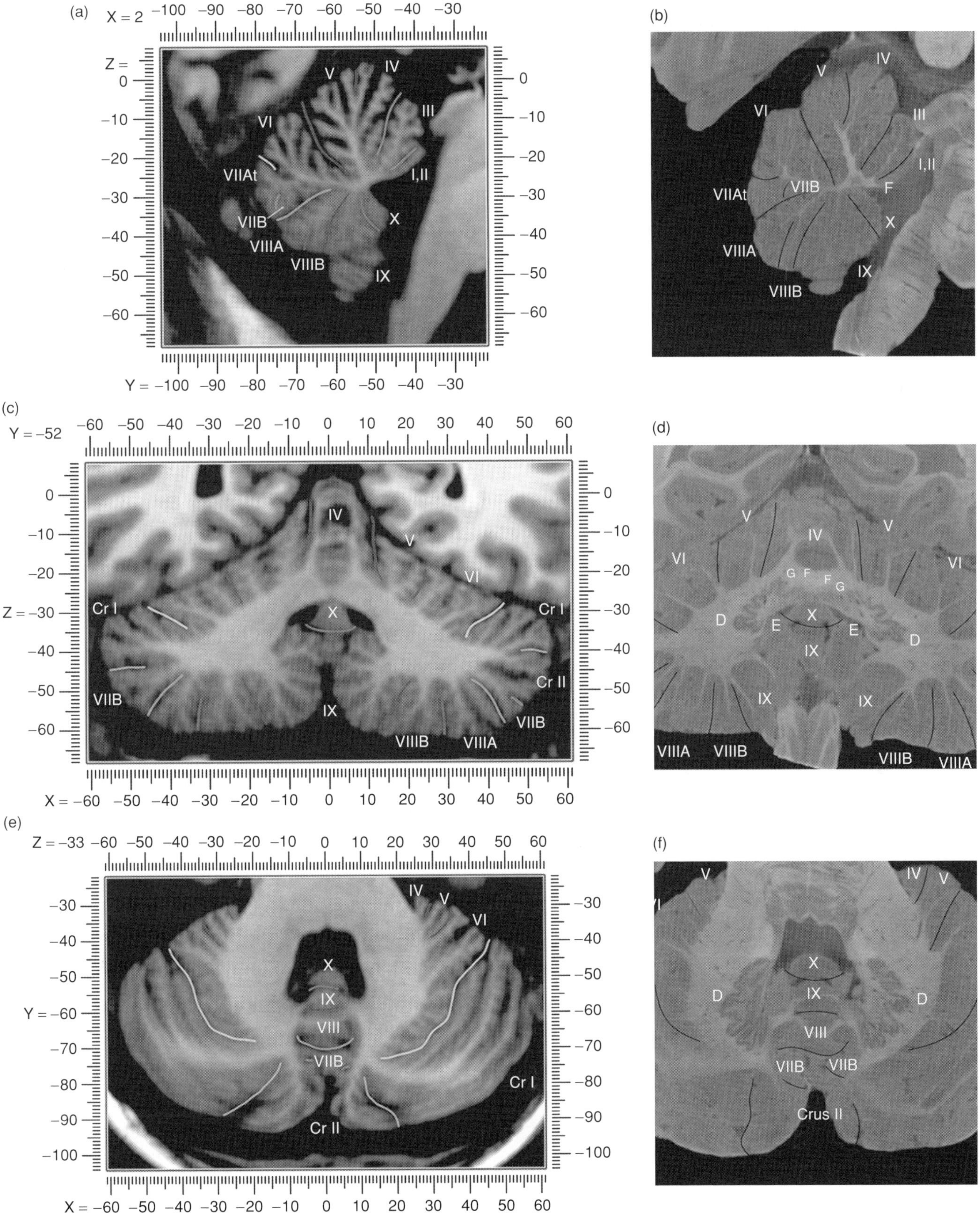

Fig. 2.4. Images of the human cerebellum on MRI (left panel) and postmortem cryosection (right panel). The cerebellum is sectioned in the sagittal plane 2mm to the right of midline in **(a)** and **(b)**; in the coronal plane 52mm behind the anterior commissure–posterior commissure (AC-PC) line in **(c)** and **(d)**; and in the transverse plane 33mm below the AC-PC line in **(e)** and **(f)**. Fissures are color coded according to the convention used in Fig. 2.2(b–h), and the lobules are designated. Deep cerebellar nuclei are identified in the cryosection brain: E, emboliform nucleus; F, fastigial nucleus; G, globose nucleus; D, dentate nucleus. (From Schmahmann et al. 2000.) (See color plate 8).

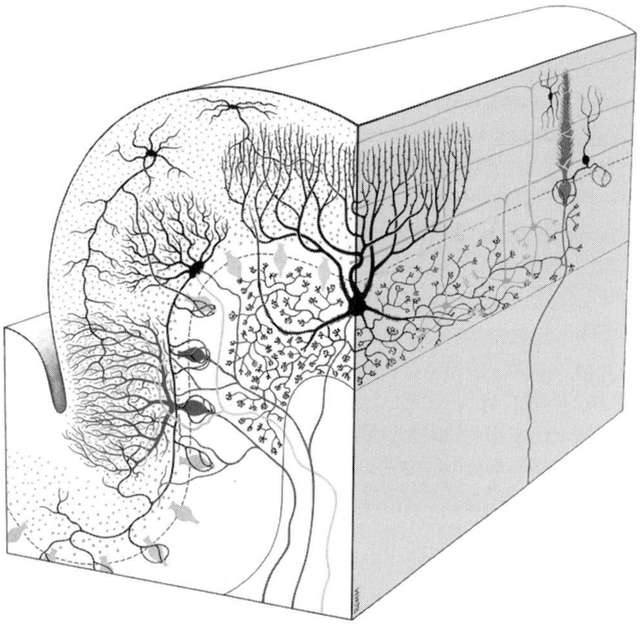

Fig. 2.5. Organization of the cerebellar cortex. A single cerebellar folium is shown sectioned in its longitudinal axis (diagram right) and transversely (left). Purkinje cells are red; superficial and deep stellate, basket and Golgi cells are black; granule cells and ascending axons and parallel fibers are yellow; mossy and climbing fibers are blue. Also shown are the glomeruli with mossy fiber rosettes, claw-like dendrites of granule cells, and Golgi axons. Lugaro and unipolar brush cells are not shown. (Diagram of Eccles, Ito, Szengothai 1967, as redrawn in Gray's Anatomy 1995.) (See color plate 9).

to precerebellar nuclei. The GABAergic Purkinje cell is the only cortical neuron that has axons leaving the cerebellar cortex. Its inhibitory output to the DCN is sculpted by the inhibitory inputs from the cerebellar cortical interneurons (basket, stellate, and Golgi cells), and recurrent Purkinje cell axon collaterals, and excitatory feedback from the DCN.

Mossy fibers provide excitatory, primarily glutamatergic, input to the Purkinje cell indirectly: they synapse on the dendritic claws of the granule cells, the axons of which provide excitatory input to the Purkinje cell dendrites. The mossy fiber termination, known as a rosette because of its large lobulated appearance, is the central component of the granule cell glomerulus (Fig. 2.6b), a complex articulation between mossy fiber rosettes, terminal arborizations of granule cell dendrites, and inhibitory feedback from descending axons of Golgi cells. The granule cell axon ascends through the granule cell layer and forms the parallel fibers, the two branches traveling in opposite directions along the folium for a distance of up to 6–8mm in the human. The orientation of the parallel fibers along the long axis of the folium is perpendicular to that of the flattened plate of the Purkinje cell dendritic tree oriented in the parasagittal plane (Fig. 2.5). This allows each granule cell to make synaptic contact with the spiny branchlets of the intermediate and distal regions of the Purkinje cell dendritic tree, on up to 300 Purkinje cells along the folium. Each Purkinje cell in turn receives synaptic inputs from approximately 200 000 parallel fibers. On its way to the distal arbors of the Purkinje cell dendritic tree, the *ascending* axon of the granule cell makes synaptic contact first with

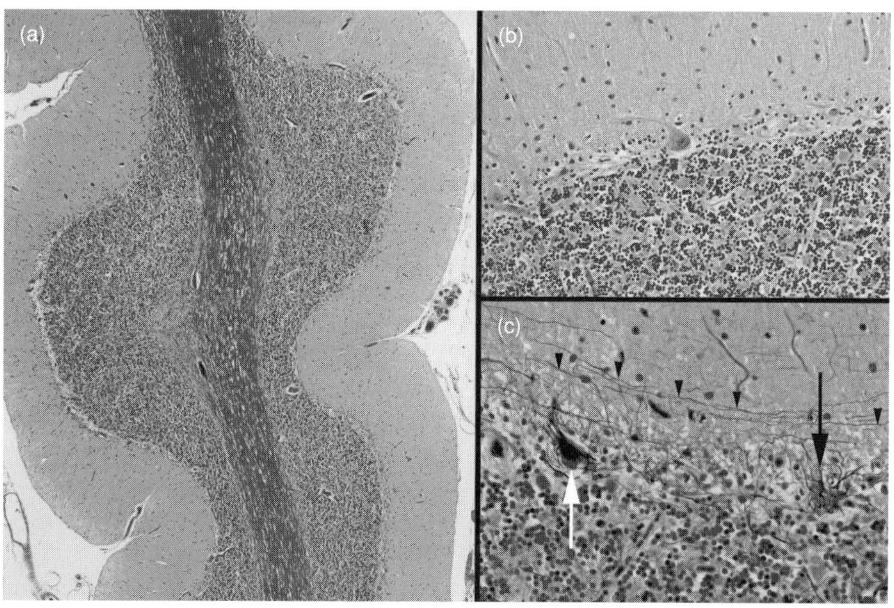

Fig. 2.6. Photomicrographs of the human cerebellar cortex. **(a)** Low power view of a cerebellar folium showing white matter (stained blue) coursing between the apposed leaves of the cerebellar cortex: granular layer innermost, Purkinje cell monolayer intermediate, and molecular layer outermost. 4× magnification, stained with hematoxylin and eosin (H&E). **(b)** The Purkinje cell layer is seen between the molecular layer (above) and the granule cell layer (below). Note the eosinophilic (pink stained) glomeruli throughout the granular layer. 20× magnification, H&E. **(c)** Cerebellar cortex derived from a patient with spinocerebellar ataxia type 7 to show axons of basket cells (arrowheads) coursing horizontally in the Purkinje cell layer, enveloping a Purkinje cell in the basket of axon terminal ramifications (white arrow) and forming an 'empty basket' around a degenerated Purkinje cell (black arrow). 40× magnification, silver stain. (Photographs courtesy of Dr. Matthew Frosch, C.S. Kubik Laboratory for Neuropathology, Massachusetts General Hospital.) (See color plate 10).

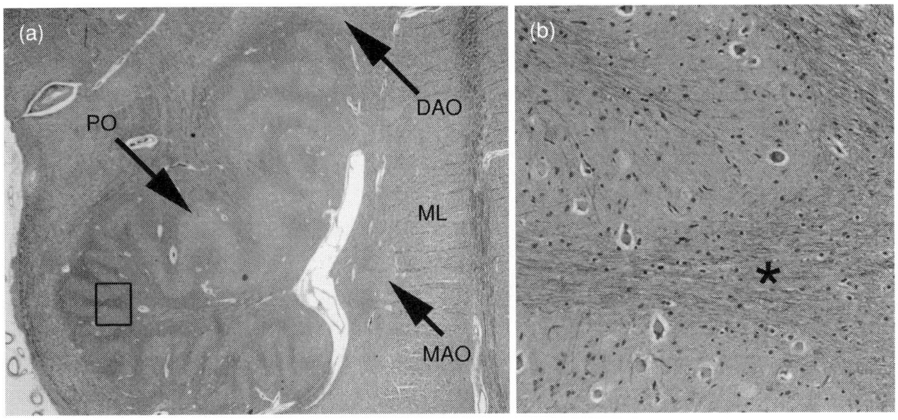

Fig. 2.7. Photomicrographs of human inferior olivary complex. **(a)** Low power view of the ventral part of the right medulla sectioned in a slightly oblique plane. 4× magnification, H&E. The principal olivary nucleus (PO), and dorsal (DAO) and medial accessory olivary nuclei (MAO) are labeled, laterally adjacent to the medial lemniscus (ML). **(b)** Higher magnification view shows neurons in the principal olive, and the hilum of the olive (asterisk) through which the olivocerebellar fibers (stained blue) course to the contralateral cerebellum. 10× magnification, H&E. (Photographs courtesy of Dr. Matthew Frosch, C.S. Kubik Laboratory for Neuropathology, Massachusetts General Hospital.) (See color plate 11).

dendrites of Golgi cells in the granular layer, and then with the spines of the proximal dendrites of Purkinje cells after it has entered the molecular layer. Approximately 20% of the granule cell synapses on a Purkinje cell are made by the ascending segment of the granule cell axon. This facilitates a more restricted influence on a single Purkinje cell than the parallel fiber-Purkinje cell synapses would allow.

The climbing fiber afferents to the Purkinje cell arise exclusively from neurons of the inferior olive (Fig. 2.7). The axons of each olivary neuron branch in the cerebellar white matter to form seven to ten climbing fibers, each of which provides extensive, excitatory synaptic contact with a single Purkinje cell, mediated principally by glutamate. They also emit collaterals to the DCN. In the lower two-thirds of the molecular layer the climbing fiber lies closely apposed to the trunk and major branches of the Purkinje cell dendritic tree, forming synapses with the stubby spines on the proximal Purkinje cell dendrites. Each varicosity of a climbing fiber synapses with several dendritic spines all arising from the same dendritic branch of the Purkinje cell, unlike the parallel fiber varicosities each of which synapses with only one or two spines on the distal branches of the Purkinje cell dendritic tree. Based on earlier connectional and functional principles, the cerebellum was considered to have three mediolateral divisions, comprising the medial, intermediate, and lateral zones. These mediolateral distinctions have been further subdivided into discrete longitudinal parasagittal zones (A, X, B, C1, C2, C3, D1, D2 from medial to lateral). These are defined by monoclonal antibody staining techniques and by the strict mediolateral topographic arrangement of the reciprocal olivocerebellar projections that link the olive with the cerebellar cortex and nuclei, and by the zonal arrangement of the corticonuclear projection (Fig. 2.8). This zonal pattern of organization of the cerebellum into multiple discrete modules is an important feature of the anatomic and functional organization of the cerebellar corticonuclear microcomplex (Tolbert et al. 1978; Courville et al. 1980; Voogd and Glickstein, 1998; Voogd 2004; Haines and Manto, 2010).

The Purkinje cell generates two very different classes of action potentials mediated by its two principal afferents. Climbing fiber input to the Purkinje cell induces a complex spike with a very low frequency of 0.5 to 2 spikes per second. This is the same rate of firing as the olivary neurons from which the climbing fiber originates. The climbing fiber input to the Purkinje cell is thought to signal the occurrence of errors. In contrast, the mossy fiber input to the Purkinje cell induces a repetitive simple spike with a frequency between 50 and 150 spikes per second. The parallel fiber input is thought to provide information about incoming signals, such as direction and speed of limb movement. In the cognitive domain the parallel fibers may provide the Purkinje cell with the context in which specific behaviors occur. These circuits are relevant to synaptic plasticity involved in learning and memory. Long-term depression (LTD) is characterized by the persistent depression of synaptic transmission from parallel fibers to the Purkinje cell that occurs when the parallel fibers are activated concurrently with the activation of climbing fibers to the same Purkinje cell. Long-term depression has also been noted in the climbing fiber-Purkinje cell synapse. Long-term potentiation (LTP) occurs in the mossy fiber–granule cell interaction.

Vascular supply

Three pairs of major arteries irrigate the cerebellum – the posterior inferior (PICA), anterior inferior (AICA), and superior cerebellar arteries (SCA). The PICAs branch off from the vertebral arteries, loop around the cerebellar tonsil and divide into at least two main branches that supply the medial and lateral aspects of the posterior lobe, the ventral parts of the cerebellar nuclei, the ICP and portions of the MCP and the medulla. The AICAs are derived from the basilar artery and irrigate the anterior aspect of the posterior lobe, part of the anterior lobe, the MCP, and the inferior aspect of the lateral pons. The SCAs are derived from the rostral basilar artery. They run along the superior aspect of the cerebellum supplying the anterior lobe and superior part of the posterior lobe, the superior aspect of the deep nuclei, SCP and rostral part of the lateral pons. There is a dorsal–ventral border zone between the SCA–PICA territories within the dentate nucleus. Venous drainage is via the superior cerebellar veins that drain to the great cerebral vein, and straight, transverse and superior petrosal sinuses; the medial inferior cerebellar veins that enter the

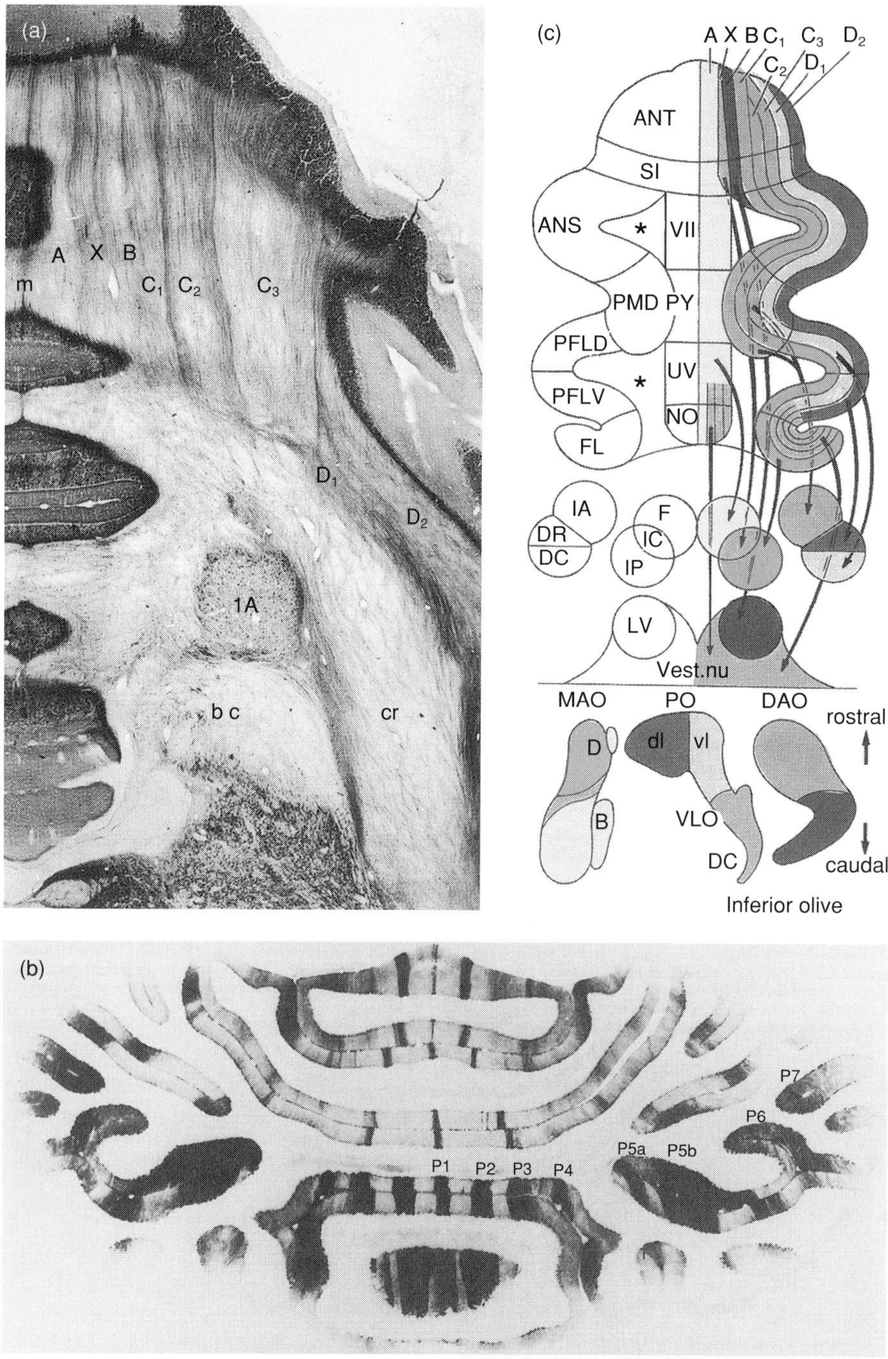

Fig. 2.8. Diagrams depicting parasagittal zones and connections in the cerebellum. **(a)** Transverse section through the anterior lobe of monkey cerebellum stained for acetylcholinesterase, showing white matter compartments. **(b)** Frontal section through the cerebellum of an adult rat to show Purkinje cells stained with immunoperoxidase for zebrin I. The immunoreactive Purkinje cells align to form parasagittal bands in the vermis and hemispheres. **(c)** Color-coded diagram showing the zonal arrangement of cerebellar corticonuclear (above) and olivocerebellar projections (below) on a flattened cerebellar cortex of the cat. Cerebellum – zones A, X, B, C1, C2, C3, D1, D2; ANS, ansiform lobule; ANT, anterior lobe; FL, flocculus; IA, anterior interposed nucleus; bc, brachium conjunctivum; cr, restiform body; NO, nodulus; P1–7, parasagittal zones in the rat cerebellum; PFL (D/V), (dorsal/ventral) paraflocculus; PMD, paramedian lobule; PY, pyramis; SI, lobulus simplex (lobule VI); UV, uvula. Cerebellar nuclei – DC, ventrocaudal dentate nucleus; DR, rostromedial dentate nucleus; IC, interstitial cell group; IP, posterior interposed nucleus; F, fastigial nucleus. Inferior olivary nucleus – B, ß cell group; D, dorsomedial cell column; DAO, dorsal accessory olive; DC, dorsal cap; dl, dorsal leaf; MAO, medial accessory olive; PO, principal olive; vl, ventral leaf; VLO, ventrolateral outgrowth. Vest. nu, vestibular nuclei; LV, lateral vestibular nucleus. ((a) and (c) from Voogd and Glickstein 1998. (b) from Leclerc et al. 1990.) (See color plate 12).

straight or sigmoid sinuses; and lateral inferior cerebellar veins that join the inferior petrosal and occipital sinuses.

Connections of the cerebellum

The cytoarchitecture of the cerebellar cortex is predictably similar in the different cerebellar areas. This paracrystalline structure of the cerebellar corticonuclear microcomplex is the basis for a number of theoretical approaches to understanding the fundamental function of the cerebellum, as we discuss later. In contrast, the connections of the cerebellum are entirely different depending on the location within the cerebellum. This is true for the cerebellar corticonuclear connections (arranged as repeating corticonuclear microcomplexes) such that the vermis and medial parts of the hemispheres are linked with the fastigial nucleus, and progressively laterally situated cortical areas are precisely linked with the globose, emboliform, and dentate nuclei. It is true also for the connections of the cerebellum with the spinal cord, brainstem, and cerebral hemispheres. A working knowledge of the fundamental features of these connections is therefore necessary in order to enhance the clinician's appreciation of the functions of the cerebellum and the clinical consequences of cerebellar lesions. We first address the afferent connections of the cerebellum that constitute the feedforward system, according to the peduncles through which they enter the cerebellum – the ICP, MCP, and SCP. The efferents from the cerebellum are then covered, according to the outputs of the different DCN (see Jansen and Brodal 1954; Courville et al. 1980; Brodal 1981; Haines et al. 1997; De Zeeuw and Cicirata 2005; Nieuwenhuys et al. 2008).

AFFERENTS ENTERING VIA THE INFERIOR CEREBELLAR PEDUNCLE

Somatosensory afferents

The central axons of primary sensory neurons that enter the spinal cord through the dorsal roots give rise to the spinocerebellar tracts (Fig. 2.9). The trunk and lower limbs are subserved by the dorsal and ventral spinocerebellar tracts, and the head, neck and upper extremities are subserved by the rostral spinocerebellar, cuneocerebellar, and trigeminocerebellar tracts.

The **dorsal spinocerebellar tract (DSCT)** arises from neurons in the nucleus dorsalis (Clarke's column) situated at the base of the dorsal horn of the spinal cord in Rexed lamina VII between T1 and L3. It travels ipsilaterally, passes through the ICP, and terminates in the hindlimb regions of the anterior lobe and paramedian lobule (lobule VIII). The DSCT conveys modality and space-specific information from muscle spindles,

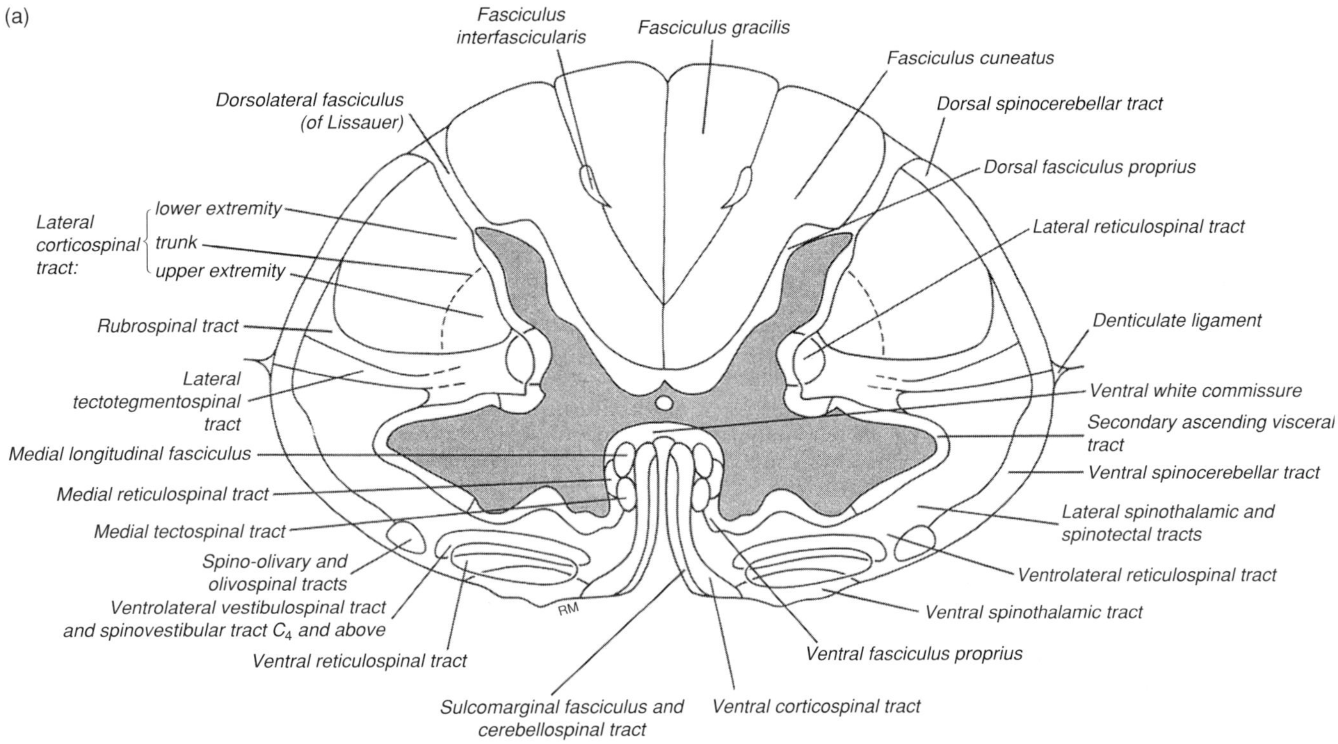

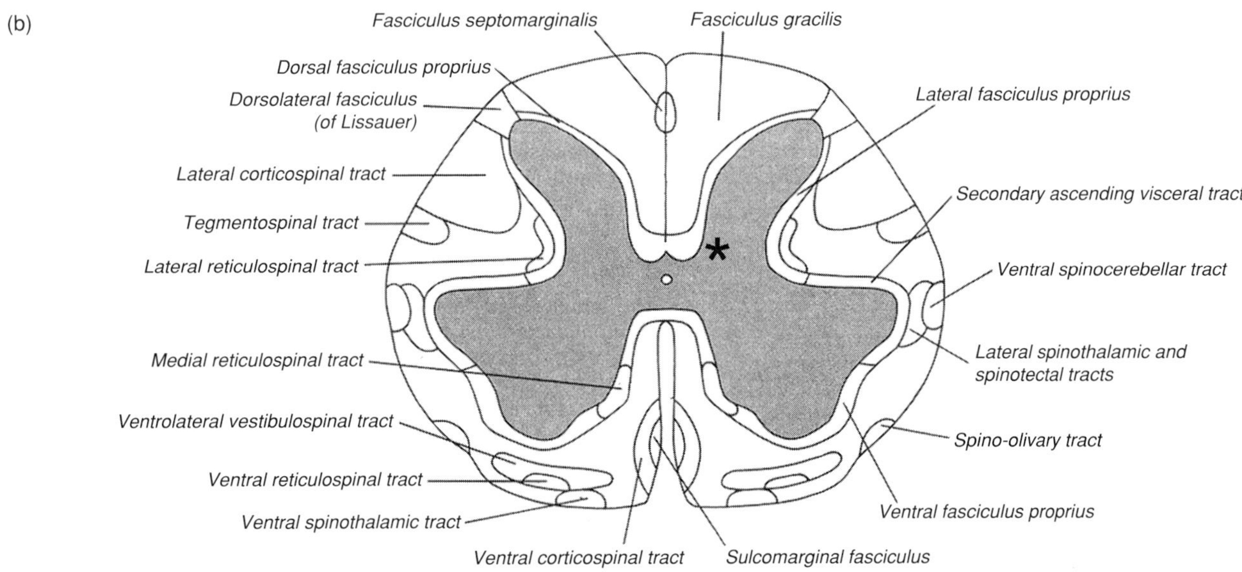

Fig. 2.9. Diagrams of the spinal cord identifying the locations of the ascending and descending tracts at **(a)** mid-cervical levels and **(b)** lumbar levels. Note the locations of the dorsal and ventral spinocerebellar tracts, the descending vestibular, reticular, tectal, and rubrospinal tracts, as well as the spino-olivary and corticospinal tracts discussed in the text. The asterisk in (b) denotes the location of Clarke's column that gives rise to the dorsal spinocerebellar tract. (From Gray's Anatomy 1995.)

tendon organs, and touch and pressure receptors in the trunk and lower limbs.

The **cuneocerebellar tract** is the equivalent of the DSCT for the neck, upper extremity, and upper trunk. This arises from the external cuneate nucleus (also, the lateral or accessory cuneate nucleus) situated lateral and rostral to the cuneate nucleus in the medulla, that receives axons from dorsal root fibers at levels C1 to T5. The cuneocerebellar fibers travel in the ICP, and convey similar types of information as found in the DSCT to the ipsilateral forelimb representation in the anterior lobe and the rostral part of the paramedian lobule.

The **rostral spinocerebellar tract** is the equivalent in the upper extremities of the ventral spinocerebellar tract (VSCT; described below with fibers that enter the cerebellum via the SCP), but unlike the VSCT it is uncrossed. The fibers in the rostral spinocerebellar tract arise in Rexed lamina VII at spinal cord levels C4 to C8, enter the ipsilateral cerebellum via both the ICP and the SCP, and terminate in the forelimb representations of the anterior lobe and paramedian lobules.

The **trigeminocerebellar tract** arises from the trigeminospinal and main sensory nuclei of the trigeminal nerve. These mossy fibers reach the cortex of the face representation in caudal lobule V and lobule VI.

Olivocerebellar afferents

The inferior olivary nuclei give rise to the climbing fiber inputs to the cerebellum. All parts of the cerebellar cortex and cerebellar nuclei receive fibers from the contralateral inferior olivary nucleus, with sharp topographic localization within a mediolateral zone and with a rostrocaudal pattern. Each cerebellar longitudinal zone (vermis, paravermis, medial and lateral hemispheres) is supplied by fibers from a particular region of the inferior olive. Collateral branches of the climbing fibers terminate also in the DCN. The topographic arrangement of the olivocerebellar projections is summarized in Fig. 2.8.

Sources of afferents to the inferior olive

The information conveyed by the olive to the cerebellum reflects the inputs that the olive receives from its various afferent sources. These inputs to the olive are topographically organized, but not with same level of precision as the olivocerebellar projections.

Spinal cord. Projections from the spinal cord are conveyed directly to the inferior olive in the crossed ventral spino-olivary tracts. Fibers in the dorsal spino-olivary tracts are also crossed but these terminate in the dorsal column nuclei that in turn project to the contralateral olive. Lumbar areas of the spinal cord project to the lateral parts of the dorsal and medial accessory olive (DAO and MAO), and these project to the leg representation in the rostral sectors of the cerebellar anterior lobe in medial and intermediate zones (A through C3). Cervical regions project medially in the nuclei, and these project to the representation of the upper extremity in the caudal part of the anterior lobe.

Red nucleus. The parvocellular component of the red nucleus (RNpc) projects via the central tegmental tract to the principal olivary nucleus that in turn projects back to the cerebellum. The RNpc can be subdivided into a dorsomedial subnucleus, and a ventrolateral and caudal portion. The dorsomedial subnucleus receives afferents from frontal eye field and premotor and prefrontal areas, and from the caudal-ventral part of the dentate nucleus linked with the medial D1 zone. It projects to the ventral lamina of the principal olive that projects back to the caudal dentate nucleus. The lateral and caudal parts of the RNpc receive somatotopically arranged afferents from primary motor and premotor regions, and from the rostral-medial dentate nucleus linked with the lateral D2 zone. It projects to the dorsal lamina and bend of the principal olive, which projects back to the rostral and dorsal dentate nucleus. The Guillain-Mollaret triangle is a circuit that links the RNpc via the central tegmental tract to the inferior olive; the olive to the cerebellar cortex and dentate nucleus through the olivocerebellar projection; and the dentate nucleus projection back to the RNpc. Lesions affecting this circuit lead to the clinical phenomenon of palatal tremor, or palatal myoclonus. Note that the magnocellular part of the red nucleus (RNmc) receives inputs from the nuclei that are the human equivalent of the cerebellar globose and emboliform nuclei. The RNmc does not project to the inferior olive, but rather to the spinal cord.

Pretectal nuclei. Projections from the nucleus of the optic tract and nuclei of the accessory optic system terminate in the dorsal cap and the ventrolateral outgrowth of the principal olivary nucleus. This input concerns optokinetic information and is relayed to the flocculonodular lobe.

Vestibular nuclei. Information from the vertical semicircular canals and otoliths is conveyed by the medial and inferior vestibular nuclei to two subnuclei of the contralateral inferior olive: the dorsomedial cell column which projects to cerebellar lobules VIII, IX and X; and the nucleus β component of the MAO that projects to lateral parts of lobules VII and VIII and medial parts of lobules IX and X.

Superior colliculus. Visual information is conveyed from the superior colliculus to the medial part of the MAO in its caudal and medial part, which then projects to the visual area in vermal lobule VII.

Cerebral cortex. Scarce projections directly to the olive from the cerebral cortex have been observed, derived exclusively from layer V of motor cortex area 4 and premotor cortex area 6. There is overlap with the somatotopic arrangement of the mossy fiber spinal inputs to the cerebellum.

Zona incerta. Unlike essentially all other sources of input to the olive, the zona incerta receives projections not only from motor and supplementary motor cortices, but also from associative regions of the cerebral cortex, including the dorsolateral and dorsomedial prefrontal, cingulate, and medial and posterior parietal areas, and the superior temporal gyrus. The projection from the zona incerta to the olive provides one of the few mechanisms whereby the climbing fiber system has access to nonmotor information.

Deep cerebellar nuclei. The interpositus nuclei project back to the inferior olivary regions (the DAO and MAO) that are linked with the anterior lobe. The dentate projections are linked to the principal olivary nucleus.

Other olivary afferents. Regions in the midbrain that have minor olivary projections include the para-oculomotor nucleus of Darkschewitsch, the interstitial nucleus of Cajal, and the Edinger-Westphal nucleus, as well as the perihypoglossal and lateral reticular nuclei and the periaqueductal gray.

Vestibulocerebellar afferents

Primary afferents from the vestibular ganglion project directly to the ventral part of vermal lobule IX (uvula) and to vermal lobule X (nodulus) as well as to lobules VIIIB and IX (corresponding to the ventral paraflocculus), and to the fastigial nucleus.

Secondary afferents from the medial and inferior vestibular nuclei terminate in regions similar to the primary afferents, plus more widespread vermal regions.

Reticulocerebellar afferents

These originate mostly from the nucleus reticularis tegmenti pontis (NRTP), the lateral reticular nucleus, and the paramedian reticular formation, and terminate in the spinal areas of the anterior lobe as mossy fibers. The NRTP receives afferents from sensorimotor cortices as well as from the posterior parietal cortex, particularly the superior parietal lobule, and from the vestibular nuclei. The lateral reticular nucleus receives inputs from the spinal cord, red nucleus and cerebral cortex, and commits its efferents through the ICP mostly to the contralateral cerebellum. The paramedian reticular nucleus situated in the medial part of the reticular formation of the medulla receives afferents from the vestibular nuclei and the somatosensory cerebral cortex and feedback from the fastigial nucleus. Projections to the cerebellum from this reticular nucleus are mostly to the vermis.

Arcuate cerebellar tract

The arcuate nucleus is situated in the medulla, ventral to the pyramidal tract. Fibers leave this nucleus and course dorsally, adjacent to the midline of the medulla, to form the striae medullares. These lie on the dorsal surface of the medulla, and separate the inferior and superior portions of the floor of the fourth ventricle. The arcuate cerebellar fibers then enter the cerebellum via the ICP and terminate in the ipsilateral flocculus (hemispheric lobule X). The arcuate nucleus is the putative homolog of the respiratory chemosensory region at the ventral medullary surface in animals, involved in central reflex chemosensitivity and cardiorespiratory activity. Neuropathological studies have shown that it is abnormal in cases of stillbirth (Matturri et al. 2002; Folkerth et al. 2008).

AFFERENTS ENTERING VIA THE MIDDLE CEREBELLAR PEDUNCLE

The corticopontocerebellar system

Each cerebral hemisphere communicates predominantly with the contralateral cerebellar hemisphere. The cerebrocerebellar circuit (Fig. 2.10) consists of a two-stage feedforward limb – the ipsilateral corticopontine projection, and the crossed pontocerebellar pathway in the MCP; and a two-stage feedback limb – the crossed cerebellothalamic pathway through the SCP, and the ipsilateral thalamocortical projection. Axons destined for the pons course in the anterior limb of the internal capsule from prefrontal regions, or the sagittal stratum and/or posterior limb of the internal capsule from posterior regions before they concentrate in the white matter above the lateral geniculate nucleus and then descend in the cerebral peduncle into the pons. Prefrontal fibers are situated most medially in the cerebral peduncle; sensorimotor fibers in an intermediate position; and those from the parietal, temporal, and occipital lobes are most laterally placed. There are relatively more prefrontopontine fibers in the cerebral peduncle of the human than there are in the monkey, reflecting the expansion and greater functional significance of the associative corticopontine projection in the human (Ramnani et al. 2006). Here we consider first the cerebral cortical projections to the pons (that arise in cortical layer Vb), then the pontocerebellar inputs that are conveyed in the MCP.

Corticopontine projections

Motor projections. These are topographically organized and more prevalent in the caudal half of the pons, situated in close proximity to traversing corticofugal fibers. Projections from the face region of the supplementary motor area (SMA) are most medial, and include the median pontine nucleus. Projections from the ventral precentral gyrus (M1 face representation) are also medial, but lateral to those from SMA to face. M1 hand projections are in medially placed curved lamellae in the mid- and caudal pons. Dorsal trunk projections are in medial and ventral locations, ventral trunk/hip projections encircle the peduncle in the caudal pons, and projections from the foot representation are heaviest caudally in laterally placed curved lamellae (Nyby and Jansen 1951; Brodal 1978; Hartmann von Monakow et al. 1981; Glickstein et al. 1985; Schmahmann et al. 2004). These observations, derived from anatomic tract tracing studies in monkeys, are supplemented by findings from an early version of voxel-based lesion symptom mapping in patients with focal small strokes (lacunes) in the pons (Schmahmann et al. 2004). This study indicated that speech in humans is represented in the rostral and medial aspect of the basis pontis. Hand coordination is medial and ventral in the rostral and mid-pons, and arm function is represented ventral and lateral to the hand. Leg coordination is in the caudal half of the pons, with lateral predominance. Gait is represented in medial and lateral locations throughout the rostral-caudal extent of the pons.

Pontine projections from cerebral association cortices. The pons also receives prominent projections from unimodal and multimodal association cortices in posterior parietal, superior temporal polymodal, and dorsolateral and medial prefrontal regions, as well as the posterior parahippocampal gyrus and the cingulate gyrus (Schmahmann and Pandya 1997a,

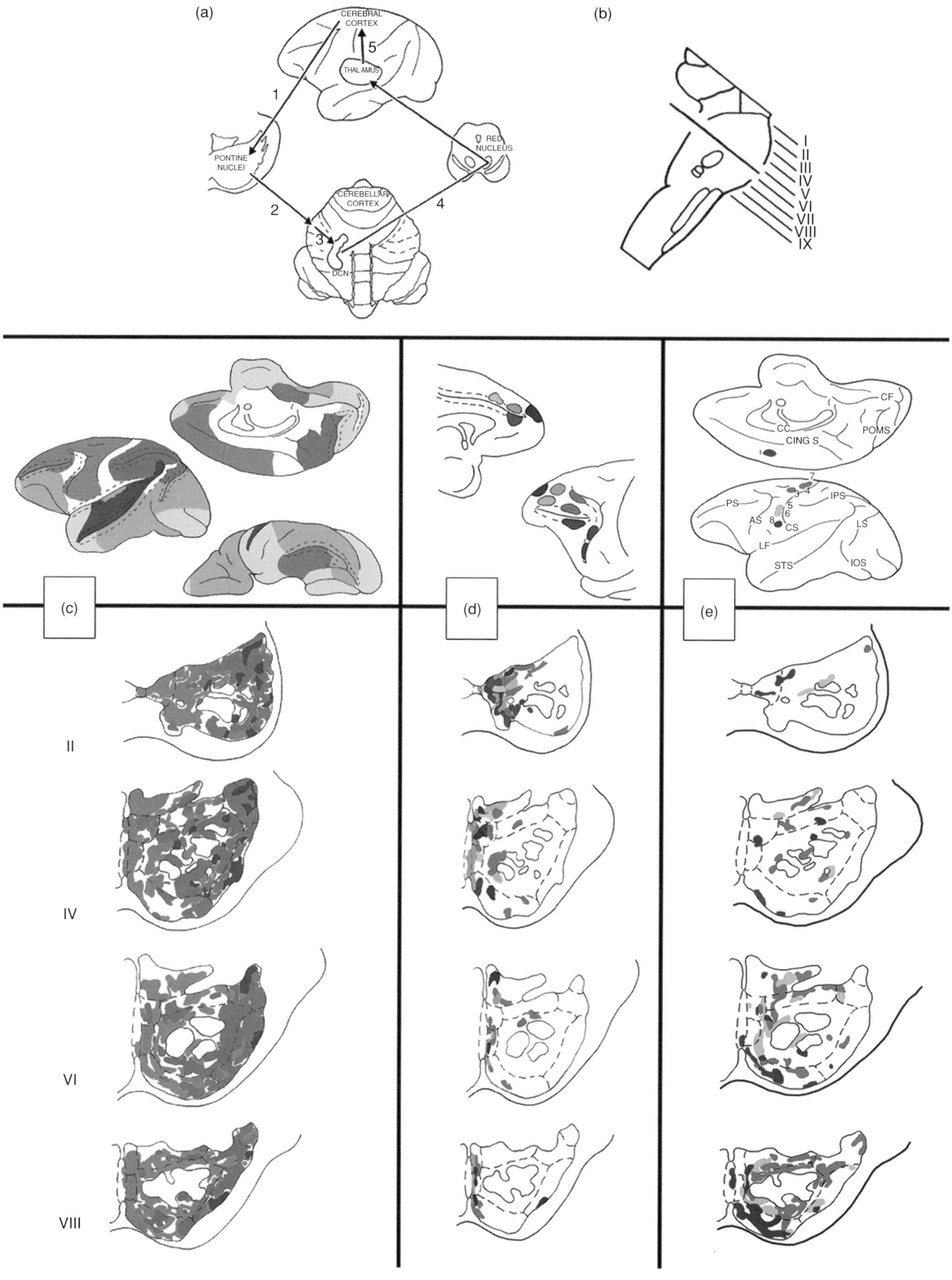
(a)
CEREBRAL CORTEX
5
THALAMUS
1
PONTINE NUCLEI
RED NUCLEUS
2
CEREBELLAR CORTEX
4
3
DCN
(b)
I
II
III
IV
V
VI
VII
VIII
IX
CF
CC
POMS
CING S
7
3
4
IPS
PS
5
6
AS
8
CS
LS
LF
STS
IOS
(c)
(d)
(e)
II
IV
VI
VIII

1997b). These connections provided the early compelling evidence that the cerebellum has access to higher order information and thus has the potential to modulate cognitive and emotional processing.

Visual projections. There is a dichotomy in the pattern of corticopontine projections according to the dorsal versus ventral streams of cognitive processing. In the visual domain, areas that are concerned with visual motion and the peripheral visual field (the 'where' pathway) have projections to pons, whereas cortical regions concerned with visual feature discrimination and the central visual field (the 'what' pathway) do not (Schmahmann and Pandya 1991, 1993). These anatomic arrangements suggest that the cerebellum plays a role in spatial awareness, and in attentional, auditory and linguistic functions subserved by the dorsal stream of cognitive processing. The pons also receives inputs from the superior colliculus to the dorsolateral pons, and to the NRTP. The tectocerebellar pathway thus uses the pontine nuclei and the NRTP as the link in its projection to the vermal visual area. Pontine inputs are also derived from the medial mammillary bodies.

Pontocerebellar projections

The corticopontine projections terminate around dendrites of the neurons in the basis pontis that constitute the pontine nuclei. These nuclei account for the characteristic ventral protuberance of the basis pontis on visual inspection of the brainstem. The mossy fiber axons of these pontine neurons cross to the contralateral side of the pons before entering the MCP and coursing to the cerebellum. The pontocerebellar projection is thus predominantly contralateral, although some mossy fiber collaterals do terminate in both cerebellar hemispheres after crossing the midline again in the cerebellar white matter.

The caudal pons (that preferentially receives motor-related inputs according to tract tracing studies in monkey) was shown through myelination (Bechterew 1885) and degeneration studies (Spitzer and Karplus 1907) to be linked with cerebellar anterior and medial areas, whereas the rostral pons (that receives the greater preponderance of projections from cerebral association areas) is linked with the lateral and caudal cerebellum. Medial parts of the caudal pons project mainly to lobule V in the anterior lobe, and the intrapeduncular nucleus projects to vermal lobule VIIIB, the paramedian lobule. These cerebellar regions contain sensorimotor representations of the upper and lower extremities. The dorsolateral pontine region and the NRTP project to the dorsal paraflocculus, uvula, and the vermal visual area, and neurons in the dorsomedial nucleus also project to the vermal visual area. Medial parts of the rostral pons project to crus I, and neurons in the medial, ventral, and lateral pons send their axons to crus II (Brodal 1979, 1982; Glickstein et al. 1994). Earlier anatomic information, together with the results of more recent transynaptic tract tracing studies using viral tracers (Dum and Strick 2003; Kelly and Strick 2003) show that the anterior lobe (particularly lobules IV and V) as well as the paramedian lobule (lobule VIII) receive afferents from pericentral motor and sensory cortices; whereas parts of lobule VI, and crus I and crus II of lobule VIIA, receive inputs from prefrontal and posterior parietal cortices.

Monoaminergic afferents

Serotonergic fibers from the raphe nuclei diffusely project to most regions in the cerebellar cortex.

AFFERENTS ENTERING VIA THE SUPERIOR CEREBELLAR PEDUNCLE

Somatosensory afferents

Somatosensory fibers enter the cerebellum through the SCP in the VSCT, and in the trigeminocerebellar tract (which also conveys fibers to the cerebellum through the ICP).

Ventral spinocerebellar tract axons arise from spinal border cells mostly in Rexed lamina VII at the dorsolateral aspect of the ventral horn of the lumbosacral spinal cord, and from other neurons in layers V through VII. The VSCT crosses to the contralateral side of the spinal cord at a level close to the cell bodies, and ascends in the contralateral ventral-lateral funiculus. At the level of the rostral pons, the VSCT fibers

Fig. 2.10. (*opposite*) Diagrammatic representations of the feedfoward limb of the corticopontine projections in rhesus monkey. **(a)** Schematic of the crossed cerebrocerebellar connections, or cerebrocerebellar loops. 1. Two-stage feedforward limb of cerebral cortex projections to the ipsilateral pontine nuclei. 2. Pontocerebellar projections through the middle cerebellar peduncle to the contralateral cerebellar hemisphere. 3. Cerebellar cortex projections to the deep cerebellar nuclei (DCN) begin the two-stage feedback limb. 4. Projections from the DCN via the contralateral red nucleus to the thalamus. 5. Thalamic projections to the same (or similar) regions of the cerebral cortex from which the corticopontine projection originated. **(b)** Plane of section through the pons from which the rostrocaudal levels II through VIII are taken in the schematics (c–e). **(c)** Composite color-coded summary diagram illustrating the distribution within selected regions of the basis pontis of projections from association and paralimbic areas shown on medial, lateral, and orbital views of the cerebral hemisphere in the prefrontal (purple), posterior parietal (blue), superior temporal (red), and parastriate and parahippocampal regions (orange), and from motor, premotor, and supplementary motor areas (SMA) (green). Other cerebral areas known to project to the pons are depicted in white. Cortical areas with no pontine projections are shown in yellow (from anterograde and retrograde studies) or gray (from retrograde studies). Dashed lines in the hemisphere diagrams represent sulcal cortices. Dashed lines in the pons diagrams represent pontine nuclei; solid lines depict corticofugal fibers. The projections are characterized by a complex mosaic of terminations in the pontine nuclei. Each cerebral cortical region has preferential sites of pontine terminations; there is interdigitation of terminations, but almost no overlap. **(d)** Color-coded summary diagram of distribution within the basis pontis of projections from the medial and lateral convexities of the prefrontal cortex. **(e)** Color-coded summary diagram of projections to the pontine nuclei from motor and supplementary motor cortices. Injection sites in the cerebral cortex in (e) (filled areas) are color-coded: SMA, red; trunk and leg, green; hand, light blue; face-hand overlapping area, dark blue. The terminations are predominantly in the caudal half of the pons; SMA projections are most medial, and the face, hand, and leg projections are progressively more laterally situated. ((a–c) from Schmahmann 1996 and Schmahmann and Pandya 1997b. (d) from Schmahmann and Pandya 1997a. (e) from Schmahmann et al. 2004.) (See color plate 13).

pass rostral to the entering trigeminal nerve and join the SCP coursing to the cerebellum where the majority of the fibers cross to the other side (i.e., hence the double crossing, thus terminating ipsilateral to the side of origin of the neurons in the spinal cord). The fibers are directed to longitudinal zones in the hindlimb representations in the anterior lobe and to a lesser extent in the paramedian lobule. The VSCT carries polysynaptic information from flexor reflex afferents that is highly integrated at the spinal level, distributes bilaterally to larger areas of the cerebellar anterior lobe than the DSCT, and appears to reflect the state of activity of the interneuron pool monitoring motor neurons.

The **trigeminocerebellar tract** arises from the mesencephalic trigeminal nucleus, and carries proprioceptive information from the face and muscles of mastication to the cerebellar cortical representation of the face in caudal lobule V and lobule VI.

Visual projections

The tectocerebellar tract carries fibers arising from the superior and inferior colliculi bilaterally, and projects to the dorsal paraflocculus, uvula, and the vermal visual area of lobule VII.

Monoaminergic system

There is a small dopaminergic input to the cerebellum arising in the substantia nigra. Noradrenergic inputs from the locus coeruleus project diffusely to the vermis and lateral hemispheres.

Efferent projections of the cerebellum: The feedback system

The vestibulocerebellum (i.e., the vermal part of the lobule IX [the uvula], and the vermal [nodulus] and hemispheric part [fl occulus] of lobule X), has direct reciprocal connections with the vestibular nuclei. In the remainder of the cerebellum, however, the efferents from the cerebellar cortex to the rest of the neuraxis are conveyed exclusively by way of the cerebellar corticonuclear projection to the DCN. This corticonuclear projection is organized in a zonal pattern conforming to parasagittal longitudinal strips such that the Purkinje cells within a defined zone, their climbing fiber innervations from the olive, and their targets within the DCN function as a cerebellar efferent module, each module operating largely independently of one another (Voogd and Bigaré 1980; Nieuwenhuys et al. 2008). The efferent connections conveyed by the DCN are outlined sequentially below.

Fastigial nucleus

Efferents from the rostral part of the fastigial nucleus traverse the ICP destined for the ipsilateral brainstem. Those from the caudal part of the fastigial nucleus cross in the cerebellum and travel in the hook bundle of Russell (the uncinate fasciculus), closely apposed to the contralateral SCP. Both rostral and caudal aspects project to the pontine and medullary reticular formation, including the nucleus reticularis gigantocellularis and nucleus reticularis pontis caudalis. They are also directed to the lateral reticular nucleus, NRTP, paramedian reticular nuclei, and to the perihypoglossal nuclei. Vestibular projections from the fastigial nucleus terminate in the medial, superior, and inferior vestibular nuclei. Deiters' lateral vestibular nucleus receives a direct projection from Purkinje cells in zone B of the anterior vermis, but not from the fastigial nucleus. The ascending crossed projections from the caudal part of the fastigial nucleus terminate in the deep and intermediate layers of the nucleus of the tractus solitarius, parabrachial nucleus, superior colliculus, pretectal area, periaqueductal gray, ventral tegmental area and interpeduncular nucleus. There are also terminations in the contralateral thalamus in the internal medullary lamina, paraventricular, paracentral, centromedian, parafascicular, central lateral and medial dorsal nuclei, as well as the ventrolateral and ventromedial thalamic nuclei. Projections to the contralateral hypothalamus arise from the fastigial nucleus as well as from the other DCN, and travel to the lateral, posterior, and dorsal hypothalamic areas and the dorsomedial and paraventricular nuclei. Efferents from the fastigial nucleus thus influence a large number of functional modules: oculomotor systems including vertical and horizontal gaze centers in the midbrain and pons; axial and limb girdle musculature (the medial motor system; Lawrence and Kuypers 1968) by way of the vestibular and reticular nuclei; autonomic centers through connections with hypothalamus and periaqueductal gray; and emotional modulation through links with limbic-related circuits in the thalamic intralaminar nucleus, and (from earlier physiologic studies) septal regions, hippocampus, and amygdala (Heath et al. 1978, 1980).

Interpositus nuclei

The posterior interpositus nucleus is equivalent to the globose nucleus in humans; and the anterior interpositus nucleus is equivalent to the emboliform.

Efferents from the interpositus nuclei exit the cerebellum via the SCP. Within the SCP, the fibers from the posterior interpositus nucleus are situated medially, the anterior interpositus nucleus fibers are intermediate, and those from the dentate nucleus are most lateral. Interpositus projections are directed to the RNmc that in turn gives rise to the rubrospinal tract; and to the ventrolateral and ventral anterior nuclei of the thalamus. Projections to the inferior olive are restricted to those olivary regions that project to the cerebellar corticonuclear zone from which the anterior and posterior interpositus nuclei feedback projections are derived. Interpositus efferents also project to the reticular formation (that gives rise to the medial and lateral reticulospinal tracts), the inferior vestibular nuclei (that give rise to the medial and lateral vestibulospinal tracts), the superior colliculus (origin of the tectospinal tract), and the contralateral inferior olive (projecting to spinal cord via the contralateral olivospinal tract).

Lateral/dentate nucleus

The lateral/dentate nucleus contributes to the Guillain-Mollaret triangle by committing efferents to the RNpc that feeds back through the central tegmental tract to the inferior olive, which in turn is linked with the cerebellum.

It has long been recognized that the dentate nucleus projects via the ventral lateral thalamic nucleus to motor areas of the cerebral cortex. Tract tracing studies of the cerebellar-thalamic-cerebral feedback circuit indicate, however, that this is an incomplete characterization. The primary motor cortex receives projections via the thalamus from dorsal portions of the dentate nucleus at mid-rostrocaudal levels and from caudal portions of the anterior interpositus nucleus where neuronal activity related to arm movement has been recorded. The premotor cortex receives input from the mid-rostrocaudal part of the dentate, ventral to the location of the M1 projecting neurons. Frontal eye field projecting neurons are located in the caudal third of the dentate that is correlated with saccadic eye movements. The dorsolateral prefrontal cortex (areas 46 and 9-lateral) receives projections from the ventral part of the dentate, and projections to the posterior parietal cortex arise from neurons in the ventral and lateral parts of the dentate nucleus (Fig. 2.11; Middleton and Strick 1994; Dum and Strick 2003; Hashimoto et al. 2010).

Functional topography in the cerebellum

The traditional schema describing three anatomic-functional divisions of the cerebellum facilitated the earlier understanding of cerebellar anatomy. It was proposed that the *vestibulocerebellum* (archicerebellum/flocculonodular lobe) has reciprocal links with vestibular nuclei either directly or indirectly, and is

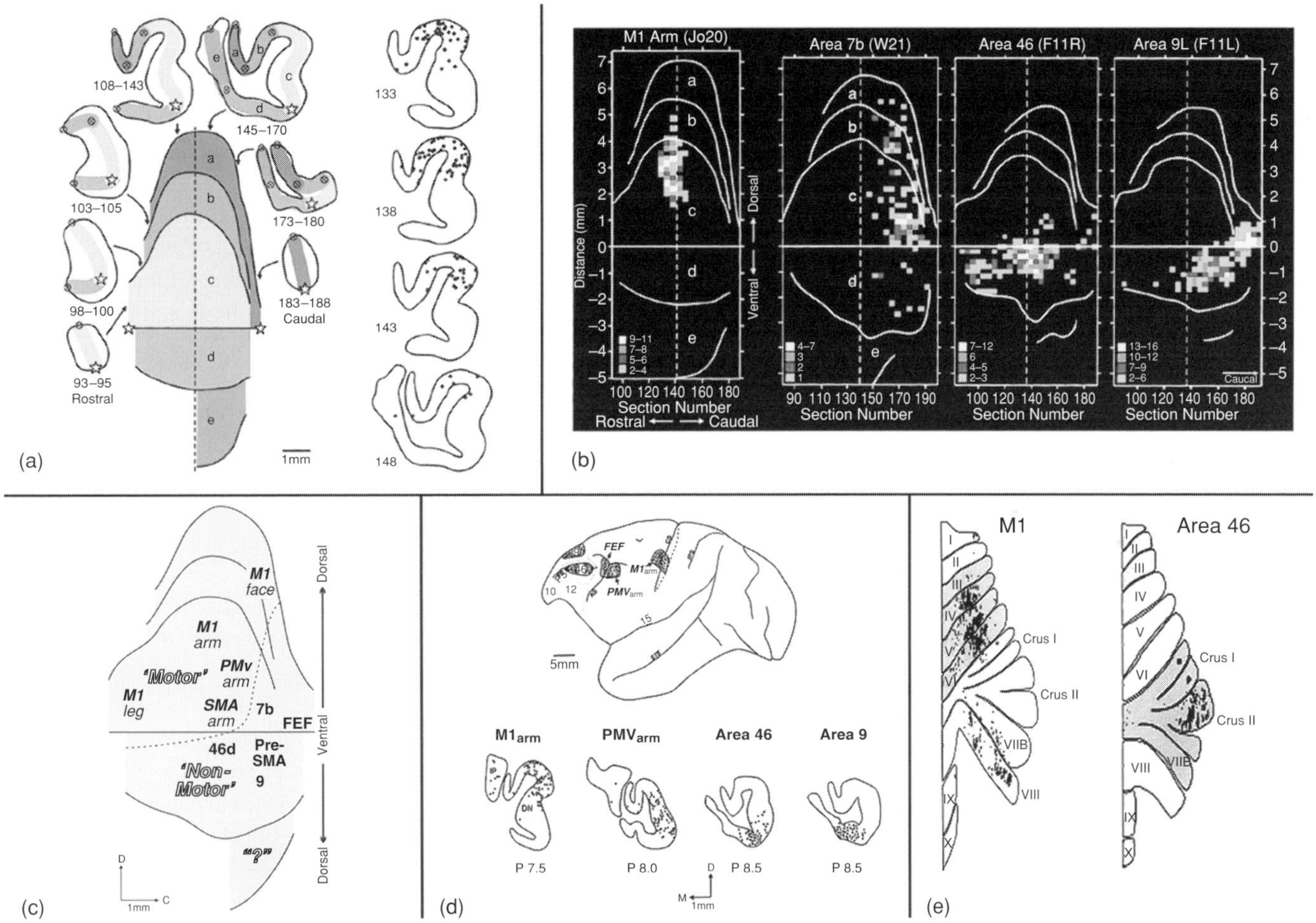

Fig. 2.11. Diagrams depicting cerebellar feedback projections to the cerebral cortex in cebus monkey. **(a)** Unfolded map of the dentate nucleus (in color) created by unfolding serial coronal sections through the nucleus. Each section is aligned to the junction of the c and d segments (open star). Dashed vertical line indicates the rostrocaudal center of the nucleus. Cross-sections of the dentate nucleus on the right show the location of 'second order' neurons (dots) labeled after transport of herpes simplex virus type 1 (HSV1) from the arm representation of M1. **(b)** Unfolded maps of the dentate nucleus illustrate the neurons labeled after virus injections into the arm representation in M1, posterior parietal cortex area 7b, and mid-dorsolateral prefrontal cortex areas 46 and 9-lateral. **(c)** Summary diagram showing the origins of dentate nucleus projections to primary motor cortex (M1) representations of the leg, arm and face; ventral premotor area (PMv); inferior parietal lobule (area 7b); and the mid-dorsolateral prefrontal cortex (areas 46 and 9L). **(d)** Lateral view of monkey brain (top) shows the locations of viral tracer injections in the M1 – arm, PMv – arm, and prefrontal cortex areas 46 and 9. The resulting retrogradely labeled neurons in the cerebellar dentate nucleus (bottom) are indicated by solid dots. **(e)** Flattened representation of cerebellum to show the folia linked with M1 motor cortex (left) and prefrontal cortex area 46 (right) using viral tracers that travel in the anterograde direction (H129 strain of HSV1) and retrograde direction (rabies virus). ((a) and (b) from Dum and Strick 2003; (c) from Strick et al. 2009; (d) from Middleton and Strick 1997; (e) from Kelly and Strick 2003.) (See color plate 14).

concerned with eye movements and equilibrium. The *spinocerebellum* (paleocerebellum) was considered to encompass most of the anterior lobe, the vermis and paravermal regions that receive cutaneous and kinesthetic afferents from spinal cord and the trigeminal nerve. The role of the vermis, linked with the fastigial nucleus, was regarded as influencing the medial motor system (postural tone, proximal muscles, reflex control) through brainstem vestibular and reticular nuclei that send descending projections to the spinal cord, and therefore important for balance and equilibrium. The paravermal areas linked with the interpositus nuclei that project to the red nucleus and primary motor cortex influence the descending lateral motor systems (flexor tone, appendicular muscles, reflex control), thus being important for the control of distal limb movements. The lateral cerebellar hemispheres that constituted the *pontocerebellum* (cerebrocerebellum or neocerebellum) receive descending input from the cerebral cortex, project through the dentate nucleus via the thalamus to motor and premotor cortices, and were thus considered important for fine motor control, motor planning, and motor learning.

This earlier approach is no longer sufficient to account for the current appreciation of the wider role of the cerebellum. It has become necessary for these organizational concepts to evolve as a result of contemporary anatomic, functional imaging and clinical investigations. Among these are the recognition that pontine projections are not confined to the cerebellar hemispheres; the spinocerebellum receives inputs from sensorimotor areas of the cerebral cortex as well as from the spinal cord; and the cerebral hemispheric connections of the cerebellum are distributed far beyond the confines of motor-related regions of the cerebral cortex.

The diverse anatomic connections of the cerebellum with the spinal cord, brainstem, and cerebral hemispheres support a role for the cerebellum in a wide array of functions, from the control of movement and posture to higher-level cognitive and affective processes. In addition to the classic cerebellar motor syndrome of dysmetria, dysarthria, and ataxia (Holmes 1939; Dow and Moruzzi 1958), lesions of the cerebellum can produce impairments in working memory, attention, linguistic and spatial processing, and emotional modulation (the cerebellar cognitive affective syndrome, Schmahmann and Sherman 1998; Levisohn et al. 2000). This wide variety of symptoms is thought to result from disruptions in the distributed neural circuits linking the cerebellum with sensorimotor, associative, and limbic/paralimbic regions of the cerebral hemispheres. Furthermore, anatomic, clinical, and functional neuroimaging studies suggest that different regions of the cerebellum are involved in these various functions – in other words, a *functional topography* exists in the cerebellum for sensorimotor (see Manni and Petrosini 2004 for review) and nonmotor functions (e.g., see Schmahmann 1991, 1996, 2004; Stoodley and Schmahmann 2009, 2010; Stoodley et al. 2010). Anatomic, clinical, and functional imaging investigations provide the evidence for this evolution in the recognition of the cerebellar role in nervous system function, as we outline below.

Anatomic connections

The anatomic basis of cerebellar functional topography is the existence of multiple cerebrocerebellar loops which connect the cerebellum with motor cortices as well as with association cortices and paralimbic regions of the cerebral hemispheres. These loops target different cerebellar regions depending on their site of origin in the cerebral cortex (Brodal 1983; Brodal and Steen 1983; Botez et al. 1985; Leiner et al. 1986; Schmahmann and Pandya 1989, 1997a, 1997b; Schmahmann 1991, 1996; Middleton and Strick 1994; Brodal and Bjaalie 1997; Hoover and Strick 1999; Kelly and Strick 2003; Schmahmann et al. 2004).

The motor cortex is linked with cerebellar lobules IV and V, with face representation extending into medial lobule VI, and lobule VIII, the second somatosensory representation in the cerebellum (Snider and Eldred 1951; Chambers and Sprague 1955a, 1955b). Lobule VII does not receive inputs from sensorimotor regions, but from prefrontal and posterior parietal cortices that are reciprocally interconnected with the hemispheric extensions of lobule VIIA, i.e., cerebellar lobules crus I and crus II (Allen and Tsukahara 1974; Hoover and Strick 1999; Kelly and Strick 2003). Physiologic and behavioral studies provide support for the postulated relationship between the cerebellar vermis and the modulation of emotion (Heath 1977; Heath et al. 1978, 1980; Schmahmann 1991, 2000).

Clinical findings

Data from clinical populations provide evidence that the cerebellar motor syndrome results from lesions principally affecting the anterior lobe, whereas cognitive deficits occur following posterior lobe damage. Additionally, converging lines of data suggest that neuropsychiatric impairments are associated with damage to the posterior vermis.

The cerebellar motor syndrome results when lesions interrupt cerebellar communication with cerebral and spinal motor systems (Holmes 1939; Schmahmann et al. 2009). Balance and gait impairment are symptoms of focal lesions such as tumors and stroke involving the fastigial nucleus, anterior lobe vermal lobules I–III, and lobules VIII and IX of the posterior lobe (Konczak et al. 2005; Schoch et al. 2006; Ilg et al. 2008). In cerebellar stroke patients, limb and gait ataxia are more strongly associated with stroke involving the SCA territory than infarcts in the PICA territory (Kase et al. 1993; Tohgi et al. 1993; Richter et al. 2007). Voxel-based morphometry of cerebellar lesions show significant correlations between the severity of ataxia and damage to the anterior lobe, including lobules II–V, with some involvement of lobule VI of the posterior lobe, supporting the idea that the anterior lobe and lobule VI are involved in sensorimotor processing (Schoch et al. 2006). Dysarthria occurs when lesions involve anterior cerebellar areas, including lobule VI (Amarenco and Hauw 1990; Amarenco et al. 1991; Ackermann et al. 1992; Urban et al. 2003). These findings provide evidence that the cerebellar motor signs of ataxia, dysmetria, and dysarthria do not result from insults to every part of the cerebellum, but from damage to sensorimotor regions located in the cerebellar anterior lobe and parts of lobule VI (Schmahmann et al. 2009). The contribution of the putative cerebellar second somatosensory area in lobule VIII (Snider and Stowell 1944; Snider 1950; Woolsey 1952; Snider and Eldred 1951) to motor function is not yet clear.

Clinical findings also support the proposal that lobules VI and VII are important for cognitive and affective processes. Cognitive impairments are associated with lesions involving lobules VI and VII (including crus I, crus II, and lobule VIIB), disrupting cerebellar modulation of cognitive loops with cerebral association cortices (e.g., Schmahmann and Sherman 1998; Exner et al. 2004; Tavano et al. 2007). Vermal damage can lead to neuropsychiatric disorders by impacting the cerebro-cerebellar limbic loops (Heath et al. 1979; Schmahmann and Sherman 1998; Schmahmann et al. 2007). In children, removal of posterior midline tumors is associated with postoperative mutism that evolves into speech and language disorders and behavioral disturbances (Pollack et al. 1995; Catsman-Berrevoets et al. 1999; Levisohn et al. 2000; Riva and Giorgi 2000; Ozgur et al. 2006). Symptoms include increased thoughtfulness, anxiety, and aggression (Richter et al. 2005), with children demonstrating evidence of both hyperspontaneous, disinhibited behavior, and hypospontaneous, flattened affect (Aarsen et al. 2004). In adults with cerebellar stroke, damage to the posterior vermis is associated with affective symptoms (Schmahmann and Sherman, 1998; Paulus et al. 2004).

Functional neuroimaging studies

Functional neuroimaging in healthy populations has helped elucidate the sensorimotor topography in the cerebellum and the functional roles of lobules VI and VII. Cerebellar activation is reported during a wide range of tasks, including higher-level tasks, even when activation due to overt responses is eliminated through subtraction analyses. A meta-analysis of functional activation patterns within the cerebellum (Stoodley and Schmahmann 2009) found evidence for activation in lobules V, VI, and VIII during sensorimotor tasks, and lateral posterior lobe (lobules VI and VII) activation during language, spatial, executive, working memory, and affective tasks. These findings are supported by functional connectivity (Fig. 2.12) and

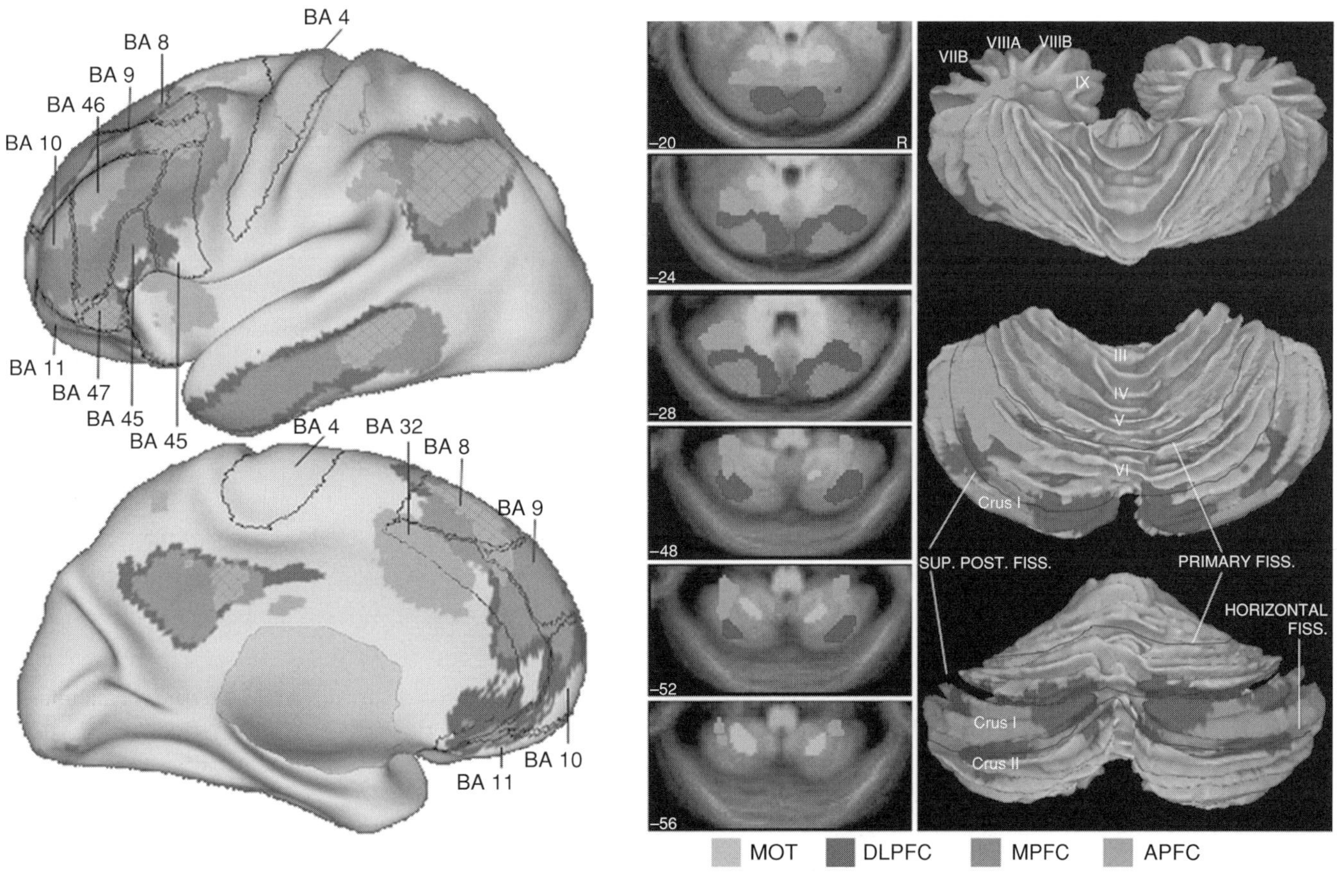

Fig. 2.12. Provisional map of human cerebellar connectivity with the frontal cortex as determined by functional connectivity MRI. Seed regions were placed in the motor cortex (MOT) shown in yellow, dorsolateral prefrontal cortex (DLPFC) in red, medial prefrontal cortex (MPFC) in orange, and anterior prefrontal cortex (APFC) in green. Correlation maps with frontal lobe and other cerebral cortical areas are shown in the cerebral hemisphere diagrams at left (hatched regions represent overlap of two correlation maps; parietal and temporal lobes not labeled); in the cerebellum in rostral-to-caudal axial sections in the middle panel; and in surface reconstructions of the cerebellum in the right panel (inverted anterior view; dorsal view; posterior view). The cerebral cortical motor correlations are in cerebellar lobules IV, V, and VIIIA; the majority of the mapped portion of the posterior cerebellum (lobules VI and crus I and crus II) is associated with prefrontal (cognitive) regions of the neocortex. Approximate borders of relevant labeled Brodmann areas (BA) are shown in the prefrontal and motor cortices. Cerebellar nomenclature as in Schmahmann et al. (1999, 2000). (Images adapted from Krienen and Buckner 2009.) (See color plate 15).

probabilistic tractography studies indicating that the cerebellum can be divided into different regions based on its connections with sensorimotor versus prefrontal and parietal cortices (Allen et al. 2005; Habas et al. 2009; Krienen and Buckner 2009; O'Reilly et al. 2010; Salmi et al. 2010).

Somatotopic representation in the human cerebellum has been demonstrated during sensorimotor tasks (Nitschke et al. 1996; Bushara et al. 2001; Grodd et al. 2001, 2005; see also Takanashi et al. 2003; Thickbroom et al. 2003), revealing a body map in the anterior lobe and lobule VI, with a second representation in lobule VIII of the posterior lobe. Movement and tactile stimulation of the hand localizes to ipsilateral lobules V and VIII (Bushara et al. 2001; Grodd et al. 2001), with leg and foot sensorimotor representations in lobules II and III (Nitschke et al. 1996). Orofacial movements activate paravermal anterior lobe regions extending into medial parts of lobule VI (Urban et al. 2003; Dresel et al. 2005).

Cerebellar lobules VI and VII are engaged during cognitive tasks (for review, see Stoodley and Schmahmann 2009). Further, the lateralization of activation patterns reflects the contralateral anatomic connections between the cerebellum and the cerebral cortex. For example, the right posterolateral cerebellum (along with the left cerebral cortex) is active during language tasks, including verbal fluency, verb-for-noun generation, semantic judgment, and word stem completion, while spatial tasks such as line bisection and mental rotation activate regions in lobules VI and crus I, and are often left-lateralized in the cerebellum. Cerebellar lobules VI and VII are active during working memory and executive function tasks, such as the Tower of London, random number generation, and complex decision-making tasks.

Affective/emotional processing involves lobules VI and VII: identifying emotional intonations produces cerebellar activation in midline lobule VII and the lateral posterior hemisphere (lobule VI bilaterally and right crus I) both during functional MRI (fMRI) (Wildgruber et al. 2005) and positron emission tomography (Imaizumi et al. 1997). Activation of the cerebellar vermis is evident in studies investigating panic (e.g., Reiman et al. 1989), sadness, and grief (Lane et al. 1997; Beauregard et al. 1998; Gundel et al. 2003). The cerebellum is also active during painful stimulation (Becerra et al. 1999; Ploghaus et al. 1999; Singer et al. 2004; Borsook et al. 2007; Moulton et al. 2010), and different cerebellar regions are involved when processing one's own pain (posterior vermis) as opposed to experiencing empathy for another's pain (lobule VI; Singer et al. 2004). Lobule VI and vermal lobule VII are consistently engaged during the presentation of emotionally salient stimuli (Stoodley and Schmahmann 2009).

Analysis of functional activation patterns in a single healthy adult performing a variety of motor and nonmotor tasks supports cerebellar functional topography at the level of a single individual (Fig. 2.13; Stoodley et al. 2010). Tapping with the right index finger activated ipsilateral cerebellar lobules IV–V

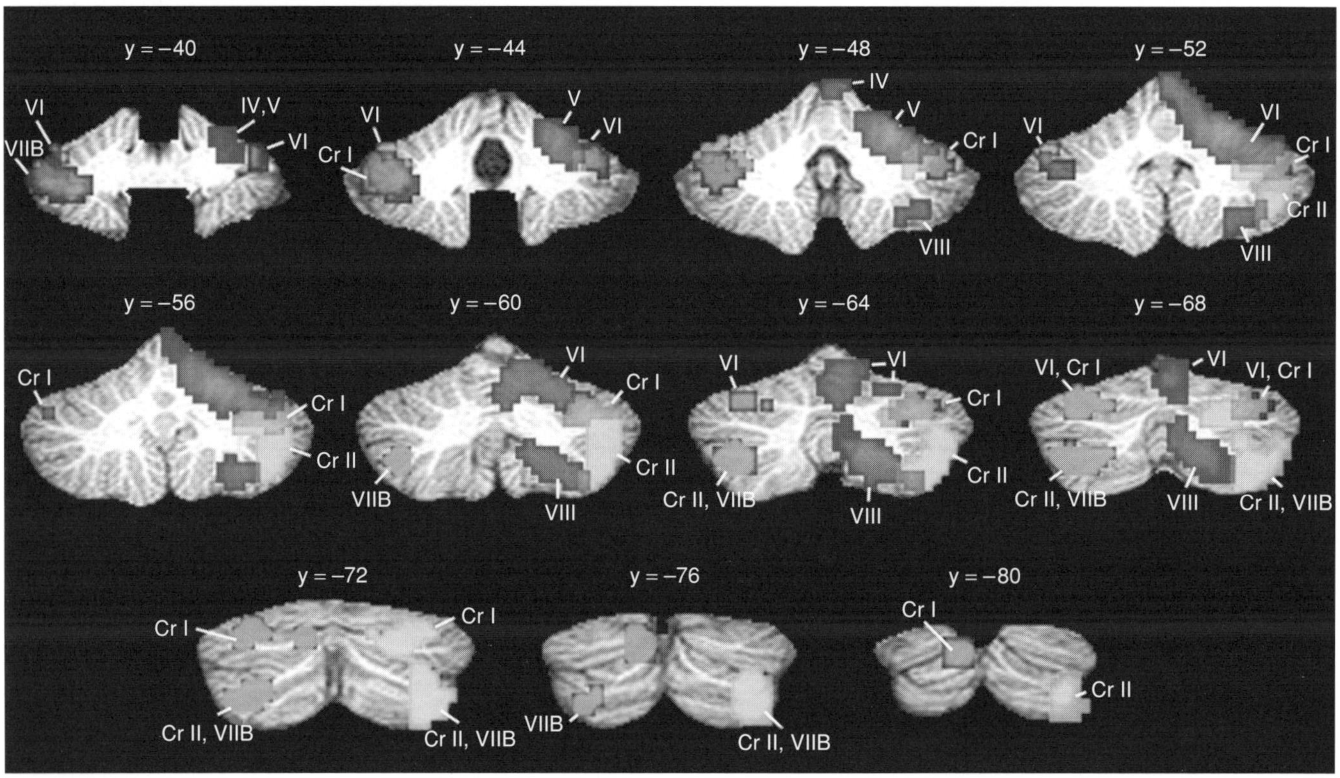

Fig. 2.13. Representative rostral (y = −44) to caudal (y = −80) coronal sections through a human cerebellum showing activation patterns in a functional magnetic resonance imaging experiment in a single individual. Tasks investigated sensorimotor function (finger tapping, shown in red), language (verb generation, blue), spatial cognition (mental rotation, green), working memory (N-back, purple), and emotional processing (viewing images from the International Affective Picture System, yellow). Cerebellar lobules are labeled according to Schmahmann et al. 1999, 2000. The right cerebellar hemisphere is shown on the right. (From Stoodley et al. 2010.) (See color plate 16).

extending into lobule VI and the second sensorimotor representation in lobule VIII. Activation during the working memory task was evident bilaterally in cerebellar lobules VII and VIIIA, as well as in right lobule VI. Verb generation activated right cerebellar lobules VI, VII, and VIIIA. Mental rotation engaged left cerebellar lobules VI, VII, and VIIIA. In this study cerebellar activation was weakest in the affective processing task for technical reasons, with small bilateral clusters in lobule VI. Notably, the anterior lobe of the cerebellum did not show activation during tasks devoid of a motor component.

Synopsis

The recognition that sensorimotor control is topographically largely separate and distinct from cognitive and emotional regulation in the cerebellum represents a major departure from earlier conventional wisdom, and necessitates a new formulation of the cerebellar role in the nervous system.

Contrasted against the essentially homogeneous architecture of the cerebellar cortex is the rich heterogeneity of the cerebellar connections with spinal cord, brainstem, and cerebral structures that we reviewed in this chapter. These circuits are the likely structural basis for putative functional subunits in the cerebellum facilitating topographic organization of its motor and cognitive functions. In this schema, the postulated functional domains in the cerebellum are the following:

- autonomic and arousal (vermis and rostral part of fastigial nucleus);
- vestibular (flocculonodular lobe and vestibular nuclei);
- oculomotor (vestibular cerebellum with vermal lobules VI and VII and the fastigial nucleus);
- limbic (vermis and caudal part of fastigial nucleus);
- sensorimotor (somatotopically arranged in the anterior lobe and adjacent part of lobule VI, second representation in lobule VIII, and interpositus nuclei); and
- cognitive (part of lobule VI, crus I and crus II of lobule VIIA, and lobule VIIB, and the ventral part of the dentate nucleus).

Lobule IX may be incorporated into the default mode network (Fox et al. 2005; Habas et al. 2009).

The model of a number of corticonuclear microcomplexes subserving different functional domains by virtue of their extracerebellar connections may extend to other parameters that we have not specifically considered here, such as cerebellar modulation of cardiovascular control.

The precise role of the cerebellum in all these functional areas remains a matter of great interest. The uniformity of cerebellar histology seems to imply that there is a computation performed in the cerebellum that holds true for the entire structure. This computation, or universal cerebellar transform (UCT), has been conceptualized as the cerebellum modulating behavior, serving as an oscillation dampener maintaining function automatically around a homeostatic baseline, smoothing out and optimizing performance in all domains according to context. This dysmetria of thought theory (Schmahmann 1991, 2000, 2004) would apply to motor performance as well as to cognitive operations. By corollary, there should be a universal cerebellar impairment (UCI), namely dysmetria. When the dysmetria involves the sensorimotor cerebellum, the various manifestations of ataxia are evident in extremity movements, eye movements, speech, and equilibrium. However, when the dysmetria involves the cognitive and/or limbic cerebellum, the result is dysmetria of thought and emotion, which manifests as the various components of the cerebellar cognitive affective syndrome. The dysmetria of thought theory is an anatomically based model in which anatomic loops subserve functional subsystems within the larger framework of the sensorimotor, associative, paralimbic, and autonomic cerebrocerebellar communication. Other approaches (see Schmahmann 1997; Strick et al. 2009) view the fundamental role of the cerebellum as being crucial for the perception and regulation of timing, context-response linkage, dynamic state estimation, control of sensory data acquisition, attentional coordination and anticipation, and the formation of internal feedforward models of behaviour.

Acknowledgments

Supported in part by RO1 MH067980, the Birmingham, MINDlink, and Sidney R. Baer Jr. Foundations. Parts of the chapter are derived from Schmahmann JD (2007) Cerebellum and Spinal Cord – Principles of Development, Anatomical Organization, and Functional Relevance. In: Brice A, Pulst S (eds). Spinocerebellar Degenerations: The Ataxias and Spastic Paraplegias. New York, Elsevier, pp. 1–60.

REFERENCES

Aarsen F, Dongen HV, Paquier P, Mourik MV, Catsman-Berrevoets C (2004) Long-term sequelae in children after cerebellar astrocytoma surgery. Neurology 62: 1311–1316.

Ackermann H, Vogel M, Petersen D, Poremba M (1992) Speech deficits in ischaemic cerebellar lesions. J Neurol 239: 223–227.

Allen G, McColl R, Barnard H, Ringe W, Fleckenstein J, Cullum C (2005) Magnetic resonance imaging of cerebellar-prefrontal and cerebellar parietal functional connectivity. Neuroimage 28: 39–48.

Allen GI, Tsukahara N (1974) Cerebrocerebellar communication systems. Physiol Rev 54: 957–1006.

Amarenco P, Chevrie-Muller C, Roullet E, Bousser M-G (1991) Paravermal infarct and isolated cerebellar dysarthria. Ann Neurol 30: 211–213.

Amarenco P, Hauw JJ (1990) Cerebellar infarction in the territory of the superior cerebellar artery: a clinicopathologic study of 33 cases. Neurology 40: 1383–1390.

Beauregard M, Leroux JM, Bergman S, Arzoumanian Y, Beaudoin G, Bourgouin P, Stip E (1998) The functional neuroanatomy of major depression: an fMRI study using an emotional activation paradigm. Neuroreport 9: 3253–3258.

Becerra LR, Breiter HC, Stojanovic M, Fishman S, Edwards A, Comite AR, et al. (1999) Human brain activation under controlled thermal stimulation and habituation to noxious heat: an fMRI study. Magn Reson Med 41: 1044–1057.

Bechterew W (1885) Zur Anatomie der Schenkel des Kleinhirns, insbesondere der Brückenarme. Neurologisches Centralblatt 4: 121–125.

Bolk L (1906) Das Cerebellum der Säugetiere. Haarlem: De Erven F. Bohn.

Borsook D, Moulton EA, Schmidt KF, Becerra LR (2007) Neuroimaging revolutionizes therapeutic approaches to chronic pain. Mol Pain 3: 25.

Botez MI, Gravel J, Attig E, Vezina JL (1985) Reversible chronic cerebellar ataxia after phenytoin intoxication: possible role of cerebellum in cognitive thought. Neurology 35: 1152–1157.
Brodal A (1981) Neurological anatomy in relation to clinical medicine, 3rd edition. Oxford, New York: Oxford University Press.
Brodal P (1978) The corticopontine projection in the rhesus monkey. Origin and principles of organization. Brain 101: 251–283.
Brodal P (1979) The pontocerebellar projection in the rhesus monkey: An experimental study with retrograde axonal transport of horseradish peroxidase. Neurosci 4: 193–208.
Brodal P (1982) Further observations on the cerebellar projections from the pontine nuclei and the nucleus reticularis tegmenti pontis in the rhesus monkey. J Comp Neurol 204: 44–55.
Brodal P (1983) Principles of organization of the corticopontocerebellar projection to crus II in the cat with particular reference to the parietal cortical areas. Neuroscience 10: 621–638.
Brodal P, Bjaalie JG (1997) Salient anatomic features of the cortico-ponto-cerebellar pathway. Prog Brain Res 114: 227–249.
Brodal P, Steen N (1983) The corticopontocerebellar pathway to crus I in the cat as studied with anterograde and retrograde transport of horseradish peroxidase. Brain Res 267: 1–17.
Bushara K, Wheat J, Khan A, Mock B, Turski P, Sorenson J, Brooks BR (2001) Multiple tactile maps in the human cerebellum. Neuroreport 12: 2483–2486.
Cajal S Ramón y (1909–1910) Histologie du système nerveux de l'homme et des vertébrés. Translated into French by L. Azoulay. Paris: Maloine. Translated into English by Swanson N, Swanson LW (1995) Histology of the nervous system of man and vertebrates. New York, Oxford University Press.
Catsman-Berrevoets C, VanDongen H, Mulder P, Gueze DP, Paquier P, Lequin M (1999) Tumour type and size are high risk factors for the syndrome of 'cerebellar' mutsim and subsequent dysarthria. J Neurol Neurosurg Psychiatry 67: 755–757.
Chambers WW, Sprague JM (1955a) Functional localization in the cerebellum. I. Organization in longitudinal cortico-nuclear zones and their contribution to the control of posture, both extrapyramidal and pyramidal. J Comp Neurol 103: 105–129.
Chambers WW, Sprague JM (1955b) Functional localization in the cerebellum. II. Somatotopic organization in cortex and nuclei. AMA Arch Neurol Psychiatry 74: 653–680.
Courville J, Montigny C de, Lamarre Y (eds) (1980) The Inferior Olivary Nucleus: Anatomy and Physiology. New York: Raven.
De Zeeuw CI, Cicirata F (eds) (2005) Creating Coordination in the Cerebellum. Progress in Brain Research vol. 148. Amsterdam: Elsevier.
Dow RS, Moruzzi G (1958) The Physiology and Pathology of the Cerebellum. Minneapolis, MN: University of Minnesota Press.
Dresel C, Castrop F, Haslinger B, Wohlschlaeger AM, Hennenlotter A, Ceballos-Baumann AO (2005) The functional neuroanatomy of coordinated orofacial movements: sparse sampling fMRI of whistling. Neuroimage 28: 588–597.
Dum RP, Strick PL (2003) An unfolded map of the cerebellar dentate nucleus and its projections to the cerebral cortex. J Neurophysiol 89: 634–639.
Eccles JC, Ito M, Szentagothai J (1967) The Cerebellum as a Neuronal Machine. New York, Heidelberg: Springer-Verlag.
Exner C, Weniger G, Irle E (2004) Cerebellar lesions in the PICA but not SCA territory impair cognition. Neurology 63: 2132–2135.
Folkerth RD, Zanoni S, Andiman SE, Billiards SS (2008) Neuronal cell death in the arcuate nucleus of the medulla oblongata in stillbirth. Int J Dev Neurosci 26: 133–140.
Foville M (1844) Traité Complet de L'Anatomie, de la Physiologie et de la pathologie Système Nerveux Cérébro-Spinal. Premiere partie. Anatomie. Atlas par MM Émile Beau et F. Bion. Paris, Fortin, Masson et cie.
Fox CA, Hillman DE, Siegesmund KA, Dutta CR (1967) The primate cerebellar cortex: A Golgi and electron microscopic study. In: Fox CA, Snider RS (eds) The Cerebellum. Progress in Brain Research. New York, Elsevier, volume 25, pp. 174–225.
Fox MD, Snyder AZ, Vincent JL, Corbetta M, Van Essen DC, Raichle ME (2005) The human brain is intrinsically organized into dynamic, anticorrelated functional networks. Proc Natl Acad Sci USA 102: 9673–9678.
Gall FJ, Spurzheim G (1810) Anatomie et Physiologie du Systeme Nerveux en general, et du Cerveau en particulier. Atlas. Paris: Chez F. Schoell.
Gray's Anatomy, 38th edition (1995) Williams PL et al. (eds). New York: Churchill Livingstone.
Glickstein M, Gerrits N, Kralj-Hans I, Mercier B, Stein J, Voogd J (1994) Visual pontocerebellar projections in the macaque. Comp Neurol 349: 51–72.
Glickstein M, May JG, Mercier BE (1985) Corticopontine projection in the macaque: the distribution of labelled cortical cells after large injections of horseradish peroxidase in the pontine nuclei. J Comp Neurol 235: 343–359.
Granziera C, Schmahmann JD, Hadjikhani N, Meyer H, Meuli R, Wedeen V, Krueger G (2009) Diffusion spectrum imaging shows the structural basis of functional cerebellar circuits in the human cerebellum in vivo. PLoS One 4(4): e5101.
Grodd W, Hulsmann E, Ackermann H (2005) Functional MRI localizing in the cerebellum. Neurosurg Clin N Am 16: 77–99.
Grodd W, Hulsmann E, Lotze M, Wildgruber D, Erb M (2001) Sensorimotor mapping of the human cerebellum: fMRI evidence of somatotopic organization. Hum Brain Mapp 13: 55–73.
Gundel H, O'Connor MF, Littrell L, Fort C, Lane RD (2003) Functional neuroanatomy of grief: an FMRI study. Am J Psychiatry 160: 1946–1953.
Habas C, Kamdar N, Nguyen D, Prater K, Beckmann CF, Menon V, Greicius MD (2009) Distinct cerebellar contributions to intrinsic connectivity networks. J Neurosci 29: 8586–8594.
Haines DE, Dietrichs E, Mihailoff GA, McDonald EF (1997) The cerebellar-hypothalamic axis: basic circuits and clinical observations. In: Schmahmann JD (ed) The cerebellum and cognition. San Diego, Academic Press. Int Rev Neurobiol 41: 83–107.
Haines DE, Manto MU (2010) Commentary on 'Hohman LB. The efferent connections of the cerebellar cortex; investigations based upon experimental extirpations in the cat. In: The cerebellum. An investigation of recent advances. association for research in nervous and mental disease, Vol. VI. Williams & Wilkins, Baltimore, 1929, pp. 445–460.' Cerebellum 9: 480–483.
Hartmann-von Monakow K, Akert K, Künzle H (1981) Projection of precentral, premotor and prefrontal cortex to the basilar pontine grey and to nucleus reticularis tegmenti pontis in the monkey (Macaca fascicularis). Schweiz Arch Neurol Neurochir Psychiatr. 129: 189–208.
Hashimoto M, Takahara D, Hirata Y, Inoue K, Miyachi S, Nambu A, et al. (2010) Motor and non-motor projections from the cerebellum to rostrocaudally distinct sectors of the dorsal premotor cortex in macaques. Eur J Neurosci 31: 1402–1413.
Heath R, Franklin D, Shraberg D (1979) Gross pathology of the cerebellum in patients diagnosed and treated as functional psychiatric disorders. J Nerv Ment Dis 167: 585–592.
Heath RG, Dempsey CW, Fontana CJ, Fitzjarrell AT (1980) Feedback loop between cerebellum and septal-hippocampal sites: its role in emotion and epilepsy. Biol Psychiatry 15: 541–556.
Heath RG, Dempsey CW, Fontana CJ, Myers WA (1978) Cerebellar stimulation: effects on septal region, hippocampus, and amygdala of cats and rats. Biol Psychiatry 13: 501–529.
Heath RG (1977) Modulation of emotion with a brain pacemamer. Treatment for intractable psychiatric illness. J Nerv Ment Dis 165: 300–317.
Holmes G (1939) The cerebellum of man. Brain 62: 1–30.
Hoover JE, Strick PL (1999) The organization of cerebellar and basal ganglia outputs to primary motor cortex as revealed by retrograde transneuronal transport of herpes simplex virus type 1. J Neurosci 19: 1446–1463.
Ikeda M, Houtani T, Ueyama T, Sugimoto T (1992) Distribution and cerebellar projections of cholinergic and corticotropin-releasing factor-containing neurons in the caudal vestibular nuclear complex and adjacent brainstem structures. Neuroscience 49: 635–651.
Ilg W, Giese MA, Gizewski ER, Schoch B, Timmann D (2008) The influence of focal cerebellar lesions on the control and adaptation of gait. Brain 131: 2913–2927.
Imaizumi S, Mori K, Kiritani S, Kawashima R, Sugiura M, Fukuda H, et al. (1997) Vocal identification of speaker and emotion activates different brain regions. Neuroreport 8: 2809–2812.
Ito M (1984) The Cerebellum and Neural Control. New York: Raven Press.

Jansen A, Brodal A (eds) (1954) Aspects of Cerebellar Anatomy. Oslo: Johan Grundt Tanum Vorlag.

Kase CS, Norrving B, Levine SR, Babikian VL, Chodosh EH, Wolf PA, Welch KM (1993) Cerebellar infarction: clinical and anatomic observations in 66 cases. Stroke 24: 76–83.

Kelly RM, Strick PL (2003) Cerebellar loops with motor cortex and prefrontal cortex of a nonhuman primate. J Neurosci. 23: 8432–44.

Konczak J, Schoch B, Dimitrova A, Gizewski E, Timmann D (2005) Functional recovery of children and adolescents after cerebellar tumour resection. Brain 128: 1428–1441.

Krienen FM, Buckner RL (2009) Segregated fronto-cerebellar circuits revealed by intrinsic functional connectivity. Cereb Cortex 19: 2485–2497.

Lane RD, Reiman EM, Bradley MM, Lang PJ, Ahern GL, Davidson RJ, Schwartz GE (1997) Neuroanatomical correlates of pleasant and unpleasant emotion. Neuropsychologia 35: 1437–1444.

Larsell O, Jansen J (1972) The Cerebellum. Minneapolis, Minnesota University Press.

Lawrence DG, Kuypers HG (1968) The functional organization of the motor system in the monkey. II. The effects of lesions of the descending brain-stem pathways. Brain 91: 15–36.

Leclerc N, Doré L, Parent A, Hawkes R (1990) The compartmentalization of the monkey and rat cerebellar cortex: Zebrin I and cytochrome oxidase. Brain Research 506: 70–78.

Leiner H, Leiner A, Dow R (1986) Does the cerebellum contribute to mental skills? Behav Neurosci 100: 443–454.

Levisohn L, Cronin-Golomb A, Schmahmann J (2000) Neuropsychological consequences of cerebellar tumour resection in children: Cerebellar cognitive affective syndrome in a paediatric population. Brain 123: 1041–1050.

Llinás R (1985) Functional significance of the basic cerebellar circuit in motor coordination. In: Bloedel JR, Dichgans J, Precht W. Cerebellar Functions. New York: Springer; 170–185.

Makris N, Schlerf JE, Hodge SM, Haselgrove C, Albaugh MD, Seidman LJ, et al. (2005) MRI-based surface-assisted parcellation of human cerebellar cortex: an anatomically specified method with estimate of reliability. Neuroimage 25(4): 1146–1160.

Manni E, Petrosini L (2004) A century of cerebellar somatotopy: a debated representation. Nat Rev Neurosci 4: 240–249.

Matturri L, Minoli I, Lavezzi AM, Cappellini A, Ramos S, Rossi L (2002) Hypoplasia of Medullary Arcuate Nucleus in Unexpected Late Fetal Death (Stillborn Infants): A Pathologic Study. Pediatrics 109: e43.

Mayo H (1827) A series of engravings intended to illustrate the structure of the brain and spinal cord in man. London: Burgess & Hill.

Middleton FA, Strick PL (1994) Anatomical evidence for cerebellar and basal ganglia involvement in higher cognitive function. Science 266: 458–461.

Middleton FA, Strick PL (1997) Cerebellar output channels. In: Schmahmann JD (ed). The Cerebellum and Cognition. Int Rev Neurobiol 41: 61–82. San Diego, CA: Academic Press.

Moulton EA, Borsook D, Schmahmann JD (2010) The Cerebellum and Pain: Passive Integrator or Active Participator? Brain Research Reviews 65(1): 14–27.

Nieuwenhuys R, Voogd J, van Huijzen C (2008) The Human Nervous System, 4th edition. New York, Springer: 807–840.

Nitschke M, Kleinschmidt A, Wessel K, Frahm J (1996) Somatotopic motor representation in the human anterior cerebellum: a high-resolution functional MRI study. Brain 119: 1023–1029.

Nyby O, Jansen J (1951) An experimental investigation of the corticopontine Projection in Macaca mulatta. Skrifter utgitt av det Norske Vedenskapsakademie: Oslo; 1. Mat Naturv Klasse. 3: 1–47.

Oertel WH (1993) Neurotransmitters in the cerebellum: Scientific aspects and clinical relevance. In: Harding AE, Deufel T (eds) Inherited Ataxias. New York, Raven Press. Adv Neurol 61: 33–75.

O'Reilly JX, Beckmann CF, Tomassini V, Ramnani N, Johansen-Berg H (2010) Distinct and overlapping functional zones in the cerebellum defined by resting state functional connectivity. Cereb Cortex 20: 953–965.

Ozgur BM, Berberian J, Aryan HE, Meltzer HS, Levy ML (2006) The pathophysiologic mechanism of cerebellar mutism. Surg Neurol 66: 18–25.

Palay S, Chan-Palay V (1974) Cerebellar Cortex: Cytology and Organization. New York: Springer-Verlag.

Paulus K, Magnano I, Conti M, Galistu P, D'Onofrio M, Satta W, Aiello I (2004) Pure post-stroke cerebellar cognitive affective syndrome: a case report. Neurol Sci 25: 220–224.

Ploghaus A, Tracey I, Gati JS, Clare S, Menon RS, Matthews PM, Rawlins JN (1999) Dissociating pain from its anticipation in the human brain. Science 284: 1979–1981.

Pollack I, Polinko P, Albright A, Towbin R, Fitz C (1995) Mutism and pseudobulbar symptoms after resection of posterior fossa tumors in children: Incidence and pathophysiology. Neurosurgery 37: 885–893.

Ramnani N, Behrens TE, Johansen-Berg H, Richter MC, Pinsk MA, Andersson JL, et al. (2006) The evolution of prefrontal inputs to the cortico-pontine system: diffusion imaging evidence from Macaque monkeys and humans. Cereb Cortex 16: 811–18.

Reiman E, Raichle M, Robins E, Mintun M, Fusselman MJ, Fox PT, Hackman KA (1989) Neuroanatomical correlates of a lactate-induced anxiety attack. Arch Gen Psychiatry 46: 493–500.

Richter S, Gerwig M, Aslan B, Wilhelm H, Schoch B, Dimitrova A, et al. (2007) Cognitive functions in patients with MR-defined chronic focal cerebellar lesions. J Neurol 254: 1193–1203.

Richter S, Schoch B, Kaiser O, Groetschel H, Dimitrova A, Hein-Kropp C, et al. (2005) Behavioral and affective changes in children and adolescents with chronic cerebellar lesions. Neurosci Lett 381: 102–107.

Riva D, Giorgi C (2000) The cerebellum contributes to higher functions during development: Evidence from a series of children surgically treated for posterior fossa tumours. Brain 123: 1051–1061.

Salmi J, Pallesen KJ, Neuvonen T, Brattico E, Korvenoja A, Salonen O, Carlson S (2010) Cognitive and motor loops of the human cerebro-cerebellar system. J Cogn Neurosci 22: 2663–76.

Schmahmann JD (1991) An emerging concept: the cerebellar contribution to higher function. Arch Neurol 48: 1178–1187.

Schmahmann JD (1996) From movement to thought: Anatomic substrates of the cerebellar contribution to cognitive processing. Hum Brain Mapp 4: 174–198.

Schmahmann JD (ed) (1997) The Cerebellum and Cognition. Int Rev Neurobiol vol 41. San Diego, CA: Academic Press.

Schmahmann JD (2000) The role of the cerebellum in affect and psychosis. J Neurolinguist 13: 189–214.

Schmahmann JD (2004) Disorders of the cerebellum: ataxia, dysmetria of thought, and the cerebellar cognitive affective syndrome. J Neuropsychiatry Clin Neurosci 16: 367–378.

Schmahmann JD, Doyon J, McDonald D, et al. (1999). Three-dimensional MRI atlas of the human cerebellum in proportional stereotaxic space. Neuroimage 10: 233–60.

Schmahmann JD, Doyon J, Toga A, Evans A, Petrides M (2000) MRI Atlas of the Human Cerebellum. San Diego, CA: Academic Press.

Schmahmann JD, Macmore J, Vangel M (2009) Cerebellar stroke without motor deficit: clinical evidence for motor and non-motor domains within the human cerebellum. Neuroscience 162: 852–861.

Schmahmann JD, Pandya DN (1989) Anatomical investigation of projections to the basis pontis from posterior parietal association cortices in rhesus monkey. J Comp Neurol 289: 53–73.

Schmahmann JD, Pandya DN (1991) Projections to the basis pontis from the superior temporal sulcus and superior temporal region in the rhesus monkey. J Comp Neurol 308: 224–248.

Schmahmann JD, Pandya DN (1993) Prelunate, occipitotemporal, and parahipppocampal projections to the basis pontis in rhesus monkey. J Comp Neurol 337: 94–112.

Schmahmann JD, Pandya DN (1997a) Anatomic organization of the basilar pontine projections from prefrontal cortices in rhesus monkey. J Neurosci 17: 438–458.

Schmahmann JD, Pandya DN (1997b). The cerebrocerebellar system. In: Schmahmann JD (ed) The Cerebellum and Cognition. San Diego, CA: Academic Press. Int Rev Neurobiol 41: 31–60.

Schmahmann J, Pandya D (2006) Fiber Pathways of the Brain. New York: Oxford University Press.

Schmahmann JD, Rosene DL, Pandya DN (2004) Motor projections to the basis pontis in rhesus monkey. J Comp Neurol 478: 248–268.

Schmahmann JD, Sherman JC (1998) The cerebellar cognitive affective syndrome. Brain 121: 561–579.

Schmahmann JD, Weilburg JB, Sherman JC (2007) The neuropsychiatry of the cerebellum – insights from the clinic. Cerebellum 6: 254–267.

Schoch B, Dimitrova A, Gizewski ER, Timmann D (2006) Functional localization in the human cerebellum based on voxelwise statistical analysis: a study of 90 patients. Neuroimage 30: 36–51.

Singer T, Seymour B, O'Doherty J, Kaube H, Dolan R, Frith C (2004) Empathy for pain involves the affective but not sensory components of pain. Science 303: 1157–1162.

Snider R, Eldred E (1951) Electro-anatomical studies on cerebro-cerebellar connections in the cat. J Comp Neurol 95: 1–16.

Snider R, Stowell A (1944) Electro-anatomical studies on a tactile system in the cerebellum of monkey (macaca mulatta). Anat Rec 88: 457.

Snider RS (1950) Recent contributions to the anatomy and physiology of the cerebellum. Arch Neurol Psychiatry 64: 196–219.

Spitzer A, Karplus JP (1907) Über experimentelle Läsionen an der Gehirnbasis. Arbeiten aus dem Neurologischen Institut 16: 348–436.

Stoodley CJ, Schmahmann JD (2009) Functional topography in the human cerebellum: a meta-analysis of neuroimaging studies. NeuroImage 44: 489–501.

Stoodley CJ, Schmahmann JD (2010) Evidence for topographic organization in the cerebellum of motor control versus cognitive and affective processing. Cortex 46: 831–844.

Stoodley CJ, Valera EM, Schmahmann JD (2010) An fMRI study of intra-individual functional topography in the human cerebellum. Behav Neurol 23: 65–79.

Strick PL, Dum RP, Fiez JA (2009) Cerebellum and nonmotor function. Annu Rev Neurosci 32: 413–434.

Takanashi M, Abe K, Yanagihara T, Sakoda S, Tanaka H, Hirabuki N, et al. (2003) A functional MRI study of somatotopic representation of somatosensory stimulation in the cerebellum. Neuroradiology 45: 149–152.

Tavano A, Grasso R, Gagliardi C, Triulzi F, Bresolin N, Fabbro F, Borgatti R (2007) Disorders of cognitive and affective development in cerebellar malformations. Brain 130: 2646–2660.

Thickbroom GW, Byrnes ML, Mastaglia FL (2003) Dual representation of the hand in the cerebellum: activation with voluntary and passive finger movement. Neuroimage 18: 670–674.

Tohgi H, Takahashi S, Chiba K, Hirata Y (1993) Cerebellar infarction: Clinical and neuroimaging analysis in 293 patients. Stroke 24: 1697–1701.

Tolbert DL, Bantli H, Bloedel JR (1978) Organizational features of the cat and monkey cerebellar nucleocortical projection. J Comp Neurol 182: 39–56.

Urban PP, Marx J, Hunsche S, Gawehn J, Vucurevic G, Wicht S, et al. (2003) Cerebellar speech representation: lesion topography in dysarthria as derived from cerebellar ischemia and functional magnetic resonance imaging. Arch Neurol 60: 965–972.

Voogd J (2004) Cerebellum and precerebellar nuclei. In: Paxinos G, Mai JK, The Human Nervous System. Second edition. Amsterdam: Elsevier Academic Press; 321–392.

Voogd J, Bigaré F (1980) Topographical distribution of olivary and cortico-nuclear fibres in the cerebellum: a review. In: Courville J (ed) The Olivary Nucleus: Anatomy and Physiology. New York: Raven; 207–234.

Voogd J, Glickstein M (1998) The anatomy of the cerebellum. Trends Cogn Sci 2: 307–313.

Wildgruber D, Riecker A, Hertrich I, Erb M, Grodd W, Ethofer T, Ackermann H (2005) Identification of emotional intonation evaluated by fMRI. NeuroImage 24: 1233–1241.

Woolsey, CN (1952) Summary of the papers on the cerebellum. Res Publ Assoc Res Nerv Ment Dis 30: 334–336.

3
Approach to the Neurological Examination of Children with Cerebellar Disorders

Peter Tsai, Katherine B. Sims, and Jeremy D. Schmahmann

In this chapter we present an approach to the clinical assessment of children with symptoms and signs suggestive of cerebellar dysfunction in order to arrive at a differential diagnosis and strategy for management. Diseases that afflict the cerebellum in childhood are frequently complex or multisystem disorders, and the evaluation should be sufficiently detailed to capture the essential features of the case. We commence with a general approach to the history and examination, and then focus particularly on the examination of the cerebellar system.

History of present illness

The history frames the differential diagnosis and focuses the physical examination. It is dependent on reliable caregivers, including parents and grandparents. The chief complaint reflects the principal problem and the caregivers' main concerns. For patients with cerebellar disease the chief complaint may be that the child is clumsy or has gait instability, abnormalities of tone, unusual eye movements, slurred speech, and/or developmental delay. Cognitive-behavioral issues may be present, as discussed in the following chapter.

The age of the child, and the nature of the symptoms at onset, direct the clinician to different etiologies. Establishing the temporal course of the evolution of the symptoms, potential triggers, exacerbating or ameliorating factors, and/or preceding or concurrent illnesses may shed light on whether deficits are episodic, static or progressive. These features will have implications for diagnosis and management.

PRESENTING SYMPTOMS

Cerebellar lesions leading to motor incoordination are located in the sensorimotor cerebellum, now known to occupy much of the anterior lobe (notably lobules III through V), part of lobule VI, and the second sensorimotor representation in lobule VIII, as well as the interconnected parts of the deep cerebellar nuclei and the white matter tracts that are afferent and efferent to these cortical areas (see Chapter 2). Depending on the precise location of the pathology, cerebellar lesions produce ataxia of gait, dysmetria of the extremities, abnormal eye movements, and/or impaired articulation (Holmes 1922; Schmahmann et al. 2009a). The history should establish whether the symptoms are axial or appendicular, whether the child ever developed the ability to sit or stand, and whether the process is unilateral or generalized. Focal cerebellar lesions result in motor deficits affecting the same side of the body. True weakness may indicate that the disease affecting the cerebellum also involves extracerebellar structures. In younger children, abnormal muscle tone – notably, floppiness – may be an early presenting feature of cerebellar disease. The presence of sensory symptoms can help establish whether the gait impairment is a reflection of a sensory ataxia, rather than a primary cerebellar process. Abnormal movements including tremor, chorea, athetosis, myoclonic movements, or seizures can occur in a range of diseases that include cerebellar pathology. It is useful to inquire about these, and have families provide videos of episodic symptoms that may not be present in the examination room.

Space-occupying lesions such as tumors in the posterior fossa can lead to obstructive hydrocephalus. In these cases, in addition to cerebellar symptoms, patients with raised intracranial pressure may experience nausea and vomiting, with headache particularly in the morning and worsened by recumbency, and with mental status changes including a decreased level of arousal. False lateralizing findings include abducens nerve (sixth cranial nerve) palsies with a subjective sense of diplopia.

Eye movement abnormalities seen in patients with cerebellar lesions may present symptomatically with diplopia, oscillopsia, or report of blurred vision. An acute or subacute presentation of an oculomotor palsy, with ataxia and areflexia, should raise the possibility of the Miller Fisher variant of an acute inflammatory demyelinating polyneuropathy.

Patients with cerebellar dysfunction may complain of dizziness, which could mean gait unsteadiness, lightheadedness caused by autonomic neuropathy or other disorders of vascular sufficiency, or true vertigo. This can be difficult to ascertain even with careful probing. Vertigo reflects dysfunction of the vestibular system from either central (cerebellar/brainstem) or peripheral etiology (vestibular nerve or labyrinthine pathology). True vertigo requires further inquiry into precipitating factors/situations, duration of episodes, and associated symptoms such as nausea, emesis, and headache. Hearing loss in this context may reflect pathology in the cerebellopontine angle. Bilateral hearing loss associated with cerebellar symptoms occurs in neurofibromatosis type 2, but may also accompany metabolic processes such as mitochondrial disorders.

Cerebellar lesions may accompany pathology in the cerebral hemispheres, and in this setting there may be clinically relevant disorders of cognition. The cerebellum is also implicated in behavioral regulation, as discussed in Chapter 4. Patients and their caregivers should be asked whether any behavioral alterations can be identified: loss of interest in previous enjoyed activities; decreased social interactions; increased irritability, tantrums, altercations with peers/family; or abnormal thought processes.

Dysarthria resulting from cerebellar lesions is characterized as 'scanning speech', with poorly modulated rate, rhythm and force, resulting in impaired cadence and volume. Cerebellar lesions can also impair verbal fluency even in the absence of dysarthria, and the phenomenon of cerebellar mutism is observed following surgical excision of vermal tumors, cerebellar hemorrhage, and inflammatory disorders (Pollack et al. 1995; Levisohn et al. 2000; Wells et al. 2008). These features should be apparent in the elicitation of the history.

Review of systems

Complete review of non-neurological systems is helpful in establishing the differential diagnosis. Gait impairment can result from labyrinthitis one of the complications of otitis media. Infectious cerebellitis or rhombencephalitis results in frank cerebellar symptoms. Acute cerebellar ataxia is common in childhood and likely has a postinfectious, immune-mediated etiology. Acute disseminated encephalomyelitis, also postinfectious or inflammatory in origin, may affect the cerebellum directly, and multiple sclerosis, sarcoidosis, and Behcet's disease may be precipitated clinically by intercurrent infections. Questions concerning skin, renal, heart, joint, gastrointestinal, and lung involvement may inform the differential diagnosis. Concerns for immunodeficiency and opportunistic infections could raise concern for ataxia-telangiectasia. Cardiac arrhythmias or thrombotic disorders would be relevant in cases of pediatric cerebellar stroke. Cerebellar disorders may have comorbid endocrinopathies related to insulin, antidiuretic hormone, steroid or thyroid dysfunction that should be considered in the review of systems. Metabolic etiologies of ataxia such as celiac disease may affect the gastrointestinal tract. Genetically inherited metabolic disorders which may have a cerebellar component include vitamin E deficiency, GM2 gangliosidosis, Niemann-Pick, type C, and ataxia-telangiectasia. Bowel and bladder habits should be discussed as diseases affecting cerebellum can involve descending brainstem tracts and spinal cord. Dysphagia occurs in cerebellar patients because of disordered control of muscles of articulation, and this may be accompanied by dysphagia with coughing or choking.

Cerebellar toxicity may also result from ingestion of medications or household toxins, and an inventory of medications in the home and in locations the child has visited can be helpful in the appropriate circumstances.

Past medical history

The cerebellar primordia and two proliferative zones develop prior to 20 weeks of gestation, and in the third trimester and first year of life, proliferation and migration from these two zones results in the bulk of cerebellar formation and development (Volpe 2009). Injuries sustained during these times can have major and persistent consequences.

Relevant maternal pregnancy health issues critical to potential cerebellar injury include hypertension, medications, and exposures to potential toxins. Birth history can provide indicators of perinatal injury suggested by decreased fetal movement, irregularities in fetal monitoring, prolonged rupture of membranes, untreated maternal fevers, maternal blood loss from placental abruption, and twin-twin transfusion as well as history of poor cry, bradycardia, poor temperature regulation, and hypotonia. Respiratory or cardiac resuscitation, infection, and other postnatal complications are also of interest.

Developmental history can help differentiate acute from static nonprogressive or degenerative processes. Cerebellar dysfunction may initially be identified in the infant by hypotonia and gross as well as fine motor delay. The development of pincer grasp, utensil use, block stacking, button or other small object manipulation, and dressing provide timelines for motor development. Development of stable reaching, hand use, midline crossing, and transfer provide other markers of cerebellar motor development. Speech may be delayed and dysarthric. Delayed or poor quality of social interactions, impairments in language, and repetitive behaviors or restricted interests may represent the behavioral manifestations of cerebellar dysfunction.

Medications

Symptoms suggestive of cerebellar dysfunction may be toxin-induced, either from inappropriate ingestion of materials or medications around the household, or from supra-therapeutic levels of prescribed medications. Review of prescribed medications for the patient and contacts should be undertaken when toxicity is suspected.

Family history

A large number of genetic and hereditary disorders affect the cerebellum. Elicitation of a family history of neurological and other disorders should include, if possible, a minimum of three generations. History elicited from grandparents can be most helpful because of their knowledge of distant relatives and prior generations, and of events during the parents' childhood of which they themselves may be unaware. The specifics of ethnic background and the possibility of consanguinity are important to ascertain.

Specific questioning may be informative regarding family members with impairments of gait, balance and speech, developmental delays, learning disabilities, mental retardation (UK: learning disability) epilepsy, autism spectrum disorders, cerebral palsy, seizure disorders, genetic diseases, or metabolic diseases including mitochondrial, endocrine, or inborn errors of metabolism may be informative. Asking about autoimmune disorders is reasonable, including multiple sclerosis and Behcet disease. Frequent miscarriages, easy bruising, clots in the extremities or pulmonary system, stroke or cardiac disease, prior to age 50, would point to possible vascular risk factors.

Social history

Educational level of the patient and family, school performance, and the home social situation may help the clinician understand the context of the illness, and frame discussion about how symptoms might impact long-term goals. A large number of infections worldwide involve structures in the posterior fossa, ranging from progressive multifocal leukoencephalopathy that occurs in patients infected with HIV, to tuberculosis, parasitic infections such as schistosomiasis and neuroboreliosis (Lyme disease) if residence is in endemic areas. The history, therefore, is informed not only by the patient's geographical environment but also by an account of recent travel. In the adolescent, a history of substances of abuse, inhalants, and other risk-taking behaviors may be pertinent.

Physical examination

The neurological examination is tailored by the nature of the chief complaint and the history, and it needs to be age appropriate. Much of the examination is performed through observation during elicitation of the history, including gait, spontaneous movement and level of activity, speech, and interest in and engagement with the examiner and environment. Examination of the younger child can be optimized by approaching the examination as a game in which the child is invited to participate. Aspects of the examination that may be less pleasant should be performed at the end, including fundoscopy, head circumference measurement, and examination of the external ear canal and oropharynx.

General examination

The general examination can provide somatic clues and is best performed systematically.

Vital signs provide an indication of acute illness, of which cerebellar dysfunction may be one component. Dizziness may rarely be caused by autonomic dysfunction in childhood and can be assessed directly by orthostatic vital sign measurement. Weight assesses in utero growth retardation (IUGR) in the newborn, failure to thrive in older patients, and is used for dosage calculation for pharmacological interventions. Macrocephaly and/or microcephaly occur in many disorders associated with cerebellar dysfunction, and thus head circumference should be measured routinely and plotted on brain growth charts at least until early adolescence. Head circumference reflects primarily brain growth, but can also be increased in bony conditions such as osteopetrosis, and in some families, large head size is a benign condition. Measurement of the parental head circumference is useful in the latter case. It should be measured three times to minimize observer error.

Examination of the head and neck includes observation of asymmetries or masses. Abnormal position of the head may suggest torticollis or tilt induced by an oculomotor palsy. Dysmorphic features of the eyes, nose, ears, lips, mouth, teeth, and jaw lead to consideration of genetic disorders. For example, a central incisor raises the possibility of holoprosencephaly which can be associated with cerebellar malformations including Dandy Walker; facial dysmorphisms and inverted nipples suggest a possible congenital disorder of glycosylation which may be associated with cerebellar findings; and the sphingolipidoses may be hinted at by frontal bossing, depressed nasal bridge, low-set ears, and/or a long philtrum.

Retinal abnormalities, optic nerve atrophy, cataracts, or colobomas provide helpful clues to diagnosis, and dedicated ophthalmological examination with a slit lamp is sometimes indicated, as in the search for Kayser-Fleischer rings in Wilson disease. External and internal structural anomalies of the ears may provide a basis for repeat ear infections and hearing loss. Inside the mouth, oral thrush might suggest immunodeficiency, vesicular lesions are a concern for herpes infection, and high arched palate occurs in neuromuscular and neurodegenerative disorders.

The cardiac examination may reveal a potential source of cardioembolic cerebellar stroke. Cardiomyopathy accompanies childhood onset Friedreich ataxia, and arrhythmias or cardiomyopathy may occur in mitochondrial diseases.

Abdominal examination may reveal organomegaly present in metabolic diseases such as the sphingolipidoses that can have cerebellar involvement. About 2–3% of patients with neuroblastoma develop opsoclonus-myoclonus syndrome (OMS), but when OMS is present the culprit is neuroblastoma in as many as 60% of children (Rothenberg et al. 2009; Krug et al. 2010); careful abdominal examination for adrenal or other masses is therefore critical. Celiac disease, an occasional cause of gluten ataxia in children (Lionetti et al. 2010), can produce cramping and nonspecific abdominal pain on examination. Posterior fossa lesions that produce nausea and vomiting need to be distinguished from primary gastrointestinal disorders. The genitourinary examination may reveal macroorchidism in patients with fragile X, and hypogonadism in the Holmes form of ataxia (Holmes 1907).

Neurocutaneous syndromes may be diagnosed on careful skin examination. Ataxia-telangiectasia has the tell-tale telangiectasias in the eye and buccal mucosa (although not always present with onset of ataxia). Up to one-third of patients with tuberous sclerosis complex may have cerebellar lesions/tubers (Ertan et al. 2009) and the cutaneous examination may reveal ash leaf spots seen best with Wood's lamp, facial angiofibromas, and shagreen patches over the nape of neck/lower back; and ungual or subungual fibromas. Cerebellar tumors do occur but are rare in neurofibromatosis type 1 (Dunn et al. 2007; Pascual-Castroviejo et al. 2010), characterized on cutaneous examination by hyperpigmented macules or café-au-lait spots. Vitiligo may be suggestive of an autoimmune (Bayreuther et al. 2008) or genetic etiology of cerebellar disease (Cohen et al. 1984; Tulinius et al. 1995). Albinism may be associated with inherited forms of ataxia such as Angelman syndrome (Smith et al. 1996; Fridman et al. 2003). Menkes disease that has prominent cerebellar pathology (Robain et al. 1988; Martínez-Granero et al. 1997) is typically associated with 'kinked' hair. The PHACES syndrome (Frieden et al. 1996; Oza et al. 2008) is a neurocutaneous disorder characterized by facial hemangiomas, with posterior fossa malformations (Dandy-Walker syndrome or variant, cerebellar hemispheric hypoplasia ipsilateral to the facial hemangioma), intra- and extracranial arterial anomalies, coarctation of the aorta, cardiac and eye abnormalities, and sternal defects.

Scoliosis occurs in a number of disorders including Chiari malformation, Joubert syndrome, and cerebellar diseases that include pathology in the spinal cord and peripheral nerves as in Friedreich ataxia. Similarly, high arches of the feet (pes cavus) may be seen in Friedreich ataxia of young onset.

Neurological examination

Much of the neurological examination, particularly in the younger child, comes from observation of the patient and his or her interaction with caregivers and the environment. The neurological examination should be seen within the context of the age of the child.

Mental status

Levels of arousal and alertness influence the rest of the neurological examination and are assessed at the outset to determine if the child interacts with the environment spontaneously, is inattentive, withdrawn, or encephalopathic. The infant by 1 month of age should fix with the eyes and track, and show interest in the environment; a child should be able to pay attention, be redirected by caregivers, make eye contact, and perform age-appropriate tasks.

Attention affects the remainder of the examination. It is assessed during the first months of life by tests of visual attention to brightly colored/contrasting objects, lights, or faces (a small mirror or colorful toy can be a convenient way to assess visual attention). The toddler should follow simple commands, and play with toys. Attention can be assessed in the preschool child by observing for hyperactivity, noting distractibility, assessing the ability to complete simple tasks, and/or the ability to follow multi-step instructions. In the older child, attention can be assessed by 'Go, No go' tasks (give thumbs up for A, nothing for B) or reversal paradigms – spelling backwards, days of the week or months of the year backwards, or digit span recall.

A child's fund of knowledge is assessed by asking them to identify and name body parts or objects, by observation of their play patterns, by asking the school-age child about what they are learning/reading, and through more detailed questions about preferred subjects, hobbies, activities, or friends. The child's ability to engage in this dialogue in a developmentally appropriate manner provides valuable information regarding cognitive function, speech patterns, receptive and expressive language, and social interaction skills. Getting down to the child's level – on the floor with a toddler or preschool child or examining an infant or shy child in a mother's lap – can facilitate the examination. Literacy can be assessed by asking the child to read an age-appropriate book or text, and follow-up questions can provide insight into reading comprehension. Writing and drawing samples evaluate literacy and the orthography, and also provide a record of change over time. Patients with cerebellar dysfunction generally have macrographia (in contrast to patients with extrapyramidal syndromes who have micrographia). Visuospatial planning can be assessed in the younger child by drawing simple (triangle, circle, and square) or intersecting shapes, and the older child may be able to attempt the more intricate Rey-Osterrieth figure. Further aspects of the cognitive and neuropsychiatric profile are discussed in Chapter 4.

Cranial nerves

Visual field testing will detect ischemic lesions of the occipital lobes which share posterior circulation vascular supply with the cerebellum. Visual acuity is impaired in late stages of Friedreich's ataxia (Fortuna et al. 2009), and in spinocerebellar ataxia type 7 particularly when it presents in childhood. Evidence on fundoscopic examination of absent venous pulsations, papilledema, or retinal hemorrhages will indicate possible raised intracranial pressure as occurs in the setting of cerebellar space-occupying lesions or trauma/hemorrhage. Optic nerve pallor or atrophy may be evident in multiple sclerosis and in hereditary diseases such as Wolfram syndrome, and some metabolic disorders such as nutritional, toxic or drug-induced amblyopia may present in childhood with cerebellar abnormalities. Metabolic disorders must be considered if one documents retinitis pigmentosa or a cherry-red spot.

Eye movements are an essential part of the cerebellar motor examination. Mass lesions or inflammatory processes may impact the cerebellum and the brainstem and/or the brainstem nuclei controlling eye movements or nerves exiting the brainstem. Supranuclear vertical gaze palsy is characteristic of Niemann-Pick type C disease, particularly the juvenile onset type, and may be the initial sign (Vanier 2010). Gaze difficulties in reading or going downstairs reflect impairment of downward gaze more than upward gaze. Characteristic findings in this disorder include abolition of all vertical voluntary saccades, paresis of downward pursuit movements and preservation of full vertical oculocephalic reflexes (Sévin et al. 2007). Ophthalmoplegia can be a hallmark of energy metabolism-mitochondrial disorders, and children with Joubert syndrome may have oculomotor apraxia (Maria et al. 1999). The PHACE syndrome includes ocular abnormalities, as well as third nerve palsy and Horner syndrome (Frieden et al. 1996; Metry et al. 2009).

Examination of eye movements in a cerebellar patient may reveal unsteady fixation in primary position (at rest) with microsaccadic oscillations and square wave jerks, ocular flutter, ocular bobbing, and opsoclonus. Pursuit eye movements may not be smooth but instead show saccadic intrusions, manifesting as jerkiness in following a moving target. This is tested by having the patient maintain fixation on the examiner's finger as it moves smoothly before the patient's eyes about an arm's length away in the horizontal and vertical directions. Abnormal saccades are characterized by overshoot (hypermetric saccade) or undershoot/catch-up (hypometric saccade). This is tested by asking the patient to look rapidly from the examiner's nose to the examiner's finger held about 20 degrees away from the midline, first to the one side then to the other, recording the performance with movements both towards and away from the midline. Patients with cerebellar dysfunction (especially with vermian involvement) can also suffer from oculomotor apraxia with difficulties in performing horizontal eye movements; patients will often move their entire head (head thrust) in order to see from side to side. To examine eye movements in children, the use of a brightly colored or contrasted object, or an object with flashing lights, can be beneficial. Faces often elicit the greatest visual attention in infants, so movement of the examiner's face or a small mirror can be effective.

Gaze-evoked nystagmus from cerebellar lesions is characterized by fast phase in the direction of eccentric gaze and a slow phase in the opposite direction, in repeating sequence. The direction of the nystagmus is determined by the direction of the fast beating phase. Downbeat nystagmus may be present in primary gaze but is usually exacerbated by down-gaze, lateral gaze, and convergence. It points to lesions of the cervicomedullary junction and results from disruption of inhibitory pathways from the flocculus to the vestibular system. It may occur in genetically inherited ataxias or it can be an isolated finding. Upbeat nystagmus often points to midline cerebellar lesions, and can also occur in the setting of a drug overdose.

The vestibulo-ocular reflex (VOR) maintains stabilization of a visualized image on the retina during head movement. This allows the healthy individual to maintain visual focus on an object despite head motion. Suppression of the VOR (VOR cancellation, or VORC) can be induced by purposefully focusing on a near object (the child's own hand, for example) during rotation of the torso and head in the horizontal plane thus allowing the distant visual world to pass by. The importance of the cerebellum for motor learning is apparent in this reflex, as cerebellar lesions interfere with cancellation or adaptation of the VOR (Yagi et al. 1981; Voogd and Barmack 2006). Failure of VOR suppression is identified by the examiner's observation of saccadic intrusions into the patient's attempt to maintain gaze on the near object during passive horizontal rotation of the head and body. Subjectively, patients experience compromised visual acuity, and dizziness that is exaggerated by movement through crowds, traveling in a moving vehicle, or when riding on escalators.

Lesions of the cerebellopontine angle may produce dysfunction of the vestibulocochlear nerve (eighth cranial nerve) – with both auditory and vestibular consequences. Impaired hearing in the infant or young child is a major cause of speech delay. Office tests of hearing integrity, including the Weber and Rinne tests, help differentiate sensorineural versus conductive hearing loss. The Weber test is performed by placing the nonvibrating end of the tuning fork at the center of the forehead – the patient should perceive the sound as coming equally from both ears. If it lateralizes to one side, this could result from conduction hearing loss on the side with the louder sound, or sensorineural hearing loss on the side with the lesser appreciation of the sound. The Rinne test will help distinguish these. The Rinne test is performed by placing the vibrating tuning fork on the mastoid process until the sound abates; the tuning fork is then immediately placed next to the external auditory canal. With normal hearing, the sound should be audible next to the ear after it has subsided at the mastoid. With conduction hearing loss, the sound persists longer through bone than air conduction (bone > air); with sensorineural hearing loss, the sound is still audible at the ear after it has disappeared at the mastoid, or in severe cases there may be no appreciation of the sound on the affected side at all. These bedside findings can be followed by formal audiological testing. Vestibular integrity is assessed by examining for nystagmus, exaggeration of precipitation of nystagmus by change in head and neck position, or by evaluation of the VORC, as discussed above.

Observation of the palate will detect palatal myoclonus that occurs in lesions of the Guillain-Mollaret triangle (red nucleus-inferior olivary complex-cerebellar deep nuclei [interpositus/dentate]). Gag and spontaneous movement of the palate should be assessed, as dysphagia is a major cause of morbidity in the cerebellar patient population.

Cerebellar dysarthria has been characterized as 'scanning speech'. This reflects the rate, rhythm and force impairments of the articulatory apparatus including tongue, mouth and palate. In the early stages of dysarthria syllables are less well articulated and cadence may be slightly irregular. This is usually apparent in conversation, and is underscored by testing recitation of days of the week or months of the year, with repeated buccal (me-me-me), palatal (go-go-go) and lingual (la-la-la) syllables, and with alternating syllables (buttercup/lollipop/pataka). Speech becomes slower as the dysarthria evolves, perhaps as a compensatory mechanism. The clarity of speech is generally improved when patients make a conscious effort to speak more slowly – a useful approach to management. The cerebellar patient may also have disordered breathing as the diaphragm and accessory muscles of respiration are under cerebellar control. Ataxic breathing with irregular inspiration and exhalation also affects the quality of speech, and problems with volume control add to the complex nature of cerebellar dysarthria. Given the cerebellar control of the muscles of deglutition, dysfunction increases the risk of aspiration in the more severely afflicted patient.

Muscular tone and bulk

Hypotonia (decreased resistance to passive manipulation of the limb or lowered resting tone) occurs in the extremities or the axial trunk of patients with cerebellar lesions. Hypotonia may be transient following acute cerebellar lesions, but in children with congenital/developmental lesions the hypotonia is usually more prominent and persistent than in adults. Tone is more complex in the spinocerebellar ataxias or other disorders that include a corticospinal component. Here there may be hypotonia but with a superimposed spastic catch when testing for pronation/supination at the elbow, even if there is not frank spasticity. In conditions such as the hereditary spastic ataxias, the tone is markedly increased particularly in the legs, reflecting the myelopathic component of the disorder.

Generalized loss of muscle bulk in the setting of ataxia raises the likelihood of nutritional, developmental or chronic neuromuscular disorders. Asymmetric decreased bulk of the limbs indicates focal developmental disorders. Hemihypertrophy of the limbs may be associated with cutaneous and cerebellar hemangiomas or hemihypertrophy (Klippel-Trénaunay-Weber syndrome; Torregrosa et al. 2000).

Muscular power

Lesions confined to the cerebellum do not cause decreased muscle power, although many patients report feeling weak and fatigued. With formal testing, the report of apparent weakness can be traced to slowness in the initiation and generation of force, but the maximum power ultimately achieved is full, unless there is extracerebellar involvement. True weakness with hypotonia and hyporeflexia points to involvement of the peripheral nervous system or gray matter of the spinal cord. The additional findings of decreased power and hyperreflexia speak to involvement of the corticospinal system in the cerebral hemispheres, brainstem and/or spinal cord.

Adventitious movements

Truncal titubation and cerebellar tremor are discussed below. Extrapyramidal movement disorders may occur in patients with cerebellar ataxia because of involvement of the basal ganglia in neurodegenerative diseases affecting the cerebellum. These include Wilson disease and neurodegeneration with iron accumulation in the brain. When the spinocerebellar ataxias (SCA) commence clinically in childhood, they frequently affect the caudate and putamen, notably SCA 1, 3, and 17, while SCA 2 and SCA 8 often have choreiform movements, torticollis, and dystonia as part of the clinical presentation. Similarly, recessively inherited ataxias with oculomotor apraxia type 1 (Coutinho and Barbot 2002) and type 2 (Anheim et al. 2009) include choreiform and dystonic postures and head tremor, and we have seen these features as the principal elementary clinical finding early in the course, with only mild peripheral neuropathy, subtle gait impairment, and disturbances in ocular pursuit.

The cerebellar motor examination

The cerebellar motor syndrome of impaired coordination and motor control is characterized by disturbances in rate, rhythm, and force of muscular contractions. The five major domains of impairment of the motor system arising from cerebellar lesions are disturbance of stance, equilibrium and gait (ataxia); impaired coordination (dysmetria) of the upper and of the lower extremities; impaired articulation (dysarthria); and eye movement abnormalities. Cerebellar tremor is also a major cause of disability. The neurological examination of the cerebellar motor system is designed to detect, characterize, and quantify these observations. Speech and eye movements were discussed above.

Truncal posture is affected with midline lesions, whereas more laterally placed lesions affect the extremities. To evaluate for truncal ataxia, the patient is examined in the seated position without leaning on any part of the chair. In infants who are able to sit, asking the parents whether the child's ability to sit has changed significantly helps assess worsening of truncal control. The patient then stands, if safe to do so, with the eyes open, and is observed for titubation – rhythmic oscillations of the head and trunk. The stance may be widened and the distance of the heels from each other can be quantified. The ability of the patient to stand in the tandem position or on one foot can be assessed. In pure cerebellar lesions the stance does not change appreciably with eyes closed, but it does become substantially more unsteady (positive Romberg sign) if there is proprioceptive deficit.

The ataxic gait of a patient with cerebellar dysfunction typically has a widened stance, is staggering, uneven and veering from side to side. It is often slowed, and displays irregular rhythm, force, and distance between steps as well as inaccurate placement of the foot and shortened stride length. Patients with unilateral lesions stumble or fall towards the affected side. The gait should be assessed when the patient ambulates in an open space such as a hallway, while performing tandem gait, and if possible, while running because this emphasizes subtle abnormalities of rhythm and stability. Having the child ambulate towards a caregiver and away from examiner can be reassuring, and asking the patient's caregiver to run with the child can facilitate this part of the examination. Asking the patient to walk around a chair, first clockwise then counter-clockwise, may identify laterality of the lesion, as the patient will stumble towards the side of the lesion – either into the chair or away from it, depending on the direction of rotation. Similarly, when marching in place with the eyes closed, the patient will tend to rotate towards the side of the lesion. For infants unable to walk, truncal instability, dysmetria of reach, or steadiness of crawl can be assessed. Ataxia will often cause parents to remark about a worsening crawl. Stressed gait testing can be performed in older children by asking them to walk on the outside of their feet, or on toes or heels. Overflow movements including posturing of the arms, hands, and sometimes facial and tongue muscles may be provoked by this maneuver, raising suspicion for extrapyramidal components to the neurological constellation.

The gait may be more complex in diseases that include pathology in noncerebellar areas as well as in the cerebellum. Spastic ataxias have unstable gait with irregular placement of the feet, but the stance may not be as wide as expected in pure cerebellar dysfunction. Spasticity may be evident both on inspection of the flexion of the hips and knees with ambulation, and with formal testing of tone. Similarly, when peripheral neuropathy, dorsal root ganglion, or posterior column involvement occurs, as in Friedreich ataxia, marked proprioceptive loss leads to a wildly high-stepping and floppy component in addition to the widened stance, impaired cadence, and inaccurate foot placement.

The term dysmetria, derived from the Greek *dys*, and *metron* (measure), has long referred to the disordered ability to regulate, judge, and control movements. (The term has subsequently also been extended to cognitive control, dysmetria of thought; Schmahmann 2004.) Dysmetria of the extremities is characterized by end-point tremor, and overshooting the target (hypermetria) or, sometimes, undershooting the target (hypometria). Patients often report that they have difficulty judging distances, the trajectory of intended movements, or the amount of force required for a particular movement. Movements are often slowed, particularly when attempting compound movements (coordinated across more than one joint). Performing movements under visual guidance only minimally improves the outcome (Day et al. 1998).

To test for postural tremor of the upper limbs, the older child is asked to extend the arms in a pronated position. With the arms held out in front of the patient, the examiner quickly displaces the arm downwards and observes for the presence and amplitude of the rebound (overshoot above the starting point of the limb). Finger-to-nose testing consists of bringing the patient's finger to his nose and then touching the examiner's finger which is held steady at a single point at arm's length in front of the patient. This is done a few times to assess both the degree of end-point tremor and the oscillations at the elbow while performing the movement. The characteristic feature of this end-point/intention tremor (or kinetic tremor) is that it increases with greater proximity to the target or the end of the voluntary movement, and the direction of the tremor is generally perpendicular to the direction of the movement. For the finger chase, or mirror test, the examiner holds her finger at arm's length from the patient and moves the finger in the horizontal and vertical directions while the patient follows the finger as rapidly and accurately as possible, pointing to, but not touching, the examiner's finger. This assesses accuracy and the degree of hyper/hypometria of the limb control. In younger children, upper extremity coordination can be tested by having the child reach out for a toy or an interesting object to attract their visual attention. It can also be informative to observe the younger child playing with toys (blocks, plastic bricks, beads and string, trains, cars) or paper and crayons during the elicitation of the history from the family. This approach facilitates the history-taking and allows observation of the requisite motor skills in a non-threatening manner that the child can enjoy. Allowing play also allows the child to relax in the examination setting and helps to build rapport, important for subsequent testing.

Dysdiadochokinesia refers to the inability to perform rapid alternating movements and in the older child can be tested by several approaches. Rapid supination and pronation of the upper extremities is tested as if turning a light bulb, or touching the palm then the dorsum of the hand on the patient's other palm, on the examiner's hand, or on the patient's thigh. Rapid and accurate tapping of the index finger on the crease of the thumb assesses distal extremity fine motor control, as one judges the rate, rhythm, and height of the index finger as it is lifted off the thumb, and accuracy of placement of the index finger on the crease of the thumb. Having the child draw a square shape in the air also allows for the evaluation of difficulty changing direction of movement.

Dysmetria is associated with dysrhythmia (inability to generate normal rhythms), and is assessed by the older child's rapid tapping of the hand on a surface as the examiner listens for disturbance in rate, rhythm, and force. The same approach is applied to the evaluation of the smoothness of rhythm generation in the legs. Dysmetric patients are unable to exert constant pressure on the examiner's hand, as the pressure is irregular and inconstant. Terms such as dysrhythmokinesia for impaired rhythm generation, and isometrataxia for the inability to maintain a constant force have been introduced; these are manifestations of impaired rate, rhythm and force, and the additional Greek-derived terms add little to the evaluation or understanding of the phenomena.

Incoordination of the lower limbs is tested traditionally by the heel-to-shin test. The older child can be asked to place the heel of one foot on the opposite knee, and run the heel down the shin. The examiner assesses the degree of proximal overshoot as the heel is placed on the knee, the presence and persistence of tremor as the heel is brought to the knee, and the accuracy of the movement of the heel down the shin. The degree to which there is slowing, jerking in the plane, or lateral movements is noted as the heel is moved down the shin. The heel-to-shin test should be performed with the patient supine, as gravity tends to minimize the findings. If this is impractical, the patient can be seated in the chair and the heel brought to the knee of the opposite leg which is held passively parallel to the ground by the examiner, thus eliminating the pull of gravity on the heel and allowing the side-to-side dysmetria to manifest more fully. Decomposition of movement is assessed with the draw-a-circle test in which the patient is asked to lie on the back, elevate the leg straight off the bed approximately 30 degrees, and draw an imaginary circle in the air. Edges on the circle indicate a problem with cerebellar control ipsilateral to the lesion. Dysrhythmia of the lower extremities is demonstrated with the patient standing on one leg while holding onto a firm structure such as the examination table, and tapping the heel of the other foot on the ground in as regular and rapid a motion as possible.

The tremor of cerebellar disorders can be dynamic or static. Dynamic end-point tremor occurs with volitional movement, is typically side-to-side, and can be seen in the arms and the legs. The static tremor of cerebellar disorders can be severely disabling, is of large amplitude, relatively slow at about 2–3Hz, and can involve all parts of the body – titubation of the head, neck and trunk, and tremor of the extremities both proximally and/or distally. Rubral tremor that occurs following lesions of the white matter tracts entering or leaving cerebellum, and following lesions of the red nucleus itself, is also generally a coarse 2–3Hz tremor with varying amplitude and frequency. It can involve one or multiple joints, move from one joint to another, change direction from the horizontal to vertical plane, and is frequently rotatory. The examiner may decrease the tremor by placing a hand on the moving joint, only to see the tremor migrate proximally or distally to another joint in the extremity. These cerebellar tremors are important to differentiate from the dynamic intention tremor, as static tremors respond more successfully to medications and even to surgical intervention.

Reflexes

The deep tendon reflexes in patients with pure cerebellar damage are either normal or slightly depressed. Hypotonia in these cases is associated with pendular reflexes. When the knee jerk is tested with the patient seated on the examination table, the leg can swing more than five times, reminiscent of the swing of the pendulum in a grandfather clock. This reflects lack of dampening or check of the leg as seen in the healthy population. Hyporeflexia or areflexia may also arise because of peripheral nerve, dorsal root ganglion or spinal cord pathology that can occur in association with the inherited ataxias. Conversely, hyperreflexia occurs in many of the inherited spinocerebellar ataxias, and in some it can be extremely exaggerated, for example, SCA 7.

Sensation

Many cerebellar ataxic disorders have accompanying sensory involvement by virtue of a peripheral neuropathy, dorsal root ganglionopathy, or posterior column dysfunction. Examining the different modalities of sensation – light touch, vibration, proprioception, pinprick, and temperature – is important to assess with particular attention to the distribution of sensory loss (e.g., distal and symmetric as in peripheral neuropathy). This part of the examination, in the infant or younger child, requires careful observation as descriptive comment by the child may not be possible.

It is also worth noting that primary sensory ataxias, particularly those with marked proprioceptive loss, may mimic aspects of the cerebellar examination. Sensory ataxias are distinguished by the sensory loss on elementary examination, and positive Romberg sign. A useful indicator of sensory ataxia of the upper extremities can be elicited in the older child by having them extend their arms in a fully supinated position. With eyes closed, the patient is asked to touch the nose. In the patient with sensory ataxia, this test is appreciably worse with eyes closed. In contrast, in the cerebellar patient, visual guidance does not improve the tremor that increases as the finger approaches its target.

Ataxia rating scales

The measurement of ataxia is useful for clinical purposes to determine the course of a patient's condition, and also, increasingly, for translational research studies of emerging therapies in the ataxic disorders. The limitations of these semi-objective scales are well recognized, but validation of the different measures provide some confidence that they are useful in the clinical setting. They have not yet been validated in young children, however. Two short versions currently in use are the 40-point Scale for the Assessment and Rating of Ataxia (SARA, Schmitz-Hübsch et al. 2006) and the 30-point Brief Ataxia Rating Scale (BARS, Schmahmann et al. 2009b). Longer versions are the 100-point International Cooperative Ataxia Rating Scale (ICARS, Trouillas et al. 1997) and the 120-point Modified ICARS (Schmahmann et al. 2009b). The BARS, SARA, and MICARS rating scales are in the appendix to this chapter. A scale specifically for Friedreich ataxia (Friedreich Ataxia Rating Scale, FARS; Subramony et al. 2005) includes noncerebellar features as well. General health, disability, and quality-of-life scales are also used in the research setting, although their utility varies in different clinical scenarios. Ataxia rating scales are supplemented by quantitative estimates of motor function including the 9-hole pegboard test, timed assessment of gait (over a distance of 25 to 50 feet according to different scales), and computer keyboard tests. Formal assessments of cerebellar motor control can be achieved in neurophysiological laboratories that assess body sway, postural adjustment, gait patterns, and extremity speed and accuracy as well as response to perturbation.

Acknowledgments

Supported in part by RO1 MH067980, the MINDlink, Birmingham, and Sidney R. Baer Jr. Foundations (JDS).

REFERENCES

Anheim M, Monga B, Fleury M, Charles P, Barbot C, Salih M, et al. (2009) Ataxia with oculomotor apraxia type 2: clinical, biological and genotype/phenotype correlation study of a cohort of 90 patients. Brain 132: 2688–2698.

Bayreuther C, Hieronimus S, Ferrari P, Thomas P, Lebrun C (2008) Auto-immune cerebellar ataxia with anti- GAD antibodies accompanied by de novo late-onset type 1 diabetes mellitus. Diabetes Metab 34: 386–388.

Cohen LE, Tanner DJ, Schaefer HG, Levis WR (1984) Common and uncommon cutaneous findings in patients with ataxia-telangiectasia. J Am Acad Dermatol 10: 431–438.

Coutinho P, Barbot C (June 11, 2002) Ataxia with Oculomotor Apraxia Type 1. In: Pagon RA, Bird TC, Dolan CR, Stephens K, editors. GeneReviews [Internet]. Seattle, WA: University of Washington, Seattle.

Day BL, Thompson PD, Harding AE, Marsden CD (1998) Influence of vision on upper limb reaching movements in patients with cerebellar ataxia. Brain 121: 357–372.

Dunn IF, Agarwalla PK, Papanastassiou AM, Butler WE, Smith ER (2007) Multiple pilocytic astrocytomas of the cerebellum in a 17-year-old patient with neurofibromatosis type I. Childs Nerv Syst 23: 1191–1194.

Ertan G, Arulrajah S, Tekes A, Jordan L, Huisman TA (2009) Cerebellar abnormality in children and young adults with tuberous sclerosis complex: MR and diffusion weighted imaging findings. J. Neuroradiol 37: 231–238.

Fortuna F, Barboni P, Liguori R, Valentino ML, Savini G, Gellera C, et al. (2009) Visual system involvement in patients with Friedreich's ataxia. Brain 132: 116–123.

Fridman C, Hosomi N, Varela MC, Souza AH, Fukai K, Koiffmann CP (2003) Angelman syndrome associated with oculocutaneous albinism due to an intragenic deletion of the P gene. Am J Med Genet A 119A: 180–183.

Frieden IJ, Reese V, Cohen D. PHACE syndrome. (1996) The association of posterior fossa brain malformations, hemangiomas, arterial anomalies, coarctation of the aorta and cardiac defects, and eye abnormalities. Arch Dermatol 132: 307–311.

Holmes G (1907) A form of familial degeneration of the cerebellum. Brain 30: 446–489.

Holmes G (1922) The Croonian Lectures on the clinical symptoms of cerebellar disease and their interpretation. Lecture II. Cerebellum 2007; 6: 148–153.

Krug P, Schleiermacher G, Michon J, Valteau-Couanet D, Brisse H, Peuchmaur M, et al. (2010) Opsoclonus-myoclonus in children associated or not with neuroblastoma. Eur J Paediatr Neurol 14: 400–409.

Levisohn L, Cronin-Golomb A, Schmahmann JD (2000) Neuropsychological consequences of cerebellar tumor resection in children: Cerebellar cognitive affective syndrome in a pediatric population. Brain 123: 1041–1050.

Lionetti E, Francavilla R, Pavone P, Pavone L, Francavilla T, Pulvirenti A, et al. (2010) The neurology of coeliac disease in childhood: what is the evidence? A systematic review and meta-analysis. Dev Med Child Neurol 52: 700–707.

Maria BL, Boltshauser E, Palmer SC, Tran TX (1999) Clinical features and revised diagnostic criteria in Joubert syndrome. J Child Neurol 14: 583–590; discussion 590–591.

Martínez-Granero MA, Hardisson D, Martínez-Bermejo A, Morales C, Gutiérrez-Molina M, Arcas-Martínez J, Pascual-Castroviejo I (1997) [Menkes' disease: anatomo-clinical presentation of a case]. Rev Neurol 25: 465–470.

Metry D, Heyer G, Hess C, Garzon M, Haggstrom A, Frommelt P, et al.; PHACE Syndrome Research Conference (2009) Consensus Statement on Diagnostic Criteria for PHACE Syndrome. Pediatrics 124: 1447–1456.

Oza VS, Wang E, Berenstein A, Waner M, Lefton D, Wells J, Blei F (2008) PHACES association: a neuroradiologic review of 17 patients. AJNR Am J Neuroradiol 29: 807–813.

Pascual-Castroviejo I, Pascual-Pascual SI, Viaño J, Carceller F, Gutierrez-Molina M, Morales C, Frutos-Martinez R (2010) Posterior fossa tumors in children with neurofibromatosis type 1 (NF1). Childs Nerv Syst 26: 1599–1603.

Pollack IF, Polinko P, Albright AL, Towbin R, Fitz C (1995) Mutism and pseudobulbar symptoms after resection of posterior fossa tumors inchildren: incidence and pathophysiology. Neurosurgery 37: 885–893.

Robain O, Aubourg P, Routon MC, Dulac O, Ponsot G (1988) Menkes disease: a Golgi and electron microscopic study of the cerebellar cortex. Clin Neuropathol 7: 47–52.

Rothenberg AB, Berdon WE, D'Angio GJ, Yamashiro DJ, Cowles RA (2009) The association between neuroblastoma and opsoclonus-myoclonus syndrome: a historical review. Pediatr Radiol 39: 723–726.

Schmahmann JD. Disorders of the cerebellum (2004) Ataxia, dysmetria of thought, and the cerebellar cognitive affective syndrome. J Neuropsych Clin Neurosci 16: 367–378.

Schmahmann JD, Gardner RC, MacMore J, Vangel M (2009b) Development of a brief ataxia rating scale (BARS) based on a modified form of the ICARS. Movement Disord 24: 1820–1828.

Schmahmann JD, MacMore J, Vangel M (2009a) Cerebellar stroke without motor deficit: Clinical evidence for motor and non-motor domains within the human cerebellum. Neuroscience 162: 852–861.

Schmitz-Hübsch T, du Montcel ST, Baliko L, Berciano J, Boesch S, Depondt C, et al. (2006) Scale for the assessment and rating of ataxia: development of a new clinical scale. Neurology 66: 1717–1720.

Sévin M, Lesca G, Baumann N, Millat G, Lyon-Caen O, Vanier MT, Sedel F (2007) The adult form of Niemann-Pick disease type C. Brain 130: 120–133.

Smith A, Wiles C, Haan E, McGill J, Wallace G, Dixon J, et al. (1996) Clinical features in 27 patients with Angelman syndrome resulting from DNA deletion. J Med Genet 33: 107–112.

Subramony SH, May W, Lynch D, Gomez C, Fischbeck K, Hallett M, et al. (2005) Measuring Friedreich ataxia: Interrater reliability of a neurologic rating scale. Neurology 64: 1261–1262.

Torregrosa A, Martí-Bonmatí L, Higueras V, Poyatos C, Sanchís A (2000) Klippel-Trenaunay syndrome: frequency of cerebral and cerebellar hemihypertrophy on MRI. Neuroradiology 42: 420–423.

Trouillas P, Takayanagi T, Hallett M, Currier RD, Subramony SH, Wessel K, Bryer A, et al. (1997) International Cooperative Ataxia Rating Scale for pharmacological assessment of the cerebellar syndrome. The Ataxia Neuropharmacology Committee of the World Federation of Neurology. J Neurol Sci 145: 205–211.

Tulinius MH, Oldfors A, Holme E, Larsson NG, Houshmand M, Fahleson P, et al. (1995) Atypical presentation of multisystem disorders in two girls with mitochondrial DNA deletions. Eur J Pediatr 154: 35–42.

Vanier MT (2010) Niemann-Pick disease type C. Orphanet J Rare Dis 5: 16.

Volpe, JJ (2009) Cerebellum of the premature infant: rapidly developing, vulnerable, clinically important. J Child Neurol 24: 1085–1104.

Voogd J, Barmack NH (2006) Oculomotor cerebellum. Prog Brain Res 151: 231–268.

Wells EM, Walsh KS, Khademian ZP, Keating RF, Packer RJ (2008) The cerebellar mutism syndrome and its relation to cerebellar cognitive function and the cerebellar cognitive affective disorder. Dev Disabil Res Rev 14: 221–228.

Yagi T, Shimizu M, Sekine S, Kamio T, Suzuki JI (1981) A new neurotological test for detecting cerebellar dysfunction. Ann N Y Acad Sci 374: 526–531.

Appendix

Brief Ataxia Rating Scale (BARS; 30-point total)

Gait

0: Normal
1: Almost normal naturally, but unable to walk with feet in tandem position
2: Walking without support, but clearly abnormal and irregular
3: Walking without support but with considerable staggering; difficulties in half-turn
4: Walking without support not possible; uses support of the wall for 10-meter test
5: Walking possible only with one cane
6: Walking possible only with two canes or with a stroller
7: Walking possible only with one accompanying person
8: Walking impossible with one accompanying person (2-person assist; wheelchair)

Knee-tibia test (decomposition of movement and intention tremor) (left and right scored)

0: Normal
1: Lowering of heel in continuous axis, but movement is decomposed in several phases, without real jerks, or abnormally slow
2: Lowering jerkily in the axis
3: Lowering jerkily with lateral movements
4: Lowering jerkily with extremely long lateral movements, or test impossible

Finger-to-nose test (decomposition and dysmetria of arm and hand) (left and right scored)

0: Normal
1: Oscillating movement of arm and/or hand without decomposition of the movement
2: Segmented movement in 2 phases and/or moderate dysmetria in reaching nose
3: Segmented movement in more than 2 phases and/or considerable dysmetria in reaching nose
4: Dysmetria preventing the patient from reaching nose

Dysarthria
0: Normal
1: Mild impairment of rate/rhythm/clarity
2: Moderate impairment of rate/rhythm/clarity
3: Severely slow and dysarthric speech
4: Speech absent or unintelligible

Oculomotor abnormalities
0: Normal
1: Slightly slowed pursuit, saccadic intrusions, hypo/hypermetric saccade, nystagmus
2: Prominently slowed pursuit, saccadic intrusions, hypo/hypermetric saccade, nystagmus

---

Scale for the Assessment and Rating of Ataxia (SARA; 40-point total)

---

1) Gait
Proband is asked (1) to walk at a safe distance parallel to a wall including a half-turn (turn around to face the opposite direction of gait) and (2) to walk in tandem (heels to toes) without support.
0: Normal, no difficulties in walking, turning and walking tandem (up to one misstep allowed)
1: Slight difficulties, only visible when walking 10 consecutive steps in tandem
2: Clearly abnormal, tandem walking >10 steps not possible
3: Considerable staggering, difficulties in half-turn, but without support
4: Marked staggering, intermittent support of the wall required
5: Severe staggering, permanent support of one stick or light support by one arm required
6: Walking >10m only with strong support (two special sticks or stroller or accompanying person)
7: Walking <10m only with strong support (two special sticks or stroller or accompanying person)
8: Unable to walk, even supported

2) Stance
Proband is asked to stand (1) in natural position, (2) with feet together in parallel (big toes touching each other) and (3) in tandem (both feet on one line, no space between heel and toe). Proband does not wear shoes, eyes are open. For each condition, three trials are allowed. Best trial is rated.
0: Normal, able to stand in tandem for >10s
1: Able to stand with feet together without sway, but not in tandem for >10s
2: Able to stand with feet together for >10s, but only with sway
3: Able to stand for >10s without support in natural position, but not with feet together
4: Able to stand for >10s in natural position only with intermittent support
5: Able to stand >10s in natural position only with constant support of one arm
6: Unable to stand for >10s even with constant support of one arm

3) Sitting
Proband is asked to sit on an examination bed without support of feet, eyes open and arms outstretched to the front.
0: Normal, no difficulties sitting >10 sec
1: Slight difficulties, intermittent sway
2: Constant sway, but able to sit >10s without support
3: Able to sit for >10s only with intermittent support
4: Unable to sit for >10s without continuous support

4) Speech disturbance
Speech is assessed during normal conversation
0: Normal
1: Suggestion of speech disturbance
2: Impaired speech, but easy to understand
3: Occasional words difficult to understand
4: Many words difficult to understand
5: Only single words understandable
6: Speech unintelligible/anarthria

5) Finger chase (rated separately for each side; score = R+L/2)
Proband sits comfortably. If necessary, support of feet and trunk is allowed. Examiner sits in front of proband and performs 5 consecutive sudden and fast pointing movements in unpredictable directions in a frontal plane, at about 50% of proband's reach. Movements have an amplitude of 30cm and a frequency of 1 movement every 2s. Proband is asked to follow the movements with his index finger, as fast and precisely as possible. Average performance of last 3 movements is rated.
0: No dysmetria
1: Dysmetria, under/overshooting target <5cm
2: Dysmetria, under/overshooting target <15cm
3: Dysmetria, under/overshooting target >15cm
4: Unable to perform 5 pointing movements

6) Nose-finger test (rated separately for each side; score = R+L/2)
Proband sits comfortably. If necessary, support of feet and trunk is allowed. Proband is asked to point repeatedly with his index finger from his nose to examiner's finger which is in front of the proband at about 90% of proband's reach. Movements are performed at moderate speed. Average performance of movements is rated according to the amplitude of the kinetic tremor.

0: No tremor
1: Tremor with an amplitude <2cm
2: Tremor with an amplitude <5cm
3: Tremor with an amplitude >5cm
4: Unable to perform 5 pointing movements

7) Fast alternating hand movements (rated separately for each side; score = R+L/2)
Proband sits comfortably. If necessary, support of feet and trunk is allowed. Proband is asked to perform 10 cycles of repetitive alternation of pro- and supinations of the hand on his/her thigh as fast and as precise as possible. Movement is demonstrated by examiner at a speed of approx. 10 cycles within 7s. Exact times for movement execution have to be taken.
0: Normal, no irregularities (performs <10s)
1: Slightly irregular (performs <10s)
2: Clearly irregular, single movements difficult to distinguish or relevant interruptions, but performs <10s
3: Very irregular, single movements difficult to distinguish or relevant interruptions, performs >10s
4: Unable to complete 10 cycles

8) Heel-shin slide (rated separately for each side; score = R+L/2)
Proband lies on examination bed, without sight of his legs. Proband is asked to lift one leg, point with the heel to the opposite knee, slide down along the shin to the ankle, and lay the leg back on the examination bed. The task is performed 3 times. Slide-down movements should be performed within 1s. If proband slides down without contact to shin in all three trials, rate 4.
0: Normal
1: Slightly abnormal, contact to shin maintained
2: Clearly abnormal, goes off shin up to 3 times during 3 cycles
3: Severely abnormal, goes off shin 4 or more times during 3 cycles
4: Unable to perform the task

Modified International Cooperative Ataxia Rating Scale (MICARS; 120-point total)
(Items 10, 11, 16, 17, 21, 22 and 26 were added to ICARS to constitute MICARS)

I. POSTURE AND GAIT DISTURBANCES (34 points)
1. Walking capacities
0: Normal
1: Almost normal naturally, but unable to walk with feet in tandem position
2: Walking without support, but clearly abnormal and irregular
3: Walking without support but with considerable staggering; difficulties in half-turn
4: Walking with autonomous support no longer possible; the patient uses the episodic support of the wall for 10-meter test
5: Walking only possible with one stick
6: Walking only possible with two special sticks or with a stroller
7: Walking only with accompanying person
8: Walking impossible, even with accompanying person (wheelchair)

2. Gait speed
0: Normal
1: Slightly reduced
2: Markedly reduced
3: Extremely Slow
4: Walking with autonomous support no longer possible

3. Standing capacities, eyes open
0: Normal: able to stand on one foot more than 10 seconds
1: Able to stand with feet together, but no longer able to stand on one foot more than 10 seconds
2: Able to stand with feet together, but no longer able to stand with feet in tandem position
3: No longer able to stand with feet together, but able to stand in natural position without support, with no or moderate sway
4: Standing in natural position without support, with considerable sway and considerable corrections
5: Unable to stand in natural position without strong support of one arm
6: Unable to stand at all, even with strong support of two arms

4. Spread of feet in natural position without support, Eyes open
0: Normal (<10cm)
1: Slightly reduced (>10cm)
2: Clearly enlarged (25cm <spread <35cm)
3: Severely enlarged (>35cm)
4: Standing in natural position impossible

5. Body sway with feet together, eyes open
0: Normal (<10cm)
1: Slight oscillations
2: Moderate oscillations (<10cm at the level of head)
3: Severe oscillations (>10cm at the level of head), threatening the upright position
4: Immediate falling

6. Body sway with feet together, eyes closed
0: Normal (<10cm)
1: Slight oscillations
2: Moderate oscillations (<10cm at the level of head)
3: Severe oscillations (>10cm at the level of head), threatening the upright position
4: Immediate falling

7. Quality of sitting position
0: Normal
1: With slight oscillations of the trunk
2: With moderate oscillations of the trunk and legs
3: With severe dysequilibirium
4: Impossible

II. KINETIC FUNCTIONS (68 points)

8. Knee-tibia test (decomposition of movement and intention tremor)
0: Normal
1: Lowering of heel in continuous axis, but the movement is decomposed in several phases, without real jerks, or abnormally slow
2: Lowering jerkily in the axis
3: Lowering jerkily with lateral movements
4: Lowering jerkily with extremely long lateral movements or test impossible

9. Action tremor in the heel-to-knee test
0: No trouble
1: Tremor stopping immediately when the heel reaches the knee
2: Tremor stopping in less than 10 seconds after reaching the knee
3: Tremor continuing for more than 10 seconds after reaching the knee
4: Uninterrupted tremor or test impossible

10. Decomposition of leg movement
0: Normal
1: Corners or edges on the circle
2: Markedly decomposed attempts at circle

11. Decomposition of leg tapping
0: Normal
1: Slightly slow and irregular
2: Clearly slow and irregular

12. Finger-to-nose test: Decomposition and dysmetria
0: No trouble
1: Oscillating movement without decomposition of the movement
2: Segmented movement in 2 phases and/or moderate dysmetria in reaching nose
3: Segmented movement in more than 2 phases and/or considerable dysmetria in reaching nose
4: Dysmetria preventing the patient from reaching nose

13. Finger-to-nose test: Intention tremor of the finger
0: No trouble
1: Simple swerve of the movement
2: Moderate tremor with estimated amplitude <10cm
3: Tremor with estimated amplitude between 10cm and 40cm
4: Severe tremor with estimated amplitude >40cm

14. Finger-finger test (action, tremor and/or instability)
0: Normal
1: Mild instability
2: Moderate oscillations of finger with estimated amplitude <10cm
3: Considerable oscillations of finger with estimated amplitude between 10 and 40cm
4: Jerky movements >40cm of amplitude

15. Pronation-supination alternating movements
0: Normal
1: Slightly irregular and slowed
2: Clearly irregular, and slowed movement, but without sway of the elbow
3: Extremely irregular, and slowed, but with sway of the elbow
4: Movement completely disorganized or impossible

16. Rebound of the arms
0: None
1: Less than 10cm
2: Greater than 10cm

17. Overshoot of the arms
0: None
1: Less than 10cm
2: Greater than 10cm

18. Drawing of Archimedes spiral on a predrawn pattern
0: Normal
1: Impairment and decomposition, the line quitting the pattern slightly, but without hypermetric swerve
2: Line completely out of the pattern with recrossings and/or hypermetric swerves
3: Major disturbances due to hypermetria and decomposition
4: Drawing completely disorganized or impossible

III. SPEECH DISORDERS (10 points)

19. Dysarthria: Fluency of speech
0: Normal
1: Mild modification of fluency
2: Moderate modification of fluency
3: Considerable slow and dysarthric speech
4: No speech

20. Dysarthria: Clarity of speech
0: Normal
1: Suggestion of slurring
2: Definite slurring, most words understandable
3: Severe slurring, speech not understandable
4: No speech

21. Dysarthria: Alternating syllables (pa-ta-ka)
0: Normal
1: Slightly irregular
2: Clearly irregular, dysrhythmic and slurred

IV. OCULOMOTOR DISORDERS (8 points)

22. Abnormal eye movements at rest
0: Absent
1: Present

23. Gaze-evoked nystagmus
0: Normal
1: Transient
2: Persistent but moderate
3: Persistent and severe

24. Abnormalities of the ocular pursuit
0: Normal
1: Slightly saccadic or slowed
2: Clearly saccadic or slowed

25. Dysmetria of the saccade
0: Absent
1: Bilateral clear overshoot or undershoot of the saccade

26. Saccadic intrusions into vestibulo-ocular reflex cancellation
0: Absent
1: Present

4
Impairments of Cognition and Emotion in Children with Cerebellar Disorders: An Approach to Recognition, Evaluation, and Treatment

Jeremy D. Schmahmann, Annah N. Abrams, and Janet C. Sherman

The clinical neurology of the cerebellum has evolved dramatically in recent years. We recognize the traditional clinical phenomenology of the cerebellar motor syndrome characterized by impairments of gait, extremity coordination, speech and oculomotor control, as discussed in Chapter 3. In addition, however, and of particular relevance to the developing nervous system, is the new field of the cognitive neuroscience of the cerebellum that has implications for diagnosis and management of children with cerebellar disorders. In this chapter we briefly review the evolution of ideas about the functions of the cerebellum, describe the neurobehavioral features that have been reported in pediatric patients with cerebellar diseases, and present an approach to the evaluation and management of these cases.

From movement to thought: Overview of the historic background

Around the time that Flourens (1824) concluded that the cerebellum is a motor control device, and long before this notion became entrenched by experimental work and clinical observations, investigators described individuals with different forms of cerebellar damage, including failure of development (agenesis) and cerebellar atrophy, who demonstrated impairments of intellectual function and emotional or psychiatric disturbances (Schmahmann 1991). Later clinical studies identified a relationship between the cerebellum and personality, aggression and emotion (Heath et al. 1979), and they linked psychosis, schizophrenia in particular, with enlargement of the fourth ventricle, smaller cerebellar vermis, and cerebellar atrophy (Moriguchi 1981; Lippmann et al. 1982). In the middle and later decades of the 20th century, patients with cerebellar cortical atrophy and what was broadly classified as olivopontocerebellar atrophy (OPCA) were found to have cognitive problems. These included impairments in verbal intelligence, visual-spatial abilities, learning and memory, and frontal system functions (Landis et al. 1974; Kish et al. 1988; Bracke-Tolkmitt et al. 1989; Botez-Marquard and Botez 1993). Tests showed deficits in strategy formation (Grafman et al. 1992) and procedural learning (Pascual-Leone et al. 1993).

Experimental studies in animals reveal that electrical potentials are activated in the cerebellum by stimulation of somatosensory, visual, and auditory cortices (Snider and Stowell 1944; Snider and Eldred 1948; Snider 1950); stimulation of deep cerebellar nuclei evokes autonomic responses (Zanchetti and Zoccolini 1954; Martner 1975), grooming, predatory attack, and sham rage (Moruzzi 1947; Reis et al. 1973); and lesions of the cerebellar anterior interpositus nucleus prevent or abolish conditional associative learning tasks (Thompson et al. 1997).

Anatomic tract tracing studies in monkeys show reciprocal connections between association areas in the cerebral cortex concerned with complex cognitive and emotional processing, and the cerebellum (Schmahmann and Pandya 1989, 1997a, 1997b; Schmahmann 1991, 1996; Middleton and Strick 1994; Kelly and Strick 2003). Functional imaging studies in healthy individuals have provided experimental support for the existence of nonmotor functions of the cerebellum. Activation of the cerebellum by cognitive tasks using this approach was first demonstrated in positron emission tomography (PET) studies of language (Petersen et al. 1989; Raichle et al. 1994). Subsequent evaluations showed cerebellar activation in a variety of nonmotor tasks including sensory processing (Gao et al. 1996), appreciation of timed intervals (Jueptner et al. 1995), anticipatory planning and prediction (shifting attention tasks) (Allen et al. 1997), verbal working memory (Desmond et al. 1997), and mental imagery (Ryding et al. 1993). Since these early studies, cerebellar activation has been found consistently on functional magnetic resonance imaging (fMRI) studies of language, working memory, visual-spatial and executive function tasks (see Stoodley and Schmahmann 2010). Moreover, functional connectivity MRI in humans (Krienen and Buckner 2009) has provided evidence in support of anatomic and physiological studies in experimental animals, showing topographic arrangement in the human cerebellum of sensorimotor versus cognitive and emotionally relevant areas (see Chapter 2).

The cerebellar cognitive affective syndrome

In earlier reports of patients with focal cerebellar lesions, language problems were noted to include agrammatism (Silveri et al. 1994), decreased verbal fluency (Molinari et al. 1997), and inability to detect one's own errors in tasks such as the verb-for-noun generation paradigm (Fiez et al. 1992). The importance of the cerebellum for nonmotor function was highlighted by the description and conceptualization of a new clinical

TABLE 4.1
Deficits that characterize the cerebellar cognitive affective syndrome (Schmahmann and Sherman 1998)

1. *Executive function.* Deficient planning, motor or ideational set-shifting, abstract reasoning, working memory and multi-tasking. Decreased verbal fluency, sometimes to the point of telegraphic speech or mutism. Perseverative ideation in thought and/or action.
2. *Spatial cognition.* Visuospatial disintegration with impaired attempts to draw or copy a diagram. Disorganized conceptualization of figures. Impaired visual-spatial memory. Simultanagnosia in some.
3. *Linguistic difficulties.* Anomia, agrammatic speech, abnormal syntactic structure, abnormal prosody.
4. *Changes in affect and personality change.* Aberrant modulation of behavior and personality with posterior lobe lesions that involve midline structures. Flattening or blunting of affect alternates or coexists with disinhibited behaviors such as overfamiliarity, flamboyant and impulsive actions, and humorous but inappropriate and flippant comments. Regressive, childlike behaviors and obsessive-compulsive traits can be observed. See Table 4.3 for the neuropsychiatric domains affected in the CCAS.

   The net effect of these disturbances in cognitive functioning is a general lowering of overall intellectual function.

syndrome, the cerebellar cognitive affective syndrome (CCAS; Schmahmann and Sherman 1998). The CCAS results from lesions of the cerebellar posterior lobe, characterized by clinically relevant deficits in executive function, visual-spatial performance, linguistic processing, and dysregulation of affect (Table 4.1).

In the original report of 20 patients, 18 demonstrated problems with executive functions, including poor working memory (in 11 of 16 tested), motor or ideational set-shifting (in 16 of 19), and perseveration of actions or drawings (in 16 of 20). Verbal fluency was impaired in 18 patients, presenting as telegraphic speech, occasionally so limited as to resemble mutism. Decreased verbal fluency was unrelated to dysarthria. Visuospatial disintegration was found in 19 patients, who were disorganized in their sequential approach to drawing, and the conceptualization of the figures was disorganized. Four patients demonstrated simultanagnosia. Naming was impaired in 13 patients, generally being spared in those with smaller lesions. Six with bilateral acute disease had agrammatic speech, and elements of abnormal syntactic structure were noted in others. Prosody was abnormal in eight patients, with tone of voice characterized by a high-pitched, whining, childish, and hypophonic quality. Mental arithmetic was deficient in 14 patients. Verbal learning and recall were mildly abnormal in 11, and visual learning and recall were impaired in four (of 13 patients in whom this was tested). Ideational apraxia was evident in two individuals.

Difficulty modulating behavior and personality style was a prominent feature of the bedside mental state examination in 15 patients, particularly those with large or bilateral infarcts in the territory of the posterior inferior cerebellar artery (PICA), and in one with surgical excision of the vermis and paravermian structures. Flattening of affect or disinhibition were manifested as overfamiliarity, flamboyant and impulsive actions, and humorous but inappropriate and flippant comments. Behavior was regressive and childlike, and obsessive-compulsive traits were occasionally observed.

Autonomic changes were a central feature in a patient with stroke involving the fastigial nucleus and paravermian cortex. This manifested as spells of hiccupping and coughing, which precipitated bradycardia and syncope.

Neuropsychological testing confirmed the observations from the bedside evaluation (Table 4.2). Deficits were more pronounced and generalized in patients with large, bilateral, or pancerebellar disorders, and particularly in those with acute onset cerebellar disease. Lesions of the posterior lobe were particularly important in the generation of the CCAS; the vermis was consistently involved in patients with pronounced affective presentations; and the anterior lobe seemed to be less involved in the generation of these cognitive and behavioral deficits. Patients with stroke improved over time, although executive function remained abnormal.

The principal features and clinical relevance of the CCAS have been emphasized and elaborated upon in subsequent clinical reports, for example, cerebellar stroke (Exner et al. 2004; Paulus et al. 2004; Yang et al. 2007; Marien et al. 2009; Baillieux et al. 2010), mass lesions (Akil et al. 2006), and superficial siderosis (van Harskamp et al. 2005; Uttner et al. 2009). Neau et al. (2000) reported cerebellar stroke patients with deficits in executive function as revealed by poor performance on phonemic and alternate categorical fluency, naming with and without interference, and a paced auditory serial addition task; and visual-spatial deficits with low scores on the Wechsler Adult Intelligence Scale-Revised Block Design. These deficits are clinically relevant; young adults (ages 18–44) with cerebellar strokes producing impaired working memory, visuospatial skills and cognitive flexibility have delayed return to the workforce because of cognitive limitations, not motor incapacity (Malm et al. 1998).

The understanding of the manifestations of the CCAS continues to evolve, as exemplified by cerebellar patients who report problems with multi-tasking, organizing their thoughts, sustaining their level of concentration and energy, and being somewhat forgetful. One with postinfectious cerebellitis developed impaired judgment, diminished insight, and inability to predict consequences of his actions. An artist with a PICA territory infarct reported loss of creativity that persisted for almost a year, no longer able to experience the flow of visual images that premorbidly characterized his artistic process. Another suffered bilateral cerebellar strokes – one in the left anterior lobe that resulted in left-sided dysmetria, and the other in the right posterior lobe and vermis. His chief complaints were executive impairments, irritability, poor impulse control, and depression.

The cerebellar cognitive affective syndrome in children

The CCAS occurs in children as well as in adults. The impact of cerebellar disorders on cognition and emotion in the pediatric

TABLE 4.2
Neuropsychological findings in the cerebellar cognitive affective syndrome grouped according to major functional category (Schmahmann and Sherman 1998)

Test	Z-score		*p*-value	*n*
	Mean	SD		
Intellectual functioning				
WAIS – Full-scale IQ	−1.0	0.123	0.0002***	13
WAIS – R Verbal IQ	−0.93	0.145	<0.0001***	15
WAIS – R Performance IQ	−1.3	0.127	0.0006***	13
Executive functioning				
Word association	−2.7	1.8	<0.0001***	16
Animal naming	−1.5	0.77	0.0002***	10
Trails A	−1.2	1.3	0.0067**	12
Trails B	−0.89	0.76	0.0030**	11
Wisconsin Card Sorting Test	−0.83	1.7	0.2205	8
Reasoning and abstraction				
Similarities	−0.42	0.99	0.1141	16
Comprehension	−0.79	0.67	0.0120*	8
Picture completion	−0.77	0.98	0.0150*	13
Arithmetic	−0.86	1.1	0.0112*	13
Picture arrangement	−1.4	0.74	<0.0001***	14
Visuospatial/visual construction				
Rey complex figure: copy	−5.9	3.2	0.0002***	13
WAIS – R Block Design	−1.2	0.90	0.0006***	12
WAIS – R Object Assembly	−0.81	0.84	0.0431*	7
Hooper Visual Orientation	−0.42	0.89	0.3038	6
Language				
Boston Naming Test BNT	−1.4	1.4	0.0047**	13
Peabody Picture Vocab.	−0.40	1.4	0.6097	4
WAIS – R Vocabulary	−0.13	1.3	0.7448	10
WAIS – R Information	−0.51	0.93	0.0501	15
Attention and orientation				
Digit span – forward	−0.51	1.3	0.1501	15
Digit span – backward	−0.61	1.2	0.0644	15
Tapping span – forward	−0.78	1.0	0.0844	7
Tapping span – backward	−0.85	0.84	0.0571	7
Digit symbol	−1.3	0.67	0.0004***	9
Stroop	0.07	0.95	0.8769	4
Memory WMS-R				
Logical memory I	−0.40	1.1	0.1756	14
Logical memory II	−0.42	0.89	0.1046	14
Visual reproduction I	−1.1	1.1	0.0038**	12
Visual reproduction II	−1.4	0.84	0.0001***	12
Rey complex figure: memory	−1.7	0.76	0.0012**	7

n = number of patients who received each test. *** $P < 0.001$; ** $P < 0.01$: * $P < 0.05$. WAIS, Wechsler Adult Intellegence Scale-Revised; WMS-R, Wechsler Memory Scale Revised.

population is now increasingly recognized, and has important clinical implications. Central nervous system tumors disproportionately affect posterior fossa structures in childhood, providing an imperative to better understand these children and define the neuropsychological and neurobehavioral consequences of these tumors on cognitive and neurobehavioral profiles. The study of Levisohn et al. (2000) first addressed this question in children who had undergone resection of cerebellar tumors but who had not received radiation therapy or methotrexate, which can adversely impact cognitive outcome. The cohort consisted of 19 children, ages 3–14, with medulloblastoma, astrocytoma, and ependymoma. Problems were noted with attention and executive function as evidenced by deficits in digit span (57% of the 14 tested), sequencing, and planning. Establishing and maintaining set was hampered in some cases by perseveration. Deficits in expressive language, present in 58% of the cohort, were characterized by brief responses, lack of elaboration, reluctance to engage in conversation, long response latencies, and word finding difficulties. Several children exhibited difficulties with language initiation and word finding difficulties even in the context of average scores on verbal tests. Deficits in confrontation naming were ameliorated with phonemic cues.

Many demonstrated difficulty with initiation of responses and with problem-solving strategies. Visual-spatial difficulties were present in 37% and were characterized by impairments in the planning and organizational aspects of tasks. Verbal memory was impaired in 33% of 15 children tested, particularly for unstructured recall of information, being able to recall only a few details from stories two paragraphs long. Story retrieval improved with multiple-choice prompts. It appeared that there was failure to organize verbal or visual-spatial material for encoding and that this impacted on retrieval of the information. The affective component of the CCAS described in the adult population was also noted in this study of children. Impaired regulation of affect was particularly evident when the damage to the cerebellum included the vermis. This manifested as irritability, impulsivity, disinhibition, and lability of affect with poor attentional and behavioral modulation.

Impaired executive functions have been reported in subsequent studies of children with cerebellar tumors, including impaired planning, sequencing, mental flexibility and hypothesis generation and testing, visual-spatial function, expressive language, and verbal memory (Karatekin et al. 2000; Grill et al. 2004; Turkel et al. 2004; Berger et al. 2005; Ronning et al. 2005; Vaquero et al. 2008). In the series of Scott et al. (2001) children with right cerebellar hemisphere tumors experienced a subsequent plateau in verbal and/or literacy skills, whereas those with left cerebellar damage were associated with delayed or impaired spatial skills. Similar phenomena were observed by Riva and Giorgi (2000) in 26 children following resection of cerebellar tumors. They noted impairments in verbal intelligence, auditory sequential memory, and language following right-sided tumors; and deficient nonverbal tasks including spatial and visual sequential memory and impaired prosody after left cerebellar hemisphere tumors. This laterality such that language deficits more frequently occur following right cerebellar lesions whereas visual-spatial impairments tend to occur with left cerebellar damage has been reported in other studies (Gottwald et al. 2004; Gross-Tsur et al. 2006; Hokkanen et al. 2006) and is consistent with the crossed connections with the cerebral cortex, and with the findings of domain-specific asymmetry in functional imaging studies of healthy individuals (Stoodley and Schmahmann 2009). This lateralized verbal-visual dichotomy appears to be less definitive following cerebellar lesions than it is following cerebral lesions, however.

As in adults, the CCAS occurs in children in the setting of stroke. In a recent study (Kossorotoff et al. 2010), five boys ages 3–14 with cerebellar infarcts were noted to have mood disturbances with a few days of outbursts of laughter and/or crying, and alternating agitation or prostration. The children experienced persistent cognitive deficits including mutism followed by anomia, and impairments in comprehension, planning, visual-spatial organization, and attention. The cognitive difficulties improved slowly and incompletely despite intensive rehabilitation, and were more disabling than the motor symptoms. This is a remarkable set of observations: the laughing and crying bear a resemblance to the phenomenon of forced laughing (*fou rire prodromique*) that occurs in basis pontine stroke (Assal et al. 2000), and the pathological laughing and crying that occurs in adults in the cerebellar form of multiple system atrophy (Parvizi et al. 2007). The cognitive more than motor residual deficits recapitulates the conclusion from an earlier study of cerebellar stroke in adults (Malm et al. 1998), and the constellation of deficits as a whole is entirely consistent with the syndrome as it manifests in adults.

Posterior fossa syndrome

More than half the children in Levisohn et al. (2000) with extensive damage to the vermis experienced the posterior fossa syndrome (PFS; Pollack et al. 1995; Sadeh and Cohen 2001). This phenomenon was described initially as pseudobulbar palsy (Wisoff and Epstein 1984); mutism without behavioral impairment (Rekate et al. 1985; Catsman-Berrevoets et al. 1992), cerebellar speech syndrome (Kingma et al. 1994); cerebellar mutism (Dietze and Mickle 1990), and cerebellar mutism and subsequent dysarthria (van Dongen et al. 1994). After a 1- to 2-day latent period of normal behavior following surgery, children developed mutism, with hypotonia and buccal and lingual apraxia. Recovery of speech ensued over many months, together with slowly improving dysarthria. The syndrome was notable also for behavioral changes including regressive personality, apathy, and poverty of spontaneous movement. Emotional lability was marked, with rapid fluctuation of emotional expression gravitating between irritability with inconsolable crying and agitation, to giggling and easy distractibility.

The PFS generally follows a surgical approach to tumor resection through the cerebellar vermis, occurring in 15–50% of patients according to different studies. The relationship between PFS and CCAS in the postoperative population has been specifically considered (Wells et al. 2008), although it should be noted that PFS, the hallmark feature of which is postoperative mutism following a delay, is not a prerequisite for the development of the intellectual and emotional deficits that comprise the CCAS, either acutely (as in stroke or tumor patients) or more chronically as occurs in destructive or degenerative lesions of the cerebellum. Further, the pediatric cerebellar stroke study of Kossorotoff et al. (2010) makes it clear that cerebellar surgery is not required to develop mutism, an observation that was evident in the original CCAS study (Schmahmann and Sherman 1998) in which the young patients with postinfectious cerebellitis developed diminished verbal fluency so severe as to approach mutism.

The affective component of the CCAS: The nature of the emotional deficits

Emotional dysregulation can be a striking aspect of the CCAS. A number of studies report that behavioral aberrations in children following cerebellar tumor resection include disinhibition, impulsivity, and irritability (Maryniak and Roszkowski 2005), dysphoria, inattention and irritability (Turkel et al. 2004), anxiety and aggression (Richter et al. 2005), hyperspontaneous, disinhibited behavior, and hypospontaneous, flattened affect (Aarsen et al. 2004). In addition to irritability and decreased ability to tolerate the company of others, the surgically induced vermal lesions that lead to postsurgical mutism and agrammatism also result in autistic features such as avoidance of physical and eye contact, complex repetitive and rhythmic rocking movements, stereotyped linguistic utterances, and lack of empathy (Riva and Giorgi 2000). Attention-deficit disorder, addiction, anorexia, uncontrolled temper tantrums, and phobias have also been described in the post-tumor resection pediatric population (Steinlin et al. 2003).

The immune-mediated opsoclonus-myoclonus syndrome (OMS) occurs in children (Turkel et al. 2006) as a postinfectious, or more commonly, as a paraneoplastic phenomenon in the setting of neuroblastoma (Gorman 2010), and it also affects adults as a paraneoplastic phenomenon (Cher et al. 1995; Ohara et al. 2007). In children OMS produces a psychiatric constellation of mood changes and inconsolable irritability with lability, aggression, and night terrors. Dysphoric mood, disinhibition and poor affect regulation, disruptive behaviors and temper tantrums occur together with the cognitive and language impairments typically seen in the CCAS. The emotional deficits in children, like the post-tumor cognitive components of the CCAS, may be persistent and clinically important (e.g., Baillieux et al. 2006; Schmahmann et al. 2007; Gorman 2010). Further, these behavioral changes have a predilection for lesions involving the vermis and paravermian regions. This is consistent with earlier clinical studies (Heath et al. 1979) and electrophysiological investigations in animals (Heath and Harper 1974) and humans (Nashold and Slaughter 1969) that led to the notion of the cerebellum as an emotional pacemaker (Heath 1977), and contemporary evidence also implicates the cerebellar vermis and fastigial nucleus as the limbic cerebellum (Schmahmann 1991, 2000, 2004).

The pediatric literature has started to explore the neuropsychiatric complications of cerebellar surgery in children. In a prospective study of children undergoing cerebellar surgery Catsman-Berrevoets and Aarsen (2010) describe the neurobehavioral deficits seen in children with PFS. In addition to mutism, most patients demonstrated irritability, whining and severe apathy, and one-third manifested autistic behaviors. In addition a wide array of behavioral abnormalities included aggression, forced crying and laughing, and compulsive presleep disorder. A few children demonstrated 'very good behavior', in contrast to their premorbid functioning. Other studies with a focus on the acute mood symptoms presenting in children with posterior fossa lesions note irritability, crying, inconsolability, withdrawn and apathetic behavior, agitation, tantrums and change in affect with lability, flatness and sadness in addition to dysphoria and distress (Turkel et al. 2004).

Cerebellar neuropsychiatry

In our continuing observations of adults and children with cerebellar lesions we have noted altered regulation of mood and personality, psychotic thinking, and behaviors that meet criteria for diagnoses of attention-deficit hyperactivity disorder, obsessive-compulsive disorder, depression, bipolar disorder, disorders on the autism spectrum, anxiety, panic, and often, atypical psychosis. Other features include a lack of initiation, apathy, and irritability. We have conceptualized these behaviors as either excessive or diminished responses to the external or internal environment. The exaggerated, positive, released, or hypermetric responses may be regarded as cognitive overshoot (Schmahmann 1998) analogous to the overshoot in the motor domain resulting from cerebellar lesions. The diminished, negative, restricted or hypometric responses may be likened to hypotonia (Holmes 1917), or to hypometric movements (undershoot) in the motor system following cerebellar lesions. Further, we conceptualize these manifestations as falling into five neuropsychiatric domains – attentional control, emotional control, social skill set, autism spectrum disorders, and psychosis spectrum disorders (Schmahmann et al. 2007) (Table 4.3). Certain manifestations, such as the social skill set negative symptoms, are reminiscent of observations regarding the cerebellar role in theory of mind studies (Brunet et al. 2000; Calarge et al. 2003), providing a clinical underpinning to this observation from experimental psychology. Some patients with acquired cerebellar lesions develop panic disorder, perhaps reflecting overshoot of anticipatory fear (Weilburg et al. 1987) resulting from cerebellar-induced emotional dyscontrol.

Neuropsychiatric features of the CCAS can be prominent in children as young as 2 years of age, presenting with impulsivity, lability, agitation, and aggression following surgery for a posterior fossa or cerebellar tumor. This is illustrated by the descriptions of the following representative cases.

Case 1

A girl aged 2 years 9 months presented to our clinic following resection of a posterior fossa ependymoma. She developed dysarthria a few days postoperatively and was ataxic, but most distressing to her parents and interfering with her care were the behavioral changes that occurred. She exhibited aggressive behavior with kicking and pulling at her intravenous lines, as well as a piercing screaming and high-pitched whining. She required multiple staff to keep her safe, and she was unable to comply with care needs in order to receive her radiation therapy. Low-dose risperidone was started twice daily and continued for the duration of her radiation therapy. Her mood and behavior dramatically improved. She was able to participate safely in treatment as well as in speech and physical therapy. The risperidone was discontinued after the completion of her radiation therapy and her mood and behavior symptoms did not reemerge. On follow-up over the past 3 years, she presents as a well-behaved and engaging child who is attending school full time and has completed kindergarten. Her behavioral issues have resolved and her speech is fluent. She continues to have some difficulty with balance and participates in physical and occupational therapy.

TABLE 4.3
Neuropsychiatric symptoms in patients with cerebellar disorders, arranged according to major domains, each with positive and negative symptoms

	Positive (exaggerated) symptoms	Negative (diminished) symptoms
Attentional control	Inattentiveness Distractibility Hyperactivity Compulsive and ritualistic behaviors	Ruminativeness Perseveration Difficulty shifting focus of attention Obsessional thoughts
Emotional control	Impulsiveness, disinhibition Lability, unpredictability Incongruous feelings, pathologic laughing/crying Anxiety, agitation, panic	Anergy, anhedonia Sadness, hopelessness Dysphoria Depression
Autism spectrum	Stereotypical behaviors Self-stimulation behaviors	Avoidant behaviors, tactile defensiveness Easy sensory overload
Psychosis spectrum	Illogical thought Paranoia Hallucinations	Lack of empathy Muted affect, emotional blunting Apathy
Social skill set	Anger, aggression Irritability Overly territorial Oppositional behavior	Passivity, immaturity, childishness Difficulty with social cues and interactions Unawareness of social boundaries Overly gullible and trusting

Case 2

A 9-year-old boy presented after gross total resection of a medulloblastoma. He was mute and had severe ataxia. During the first 2 weeks postoperatively, he exhibited severe behavioral challenges including agitation, mood lability, and irritability. Initially his mood symptoms were attributed to therapy with dexamethasone; however, with the discontinuation of dexamethasone these symptoms continued unabated. His parents did not want to start a standing medication for the behavior and preferred the use of benzodiazepines on an as-needed basis. Lorazepam 0.5mg was given on an as-needed basis with good benefit. His irritability and agitation calmed after each dose of lorazepam. Over time his behavior improved significantly and the lorazepam was discontinued. He slowly regained his speech; however, he remained ataxic. Unfortunately his tumor recurred and he died 22 months after initial surgery.

Case 3

A 10-year-old boy presented after gross total resection of a medulloblastoma. He was mute, ataxic, and disinhibited with labile mood, irritability, and aggression. Some of his behavior was attributed to pain and initially he was given intravenous morphine, but the mood symptoms persisted. Atypical antipsychotics were offered, but his parents refused and he was given lorazepam on an as-needed basis. Although this was helpful, he remained irritable and labile for about 1 month post-surgery before returning to baseline. He regained some speech although it remained dysarthric and his balance improved to the point that he could ambulate with a walker. Over time, his speech and behavior have improved, but not to premorbid functioning levels, and his balance remains challenging.

Over the years, a number of parents in our clinic have confided that their child's behavioral changes following surgery have been the most difficult aspect of their treatment for a brain tumor. In particular they note that their child is no longer the person they knew and feel unable to understand and manage their child's situation. As one teenage boy who recovered from PFS over the course of a few months following surgery shared: 'I felt locked in. I knew what I wanted to say, but couldn't say it. And now that I can speak and my mood is better, I know that the person you initially met wasn't me.'

Little has been written about the clinical management of the neuropsychiatric symptoms in this patient population. One retrospective study found that carbamazepine was helpful for decreasing the marked dysphoria (Turkel et al. 2004). The Children's Oncology Group is currently enrolling children with cerebellar mutism syndrome in a study that uses risperidone with the initial goal of improving expressive language and a secondary goal of improving receptive language and mood and behavior symptoms. We have found risperidone to be helpful in managing the acute mood symptoms seen in children with the CCAS. Benzodiazepines have been used as well, but may lead to sedation, which can interfere with a child's ability to participate in rehabilitation therapies critical to their recovery.

The deficits in intellect and emotion that characterize the CCAS and that accompany the mutism of PFS were initially thought to be transient. More recent reports indicate that significant psychological sequelae persist in these children, and have a significant impact on overall level of function. Children who developed PFS following surgery for medulloblastoma were at increased risk 7–21 months following surgery for withdrawn behavior, internalizing and social problems as well as obsessive-compulsive behaviors compared to children who had the same diagnosis and treatment, but no PFS postoperatively (Wolff et al. 2007). This study exemplifies the growing need to be aware of the neuropsychiatric manifestations that may develop following resection of cerebellar tumors, and that there are medications available to treat them.

In a study of the protracted effects of postoperative cerebellar mutism, 22 children who had surgical resection of cerebellar embryonal tumors and who developed mutism were compared at 1-year follow-up with matched controls whose treatment for these tumors was similar but who did not develop cerebellar mutism (Palmer et al. 2010). On the neuropsychological evaluation performed 1 year after the completion of treatment, the patients who had experienced mutism scored significantly lower on tests of processing speed, attention, working memory, executive processes, cognitive efficiency, reading, spelling, and math. Thus, while the mutism may improve, the cognitive difficulties can persist.

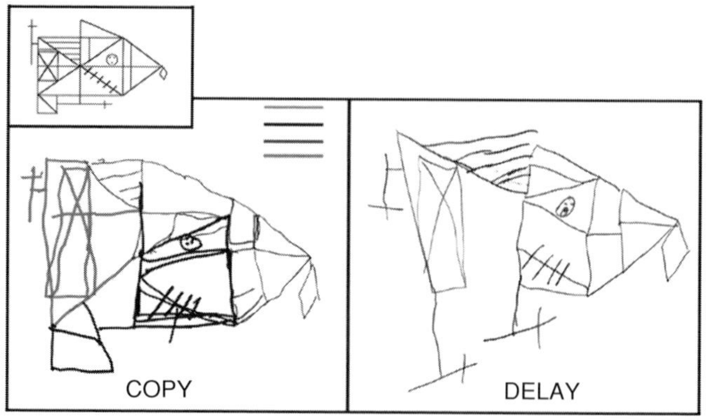

Fig. 4.1. Copy and 5-minute delayed recall of the Rey-Osterrieth figure by a 15-year-old boy with cerebellar agenesis. (See color plate 17).

Cerebellar lesions impair cognition in the developing brain

The developing nervous system appears to require an intact cerebellum for normal intellectual and social/emotional function as well as for motor skill. The cerebellum has a protracted developmental trajectory, reaching its peak volume later than the cerebrum. Phylogenetically more recent cerebellar regions (the lateral hemispheres engaged in cognitive processing) mature particularly late (Tiemeier et al. 2010). This renders the cerebellum vulnerable to environmental influences, and is clinically relevant in infants born pre-term, as the rapid rate of growth of the cerebellum during late gestation is impeded by the pre-term birth (Limperopoulos et al. 2005a). Adolescents who had been born very preterm (<33 weeks' gestation) have reduced cerebellar volumes, and deficits in executive, visual-spatial and language skills including impaired reading (Allin et al. 2001). With the ability to successfully deliver infants at earlier gestational age, the number of children with these problems is likely to increase.

Malformations, agenesis, and hypoplasia of the cerebellum are associated with a range of motor, linguistic, intellectual, and emotional manifestations (Chheda et al. 2002; Richter et al. 2005; Gross-Tsur et al. 2006; Tavano et al. 2007). Gardner and others (2001) reported delayed milestones, mild motor impairments, and intellectual disability in three patients with varying degrees of cerebellar agenesis. Chheda et al. (2002) found that near-complete or partial cerebellar agenesis in 6 children was accompanied by behavioral and motor deficits. The severity and range of the motor, cognitive, and psychiatric impairments were greater in those with more pronounced agenesis. The children presented with gross and fine motor delay, oral motor apraxia, impaired saccades and vestibulo-ocular reflex cancellation, clumsiness, and mild ataxia. Behavioral features included autistic-like stereotypical performance, obsessive rituals, and difficulty understanding social cues. Tactile defensiveness (avoidance of, and adverse reaction to touch), was a prominent feature in four children. Executive impairments included perseveration, disinhibition, and poor abstract reasoning, working memory and verbal fluency. Spatial cognition was impaired for perceptual organization, visual-spatial copying, and recall (Fig. 4.1). Some children presented with expressive language delay as the principal manifestation, in two instances so severe as to require instruction in sign language. Impaired prosody was evident in all cases, and over-regularization of past tense verbs was noted. In longitudinal follow-up, extensive rehabilitation enhanced motor, linguistic, and cognitive performance.

Children with cerebellar hypoplasia and nonprogressive cerebellar ataxia struggle with cognitive and emotional deficits conforming to the description of the CCAS (Steinlin et al. 1998, 1999). The IQ is decreased in these cases, with decreased alertness and sustained attention, and marked difficulties with visuoconstructive tasks and visual perception. Further, autistic features and speech delay, together with ataxia, hypotonia, and ocular signs, correctly predict 86% of children with cerebellar hypoplasia (Wassmer et al. 2003).

As discussed elsewhere in this volume, children with malformations of the cerebellum may have cognitive and emotional deficits in addition to the motor disorders, as seen in rhombencephalosynapsis, Joubert syndrome, some cases of Dandy-Walker syndrome, and Chiari malformations, among others. Many of these congenital malformations of the cerebellum are accompanied by cerebral lesions that rightly may be regarded as the proximate cause of the intellectual limitations. The instances of pure cerebellar dysfunction associated with the CCAS (e.g., cerebellar agenesis, stroke, hemorrhage, tumor) raise the possibility that patients with complex malformation syndromes may be experiencing a cognitive double-hit arising from the combination of impaired cerebral as well as cerebellar function. Some patients present the conundrum of a dysmorphic-appearing cerebellum on brain imaging but without accompanying overt motor or cognitive manifestations, as exemplified by patients with mega cisterna magna in whom the cerebellum is small, but who are not clinically affected. Further study of these cases is warranted.

The recognition that cerebellum appears to have a trophic influence on the development of interconnected brain systems subserving higher order function is of great interest and it also has practical implications for diagnosis and management. Even at the level of gross morphology, early damage to cerebellar hemispheres results in volume loss in the contralateral cerebral hemisphere (Dow and Moruzzi 1958; Limperopoulos et al. 2005b), a phenomenon that harks back to the early descriptions by Gudden and von Monakow of sustaining projections (see Schmahmann and Pandya 2006), and which appears to be clinically significant.

The cerebellum in psychiatric disease

It is worth emphasizing that the neuropsychiatric manifestations of cerebellar disease are not always accompanied by overt cerebellar motor dysfunction. Reports in the 1800s noted deviant and aberrant behaviors in individuals with cerebellar anomalies (Schmahmann 1991). Later clinical observers (Cooper et al. 1978; Heath et al. 1979) noted a relationship between the cerebellum and personality, aggression, and emotion, suggesting a causal link between cerebellar structural abnormalities and psychosis. The connections of the cerebellum with brain circuits implicated in psychiatric illness, and notably in early infantile autism and schizophrenia, are particularly important in this regard (Watson 1978; Frick 1982; Snider 1982; Schmahmann 1991, 2000, 2001).

Early damage to the cerebellar vermis is particularly relevant for the later emergence of neuropsychiatric phenomena. Vermal regions are among the brain areas showing structural differences in autism spectrum disorders (Courchesne et al. 1988; Bauman and Kemper 2005; Penn 2006); preterm infants with cerebellar hemorrhage in the vermis have pervasive developmental disorder and diagnostic scores on autism screening questionnaires (Limperopoulos et al. 2007); the vermis has been implicated in psychoneurotic symptoms following early childhood trauma, and in addictive behaviors that underlie substance abuse (Anderson et al. 2002, 2006); and morphometric studies reveal reduced size of the posterior vermis (lobules VIII–X) in attention-deficit hyperactivity disorder (Berquin et al. 1998; Mostofsky et al. 1998; Castellanos et al. 2001). Surgically induced vermal lesions in children with tumors are associated with a range of neurobehavioral abnormalities including autistic features such as avoidance of physical and eye contact, complex repetitive and rhythmic rocking movements, stereotyped linguistic utterances, and lack of empathy (Levisohn et al. 2000; Riva and Giorgi 2000).

Individuals with early infantile autism, once classified as juvenile schizophrenia, have enlarged fourth ventricles, loss of Purkinje cells in the lateral and inferior cerebellar cortex, and abnormal or reduced numbers of neurons in the deep cerebellar nuclei (Williams et al. 1980; Bauman and Kemper 1985; Ritvo et al. 1986; Kemper and Bauman 1998). Vermal (Courchesne et al. 1988) and hemispheric atrophy (Murakami et al. 1989) are evident on some MRI studies of individuals with autism, although these findings remain controversial (Rapin 1999). Pathological findings are present in other brain regions in autism, particularly in the limbic system, and thus it remains to be established which anatomic-pathological features are most closely associated with the autistic features, and whether these pathological findings cause the behavioral aberrations. The finding of autistic behaviors in more than 40% of preterm children who suffered prenatal cerebellar hemorrhage (Limperopoulos et al. 2007) provides support for a causal link between cerebellar damage and autistic manifestations.

There is now also a sizeable literature examining structural and functional imaging observations in cerebellum in schizophrenia, depression, bipolar disorder, panic and obsessive-compulsive disorder (see Konarski et al. 2005; Hoppenbrouwers et al. 2008; Picard et al. 2008; Wolf et al. 2009). These observations build upon early reports suggesting that the vermis and fastigial nucleus in patients and monkeys play a role in emotion, aggression, and psychosis (Snider 1950; Reis et al. 1973; Heath 1977; Berman et al. 1978; Cooper et al. 1978). The definition of the five domains of neuropsychiatric impairments arising from lesions of cerebellum – attentional control, emotional control, social skill set, autism spectrum disorders, and psychosis spectrum disorders – provides a clinical framework within which to consider the role of the cerebellum in psychiatric illness. The implications of a cerebellar role in the pathophysiology of mental illness are far-reaching, and include new approaches to treatment.

Cognition in ataxic disorders

The recognition of the CCAS in patients with focal lesions of the cerebellum has led to a greater appreciation of the higher order deficits in patients with neurodegenerative ataxia. It is important to recognize these impairments in patients with cerebellar ataxia in order to treat clinical symptoms and enhance quality of life. From the perspective of defining the role of the cerebellum in nonmotor function, however, it is prudent to be cautious when drawing conclusions in these disorders, because the neuropathology frequently extends beyond the cerebellum into the brainstem, basal ganglia, thalamus, and sometimes, the cerebral cortex.

There is some degree of cognitive change at different stages in most of the spinocerebellar ataxias (SCAs) (Geschwind 1999). Impaired executive functions, deficits in verbal short-term memory, and mild generalized cognitive impairment (Burk et al. 2001) have been documented in SCA 1 (CAG repeat on chromosome 6). Patients with SCA 2 (triplet repeat on chromosome 12) may develop poor memory, concentration problems, impairments of conceptual reasoning, and frontal-executive dysfunction on tests of verbal fluency and the Luria test of motor set switching, as well as emotional instability and impulsivity (Gambardella et al. 1998; Storey et al. 1999). Individuals with Machado-Joseph disease or SCA 3 (CAG expansion on chromosome 14) demonstrate deficits in visual and verbal attention, verbal fluency, and planning and strategy tests such as the Wisconsin Card Sort Test (Zawacki et al. 2002). Cognitive deficits are noted in SCA 6 (CAG expansion in the *CACNA1A* [alpha-1A-(P/Q-type) voltage-dependent Ca channel] gene on chromosome 19p13) in which the pathology is predominantly in the cerebellar cortex with degeneration of Purkinje cells and, to a lesser degree, the granule cells, deep cerebellar nuclei, and brainstem (Sasaki et al. 1998; Ishikawa et al. 1999; Gierga et al. 2009). Neuropsychological investigations reveal significant impairments in executive function involving skills of cognitive flexibility, inhibition of response, verbal reasoning, and abstraction (Cooper et al. 2010) as well as verbal fluency, and immediate visual memory (Suenaga et al. 2008). In one large family with SCA 7 (Horton et al. 2011), office-based mental state testing revealed impairments in executive functions including working memory (reverse digit span, serial 7 subtraction) and abstract reasoning (Similarities Test), deficits in both semantic and phonemic fluency, and mild impairments in free recall on tests of episodic memory. Tests of emotion attribution have been reported to be abnormal also in SCA 7 (Sokolovsky et al. 2010). In SCA 8, consistent features include deficits in attention, information processing, and executive functions (Lilja et al. 2005). In SCA 13 (chromosome 19), moderate mental retardation (UK: learning disability) (IQ 62–76) occurs in association with a progressive childhood-onset cerebellar motor syndrome and developmental delay (Herman-Bert et al. 2000). Dementia is part of the diagnosis in SCA 17 with a CAG repeat on chromosome 6 (dementia, psychosis, dystonia, chorea, and seizures; Koide et al. 1999; Nakamura et al. 2001), and it may resemble the phenotype of Huntington disease (Mariotti et al. 2007). Dementia also occurs in SCA 21 (ataxia with hyporeflexia, akinesia, rigidity, and cognitive impairment in French kindred, with linkage to chromosome 7; Devos et al. 2001).

In Friedreich ataxia much of the pathology is located outside the cerebellum and the extent of neuropsychological impairment has been studied with varying results. Some have reported relative preservation of the cognitive skill set (White et al. 2000), while others describe impairments on tests of visual-perceptual and visual-constructive abilities, slowed information processing speed, decreased sustained attention, reduced verbal span, deficits in letter fluency, and impaired acquisition and consolidation of verbal information (Wollmann et al. 2002). In the patients of Mantovan et al. (2006) IQ was preserved, but patients demonstrated concrete thinking leading to impaired concept formation, executive deficits (reduced digit span, difficulties with mental control including complex planning and sequencing), reduced verbal span and deficits in verbal fluency, and poor visuospatial reasoning and memory. Increased irritability, poor impulsive control, or blunting of affect was also noted.

Mechanisms of the cerebellar contribution to cognition and emotion

Earlier investigators regarded the cerebellum as the great modulator of neurological function (Snider 1950; Heath 1977). The fundamental mechanism by which the cerebellum modulates movement, intellect and emotion remains a matter of debate (e.g., Bower 1997; Ito 1997; Ivry 1997; Molinari et al. 2008). Our dysmetria of thought theory (Schmahmann 1991, 1996, 2000; Schmahmann and Sherman 1998; Schmahmann and Pandya 2008) is based upon two complementary facts of anatomic organization. First, cerebellar histology is essentially uniform throughout. This enables a computation we have termed the Universal Cerebellar Transform (UCT), allowing the cerebellum to modulate behavior, acting as an oscillation dampener maintaining function in equilibrium around a homeostatic baseline and smoothing out performance, modifying it according to context. It does so automatically, and without conscious awareness. Second, the specificity of anatomical connections between cerebellum and spinal cord, brainstem, and cerebral hemispheres facilitates functional topography within the cerebellum. Thus, in the same way that the cerebellum regulates the rate, force, rhythm, and accuracy in the motor domain, so does it regulate the speed, capacity, consistency, and appropriateness of cognitive and emotional processes. If the UCT is the essential functional contribution that cerebellum makes to the distributed neural system, then by corollary, there should be a Universal Cerebellar Impairment – namely, dysmetria (the Greek term originally used to designate motor incoordination). When the motor cerebellum is damaged the dysmetria manifests as ataxia of extremity movements, eye movements, speech and equilibrium. When the lesion is in the cognitive (posterior) cerebellum, the result is dysmetria of thought, or cognitive dysmetria, which manifests as the various components of the CCAS. When the limbic (midline) cerebellum is damaged, the dysmetria of emotional control manifests predominantly as neuropsychiatric impairments. Studies employing the contemporary methods of cognitive neuroscience are under way in a number of centers to attempt to define whether the UCT indeed exists, and the precise nature of the computation that defines the transform (Miall et al. 1993; Ivry 1997; Thach 1997; Nixon and Passingham 2001; Doyon et al. 2002; Dreher and Grafman 2002; Molinari et al. 2002). The notion embodied in the dysmetria of thought theory, namely, that the cerebellum performs its unique computations in a topographically precise manner on diverse streams of information relating to almost all aspects of behavior, has brought to life the ideas and contributions of earlier investigators such as Snider (1950), Dow (1974), and Heath (1977) and opened the way to a new era of cognitive neuroscience.

Approach to clinical evaluation

The mental state examination at the bedside forms part of the neurological examination, as discussed in Chapter 3. The nature of the testing is dictated by the age of the child. As is evident from the pattern of deficits in the CCAS, in the older child who can cooperate, particular attention should be paid to working memory (reverse digit span, mental arithmetic), verbal fluency (phonemic usually more affected than semantic), free recall of episodic memory, and visual-spatial function (clock drawing, person, 3-D cube, copy and recall of complex shapes). The memory of patients with cerebellar dysfunction resembles that following other subcortical lesions that improve with cueing (clues or multiple choice). True memory loss does not result from isolated cerebellar damage but more likely reflects lesions in other cortical-subcortical memory circuits.

The mental status examination of the young child involves both close observation and interaction with the child as well as history and observations obtained from the parents and staff. The assessment of the child is usually accomplished by actively engaging the child in developmentally appropriate activities and a task that has been previously mastered by the child such as drawing, coloring or building with plastic bricks. For children with CCAS who may have limited speech this allows for assessment of their ability to understand and comprehend directions as well as their ability to work on a task (i.e., initiate, persist on task). During this active engagement with the child it is also possible to observe and assess the child's mood and behavior at a particular point in time. It is important to note that these can fluctuate, and the interaction provides an objective data point on which to expand with subsequent examinations. If the child's behavior and/or mood preclude engaging in an activity, the examination is based on observation and the history typically obtained through speaking with the child's parents or caregivers.

When documenting the examination, descriptive language is needed to fully appreciate the observed behaviors and should include not only the lack of speech or the dysarthric quality of the speech, but also the pitch of the sounds (such as screeching or whining speech). Similarly, it is important to observe and describe the intensity, frequency and duration of the behavioral symptoms, and include the range of neuropsychiatric symptoms associated with cerebellar disease such as irritable, labile, agitated, crying, sad, withdrawn, apathetic, yelling, tantruming, and inconsolable. Bizarre or psychotic behavior should also be noted.

In children it is important to document developmental milestones that were achieved previously and assess whether the child has regressed since the development of CCAS. It is not uncommon to see regression in tasks and behavior such as reverting to using a sippy cup or needing to use diapers.

Neuropsychological evaluation

These observations can be further assessed by neuropsychological tests designed to more formally detect and characterize areas of weakness and strength across multiple cognitive domains. Definition of these aspects of the child's performance is critical to understanding the nature and severity of the cognitive and emotional manifestations, and to planning the range and intensity of cognitive and educational rehabilitation services needed to maximize the child's overall level of function. This is necessary both in the healthcare environment and in the school system.

Based on descriptions of the range of cognitive, behavioral, and emotional difficulties manifested by children with cerebellar disorders, and the fact that these can manifest differently at different stages of development, it is important that the neuropsychologist approach the evaluation of children with these disorders appreciating the need to fully evaluate a range of functions using tests that have appropriate developmental norms. A complete neuropsychological evaluation of children with cerebellar disorders needs to go well beyond assessing a child's intellectual and academic functioning and must also include measures that address the child's functioning within the domains of attention (including sustained attention, working memory, selective attention), executive functioning (planning, organization, initiation, shift of set, inhibition, abstract reasoning), language (expressive and receptive language at single word, sentence and discourse levels), visuospatial abilities (perceptual abilities, construction abilities), memory (in both verbal and visual domains and assessing all stages of memory), motor functions (i.e., fine motor coordination, motor speed), emotional/psychiatric functioning (including a determination of whether the child exhibits mood disorders, anxiety disorders, psychotic thinking), and behavioral impairments (including measures of attention-deficit hyperactivity disorder symptomatology, behavioral dysregulation, and assessment of autistic behaviors).

In selecting appropriate measures for children with cerebellar disorders, it is important to appreciate that motor functions and expressive speech may be impaired, requiring the neuropsychologist to choose tests in which the child is able to demonstrate his or her comprehension and reasoning skills without interference from difficulties with response output. It is also important to ensure that those areas that have been identified as particularly vulnerable in children with cerebellar disorders, including the cognitive components of executive dysfunction, language impairment and visuospatial difficulties, and the behavioral and affective components that can manifest as behavioral dysregulation and emotional problems are always included in the evaluation.

The neuropsychological evaluation is a critical aspect of these children's care as it can help parents and teachers appreciate the range of difficulties that children with cerebellar disorders may experience, as well as their areas of strength. As described above, it is often the child's behavioral changes and not their motor difficulties that are most distressing to parents of these children and to children themselves. Helping a parent understand that their child's cognitive, affective, and behavioral changes are due to cerebellar dysfunction can help not only with raising the level of understanding, but also to modify how a parent, caregiver or teacher approaches and addresses a child's difficulties. Also, providing detailed information about a child's areas of cognitive strengths and weaknesses, their behavioral and emotional functioning, and the impact that their underlying cerebellar disorder has on their academic functioning is essential in determining the types of educational placement and services that will be most helpful in promoting the child's success in school.

In Table 4.4 we provide a guide to tests that are helpful in identifying the range of cognitive, affective, and emotional difficulties that a child with cerebellar disorder may display. The table is meant as a comprehensive, though not exhaustive, list organized into the important domains that are affected in

TABLE 4.4
Neuropsychological tests for the assessment of children with cerebellar disorders†

Domain and measure	Age range‡	Description of measure
Cognitive		
Developmental/intellectual abilities		
• Bayley Scales of Infant and Toddler Development – 3rd edition[1]	0:16–42:15 months	General measure of cognitive, language, motor, social-emotional, and adaptive skills
• Differential Ability Scales – 2nd edition (DAS-II)[2]	2:6–17:11	General conceptual abilities in verbal, nonverbal reasoning domains; also includes diagnostic measures of school readiness, working memory, and processing speed
• Mullen Scales of Early Learning[3]	1:30–68:30 months	Gross motor, visual reception, fine motor, language
• Neuropsychological Test of Development for Children – 2nd edition (NEPSY-2)[4]	3:0–16:11	Includes measures in the domains of attention, executive functioning, language, memory/learning, sensorimotor, social perception, and visuospatial processing
• Leiter International Performance Scale–Revised[5]	2:0–20:11	Provides a measure of nonverbal intelligence, visuospatial memory and attention
• Stanford-Binet Intelligence Scales – 5th edition[6]	2:0–89:11 years	Fluid and quantitative reasoning, knowledge, visual-spatial, and working memory
Wechsler scales: *		
• Wechsler Preschool and Primary Scale of Intelligence – 3rd edition (WPPSI-III)[7]	2:6–7:3	Verbal, nonverbal, processing speed, and expressive and receptive vocabulary
• Wechsler Intelligence Scales for Children – 4th edition (WISC-IV)[8]	6:0–16:11	Verbal comprehension, perceptual reasoning, working memory and processing speed
• Wechsler Adult Intelligence Scale – 4th edition (WAIS-IV)[9]	16:0–90:11	
Attention		
Sustained attention:		
• Conners' Continuous Performance Test–Kiddie (CPT-K)[10]*	4:0–5:11	Computerized task requiring monitoring of visual targets (pictures at kiddie level; letters at older level)
• Conners' Continuous Performance Test – 2nd edition (CPT-II)[11]*	6:0–55+	
Visual search:		
• WISC-IV/WAIS-IV Symbol Search[8,9]	6:0–90:11	Tests requiring visual detection of targets from an array
• Delis-Kaplan Executive Function System (D-KEFS) Trails 1: Visual Scanning[12]	8:0–89	
Attention span:		
• Verbal and visual span tasks (WISC-IV, Children's Memory Scale (CMS), DAS-II, Wide Range Assessment of Memory and Learning (WRAML2))[2,8,13,14]*	2:6–85+	Repetition of sequences of digits or spatial locations of increasing length
Selective attention:		
• NEPSY-II Auditory Attention and Response Set[4]	5:0–16:11	Auditory continuous performance test that measures selective and sustained attention as well as response inhibition
Sequencing:		
• D-KEFS Trails (conditions 2 and 3)[12]	8:0–89	Visual sequencing of number and/or letters
• CMS Sequences[13]	5:0–16:11	Rapid oral production of familiar and novel sequences
Executive functioning		
Working memory:		
• WISC-IV/WAIS-IV Digit Span (Backward, Sequencing), Arithmetic, Letter-Number Sequencing[8,9]*	5:0–16:11	Measures require child to hold information in mind and mentally manipulate it
Initiation of behavior:		
• D-KEFS Verbal Fluency: Letter Fluency, Category Fluency[12]*	3:0–89	Rapid generation of verbal responses based on either an initial letter or semantic cue;
• NEPSY-II Word Generation: Initial Letter, Semantic[4]*		Rapid generation of novel designs
• Design Fluency (D-KEFS, NEPSY-II)[4,12]*		
Cognitive flexibility (shift of set):		
Switching Tests:		
• D-KEFS Trails (Condition 4: Number-Letter)[12]*	6:6–89	Measures require child to alternate between two response sets or stimuli or to generate alternative solutions to problems
• D-KEFS Verbal Fluency: Category Switching[12]*		
• D-KEFS Design Fluency: Switching[12]*		
Sorting Tests:		
• D-KEFS Sorting Test[12]		
• NEPSY-II Animal Sorting[4]		
• Wisconsin Card Sorting Test[15]*		

TABLE 4.4
(continued)

Domain and measure	Age range‡	Description of measure
Inhibition: • D-KEFS Color Word Interference[12]* • NEPSY-II Inhibition[4] • CPT-II[11]* • NEPSY-II Statue[4]	3:0–89	Measures that assess inhibitory processes, typically requiring inhibition to an automatic or prepotent response
Planning and organization: • Rey-Osterrieth Complex Figure Test[16]* • NEPSY Clocks[4]	6:0–89	Measures that allow the examiner to assess how the child goes about organizing or planning a task
Memory Visual memory: • CMS[13] • WRAML-2[14]* • Wechsler Memory Scale-IV (WMS-IV)[17]* • NEPSY-II[4] • Rey Complex Figure Test: Incidental, Delayed Recall[16]* • Differential Ability Scale (DAS II): Recall of Designs, Recall of Objects[2]	4:0–89:11	Measures of that assess encoding, storage and retrieval of visual information (e.g., designs, pictures) by including measures of immediate and delayed recall and recognition
Verbal memory: • CMS[13] • WMS-IV[17] • WRAML-2[14]* • NEPSY-II[4] • California Verbal Learning Test (CVLT-C, CVLT-2)[18,19]*	5:0–89	Measures that assess encoding, storage and retrieval of verbal information (e.g., stories, designs) by including measures of immediate and delayed recall and recognition. The CVLT also allows for assessment of learning strategies
Language Receptive language: • MacArthur Communicative Development Inventories[20] • Clinical Evaluation of Language Fundamentals-4 (CELF-4)[21]* • Peabody Picture Vocabulary Test – 4th edition (PPVT-4)[22]* • Receptive One-Word Picture Vocabulary Test – 2nd edition[23]* • Receptive-Expressive Emergent Language Scale – 3rd edition[24] • Test of Auditory Conceptualization of Language – 3rd edition (TACL-3)[25]	Birth–90+	Assessment of comprehension of language at lexical, morphological and sentence levels with measures at early years based on parent report
Expressive language: • CELF-4[21]* • Expressive One-Word Picture Vocabulary Test[26]* • Expressive Vocabulary Test – 2nd edition (EVT-2)[27]* • Boston Naming Test[28]* • NEPSY-II Oromotor Sequences[4] • Preschool Language Scale – 4th edition (PLS-4)[29]	Birth–90+	Assessment of language expression at lexical, morphological and sentence levels; measures at early years based on parent report
Pragmatic language: CELF-4 Pragmatics Profile[21]	5:0–21:11	Profile completed by examiner, parent or teacher in order to identify verbal and nonverbal pragmatic deficits important in social and academic settings
Phonological processing: • NEPSY-II: Phonological Processing, Speeded Naming[4] • Comprehensive Test of Phonological Processing (CTOPP)[30]	3:0–24:11	Assessment of phonological awareness, phonological decoding, production and rapid naming
Visual-motor/visual spatial Visual construction/organization: • Developmental Test of Visual-Motor Integration – 6th edition (VMI-6)[31]* • Rey-Osterrieth Complex Figure Test[16]* • Developmental Test of Visual Perception–2 (DTVP-2), Adolescent and Adult version (DTVP-A)[32]	2:0–89:11	Visual perception/visual-motor coordination, visuospatial organization (Rey)

TABLE 4.4
(*continued*)

Domain and measure	Age range‡	Description of measure
Visual-perceptual: • Motor Free Visual Perception Test – 3rd edition[33]* • NEPSY-II Arrows[4] • DTVP-2, DTVP-A[32]	4:0–90+	Visual perception, visual-motor, and eye-hand coordination, spatial relations, visual discrimination, closure, memory, and figure-ground
Sensorimotor Fine motor coordination and speed: • Purdue Pegboard Test[34]* • Grooved Pegboard Test[35]* • NEPSY-II: Fingertip Tapping[4]	2:6–70	Assess fine motor coordination with each hand (all tests) and bilateral coordination (Purdue)
Motor planning and sequencing: • NEPSY-II Manual Motor Sequences[4]	3:0–12:11	Assess ability to learn and automatize series of hand movements
Academic skills/readiness Readiness: • Bracken Basic Concept Scale – 3rd edition[36] • Slosson Test of Reading Readiness[37]	2:6–7:11	Knowledge of concept categories (e.g., numbers; shapes) and visual, auditory and cognitive skills underlying reading readiness
Academic achievement: • Wechsler Individual Achievement Test – 3rd edition (WIAT-III)[38] • Wide Range Achievement Test – 4th edition (WRAT-4)[39] • Woodcock Johnson III Tests of Achievement[40] Social perception/emotional regulation (A)	2:0–90+	Assess academic skills in a broad range of domains including reading, spelling, written expression and math
Social affect and perception: • NEPSY-II: Affect Recognition, Theory of Mind, Memory for Faces[4]*	3:0–16:11	Ability to recognize and remember faces, and to perceive and comprehend affect and mental functions including belief, intention, deception, imagination and pretending
Self, parent and teacher scales of behavior and emotional problems: • Behavior Assessment System for Children – 2nd edition (BASC-2)[41]* • Achenbach Child Behavior Checklist[42]	2:0–25:11	Rating scales of attention, behavior, emotional and adaptive problems
Self, parent and teacher report of psychiatric symptoms: • Early Childhood Inventory–4[43]* • Child Symptom Inventory–4[44]* • Adolescent Symptom Inventory–4[45]*	3:0–18:11	Screens for DSM-IV emotional and behavioral disorders; parent and teacher report
Depression rating scales: • Childhood Depression Inventory[46] • Reynolds Adolescent Depression Scale[47]	7:0–20:11	Self-report measures to assess depressive symptomatology in children and adolescents
Projective measures: • Draw-A-Person Tests (e.g., McCarthy Scales of Children's Abilities)[48] • Robert's Apperception Test[49] • Rorschach Inkblot Test[50]	2:6– adulthood	Assess self-concept, personality, personal adjustment and emotional functioning
Behavior/developmental disorders *Adaptive functioning*		
• Adaptive Behavior Assessment System – 2nd edition (ABAS-II) Parent Form, Teacher/Day Care Provider Form[51]	Birth–21:11 2:0–21:11	Conceptual, social, and practical skills areas
• Scales of Independent Behavior–Revised (SIB-R)[52]*	Birth–80+	Motor, language, social, daily living and community living skills; maladaptive behavior; parent report
• Vineland Adaptive Behavior Scale – 2nd edition[53]*	Birth–90:11	Communication, socialization, and daily living. Motor skills before age 6
Self, parent and teacher scales of behavior and emotional problems: • Behavior Assessment System for Children – 2nd edition (BASC-2)[41]* • Achenbach Child Behavior Checklist[42]	2:0–25:11	Assess attention, behavior, emotional and adaptive problems

TABLE 4.4
(continued)

Domain and measure	Age range‡	Description of measure
Attention/dysexecutive behaviors		
Self, parent and teacher rating scales of executive functioning:		
• Behavior Rating Inventory of Executive Function (BRIEF)[54]*	2:0–18:11	Assess inhibition, shifting, emotional control, working memory, and planning/organizing
Parent and teacher ratings of attention and behavior problems:		
• Conners' Parent Rating Scale–Revised[55]* Autism spectrum disorders	3:0–17:11	Parent and teacher scales of attention and behavior problems
Observational and rating scales related to autism and Asperger syndrome:		
• Autism Diagnostic Observation Schedule (ADOS)[56]	Toddler–Adult	Assesses behaviors characteristic of autism and pervasive developmental disorder
• Gilliam Asperger's Disorder Scale (GADS)[57]*	3:0–22:11	Parent and Teacher ratings that assess social interaction; restricted patterns of behavior, cognitive patterns, pragmatic skills; stereotyped behavior, and communication disorders
• Gilliam Autism Rating Scale–2 (GARS-2)[58]*		

* Asterisks denote tests that are particularly sensitive to the impairments that characterize the CCAS.
† Please see text regarding recommendation for a flexible approach to testing based on the child's developmental stage, medical history and presentation.
‡ Other than when months are specified, age ranges refer to years. Note that for many of the domains, age ranges provided refer to the entire cluster of tests provided, with each individual test having norms for different age ranges.
1: Bayley 2005, 2: Elliot 2007, 3: Mullen 1995, 4: Korkman et al. 2007, 5: Roid and Miller 1997, 6: Roid 2003, 7: Wechsler 2002, 8: Wechsler 2003, 9: Wechsler 2008, 10: Conners 2006, 11: Conners 2004, 12: Delis et al. 2001, 13: Cohen 1997, 14: Sheslow and Adams 2003, 15: Heaton et al. 1993, 16: Meyers and Meyers 1995, 17: Wechsler 2009b, 18: Delis et al. 1994, 19: Delis et al. 2000, 20: Fenson et al. 1994, 21: Semel et al. 2003, 22: Dunn and Dunn 2007, 23: Brownell 2000b, 24: Bzoch et al. 2003, 25: Carrow-Woolfork 1999, 26: Brownell 2000a, 27: Williams 2007, 28: Goodglass and Kaplan 2000, 29: Zimmerman et al. 2002, 30: Wagner et al. 1999, 31: Beery and Beery 2004, 32: Hammill et al. 1993, 33: Colarusso and Hammill 2003, 34: Tiffin 1968, 35: Lewis and Rennick 1979, 36: Bracken 1998, 37: Perry and Vitali 1991, 38: Wechsler 2009a, 39: Wilkinson and Robertson 2006, 40: Woodcock et al. 2001, 41: Reynolds and Kamphaus 2004, 42: Achenbach and Rescorla 2001, 43: Sprafkin and Gadow 2000, 44: Gadow and Sprafkin 2002, 45: Gadow and Sprafkin 2008, 46: Kovacs 1992, 47: Reynolds 2002, 48: McCarthy 1972, 49: McArthur and Roberts 1982, 50: Exner Jr. 1990, 51: Harrison and Oakland 2003, 52: Bruininks et al. 1996, 53: Sparrow et al. 2005, 54: Gioia et al. 2000, 55: Conners 1997, 56: Lord et al. 2002, 57: Gilliam 2001, 58: Gilliam 2006.

children with cerebellar disorders, including cognitive, affective, academic, and behavioral emotional functioning. It is, of course, important to note that children with cerebellar disorders vary in the severity of their symptoms and signs. The neuropsychologist should have a flexible approach to choosing tests that are most appropriate, taking into account the individual child's particular developmental stage, medical history, and presenting concerns. While a delineation of a child's cognitive and behavioral strengths and weaknesses is best accomplished through a comprehensive examination, in Table 4.1 those tests that have previously been identified as particularly sensitive to the types of impairments seen in CCAS are indicated with an asterisk. Also, as children can present with cerebellar disorders at various ages, the table includes the age range for normative data available for tests within the different domains.

Approach to management

Knowledge of the characteristic features of the CCAS provides an opportunity for counseling and education, fulfilling the family and the patient's need-to-know imperative. It is helpful to families to know that the nonmotor consequences of their child's disorder are not necessarily a psychological reaction to the more traditional motor impairments, but could well be part of the disease itself. It is also prudent to alert families of infants who have sustained cerebellar damage, for example, to be vigilant for the development of neurocognitive deficits, because the cerebellar disruption has effects on behavior that extend beyond motor control. Further, as we have seen in our patients with cerebellar agenesis, hypoplasia, and post-tumor resection, the nature of the cognitive and neuropsychiatric manifestation may change with time, for reasons likely related to the neurobiology of the developing nervous system, as well as to the changing psychosocial environment of the growing child. This informed, honest, and open approach by caregivers facilitates therapeutic intervention by cognitive and behavioral therapy for previously unrecognized emotional disturbances in cerebellar patients. Early studies of cognitive rehabilitation in CCAS appear promising, particularly for the executive dysfunction (Schweizer et al. 2008). Moreover, ongoing physical, occupational, and speech therapy in the child with cerebellar disease as well as appropriate school placement and services is imperative. In our anecdotal experience, children with developmental delay on the basis of static lesions such as cerebellar hypoplasia and agenesis continue to make strides when the motor, cognitive, social, and emotional consequences of the lesions are dealt with early and consistently.

Recognizing the neuropsychiatric manifestations in patients with cerebellar dysfunction also opens the way to the use of available pharmacological agents that treat neurobehavioral and neuropsychiatric symptoms. In our experience the use of atypical antipsychotics such as risperidone have been helpful in managing severe mood lability and atypical psychosis. The use of benzodiazepines, such as lorazepam and clonazepam, has alleviated anxiety, panic, and some mood symptoms. However, prospective studies of these and other pharmacological treatments of the CCAS have not yet been performed.

Earlier investigators (Riklan et al. 1974; Heath 1977) reported that electrical stimulation of the cerebellum resulted in successful treatment of behavioral disorders including aggression and psychosis. We have suggested that applying repetitive transcranial magnetic stimulation to the limbic cerebellum in the vermis may improve psychiatric disorders such as schizophrenia by upregulating cerebellar modulation of cerebrocerebellar circuits engaged in cognition and emotion (Schmahmann et al. 2007; Hoppenbrouwers et al. 2008). Our preliminary results using intermittent theta burst stimulation in eight patients with refractory schizophrenia provide support for this contention, resulting in improvements in mood as well as in tests of attention (Demirtas-Tatlidede et al. 2010).

Conclusions

The cerebellar role in cognitive, affective, and emotional functioning has clinical relevance for children with cerebellar disorders. We have presented an overview of the cognitive and neuropsychiatric manifestations that characterize the cerebellar cognitive affective syndrome which results from a wide range of clinical conditions, and we have described an approach to the recognition, assessment, diagnosis, and management of these manifestations. As the field of cognitive neuroscience focusing on the cerebellum matures, it may be expected that the clinical understanding and treatment of patients with neurobehavioral manifestations of cerebellar dysfunction will continue to improve.

Acknowledgments

Supported in part by RO1 MH067980, the Birmingham, MINDlink, and Sidney R. Baer Jr. Foundations. Parts of this chapter are derived from Schmahmann (2005, 2011). The assistance of Jason MacMore and Sarah Mancuso is gratefully acknowledged.

REFERENCES

Aarsen FK, Van Dongen HR, Paquier PF, Van Mourik M, Catsman-Berrevoets CE (2004) Long-term sequelae in children after cerebellar astrocytoma surgery. Neurology 62: 1311–1316.

Achenbach T, Rescorla L (2001) Manual for the ASEBA School-Age Forms & Profiles. Burlington, VT: University of Vermont, Research Center for Children, Youth, & Families.

Akil H, Statham PF, Gotz M, Bramley P, Whittle IR (2006) Adult cerebellar mutism and cognitive-affective syndrome caused by cystic hemangioblastoma. Acta Neurochir (Wien) 148: 597–598.

Allen G, Buxton RB, Wong EC, Courchesne E (1997) Attentional activation of the cerebellum independent of motor involvement. Science 275: 1940–1943.

Allin M, Matsumoto H, Santhouse AM, Nosarti C, AlAsady MH, et al. (2001) Cognitive and motor function and the size of the cerebellum in adolescents born very pre-term. Brain 124(Pt 1): 60–66.

Anderson CM, Maas LC, Frederick B, Bendor JT, Spencer TJ, et al. (2006) Cerebellar vermis involvement in cocaine-related behaviors. Neuropsychopharmacology 31: 1318–1326.

Anderson CM, Teicher MH, Polcari A, Renshaw PF (2002) Abnormal T2 relaxation time in the cerebellar vermis of adults sexually abused in childhood: potential role of the vermis in stress-enhanced risk for drug abuse. Psychoneuroendocrinology 27: 231–244.

Assal F, Valenza N, Landis T, Hornung JP (2000) Clinicoanatomical correlates of a Fou rire prodromique in a pontine infarction. J Neurol Neurosurg Psychiatry 69: 697–698.

Baillieux H, De Smet HJ, Lesage G, Paquier P, De Deyn PP, Mariën P (2006) Neurobehavioral alterations in an adolescent following posterior fossa tumor resection. Cerebellum 5: 289–295.

Baillieux H, De Smet HJ, Dobbeleir A, Paquier PF, De Deyn PP, Mariën P (2010) Cognitive and affective disturbances following focal cerebellar damage in adults: A neuropsychological and SPECT study. Cortex 46: 869–879.

Bauman M, Kemper T (1985) Histoanatomic observations of the brain in early infantile autism. Neurology 35: 866–874.

Bauman ML, Kemper TL (2005) Neuroanatomic observations of the brain in autism: a review and future directions. Int J Dev Neurosci 23: 183–187.

Bayley N (2005) Bayley Scales of Infant and Toddler Development: Administration Manual, 3rd edition). San Antonio, TX: Harcourt Assessment.

Beery KE, Beery NA (2004) The Beery-Buktenica Developmental Test of Visual-Motor Integration: Administration, scorng, and teaching manual, 5th edition. Minneapolis, MN: NCS Pearson.

Berger A, Sadeh M, Tzur G, Shuper A, Kornreich L, et al. (2005) Task switching after cerebellar damage. Neuropsychology 19: 362–370.

Berman AF, Berman D, Prescott JW (1978) The effect of cerebellar lesions on emotional behavior in the rhesus monkey. In: The Cerebellum, Epilepsy and Behavior (Cooper IS, Riklan M and Snider RS, eds). New York: Plenum Press; 277–284.

Berquin PC, Giedd JN, Jacobsen LK, Hamburger SD, Krain AL, Rapoport JL, Castellanos FX (1998) Cerebellum in attention-deficit hyperactivity disorder: a morphometric MRI study. Neurology 50: 1087–1093.

Botez-Marquard T, Botez MI (1993) Cognitive behavior in heredodegenerative ataxias. Eur Neurol 33: 351–357.

Bower JM (1997) Control of sensory data acquisition. In: Schmahmann JD, eds. Cerebellum and Cognition. San Diego, CA: Academic Press; 489–513.

Bracken B (1998) Bracken Basic Concept Scale-Revised: Examiner's Manual. San Antonio, TX: Psychological Corporation.

Bracke-Tolkmitt R, Linden A, Canavan A, Rockstroh B, Scholz E, et al. (1989) The cerebellum contributes to mental skills. Behav Neurosci 103: 442–446.

Brownell R (2000a) Expressive One-Word Picture Vocabulary Test: Manual (3rd ed). Novato, CA: Academic Therapy Publications.

Brownell R (2000b) Receptive One-Word Picture Vocabulary Test (2nd ed). Novato, CA: Academic Therapy Publications.

Bruininks RH, Woodcock RW, Weatherman RF, Hill BK (1996) Scales of Independent Behavior – Revised. Chicago: Riverside.

Brunet E, Sarfati Y, Hardy-Bayle MC, Decety J (2000) A PET investigation of the attribution of intentions with a nonverbal task. Neuroimage 11: 157–166.

Burk K, Bosch S, Globas C, Zuhlke C, Daum I, et al. (2001) Executive dysfunction in spinocerebellar ataxia type 1. Eur Neurol 46: 43–48.

Bzoch KR, League R, Brown VL (2003) Receptive-Expressive Emergent Language Test (3rd ed). Los Angeles, CA: Western Psychological Services.

Calarge C, Andreasen NC, O'Leary DS (2003) Visualizing how one brain understands another: a PET study of theory of mind. Am J Psychiatry 160: 1954–1964.

Carrow-Woolfork E (1999) Test of Auditory Conceptualization of Language: Examiner's manual, 3rd edition. Austin, TX: PRO-ED, Inc.

Castellanos FX, Giedd JN, Berquin PC, Walter JM, Sharp W, et al. (2001) Quantitative brain magnetic resonance imaging in girls with attention-deficit/hyperactivity disorder. Arch Gen Psychiatry 58: 289–295.

Catsman-Berrevoets CE, Aarsen FK (2010) The spectrum of neurobehavioural deficits in the Posterior Fossa Syndrome in children after cerebellar tumour surgery. Cortex 46: 933–946.

Catsman-Berrevoets CE, van Dongen HR, Zwetsloot CP (1992) Transient loss of speech followed by dysarthria after removal of posterior fossa tumour. Dev Med Child Neurol 34: 1102–1109.

Cher LM, Hochberg FH, Teruya J, Nitschke M, Valenzuela RF, et al. (1995) Therapy for paraneoplastic neurologic syndromes in six patients with protein A column immunoadsorption. Cancer 75: 1678–1683.

Chheda M, Sherman J, Schmahmann JD (2002) Neurologic, psychiatric and cognitive manifestations in cerebellar agenesis. Neurology 58(Suppl 3): 356.

Cohen M (1997) Children's Memory Scale. San Antonio, TX: The Psychological Corporation.

Colarusso RP, Hammill DD (2003) Motor-Free Visual Perception Test: Manual (3rd ed). Novato, CA: Academic Therapy.

Conners C (1997) Conners' Rating Scales – Revised. North Tonawanda, NY: Multi-Health Systems.

Conners C (2004) Conners' Continuous Performance Test (2nd ed). North Tonawanda, NY: Multi-Health Systems, Inc.

Conners CK (2006) Conners' Kiddie Continuous Performance Test: Technical guide and software manual. North Tonawanda, NY: Multi-Health Systems.

Cooper FE, Grube M, Elsegood KJ, Welch JL, Kelly TP, et al. (2010) The contribution of the cerebellum to cognition in Spinocerebellar Ataxia Type 6. Behav Neurol 23: 3–15.

Cooper IS, Riklan M, Amin I and Cullinan T (1978) A long-term follow-up study of cerebellar stimulation for the control of epilepsy. In: Cooper IS, eds. Cerebellar Stimulation in Man. New York: Raven Press; 19–38.

Courchesne E, Yeung-Courchesne R, Press GA, Hesselink JR, Jernigan TL (1988) Hypoplasia of cerebellar vermal lobules VI and VII in autism. N Engl J Med 318: 1349–1354.

Delis DC, Kramer JH, Kaplan E, Ober BA (1994) California Verbal Learning Test – Children's Version. San Antonio, TX: Psychological Corporation.

Delis D, Kramer J, Kaplan E, Ober B (2000) California Verbal Learning Test – Adult Version (2nd ed). San Antonio, TX: The Psychological Corporation.

Delis D, Kaplan E, Kramer J (2001) Delis-Kaplan Executive Function System: Examiner's manual. San Antonio, TX: The Psychological Corporation.

Demirtas-Tatlidede A, Freitas C, Cromer JR, Safar L, Ongur D, et al. (2010) Safety and proof of principle study of cerebellar vermal theta burst stimulation in refractory schizophrenia. Schizophr Res 124: 91–100.

Desmond JE, Gabrieli JD, Wagner AD, Ginier BL, Glover GH (1997) Lobular patterns of cerebellar activation in verbal working-memory and finger-tapping tasks as revealed by functional MRI. J Neurosci 17: 9675–9685.

Devos D, Schraen-Maschke S, Vuillaume I, Dujardin K, Naze P, et al. (2001) Clinical features and genetic analysis of a new form of spinocerebellar ataxia. Neurology 56: 234–238.

Dietze DD, Jr, Mickle JP (1990) Cerebellar mutism after posterior fossa surgery. Pediatr Neurosurg 16: 25–31; discussion 31.

Dow RS (1974) Some novel concepts of cerebellar physiology. Mt Sinai J Med 41: 103–119.

Dow RS, Moruzzi G (1958) The Physiology and Pathology of the Cerebellum. Minneapolis, MN: University of Minnesota Press.

Doyon J, Song AW, Karni A, Lalonde F, Adams MM, et al. (2002) Experience-dependent changes in cerebellar contributions to motor sequence learning. Proc Natl Acad Sci U S A 99: 1017–1022.

Dreher JC, Grafman J (2002) The roles of the cerebellum and basal ganglia in timing and error prediction. Eur J Neurosci 16: 1609–1619.

Dunn LM, Dunn DM (2007) Peabody Picture Vocabulary Test: Manual. Minneapolis, MN: NCS Pearson.

Elliot CD (2007) Differential Ability Scales: Administration and scoring manual, 2nd edition. San Antonio, TX: Harcourt Assessment.

Exner C, Weniger G, Irle E (2004) Cerebellar lesions in the PICA but not SCA territory impair cognition. Neurology 63(11): 2132–2135.

Exner Jr, J (1990) A Rorschach Workbook For the Comprehensive System, 3rd edition. Asheville, NC: Rorschach Workshops.

Fenson L, Dale PS, Reznick DT, Bates E, Hartung JP, et al. (1994) MacArthur Communicative Development Inventories: User's guide and technical manual. San Diego, CA: Singular.

Fiez JA, Petersen SE, Cheney MK, Raichle ME (1992) Impaired non-motor learning and error detection associated with cerebellar damage. A single case study. Brain 115 (Pt 1): 155–178.

Flourens P (1824) Recherches experimentales sur les proprietes et les fonctions du systseme nerveux, dans les animaux vertebres. Paris: Crevot.

Frick RB (1982) The ego and the vestibulocerebellar system: some theoretical perspectives. Psychoanal Q 51: 93–122.

Gadow K, Sprafkin J (2002) Child Symptom Inventory 4. Stony Brook, NY: Checkmate Plus.

Gadow K, Sprafkin J (2008) Adolescent Symptom Inventory 4. Stony Brook, NY: Checkmate Plus.

Gambardella A, Annesi G, Bono F, Spadafora P, Valentino P, et al. (1998) CAG repeat length and clinical features in three Italian families with spinocerebellar ataxia type 2 (SCA2): early impairment of Wisconsin Card Sorting Test and saccade velocity. J Neurol 245: 647–652.

Gao JH, Parsons LM, Bower JM, Xiong J, Li J, et al. (1996) Cerebellum implicated in sensory acquisition and discrimination rather than motor control. Science 272: 545–547.

Gardner RJ, Coleman LT, Mitchell LA, Smith LJ, Harvey AS, et al. (2001) Near-total absence of the cerebellum. Neuropediatrics 32: 62–68.

Geschwind DH (1999) Focusing attention on cognitive impairment in spinocerebellar ataxia. Arch Neurol 56: 20–22.

Gierga K, Schelhaas HJ, Brunt ER, Seidel K, Scherzed W, et al. (2009) Spinocerebellar ataxia type 6 (SCA6): neurodegeneration goes beyond the known brain predilection sites. Neuropathol Appl Neurobiol 35: 515–527.

Gilliam JE (2001) Gilliam Asperger's Disorder Scale: Examiner's manual. Austin, TX: PRO-ED.

Gilliam JE (2006) Gilliam Autism Rating Scale: Examiner's manual, 2nd edition. Austin, TX: PRO-ED.

Gioia G, Isquith P, Guy S, Kenworthy L (2000) Behavior Rating Inventory of Executive Function. Odessa, FL: Psychological Assessment Resources.

Goodglass H, Kaplan E (2000) Boston Naming Test. Philadelphia: Lippincott Williams & Wilkins.

Gorman MP (2010) Update on diagnosis, treatment, and prognosis in opsoclonus-myoclonus-ataxia syndrome. Curr Opin Pediatr 22: 745–750.

Gottwald B, Wilde B, Mihajlovic Z, Mehdorn HM (2004) Evidence for distinct cognitive deficits after focal cerebellar lesions. J Neurol Neurosurg Psychiatry 75: 1524–1531.

Grafman J, Litvan I, Massaquoi S, Stewart M, Sirigu A, et al. (1992) Cognitive planning deficit in patients with cerebellar atrophy. Neurology 42: 1493–1496.

Grill J, Viguier D, Kieffer V, Bulteau C, Sainte-Rose C, et al. (2004) Critical risk factors for intellectual impairment in children with posterior fossa tumors: the role of cerebellar damage. J Neurosurg 101(2 Suppl): 152–158.

Gross-Tsur V, Ben-Bashat D, Shalev RS, Levav M, Sira LB (2006) Evidence of a developmental cerebello-cerebral disorder. Neuropsychologia 44: 2569–2572.

Hammill DD, Pearson NA, Voress JK (1993) Developmental Test of Visual Perception: Examiner's manual, 2nd edition. Austin, TX: PRO-ED.

Harrison P, Oakland, T (2003) Adaptive Behavior Assessment System, 2nd edition. San Antonio, TX: NCS Pearson.

Heath RG (1977) Modulation of emotion with a brain pacemaker. Treatment for intractable psychiatric illness. J Nerv Ment Dis 165: 300–317.

Heath RG, Harper JW (1974) Ascending projections of the cerebellar fastigial nucleus to the hippocampus, amygdala, and other temporal lobe sites: evoked potential and histological studies in monkeys and cats. Exp Neurol 45: 268–287.

Heath RG, Franklin DE, Shraberg D (1979) Gross pathology of the cerebellum in patients diagnosed and treated as functional psychiatric disorders. J Nerv Ment Dis 167: 585–592.

Heaton RK, Chelune GJ, Talley JL, Kay GG, Curtiss G. (1993) Wisconsin Card Sorting Test Manual – Revised and Expanded. Lutz, FL: Psychological Assessment Resources.

Herman-Bert A, Stevanin G, Netter JC, Rascol O, Brassat D, et al. (2000) Mapping of spinocerebellar ataxia 13 to chromosome 19q13.3-q13.4 in a family with autosomal dominant cerebellar ataxia and mental retardation. Am J Hum Genet 67: 229–235.

Hokkanen LS, Kauranen V, Roine RO, Salonen O, Kotila M (2006) Subtle cognitive deficits after cerebellar infarcts. Eur J Neurol 13: 161–170.

Holmes G (1917) The symptoms of acute cerebellar injuries due to gunshot wounds. Brain 40: 461–535.

Hoppenbrouwers SS, Schutter DJ, Fitzgerald PB, Chen R, Daskalakis ZJ. (2008) The role of the cerebellum in the pathophysiology and treatment of neuropsychiatric disorders: a review. Brain Res Rev 59: 185–200.

Horton LC, Frosch MP, Schmahmann JD (2011) Spinocerebellar Ataxia Type 7 (SCA7): A 13-year Longitudinal Study of Clinical Course,

Neuropathological Features, and Phenotype-Genotype Correlations. 63rd Annual Meeting of the American Academy of Neurology. Honolulu, HI.
Ishikawa K, Watanabe M, Yoshizawa K, Fujita T, Iwamoto H, et al. (1999) Clinical, neuropathological, and molecular study in two families with spinocerebellar ataxia type 6 (SCA6). J Neurol Neurosurg Psychiatry 67: 86–89.
Ito M (1997) Cerebellar microcomplexes. In: Schmahmann JD, eds. Cerebellum and Cognition. San Diego, CA: Academic Press; 475–489.
Ivry R (1997) Cerebellar timing systems. In: Schmahmann JD, eds. Cerebellum and Cognition. San Diego, CA: Academic Press; 555–573.
Jueptner M, Rijntjes M, Weiller C, Faiss JH, Timmann D, et al. (1995) Localization of a cerebellar timing process using PET. Neurology 45: 1540–1545.
Karatekin C, Lazareff JA, Asarnow RF (2000) Relevance of the cerebellar hemispheres for executive functions. Pediatr Neurol 22: 106–112.
Kelly RM, Strick PL (2003) Cerebellar loops with motor cortex and prefrontal cortex of a nonhuman primate. J Neurosci 23: 8432–8444.
Kemper TL, Bauman M (1998) Neuropathology of infantile autism. J Neuropathol Exp Neurol 57: 645–652.
Kingma A, Mooij JJ, Metzemaekers JD, Leeuw JA (1994) Transient mutism and speech disorders after posterior fossa surgery in children with brain tumours. Acta Neurochir (Wien) 131: 74–79.
Kish SJ, el-Awar M, Schut L, Leach L, Oscar-Berman M, et al. (1988) Cognitive deficits in olivopontocerebellar atrophy: implications for the cholinergic hypothesis of Alzheimer's dementia. Ann Neurol 24: 200–206.
Koide R, Kobayashi S, Shimohata T, Ikeuchi T, Maruyama M, et al. (1999) A neurological disease caused by an expanded CAG trinucleotide repeat in the TATA-binding protein gene: a new polyglutamine disease? Hum Mol Genet 8: 2047–2053.
Konarski JZ, McIntyre RS, Grupp LA, Kennedy SH (2005) Is the cerebellum relevant in the circuitry of neuropsychiatric disorders? J Psychiatry Neurosci 30: 178–186.
Korkman M, Kirk U, Kemp S (2007) Neuropsychological Test of Development for Children (NEPSY): Clinical and interpretive manual, 2nd edition. San Antonio, TX: Harcourt Assessment.
Kossorotoff M, Gonin-Flambois C, Gitiaux C, Quijano S, Boddaert N, et al. (2010) A cognitive and affective pattern in posterior fossa strokes in children: a case series. Dev Med Child Neurol 52: 626–631.
Kovacs M (1992) Children's Depression Inventory. North Tonawanda, NY: Multi-Health Systems.
Krienen FM, Buckner RL (2009) Segregated fronto-cerebellar circuits revealed by intrinsic functional connectivity. Cereb Cortex 19: 2485–2497.
Landis DM, Rosenberg RN, Landis SC, Schut L, Nyhan WL (1974) Olivopontocerebellar degeneration. Clinical and ultrastructural abnormalities. Arch Neurol 31: 295–307.
Levisohn L, Cronin-Golomb A, Schmahmann JD (2000) Neuropsychological consequences of cerebellar tumour resection in children: cerebellar cognitive affective syndrome in a paediatric population. Brain 123 (Pt 5): 1041–1050.
Lewis RS, Rennick PM (1979) Manual for the Repeatable Cognitive-Perceptual-Motor Battery. Clinton Township, MI: Ronald F. Lewis.
Lilja A, Hamalainen P, Kaitaranta E, Rinne R. (2005) Cognitive impairment in spinocerebellar ataxia type 8. J Neurol Sci 237: 31–38.
Limperopoulos C, Bassan H, Gauvreau K, Robertson RL, Jr., Sullivan NR, et al. (2007) Does cerebellar injury in premature infants contribute to the high prevalence of long-term cognitive, learning, and behavioral disability in survivors? Pediatrics 120: 584–593.
Limperopoulos C, Soul JS, Gauvreau K, Huppi PS, Warfield SK, et al. (2005a) Late gestation cerebellar growth is rapid and impeded by premature birth. Pediatrics 115: 688–695.
Limperopoulos C, Soul JS, Haidar H, Huppi PS, Bassan H, et al. (2005b) Impaired trophic interactions between the cerebellum and the cerebrum among preterm infants. Pediatrics 116: 844–850.
Lippmann S, Manshadi M, Baldwin H, Drasin G, Rice J, et al. (1982) Cerebellar vermis dimensions on computerized tomographic scans of schizophrenic and bipolar patients. Am J Psychiatry 139: 667–668.
Lord C, Rutter M, DiLavore PC, Risi S (2002) Autism diagnostic observation schedule. Los Angeles: Western Psychological Services.
Malm J, Kristensen B, Karlsson T, Carlberg B, Fagerlund M, et al. (1998) Cognitive impairment in young adults with infratentorial infarcts. Neurology 51: 433–440.
Mantovan MC, Martinuzzi A, Squarzanti F, Bolla A, Silvestri I, et al. (2006) Exploring mental status in Friedreich's ataxia: a combined neuropsychological, behavioral and neuroimaging study. Eur J Neurol 13: 827–835.
Marien P, Baillieux H, De Smet HJ, Engelborghs S, Wilssens I, et al. (2009) Cognitive, linguistic and affective disturbances following a right superior cerebellar artery infarction: a case study. Cortex 45: 527–536.
Mariotti C, Alpini D, Fancellu R, Soliveri P, Grisoli M, et al. (2007) Spinocerebellar ataxia type 17 (SCA17): oculomotor phenotype and clinical characterization of 15 Italian patients. J Neurol 254: 1538–1546.
Martner J (1975) Cerebellar influences on autonomic mechanisms. An experimental study in the cat with special reference to the fastigial nucleus. Acta Physiol Scand Suppl 425: 1–42.
Maryniak A, Roszkowski M (2005) Cognitive and affective disturbances in children after surgical treatment of cerebellar tumors. Neurol Neurochir Pol 39: 202–206.
McArthur DS, Roberts GE (1982) Roberts Apperception Test for Children. Los Angeles, CA: Western Psychological Services.
McCarthy D (1972) Manual for the McCarthy Scales of Children's Abilities. Cleveland, OH: The Psychological Corporation.
Meyers J, Meyers K. (1995) Rey Complex Figure Test and Recognition Trial: Professional manual. Lutz, FL: Psychological Assessment Resources.
Miall RC, Weir DJ, Wolpert DM, Stein JF (1993) Is the cerebellum a smith predictor? J Mot Behav 25: 203–216.
Middleton FA, Strick PL (1994) Anatomical evidence for cerebellar and basal ganglia involvement in higher cognitive function. Science 266: 458–461.
Molinari M, Chiricozzi FR, Clausi S, Tedesco AM, De Lisa M, et al. (2008) Cerebellum and detection of sequences, from perception to cognition. Cerebellum 7: 611–615.
Molinari M, Filippini V, Leggio MG (2002) Neuronal plasticity of interrelated cerebellar and cortical networks. Neuroscience 111: 863–870.
Molinari M, Leggio MG, Solida A, Ciorra R, Misciagna S, et al. (1997) Cerebellum and procedural learning: evidence from focal cerebellar lesions. Brain 120 (Pt 10): 1753–1762.
Moriguchi I (1981) A study of schizophrenic brains by computerized tomography scans. Folia Psychiatr Neurol Jpn 35: 55–72.
Moruzzi G (1947) Sham rage and localized autonomic responses elicited by cerebellar stimulation in the acute thalamic cat. In, eds. Proc. XVII Internat. Congress Physiol. Oxford. 114–115.
Mostofsky SH, Reiss AL, Lockhart P, Denckla MB (1998) Evaluation of cerebellar size in attention-deficit hyperactivity disorder. J Child Neurol 13: 434–439.
Mullen E. (1995) Mullen Scales of Early Learning: Manual. Circle Pines, MN: AGS Publishing.
Murakami N, Yoshida M, Hashizume Y, Muroga T and Takahashi A (1989) [A nosological study of a patient showing ataxia & lower motor neuron involvement]. Rinsho Shinkeigaku 29: 1116–1121.
Nakamura K, Jeong SY, Uchihara T, Anno M, Nagashima K, et al. (2001) SCA17, a novel autosomal dominant cerebellar ataxia caused by an expanded polyglutamine in TATA-binding protein. Hum Mol Genet 10: 1441–1448.
Nashold BS, Jr, Slaughter DG (1969) Effects of stimulating or destroying the deep cerebellar regions in man. J Neurosurg 31: 172–186.
Neau JP, Arroyo-Anllo E, Bonnaud V, Ingrand P, Gil R (2000) Neuropsychological disturbances in cerebellar infarcts. Acta Neurol Scand 102: 363–370.
Nixon PD, Passingham RE (2001) Predicting sensory events. The role of the cerebellum in motor learning. Exp Brain Res 138: 251–257.
Ohara S, Iijima N, Hayashida K, Oide T, Katai S (2007) Autopsy case of opsoclonus-myoclonus-ataxia and cerebellar cognitive affective syndrome associated with small cell carcinoma of the lung. Movement Disord 22: 1320–1324.
Palmer SL, Hassall T, Evankovich K, Mabbott DJ, Bonner M, et al. (2010) Neurocognitive outcome 12 months following cerebellar mutism syndrome in pediatric patients with medulloblastoma. Neuro Oncol 12: 1311–1317.
Parvizi J, Joseph J, Press DZ, Schmahmann JD (2007) Pathological laughter and crying in patients with multiple system atrophy-cerebellar type. Mov Disord 22: 798–803.

Pascual-Leone A, Grafman J, Clark K, Stewart M, Massaquoi S, et al. (1993) Procedural learning in Parkinson's disease and cerebellar degeneration. Ann Neurol 34: 594–602.

Paulus KS, Magnano I, Conti M, Galistu P, D'Onofrio M, et al. (2004) Pure post-stroke cerebellar cognitive affective syndrome: a case report. Neurol Sci 25: 220–224.

Penn HE (2006) Neurobiological correlates of autism: a review of recent research. Child Neuropsychol 12: 57–79.

Perry LA, Vitali GJ (1991) Slosson Test of Reading Readiness: Manual. East Aurora, NY: Slosson Educational Publications.

Petersen SE, Fox PT, Posner MI, Mintun M, Raichle ME (1989) Positron emission tomographic studies of the processing of single words. J Cognit Neurosci 1: 153–170.

Picard H, Amado I, Mouchet-Mages S, Olie JP, Krebs MO (2008) The role of the cerebellum in schizophrenia: an update of clinical, cognitive, and functional evidences. Schizophr Bull 34: 155–172.

Pollack IF, Polinko P, Albright AL, Towbin R, Fitz C (1995) Mutism and pseudobulbar symptoms after resection of posterior fossa tumors in children: incidence and pathophysiology. Neurosurgery 37: 885–893.

Raichle ME, Fiez JA, Videen TO, MacLeod AM, Pardo JV, et al. (1994) Practice-related changes in human brain functional anatomy during nonmotor learning. Cereb Cortex 4: 8–26.

Rapin I (1999) Autism in search of a home in the brain. Neurology 52: 902–904.

Reis DJ, Doba N, Nathan MA (1973) Predatory attack, grooming, and consummatory behaviors evoked by electrical stimulation of cat cerebellar nuclei. Science 182: 845–847.

Rekate HL, Grubb RL, Aram DM, Hahn JF, Ratcheson RA (1985) Muteness of cerebellar origin. Arch Neurol 42: 697–698.

Reynolds CR, Kamphaus RW (2004) Behavior Assessment System for Children: Manual, 2nd edition. Circle Pines, MN: AGS Publishing.

Reynolds W (2002) Reynolds Adolescent Depression Scale, 2nd edition. Lutz, FL: Psychological Assessment Resources.

Richter S, Dimitrova A, Maschke M, Gizewski E, Beck A, et al. (2005) Degree of cerebellar ataxia correlates with three-dimensional mri-based cerebellar volume in pure cerebellar degeneration. Eur Neurol 54: 23–27.

Riklan M, Marisak I, Cooper IS (1974) Psychological studies of chronic cerebellar stimulation in man. In: Cooper IS, Riklan M and Snider RS, eds. The Cerebellum, Epilepsy and Behavior. New York: Plenum Press; 285–342.

Ritvo ER, Freeman BJ, Scheibel AB, Duong T, Robinson H, et al. (1986) Lower Purkinje cell counts in the cerebella of four autistic subjects: initial findings of the UCLA-NSAC Autopsy Research Report. Am J Psychiatry 143: 862–866.

Riva D, Giorgi C (2000) The cerebellum contributes to higher functions during development: evidence from a series of children surgically treated for posterior fossa tumours. Brain 123 (Pt 5): 1051–1061.

Roid GH (2003) Stanford Binet Intelligence Scales: Examiner's manual, 5th edition. Itasca, IL: Riverside.

Roid G, Miller L (1997) Leiter International Performance Scale – Revised: Examiner's manual. In: Roid G and Miller L, eds. Leiter International Performance Scale-Revised. Wood Dale, IL: Stoelting Co.

Ronning C, Sundet K, Due-Tonnessen B, Lundar T, Helseth E (2005) Persistent cognitive dysfunction secondary to cerebellar injury in patients treated for posterior fossa tumors in childhood. Pediatr Neurosurg 41: 15–21.

Ryding E, Decety J, Sjoholm H, Stenberg G, Ingvar DH (1993) Motor imagery activates the cerebellum regionally. A SPECT rCBF study with 99mTc-HMPAO. Brain Res Cogn Brain Res 1: 94–99.

Sadeh M, Cohen I (2001) Transient loss of speech after removal of posterior fossa tumors – one aspect of a larger neuropsychological entity: the cerebellar cognitive affective syndrome. Pediatr Hematol Oncol 18: 423–426.

Sasaki H, Kojima H, Yabe I, Tashiro K, Hamada T, et al. (1998) Neuropathological and molecular studies of spinocerebellar ataxia type 6 (SCA6). Acta Neuropathol 95: 199–204.

Schmahmann J (1991) An emerging concept. The cerebellar contribution to higher function. Arch Neurol 48: 1178–1187.

Schmahmann JD (1996) From movement to thought: Anatomic substrates of the cerebellar contribution to cognitive processing. Human Brain Mapping 4: 174–198.

Schmahmann JD (1998) Dysmetria of thought. Clinical consequences of cerebellar dysfunction on cognition and affect. Trends in Cognitive Sciences 2: 362–370.

Schmahmann JD (2000) The role of the cerebellum in affect and psychosis. Journal of Neurolinguistics 13: 189–214.

Schmahmann JD (2001) The cerebellar cognitive affective syndrome: Clinical correlations of the dysmetria of thought hypothesis. Int Rev Psychiatry 13: 313–322.

Schmahmann JD (2004) Disorders of the cerebellum: ataxia, dysmetria of thought, and the cerebellar cognitive affective syndrome. J Neuropsychiatry Clin Neurosci 16: 367–378.

Schmahmann JD (2005) Cerebellar motor and cognitive functions. In: Leiguardia R, Freund H-J, Jeannerod M, Hallett M (eds) Higher Order Motor Disorders: from Neuroanatomy and Neurobiology to Clinical Neurology. Oxford: Oxford University Press; 105–121.

Schmahmann JD (2012, in press) Cerebellum. In: Arciniegas DB, Anderson CA, Filley CM (eds). Behavioral Neurology and Neuropsychiatry. Cambridge: Cambridge University Press.

Schmahmann JD, Pandya DN (1989) Anatomical investigation of projections to the basis pontis from posterior parietal association cortices in rhesus monkey. J Comp Neurol 289: 53–73.

Schmahmann JD, Pandya DN (1997a) Anatomic organization of the basilar pontine projections from prefrontal cortices in rhesus monkey. J Neurosci 17: 438–458.

Schmahmann J, Pandya D (2006) Fiber Pathways of the Brain. New York: Oxford University Press.

Schmahmann JD, Pandya DN (1997b) The cerebrocerebellar system. Int Rev Neurobiol 41: 31–60.

Schmahmann JD, Pandya DN (2008) Disconnection syndromes of basal ganglia, thalamus, and cerebrocerebellar systems. Cortex 44: 1037–1066.

Schmahmann JD, Sherman JC (1998) The cerebellar cognitive affective syndrome. Brain 121(Pt 4): 561–579.

Schmahmann JD, Weilburg JB, Sherman JC (2007) The neuropsychiatry of the cerebellum – insights from the clinic. Cerebellum 6: 254–267.

Schweizer TA, Levine B, Rewilak D, O'Connor C, Turner G, et al. (2008) Rehabilitation of executive functioning after focal damage to the cerebellum. Neurorehabil Neural Repair 22: 72–77.

Scott RB, Stoodley CJ, Anslow P, Paul C, Stein JF, et al. (2001) Lateralized cognitive deficits in children following cerebellar lesions. Dev Med Child Neurol 43: 685–691.

Semel E, Wiig E, Secord W (2003) Clinical Evaluation of Language Fundamentals, 3rd edition. San Antonio, TX: The Psychological Corporation.

Sheslow D, Adams W (2003) Wide Range Assessment of Memory and Learning: Administration and technical manual (2nd ed). Lutz, FL: Psychological Assessment.

Silveri MC, Leggio MG, Molinari M (1994) The cerebellum contributes to linguistic production: a case of agrammatic speech following a right cerebellar lesion. Neurology 44: 2047–2050.

Snider RS, Eldred E (1948) Cerebral projections to the tactile, auditory and visual areas of the cerebellum. Anat Rec 100: 714.

Snider RS (1950) Recent contributions to the anatomy and physiology of the cerebellum. Arch Neurol Psychiat 64: 196–219.

Snider RS (1982) Cerebellar pathology in schizophrenia – cause or consequence? Neurosci Biobehav Rev 6: 47–53.

Snider RS, Stowell A (1944) Receiving areas of the tactile, auditory, and visual systems in the cerebellum. J Neurophysiol 7: 331–357.

Sokolovsky N, Cook A, Hunt H, Giunti P, Cipolotti L (2010) A preliminary characterisation of cognition and social cognition in spinocerebellar ataxia types 2, 1, and 7. Behav Neurol 23: 17–29.

Sparrow SS, Cicchetti DV, Balla DA (2005) Vineland Adaptive Behavior Scales: Survey forms manual, 4th edition. Circle Pines, MN: AGS Publishing.

Sprafkin J, Gadow KD (2000) Early Childhood Inventory: Screening manual, 4th edition. Stony Brook, NY: Checkmate Plus.

Steinlin M, Imfeld S, Zulauf P, Boltshauser E, Lovblad KO, et al. (2003) Neuropsychological long-term sequelae after posterior fossa tumour resection during childhood. Brain 126(Pt 9): 1998–2008.

Steinlin M, Zangger B, Boltshauser E (1998) Non-progressive congenital ataxia with or without cerebellar hypoplasia: a review of 34 subjects. Dev Med Child Neurol 40: 148–54.

Steinlin M, Styger M, Boltshauser E. (1999) Cognitive impairments in patients with congenital nonprogressive cerebellar ataxia. Neurology. 53: 966–73.

Stern TA, Rosenbaum JF, Fava M, Biederman J, Rauch SL (eds) Comprehensive Clinical Psychiatry. Philadelphia, PA: Mosby/Elsevier; 103–119.

Stoodley CJ, Schmahmann JD (2009) Functional topography in the human cerebellum: a meta-analysis of neuroimaging studies. Neuroimage 44: 489–501.

Stoodley CJ, Schmahmann JD (2010) Evidence for topographic organization in the cerebellum of motor control versus cognitive and affective processing. Cortex 46: 831–844.

Storey E, Forrest SM, Shaw JH, Mitchell P, Gardner RJ (1999) Spinocerebellar ataxia type 2: clinical features of a pedigree displaying prominent frontal-executive dysfunction. Arch Neurol 56: 43–50.

Suenaga M, Kawai Y, Watanabe H, Atsuta N, Ito M, et al. (2008) Cognitive impairment in spinocerebellar ataxia type 6. J Neurol Neurosurg Psychiatry 79: 496–499.

Tavano A, Grasso R, Gagliardi C, Triulzi F, Bresolin N, et al. (2007) Disorders of cognitive and affective development in cerebellar malformations. Brain 130(Pt 10): 2646–2660.

Thach WT (1997) Context-response linkage. Int Rev Neurobiol 41: 599–611.

Thompson RF, Bao S, Chen L, Cipriano BD, Grethe JS, et al. (1997) Associative learning. Int Rev Neurobiol 41: 151–189.

Tiemeier H, Lenroot RK, Greenstein DK, Tran L, Pierson R, et al. (2010) Cerebellum development during childhood and adolescence: a longitudinal morphometric MRI study. Neuroimage 49: 63–70.

Tiffin J (1968) Purdue Pegboard: Examiner Manual. Chicago: Science Research Associates.

Turkel SB, Brumm VL, Mitchell WG, Tavare CJ (2006) Mood and behavioral dysfunction with opsoclonus-myoclonus ataxia. J Neuropsychiatry Clin Neurosci 18: 239–241.

Turkel SB, Shu Chen L, Nelson MD, Hyder D, Gilles FH, et al. (2004) Case series: acute mood symptoms associated with posterior fossa lesions in children. J Neuropsychiatry Clin Neurosci 16: 443–445.

Uttner I, Tumani H, Arnim C, Brettschneider J (2009) Cognitive impairment in superficial siderosis of the central nervous system: a case report. Cerebellum 8: 61–63.

van Dongen HR, Catsman-Berrevoets CE, van Mourik M (1994) The syndrome of 'cerebellar' mutism and subsequent dysarthria. Neurology 44: 2040–2046.

van Harskamp NJ, Rudge P, Cipolotti L (2005) Cognitive and social impairments in patients with superficial siderosis. Brain 128(Pt 5): 1082–1092.

Vaquero E, Gomez CM, Quintero EA, Gonzalez-Rosa JJ and Marquez J. (2008) Differential prefrontal-like deficit in children after cerebellar astrocytoma and medulloblastoma tumor. Behav Brain Funct 4: 18.

Wagner R, Torgesen JK, Rashotte CA (1999) Comprehensive Test of Phonological Processing: Examiner's manual. Austin, TX: PRO-ED.

Wassmer E, Davies P, Whitehouse WP, Green SH (2003) Clinical spectrum associated with cerebellar hypoplasia. Pediatr Neurol 28: 347–351.

Watson PJ (1978) Nonmotor functions of the cerebellum. Psychol Bull 85: 944–967.

Wechsler D (2002) Wechsler Preschool and Primary Scale of Intelligence: Administration and scoring manual, 3rd edition. San Antonio, TX: Psychological Corporation.

Wechsler D (2003) Wechsler Intelligence Scales for Children: Administration and scoring manual, 4th edition. San Antonio, TX: Psychological Corporation.

Wechsler D (2008) Wechsler Adult Intelligence Scale: Administration and scoring manual, 4th edition. San Antonio, TX: NCS Pearson.

Wechsler D (2009a) Wechsler Individual Achievement Test: Examiner's Manual, 3rd edition. San Antonio, TX: NCS Pearson.

Wechsler D (2009b) Wechsler Memory Scale: Administration and scoring manual, 4th edition. San Antonio, TX: NCS Pearson.

Weilburg JB, Bear DM, Sachs G (1987) Three patients with concomitant panic attacks and seizure disorder: possible clues to the neurology of anxiety. Am J Psychiatry 144: 1053–1056.

Wells EM, Walsh KS, Khademian ZP, Keating RF, Packer RJ (2008) The cerebellar mutism syndrome and its relation to cerebellar cognitive function and the cerebellar cognitive affective disorder. Dev Disabil Res Rev 14: 221–228.

White M, Lalonde R, Botez-Marquard T (2000) Neuropsychologic and neuropsychiatric characteristics of patients with Friedreich's ataxia. Acta Neurol Scand 102: 222–226.

Wilkinson G, Robertson G (2006) Wide Range Achievement Test 4 professional manual. Lutz, FL: Psychological Assessment Resources.

Williams KT (2007) Expressive Vocabulary Test: Manual, 2nd edition. Minneapolis, MN: NCS Pearson.

Williams RS, Hauser SL, Purpura DP, DeLong GR, Swisher CN (1980) Autism and mental retardation: neuropathologic studies performed in four retarded persons with autistic behavior. Arch Neurol 37: 749–753.

Wisoff JH, Epstein FJ (1984) Pseudobulbar palsy after posterior fossa operation in children. Neurosurgery 15(5): 707–709.

Wolf U, Rapoport MJ, Schweizer TA (2009) Evaluating the affective component of the cerebellar cognitive affective syndrome. J Neuropsychiatry Clin Neurosci 21: 245–253.

Wolff JE, Huttermann U, Askins MA (2007) Quantifying health status outcomes in pediatric medulloblastoma patients. Anticancer Res 27(1B): 523–529.

Wollmann T, Barroso J, Monton F, Nieto A. (2002) Neuropsychological test performance of patients with Friedreich's ataxia. J Clin Exp Neuropsychol 24: 677–686.

Woodcock R, McGrew K, Mather N (2001) Woodcock-Johnson III Tests of Achievement. Itasca, IL: Riverside Publishing.

Yang Y, Kim JE, Lee JS, Kim S (2007) Akinetic Mutism and Cognitive-Affective Syndrome Caused by Unilateral PICA Infarction. J Clin Neurol 3: 192–196.

Zanchetti A, Zoccolini A (1954) Autonomic hypothalamic outbursts elicited by cerebellar stimulation. J Neurophysiol 17: 475–483.

Zawacki TM, Grace J, Friedman JH, Sudarsky L (2002) Executive and emotional dysfunction in Machado-Joseph disease. Mov Disord 17: 1004–1010.

Zimmerman IL, Steiner VG, Pond RE (2002) Preschool Language Scale: Examiner's manual, 4th edition. San Antonio, TX: Psychological Corporation.

Part 3
Imaging of the Cerebellum

5
Prenatal Cerebellar Imaging

Daniel A. Doherty and Deborah Levine

This chapter focuses on prenatal imaging of the posterior fossa and the relationship between prenatal imaging findings and postnatal outcomes. Over the past 25 years, prenatal imaging has improved remarkably, allowing the detailed visualization of brain anatomy by ultrasound and MRI (Fig. 5.1). Despite these advances, little systematic data exist describing postnatal outcomes in fetuses with abnormal posterior fossa imaging. Accurate imaging data correlated with postnatal outcome is critical, since this information is often used to decide whether to continue or terminate a pregnancy. In addition to the inherent limitations in imaging the fetal brain, existing outcome studies suffer from diverse case definitions, small numbers, short duration of follow-up, retrospective study design and lack of standardized neurodevelopmental assessments. Nonetheless, it

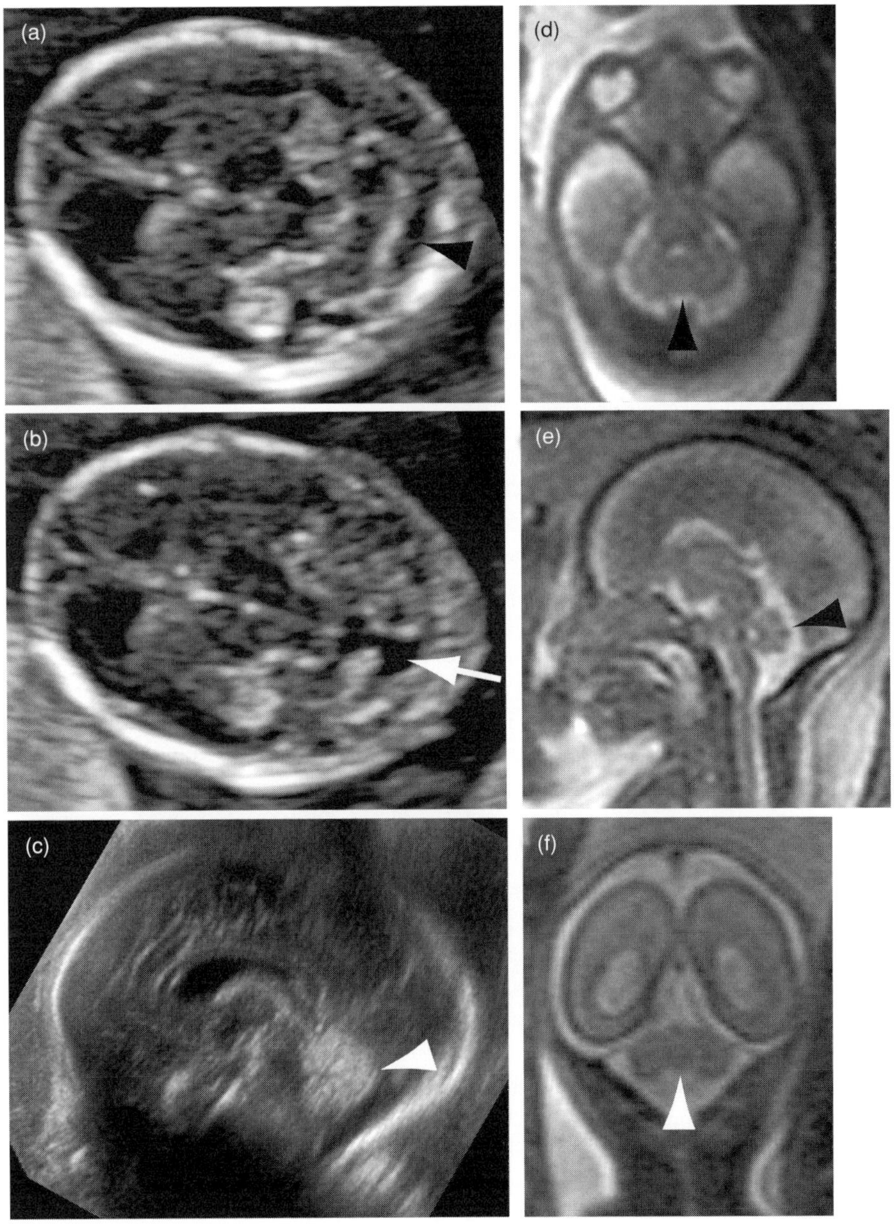

Fig. 5.1. Normal imaging. **(a)** Ultrasound: View through cerebellum at 15 weeks demonstrating the normal appearance of the cerebellar hemispheres and vermis (arrowhead). **(b)** Ultrasound: In the same fetus, angling the probe more inferiorly in the posterior fossa identifies an apparent keyhole deformity with asymmetry of the cerebellar hemispheres, demonstrating the importance of appropriate scanning plane in the fetus. This is a normal fetus, but the images in (b) can be misinterpreted as showing an abnormality due to obliquity of the scanning plane. **(c)** Ultrasound: sagittal view demonstrating a normal vermis in a 35-week fetus (arrowhead). **(d–f)** MRI: axial (d), sagittal (e) and coronal (f) views of a 22-week fetus: demonstrating normal sized vermis with normal foliation pattern (arrowheads). Note normal cerebellar hemispheres flanking the vermis in (d) and (f), as well as normal pons in (e).

is essential to provide the most accurate information possible to support pregnancy decision-making and/or preparation for the birth of an affected child.

Classification

Clinical classification schemes group similar disorders to guide diagnostic work-up, inform prognosis, and define recurrence risk. Specific diagnostic categories are also essential for research studies to identify the underlying causes of posterior fossa malformations. Several classification schemes for midbrain-hindbrain malformations have been proposed based on postnatal imaging findings, inheritance pattern, clinical characteristics, genetic diagnosis, and inferences from normal brain development (Ramaekers et al. 1997; Niesen 2002; Patel and Barkovich 2002; Parisi and Dobyns 2003; Barkovich et al. 2007, 2009). While a developmental/genetic approach to classification is preferred (Barkovich et al. 2009), it is challenging to translate the advances in postnatal classification/diagnosis to the prenatal period, mainly due to the immaturity of the fetal brain, changing appearance of some anomalies over time, and limitations in prenatal imaging.

Historically, the vast majority of the prenatal literature has used three categories to describe prenatal posterior fossa imaging abnormalities (PFA): Dandy-Walker malformation (DWM), Dandy-Walker variant (DWV), and mega cisterna magna (MCM); however, these categories are variably defined in the literature and do not provide very specific information regarding further diagnostic work-up, prognosis, and recurrence risk. Some authors have proposed that PFA represent a continuum, 'Dandy-Walker complex' (Barkovich et al. 1989), rather than distinct categories; however, it is likely that the spectrum of PFA represent overlapping phenotypic expressions of a large number of distinct disorders. Although a prenatal classification scheme cannot approach the sophistication of postnatal distinctions, a clinically useful prenatal classification scheme must rely on the limited imaging information available relatively early in gestation to guide additional work-up and provide prognostic information. While distinguishing classic examples of different malformations is relatively straightforward, when the appearance is not classic, these categories blend into each other. Much of the time, these distinct disorders cannot be distinguished in utero, so we advocate a descriptive approach similar to that proposed by Guibaud and des Portes (2006), combined with assigning a diagnostic category. We agree with these authors that standardized nomenclature should be used to describe complete or partial absence of structures (agenesis), small size of intact structures (hypoplasia), and volume loss pre-existing structures (atrophy).

To improve on the traditional three categories for prenatal PFA, while maintaining a link to the existing outcome studies, we propose the following categories based on the distinctions that can be made by prenatal imaging (similar to those proposed by Malinger et al. 2009): DWM, cerebellar vermis hypoplasia (CVH, historically termed DWV), pancerebellar hypoplasia, pontocerebellar hypoplasia (PCH), MCM, cerebellar dysplasia, unilateral cerebellar hypoplasia, arachnoid/Blake's pouch cyst, and Chiari type I and Chiari type II (Table 5.1). Most of these imaging categories include known genetic or environmental causes (Table 5.2) that cannot always be easily distinguished early in gestation. Additional imaging findings, family history, and genetic testing can aid in identifying genetic causes. When available, the most specific genetic diagnosis or environmental cause should be used for counseling pregnant women; however, the imaging appearance and the underlying etiology likely make independent contributions to the risk of abnormal postnatal outcome and both should be considered.

DWM (Fig. 5.2) is defined by hypoplasia and upward rotation of the cerebellar vermis, dilation of the fourth ventricle in direct communication with a posterior fossa fluid collection, and enlargement of the posterior fossa (Sutton 1887; Dandy and Blackfan 1914; Taggart and Walker 1942). Hydrocephalus and other brain malformations such as agenesis of the corpus callosum can also occur. While mutations affecting *ZIC1/ZIC4* (Grinberg et al. 2004) and *FOXC1* (Aldinger et al. 2009) have been specifically associated with DWM, it can occur in patients with a variety of chromosomal abnormalities and genetic syndromes. The recurrence risk is low (1–5%) and most cases remain unexplained (Murray et al. 1985; Bordarier and Aicardi 1990). Although DWM is the most distinctive of the PFA and clear diagnostic criteria have been proposed, prior prenatal studies have used diverse criteria (see Outcomes studies, below).

CVH (Fig. 5.3). DWV refers to an even more variable spectrum of patients with varying criteria including aplasia/hypoplasia of vermis, connection between the fourth ventricle and cisterna magna, presence of a posterior fossa cyst, and splaying of the hemispheres (Estroff et al. 1992; Keogan et al. 1994; Ulm et al. 1997; Aletebi and Fung 1999; Ecker et al. 2000). The term DWV is so problematic (due to poor specificity and variable outcomes) that many have recommended discontinuing its use in favor of the more descriptive category of cerebellar vermis hypoplasia (CVH); however, measurements quantifying CVH have not been validated with respect to postnatal outcome. CVH should prompt careful imaging for features of Joubert/Meckel syndromes including occipital encephalocele, polydactyly, and echogenic/cystic kidneys. In some cases as early as 22 weeks estimated gestational age, Joubert syndrome can be distinguished by the presence of the 'molar tooth sign' that results from vermis hypoplasia in combination with thick, horizontally oriented superior cerebellar peduncles (Fig. 5.3a,b; Maria et al. 1997; Fluss et al. 2006; Saleem and Zaki 2010) while in other cases (Fig. 5.3c,d) Joubert syndrome may be more difficult to distinguish from other disorders such as very low density lipoprotein receptor-(VLDLR)-associated cerebellar hypoplasia (Fig. 5.3e,f) or CVH of unknown cause (Fig. 5.3g,h). While it is possible to identify the molar tooth sign in some fetuses before 25 weeks' gestation, the reliability of fetal imaging for the diagnosis of Joubert syndrome is not known. In the absence of additional imaging features or a family history, prenatal genetic testing for fetuses with CVH is problematic,

TABLE 5.1
Categories of fetal posterior fossa imaging abnormalities

Diagnostic categories	Hemispheres	Vermis size	Vermis angle	Tentorium	CM size	Pons	Syndromes	Etiologies[1]	Associated findings
Dandy-Walker malformation	Splayed, +/– compressed +/– small	Small or absent	Elevated if vermis present	Elevated	Increased	Normal	Multiple, none typical	*FOXC1*, *ZIC1/ZIC4* del	Agenesis of the corpus callosum, hydrocephalus
Cerebellar vermis hypoplasia/aplasia (formerly Dandy-Walker variant = DWV)	Normal	Small	Variably elevated	Normal	Normal	Normal	Joubert, Meckel	*OPHN1*, Joubert/ Meckel genes, *VLDLR*, *PMM2* (CDG type 1)	Polydactyly, encephalocele, echogenic, cystic kidneys, 'molar tooth sign' late in gestation
Pancerebellar hypoplasia	Small	Small	Normal	Normal or depressed	Normal to increased	Normal	Walker Warburg, Cockayne	CMV, *POMT1*, *ERCC6*, *ERCC8*, *RELN*	Decreased cerebral volume, calcifications, hydrops, lissencephaly, PMG, kinked brainstem
Unilateral cerebellar hypoplasia	One small	+/– small or dysplastic	Normal or elevated	Normal	Normal	Normal or contralateral hypoplasia	PHACE	vascular insult, hemorrhage, infection	Other features of in utero infection
Rhombencephalo-synapsis	Fused	Absent (no midline fluid)	NA	Normal	Normal	Normal	Gomez-Lopez-Hernandez	Unknown	Absent septum, limb, kidney, cardiac and/or vertebral anomalies, holoprosencephaly, ventriculomegaly
Pontocerebellar hypoplasia (PCH)	Small	Small	Normal	Normal or depressed	Normal to increased	Small	Pontocerebellar hypoplasias	*TSEN2*, *TSEN34*, *TSEN54*, *RARS2*, *VRK1*, *PMM2* (CDG type 1), metabolic disorders	No prenatal (can be progressive)
Mega cisterna magna (MCM) axial diameter >10mm	Normal	Normal	Normal	Normal	Increased	Normal	ND	Normal variant	Normal appearing cerebellum and brainstem with enlarged cisterna magna
Cerebellar dysplasia	+/– Small	+/– Small	Normal	Normal	Normal	Normal	ND	*RELN*, *TUBA1A*	Lissencephaly
Cysts Arachnoid cyst Blake's pouch cyst	+/– Compressed, +/– Asymmetric	+/– Compressed	+/– Elevated	+/– Elevated	+/– Increased	Normal, +/– Compressed	ND	None or unknown	Mass effect can change over time. Arachnoid cysts can be off-midline
Chiari type I malformation	+/– Low position	Low position	NA	Normal or low	Normal or small	Normal	Occasional in multiple syndromes	None	None typically
Chiari type II malformation	Compressed, wrapped around brainstem	Difficult to assess vermis secondary to low position	NA	+/– Low position	Small	Normal	Occasional in Waardenburg and other syndromes	Multifactorial, occasionally with chromosomal abnormalities	Open neural tube defect, 'lemon' and 'banana' signs

[1] Most, if not all, categories have been associated with chromosomal abnormalities with the possible exception of arachnoid and Blake's pouch cysts.
CM, cisterna magna; CMV, cytomegalovirus infection; CDG, congenital disorders or glycosylation; NA, not applicable; ND, none documented; PHACE, Posterior fossa malformations, Hemangiomas, Arterial anomalies, Coarctation of the aorta and cardiac defects, Eye abnormalities; PMG, polymicrogyria.

TABLE 5.2
Selected differential diagnosis for conditions associated with abnormal fetal posterior fossa fluid collection

Diagnosis/clinical category	INH	RR	Other prenatal features (often variable)	Outcome
Mendelian: known single genes				
Joubert syndrome *AHI1 ARL13B CC2D2A CEP290 INPP5E NPHP1 OFD1 RPGRIP1L TMEM67 TMEM216 TCTN1, TCTN2, KIF7*	AR	25%	Polydactyly, encephalocele, echogenic or cystic kidneys, thickened nuchal fold	Variable, little overlap with unaffected, risk of retinal, renal and liver disease
Smith-Lemli-Opitz syndrome *DHCR7*	AR	25%	Variable: microcephaly, VM, micrognathia, cleft palate, nuchal thickening, clenched hands, valgus feet, syndactyly, polydactyly, cardiac abnormalities, renal abnormalities, growth restriction	Variable, but often poor with substantial brain involvement
Congenital disorders of glycosylation type 1a *PMM2*	AR	25%	None	Variable intellectual disability and ataxia, minimal overlap with unaffected
Walker-Warburg syndrome *POMT1 POMPT2 FKRP LARGE FCMD*	AR	25%	VM, lissencephaly, ACC, microphthalmia, cleft lip	Severe disability, early mortality with substantial brain involvement
Meckel syndrome *MKS1 CEP290 TMEM67 CC2D2A TMEM216 RPGRIP1L B9D1 TCTN2*	AR	25%	Polydactyly, encephalocele, enlarged echogenic kidneys	Severe disability, early mortality with substantial brain involvement
Cerebro-ocular-facial/Cockayne syndrome *ERCC2, ERCC5. ERCC1*	AR	25%	IUGR, microcephaly	Severe disability, early mortality with substantial brain involvement
OPHN1-associated cerebellar hypoplasia	XL	25%	None	Intellectual disability common in males
VLDLR-associated cerebellar hypoplasia	AR	25%	None	Ataxia and moderate to severe intellectual disability
Pontocerebellar hypoplasia *TSEN2, TSEN34, TSEN54, RARS2, VRK1, PMM2* (CDGS type 1), metabolic disorders	AR	25%	None (late cerebellar volume loss)	Severe disability, early mortality with substantial brain involvement
Chromosomal				
Trisomies, triploidy	NA	LOW	Multiple morphological abnormalities, growth restriction	Generally poor with substantial brain involvement
Velocardiofacial syndrome (del22q11)	AD	VAR[1]	Facial abnormalities	Variable, overlap with unaffected
Other duplications, deletions and translocations	NA	VAR[2]	Multiple morphological abnormalities, growth restriction	Variable, generally poor with substantial brain involvement
Turner syndrome (45,X and rearrangements)	NA	LOW	Cystic hygroma, cardiac abnormalities, growth restriction	Variable, overlap with unaffected
Environmental				
Cytomegalovirus	NA	LOW	Other signs of prenatal infection: echogenic bowel, hydrops, periventricular calcifications, growth restriction	Variable but poor with substantial brain involvement, hearing loss (common), visual impairment (less common)
Rubella virus	NA	LOW	Other signs of prenatal infection	Generally poor with substantial brain involvement
Ethyl alcohol	NA	VAR[3]	IUGR	Generally poor with substantial brain involvement
Clinical categories				
DW malformation, isolated	Sporadic	1–5%[4]	ACC	Variable[5]
Vermis hypoplasia	UNK	UNK[6]	Variable	Variable
PHACE syndrome	UNK ?XL	UNK	Cardiac abnormalities	Variable, overlap with unaffected
Arachnoid cyst	sporadic	LOW	None	Good w/out hydrocephalus or other diagnosis
Blake's pouch cyst	sporadic	LOW	None	Good w/out hydrocephalus or other diagnosis
Mitochondrial disorders	VAR[7]	VAR[7]	None	Variable, overlap with unaffected

[1] Low if de novo, 50% if present in parent.
[2] Depends on specific rearrangement.
[3] Depends on alcohol exposure to subsequent pregnancies.
[4] Murray et al. 1985.
[5] Depends on treatment of hydrocephalus and possibly the degree of vermis dysplasia (Boddaert et al. 2003, Klein et al. 2003).
[6] Can show autosomal recessive, autosomal dominant and X-linked inheritance.
[7] Depends on whether mutation is nuclear or mitochondrial.
ACC, agenesis of the corpus callosum; AR, autosomal recessive; AD, autosomal dominant; DW, Dandy-Walker; INH, inheritance pattern; IUGR, intrauterine growth restriction; NA, not applicable, PHACE, Posterior fossa malformations, Hemangiomas, Arterial anomalies, Coarctation of the aorta and cardiac defects, and Eye abnormalities; RR, recurrence risk; UNK, unknown; VAR, variable inheritance or recurrence risk; VM, ventriculomegaly; XL = X-linked.

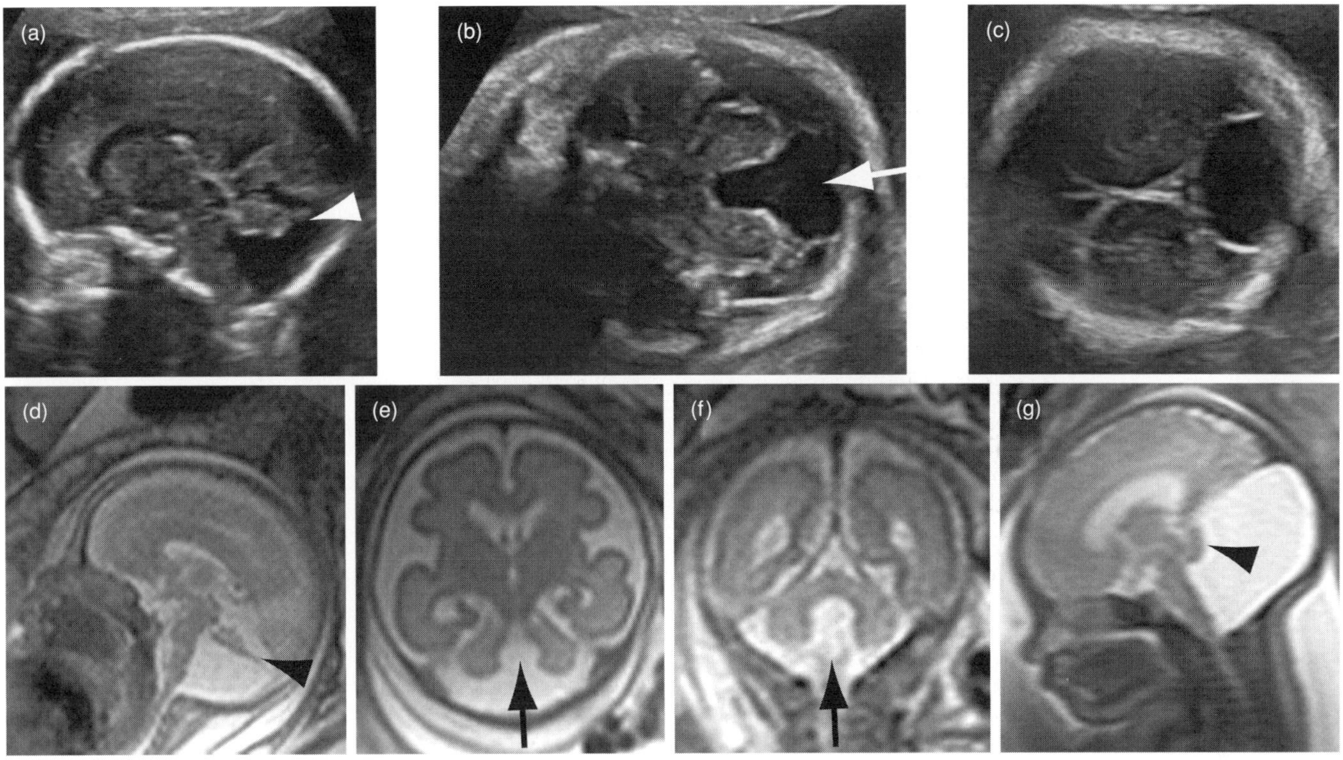

Fig. 5.2. Dandy-Walker malformation. **(a)** Ultrasound: sagittal view showing mildly enlarged posterior fossa, small/upturned vermis (arrowhead) and posterior fossa fluid collection. **(b)** Ultrasound: transcerebellar view showing posterior fossa fluid collection and splaying of the verebellar hemispheres (arrow). **(c)** Ultrasound: steeper angle posterior coronal image showing posterior fossa fluid collection. **(d)** MRI: sagittal T2-weighted image shows elevated vermis (arrowhead) and enlarged cistern magna. **(e, f)** MRI: axial (e) and coronal (f) images show splaying of cerebellar hemispheres (arrows). **(g)** MRI: sagittal image shows a small amount of cerebellar tissue in the midline with a grossly enlarged posterior fossa and elevated tentorium. (a–f) 29-week fetus. (g) 36-week fetus.

because of the large number of genes associated with Joubert/Meckel syndrome and other entities associated with CVH such as *VLDLR*-associated cerebellar hypoplasia (*VLDLR* is the very-low-density lipoprotein receptor gene).

Cerebellar hypoplasia (Fig. 5.4a) is not well defined and encompasses a broad spectrum that overlaps with normal. It is frequently seen in fetuses with trisomy 21. A number of normal fetal reference ranges for cerebellar size have been published (Hill et al. 1991; Sarno et al. 1992; Meyer et al. 1993; Snijders and Nicolaides 1994; Persutte et al. 1997; Winter et al. 2000; Hashimoto et al. 2001; Vinkesteijn et al. 2001; Serhatlioglu et al. 2003; Chavez et al. 2003, 2004, 2006; Sherer et al. 2007). The clinical impact of measurements 2 or 3 standard deviations below the mean with otherwise normal anatomy is unknown. Unilateral cerebellar hypoplasia (Fig. 5.4b,c,d) can be associated with in utero infection, vascular insults, and PHACE syndrome (see Chapter 30) (Metry et al. 2009).

PCH (Fig. 5.4e–h) includes fetuses with decreased size of the pons and cerebellum. PCH is often progressive and often becomes apparent only late in gestation, and the pons hypoplasia can be difficult to identify. Several subtypes have been identified in children, but cannot be distinguished prenatally. Patients with PCH type 1 exhibit spinal muscular atrophy while patients with type 2 exhibit a characteristic movement disorder (Barth 1993, 2000). Type 2 and the more severe type 4 are caused by mutations in the tRNA endonuclease genes, and PCH has also been reported in patients with elevated lactate (*RARS2* mutations), congenital disorders of glycosylation type 1a (*PMM2* mutations) and in patients with lissencephaly caused by mutations in the *RELN*, *POMGnT1*, *POMT1* and *FCMD* genes (Kobayashi et al. 1998; Hong et al. 2000; Yoshida et al. 2001; de Bernabe et al. 2003; Edvardson et al. 2007; Budde et al. 2008). Many patients with PCH do not fit into these established categories (Rudnik-Schoneborn et al. 2003).

MCM (Fig. 5.5) is diagnosed when the cisterna magna measures greater than 10mm on oblique axial images (through the suboccipital bregmatic plane) and the remainder of the posterior fossa anatomy appears normal (Mahony et al. 1984; Nyberg et al. 1991). Isolated MCM is thought to be a normal variant; however, MCM can be seen in association with other CNS abnormalities, extra-CNS malformations, chromosomal disorders, and genetic syndromes.

Arachnoid and **Blake's pouch cysts** can cause elevation of the vermis, an anomaly included in the Dandy-Walker spectrum. Arachnoid cysts are enclosed by the pia and arachnoid layers of the meninges, do not communicate directly with the ventricular system and often occur off the midline (Fig. 5.6). Blake's pouch cysts are thought to result from incomplete

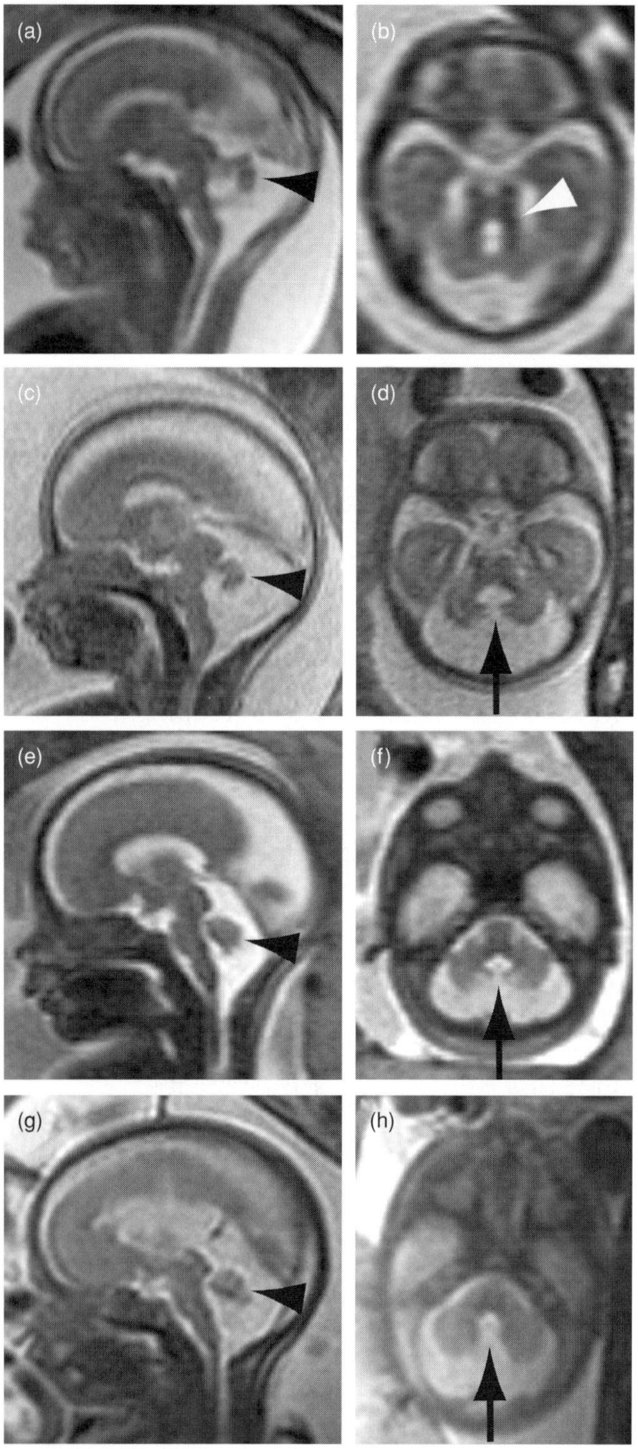

Fig. 5.3. Vermis hypoplasias. **(a–d)** MRI of fetuses with Joubert syndrome at 22 (a, b) and 24 (c, d) weeks showing vermis hypoplasia with elevation of the roof of the fourth ventricle (black arrowheads), horizontally oriented thick superior cerebellar peduncles (white arrowhead) and apparent connection between the fourth ventricle and the cisterna magna (arrow). **(e, f)** MRI of a 26-week fetus with VLDLR-associated cerebellar hypoplasia showing vermis hypoplasia (arrowhead) and apparent connection between the fourth ventricle and cisterna magna (arrow) in a small posterior fossa. **(g, h)** Vermis hypoplasia and apparent connection between the fourth ventricle and cisterna magna (arrow) with a normal-size posterior fossa in a 27-week fetus with agenesis of the corpus callosum, unknown cause.

fenestration of the foramen of Magendie into the cisterna magna. Blake's pouch cysts extend from the fourth ventricle in the midline and sometimes contain choroid plexus (Nelson et al. 2004). Cysts are important to distinguish from other abnormalities, since they are infrequently associated with other anomalies. Often, it is not possible (and likely not important) to distinguish between arachnoid and Blake's pouch cysts, although Blake's pouch cysts are most often midline and can contain choroid plexus (Nelson et al. 2004).

Chiari type I malformation is characterized by inferior ectopia of the cerebellar tonsils without other cerebellar or brainstem anomalies. Chiari type I has rarely been diagnosed prenatally (Iruretagoyena et al. 2010) and postnatally it can be associated with headache and/or neck pain, although it is also seen in asymptomatic patients (Aitken et al. 2009). While Chiari type I is most commonly seen in isolation, it can be associated with skin-covered spinal dysraphism and a variety of genetic conditions. **Chiari type II** is characterized by a small posterior fossa, small to absent cisterna magna, herniation of posterior fossa contents (vermis, tonsils, and/or brainstem) and beaked tectum (Fig. 5.7). It is seen almost exclusively in patients with open neural tube defects, and subsets of patients also have corpus callosum and cortical abnormalities. Of note, the intracranial findings of Chiari type II malformation (the 'lemon' sign, where the frontal bones are slightly indented, best seen in the mid-second trimester, and 'banana' sign where the cerebellum is wrapped around the midbrain) should prompt a careful assessment of the brain and spine for additional abnormalities, particularly an open neural tube defect (Van den Hof et al. 1990). The 'banana' sign is highly specific for neural tube defects, while the 'lemon' sign can be seen in normal fetuses. When a neural tube defect is identified, amniocentesis for karyotype should be considered, and if the diagnosis of an open neural tube defect is in doubt, amniotic fluid alpha-fetoprotein and acetylcholinesterase can be used as confirmatory tests.

Prevalence

Little prevalence data exists for PFAs because of the relative rarity of the many different diagnostic entities in this group of disorders and the diverse diagnostic criteria used. The postnatal prevalence of Dandy-Walker malformation has been estimated to be ~1/30 000 (Hirsch et al. 1984). This estimate is likely to be inaccurate as it is extrapolated from the prevalence of DWM in several cases series of patients with hydrocephalus and a hydrocephalus prevalence of ~1%. The birth prevalence based on Metropolitan Atlanta Congenital Defects Program data has been quoted as 1/5000 (Parisi and Dobyns 2003); however, the primary data for this estimate has not been published. Nonetheless, the prenatal prevalence is almost certainly much higher than the postnatal prevalence, due to in utero demise of fetuses with DWM. The best prenatal data come from Long et al. (2006) who found prevalences of 1/11 574 and 1/8268 births for DWM/V and MCM, respectively, in a large birth defects registry.

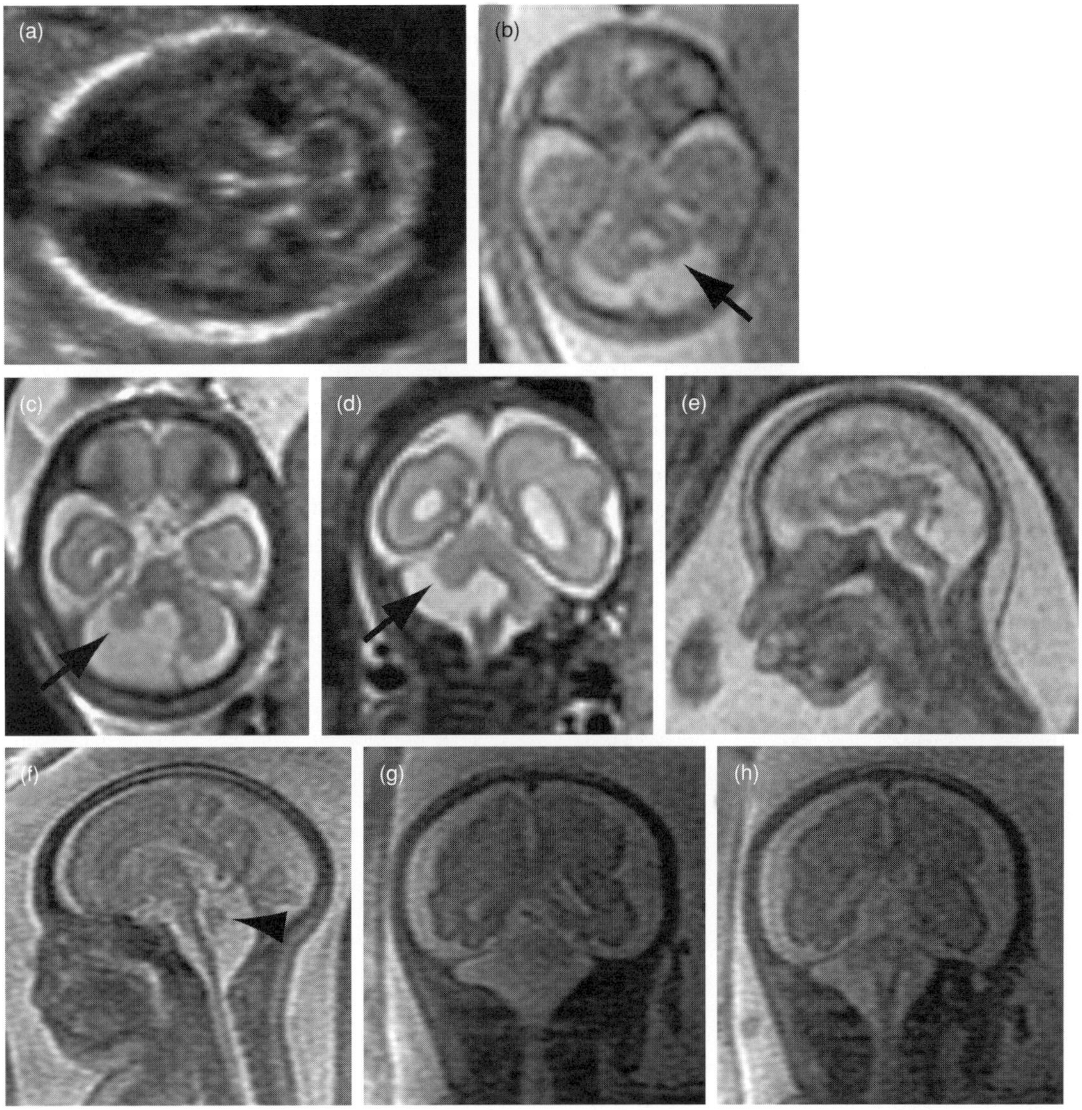

Fig. 5.4. Cerebellar and pontocerebellar hypoplasia. **(a)** Ultrasound: transcerebellar view of cerebellar hypoplasia in an 18-week fetus with trisomy 21. The cerebellar diameter was 2 standard deviations below expected but otherwise appears normal. **(b)** MRI: Unilateral cerebellar hypoplasia (arrow) in a 22 week fetus carried by a woman with presumed viral infection. **(c, d)** MRI: axial (c) and coronal (d) views of unilateral cerebellar hypoplasia (arrow) in a fetus with PHACE syndrome. Note the abnormal supratenotorial appearance of the brain with abnormal cortical development. The baby developed a large segmental hemangioma over the right orbit/cheek and postnatal imaging identified absent right internal carotid artery and aberrant right subclavian arteries. **(e)** MRI: sagittal view of a kinked midbrain and brainstem in a fetus with pan-cerebellar hypoplasia of unknown cause. **(f–h)** MRI: sagittal (f) and coronal (g, h) views of pons and cerebellum hypoplasia/atrophy (arrowhead) in a 32-week fetus due to mutations in the *TSEN54* gene. The imaging findings were confirmed postnatally.

Fig. 5.5. Mega cisterna magna. **(a, b)** Transcerebellar ultrasound view (a) and sagittal MRI (b) of isolated mega cisterna magna in a 29-week fetus. Note normal size and foliation of cerebellar vermis (arrowhead).

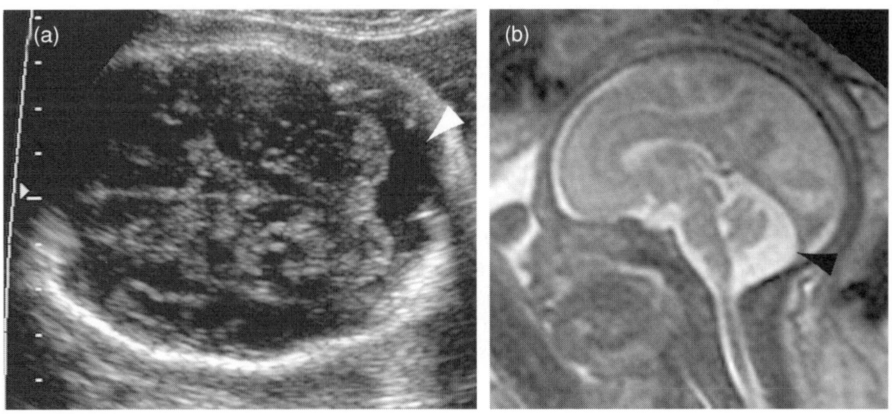

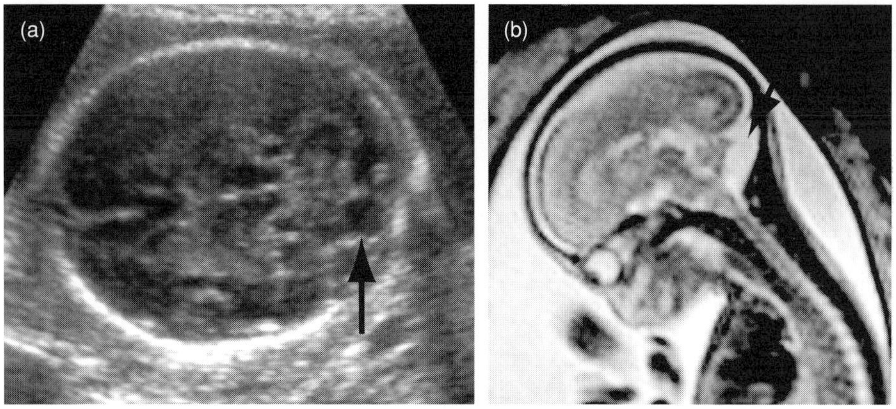

Fig. 5.6. Arachnoid cyst. **(a, b)** Transcerebellar ultrasound view (a) and sagittal MRI (b) of an arachnoid cyst in a 23-week fetus. Note the mass effect on the cerebellum.

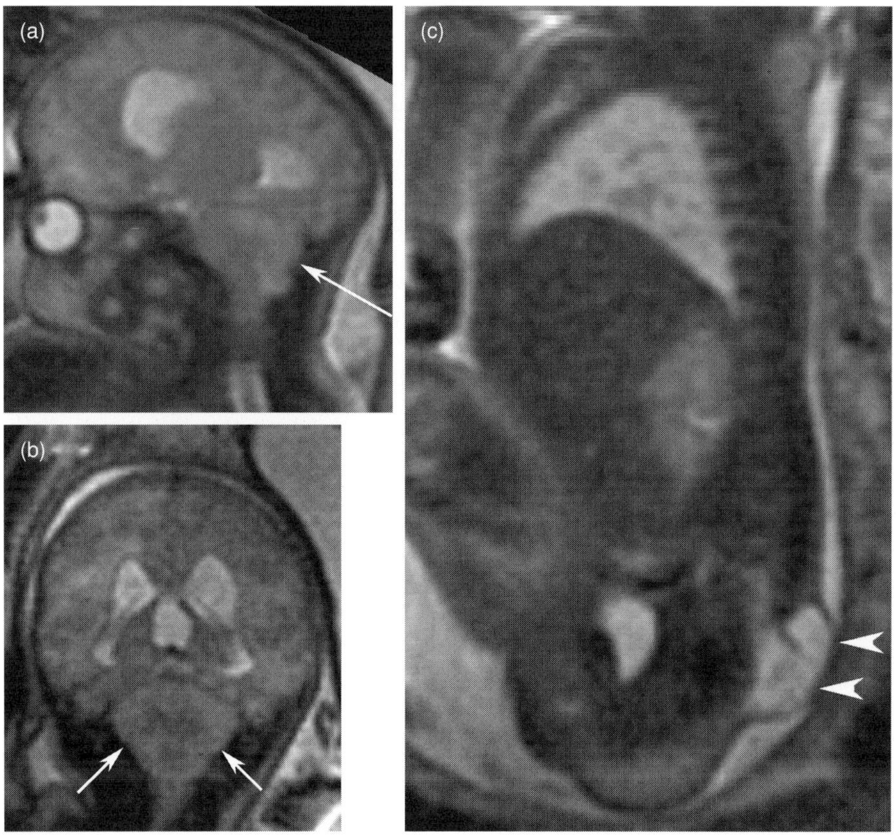

Fig. 5.7. Chiari II malformation. **(a, b)** MRI: sagittal (a) and coronal (b) views of the crowded posterior fossa with inferior ectopia of the cerebellum (arrows). Note that the fourth ventricle and cisterna magna are not visible. **(c)** Cystic lumbosacral myelomeningocele lesion in the same fetus (arrowheads).

Diagnostic evaluation

Ultrasound

The vast majority of pregnancies in Western countries are screened for abnormalities using ultrasound between 16 and 20 weeks' gestation. Traditionally, the standard evaluation of the posterior fossa has consisted of the transcerebellar view to examine the cerebellar hemispheres, vermis, and cisterna magna (American College of Radiology 2007). The normal cerebellum can be visualized in the axial plane by ultrasound after 14 weeks' gestation (Fig. 5.1a). Transcerebellar diameter is a good marker for gestational age and charts of normal cerebellar size (Hill et al. 1991; Sarno et al. 1992; Meyer et al. 1993; Snijders and Nicolaides 1994; Persutte et al. 1997; Winter et al. 2000; Hashimoto et al. 2001; Vinkesteijn et al. 2001; Nyberg et al. 2002; Serhatlioglu et al. 2003; Chavez et al. 2003, 2004, 2006; Sherer et al. 2007), normal vermis size (Goldstein et al. 2001; Malinger et al. 2001; Zalel et al. 2002; Vinals et al. 2005), and cisterna magna size (Steiger et al. 1995; Serhatlioglu et al. 2003; Koktener et al. 2007) have been published elsewhere. While PFA can be suspected during the first trimester (Nizard et al. 2005) anatomic abnormalities of the vermis cannot be reliably identified by ultrasound until after the vermis is expected to 'cover' the fourth ventricle between 16 and 18 weeks' gestation. Prior to that age, an apparent connection between the fourth ventricle and cisterna magna can be seen in typically developing fetuses. Bromley et al. (1994) demonstrated this connection in 56% of otherwise normal appearing euploid fetuses at 14 weeks' gestation and 6% at 17 weeks. Using the appropriate transducer angle is vital, as too steep an imaging plane may lead to overdiagnosis of vermis hypoplasia because the vermis does not extend as inferiorly as the cerebellar hemispheres, particularly before 18 weeks' gestation (Fig. 5.1b). Imaging the cerebellum in a plane with the septum pellucidum ensures that the scanning angle is not too steep.

In addition to the standard views of fetal anatomy recommended in practice guidelines (American College of Radiology 2007) the fetal face and extremities should be assessed in detail. Evaluation of the brain should include views of both lateral ventricles, examination of the cerebral cortex, and midline imaging to assess the size and position of the vermis as well as the corpus callosum. If the fetus is in cephalic position, transvaginal imaging of the fetal head is often helpful for a more detailed assessment of intracranial anatomy. Although difficult to acquire, sagittal views are essential for the evaluation of suspected PFA (Fig. 5.1c). Several papers suggest that three-dimensional ultrasound imaging aids in characterization of the vermis, but whether three-dimensional ultrasound adds clinically useful information has not been fully evaluated (Paladini and Volpe 2006; Vinals et al. 2007; Zalel et al. 2009), and we have not found three-dimensional ultrasound more helpful than acquiring two-dimensional sagittal images.

Fetal magnetic resonance imaging

Multiple studies have shown that MRI adds additional information beyond that available with ultrasound in fetuses with CNS abnormalities (Levine et al. 1997; Morris et al. 2007). This is particularly true for assessment of the fetal cerebellum (with the exception of Chiari type II malformations where spinal assessment by ultrasound is typically sufficient for diagnosis). Fetal MRI provides many advantages over ultrasound evaluation: image quality is much less dependent on fetal position and maternal body habitus, and fetal MRI demonstrates details of the brainstem and cortical brain anatomy better than ultrasound alone (Levine and Barnes 1999; Glenn et al. 2005). Fetal MRI should be performed with T2-weighted single-shot fast-spin imaging technique in three orthogonal planes through the fetal head (American College of Radiology 2010). T1-weighted imaging may supply additional information regarding hemorrhage. Diffusion-weighted imaging is used in some centers, but the additional information provided by this technique is limited.

The timing is governed by the clinical situation. In general, fetal MRI should be performed as late in gestation as possible to provide the information required. For instance, if a pregnant woman is deciding whether to terminate or continue a pregnancy, the MRI should be performed as late in the second trimester as possible, leaving adequate time for counseling and decision-making. If the information is required to prepare for the birth of an affected child, it may be better to wait until the third trimester when the brain is larger and more developed. Alternatively, earlier imaging may be warranted to reduce the stress associated with diagnostic uncertainty.

Measurements

Well-accepted standardized linear measurements of posterior fossa structures are limited to the transcerebellar diameter and cisterna magna. Other measurements are emerging, such as vermis height, vermis width, vermis area, and fastigial angle (Garel 2004; Vinals et al. 2005; Robinson et al. 2007; Tepper et al. 2009; Tilea et al. 2009; Zalel et al. 2009) but the clinical significance of these measurements has not been well evaluated. The reproducibility of these measures and their accuracy in predicting abnormal outcome have also not been adequately assessed.

Additional malformations and genetic conditions

When a fetus is diagnosed with a PFA, it is essential to perform a comprehensive evaluation including maternal health (pregnancy infections, teratogenic exposures – hyperthermia, radiation, alcohol, medications, and trauma), family history of any birth defects and meticulous imaging for additional CNS and extra-CNS abnormalities. Associated imaging abnormalities can provide clues to a specific diagnostic category to guide gene testing or additional laboratory work-up for congenital infections. Genetic defects are common: more than 100 diagnostic entities have been reported in association with fetal PFA, including chromosomal abnormalities, Mendelian disorders such as Joubert and Meckel syndromes, as well as a wide variety of disorders without known cause (Table 5.1). PFA may also be associated with teratogens, diabetes, infection, or hemorrhage. Despite these known causes, the etiology is not identified in the majority of fetuses. Additional abnormalities and/or genetic defects in fetuses with PFA are correlated with poorer outcomes (see Outcomes section below). In particular, pontine hypoplasia, kinking of the brainstem (Fig. 5.4e), cortical malformations, microcephaly, cerebellar atrophy (on serial imaging), and nonobstructive polyhydramnios are associated with poor outcomes.

Correlation with postnatal imaging and pathology

In a study by Limperopoulos et al. (2006), postnatal imaging did not confirm the prenatal diagnosis of inferior vermian hypoplasia in 32% of 19 live-born cases. In a second study of 60 fetuses with PFAs, Limperopoulos et al. (2008) found complete concordance between fetal and postnatal MRI in 23 of 39 fetuses that survived and had a postnatal MRI. No concordance data was presented for 18 terminated fetuses (most with additional malformations) and 3 infants who were not evaluated by postnatal MRI. Discrepancies included prenatal findings not confirmed postnatally (inferior vermian hypoplasia and MCM), as well as postnatal findings not identified prenatally (heterotopias, brainstem hypoplasia, lissencephaly, cerebellar hypoplasia, and hemorrhage).

In general, concordance between fetal imaging and autopsy findings is high (Carroll et al. 2000; Sankar and Phadke 2006) both for CNS and extra-CNS malformations. PFA are a notable exception. Carroll et al. (2000) found discordance in 8 of 14 fetuses while Phillips et al. (2006) found that 26 of 44 well-imaged Dandy-Walker spectrum malformations could not be confirmed by fetal pathology. Phillips et al. (2006) found better concordance between prenatal imaging and pathological diagnosis in fetuses with a 'keyhole' rather than 'trapezoid'-shaped connection between the fourth ventricle and cisterna magna; however, this distinction does not always appropriately categorize fetuses (Fig. 5.3d,f). While these studies emphasize the limitations of prenatal imaging, abnormal imaging findings may still reflect abnormal brain development that is not well assessed on routine pathological evaluation and, therefore, such imaging findings may still be associated with abnormal neurodevelopmental outcome.

Due to changes in appearance over time of many PFAs, we strongly advocate confirmation of prenatal imaging findings by postnatal MRI. It is our practice to perform the postnatal MRI during the first week after birth without sedation. Recently fed and tightly swaddled neonates will hold still for long enough to acquire a full brain MRI including axial, sagittal, and coronal planes, as well as T1, T2, T2 FLAIR, and diffusion sequences.

Multidisciplinary evaluation

Given the complexity of the differential diagnosis of PFA and the sometimes complex medical needs, a multidisciplinary team with expertise in prenatal ultrasound, fetal and pediatric neuroradiology, maternal-fetal medicine, pediatric genetics, neonatology, and pediatric neurology/developmental medicine is often required to adequately evaluate and counsel women carrying these fetuses. Additional specialists may be required to manage other medical issues such as hydrocephalus, cleft lip/palate as well as urogenital, cardiac or limb malformations. In the absence of a family history or characteristic imaging features to guide testing for a specific disorder, screening genetic testing should be performed. Traditionally, a karyotype has been the study of choice and remains the study recommended by the American College of Obstetrics and Gynecology (2009). Array comparative genomic hybridization has the potential to provide a genetic diagnosis in a higher proportion of fetuses compared to karyotype (Le Caignec et al. 2005; Van den Veyver et al. 2009; Valduga et al. 2010) because it identifies much smaller chromosome deletions and duplications. The major drawback is the identification of variants where the implications are not well understood. As the spectrum of copy number variation becomes better documented, this will become less of an issue, and array comparative genomic hybridization will likely become the preferred test, at least for fetuses with major malformations (reviewed in Fruhman and Van den Veyver 2009). Rarely, specific gene testing is indicated, either because the imaging findings are highly characteristic for a particular disorder or, more commonly, when there is a history of a prior affected child.

Outcome studies

The medical literature is replete with case reports and small case series documenting adverse neurodevelopmental and medical outcomes in fetuses with abnormal posterior fossa imaging findings. More recent data has expanded the repertoire of disabilities to include behavioral and social impairments including attention problems and autism (Holroyd et al. 1991; Schaefer et al. 1996; Ciesislski et al. 1997; Ozonoff et al. 1999; Townsend et al. 1999; Schoch et al. 2004; Courchesne et al. 2005; Gross-Tsur et al. 2006). For fetuses with severely abnormal brain imaging findings, multiple malformations and/or a chromosome defect known to be associated with a poor prognosis, this data is adequate for prenatal counseling. In the vast majority of cases, the imaging findings are more subtle and the prognosis much less clear. To date, prospective outcome studies to determine the prevalence of fetal PFA and characterize the spectrum of neurodevelopmental disabilities in children with prenatally diagnosed PFA are lacking. Nonetheless, once an imaging abnormality is identified, a pregnant woman must be counseled as accurately as possible using the available information, particularly if pregnancy termination is being considered.

Bolduc and Limperopoulos (2009) recently summarized neurodevelopmental outcomes in children with cerebellar malformations based on pre- and postnatally ascertained patients; however, data on outcomes in postnatally ascertained patients cannot be extrapolated to prenatal cases, because the vast majority of postnatal patients are imaged to evaluate existing medical or developmental problems. Therefore, we restricted our systematic review of the medical literature to English language papers that reported outcomes (at fetal demise, birth or later) for fetuses with PFA diagnosed prenatally. To reduce ascertainment bias, only papers that reported the entire experience at a center(s) rather than selected cases were included. We excluded fetuses with Chiari type II malformation and occipital encephalocele since these malformations are not generally included in PFA outcome studies. We selected 20 papers that met criteria after reviewing more than 1000 abstracts in PubMed, identified using search terms for ultrasound, pregnancy, fetus, posterior fossa, cerebellum, vermis, brainstem, Dandy-Walker, cisterna magna, and MRI (Table 5.3). Since we did not have access to the primary imaging data, we adopted the diagnostic categories used by the authors. We identified 6 papers on fetuses with MCM, uniformly defined as an anterior-posterior diameter of the cisterna magna more than 10mm, although details of how this measurement was performed were not always given (Comstock and Boal 1985; Nyberg et al. 1991; Haimovici et al. 1997; Ek et al. 1998; Long et al. 2006; Forzano et al. 2007). Definitions for Dandy-Walker malformation (10 papers) (Pilu et al. 1986a; Nyberg et al. 1988; Russ et al. 1989; Cornford and Twining 1992; Chang et al. 1994; Ulm et al. 1997; Aletebi and Fung 1999; Ecker et al. 2000; Kolble et al. 2000; Harper et al. 2007) were diverse (Table 5.3), while Dandy-Walker variant was defined nonspecifically as vermis hypoplasia and/or an apparent connection between the fourth ventricle with infrequent mention of posterior fossa size (7 papers) (Estroff et al. 1992; Chang et al. 1994; Keogan et al. 1994; Blazer et al. 1997; Ulm et al. 1997; Ecker et al. 2000; Harper et al. 2007). In more recent studies, DWM and DWV have been merged into a single category (3 papers) (Has et al. 2004; Long et al. 2006; Forzano et al. 2007) as suggested

TABLE 5.3
Variable definitions of Dandy-Walker malformation and Dandy-Walker variant used in fetal outcome studies

Paper	N	Imaging criteria					
		Vermis a/hypoplasia	4V-CM connection	PF cyst	Large PF	Hydrocephalus	Splayed hemispheres
Dandy-Walker malformation (DWM)							
Pilu 1986	5	+	+	+	0	+/–	0
Nyberg 1988	7	+	0	+	0	+/–	0
Russ 1989	15	+	+	+	+	0	+
Cornford 1992	3	+	+	+	+	0	+
Chang 1994[1]	28	+	+	0	0	0	0
Ulm 1997	24	+	+	0	(+)	0	0
Aletebi 1999	13	+	0	+	0	+	0
Kölble 2000	10	+	(+)	+	+	0	0
Ecker 2000	50	+	(+)	+	0	0	+
Harper 2007	15	+	0	+	0	0	0
Total	170	10/10	7/10	8/10	4/10	1/10	3/10
Dandy-Walker variant (DWV)							
Estroff 1992	17	+	+	0	0	0	0
Keogan 1994	9	0	+	0	0	0	0
Chang 1994[1]	37	+	+	0	0	0	0
Ulm 1997	4	+	+	0	0	0	0
Ecker 2000	49	+	+	0	0	0	0
Harper 2007	40	+	+	–	–	0	0
Total	156	6/7	5/7	1/7	0/7	0/7	0/7

[1] Chang et al. (1994) divided their cases into two categories (complete versus partial absence of the vermis) that we assigned to DWM and DWV respectively.
+, documented present; –, documented not present; (+), inferred but not directly stated; +/–, allowed but not required; 0, not documented; 4V, fourth ventricle; CM, cistern magna; PF, posterior fossa.

TABLE 5.4
Quality of outcome data for Dandy-Walker malformation studies

Paper	Shortest FU >2y	Standardized assessments	Physician/parent report	NDV outcome	Mortality	Autopsy	Postnatal imaging	Medical issues
Pilu 1986	–	NA	NA	NA	+	+	+	+
Nyberg 1988	–	–	–	–	+	+	+	+
Russ 1989	–	–	–	+	+	+	–	+
Cornford 1992	–	–	0	+	+	+	–	+
Chang 1994	–	–	+	+	+	+	+	+
Ulm 1997	–	–	+	+	+	–	–	+
Aletebi 1999	+	+	0	+	+	+	+	+
Kölble 2000	–	–	+	+	+	+	+	+
Ecker 2000	–	–	–	+	+	+	–	+
Harper 2007	–	NA	NA	NA	+	–	+	–

+, documented present; –, documented not present; 0, not documented; NA, not applicable usually due to short duration of follow-up; FU, follow-up; NDV, neurodevelopmental.

by Barkovich et al. (1989). Of note, no published studies in our review included fetal MRI, probably because of the relatively recent availability of this imaging modality.

In general, the published studies are limited by diverse inclusion criteria, small numbers of patients, lack of comparison group and infrequent use of fetal MRI, as well as high termination rates, short postnatal follow-up and lack of standardized outcome measures (Table 5.4). For instance, the largest study to date includes 50 fetuses with DWM and DWV, but reports outcomes for only 3 and 13 live-born fetuses respectively, because of demise and unknown outcome (Ecker et al. 2000). Retrospective study design and ascertainment bias due to other imaging abnormalities may skew the results (usually to more severe outcomes) as well (Pilu et al. 1986a; Nyberg et al. 1988; Russ et al. 1989; Cornford and Twining 1992; Chang et al. 1994; Ulm et al. 1997; Aletebi and Fung 1999; Ecker et al. 2000; Kolble et al. 2000). These limitations contribute substantially to the inconsistencies in outcomes reported for children with prenatally diagnosed PFAs.

Despite these limitations, some conclusions can be drawn. All diagnostic categories are associated with a high risk of having other imaging abnormalities (Table 5.5) and an abnormal karyotype, although the risk of an abnormal karyotype is substantially lower with isolated malformations (Table 5.6).

TABLE 5.5
Additional central nervous system and non-central nervous system malformations commonly identified in fetuses with posterior fossa abnormalities

	N	% isolated	% other CNS findings[1]	% other non-CNS findings[2]
MCM	146	62	7	33
DWV	161	32	24	49
DWM/V	81	33	19	56
DWM	150	30	32	61

[1] CNS findings in addition to PFA and ventriculomegaly.
[2] Likely selection bias for fetuses with other abnormalities. MCM, mega cisterna magna; DWV, Dandy-Walker variant; DWM, Dandy-Walker malformation.

TABLE 5.6
Abnormal karyotypes are commonly identified in fetuses with non-isolated posterior fossa abnormalities

	% abnormal karyotype			
	All fetuses	*N*	Isolated	*N*
MCM	49	47	>14[1]	<14
DWV	43	108	18[2]	11
DWM/V	27	83	33	6
DWM	35	111	6	18

[1] In Long et al. (2006), two fetuses with isolated MCM had chromosomal abnormalities (Trisomy 21 and mosaic trisomy 7q monosomy t9p) without information on how many of the seven fetuses tested had isolated versus non-isolated MCM.
[2] One additional fetus with isolated DWV had an abnormal karyotype without information on how many pregnancies were tested (10 total in the series).

Providing risk estimates for abnormal neurodevelopmental outcome is more difficult because of the large number of pregnancies terminated and children lost to follow-up; therefore, the percentage of fetuses with abnormal postnatal outcome is given as a range to illustrate the uncertainty: the lower number assumes that all fetuses terminated and lost to follow-up were normal, while the higher number assumes that all of these fetuses had an abnormal outcome. Neither of these extremes represents reality, so the true prevalence of normal outcome is somewhere in between, with highest risk in fetuses classified as having DWM and lowest risk in those with MCM (Table 5.7). Restricting the data to fetuses that were not terminated gives narrower ranges, but these results are likely to be skewed toward better outcomes since more severely affected pregnancies are likely to have been terminated. Fetuses without additional CNS or extra-CNS abnormalities have a lower risk of abnormal neurodevelopmental outcome, and isolated MCM may confer no increased risk over fetuses without PFA (Table 5.8).

Although not included in this systematic analysis, several other papers raise important issues. Pilu et al. (1992) demonstrated that transcerebellar diameter measurement is not a sensitive method for identifying PFA. Ulm et al. (1997) suggest that diagnosis earlier in gestation is associated with increased additional abnormalities, abnormal karyotype, and higher risk of adverse outcome; these conclusions have not been evaluated in other studies. Limperopoulos et al. (2006) evaluated infants

TABLE 5.7
Outcomes in fetuses with posterior fossa abnormalities (with or without other imaging findings)[1]

Diagnosis	All fetuses			Fetuses not terminated	
	N	% TOP (range)	% abnormal outcome[2]	*N*	% abnormal outcome[3]
MCM	117	16 (0–30)	32–56	98	38–48
DWV	161	34 (0–100)	30–78	107	44–67
DWM/V	159	66 (56–81)	30–97	54	89–91
DWM	170	54 (14–75)	34–98	79	72–96

[1] Aletebi and Fung 1999, Blazer et al. 1997, Chang et al. 1994, Comstock and Boal 1985, Cornford and Twining 1992, Ecker et al. 2000, Ek et al. 1998, Estroff et al. 1992, Haimovici et al. 1997, Has et al. 2004, Keogan et al. 1994, Kolble et al. 2000, Long et al. 2006, Nyberg et al. 1988, 1991, Pilu et al. 1986b, Russ et al. 1989, Ulm et al. 1997.
[2] Lower number assumes that fetuses terminated and lost to follow-up developed normally, higher number assumes that fetuses terminated and lost to follow-up developed abnormally.
[3] Lower number assumes that fetuses lost to follow-up developed normally, higher number assumes that fetuses lost to follow-up developed abnormally.
TOP, termination of pregnancy.

TABLE 5.8
Outcomes in fetuses with isolated posterior fossa abnormalities (without other central nervous system and non-central nervous system findings)

Diagnosis	All fetuses			Fetuses not terminated	
	N	% TOP (range)	% abnormal outcome[1]	*N*	% abnormal outcome[2]
MCM	90	3 (0–40)	6–33	87	6–31
DWV	43	7 (20–100)	28–49	40	30–45
DWM/V	27	56 (31–79)	11–96[3]	12	25–92
DWM	30	73 (0–100)	13–97[3]	8	50–87

[1] Lower number assumes that fetuses terminated and lost to follow-up developed normally, higher number assumes that fetuses terminated and lost to follow-up developed abnormally.
[2] Lower number assumes that fetuses lost to follow-up developed normally, higher number assumes that fetuses lost to follow-up developed abnormally.
[3] Very broad ranges due to high termination rates.

with a prenatal diagnosis of inferior vermian hypoplasia and found that the prenatal diagnosis was frequently not confirmed on postnatal imaging. While this study clearly demonstrates that inferior vermian hypoplasia is frequently not confirmed by postnatal imaging, it has two significant limitations: (1) it is not possible to know whether the prenatal imaging findings would have been confirmed in the pregnancies that were terminated; (2) it does not evaluate whether there is an increased risk of abnormal outcome in these fetuses, even if the postnatal imaging is considered normal. To our knowledge, no series has been reported in which MRI was performed on all or most fetuses. It may be that MRI will improve the ability to differentiate fetuses with higher and lower risk of adverse outcome. In fact Boddaert et al. (2003) published a small series of children with DWM, indicating that the presence of more normal vermis landmarks is associated with a better outcome.

Counseling

Prenatal counseling is a complex topic outside the scope of this chapter and well addressed in other resources (Uhlmann et al. 2009); however, a number of specific points warrant mention. While this review provides specific numbers for the risk of abnormal neurodevelopmental outcome, these numbers should be used with extreme caution when counseling individual pregnant women. The ranges are broad, and study populations in the medical literature may or may not reflect the situation for a given fetus. How information is framed also makes a difference in how information is perceived by the pregnant woman. For instance, a 20% chance of a poor outcome sounds very different from an 80% chance of a normal outcome, despite being exactly the same objective information. For most women, decision-making relies on a combination of the magnitude of the risk combined with the specific abnormalities and their severity, data not adequately presented in the literature. Rather than giving specific estimates, it is often more effective to explore the woman's tolerance for having a child with particular types of disability, as well as her tolerance for terminating a pregnancy that might result in the birth of a healthy child. When a woman expresses a strong preference about their tolerance for different risks, the decision can become clearer, even with the limited data available. When the woman's preferences are less clear, the decision-making process is more difficult, and it is important to make sure that the woman has received all of the information she needs, appropriate decision-making assistance, ample emotional support, and adequate time for deliberation.

Conclusions

Despite remarkable advances in fetal imaging, prenatal diagnosis, prognostication and counseling for women carrying fetuses with PFA is fraught with difficulty. Current clinical practice based on subjective diagnosis combined with the limited information in the literature leads to high patient anxiety, additional diagnostic evaluation including amniocentesis, and sometimes termination of fetuses with imaging findings that are likely to represent normal variation. In addition, although multiple specific genetic causes for hindbrain malformations have been identified, no genetic diagnosis is identified in a substantial number of prenatal cases, especially in the absence of a family history. Nonetheless, counseling is required to allow for pregnancy decision-making, reduce anxiety (when possible), and/or prepare for the birth of an affected child. The medical literature has numerous limitations including diverse case definitions, short duration of follow-up, high termination rates, non-standardized outcome measures, lack of postnatal imaging, retrospective data collection, and small numbers. Despite these limitations, it appears that several isolated imaging findings (MCM, posterior fossa arachnoid or Blake's pouch cysts) are associated with no or small increased risk of abnormal neurodevelopmental outcome. Other imaging findings are associated with substantially greater risk, especially in association with other imaging abnormalities and/or genetic defects. While fetal MRI is likely to aid in diagnosis and prognostication, its role in predicting outcome for fetuses with PFA has not been systematically demonstrated. Multidisciplinary follow-up after birth or fetal autopsy is recommended to maximize the chance of identifying a specific diagnosis and to provide recurrence risk counseling. Prospective studies of systematically imaged fetuses evaluated with standardized postnatal outcome measures are required to provide adequate information for women carrying fetuses with PFA.

REFERENCES

ACOG (2009) ACOG Committee Opinion No. 446: array comparative genomic hybridization in prenatal diagnosis. Obstet Gynecol 114: 1161–1163.

Aitken LA, Lindan CE, Sidney S, Gupta N, Barkovich AJ, Sorel M & Wu, YW (2009) Chiari type I malformation in a pediatric population. *Pediatr* Neurol 40: 449–454.

Aldinger KA, Lehmann OJ, Hudgins L, Chizhikov VV, Bassuk AG, Ades LC, et al. (2009) FOXC1 is required for normal cerebellar development and is a major contributor to chromosome 6p25.3 Dandy-Walker malformation. Nat Genet 41: 1037–1042.

Aletebi FA, Fung KF (1999) Neurodevelopmental outcome after antenatal diagnosis of posterior fossa abnormalities. J Ultrasound Med 18: 683–689.

American College of Radiology (2007) ACR practice guideline for the performance of antepartum obstetrical ultrasound. ACR practice guidelines and technical standards. Philadelphia, PA: American College of Radiology.

American College of Radiology (2010) ACR practice guideline for the safe and optimal performance of fetal magnetic resonance imaging (MRI). ACR practice guidelines and technical standards. Reston, VA: American College of Radiology.

Barkovich AJ, Kjos BO, Norman D, Edwards MS (1989) Revised classification of posterior fossa cysts and cystlike malformations based on the results of multiplanar MR imaging. AJR Am J Roentgenol 153: 1289–300.

Barkovich AJ, Millen KJ, Dobyns WB (2007) A developmental classification of malformations of the brainstem. Ann Neurol 62: 625–639.

Barkovich AJ, Millen KJ, Dobyns WB (2009) A developmental and genetic classification for midbrain-hindbrain malformations. Brain 132: 3199–3230.

Barth PG (1993) Pontocerebellar hypoplasias. An overview of a group of inherited neurodegenerative disorders with fetal onset. Brain Dev 15: 411–422.

Barth PG (2000) Pontocerebellar hypoplasia – how many types? Eur J Paediatr Neurol 4: 161–162.

Blazer S, Berant M, Sujov PO, Zimmer EZ, Bronshtein M (1997) Prenatal sonographic diagnosis of vermal agenesis. Prenat Diagn 17: 907–911.

Boddaert, N, Klein O, Ferguson N, Sonigo P, Parisot D, Hertz-Pannier L, et al. (2003) Intellectual prognosis of the Dandy-Walker malformation in children: the importance of vermian lobulation. Neuroradiol 45: 320–324.

Bolduc ME, Limperopoulos C (2009) Neurodevelopmental outcomes in children with cerebellar malformations: a systematic review. Dev Med Child Neurol 51: 256–267.

Bordarier C, Aicardi J (1990) Dandy-Walker syndrome and agenesis of the cerebellar vermis: diagnostic problems and genetic counselling. Dev Med Child Neurol 32: 285–294.

Bromley B, Nadel AS, Pauker S, Estroff JA, Benacerraf BR (1994) Closure of the cerebellar vermis: evaluation with second trimester US. Radiology 193: 761–763.

Budde BS, Namavar Y, Barth PG, Poll-The BT, Nurnberg G, Becker C, et al. (2008) tRNA splicing endonuclease mutations cause pontocerebellar hypoplasia. Nat Genet 40: 1113–1118.

Carroll SG, Porter H, Abdel-Fattah S, Kyle PM, Soothill PW (2000) Correlation of prenatal ultrasound diagnosis and pathologic findings in fetal brain abnormalities. Ultrasound Obstet Gynecol 16: 149–153.

Chang MC, Russell SA, Callen PW, Filly RA, Goldstein, RB (1994) Sonographic detection of inferior vermian agenesis in Dandy-Walker malformations: prognostic implications. Radiology 193: 765–770.

Chavez MR, Ananth CV, Smulian JC, Lashley S, Kontopoulos EV, Vintzileos AM (2003) Fetal transcerebellar diameter nomogram in singleton gestations with special emphasis in the third trimester: a comparison with previously published nomograms. Am J Obstet Gynecol 189: 1021–1025.

Chavez MR, Ananth CV, Smulian JC, Yeo L, Oyelese Y, Vintzileos AM (2004) Fetal transcerebellar diameter measurement with particular emphasis in the third trimester: a reliable predictor of gestational age. Am J Obstet Gynecol 191: 979–984.

Chavez MR, Ananth CV, Kaminsky LM, Smulian JC, Yeo L, Vintzileos AM (2006) Fetal transcerebellar diameter measurement for prediction of gestational age in twins. Am J Obstet Gynecol 195: 1596–1600.

Ciesislski KT, Harris RJ, Hart BL (1997) Cerebellar hypoplasia and frontal lobe cognitive deficits in disorders of early childhood. Neuropsychologia 35: 643–655.

Comstock CH, Boal DB (1985) Enlarged fetal cisterna magna: appearance and significance. Obstet Gynecol 66: 25S–28S.

Cornford E, Twining P (1992) The Dandy-Walker syndrome: the value of antenatal diagnosis. Clin Radiol 45: 172–174.

Courchesne E, Redcay E, Morgan JT, Kennedy DP (2005) Autism at the beginning: microstructural and growth abnormalities underlying the cognitive and behavioral phenotype of autism. Dev Psychopathol 17: 577–597.

Dandy WE, Blackfan KD (1914) Internal hydrocephalus: an experimental, clinical, and pathological study. Am J Dis Child 8: 406–482.

de Bernabe DB, van Bokhoven H, van Beusekom E, Van den Akker W, Kant S, Dobyns WB, et al. (2003) A homozygous nonsense mutation in the fukutin gene causes a Walker-Warburg syndrome phenotype. J Med Genet 40: 845–848.

Ecker JL, Shipp TD, Bromley B, Benacerraf B (2000) The sonographic diagnosis of Dandy-Walker and Dandy-Walker variant: associated findings and outcomes. Prenat Diagn 20: 328–332.

Edvardson S, Shaag A, Kolesnikova O, Gomori JM, Tarassov I, Einbinder T, et al. (2007) Deleterious mutation in the mitochondrial arginyl-transfer RNA synthetase gene is associated with pontocerebellar hypoplasia. Am J Hum Genet 81: 857–862.

Ek S, Anadakumar C, Wong YC, Chau TM, Gole LA, Malarvishy G (1998) Enlargement of cisterna magna as an indicator of chromosomal abnormalities in a low-risk Asian population. J Perinat Med 26: 325–327.

Estroff JA, Scott MR, Benacerraf BR (1992) Dandy-Walker variant: prenatal sonographic features and clinical outcome. Radiology 185: 755–758.

Fluss J, Blaser S, Chitayat D, Akoury H, Glanc P, Skidmore M, Raybaud C (2006) Molar tooth sign in fetal brain magnetic resonance imaging leading to the prenatal diagnosis of Joubert syndrome and related disorders. J Child Neurol 21: 320–324.

Forzano F, Mansour S, Ierullo A, Homfray T, Thilaganathan B (2007) Posterior fossa malformation in fetuses: a report of 56 further cases and a review of the literature. Prenat Diagn 27: 495–501.

Fruhman G, Van den Veyver IB (2010) Applications of array comparative genomic hybridization in obstetrics. Obstet Gynecol Clin North Am 37: 71–85.

Garel C (2004) MRI of the Fetal Brain Normal Development and Cerebral Pathologies. Berlin: Springer.

Glenn OA, Goldstein RB, Li KC, Young SJ, Norton ME, Busse RF, et al. (2005) Fetal magnetic resonance imaging in the evaluation of fetuses referred for sonographically suspected abnormalities of the corpus callosum. J Ultrasound Med 24: 791–804.

Goldstein I, Tamir A, Reece EA (2001) The fetal superior cerebellar vermian width in normal, growth-restricted and macrosomic fetuses. J Matern Fetal Med 10: 23–27.

Grinberg I, Northrup H, Ardinger H, Prasad C, Dobyns WB, Millen KJ (2004) Heterozygous deletion of the linked genes ZIC1 and ZIC4 is involved in Dandy-Walker malformation. Nat Genet 36: 1053–1055.

Gross-Tsur V, Ben-Bashat D, Shalev RS (2006) Evidence of a developmental cerebrello-cerebral disorder. Neuropsychologia 44: 2569–2572.

Guibaud L, des Portes V (2006) Plea for an anatomical approach to abnormalities of the posterior fossa in prenatal diagnosis. Ultrasound Obstet Gynecol 27: 477–481.

Haimovici JA, Doubilet PM, Benson CB, Frates MC (1997) Clinical significance of isolated enlargement of the cisterna magna (>10mm) on prenatal sonography. J Ultrasound Med 16: 731–734; quiz 735–736.

Harper T, Fordham LA, Wolfe HM (2007) The fetal Dandy Walker complex: associated anomalies, perinatal outcome and postnatal imaging. Fetal Diagn Ther 22: 277–281.

Has R, Ermis H, Yuksel A, Ibrahimoglu L, Yildirim A, Sezer HD, Basaran S (2004) Dandy-Walker malformation: a review of 78 cases diagnosed by prenatal sonography. Fetal Diagn Ther 19: 342–347.

Hashimoto K, Shimizu T, Shimoya K, Kanzaki T, Clapp JF, Murata Y (2001) Fetal cerebellum: US appearance with advancing gestational age. Radiology 221: 70–74.

Hill LM, Martin JG, Fries J, Hixson J (1991) The role of the transcerebellar view in the detection of fetal central nervous system anomaly. Am J Obstet Gynecol 164: 1220–1224.

Hirsch JF, Pierre-Kahn A, Renier D, Sainte-Rose C, Hoppe-Hirsch E (1984) The Dandy-Walker malformation. A review of 40 cases. J Neurosurg 61: 515–522.

Holroyd S, Reiss AL, Bryan RN (1991) Autistic features in Joubert syndrome: a genetic disorder with agenesis of the cerebellar vermis. Biol Psychiatry 29: 287–294.

Hong SE, Shugart YY, Huang DT, Shahwan SA, Grant PE, Hourihane JO, et al. (2000) Autosomal recessive lissencephaly with cerebellar hypoplasia is associated with human RELN mutations. Nat Genet 26: 93–96.

Iruretagoyena JI, Trampe B, Shah D (2010) Prenatal diagnosis of Chiari malformation with syringomyelia in the second trimester. J Matern Fetal Neonatal Med 23: 184–186.

Keogan MT, DeAtkine AB, Hertzberg BS (1994) Cerebellar vermian defects: antenatal sonographic appearance and clinical significance. J Ultrasound Med 13: 607–611.

Klein O, Pierre-Kahn A, Boddaert N, Parisot D, Brunelle F (2003) Dandy-Walker malformation: prenatal diagnosis and prognosis. Childs Nerv Syst 19: 484–489.

Kobayashi K, Nakahori Y, Miyake M, Matsumura K, Kondo-Iida E, Nomura Y, et al. (1998) An ancient retrotransposal insertion causes Fukuyama-type congenital muscular dystrophy. Nature 394: 388–392.

Koktener A, Dilmen G, Kurt A (2007) The cisterna magna size in normal second-trimester fetuses. J Perinat Med 35: 217–219.

Kolble N, Wisser J, Kurmanavicius J, Bolthauser E, Stallmach T, Huch A, Huch R (2000) Dandy-walker malformation: prenatal diagnosis and outcome. Prenat Diagn 20: 318–327.

Le Caignec C, Boceno M, Saugier-Veber P, Jacquemont S, Joubert M, David A, et al. (2005) Detection of genomic imbalances by array based comparative genomic hybridisation in fetuses with multiple malformations. J Med Genet 42: 121–128.

Levine D, Barnes PD (1999) Cortical maturation in normal and abnormal fetuses as assessed with prenatal MR imaging. Radiology 210: 751–758.

Levine D, Barnes PD, Madsen JR, Li W, Edelman RR (1997) Fetal central nervous system anomalies: MR imaging augments sonographic diagnosis. Radiology 204: 635–642.

Limperopoulos C, Robertson RL, Estroff JA, Barnewolt C, Levine D, Bassan H, du Plessis AJ (2006) Diagnosis of inferior vermian hypoplasia by fetal magnetic resonance imaging: potential pitfalls and neurodevelopmental outcome. Am J Obstet Gynecol 194: 1070–1076.

Limperopoulos C, Robertson RL Jr, Khwaja OS, Robson CD, Estroff JA, Barnewolt C, et al. (2008) How accurately does current fetal imaging identify posterior fossa anomalies? AJR Am J Roentgenol 190: 1637–1643.

Long A, Moran P, Robson S (2006) Outcome of fetal cerebral posterior fossa anomalies. Prenat Diagn 26: 707–710.

Mahony BS, Callen PW, Filly RA, Hoddick WK (1984) The fetal cisterna magna. Radiology 153: 773–776.

Malinger G, Ginath S, Lerman-Sagie T, Watemberg N, Lev D, Glezerman M (2001) The fetal cerebellar vermis: normal development as shown by transvaginal ultrasound. Prenat Diagn 21: 687–692.

Malinger G, Lev D, Lerman-Sagie T (2009) The fetal cerebellum: pitfalls in diagnosis and management. Prenat Diagn 29: 372–380.

Maria BL, Hoang KB, Tusa RJ, Mancuso AA, Hamed LM, Quisling RG, et al. (1997) 'Joubert syndrome' revisited: key ocular motor signs with magnetic resonance imaging correlation. J Child Neurol 12: 423–430.

Metry D, Heyer G, Hess C, Garzon M, Haggstrom A, Frommelt P, et al. (2009) Consensus Statement on Diagnostic Criteria for PHACE Syndrome. Pediatrics 124: 1447–1456.

Meyer WJ, Gauthier DW, Goldenberg B, Santolaya J, Sipos J, Cattledge F (1993) The fetal transverse cerebellar diameter/abdominal circumference ratio: a gestational age-independent method of assessing fetal size. J Ultrasound Med 12: 379–382.

Morris JE, Rickard S, Paley MN, Griffiths PD, Rigby A, Whitby EH (2007) The value of in-utero magnetic resonance imaging in ultrasound diagnosed foetal isolated cerebral ventriculomegaly. Clin Radiol 62: 140–144.

Murray JC, Johnson JA, Bird TD (1985) Dandy-Walker malformation: etiologic heterogeneity and empiric recurrence risks. Clin Genet 28: 272–283.

Nelson, MD, Jr., Maher, K & Gilles, FH (2004) A different approach to cysts of the posterior fossa. Pediatr Radiol 34: 720–732.

Niesen CE (2002) Malformations of the posterior fossa: current perspectives. Sem Pediatr Neurol 9: 320–334.

Nizard J, Bernard JP, Ville Y (2005) Fetal cystic malformations of the posterior fossa in the first trimester of pregnancy. Fetal Diagn Ther 20: 146–151.

Nyberg DA, Cyr DR, Mack LA, Fitzsimmons J, Hickok D, Mahony BS (1988) The Dandy-Walker malformation prenatal sonographic diagnosis and its clinical significance. J Ultrasound Med 7: 65–71.

Nyberg DA, Mahony BS, Hegge FN, Hickok D, Luthy DA, Kapur R (1991) Enlarged cisterna magna and the Dandy-Walker malformation: factors associated with chromosome abnormalities. Obstet Gynecol 77: 436–442.

Nyberg DA, McGahan JP, Pretorius DH, Pilu G (2002) Diagnostic Imaging of Fetal Anomalies. Philadelphia, PA: Lippincott Williams & Wilkins.

Ozonoff S, Williams BJ, Gale S, Miller JN (1999) Autism and autistic behavior in Joubert syndrome. J Child Neurol 14: 636–641.

Paladini D, Volpe P (2006) Posterior fossa and vermian morphometry in the characterization of fetal cerebellar abnormalities: a prospective three-dimensional ultrasound study. Ultrasound Obstet Gynecol 27: 482–489.

Parisi MA, Dobyns WB (2003) Human malformations of the midbrain and hindbrain: review and proposed classification scheme. Mol Genet Metab 80: 36–53.

Patel S, Barkovich A (2002) Analysis and classification of cerebellar malformations. AJNR Am J Neuroradiol 23: 1074–1087.

Persutte WH, Coury A, Hobbins JC (1997) Correlation of fetal frontal lobe and transcerebellar diameter measurements: the utility of a new prenatal sonographic technique. Ultrasound Obstet Gynecol 10: 94–97.

Phillips JJ, Mahony BS, Siebert JR, Lalani T, Fligner CL, Kapur RP (2006) Dandy-Walker malformation complex: correlation between ultrasonographic diagnosis and postmortem neuropathology. Obstet Gynecol 107: 685–693.

Pilu G, Goldstein I, Reece EA, Perolo A, Foschini MP, Hobbins JC, Bovicelli L (1992) Sonography of fetal Dandy-Walker malformation: a reappraisal. Ultrasound Obstet Gynecol 2: 151–157.

Pilu G, Romero R, De Palma L, Rizzo N, Jeanty P, Copel JA, et al. (1986a) Antenatal diagnosis and obstetric management of Dandy-Walker syndrome. J Reprod Med 31: 1017–1022.

Pilu G, Romero R, Reece EA, Jeanty P, Hobbins JC (1986b) The prenatal diagnosis of Robin anomalad. Am J Obstet Gynecol 154: 630–632.

Ramaekers VT, Heimann G, Reul J, Thron A, Jaeken J (1997) Genetic disorders and cerebellar structural abnormalities in childhood. Brain 120: 1739–1751.

Robinson AJ, Blaser S, Toi A, Chitayat D, Halliday W, Pantazi S, et al. (2007) The fetal cerebellar vermis: assessment for abnormal development by ultrasonography and magnetic resonance imaging. Ultrasound Q 23: 211–223.

Rudnik-Schoneborn S, Sztriha L, Aithala GR, Houge G, Laegreid LM, Seeger J, et al. (2003) Extended phenotype of pontocerebellar hypoplasia with infantile spinal muscular atrophy. Am J Med Genet A 117: 10–17.

Russ PD, Pretorius DH, Johnson MJ (1989) Dandy-Walker syndrome: a review of fifteen cases evaluated by prenatal sonography. Am J Obstet Gynecol 161: 401–406.

Saleem SN, Zaki MS (2010) Role of MR imaging in prenatal diagnosis of pregnancies at risk for Joubert syndrome and related cerebellar disorders. AJNR Am J Neuroradiol 31: 424–429.

Sankar VH, Phadke SR (2006) Clinical utility of fetal autopsy and comparison with prenatal ultrasound findings. J Perinatol 26: 224–229.

Sarno AP, Rose GS, Harrington RA (1992) Coronal transcerebellar diameter: an alternate view. Ultrasound Obstet Gynecol 2: 158–161.

Schaefer GB, Thompson JN, Bodensteiner JB, McConnell JM, Kimberling WJ, Gay CT, et al. (1996) Hypoplasia of the cerebellar vermis in neurogenetic syndromes. Ann Neurol 39: 382–385.

Schoch B, Gorissen B, Richter S, Ozimek A, Kaiser O, Dimitrova A, et al. (2004) Do children with focal cerebellar lesions show deficits in shifting attention? J Neurophysiol 92: 1856–1866.

Serhatlioglu S, Kocakoc E, Kiris A, Sapmaz E, Boztosun Y, Bozgeyik Z (2003) Sonographic measurement of the fetal cerebellum, cisterna magna, and cavum septum pellucidum in normal fetuses in the second and third trimesters of pregnancy. J Clin Ultrasound 31: 194–200.

Sherer DM, Sokolovski M, Dalloul M, Pezzullo JC, Osho JA, Abulafia O (2007) Nomograms of the axial fetal cerebellar hemisphere circumference and area throughout gestation. Ultrasound Obstet Gynecol 29: 32–37.

Snijders RJ, Nicolaides KH (1994) Fetal biometry at 14–40 weeks' gestation. Ultrasound Obstet Gynecol 4: 34–48.

Steiger RM, Porto M, Lagrew DC, Randall R (1995) Biometry of the fetal cisterna magna: estimates of the ability to detect trisomy 18. Ultrasound Obstet Gynecol 5: 384–390.

Sutton JB (1887) The lateral recesses of the fourth ventricle: their relation to certain cysts and tumors of the cerebellum and to occipital meningocele. Brain 9: 352–361.

Taggart JK, Walker AE (1942) Congenital atresia of the foramens of Luschka and Magendie. Arch. Neurol. Psychiatry 48: 583–612.

Tepper R, Kidron D, Hershkovitz R (2009) Sonographic measurements of the fetal fastigium between 20 and 40 weeks' gestation. J Ultrasound Med 28: 1657–1661.

Tilea B, Alberti C, Adamsbaum C, Armoogum P, Oury JF, Cabrol D, et al. (2009) Cerebral biometry in fetal magnetic resonance imaging: new reference data. Ultrasound Obstet Gynecol 33: 173–181.

Townsend, J, Courchesne E, Covington J, Westerfield M, Harris NS, Lyden P, et al. (1999) Spatial attention deficits in patients with acquired or developmental cerebellar abnormality. J Neurosci 19: 5632–5643.

Uhlmann WR, Schuette JL, Yashar B (2009) A Guide to Genetic Counseling. Hoboken, NJ: Wiley-Blackwell.

Ulm B, Ulm MR, Deutinger J, Bernaschek G (1997) Dandy-Walker malformation diagnosed before 21 weeks of gestation: associated malformations and chromosomal abnormalities. Ultrasound Obstet Gynecol 10: 167–170.

Valduga M, Philippe C, Bach Segura P, Thiebaugeorges O, Miton A, Beri M, et al. (2010) A retrospective study by oligonucleotide array-CGH analysis in 50 fetuses with multiple malformations. Prenat Diagn 30: 333–341.

Van den Hof MC, Nicolaides KH, Campbell J, Campbell S (1990) Evaluation of the lemon and banana signs in one hundred thirty fetuses with open spina bifida. Am J Obstet Gynecol 162: 322–327.

Van den Veyver IB, Patel A, Shaw CA, Pursley AN, Kang SH, Simovich MJ, et al. (2009) Clinical use of array comparative genomic hybridization (aCGH) for prenatal diagnosis in 300 cases. Prenat Diagn 29: 29–39.

Vinals F, Munoz M, Naveas R, Shalper J, Giuliano A (2005) The fetal cerebellar vermis: anatomy and biometric assessment using volume contrast imaging in the C-plane (VCI-C). Ultrasound Obstet Gynecol 26: 622–627.

Vinals F, Munoz M, Naveas R, Giuliano A (2007) Transfrontal three-dimensional visualization of midline cerebral structures. Ultrasound Obstet Gynecol 30: 162–168.

Vinkesteijn AS, Jansen CL, Los FJ, Mulder PG, Wladimiroff JW (2001) Fetal transcerebellar diameter and chromosomal abnormalities. Ultrasound Obstet Gynecol 17: 502–505.

Winter TC, Ostrovsky AA, Komarniski CA, Uhrich SB (2000) Cerebellar and frontal lobe hypoplasia in fetuses with trisomy 21: usefulness as combined US markers. Radiology 214: 533–538.

Yoshida A, Kobayashi K, Manya H, Taniguchi K, Kano H, Mizuno M, et al. (2001) Muscular dystrophy and neuronal migration disorder caused by mutations in a glycosyltransferase, POMGnT1. Dev Cell 1: 717–724.

Zalel Y, Seidman DS, Brand N, Lipitz S, Achiron R (2002) The development of the fetal vermis: an in-utero sonographic evaluation. Ultrasound Obstet Gynecol 19: 136–139.

Zalel Y, Yagel S, Achiron R, Kivilevich Z, Gindes L (2009) Three-dimensional ultrasonography of the fetal vermis at 18 to 26 weeks' gestation: time of appearance of the primary fissure. J Ultrasound Med 28: 1–8.

6 Neuroimaging of the Posterior Fossa

Thierry A.G.M. Huisman

For many decades the cerebellum has been neglected by mainstream neuroradiology and neuroradiological research. Most of the research has focused on the supratentorial brain. More recently, research groups have begun using high-end anatomic and functional non-invasive imaging techniques (Manto 2008; Timmann et al. 2010) to unravel the mystery of the cerebellum.

Classic, anatomic imaging techniques such as ultrasonography, computed tomography (CT), and magnetic resonance imaging (MRI) can easily depict the cerebellar macro-anatomy. The cerebellum consists of a midline vermis, three pairs of cerebellar peduncles (inferior, middle, and superior), two lateral hemispheres with about 260 folia and four pairs of gray matter nuclei (dentate, emboliform, globose, and fastigial nuclei). The anatomic imaging techniques are however limited for the functional exploration of the cerebellum. Many of the functional cerebellar processes are highly complex and poorly or incompletely understood.

Given the complex functional processes and unique cerebellar circuitry, it is evident that high resolution anatomic imaging should be combined with functional imaging sequences to better understand the normal and abnormal cerebellum.

In the current chapter all clinically available imaging modalities including ultrasonography, CT, and anatomic and functional MRI will be discussed.

Ultrasonography

Ultrasound examination of the neonatal brain is a well-established technique that allows safe study of the neonatal brain without using ionizing radiation (Daneman et al. 2006; Steggerda et al. 2009; van Wezel-Meijler et al. 2010). In addition, ultrasound studies rarely require patient sedation, can be performed at the bedside, are relatively inexpensive, and can be repeated as often as necessary (serial imaging). Ultrasound studies take advantage of the various fontanels that serve as acoustic windows to explore the cranial vault. Image quality is highly dependent on the skills of the sonographer and the chosen imaging technique. Studies should take advantage of high resolution, real-time 2D and 3D ultrasound machines, multi-frequency transducers or different frequency transducers (5, 7.5, and 10MHz), an optimal match between the footprint of the transducer and the size of the fontanel, and a meticulous technique with optimized imaging settings (Daneman et al. 2006). It goes without saying that the sonographer should be familiar with normal and abnormal anatomy. Typically the anterior fontanel is used to study the brain in predefined coronal and sagittal planes (Fig. 6.1a,b). The close proximity of the supratentorial brain to the transducer allows detailed imaging of the ventricular system and periventricular white matter. The subarachnoid space, cortex, and immediate subcortical white matter can be studied in even higher detail using high frequency linear transducers.

Detailed evaluation of the posterior fossa structures is however limited via the anterior fontanel. The larger distance between the transducer and the posterior fossa reduces image quality. In addition, the echogenic tentorium and vermis further impede image detail. However, by taking advantage of the additional fontanels closer to the posterior fossa, such as the mastoid and posterior fontanels, detailed images of the posterior fossa and its contents can be achieved (Steggerda et al. 2009; van Wezel-Meijler et al. 2010).

The mastoid fontanel is located at the junction of the parietal, temporal, and occipital bones (Steggerda et al. 2009; van Wezel-Meijler et al. 2010). Typically multilevel axial and coronal images are obtained covering the entire brainstem and cerebellum (Fig. 6.1c,d). The posterior fontanel is located at the junction of the lambdoid and sagittal suture and is well suited to study the occipital lobes and posterior fossa. In addition, the transosseous approach through the thin temporal bone about 1cm superior to the external auditory may be considered for additional imaging.

On sagittal images the vermis is recognized as a hyperechogenic structure immediately posterior to the hypoechogenic triangular-shaped fourth ventricle. The adjacent posterior brainstem and mesencephalon are mildly hypoechogenic while the anterior located pons appears mildly hyperechogenic. The hyperechogenic signal of the vermis and pons result from the densely packed white matter tracts that run in an axial (left to right) plane, perpendicular to the course of the ultrasound waves. On more lateral sagittal views the cerebellar hemispheres are characterized by a hyperechogenic cortex surrounding the mildly hypoechogenic cerebellar white matter. Dorsally and inferior to the cerebellum, a hypoechogenic cerebrospinal fluid (CSF) collection is usually noted (cisterna magna). Axial images through the brainstem (via the mastoid fontanel) typically show the posterior pons as mildly hyperechogenic (descending corticospinal tracts) while the anterior pons is heterogeneous hypo-hyperechogenic. The cerebellar fissures appear hyperechogenic, likely to be due to reflections of the arachnoidea and pia mater.

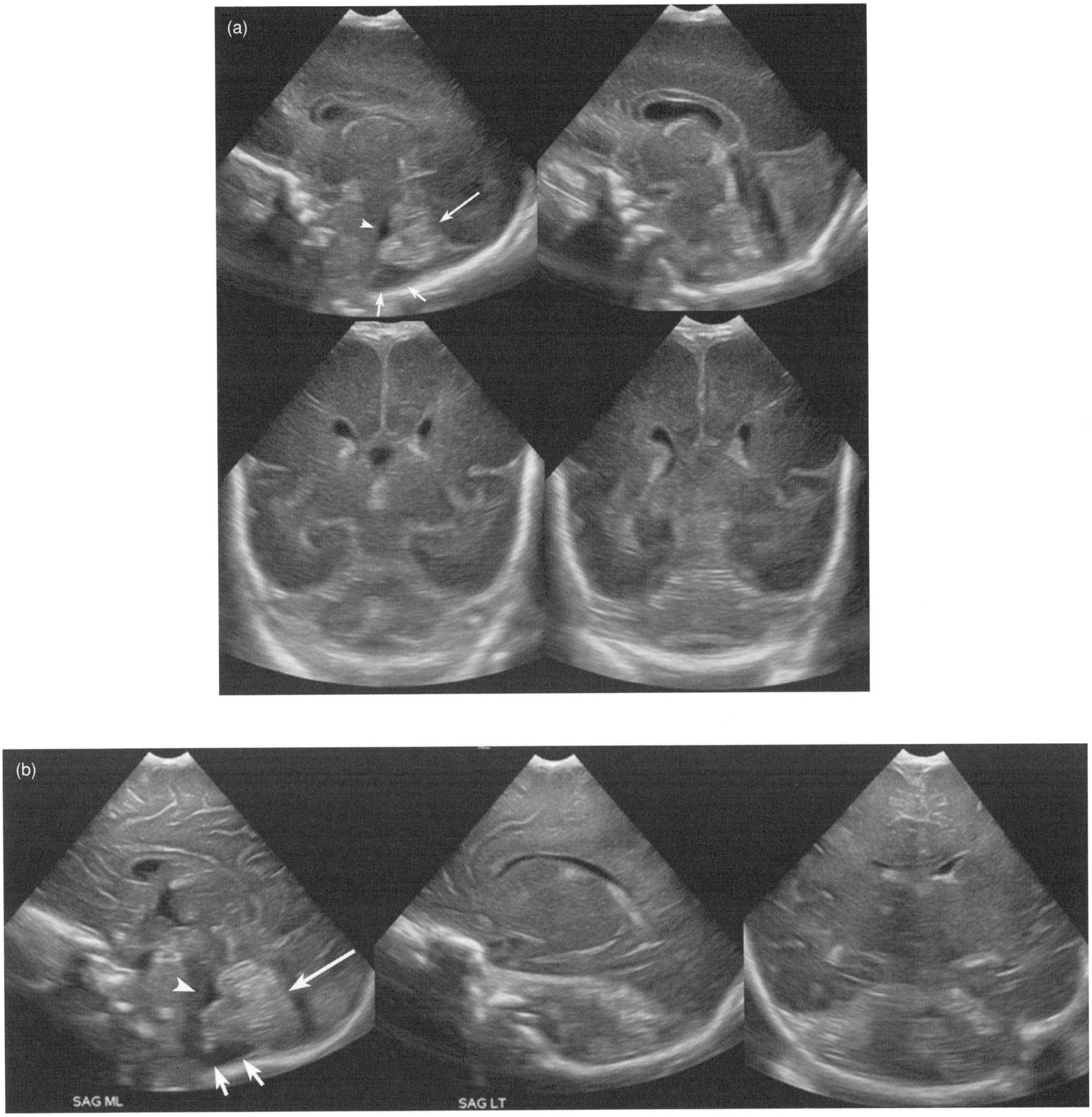

Fig. 6.1(a, b). High resolution sagittal and coronal ultrasonography of the brain in **(a)** a preterm and **(b)** a term neonate scanned through the anterior fontanel. The midline vermis appears hyperechogenic on sagittal views (large arrow), the fourth ventricle is filled with hypoechogenic cerebrospinal fluid (CSF) (arrowhead), and the cerebral cortex is mildly hyperechogenic compared to the hypoechogenic cerebellar white matter. The cisterna magna is filled with hypoechogenic CSF (small arrows). The cerebral surface is smooth in the preterm neonate; the sulcal pattern is more complex in the term neonate.

Multiple lesions can be depicted in the neonatal cerebellum if the appropriate technique and acoustic window is used (Daneman et al. 2006). This may include intraventricular hemorrhage, ventricular dilatation, acquired cerebellar lesions (e.g. hemorrhage, ischemia, and abscess) as well as a variety of congenital malformations (e.g., Dandy-Walker, Chiari type II) (Fig. 6.2).

Computed tomography

Computed tomography is frequently considered to be the first-line imaging modality in children who present with a sudden onset of neurologic symptoms, in children who have suffered an acute trauma, and in children with skull base and craniocervical junction anomalies. Modern helical CT units allow study of the entire brain and skull within a few seconds,

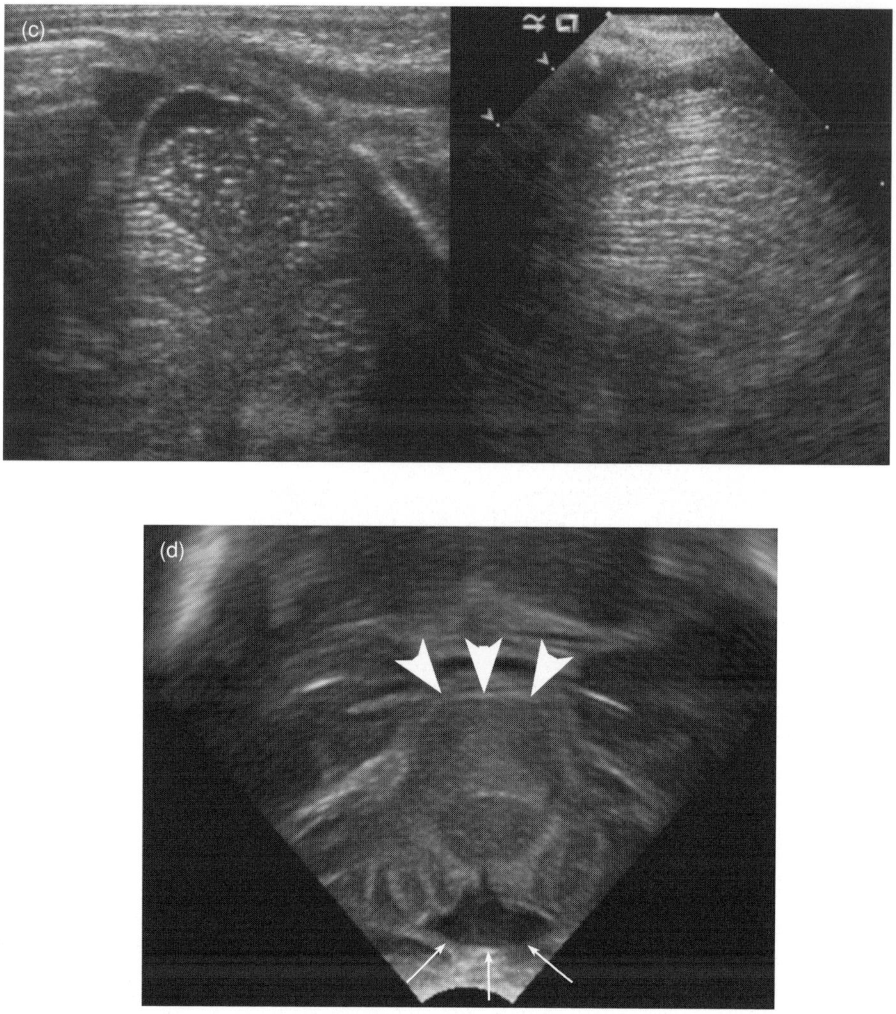

Fig. 6.1(c, d). **(c)** High resolution axial and coronal ultrasonography in a term neonate through the temporal fontanel shows the typical parallel course of the cerebellar fissures. **(d)** The temporal fontanel also allows detailed visualization of the pons (arrowheads) and lower brainstem in an axial plane. The brainstem is seen anteriorly to the caudal extension of the slightly hyperechogenic, slit-like fourth ventricle. A mildly prominent midline, dorsally located mega cisterna magna (arrows) is seen outlining the inferior cerebellar hemispheres.

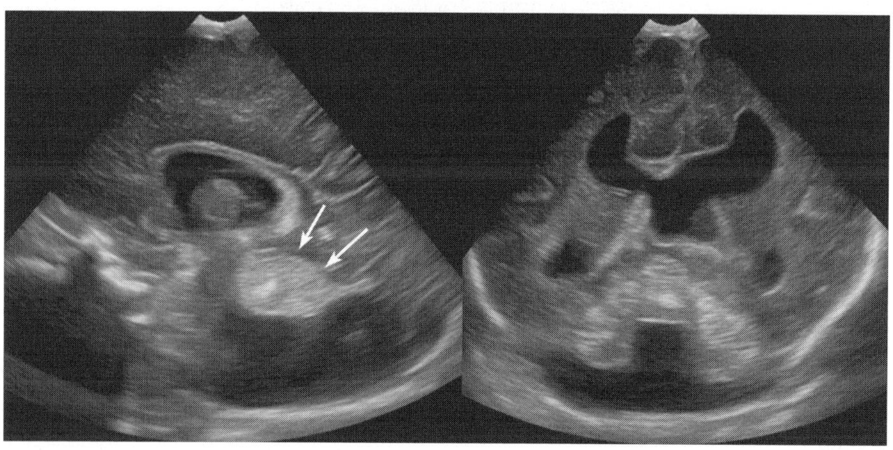

Fig. 6.2. Sagittal and coronal ultrasonography of the brain in a neonate with a Dandy-Walker malformation. The hypoplastic vermis is hyperechogenic and appears rotated upwards (arrows); the fourth ventricle is enlarged and extends dorsally. Mild supratentorial hydrocephalus is seen with thin corpus callosum.

frequently obviating the need for sedation in young children. In addition, the acquired volume datasets allow reconstruction of both the soft tissues and the skull in multiple secondary planes as well as three-dimensionally (Fig. 6.3a,b,c). Despite the fact that multiple hard and software approaches have been developed to reduce or limit radiation dose, CT still poses a significant radiation burden for the pediatric population. The child's brain and in particular the pediatric eye lens are more susceptible to the deleterious effects of radiation than the adult brain and eye lenses. CT should consequently be used with caution and alternative imaging modalities including ultrasonography and MRI should be used whenever possible.

On CT, the cerebellar white matter typically appears hypodense in comparison with the mildly hyperdense

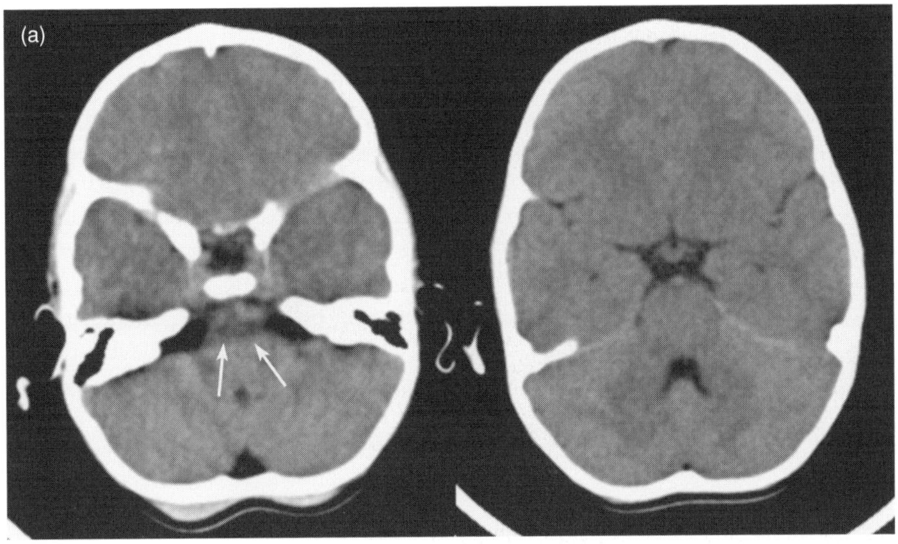

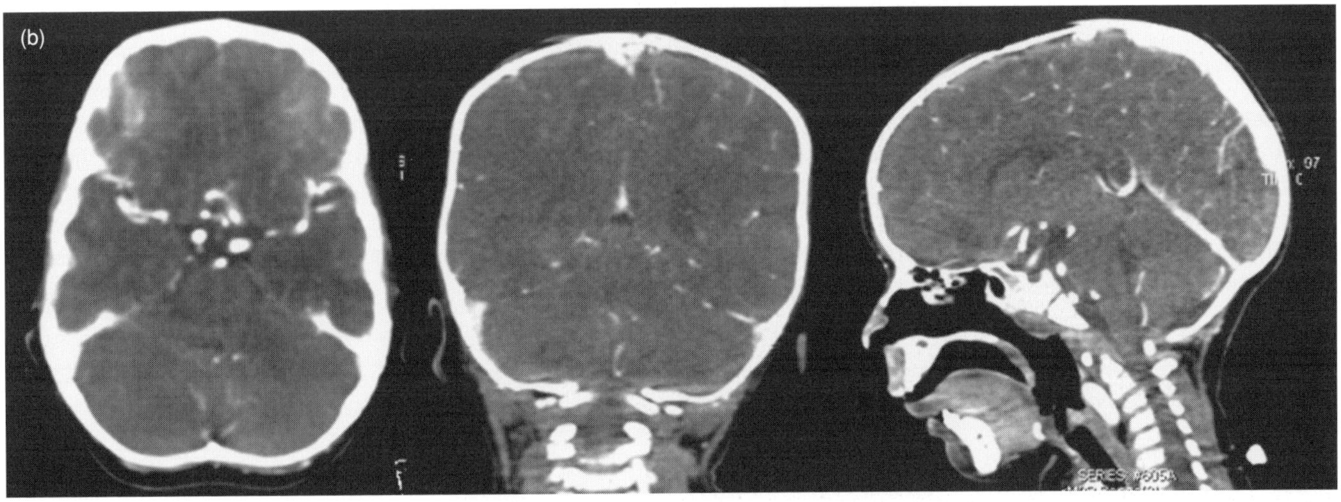

Fig. 6.3(a, b). Pre-contrast **(a)** and postcontrast **(b)** CT study of the posterior fossa. The cerebellar cortex and vermis appear slightly hyperdense in relation to the cerebellar white matter. The fourth ventricle is filled with hypodense cerebrospinal fluid. Beam-hardening artifacts originating from the petrous bone obscure brainstem imaging detail **(a)** (arrows). On contrast-enhanced CT the dural sinuses are hyperdense as well as the circulus arteriosus Willisi. Volume acquisition allows secondary multiplanar, coronal and sagittal reconstructions **(b)**.

Fig. 6.3(c). Three-dimensional surface shaded reconstruction of a CT dataset allows detailed study of the skull and skull base as well as the craniocervical junction. (See color plate 18).

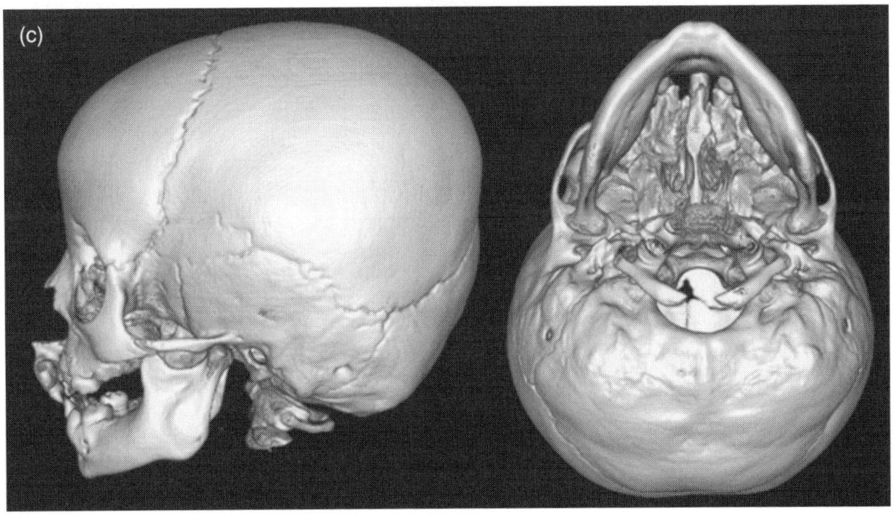

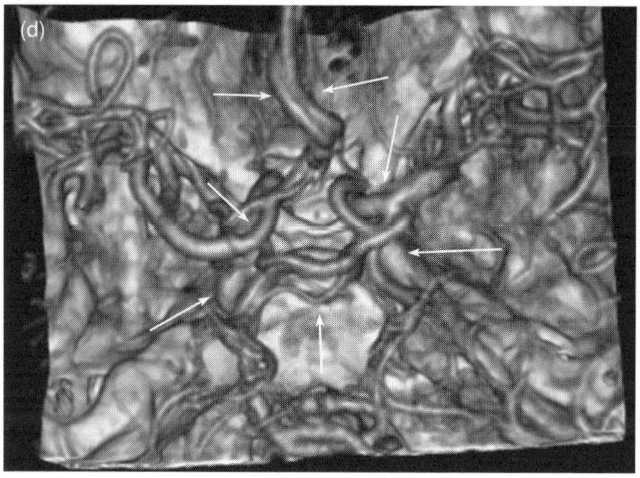

Fig. 6.3(d). Three-dimensional reconstruction of a contrast-enhanced CT angiography. The circulus arteriosus Willisi is seen from above, projected on the osseous skull base (arrows). (See color plate 19).

cerebellar cortex and brainstem. With ongoing brain maturation the density of the white matter increases slightly; however, the cortex will remain hyperdense in relation to the cerebellar white matter. The CSF in the fourth ventricle as well as in the basal cisterns appears hypodense on CT. The cerebellar tentorium and dural sinuses may appear slightly hyperdense, in particular in neonates with high-density fetal hemoglobin (HbF) and low hematocrit levels. The current spatial resolution and contrast-to-noise ratio of CT usually do not allow identification of the dentate nuclei or cranial nerves as separate anatomic structures. Contrast-enhanced sequences are rarely necessary. If a focal lesion is identified in the posterior fossa, most frequently dedicated MRI will follow. If indicated, CT angiography (e.g., to exclude an aneurysm) or CT venography (e.g., to exclude a dural sinus thrombosis) may be performed (Fig. 6.3d,e). MR angiography or MR venography should however be considered as a radiation-free alternative.

CT of the posterior fossa may be challenging because of CT-specific streak artifacts that may obscure or mimic pathology (Fig. 6.3a). Streak artifacts result from beam hardening and nonlinear partial volume effects caused by the compact, highly complex osseous skull base (Jones et al. 2001). Multidetector helical CT with thin collimation and adequate denoising filters may improve image detail in the posterior fossa.

Newer developments including cerebral perfusion CT and positron emission tomography CT (PET-CT) may increase the sensitivity and specificity of CT. However, the inherent additional radiation dose requires careful consideration of whether to use these techniques in children (Hoeffner et al. 2004; Kim et al. 2010). Consequently few studies have evaluated the value of these CT-based techniques for pediatric posterior fossa pathologies, especially as most questions can be answered without radiation and frequently in higher detail by the various MRI techniques.

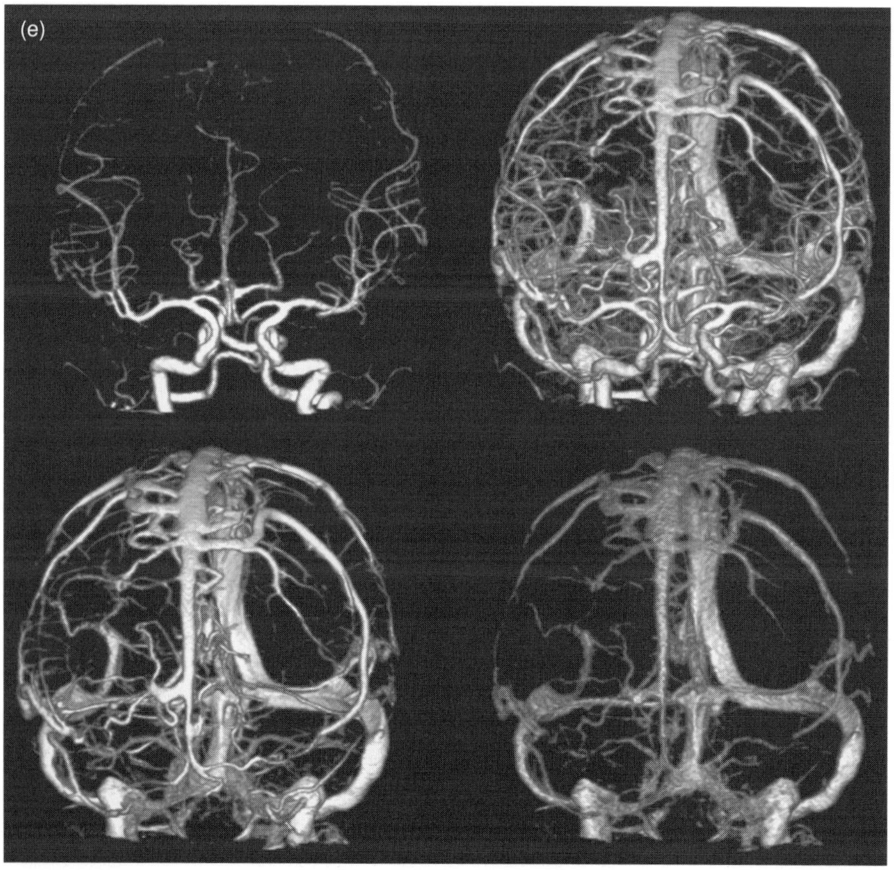

Fig. 6.3(e). Dynamic, multiphase contrast-enhanced CT angiography of the cerebral vasculature with reconstruction of the arterial, arteriovenous, venous, and late venous phase. (Courtesy of Dr Diego San Milan Ruiz, Johns Hopkins School of Medicine, Baltimore.)

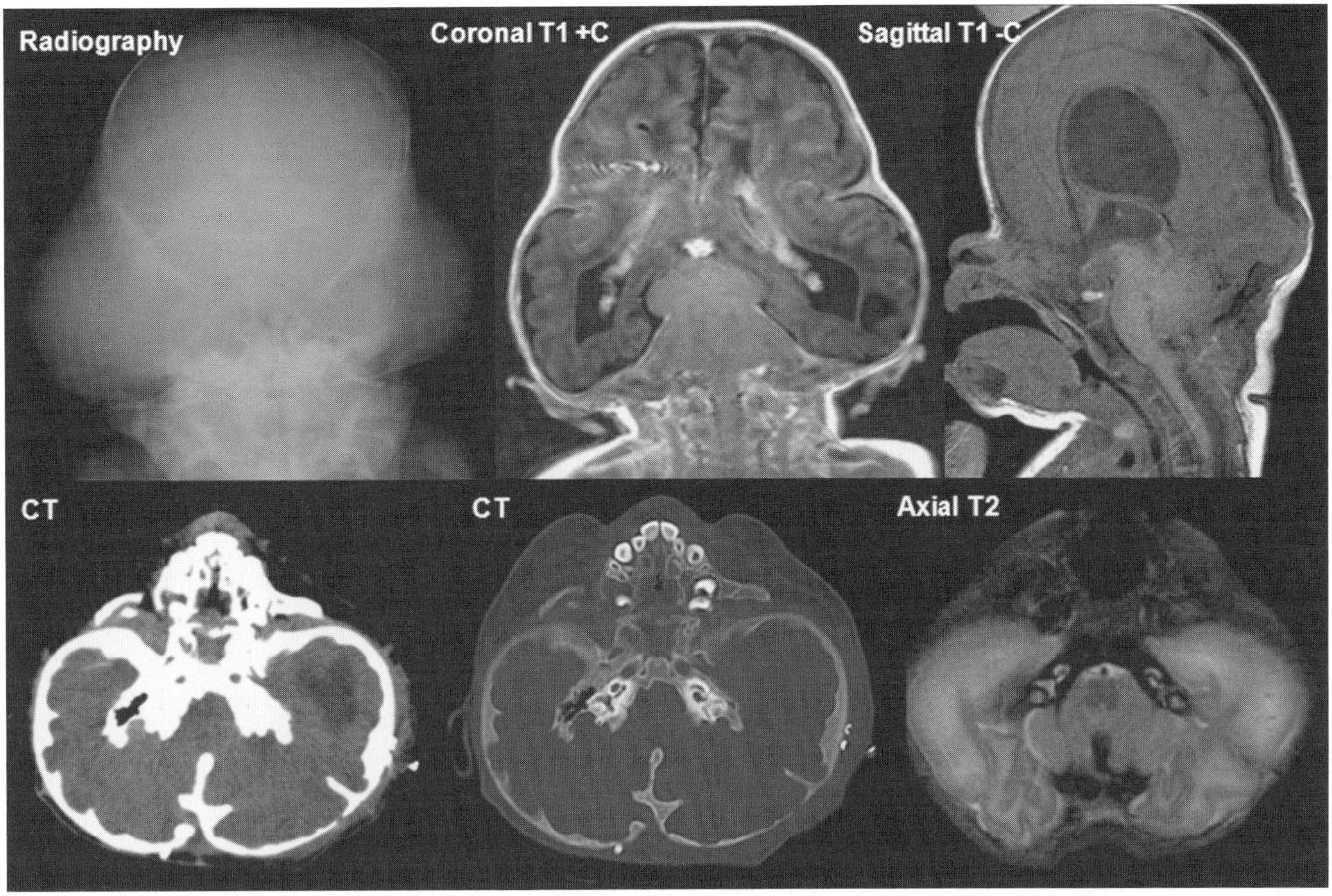

Fig. 6.4. Multimodality imaging of a child with cloverleaf deformity of the skull. Conventional radiography, MRI, and CT show the degree of osseous malformation and resultant deformation of the brain. CT shows in exquisite detail the skull base deformity with basal impression.

CT remains a valuable adjunct to MRI in pathologies that simultaneously affect the osseous skull and brain (Fig. 6.4) as well as in malformations/pathologies affecting the inner and middle ear.

Magnetic resonance imaging

Magnetic resonance imaging has revolutionized pediatric neuroimaging. The lack of radiation, the high spatial resolution, the different image contrasts (T1, T2, and T2*) that can be generated, the multiplanar capabilities, and the combined anatomic and functional information that can be collected in one study make MRI exquisitely well suited for pediatric neuroimaging. There are of course also some limitations, like the long acquisition times, the limited access to the patient inside the bore of the MRI scanner, absolute MRI contraindications (e.g., pacemaker, cochlear implant), the high costs, and the fact that an MRI scanner is not always available. Nevertheless, the many benefits usually outweigh the disadvantages. MRI should especially be considered if ultrasonography or CT cannot explain the neurologic symptoms adequately and when multiple follow-up examinations are anticipated.

Moreover, MRI has proven to be especially helpful in studying the pediatric posterior fossa because imaging detail is not obscured by beam-hardening artifacts from the skull base, as seen in CT. Consequently, MRI allows study of the complex normal and abnormal posterior fossa anatomy and the internal neuro-architecture of the cerebellum and brainstem in exquisite detail (Figs 6.5 and 6.6).

In addition, the toolbox of MRI for imaging the posterior fossa is full of multiple anatomic and functional sequences. Most anatomic imaging relies on high resolution T1 and T2-weighted sequences. In particular, T2-weighted sequences render high-quality anatomic images. The macro-anatomy is well displayed as well as the internal architecture with identification of the cerebellar white and gray matter, cerebellar cortex, dentate nuclei, and many of the various nuclei within the brainstem. Care should be taken that the spatial resolution is optimized by using a small field of view, high matrix, and thin slices. In addition, the sequence variables such as the repetition and echo time (TR, TE) as well as the MR pulse profile and shimming of the magnetic field should be optimized to enhance the signal-to-noise ratio as well as the contrast-to-noise ratio. Depending on the encountered pathologies, various sequences will give the most sensitive and specific information. T1-weighted sequences are beneficial for recognition of hemorrhages and fat and identification of contrast-enhancing pathologies such as neoplasms,

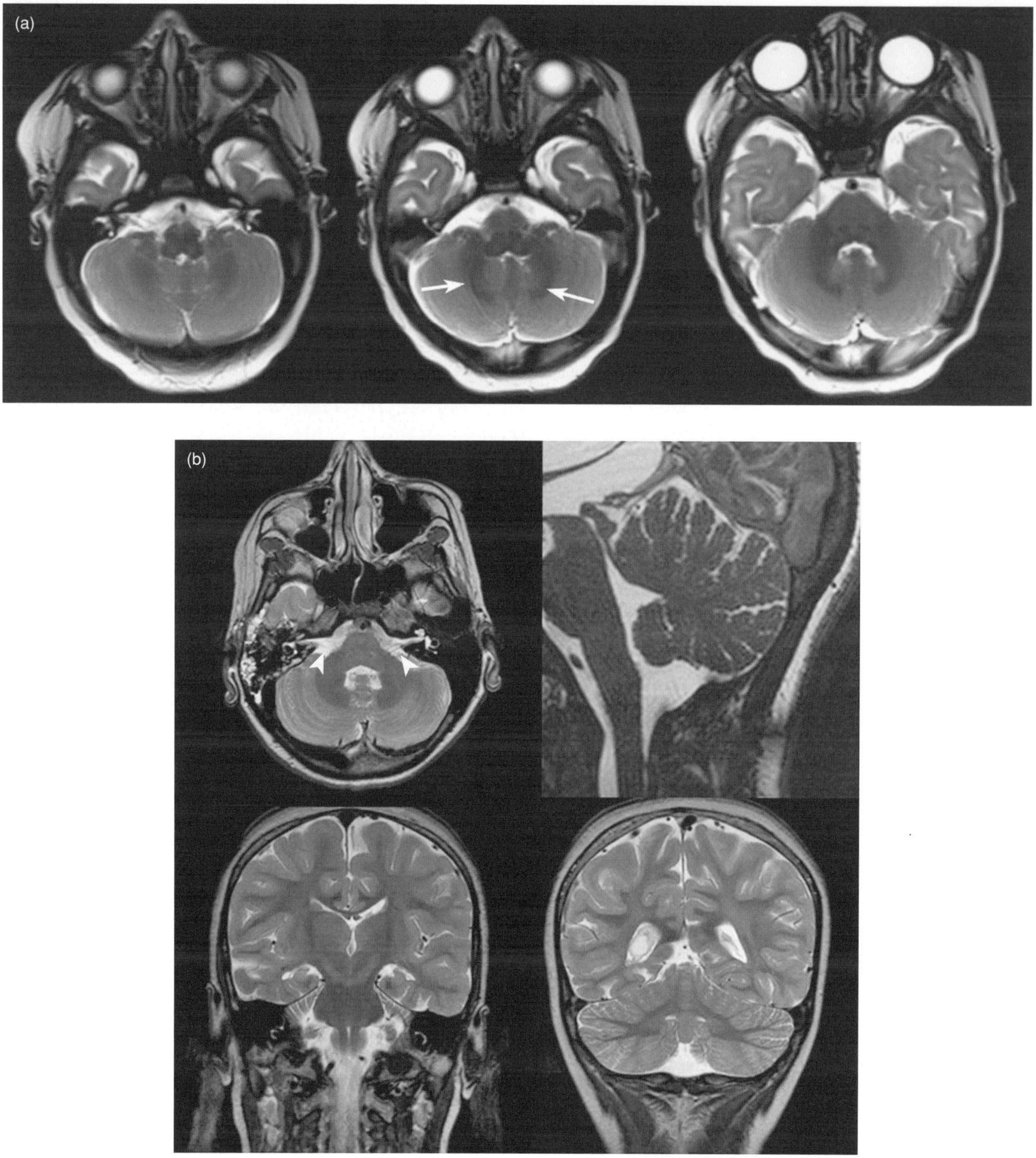

Fig. 6.5. (a) Axial T2-weighted MRI of a neonatal cerebellum and brainstem and **(b)** triplanar T2-weighted MRI of an infant show the cerebellar, vermian, and brainstem anatomy in high detail. The cerebellar cortex is hyperintense in relation to the cerebellar white matter. The dentate nuclei (arrows) and various brainstem nuclei are seen as mildly hypointense structures. The vestibulo-cochlear nerve is outlined by T2-hyperintense cerebrospinal fluid in the cerebello-pontine cistern (arrowheads). Ultrathin sagittal, heavily T2-weighted image shows the vermian fissures and the Sylvian aqueduct in detail.

abscesses, or infarctions. If focal hemorrhages or calcifications are suspected, additional T2*-weighted sequences including the recently developed susceptibility-weighted imaging should be added to the standard T1- and T2-weighted imaging. In a structural abnormality is to be studied, high resolution T2-weighted sequences should be used. High resolution, thin-sliced heavily T2-weighted acquisitions like the 'constructive interference in steady state' sequence take advantage of the high

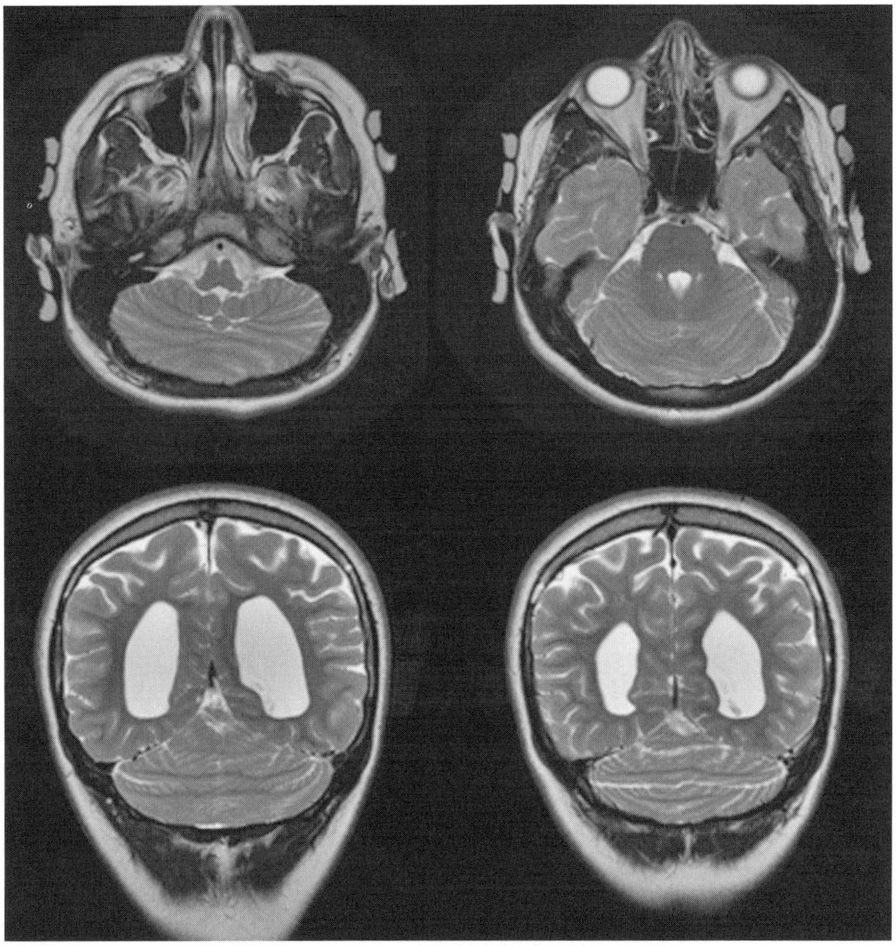

Fig. 6.6. Example of an abnormal axial and coronal T2-weighted MRI in a child with rhombencephalosynapsis. The vermis is absent, the cerebellar white matter is fused with an uninterrupted horizontal course of the cerebellar fissures, the dentate nuclei are fused, and the fourth ventricle is malformed. Mild supratentorial hydrocephalus.

difference in signal intensity between CSF and neuronal structures to outline/identify small anatomic structures such as the cranial nerves or the cerebellar folia. Focal lesions or anatomically complex pathologies should preferably be examined in multiple imaging planes. Standardized axial, sagittal, and coronal sequences should be measured along predefined landmarks. It goes without saying that the physician should be familiar with the embryology, anatomy, and ongoing normal maturation of the pediatric brain on MRI. Progressing myelination and fiber packing will continuously change the signal intensities of the cerebellar white matter and brainstem both on T1- and T2-weighted imaging.

Depending on the clinical presentation, suspected diagnosis or encountered pathology, various additional functional MRI sequences may be considered. In functional MR imaging, differences in signal intensity are directly or indirectly related to or resulting from various functional or dynamic processes within the brain. This may include diffusion of protons or water molecules (diffusion-weighted or diffusion tensor imaging, DWI/DTI); neurometabolic processes (^{1}H magnetic resonance spectroscopy, ^{1}H-MRS); blood flow (MR angiography (MRA), MR-venography (MRV)); tissue perfusion (perfusion-weighted imaging, PWI); and CSF flow (phase contrast flow studies). Detailed clinical data with a precise question including information about the suspected diagnosis will guide the MRI examination and help to determine which sequences should be measured. In pediatric neuroradiology, standard protocols are rarely used. Ideally, the pediatric neuroradiologist guides the study on site in real time and decides which sequences should be added to the standard imaging protocol to answer the clinical questions.

Diffusion-weighted and diffusion tensor imaging

Diffusion-weighted imaging (DWI) is a relatively new functional MR sequence that generates tissue contrast based on differences in the diffusion properties of protons ($^{+}$H) within tissue. Depending on the given micro-structural properties, these protons will differ in their mobility and diffusion characteristics. Protons within the CSF, for example, have a higher mobility than those within the white or gray matter of the brain. By adding diffusion gradients to the MR pulse sequence, the difference in diffusion characteristics is translated into differences in MR signal intensity. Similar to conventional T1- and T2-weighted MR images, these differences in signal intensities can be displayed as two-dimensional DWI images (Huisman 2003) (Fig. 6.7a).

In addition to the DWI images, post-processing of the imaging data allow the calculation of a map of *apparent diffusion coefficients* (ADC) (Fig 7a). ADC quantifies the magnitude of diffusion within the brain and is expressed in mm^2/s. Areas with a high ADC value (e.g., CSF) are displayed with a high signal intensity (bright) on the ADC maps while areas with a low ADC value (e.g., brain tissue) are displayed with a low signal intensity (dark). A major advantage of ADC maps compared to DWI images is that ADC calculations/maps only represent signal intensities related to the local water mobility/diffusion and are not contaminated by any other physical phenomenon such as, for example, T2 relaxation. Calculation of the ADC maps allows quantitative study of normal brain maturation. Multiple studies have shown that the ADC values show a continuous drop from the neonatal period towards adolescence (Schneider et al. 2004). These ADC changes are related to multiple developmental processes including progressing white matter myelination, fiber packing, and progressively decreasing overall water content of the brain. In addition, DWI/ADC analyses have proven to identify many pathologic processes early, even before conventional T1/T2-weighted MRI shows disease. DWI/ADC has especially revolutionized the early detection of ischemic brain injury. Cytotoxic edema occurs early (within minutes of vessel occlusion) within the core of ischemic injury and results from a shift of water from the extracellular space to the intracellular space. The resulting narrowed and more tortuous extracellular space reduces overall water mobility which is picked up by DWI before conventional T1/T2-weighted imaging shows pathology. The restricted diffusion is characterized by low ADC values on the ADC maps. Because the overall water content does not change in the early minutes of ischemia, T1- and T2-weighted imaging remains unremarkable. The fact that DWI/ADC maps show pathology before tissue injury becomes apparent on conventional T1/T2-weighted MRI is essential for the very early treatment of ischemia in order to limit irreversible neurologic deficits. With progressing duration of ischemia (>2 hours), signal changes will eventually also become apparent on T1- and T2-weighted MRI because of an increasing total water content due to increasing vascular permeability with resultant vasogenic edema. DWI gives valuable information about the timing of ischemic injury. The ADC values follow a well-defined time course. After the initial ADC drop (in the acute phase of ischemia), the ADC values will gradually increase over several days. The ADC

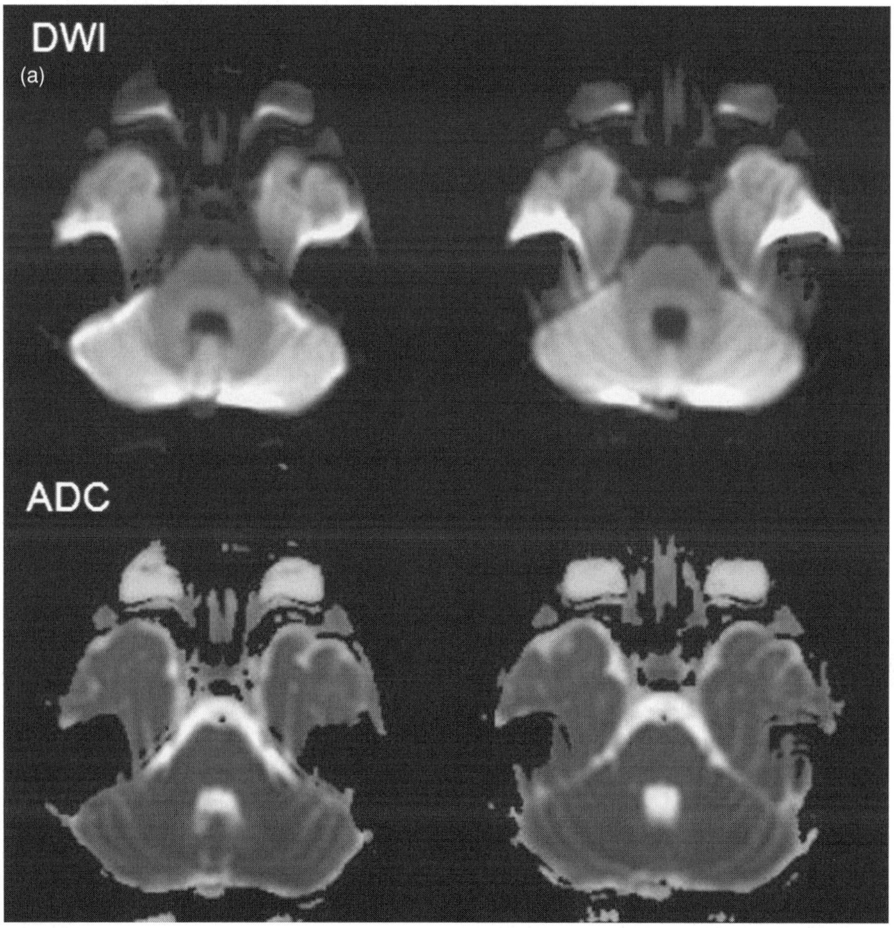

Fig. 6.7. Axial diffusion tensor imaging of the cerebellum and brainstem. **(a)** Diffusion-weighted (DWI), apparent diffusion coefficient (ADC) show only minimal differences in diffusion between gray and white matter. The high water mobility in the cerebrospinal fluid explains the DWI hypointensity and high ADC value/signal. **(b)** Fractional anisotropy (FA) maps reveal the complex internal architecture within the brainstem and cerebellum. A high degree of anisotropic diffusion is seen within the tightly packed white matter tracts in the brainstem and cerebellar peduncles. **(c)** Color-coded FA maps show the predominant diffusion direction, course of the various white matter tracts (green: anterior-posterior; red: left-right; blue: superior-inferior). (See color plate 20).

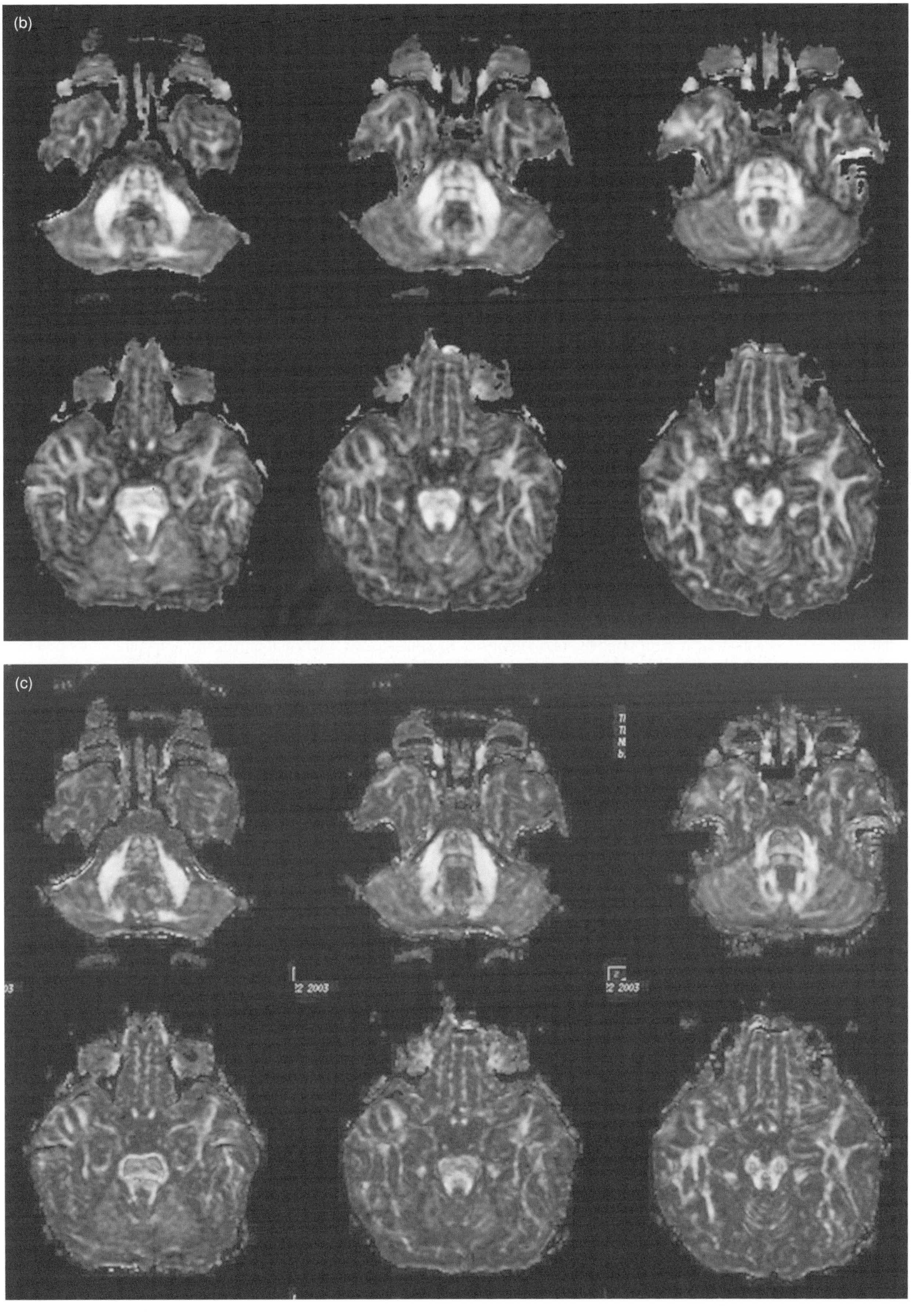

Fig. 6.7. (*continued*)

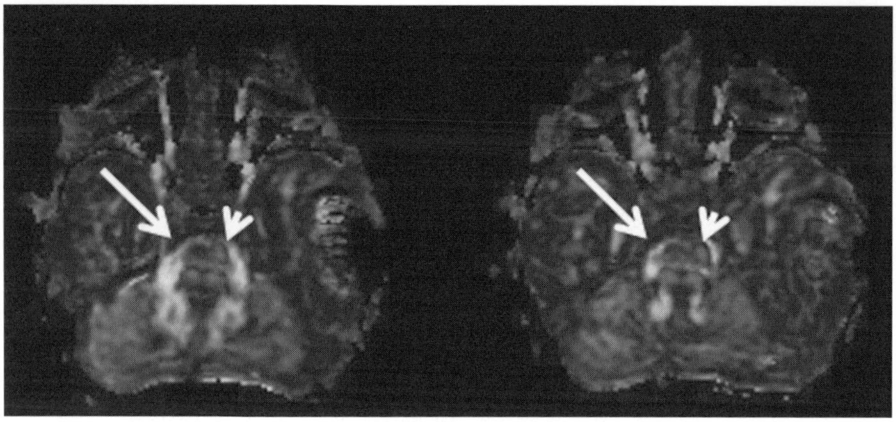

Fig. 6.8. Example of a pathologic color-coded fractional anisotropy (FA) map. The descending corticospinal tract (blue) is absent on the right (large arrow) due to a large supratentorial infarction in the ipsilateral motor cortex. The left corticospinal tract (arrowhead) is preserved and can easily be depicted. (See color plate 21).

values initially increase because of the developing vasogenic edema which widens the extracellular space, and later because of progressive cell lysis and tissue resorption. This results in a typical pseudo-normalization of the ADC values after 7–10 days, followed by a steady increase up to ADC values similar to those of CSF (cystic transformation of the infarction). The exact time course is dependent on multiple additional factors including location and size of infarction, acute versus chronic injury, degree of collateral circulation, and treatment, to mention a few.

As well as the early identification of ischemic injury, DWI/ADC analysis also allows quantification of ongoing tissue injury in multiple other disease processes including inflammatory, metabolic, and neoplastic diseases. The quantitative analysis of the ADC maps may give valuable data to monitor disease progression or treatment results.

Diffusion tensor imaging (DTI) is a further development of DWI in which the three-dimensional shape of diffusion is sampled by using multiple diffusion sensitizing gradients along at least six different, orthogonal directions in space. In addition to the calculation of the magnitude of overall diffusion (ADC), this technique also allows characterization of the three-dimensional shape of diffusion in detail. Diffusion is consequently represented by three eigenvectors that are perpendicular to each other. The lengths of the individual eigenvectors represent the maximal diffusion (magnitude) along the respective three axes in space, and are known as eigenvalues (λ_1, λ_2, λ_3). If diffusion is equal in all directions, as in CSF, diffusion is isotropic: $\lambda_1=\lambda_2=\lambda_3$). If there is a predominant direction of diffusion, for example along fiber tracts, the eigenvector/eigenvalue along the main axis of this fiber tract is significantly larger than the eigenvectors/eigenvalues perpendicular to the main axis of the fiber tract (anisotropic diffusion: $\lambda_1>\lambda_2/\lambda_3$). By calculating the proportion of anisotropic diffusion relative to the overall diffusion, a measurement of tissue directionality/anisotropy is achieved. A typical scalar of anisotropic diffusion is the *'fractional anisotropy'* index. The fractional antistropy value ranges between 0 (maximal isotropic diffusion) and 1 (maximal anisotropic diffusion). These values can again be displayed as a two-dimensional map (fractional antistropy map) representing the spatial distribution of anisotropic diffusion (Fig. 6.7b). Similar to the changes of the ADC values with progressing brain maturation, fractional antistropy values also allow study of ongoing brain development. ADC and fractional antistropy data study partially overlapping, partially differing components of brain development. The fractional antistropy values increase significantly during the first decades of life, especially along the white matter tracts due to progressive myelination and fiber packing (Schneider et al. 2004). Moreover, the DTI dataset analysis also allows graphic display of the principal direction of diffusion within each voxel. Typically color-coded fractional antistropy maps are generated in which green indicates predominant left-right, blue superior-inferior, and red anterior-posterior diffusion (Fig. 6.7c). These color-coded maps help to identify normal and abnormal or injured fiber tracts within the brainstem and cerebellum (Fig. 6.8).

Finally, complex post-processing techniques are used to reconstruct the course of major fiber tracts within the brain from the DTI datasets. These *tractography* studies are especially helpful to better understand complex brain malformations and may shed light into normal and abnormal neuronal circuitry as well as neuronal plasticity and connectivity (Vulliemoz et al. 2005; Poretti et al. 2007; Juranek and Salman 2010) (Fig. 6.9).

Mori and colleagues have developed a normative atlas of brain maturation for the different age groups based on the DWI/DTI datasets (Mori et al. 2005).

High-end DWI/DTI studies of the posterior fossa require optimized protocols, especially for young neonates because the dense skull base and air/bone interface distort the magnetic field homogeneity, resulting in artifact-loaded or distorted DWI/ADC/FA maps. Ongoing developments in equipment and software continue to increase the quality of DWI/DTI datasets. DWI/DTI measurements profit from a high signal-to-noise ratio which is offered by higher magnetic field strengths. The progressive availability of 3T (tesla) MRI scanners in clinical routine further enhances the quality of the DWI/DTI data.

Magnetic resonance angiography and venography

Magnetic resonance angiography (MRA) and venography (MRV) allows study of the macro-vasculature of the brain (Figs 6.10

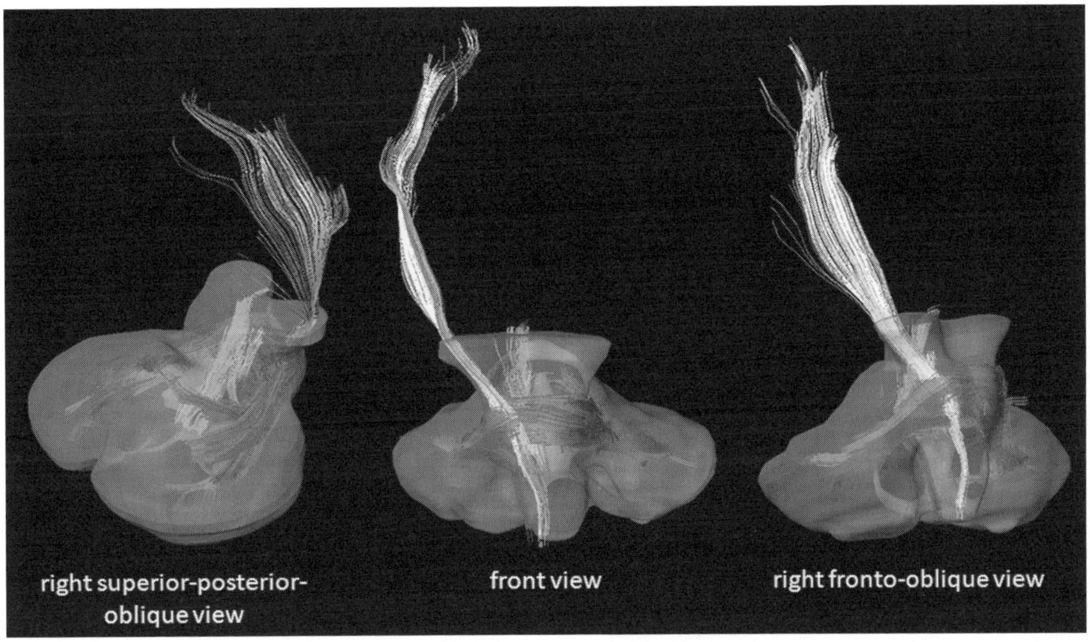

Fig. 6.9. Color-coded multiplanar, three-dimensional reconstruction of various fiber tracts (tractography) within the brainstem and cerebellum from a diffusion tensor dataset. The corticospinal, corticobulbar, and corticopontine tracts, the medial lemniscus, the inferior, middle, and superior cerebellar tract, and transverse pontine fibers are displayed. (Courtesy of Dr Kenichi Oishi, Johns Hopkins Hospital, Baltimore, USA.) (See color plate 22).

and 6.11). Various techniques are available including two- and three-dimensional time-of-flight and phase contrast techniques (Huisman et al. 2010). In addition, fast, multiphase contrast-enhanced angiographic sequences have been developed that allow to study the brain vasculature similar to conventional catheter angiography. Within one acquisition, multiple contrast phases including an arterial, venous, or late venous phase are measured (Fig. 6.10c). Depending on the pathology to be studied, the optimal technique has to be chosen and adapted. Three-dimensional datasets allow multiplanar detailed reconstructions similar to CT angiography. A major advantage compared to CT angiography is that no overlying bony structures obscure the vascular detail, making MRA/MRV exquisitely well suited to study of the vertebrobasilar system in the posterior fossa.

Perfusion-weighted imaging

Perfusion-weighted imaging (PWI) maps the micro-perfusion of brain tissue topographically (Huisman and Sorensen 2004). Depending on the chosen technique, various hemodynamic maps can be calculated including maps of cerebral blood flow, cerebral blood volume, mean transit time, and time to peak (Fig. 6.12). Currently two clinically approved techniques are available: dynamic susceptibility-weighted contrast-enhanced PWI and arterial spin labeling (ASL). The contrast-enhanced technique combines ultrafast, serial MR imaging with a rapid bolus injection of intravenous paramagnetic MR contrast agent (gadolinium). During the first pass of the contrast through the brain, the high concentration of the paramagnetic gadolinium in the microvasculature will distort the local, microscopic magnetic field with resulting signal loss. The magnitude, onset, duration, and recovery of the observed MR signal loss gives information about the brain perfusion. A major advantage is that this robust technique allows study of the entire brain with calculation of multiple hemodynamic maps within a single, fast MR scan. The major disadvantage, however, is the need for injection of gadolinium-based contrast agents which have been linked to an increased risk of nephrogenic systemic fibrosis in patients with renal failure. In addition, data acquisition is limited to one contrast injection. If the imaging data should be degraded by patient motion, no immediate second run is possible.

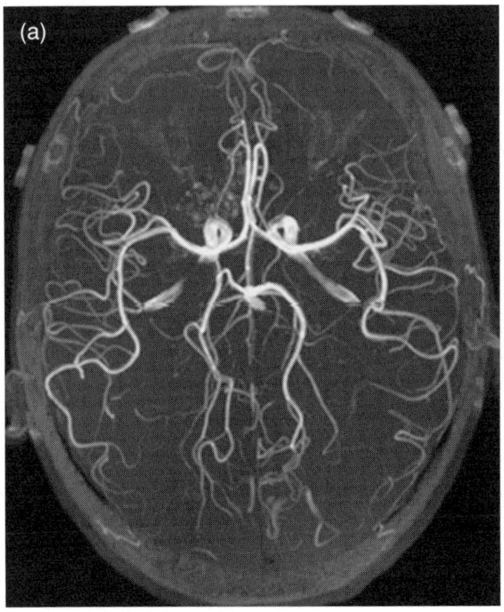

Fig. 6.10(a). Three-dimensional time-of-flight MR angiography of the circulus arteriosus Willisi. All major vessels (anterior, middle, and posterior cerebral artery) are seen in detail.

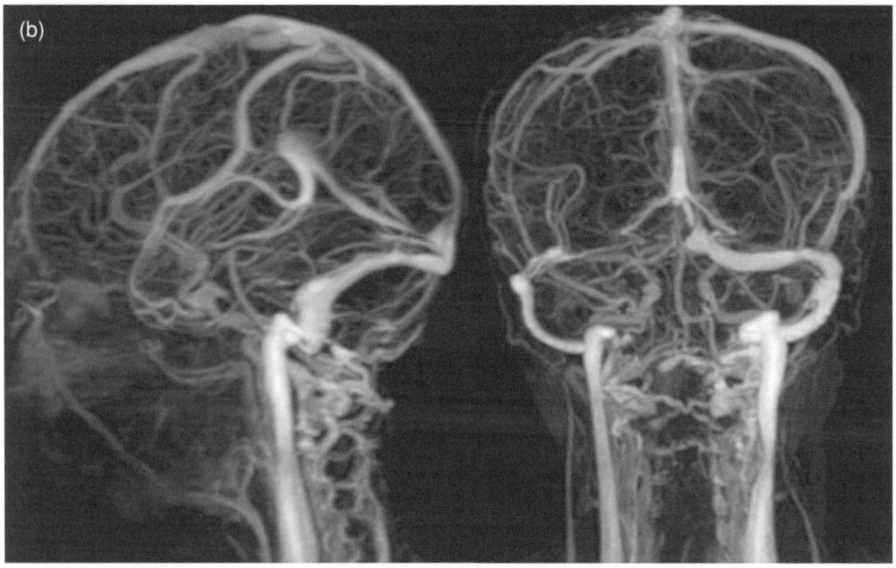

Fig. 6.10(b). Contrast-enhanced MR venography in sagittal and coronal projection. The entire superficial and deep venous system as well as the epidural spinal venous plexus is seen. The arterial circle of Willis is faintly seen superimposed by the venous system.

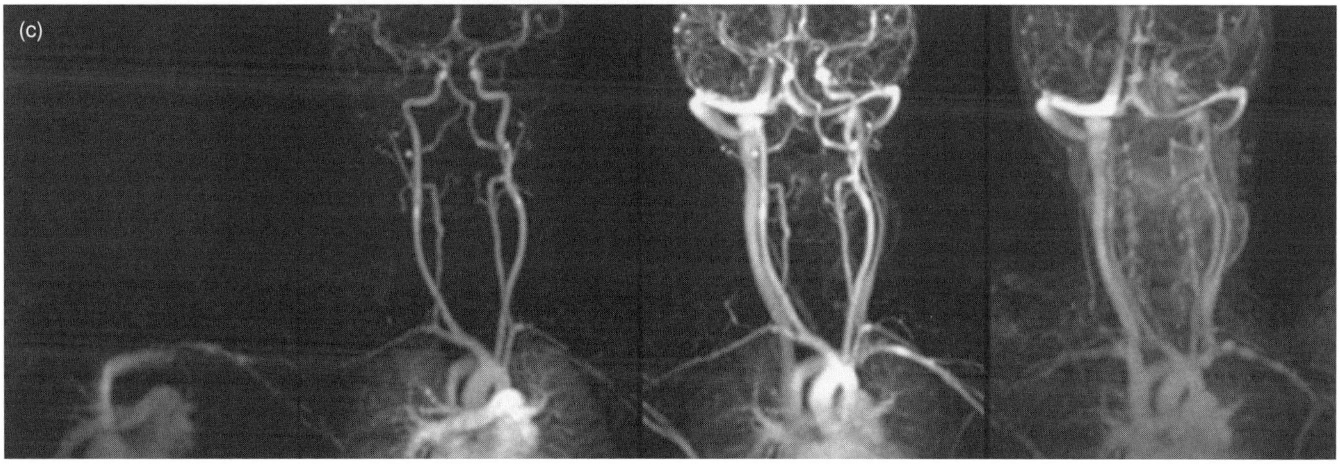

Fig. 6.10(c). Multiphase, dynamic contrast-enhanced MR venography of the head and neck vessels renders various arterial and venous phases for one contrast injection.

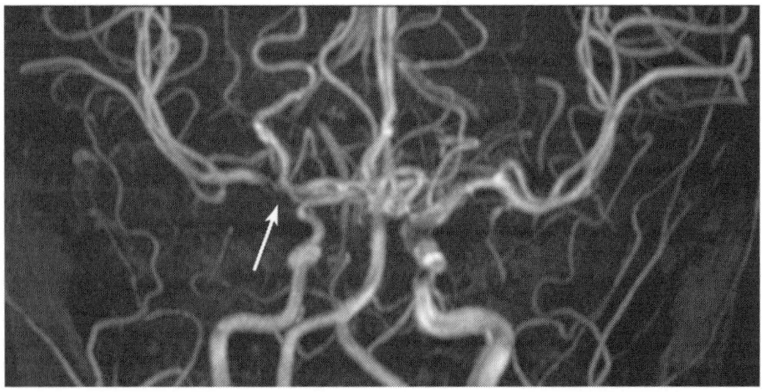

Fig. 6.11. Example of a pathologic time-of-flight MR angiography of the circle of Willis. In this young patient with neurofibromatosis type 1, the proximal right middle cerebral artery (MCA) is highly stenotic (arrow). Additional stenoses are seen in the left MCA and distal internal carotid arteries.

Alternatively, ASL allows the study of brain perfusion. This technique takes advantage of an intrinsic 'contrast agent'. The protons within the flowing blood are magnetically labeled by a saturation pulse positioned over the arteries feeding the brain. After repeating the MR sequence without the saturation pulse, subtraction of both datasets gives information about brain perfusion. Major advantages of this approach are that no contrast has to be injected and the sequence can be repeated as often as necessary. In addition, by selectively saturating individual vessels, the different vascular territories can be studied.

It is likely that ASL will eventually replace contrast-enhanced PWI, not only because no contrast injection is necessary, but also because the selective labeling of the different vessels by ASL allows study of the unique vascular supply of the posterior fossa. The basilar artery is the only major vessel in the human body that arises from an arterial confluence (left and right vertebral arteries). A recent ASL study took advantage of the selective labeling of the vertebral arteries to study the posterior circulation hemodynamics (Kansagra and Wong 2008). ASL data showed that there is little mixing of vertebral artery blood in the basilar artery. ASL also showed that the cerebellar supply is primarily from the ipsilateral vertebral artery and that the vertebral arteries contribute unequally to

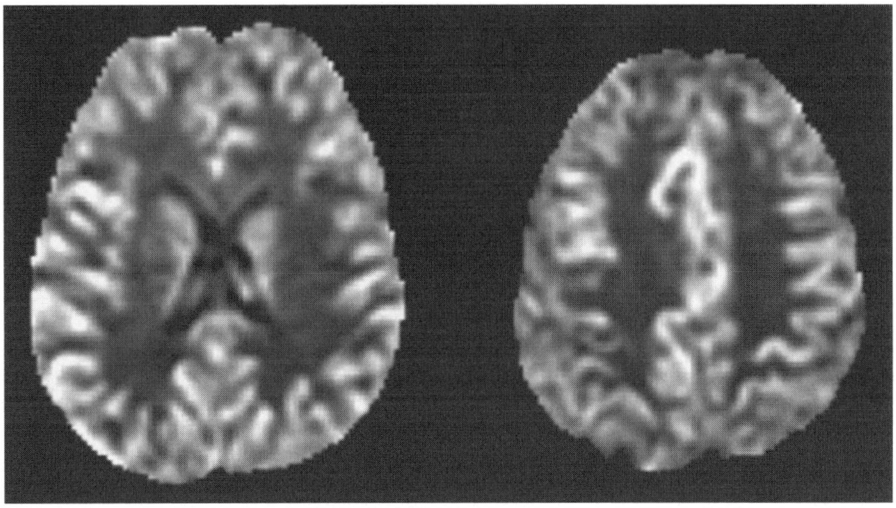

Fig. 6.12. Example of a cerebral blood flow (CBF) map generated from a dynamic contrast-enhanced perfusion-weighted MR study. The cortex and central gray matter have a significantly higher perfusion (hyperintense) than the white matter (hypointense).

the total vertebrobasilar flow. This unique anatomic feature may be of importance for vascular pathologies affecting the cerebellum and brainstem.

PWI has proven to be helpful in identifying regions of critical perfusion in acute and chronic ischemia. By combining the information gathered by PWI and DWI/DTI, PWI can identify tissue at risk for infarction. The area of restricted diffusion as seen on DWI/DTI in patients with acute ischemia is believed to represent the irreversible core of infarction. PWI usually shows a matching area of hypoperfusion (PWI-DWI match). PWI may however show an area of hypoperfusion larger than the area of restricted diffusion (PWI-DWI mismatch) which is believed to represent the penumbra surrounding the core of infarction. The penumbra is a region of hypoperfused, viable brain tissue at risk for ischemic injury if no immediate treatment is initiated.

In addition to the early identification of regions with impaired perfusion due to vascular diseases, PWI may provide valuable information for a better understanding of complex functional cerebellar syndromes due to cerebellar hypoperfusion. The link between hypoperfusion of the left cerebellar hemisphere and cerebellar mutism was shown as early as 1996 using single photon emission CT (Ersahin et al. 1996). In 1998, Germano showed that reversible cerebral perfusion alterations were also encountered in children with transient mutism after posterior fossa surgery (Germano et al. 1998). More recently, single-photon emission computed tomography (SPECT) studies showed that perfusion impairments involving the insula, temporal cortex, medial prefrontal cortex, anterior cingulate gyrus, and hippocampus are noted in patients with infantile autism (Ohnishi et al. 2000). The results of these studies show that the hemodynamic exploration of the cerebellum is vital for the better understanding of functional cerebellar disorders. Because PWI does not use any ionizing radiation, this technique should replace SPECT studies wherever possible. Recently, a PWI study showed that injury/interruption of the proximal efferent cerebellar pathway due to posterior fossa tumor surgery results in a global supratentorial cortical hypoperfusion with frontal predominance. These findings support the proposal that this reverse cerebello-cerebral diaschisis with resulting transsynaptic disruption of cerebellar input toward the cerebral cortex in areas critical to many neurocognitive and executive functions may lead to the complex posterior fossa syndrome (mutism, cognitive impairment, emotional lability) (Miller et al. 2010).

^{1}H Magnetic resonance spectroscopy

^{1}H Magnetic resonance spectroscopy (MRS) is a functional MRI tool that allows study of brain metabolites non-invasively both qualitatively as well as quantitatively (Costa et al. 2002). Various MRS sequences are currently available taking advantage of either a single voxel or multivoxel approach including quantitative multislice spectroscopic imaging. The metabolites that are typically studied include *N*-acetylaspartate (NAA), believed to be a marker of neuronal density and integrity; choline (Cho) as a marker of membrane turnover; and creatine (Cr)/phosphocreatine (PCr) as a marker of cellular energy metabolism (Fig. 6.13). In addition, lactate may be identified as a marker of anaerobic metabolism due to, for example, tissue necrosis, infection or ischemia. Depending on the chosen magnetic field strength and MRS parameter, many more low-molecular-weight metabolites can be identified including glutamine, glutamate, myoinositol, glycine, scylloinositol, to mention a few.

Qualitative and quantitative MRS has become a valuable adjunct to conventional MRI in studying and monitoring a variety of diseases affecting the supratentorial brain. Age-related normative metabolite ratios and concentrations have been collected for the supratentorial gray and white matter. Few studies, however, have focused on the cerebellum and brainstem (Jacobs et al. 2001; Costa et al. 2002; Mascalchi et al. 2002a). One major reason is that MRS of the posterior fossa is technically challenging. The densely ossified skull base, air within the sphenoid sinus, and mastoid air cells result in a significant magnetic field inhomogeneity and difficult shimming. In addition, the smaller size of the cerebellum and brainstem require smaller voxel sizes to prevent contamination by adjacent

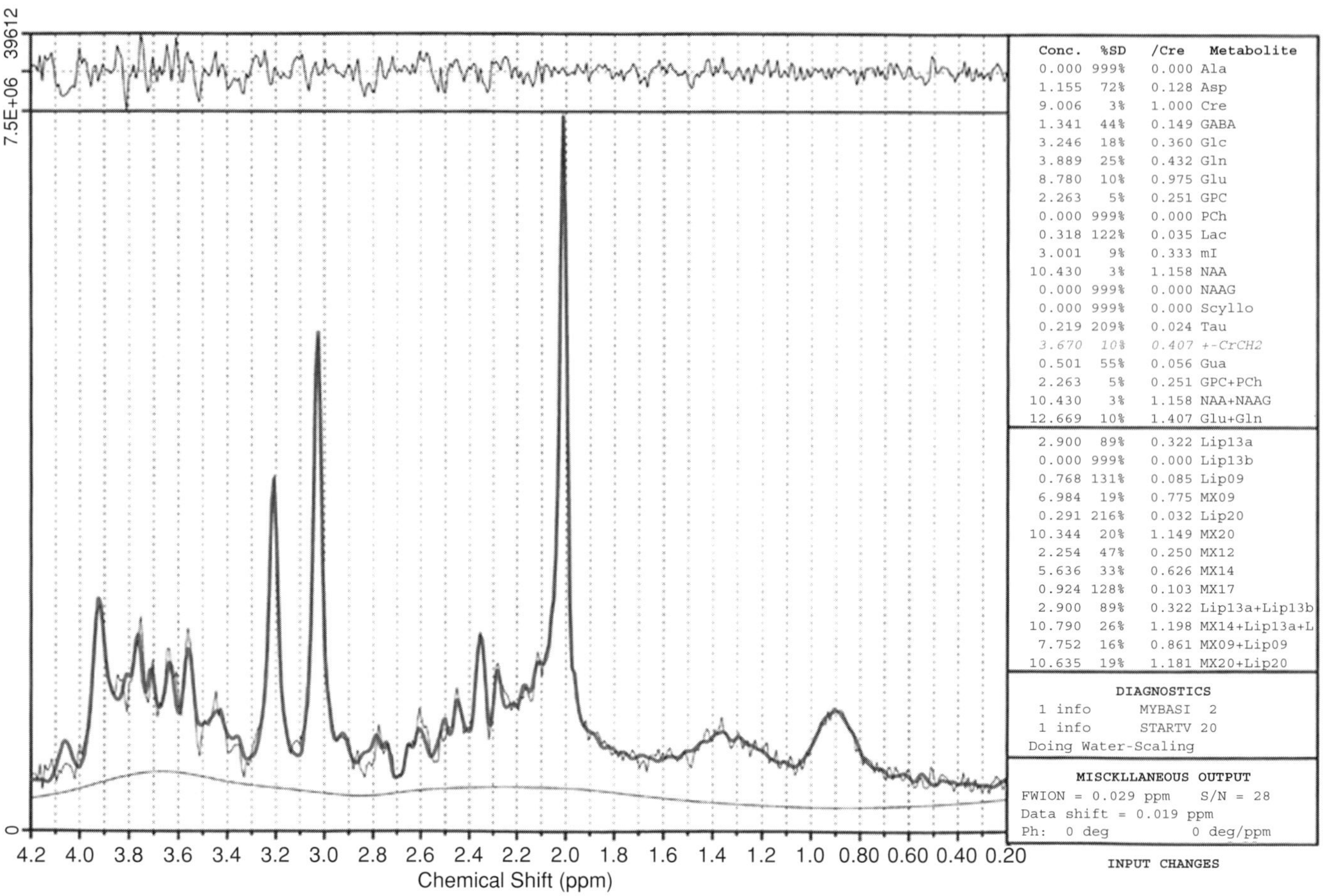

Fig. 6.13. [1]H Magnetic resonance spectroscopy of the cerebellar white matter. The dominant peak is *N*-acetylaspartate (at 2ppm). Additional peaks are creatine and choline. The metabolite concentration is calculated from the normalized surface area underneath the peak. (See color plate 23).

CSF, bone marrow within the skull base, or subcutaneous fat. Moreover, in the posterior fossa, pulsation artifacts from the major vessels, CSF pulsations, and brain motion are more pronounced compared to the supratentorial compartment. All these factors decrease the signal-to-noise ratio and consequently spectral resolution. However, with increasing magnetic field strength, ongoing developments in MR hardware and software and optimized MRS sequences, more MRS data of the cerebellum and brainstem are becoming available. A detailed knowledge of the normal regional distribution and concentration of metabolites is essential to correctly identify neurologic diseases affecting the brainstem and cerebellum.

Several recent studies have shown that the concentrations of several major metabolites differ significantly between the cerebellum/brainstem and the supratentorial brain (Jacobs et al. 2001; Mascalchi et al. 2002a). In addition, significant regional differences were noted within the different posterior fossa structures. Jacobs et al. identified significantly higher levels of Cr in the cerebellum (8.9 SD 2.1mM/L) compared to the parieto-occipital gray (5.7 SD 1.1mM/L) and occipital white matter (5.3 SD 1.3mM/L). Cr concentration was highest in the cerebellar vermis (8.8 SD 1.7mM/L) and hemispheres (8.9 SD 2.1mM/L) and lowest in the pons (4.3 SD 1.1mM/L). Mascalchi et al. found even higher Cr concentrations in the dentate nucleus (13.5 SD 1.9mM/L). The high Cr concentration within the cerebellum is best explained by the different cellular composition of the cerebellar cortex compared to the supratentorial cortex. In contrast to the six-layer neocortex, the cerebellar cortex consists of three layers (external molecular, Purkinje cell, and inner granular layer). The high levels of Cr are believed to be linked to the high energy demand of the abundant Purkinje cells.

Cho concentration also proved to be significantly higher in the cerebellar vermis (2.3 SD 0.4mM/L), cerebellar hemispheres (2.2 SD 0.6mM/L), and pons (2.2 SD 0.5mM/L) compared to the parieto-occipital gray (1.3 SD 0.3mM/L) and occipital white matter (1.4 SD 0.3mM/L).

With the exception of the pons, Jacobs et al. did not find significant regional differences for the NAA concentrations between the cerebellum and supratentorial brain (Jacobs et al. 2001). In this study, the NAA concentration in the pons proved to have the highest value (8.3 SD 0.9mM/L), which is best explained by the tightly packed white matter tracts in the pons. Mascalchi et al. confirmed the high NAA values in the pons but also showed high NAA concentrations in the dentate nucleus (14.3 SD 1.6mM/L) (Mascalchi et al. 2002a).

These absolute metabolite concentrations show that comparing supra- and infratentorial metabolite ratios (NAA/Cr,

Cho/Cr) should be approached with caution. The identified regional variance in Cr concentrations limits the significance of these ratios if the supra- and infratentorial brain are compared.

Few studies have focused on age-dependent changes in infratentorial metabolites. Costa noticed a tendency of the NAA/Cr ratio to increase with age in the cerebellum (Costa et al. 2002). This is supported by an in vitro study by Nishina et al. who showed that both NAA and Cr levels increased three- to four-fold from the fetal period to childhood (Nishina et al. 1999).

Familiarity with the exact metabolite concentrations/ratios and their regional variance within the cerebellum and brainstem allows identification of various neurologic diseases affecting the cerebellum and brainstem. Several case reports and small case series have recently been published. Mascalchi et al. (2002b) identified a reduced NAA/Cr and Cho/Cr ratio in children with olivo-ponto-cerebellar atrophy (OPCA) as well as a correlation between the pontine NAA/Cr ratio and degree of disability in children with OPCA. Boddaert et al. identified high lactate levels in the dentate nucleus of 11 children with cerebellar ataxia, in whom subsequent tests diagnosed mitochondrial respiratory chain deficiency (Boddaert et al. 2008). Öz et al. showed in a mouse model that various neurometabolites were significantly different in spinocerebellar ataxia type 1 (SCA1) mice at 6 weeks, prior to major pathologic and neurologic changes (Öz et al. 2010). They also showed that alterations in NAA, myoinositol and glutamate progressively worsened and were significantly correlated with disease progression as assessed by histology. They concluded that their study demonstrates that presymptomatic and progressive neurodegeneration in SCA1 can be non-invasively monitored using MRS.

Future prospective studies with optimized MRS sequences will probably give valuable additional metabolic information in cerebellar diseases.

Functional magnetic resonance imaging

Functional MRI (fMRI) is an imaging technique that allows non-invasive mapping of various functional events within the brain. The technique takes advantage of the tight functional coupling between brain perfusion and cortical activity. Cortical areas that are activated receive a surplus of oxygenated blood overshooting the oxygen extraction rate, resulting in a local reduction of deoxyhemoglobin. This change of deoxyhemoglobin can be mapped topographically by optimized fast T2*-weighted MRI sequences. Deoxyhemoglobin serves as an endogenous contrast agent on so-called 'blood oxygenation level dependent' (BOLD) MRI sequences. The paramagnetic properties of deoxyhemoglobin result in a small local T2* signal loss that can be mapped by MRI. These BOLD-related signal changes are subsequently superimposed on high resolution three-dimensional anatomic MR imaging data. A major advantage of this technique is that various complex functional centers, processes, and networks can be studied non-invasively without the use of ionizing radiation or the necessity for injection of contrast agents. In addition, by combining the functional data with high resolution imaging sequences, function can be precisely localized to the various anatomic regions. A disadvantage is that, despite the fact that the fastest available fMRI sequences are being used, the temporal resolution is limited. This can however be overcome by simultaneous EEG-fMRI measurements which combine the high temporal resolution of electroencephalography (EEG) with the high spatial resolution of fMRI. Nowadays, powerful post-processing algorithms extract artifact-free EEG data from the EEG-fMRI acquisitions.

Compared to the supratentorial brain, significantly fewer studies have focused on the cerebellum and brainstem. fMRI studies have confirmed the presence of somatotopically organized anterior and posterior skeletomotor areas with eye movement activity centered in the oculomotor vermis. A recent meta-analysis of neuroimaging studies discussed the functional topography of the human cerebellum as reported in several studies (Stoodley and Schmahmann 2009). In summary, there appears to be an anterior sensorimotor versus posterior cognitive/emotional dichotomy in the human cerebellum. Moreover, the deep cerebellar nuclei, in particular the dentate nucleus as the leading output channel of the cerebellum and neocerebellar cortex, has been shown to be preferentially involved in sensorimotor (exploratory movements), procedural memory such as motor skill acquisition, and emotional and cognitive functions because of its interconnections with the sensorimotor and associative cortices. These executive and affective networks are at least partially devoted to attention, working memory, procedural reasoning, and salience detection (Habas 2010). Currently, fMRI is not able to adequately differentiate between the various deep cerebellar nuclei. The fastigial and globose/emboliform nuclei are too small to be adequately differentiated from the large dentate nuclei. In addition, the activation of these additional deep cerebellar nuclei is too weak to be detected with a statistically significant threshold. Future equipment and software developments and higher field strengths may shed more detailed light into the functional significance of these nuclei as well as the cerebellar activation in motor and cognitive tasks.

Phase contrast magnetic resonance imaging of cerebrospinal fluid flow

Phase contrast MRI is a flow-sensitive sequence that allows study of the direction, amplitude/magnitude, and pulsatility of CSF flow within the cranial vault (Fig. 6.14). This sequence is similar to the PC-MRA sequence. PC flow studies are especially helpful for study of the CSF flow within the posterior fossa and at the craniocervical junction. The Monro-Kellie doctrine, in which it is stated that the skull is rigid and the volume of the intracranial space is constant, explains that during cardiac systole the systolic arterial pulse wave entering the cranial vault induces a compensatory displacement of CSF from the intracranial vault into the spinal canal. Conversely, during diastole, CSF will flow back into the cranial vault due to the elastic recoil of the spinal dura. Consequently, at the craniocervical junction, a bidirectional CSF flow is present

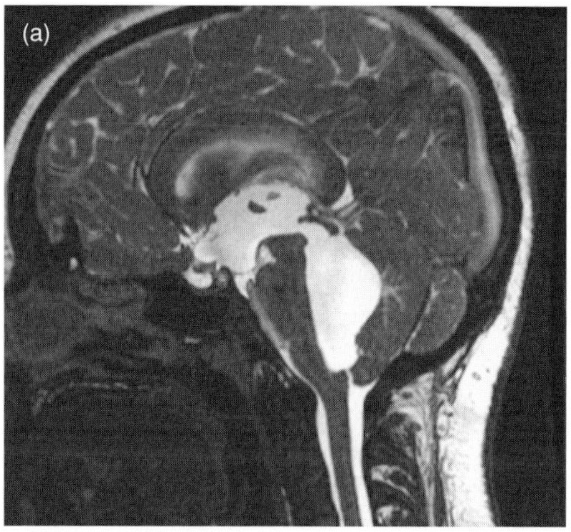

Fig. 6.14. (a) Thin-sliced heavily T2-weighted sagittal MRI of the posterior fossa with low-lying cerebellar tonsils and mildly dilated fourth and third ventricle as well as Sylvian aqueduct. **(b)** Phase-contrast cerebrospinal fluid (CSF) studies show on the magnitude images (left image) high CSF flow (hyperintense) along the anterior contour of the brainstem as well as anterior and posterior to the spinal cord. The phase images (middle and right image) show alternating hyper- and hypointense flow along the anterior brainstem and spinal cord, indicating bidirectional CSF flow. The flow within the fourth ventricle is unchanged slightly heterogeneous hypointense, indicating unidirectional, slightly turbulent CSF flow.

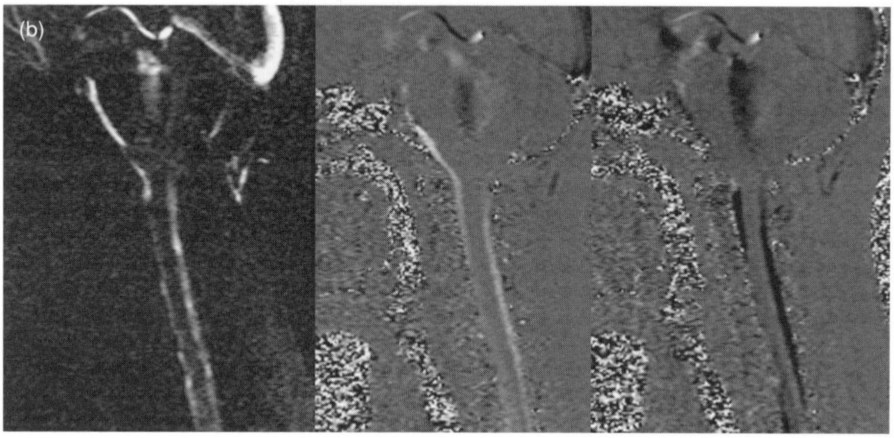

(Alperin et al. 2001). Various posterior fossa pathologies, including malformations such as the Chiari I malformation in which the downward displaced tonsils act as pistons, may limit this CSF flow, with resulting neurologic symptoms including headache, ataxic gait or sensory deficits and hydrocephalus or hydromyelia/syringomyelia. This technique has proven to be fast and reliable. The generated physiologic data may solidify the causal relationship between obstructed/impaired CSF flow at the craniocervical junction and neurologic symptoms. In addition, PC flow studies allow visualization of CSF flow at the Sylvian aqueduct or patency of a third ventriculostomy.

REFERENCES

Alperin N, Kulkarni K, Roitberg B, Loth F, Pandian NK, Mafee MF, et al. (2001) Analysis of magnetic resonance imaging-based blood and cerebrospinal fluid flow measurements in patients with Chiari I malformation: a system approach. Neurosurg Focus 11: 1–10.

Boddaert N, Romano S, Funalot B, Rio M, Sarzi E, Lebre AS, et al. (2008) 1H MRS spectroscopy evidence of cerebellar high lactate in mitochondrial respiratory chain deficiency. Molec Genet Metab 93: 85–88.

Costa MOR, Lacerda MTC, Otaduy MCG, Cerii GG, da Costa Leite C (2002) Proton magnetic resonance spectroscopy: normal findings in the cerebellar hemisphere in childhood. Pediatr Radiol 32: 787–792.

Daneman A, Epelman M, Blaser S, Jarrin JR (2006) Imaging of the brain in full-term neonates: does sonography still play a role? Pediatr Radiol 36: 636–646.

Ersahin Y, Mutluer S, Cagli S, Duman Y (1996) Cerebellar mutism: report of seven cases and review of the literature. Neurosurgery 28: 60–66.

Germano A, Baldari S, Caruso G, Caffo M, Montemagno G, Cardia E, Tomasello F (1998) Reversible cerebral perfusion alterations in children with transient mutism after posterior fossa surgery. Child's Nerv Syst 14: 114–119.

Habas C (2010) Functional imaging of the deep cerebellar nuclei: a review. Cerebellum 9: 22–28.

Hoeffner EG, Case I, Jain R, Gujar SK, Shah GV, Deveikis JP, et al. (2004) Cerebral perfusion CT: technique and clinical applications. Radiology 231: 632–644.

Huisman TA (2003) Diffusion-weighted imaging: basic concepts and application in cerebral stroke and head trauma. Eur Radiol 13: 2283–2297.

Huisman TA, Sorensen AG (2004) Perfusion-weighted magnetic resonance imaging of the brain: techniques and application in children. Eur Radiol 14: 59–72.

Huisman TA, Singhi S, Pinto P (2010) Non-invasive imaging of intracranial pediatric vascular lesions. Child Nerv Syst 26(10): 1275–1295.

Jacobs MA, Horska A, van Zijl PCM, Barker PB (2001) Quantitative proton MR spectroscopic imaging of normal human cerebellum and brain stem. Magn Reson Med 46: 699–705.

Jones TR, Kaplan RT, lane B, Atlas SW, Rubin GD (2001) Single- versus multi-detector row CT of the brain: Quality assessment. Radiology 219: 750–755.

Juranek J, Salman MS (2010) Anomalous development of brain structure and function in spina bifida myelomeningocele. Dev Disabil Res Rev 16: 23–30.

Kansagra AP, Wong EC (2008) Mapping of vertebral artery perfusion territories using arterial spin labeling MRI. J Magn Reson Imaging 28: 762–766.

Kim S, Salamon N, Jackson HA, Bluemi S, Panigraphy A (2010) PET imaging in pediatric neuroradiology: current and future applications. Pediatr Radiol 40: 82–96.

Manto M (2008) The cerebellum, cerebellar disorders, and cerebellar research-Two centuries of discoveries. Cerebellum 7: 505–516.

Mascalchi M, Brugnoli R, Guerrini L, Belli G, Nistri M, Politi LS, et al. (2002a) Single-voxel long TE 1H –MR spectroscopy of the normal brainstem and cerebellum. J Magn Reson Imaging 16: 532–537.

Mascalchi M, Cosottini M, Lolli F, Salvi F, Tessa CV, Macucci M, et al. (2002b) Proton MR spectroscopy of the cerebellum and pons in patients with degenerative ataxia. Radiology 223: 371–378.

Miller NG, Reddick WE, Kocak M, Glass JO, Loebel U, Morris N, et al. (2010) Cerebellocerebral diaschisis is the likely mechanism of postsurgical posterior fossa syndrome in pediatric patients with midline cerebellar tumors. AJNR Am J Neuroradiol 31: 288–294.

Mori S, Wakana S, Nagae-Poetscher LM, van Zijl PCM (2005) MRI Atlas of Human White Matter. Amsterdam, Oxford: Elsevier.

Nishina M, Kato T, Ito M, Takashima S (1999) In vitro high resolution proton magnetic resonance study of human cerebellar development during the period from the fetus to childhood. Physiol Chem Phys Med NMR 31: 103–108.

Ohnishi T, Matsuda H, Hashimoto T, Kunihiro T, Nishikawa M, Uema T, Sasaki M (2000) Abnormal regional cerebral blood flow in childhood autism. Brain 123: 1838–1844.

Öz G, Nelson CD, Koski DM, Henry P-G, Marjanska M, Deelchand DK, et al. (2010) Noninvasive detection of pre-symptomatic and progressive neurodegeneration in a mouse model of spinocerebellar ataxia type 1. J Neurosci 30(10): 3831–3838.

Poretti A, Boltshauser E, Loenneker T, Valente EM, Brancati F, Il'yasov K, Huisman TA (2007) Diffusion tensor imaging in Joubert syndrome. AJNR Am J Neuroradiol 28: 1929–1933.

Schneider JF, Il'Yasov KA, Hennig J, Martin E (2004) Fast quantitative diffusion-tensor imaging of cerebral white matter from the neonatal period to adolescence. Neuroradiology 46: 258–266.

Steggerda SJ, Leijser LM, Walther FJ, van Wezel-Meijler G (2009) Neonatal cranial ultrasonography: how to optimize its performance. Early Hum Dev 85: 93–99.

Stoodley CJ, Schmahmann JD (2009) Functional topography in the human cerebellum: a meta-analysis of neuroimaging studies. Neuroimage 15: 489–501.

Timmann D, Drepper J, Frings M, Maschke M, Richter S, Gerwig M, Kolb FP (2010) The human cerebellum contributes to motor, emotional and cognitive associative learning. A review. Cortex 46: 845–857.

Van Wezel-Meijler G, Steggerda SJ, Leijser LM (2010) Cranial ultrasonography in neonates: Role and limitations. Semin Perinatol 34: 28–38.

Vulliemoz S, Raineteau O, Jabaudan D (2005) Reaching beyond the midline: why are human brains cross wired? Lancet Neurol 4: 87–98.

Part 4
Malformations

Introductory comments

Eugen Boltshauser

In Part 4, Malformations, a number of classic, newly described, and rare malformations are discussed. We are fully aware that the delineation and allocation of some chapters is arbitrary and open to criticism.

Some malformations (e.g., Joubert syndrome and related disorders) are genetically determined, but we have not grouped these conditions in Part 5 on Genetic and Metabolic Disorders. In contrast, pontocerebellar hypoplasias (most are genetically based) are not grouped among the malformations, as they are prenatal-onset degenerative disorders.

Other malformations (e.g., cerebellar agenesis, hypoplasia, dysplasia) may result from a primary developmental process or a secondary disruption; they are discussed among malformations with a reference note in the chapter on disruptions, if appropriate.

We have included a chapter on nonprogressive congenital ataxia (NPCA) in this part although neuroimaging is often normal, while some patients have cerebellar hypoplasia. Because of lack of awareness and these potentially misleading normal images, NPCA is underdiagnosed although it is more prevalent in clinical practice than any defined cerebellar malformation.

The delineation of some malformations (e.g., cerebellar hypoplasia, Dandy-Walker malformation) is still controversial. This problem of definition and classification is aggravated by recent observations that some mutations (e.g., *FOXC1*) can be associated with a spectrum (e.g., cerebellar hypoplasia, mega cisterna magna, Dandy Walker-malformation), rendering image-based classification in this context very problematic (Aldinger et al. 2009).

We felt unable to follow existing classification schemes. In our view the proposal suggested by Patel and Barkovich (2002) used the term dysplasia too broadly and included disruptions as well. The classification by Parisi and Dobyns (2003) included new genetic insights, but remained basically imaging based. They stressed the importance of considering anomalies of the brainstem as well. The recently suggested 'developmental and genetic classification' (Barkovich et al. 2009) is certainly a major step forward. It includes updated genetic (human and mouse mutants) information. The classification is designed to be flexible to allow modifications when new embryological progress or new malformations are discovered. However, this classification is difficult to use in practice (e.g., cerebellar hypoplasia can result from different processes and is grouped in various categories). In summary, our practical everyday diagnostic work-up still relies mainly on a pattern recognition neuroimaging approach.

The sequence of chapters in this part is somewhat arbitrary. We aimed to start with malformations associated with a 'small cerebellum' (e.g., agenesis, hypoplasia). Nonprogressive cerebellar ataxia follows hypoplasia, as some patients have cerebellar hypoplasia. Subsequent chapters deal with predominantly 'small vermis' (e.g., Dandy-Walker malformation, Joubert syndrome), 'dysplastic cerebellum' (e.g., dysplasia, cerebellar cysts), and 'large cerebellum'. Chiari type I and type II malformations are historically related and are therefore discussed consecutively, although the pathogenesis is quite different. Finally, chapters describing malformations chiefly affecting the brainstem (e.g., disconnection, pontine tegmental cap dysplasia) are presented.

Glossary

Cerebellar agenesis

Cerebellar agenesis implies near-complete absence of cerebellar structures. This term does not comprise pathogenesis, may be a primary malformation or a disruption. Remarkably, the size of the posterior fossa may be enlarged.

Cerebellar atrophy

Cerebellar atrophy implies loss of cerebellar parenchyma. Cerebellar atrophy may result from a genetic or metabolic disease, or may be acquired (intoxication, inflammation). Cerebellar atrophy can occasionally be 'superimposed' on cerebellar hypoplasia (in congenital disorders of glycosylation). In infants with severe neurological impairment progressive cerebellar atrophy, as demonstrable by MRI, is not accompanied by obvious clinical deterioration (progressive encephalopathy with oedema, hypsarrhythmia and optic atrophy (PEHO) syndrome, infantile vanishing white matter disease). On neuroimaging cerebellar atrophy is not always distinguishable from variants of 'static' cerebellar hypoplasia with small cerebellar volume and enlarged interfolial spaces.

Cerebellar dysplasia

The term cerebellar dysplasia implies a deranged development of the cerebellar tissue resulting in abnormal cerebellar foliation and fissuration. However, not only the cerebellar cortex is affected, but also the architecture of the cerebellar white matter. Cerebellar dysplasia includes a heterogeneous spectrum of different neuroimaging findings, clinical presentations, and etiologies leading to a purely descriptive definition.

Cerebellar hypoplasia

The term cerebellar hypoplasia implies a reduced cerebellar volume. It is not (necessarily) conclusive for its pathogenetic mechanism. It can result from a malformative as well as from a disruptive process. The size of the posterior fossa may be normal or reduced. In some patients with a static course the interfoliar spaces are enlarged, mimicking cerebellar atrophy.

Disruption

Disruptions are defined as morphological defects of an organ, part of an organ, or a larger region of the body resulting from an extrinsic breakdown of, or an interference with, an originally normal developmental process. It may well be that genetic factors contribute to the susceptibility to disruptions.

Malformation

Malformations are defined as morphological defects of an organ, part of an organ, or a larger region of the body resulting from an intrinsically abnormal developmental process.

Nonprogressive congenital ataxia

Nonprogressive congenital ataxia (NPCA) implies ataxia evident in an early (usually infancy) developmental stage. Obvious signs of ataxia are preceded by hypotonia and delayed motor milestones.

Pontocerebellar hypoplasias

In clinical practice the use of the term pontocerebellar hypoplasia (PCH) is not uniform. It is often used in a descriptive manner to imply that the volume of the cerebellum and the pons are reduced, generally in a nonspecific way. On the other hand it is used in the context of so-called pontocerebellar hypoplasia, as previously conceptualized by Peter Barth. However, in the last sense, PCH are not 'static' malformations, but early (prenatal)-onset degenerative disorders.

REFERENCES

Aldinger KA, Lehmann OJ, Hudgins L, Chizhikov VV, Bassuk AG, Ades LC, Krantz ID, Dobyns WB, Millen KJ (2009) FOXC1 is required for normal cerebellar development and is a major contributor to chromosome 6p25.3 Dandy-Walker malformation. Nat Genet 41: 1037–1042.

Barkovich AJ, Millen KJ, Dobyns WB (2009) A developmental and genetic classification for midbrain-hindbrain malformations. Brain 132: 3199–3230.

Parisi MA, Dobyns WB (2003) Human malformations of the midbrain and hindbrain: review and proposed classification scheme. Mol Genet Metab 80: 36–53.

Patel S, Barkovich AJ (2002) Analysis and classification of cerebellar malformations. AJNR Am J Neuroradiol 23: 1074–1087.

7
Cerebellar Agenesis

Andrea Poretti, Eugen Boltshauser, and Jeremy D. Schmahmann

Cerebellar agenesis is an extremely rare condition characterized by absence of the cerebellum. Cerebellar agenesis was first described by Combettes (1831) and later by Ferrier (1876). The term cerebellar agenesis itself is problematic for two reasons. First, the majority of reported patients have at least some remnants of cerebellar tissue (Boyd 1940; Rubinstein and Freeman 1940; Glickstein 1994; Gardner et al. 2001; Caroppo et al. 2009; Boyd 2010), and so the condition is usually near-complete in its most fully developed form. Second, the condition appears to result from at least two distinct pathophysiological mechanisms. One is likely to be genetically mediated and is often associated with other brain malformations, hence complex cerebellar agenesis. The other results from disruptive causes – the result of intrauterine or neonatal injury to the developing cerebellum, and usually presents with isolated cerebellar agenesis together with secondary involvement of precerebellar brainstem nuclei (pons and inferior olive). Reports in the era of computerized axial tomography (CT) and magnetic resonance imaging (MRI) have described the disorder antemortem, accounting for a total of perhaps more than 40 in vivo cases published to date (Wang et al. 1983; Sener and Jinkins 1993; Sener 1995; van Hoof and Wilmink 1996; Van Coster et al. 1998; Velioglu et al. 1998; Hoveyda et al. 1999; Chheda et al. 2002; Timmann et al. 2003; Zafeiriou et al. 2004; Titomanlio et al. 2005; Tortori-Donati et al. 2005; Saito et al. 2006; Tavano et al. 2007; Alkan et al. 2009; Huissoud et al. 2009; Poretti et al. 2009; Tutak et al. 2009; Jacob and Goez 2011; and S Cirak et al., personal communication 2005).

Etiology

Genetic etiology

A genetic etiology of cerebellar agenesis may be suspected if there are associated dysmorphic features on general examination, developmental anomalies of other neural structures, or inherited endocrine disorders. Mutations in the pancreas transcription factor 1α (*PTF1A*) gene on chromosome 10p13-p12.1 (MIM #607194) were identified in a large family with both cerebellar agenesis and neonatal diabetes (Sellick et al. 2004; Tutak et al. 2009). This gene plays a major role in cerebellar neurogenesis and pancreatic development (Kumar and Melton 2003). It encodes a basic helix-loop-helix transcription factor that has been shown to be expressed in progenitor cells in the ventricular zone of the dorsal aspect of rhombomere 1 (Millen and Gleeson 2008). Its protein product is essential for the generation of GABAergic cells in the cerebellum (Purkinje cells and interneurons) (Hoshino et al. 2005). In the absence of *PTF1A*, the failure to generate GABAergic neurons leads to massive prenatal death of all cerebellar glutamatergic neurons because of the absence of their GABAergic synaptic partners (Hoshino et al. 2005; Millen and Gleeson 2008). Thus, just as accentuated apoptosis can cause cerebral hypoplasia, it can also result in cerebellar hypoplasia or cerebellar agenesis (Kaindl et al. 2006; Takano et al. 2006; Millen and Gleeson 2008). In humans, mutations of the *PTF1A* gene results not only in cerebellar agenesis, but also in neonatal diabetes mellitus (due to pancreatic agenesis), dysmorphic signs (triangular face, small chin, low-set ears, little subcutaneous fat, joint stiffness), and irregular respiration (Hoveyda et al. 1999; Sellick et al. 2004 Tutak et al. 2009). Additionally, these children have low birthweight, probably reflecting the absence of insulin which, in the healthy infant, acts as a growth factor.

Zaferiou et al. reported the combination of cerebellar agenesis and diabetes insipidus in a 7-year-old girl (Zafeiriou et al. 2004). To our knowledge, this combination has not otherwise been reported, and thus may be coincidental. Diabetes insipidus occurs only rarely in association with cerebellar disorders, as in Wolfram syndrome (DIDMOAD – diabetes insipidus, diabetes mellitus, optic atrophy and deafness with cerebellar and brainstem atrophy; Minton et al. 2003), but this patient did not manifest the other features of that syndrome.

Wang et al. reported a 13-year-old girl with cerebellar agenesis and an organoid nevus (or linear nevus sebaceus) on her scalp (Wang et al. 1983). Gross structural abnormalities of the cerebrum or cranium consisting mainly of hemimegalencephaly, hemimegacranium, or enlargement of one lateral ventricle has frequently been observed (72%) in the linear nevus sebaceus syndrome (van de Warrenburg et al. 1998). To our knowledge, however, cerebellar abnormalities are not encountered in this syndrome.

An X-linked inherited origin of cerebellar agenesis was proposed on the basis of two male siblings who died shortly after birth with congenital hydrocephalus, one of whom had cerebellar agenesis and absence of the foramina of Luschka and Magendie (Riccardi and Marcus 1978).

Some earlier reports of complete cerebellar agenesis are likely also to represent genetically mediated disorders that were incompatible with life. The cases reported by Warrington and Monsarrat (1902) and Priestley (1920) had hydrocephalus

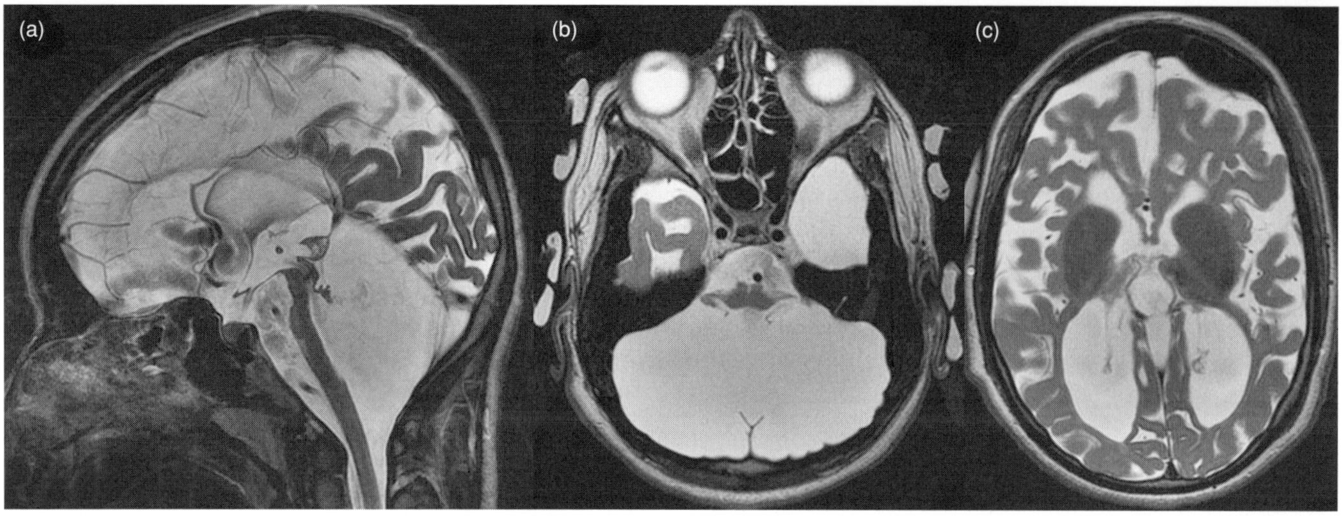

Fig. 7.1. Cerebellar agenesis in a 15-year-old girl. **(a)** Sagittal T2-weighted MRI showing an empty enlarged posterior fossa; the cerebellar structures are almost absent except for a rudimentary structure projecting posterior to the inferior colliculi, and the pons is markedly hypoplastic. **(b)** Axial T2-weighted MRI demonstrating minute cerebellar tissue projecting lateral to the brainstem and an enlarged posterior fossa; **(c)** Supratentorial T2-weighted MRI revealing loss of the white matter. (Reprinted with permission from Poretti A et al. Eur J Paediatr Neurol 2009; 13: 397–40.)

and spina bifida. Both cases of Hamilton and Grafe (1994) had multiple somatic and neurological malformations, with additional features of hydrocephalus in one and microcephaly in the other. These cases succumbed in infancy (or gestation was terminated), and are entirely different from patients with isolated cerebellar agenesis who live to adulthood, and whose cerebellar agenesis probably results from disruption.

Disruptive etiology

Isolated cerebellar agenesis seems to represent the most severe form of cerebellar disruption such as a haemorrhage, ischaemia, or infection that occurs during gestation or the perinatal period, after the cerebellum has already developed. We reported a child in whom fetal ultrasound demonstrated normal cerebellar anatomy at 18 and 22 gestational weeks, respectively, but cerebellar agenesis was identified at 12 months of age when the patient was referred for developmental delay (Poretti et al. 2009). This case is a clear example of an intrauterine disruption. In another case, a girl with cerebellar agenesis had additional extensive cerebral white matter loss reminiscent of periventricular leukomalacia, with a clinical presentation of spastic quadriplegia cerebral palsy and secondary microcephaly. This case also represents an acquired, not hereditary lesion (Fig. 7.1c) (Poretti et al. 2009). Recently, Mohila et al. (2010) reported cerebellar agenesis in a newborn with neonatal alloimmune thrombocytopenia, diffuse body ecchymoses, petechiae, and arthrogryposis at birth. She died on day 3 because of multisystem organ failure and disseminated intravascular coagulopathy. Neuropathological findings revealed cerebellar loss, atrophic pons and medulla with prominent pyramidal tracts and absent olivary nuclei, acute and chronic germinal matrix haemorrhages, and extensive haemosiderin deposition in the posterior fossa. These observations support a disruptive etiology of cerebellar agenesis. Unilateral cerebellar aplasia may be the result of a unilateral disruptive event, and a bilateral disruptive event may similarly be considered as the underlying cause of near-total cerebellar agenesis (Poretti et al. 2010). This conclusion receives support from the MRI report of a rudimentary brainstem and cerebellar primordium resembling cerebellar agenesis in a case of anencephaly (Calzolari et al. 2004).

Neuroimaging and neuropathology

The characteristic finding in cerebellar agenesis is the minute remnant of cerebellar tissue that probably corresponds to the middle cerebellar peduncles (MCPs), anterior vermal lobules (particularly vermal lobule III), or flocculi (Figs 7.1 and 7.2). The volume of the posterior fossa is variable, mostly of normal or increased size, but cases with reduced volume have been also reported (Sener and Jinkins 1993). We have observed increased volume of an empty skull not only in cerebellar agenesis, but also in hemi-hydranencephaly, and we speculate that cerebrospinal fluid (CSF) pulsations may be responsible. It has also been proposed that posthaemorrhagic obstruction of CSF drainage from the developing fourth ventricle explained enlargement of the posterior fossa in a case with posthaemorrhagic cerebellar disruption affecting the vermis and both cerebellar hemispheres (Limperopoulos et al. 2010). In cases of isolated cerebellar agenesis, there is secondary brainstem involvement, with marked pontine hypoplasia and absence of the protuberance of the inferior olives (Fig. 7.1), reflecting retrograde loss of the nuclei of the basis pontis and therefore of the pontocerebellar fibers; and retrograde loss also of the neurons of the inferior olive that provide the olivocerebellar projection. These neuroimaging findings are corroborated by neuropathological reports (Baker and Graves 1931; Boyd 1940;

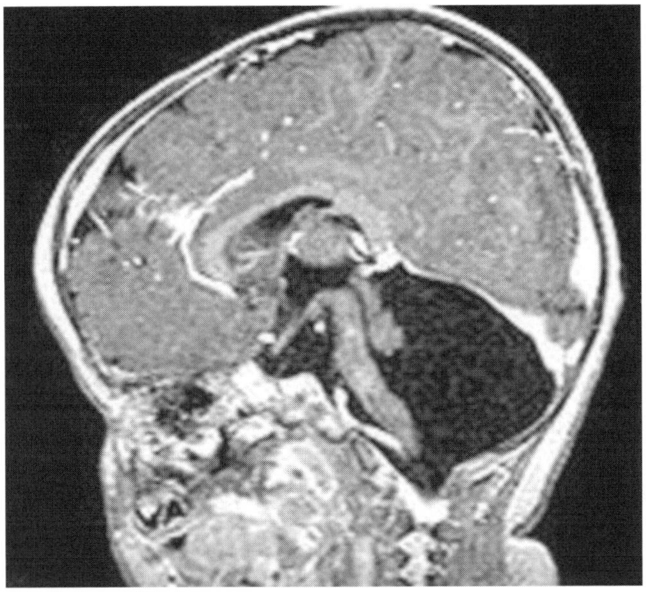

Fig. 7.2. Cerebellar agenesis in a 1-year-old child with normal cerebellar anatomy on the routine ultrasound at 18 and 22 gestational weeks, respectively: sagittal T1-weighted MRI of suboptimal quality revealing an enlarged fossa posterior, marked hypoplasia of the pons, and almost complete absence of cerebellar structures except for remnants located in the anterior vermal area. (Reprinted with permission from Poretti A et al. Eur J Paediatr Neurol 2009; 13: 397–407.)

Rubinstein and Freeman 1940; Stewart 1956; Glickstein 1994; Leestma and Torres 2000; Boyd 2010).

Supratentorial abnormalities such as fused thalami may be detected in cases of genetically determined cerebellar agenesis (Van Coster et al. 1998).

Prenatal diagnosis of cerebellar agenesis is possible. In one case ultrasound at 23 weeks of gestation revealed absence of cerebellar structures with a normal brainstem but reduced volume of the posterior fossa. These findings were confirmed at autopsy following medical termination of pregnancy at 25 weeks of gestation (Huissoud et al. 2009).

Diagnosis

The diagnosis of cerebellar agenesis is made by the typical MRI findings pre- or postnatally. Newborns with cerebellar agenesis should be evaluated for diabetes mellitus; the association of cerebellar agenesis with neonatal diabetes mellitus is suggestive of a mutation in the *PTF1A* gene.

Differential diagnosis

The critical differential diagnostic consideration is between isolated cerebellar agenesis (partial or near-complete) that probably represents a disruption, from complex cerebellar agenesis that is part of a syndromic or neurodevelopmental disorder likely to be of genetic origin, which may include dysmorphic features on the general examination, endocrine disorders (such as diabetes) on metabolic screens, and morphological abnormalities of the corpus callosum, cerebral hemispheres, or spinal cord on neuroimaging.

The small cerebellum in nonprogressive cerebellar ataxia (Steinlin et al. 1999), progressive neurodegenerative conditions such as infantile-onset spinocerebellar ataxia (IOSCA), and the genetically determined spectrum of pontocerebellar hypoplasias (Maricich et al. 2011) are also readily distinguished from cerebellar agenesis by the presence in these neurodegenerative conditions or malformations of a small, abnormal cerebellum, rather than the missing cerebellum that characterizes cerebellar agenesis. The pontocerebellar hypoplasias and IOSCA also have a hypoplastic or atrophic brainstem, frequently together with dysmorphic phenotype and abnormal morphology of the cerebral hemispheres. The essential, distinguishing feature of cerebellar agenesis, however, is that the cerebellum is absent, either in part, or (almost) completely. This is a quite different neuroimaging picture than in these other infantile-onset disorders.

Clinical features

To our knowledge, almost all patients with cerebellar agenesis have been symptomatic. A female described by Sener and Jinkins (1993) appeared to be asymptomatic, but a detailed clinical description of the case was not provided. The clinical presentation of cerebellar agenesis appears to be quite heterogeneous, ranging from early death in presumed genetically mediated complex cerebellar agenesis to variable degrees of cerebellar dysfunction including cognitive impairment in cases of isolated cerebellar agenesis following disruption.

Cerebellar agenesis together with infantile diabetes mellitus may be lethal in the first 2 months of life. Patients with this constellation have succumbed to sepsis and recurrent bouts of apnea. The syndrome may be apparently sporadic (Van Coster et al. 1998), inherited as a recessive disorder as described in a highly consanguineous family (Hoveyda et al. 1999), or the presenting manifestation of the known recessively inherited *PTF1A* gene disorder as described in a Turkish infant (Tutak et al. 2009).

The clinical findings of eight patients with isolated cerebellar agenesis with secondary pontine and olivary involvement have been reported in detail (Wang et al. 1983; Velioglu et al. 1998; Timmann et al. 2003; Zafeiriou et al. 2004; Titomanlio et al. 2005; Jacob and Goez 2011; and S Cirak et al., personal communication 2005). At the last reported follow-up the median age of these patients was 13 years (mean 17.1 years, range 1.6–59 years). In all patients there was evidence of motor incapacity, although all patients older than 2 years of age achieved independent walking. All patients had truncal ataxia, four had limb ataxia with dysmetria, intention tremor, and muscular hypotonia, three had dysarthria and head nodding, and one had microcephaly and spasticity of the lower extremities. Dexterity was studied in one adult with cerebellar agenesis who generated greater grasping forces compared to healthy controls, and who showed impairment of the predictive adjustment of grasping forces to the differential loading requirements of movement direction (Nowak et al. 2007). Ocular motor abnormalities were found in six patients: squint and nystagmus in four (gaze-evoked nystagmus in three and periodic alternating nystagmus in one patient), saccadic intrusions into smooth pursuit eye movements in three, and hypometric saccades in one.

Cognitive outcome has been reported in five cases with isolated cerebellar agenesis (Wang et al. 1983; Velioglu et al. 1998; Zafeiriou et al. 2004; Titomanlio et al. 2005; Richter et al. 2005). Normal cognitive development has been reported only in one patient, although no intelligence quotient (IQ) results were documented (Velioglu et al. 1998). The other patients had impaired cognitive functions: one had mild mental retardation (UK: learning disability) (although no standardized outcome measures were used), and attended a normal school (Titomanlio et al. 2005), one had a developmental quotient according to the Griffith scale of 60 at the age of 7 years (Zafeiriou et al. 2004), one a full-scale IQ of 50 (Wang et al. 1983), and one a full-scale IQ of 66 (Richter et al. 2005). Detailed neuropsychological assessment in a 59-year-old woman (Timmann et al. 2003; Richter et al. 2005) showed mild to moderate deficits in planning behavior, visuospatial abilities, visual memory, attention, speech comprehension, verbal learning, and declarative memory. No significant affective symptoms were observed.

The patient with near-complete cerebellar agenesis described by Tavano et al. (2007) is reminiscent of our own experience of patients with this rare syndrome (Chedda et al. 2002; others not yet published). Their case was severely compromised early in life, but with life-long remediation and rehabilitation he showed considerable gains. As an infant he had marked hypotonia. He sat at age 2, crawled at age 5, walked with assistance at age 10 and walked independently only at age 22. (Other cases have achieved independent ambulation earlier than this, around ages 5 to 7). He uttered his first words after age 2, single word sentences age 7, and short context-related sentences at age 12. He was initially withdrawn, showed autistic traits with stereotyped and repetitive rituals, and avoided contact with others. Emotional fragility, passivity, and impaired socialization persisted until adolescence. By the time he reached age 34 he had moderate gait ataxia, mild extremity dysmetria and intention tremor. He showed persistent cognitive deficits into the mildly retarded range (VIQ = 72, PIQ = 67, FIQ = 69) with particular deficits in selective attention, visuospatial organization, and spatial and procedural memory. Verbal memory was relatively preserved. Linguistic function had improved to the point of allowing him to communicate effectively despite dysphonic voice, morphosyntactic errors, and impaired word choice as well as persistent deficits in comprehension of complex sentences. He displayed a more normal affect, and improved interpersonal interactions (Tavano et al. 2007). No two patients are identical, but this pattern of improved function over the years, with motor deficits becoming less persistent and clinically meaningful than the cognitive or psychosocial issues, appears to be a consistent theme in the long-term course of these patients with cerebellar agenesis.

Approaches to management

The treatment of cerebellar agenesis is symptomatic and includes protracted and focused physical, occupational, and speech therapy over a period of years directed at improving motor and cognitive development. Accommodations in the school setting are required to enable patients with cerebellar agenesis to benefit from the educational process, supporting them in areas of cognitive impairment and nurturing the skill sets that are relatively well preserved. Speech delay may require alternative approaches in the early years. Some patients with cerebellar agenesis (as also in those with nonprogressive cerebellar ataxia; Steinlin et al. 1999) benefit from instruction in sign language until the verbal linguistic skills develop at the age of 5 or 6 years. Those with gross motor delay and gait instability may do well with service dogs – this enhances the child's motor skills and gait, and promotes the social acceptance among their peers that can be challenging in the early school years. Close monitoring for potential cognitive and neuropsychiatric interventions can prevent avoidable complications over the long term.

Outcome

Essentially all patients with near-complete isolated cerebellar agenesis with secondary involvement of brainstem precerebellar nuclei reported in the literature and in our own collective experience have been symptomatic. Motor deficits are present in all, but the degree of involvement of gait, extremity, speech, and ocular motor control is variable, depends on the degree to which there is any preserved cerebellar tissue, and perhaps most importantly, improves with time, possibly aided by persistent physical and other rehabilitation intervention strategies (Tavano et al. 2007; personal experience of the authors). Although walking is delayed occasional patients with cerebellar agenesis achieve independent walking. Patients with cerebellar agenesis demonstrate the range of intellectual, psychosocial, and neuropsychiatric impairments that conform to the various aspects of the cerebellar cognitive affective syndrome, including deficits in executive, visuospatial, linguistic (both expressive and receptive), and affective functions (Schmahmann and Sherman 1998; Levisohn et al. 2000). Their neuropsychiatric features conform to those reported in Schmahmann et al. (2007) including impairments in the domains of attention control, emotional control, social skill set, autism spectrum disorders, and psychosis spectrum disorders (see Chapter 4). Like the motor syndrome, the range and severity of the cognitive deficits is quite variable. The higher order deficits, like the motor incapacity, also tend to improve with time and with focused rehabilitation strategies. Adult patients with near-complete cerebellar agenesis may live semi-independently with supervision, holding down positions of employment that place few demands on fine motor or complex cognitive skill sets.

Acknowledgments

Supported in part by RO1 MH067980, the Birmingham and MINDlink Foundations (JDS).

REFERENCES

Alkan O, Kizilkilic O, Yildirim T (2009) Malformations of the midbrain and hindbrain: a retrospective study and review of the literature. Cerebellum 8: 355–365.

Baker RC, Graves GO (1931) Cerebellar agenesis. Arch Neurol Psychiat 25: 548–555.

Boyd CA (2010) Cerebellar agenesis revisited. Brain 133: 941–944.

Boyd JD (1940) A case of neocerebellar hypoplasia. J Anat 74: 557.

Calzolari F, Gambi B, Garani G, Tamisari L (2004) Anencephaly: MRI findings and pathogenetic theories. Pediatr Radiol 34: 1012–1016.

Caroppo P, Orsi L, D'Agata F, Baudino B, Boghi A, Avidano F, et al. (2009) Neuropsychological and functional study in a case of partial cerebellar agenesis. Neurocase 15: 373–383.

Chedda MG, Sherman JC, Schmahmann J (2002) Neurologic, psychiatric, and cognitive manifestations in cerebellar agenesis. Neurology 58(suppl. 3): A356.

Combettes M (1831) Absence complète du cervelet, des pédoncules postérieurs et de la protuberance cèrèbrale chez une jeune fille morte dans la onzième année. Bull Soc Anat Paris 5: 148–157.

Ferrier D (ed.) (1876) Functions of the cerebellum. In: The Functions of the Brain. London: Smith Elder.

Gardner RJ, Coleman LT, Mitchell LA, Smith LJ, Harvey AS, Scheffer I.E., et al. (2001) Near-total absence of the cerebellum. Neuropediatrics 32: 62–68.

Glickstein M (1994) Cerebellar agenesis. Brain 117: 1209–1212.

Hamilton RL, Grafe MJ (1994) Complete absence of the cerebellum: a report of two cases. Acta Neuropathol 88: 258–261.

Hoshino M, Nakamura S, Mori K, Kawauchi T, Terao M, Nishimura YV, et al. (2005) Ptf1a, a bHLH transcriptional gene, defines GABAergic neuronal fates in cerebellum. Neuron 47: 201–213.

Hoveyda N, Shield JP, Garrett C, Chong WK, Beardsall K, Bentsi-Enchill E, et al. (1999) Neonatal diabetes mellitus and cerebellar hypoplasia/agenesis: report of a new recessive syndrome. J Med Genet 36: 700–704.

Huissoud C, Rudigoz RC, Bisch C, Brahimi P, Alias F, Tixier H, Guibaud L (2009) Complete cerebellar agenesis: a very rare abnormality of the posterior fossa. Ultrasound Obstet Gynecol 33: 730–731.

Jacob FD, Goez HR (2011) Preservation of language in the ataxic infant in a case of cerebellar agenesis. Can J Neurol Sci 38: 143–144.

Kaindl AM, Asimiadou S, Manthey D, Hagen MV, Turski L, Ikonomidou C (2006) Antiepileptic drugs and the developing brain. Cell Mol Life Sci 63: 399–413.

Kumar M, Melton D (2003) Pancreas specification: a budding question. Curr Opin Genet Dev 13: 401–407.

Leestma JE, Torres JV (2000) Unappreciated agenesis of cerebellum in an adult: case report of a 38-year-old man. Am J Forensic Med Pathol 21: 155–161.

Levisohn L, Cronin-Golomb A, Schmahmann JD (2000) Neuropsychological consequences of cerebellar tumour resection in children: cerebellar cognitive affective syndrome in a paediatric population. Brain 123:1041–1050.

Limperopoulos C, Folkerth R, Barnewolt CE, Connolly S, du Plessis AJ (2010) Posthemorrhagic cerebellar disruption mimicking Dandy-Walker malformation: fetal imaging and neuropathology findings. Semin Pediatr Neurol 17: 75–81.

Maricich SM, Aqeeb KA, Moayedi Y, Mathes EL, Patel MS, Chitayat D, et al. (2011) Pontocerebellar hypoplasia: review of classification and genetics, and exclusion of several genes known to be important for cerebellar development. J Child Neurol 26: 288–294.

Millen KJ, Gleeson JG (2008) Cerebellar development and disease. Curr Opin Neurobiol 18: 12–19.

Minton JA, Rainbow LA, Ricketts C, Barrett TG (2003) Wolfram syndrome. Rev Endocr Metab Disord 4: 53–59.

Mohila CA, Kubicka ZJ, Ornvold KT, Harris BT (2010) Cerebellar loss and brain-stem atrophy associated with neonatal alloimmune thrombocytopenia in a discordant twin. Pediatr Dev Pathol 13: 55–62.

Nowak DA, Timmann D, Hermsdorfer J (2007) Dexterity in cerebellar agenesis. Neuropsychologia 45: 696–703.

Poretti A, Prayer D, Boltshauser E (2009) Morphological spectrum of prenatal cerebellar disruptions. Eur J Paediatr Neurol 13: 397–407.

Poretti A, Limperopoulos C, Roulet-Perez E, Wolf NI, Rauscher C, Prayer D, et al. (2010) Outcome of severe unilateral cerebellar hypoplasia. Dev Med Child Neurol 52: 718–724.

Priestley DP (1920) Complete absence of the cerebellum. Lancet 2: 1302.

Riccardi VM, Marcus ES (1978) Congenital hydrocephalus and cerebellar agenesis. Clin Genet 13: 443–447.

Richter S, Dimitrova A, Hein-Kropp C, Wilhelm H, Gizewski E, Timmann D (2005) Cerebellar agenesis II: motor and language functions. Neurocase 11: 103–113.

Rubinstein HS, Freeman W (1940) Cerebellar agenesis. J Nerv Ment Dis 92: 489–502.

Saito Y, Kawashima Y, Kondo A, Chikumaru Y, Matsui A, Nagata I, Ohno K (2006) Dysphagia-gastroesophageal reflux complex: complications due to dysfunction of solitary tract neucleus-mediated vago-vagal reflex. Neuropediatrics 37: 115–120.

Schmahmann JD, Sherman JC (1998) The cerebellar cognitive affective syndrome. Brain 121: 561–579.

Schmahmann JD, Weilburg JB, Sherman JC (2007) The neuropsychiatry of the cerebellum – insights from the clinic. Cerebellum 6: 254–267.

Sellick GS, Barker KT, Stolte-Dijkstra I, Fleischmann C, Coleman RJ, Garrett C, et al. (2004) Mutations in PTF1A cause pancreatic and cerebellar agenesis. Nat Genet 36: 1301–1305.

Sener RN, Jinkins JR (1993) Subtotal agenesis of the cerebellum in an adult. MRI demonstration. Neuroradiology 35: 286–287.

Sener RN (1995) Cerebellar agenesis versus vanishing cerebellum in Chiari II malformation. Comput Med Imaging Graph 19: 491–494.

Steinlin M, Styger M, Boltshauser E (1999) Cognitive impairments in patients with congenital non-progressive cerebellar ataxia. Neurology 53: 966–973.

Stewart RM (1956) Cerebellar agenesis. J Mental Sciences 102: 67–77.

Takano T, Akahori S, Takeuchi Y, Ohno M (2006) Neuronal apoptosis and gray matter heterotopia in microcephaly produced by cytosine arabinoside in mice. Brain Res 1089: 55–66.

Tavano A, Grasso R, Gagliardi C, Triulzi F, Bresolin N, Fabbro F, Borgatti R (2007) Disorders of cognitive and affective development in cerebellar malformations. Brain 130: 2646–2660.

Timmann D, Dimitrova A, Hein-Kropp C, Wilhelm H, Dorfler A (2003) Cerebellar agenesis: clinical, neuropsychological and MR findings. Neurocase 9: 402–413.

Titomanlio L, Romano A, Del Giudice E (2005) Cerebellar agenesis. Neurology 64: E21.

Tortori-Donati P, Rossi A, Biancheri R (2005) Cerebellar agenesis. In: Pediatric Neuroradiology (ed. P Tortori-Donati). Berlin: Springer; 162–163.

Tutak E, Satar M, Yapicioglu H, Altintas A, Narli N, Herguner O, Byram Y (2009) A Turkish newborn infant with cerebellar agenesis/neonatal diabetes mellitus and PTF1A mutation. Genet Couns 20: 147–152.

Van Coster RN, De Praeter CM, Vanhaesebrouck PJ, Leroy JG (1998) MRI findings in a neonate with cerebellar agenesis. Pediatr Neurol 19: 139–142.

van de Warrenburg BP, van Gulik S, Renier WO, Lammens M, Doelman JC (1998) The linear naevus sebaceus syndrome. Clin Neurol Neurosurg 100: 126–132.

van Hoof SC, Wilmink JT (1996) Cerebellar agenesis. J Belge Radiol 79: 282.

Velioglu SK, Kuzeyli K, Zzmenoglu M (1998) Cerebellar agenesis: a case report with clinical and MR imaging findings and a review of the literature. Eur J Neurol 5: 503–506.

Wang PJ, Maeda Y, Izumi T, Yajima K, Hara M, Kobayashi N, Fukuyama Y (1983) An association of subtotal cerebellar agenesis with organoid nevus – a possible new variety of neurocutaneous syndrome. Brain Dev 5: 503–508.

Warrington WB, Monsarrat K (1902) A case of arrested development of the cerebellum and its peduncles with spina bifida and other developmental peculiarities in the cord. Brain 25: 444–478.

Zafeiriou DI, Vargiami E, Boltshauser E (2004) Cerebellar agenesis and diabetes insipidus. Neuropediatrics 35: 364–367.

8
Cerebellar Hypoplasia

Andrea Poretti and Eugen Boltshauser

Cerebellar hypoplasia includes a group of developmental disorders of the cerebellum and implies a cerebellum with normal or near normal shape, but reduced volume (Figs 8.1 and 8.2) (see Checklists, Table 14) (Boltshauser 2004; Poretti et al. 2008b). Cerebellar hypoplasia is mostly symmetric, but occasionally unilateral or markedly asymmetric cerebellar hemispheres can be seen, particularly as a residual change after a disruptive prenatal cerebellar insult, most likely haemorrhagic (Poretti et al. 2010).

Cerebellar hypoplasia should be distinguished from *cerebellar atrophy* (CA) which implies loss of cerebellar parenchyma with secondary enlargement of the cerebellar interfolial spaces (Poretti et al. 2008b). Distinguishing cerebellar agenesis from cerebellar hypoplasia does not seem difficult in theory, but can be problematic or impossible in practice based on a single examination. In patients with nonprogressive congenital ataxia (i.e., with an obviously longstanding static situation) enlarged cerebellar sulci can be seen mimicking CA (Figs 8.3 and 8.4) (Margari et al. 2004; Yapici and Eraksoy 2005; Donald et al. 2006; Turkmen et al. 2006; Lamonica et al. 2010). In these cases separation of CA from cerebellar hypoplasia is thus not always possible. Additionally, atrophy can be superimposed on hypoplasia, as documented in some patients with congenital disorder of glycosylation.

Generally there is poor correlation between neuroimaging findings (particularly the degree of cerebellar hypoplasia) and both neurological signs and cognitive impairment. In genetic causes of cerebellar hypoplasia there is often considerable variability in neuroimaging and clinical presentation. Additionally, similar imaging patterns can have different etiologies. Therefore, the presence of CH is not (necessarily) indicative of a specific pathogenetic mechanism.

Hypoplasia may affect the cerebellum globally (most commonly) or selectively involve either the vermis with sparing of the lateral hemispheres (*paleocerebellar hypoplasia*) or one or both hemispheres sparing the vermis (*neocerebellar hypoplasia*).

Cerebellar hypoplasia can result from several aetiologies including prenatal infections (particularly cytomegalovirus), prenatal exposure to teratogens (e.g., retinoic acid), chromosomal aberrations, metabolic disorders, genetic (isolated) cerebellar hypoplasia, genetic (complex) malformations, migration disorders, some forms of congenital muscular dystrophies, and pontocerebebellar hypoplasia. Therefore, cerebellar hypoplasia can result from primary genetic causes as well as from secondary (i.e., prenatally acquired) events. The distinction between primary developmental processes and secondary disruptive lesions is of utmost importance for pathogenetic considerations and genetic counselling.

In this chapter we will discuss some general points about the clinical manifestation of cerebellar hypoplasia and selective disorders causing cerebellar hypoplasia which are not included elsewhere in the book. We will categorize cerebellar hypoplasia into (1) unilateral cerebellar hypoplasias, (2) predominantly midline hypoplasias with mainly vermis involvement, (3) global cerebellar hypoplasias with involvement of both vermis and hemispheres, and (4) pontocerebellar hypoplasias. This simplified categorization is based on the neuroimaging pattern as in the practical 'everyday' approach, not on the underlying pathogenetic mechanisms.

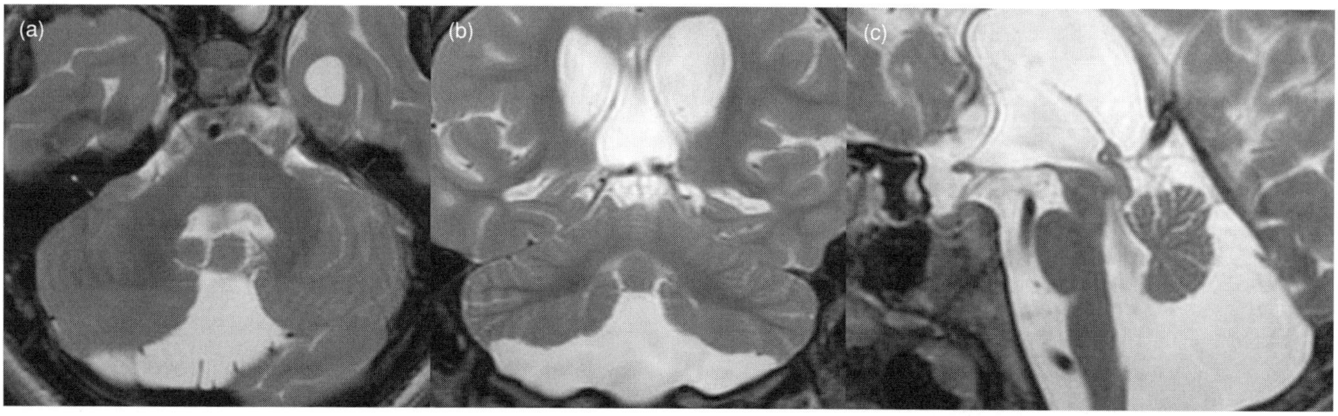

Fig. 8.1. Cerebellar hypoplasia in a 17-year-old boy with seizures. **(a)** Axial, **(b)** coronal, and **(c)** midsagittal T2-weighted MRI showing reduced cerebellar volume but near normal structure, cavum Vergae, and reduced periventricular white matter bilaterally.

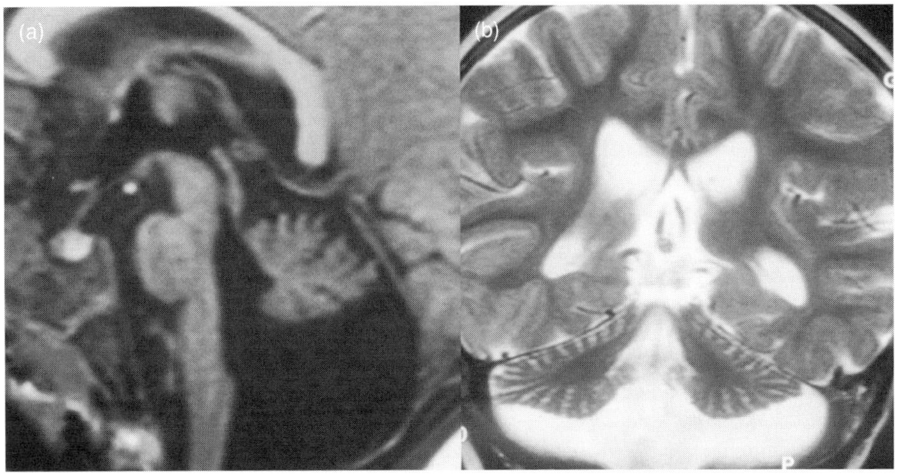

Fig. 8.2. Cerebellar hypoplasia in a 5-year-old child with marked developmental delay. **(a)** Sagittal T1-weighted and **(b)** coronal T2-weighted images show reduced cerebellar volume and mild enlargement of the interfoliar spaces. (Reprinted with permission from Poretti A et al., Eur J Paediatr Neurol 2008; 12: 155–167.)

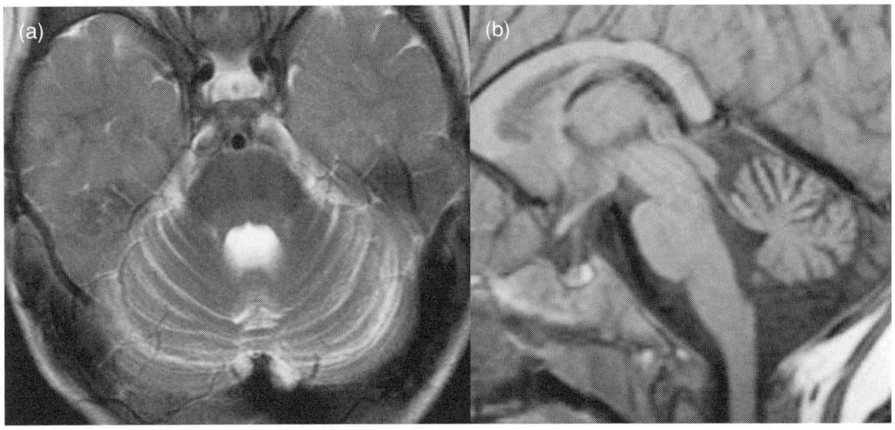

Fig. 8.3. Child aged 5 years with nonprogressive cerebellar ataxia. **(a)** Axial and **(b)** midsagittal T2-weighted MRI presenting normal size of the cerebellum, but enlarged interfolial spaces mimicking cerebellar atrophy. (Reprinted with permission from Poretti A et al., Eur J Paediatr Neurol 2008; 12: 155–167.) MRI at 3 years was identical.

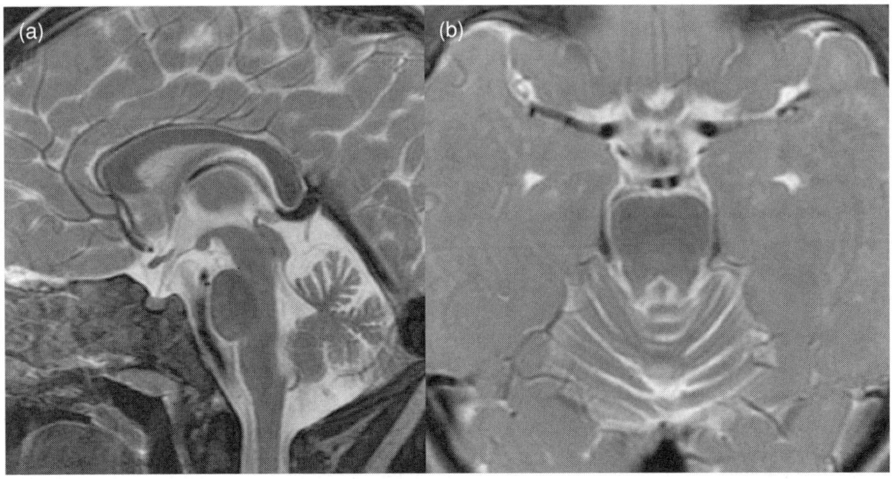

Fig. 8.4. Child aged 17 months with truncal and limb ataxia. **(a)** Midsagittal and **(b)** axial T2-weighted MRI demonstrating enlarged interfolial spaces.

Clinical spectrum associated with cerebellar hypoplasia: General remarks

Different forms of cerebellar hypoplasia differ in their clinical presentation, which may cover a broad phenotypic spectrum. The clinical presentation of cerebellar hypoplasia may depend on associated supratentorial abnormalities (e.g., in children with cerebellar hypoplasia and lissencephaly due to a mutation in the *RELN* or *LIS1* gene) and some clinical symptoms can be found in particular disorders with cerebellar hypoplasia, but they are unrelated to cerebellar hypoplasia (e.g., aniridia in Gillespie syndrome).

In general, children with cerebellar hypoplasia present with early muscular hypotonia and developmental delay (commonly global, not only in motor skills) and show classic cerebellar signs at a later stage (Wassmer et al. 2003, Bolduc and Limperopoulos 2009). Overall reported neurological findings include truncal ataxia (49–93%), muscular hypotonia (may be mild, but more commonly is moderate to severe) (47–49%), ocular signs including nystagmus (several types such as gaze-evoked, rebound, down-beat, up-beat, and periodic alternating nystagmus), strabismus, or ocular movement disorders (saccadic intrusions into ocular pursuit, hypo- or hypermetric saccades, ocular motor apraxia) (40–46%), dysarthria (38%), intention tremor (as sign of limb ataxia, which is present particularly if the cerebellar hemispheres are involved) (9–35%), muscular hypertonia (29%), and microcephaly (20%) (Wassmer et al. 2003; Yapici and Eraksoy 2005; Tavano et al. 2007). Seizures (particularly partial seizures) had a higher occurrence in comparison with the general population. Seizures have been reported in 28–56% of patients in different studies (Wassmer et al. 2003; Ventura et al. 2006).

Developmental delay or cognitive impairment was found in at least two-thirds of patients (66–100%) (Wassmer et al. 2003; Yapici and Eraksoy 2005; Ventura et al. 2006; Tavano et al. 2007), and over one-third had severe impairments (Tavano et al. 2007). Speech and/or language disorders were frequent (about half of the patients) and of variable degree ranging from mild impairment to total absence of expressive language development (Wassmer et al. 2003; Tavano et al. 2007). Furthermore, 5–20% of children were reported to present with autistic features (Wassmer et al. 2003; Tavano et al. 2007) and about 40% had other psychiatric problems including pervasive developmental disorders, obsessive-compulsive disorder, and attention-deficit hyperactivity disorder (Tavano et al. 2007). The contribution of the cerebellum to nonmotor functions was shown first by Schmahmann and Sherman in adults with acquired focal cerebellar strokes (see Chapters 2, 3, and 4) (Schmahmann and Sherman 1998). The involvement of the cerebellum in nonmotor functions was also documented in children with acquired lesions such as benign cerebellar tumours (Levisohn et al. 2000; Riva and Giorgi 2000; Steinlin et al. 2003; Aarsen et al. 2009; De Smet et al. 2009) or prenatal cerebellar disruptions (Poretti et al. 2009d) as well as those with primary cerebellar disorders such as congenital ataxia (Steinlin et al. 1999), Joubert syndrome (Steinlin et al. 1997; Poretti et al. 2009b), and rhombencephalosynapsis (Poretti et al. 2009a). Schmahmann and Sherman coined the term *cerebellar cognitive affective syndrome* in view of the following observations: disturbance of executive function, including poor planning; visuospatial disorganization and impaired visuospatial memory; personality change with blunting of affect or disinhibited and inappropriate behaviour; difficulty with interpreting and producing logical sequences; language difficulties including dysprosody, mild anomia, and agrammatism (Schmahmann and Sherman 1998).

Unilateral cerebellar hypoplasia

Unilateral cerebellar hypoplasia (UCH) (see Checklists, Table 15) is a rare finding encompassing a spectrum ranging from complete aplasia (unilateral absence of one cerebellar hemisphere) through subtotal asymmetric hypoplasia to mild asymmetry in the size of the cerebellar hemispheres (Poretti et al. 2009d, 2010).

UCH is of prenatal origin and represents a residual change after a disruptive prenatal cerebellar insult, most likely haemorrhagic (see Chapter 30) (Boltshauser et al. 1996; Poretti et al. 2010). A less severe form of UCH can be found together with cerebellar clefts, another form of prenatal cerebellar disruption (see Chapter 30) (Poretti et al. 2008a, 2009c).

Additionally, UCH has been inconsistently reported in PHACE(S) syndrome (MIM 606519) (Metry et al. 2009). PHACES is an acronym for a neurocutaneous syndrome encompassing posterior fossa brain malformations, haemangiomas of the face (large or complex), arterial anomalies, cardiac anomalies, eye abnormalities, and sternal clefting or supraumbilical raphe. Facial haemangiomas are considered the identifying feature, while cerebellar abnormalities are the most common intracranial finding. These include Dandy-Walker malformation, cerebellar hypoplasia, UCH, vermis hypoplasia, or cerebellar dysplasia (Fig. 8.5) (Rossi et al. 2001; Bhattacharya et al. 2004; Church and Lowe 2006).

Cerebellar hypoplasias with prominent midline (vermis) involvement

Cerebellar hypoplasias with prominent midline (vermis) involvement (see Checklists, Table 14) include:

- Dandy-Walker malformation (see Chapter 10).
- Joubert syndrome and related disorders (JSRD) (see Chapter 11).

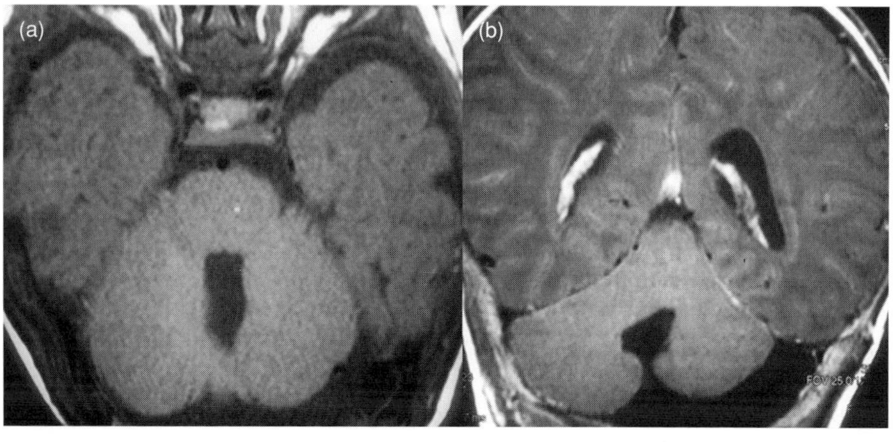

Fig. 8.5. Cerebellar hypoplasia in a child with PHACES syndrome. **(a)** Axial and **(b)** coronal T1-weighted MRI revealing hypoplasia of the cerebellar vermis and a slightly asymmetric mild hypoplasia of the cerebellar hemispheres.

- Rhombencephalosynapsis and Gómez-López-Hernández syndrome (see Chapter 16).
- Pontine tegmental cap dysplasia (see Chapter 20).
- Tectocerebellar dysraphism with occipital meningoencephalocele (see Chapter 21).

Deletions or duplications in the *FOXC1* gene on chromosome 6p25.3 are associated with a spectrum of cerebellar and posterior fossa malformations including cerebellar vermis hypoplasia (CVH), Dandy-Walker malformation, and mega cisterna magna (Aldinger et al. 2009). Aldinger et al. demonstrated a mesenchymal expression of this gene in the posterior fossa, highlighting a role for mesenchyme-neuroepithelium interactions in the mid-hindbrain during early embryogenesis. The authors hypothesized that genes with primary cerebellar expression (such as *CASK* or *OPHN1*) will be associated with CVH or diffuse cerebellar hypoplasia, whereas genes with posterior fossa mesenchymal expression will be associated with the complete spectrum of malformations (Aldinger et al. 2009).

CVH has been reported in 'Joubert-like syndromes'. Janecke et al. reported two affected children and one fetus with morning glory disc anomaly, cystic dysplastic kidneys, developmental delay, and abnormal breathing pattern (Janecke et al. 2004). These patients did not have evidence of hepatic involvement and the molar tooth sign was not present. A distinct syndrome resembling COACH syndrome (cerebellar vermis hypoplasia, oligophrenia, ataxia, coloboma, and hepatic fibrosis) has been suggested by these authors. Kroes et al. reported two brothers and a maternal half-brother with muscular hypotonia, cognitive impairment, ocular abnormalities with impaired vision and colobomas, a breathing pattern compatible with JSRD, and CVH (Kroes et al. 2005). The molar tooth sign was not present. The authors proposed a new X-linked mental retardation (UK: learning disability) syndrome with features overlapping with JSRD and suggested the name *X-linked cerebral-cerebellar-coloboma syndrome*.

In *congenital ocular motor apraxia type Cogan* (COMA) isolated hypoplasia of the inferior cerebellar vermis has been inconsistently reported (Sargent et al. 1997; Kondo et al. 2007). Neuroimaging in COMA may be also normal or show other abnormalities such as agenesis of the corpus callosum or brainstem dysgenesis (Whitsel et al. 1995; Sargent et al. 1997; Kondo et al. 2007). COMA is characterized by an inability to initiate voluntary horizontal saccades (Kondo et al. 2007; Orssaud et al. 2009). Children with COMA typically present with attenuated visual responses during early infancy and head-thrusting movements in the horizontal direction, which compensate the ocular movement abnormalities (Kondo et al. 2007; Orssaud et al. 2009). Children with COMA can additionally present with ataxia (mostly truncal) and cognitive impairment of different degrees (Steinlin et al. 1990; Marr et al. 2005; Kondo et al. 2007). A correlation between neuroimaging findings and clinical symptoms is not present.

Gillespie syndrome (MIM #206700) is an autosomal recessive disorder characterized by aniridia, nonprogressive cerebellar ataxia, and variable degrees of cognitive impairment (Donald et al. 2006; Marien et al. 2008). Cerebellar hypoplasia, particularly affecting the vermis, has been reported in the majority of cases (Marien et al. 2008). In a few patients, additional abnormalities such as diffuse white matter changes, diffuse atrophy of the cerebral hemispheres and brainstem, and frontal cortical atrophy have been reported (Marien et al. 2008). In some patients a mutation in the *PAX6* gene was found (Graziano et al. 2007).

Acrocallosal syndrome (MIM #200990) is an autosomal recessive inherited syndrome characterized by agenesis of the corpus callosum, macrocephaly, hypertelorism, pre- and post-axial polydactyly, and severe cognitive and motor impairment (Koenig et al. 2002). In one patient, a mutation in the *GLI3* gene was found (Elson et al. 2002). Cerebellar hypoplasia mostly affecting the vermis has been reported in two cases (Koenig et al. 2002; Fernandez et al. 2008).

The role of the cerebellum (and particularly of the vermal lobules VI and VII) in *autism* has been discussed in many studies (Amaral et al. 2008; Steinlin 2008; Hallahan et al. 2009). However, there is no clear and consistent pathology that has emerged for autism (Amaral et al. 2008). The size of the vermis appears to be slightly smaller in some children with autism (Courchesne et al. 1994; Kaufmann et al. 2003), but a larger vermis has been also reported (Courchesne et al. 1994). Moreover, it seems that the time course of brain development rather than the final product is most disturbed in autism. In this context, CVH is not a neuroanatomical marker for autism.

Global cerebellar hypoplasia

Global cerebellar hypoplasia (see Checklists, Table 14) refers to involvement of both vermis and cerebellar hemispheres. We categorize the different disorders associated with global cerebellar hypoplasia according to their aetiology.

GLOBAL CEREBELLAR HYPOPLASIA IN PRENATAL INFECTIONS

Cerebellar hypoplasia can be seen following prenatal infections, particularly cytomegalovirus (CMV), representing a disruption (Barkovich and Lindan 1994; de Vries et al. 2004; van der Knaap et al. 2004; Poretti et al. 2009d; Fink et al. 2010). Global cerebellar hypoplasia in prenatal CMV infection is discussed in Chapter 30 about prenatal cerebellar disruptions.

In animals, cerebellar hypoplasia has been reported in various species following prenatal infections due to different viruses, such as Aino virus in calves or parvovirus in cats (Tsuda et al. 2004; Aeffner et al. 2006).

GLOBAL CEREBELLAR HYPOPLASIA AFTER PRENATAL EXPOSURE TO TERATOGENS

Global cerebellar hypoplasia has been reported after prenatal exposure to *anticonvulsant drugs*, *alcohol*, or *cocaine*.

Squier et al. reported an infant with dysmorphic features and intractable seizures born to an epileptic mother who had taken *phenytoin* and *sodium valproate* throughout pregnancy (Squier et al. 1990). Computed tomography showed cerebral and cerebellar underdevelopment, and postmortem examination revealed a small brain with cerebellar hypoplasia.

Alcohol is a frequent toxic and teratogenic factor in the developing fetal brain. The cerebellum appears to be a specific target of alcohol teratogenesis. Decreased surface area and volume of the cerebellum have been described repeatedly in children with fetal alcohol syndrome as well as in nondysmorphic children with prenatal alcohol exposure (Bookstein et al. 2006; Norman et al. 2009).

Bellini et al. reported a female infant born after 37 weeks of gestation to a mother with occasional *cocaine* abuse during the first and second trimester of pregnancy (Bellini et al. 2000). Clinical examination showed microcephaly, overlapping sutures, occipital bone prominence, and scalp rugae. MRI revealed enlargement of lateral ventricles and extracerebral spaces, severe reduction of cerebral parenchyma, generalized hypoplasia of the white matter and pontomesencephalic region, diffuse anomalies of migration and gyration, and global cerebellar hypoplasia. These findings are compatible with a diagnosis of fetal brain disruption sequence. Vascular pathogenesis later on in gestation has been proposed and this hypothesis is compatible with the proven vasoconstricting action of cocaine (Chen et al. 1996).

Global cerebellar hypoplasia in chromosomal abnormalities

Global cerebellar hypoplasia has been reported as an inconsistent neuroimaging finding in children or fetuses with chromosomal abnormalities. Trisomies 13 and 18 are the chromosomal abnormalities most consistently associated with cerebellar hypoplasia (Rosati and Guariglia 1999; Lin et al. 2006). Other less constant associations include trisomy 21 (Rosati and Guariglia 1999), trisomy 9, partial trisomy 12q and monosomy 21q (Chen et al. 2006), trisomy 17 mosaicism (Terhal et al. 2004), monosomy 1p36 (Campeau et al. 2008), and ring chromosome 6 (Andrieux et al. 2005).

Global cerebellar hypoplasia in metabolic disorders

Many metabolic disorders lead to cerebellar atrophy, cerebellar white matter and/or cerebellar nuclei involvement, but cerebellar hypoplasia is only rarely encountered (Steinlin et al. 1998). Typically, cerebellar hypoplasia has been reported in adenylosuccinase deficiency and occasionally in Smith-Lemli-Opitz syndrome, Zellweger syndrome, nonketotic hyperglycinemia, molybdenum cofactor deficiency, isolated sulphite oxidase deficiency, and some mitochondrial disorders (Steinlin et al. 1998).

Adenylosuccinase deficiency (MIM #103050), an extremely rare disorder of the purine metabolism, is reported to be associated with mild cerebellar hypoplasia at an early stage and with cerebellar atrophy and periventricular white matter abnormalities at a late stage (Edery et al. 2003). The clinical manifestation includes muscular hypotonia, severe developmental delay, autistic features, and epileptic seizures (Spiegel et al. 2006).

Smith-Lemli-Opitz syndrome (SLO) (MIM #270400) is an autosomal recessively inherited disorder of the cholesterol biosynthesis and it is caused by mutations in the gene encoding sterol delta-7-reductase mapping to chromosome 11q12-q13 (Kelley and Hennekam 2000). The clinical manifestation includes cognitive impairment (97%), anteverted nares (90%), postnatal growth retardation (85%), syndactyly of the second and third toe (85%), microcephaly (80%), ambiguous genitalia in males (74%), ptosis (69%), cleft palate (51%), congenital heart defects (50%) (Kelley and Hennekam 2000). SLO may be associated with variable degrees of cerebellar hypoplasia (Caruso et al. 2004). Additional neuroimaging findings include corpus callosum hypoplasia, arachnoid cysts, and holoprosencephaly (Caruso et al. 2004).

Zellweger syndrome (MIM #214100) is an autosomal recessively inherited disorder of the biogenesis of peroxisomes due to mutations in at least 13 different *PEX* genes (Baumgartner and Saudubray 2002). Zellweger syndrome is characterized by presentation in the neonatal period with profound hypotonia, characteristic facies, seizures, inability to feed, liver cysts with hepatic dysfunction, and chondrodysplasia punctata (Baumgartner and Saudubray 2002). Typical neuroimaging findings include abnormal gyration pattern such as polymicrogyria and pachygyria, cerebellar leukencephalopathy (more pronounced with increasing age of patients), germinolytic cysts, heterotopias, and cerebral atrophy (Weller et al. 2008). Cerebellar hypoplasia is an occasional finding (Lindhard et al. 1993).

Nonketotic hyperglycinemia (MIM #605899) is an autosomal recessive disorder characterized by accumulation of large amounts of glycine in body fluids due to mutations in several genes in the mitochondrial glycine cleavage system (Applegarth and Toone 2004). Most patients have the neonatal phenotype, presenting in the first few days of life with lethargy, hypotonia, and myoclonic jerks, and progressing to apnea, and often to death (Applegarth and Toone 2004). Those who regain spontaneous respiration develop intractable seizures and profound cognitive impairment (Applegarth and Toone 2004). Typical neuroimaging findings are agenesis or abnormalities of the corpus callosum, delayed myelination, and white matter oedema (Shah et al. 2005). Cerebellar hypoplasia has been occasionally reported (Shah et al. 2005).

Molybdenum cofactor deficiency (MIM #252150) and *isolated sulfite oxidase deficiency* (MIM #272300) are autosomal recessive disorders of the catabolism of sulphur-containing aminoacids (Sass et al. 2010). The accumulated sulphites are toxic for brain mitochondria. Energy deficit seems to be the underlying pathomechanism. The clinical presentation is typically in the first days of life with feeding difficulties, vomiting, and intractable seizures. The neuroimaging findings show temporal alterations and include initially global cerebral oedema and later cystic encephalomalacic changes in the subcortical white matter and signal abnormalities in the basal ganglia (Hoffmann et al. 2007, Sass et al. 2010). Abnormalities in the posterior fossa have been reported in several patients and include cerebellar hypoplasia, mega cisterna magna, and pontine hypoplasia (Hoffmann et al. 2007, Carmi-Nawi et al. 2011).

In *mitochondrial disorders* cerebellar atrophy is common, but cerebellar hypoplasia is rather unusual (Saneto et al. 2008). Cerebellar hypoplasia has been occasionally reported in respiratory chain disorders such as Leigh disease (Lincke et al. 1996), MELAS syndrome (Steinlin et al. 1998), and pyruvate dehydrogenase deficiency.

Cerebellar hypoplasia has been reported in one patient with *mucopolysaccharidosis type I* (Gabrielli et al. 1992).

GLOBAL CEREBELLAR HYPOPLASIA IN MIGRATIONAL DISORDERS
Global cerebellar hypoplasia can be found in several migrational disorders including lissencephaly, polymicrogyria, and periventricular nodular heterotopias (Guerrini et al. 2008; Barkovich et al. 2009; Verrotti et al. 2010).

In lissencephaly, global cerebellar hypoplasia is typically found in *RELN*, *VLDLR*, and *TUBA1A* mutations, but it was also reported in *LIS1*, *DCX*, and *ARX* mutations as well as in lissencephaly forms with unknown genetic background (Ross et al. 2001; Jissendi-Tchofo et al. 2009).

Lissencephaly with cerebellar hypoplasia has been associated with mutations of the *reelin (RELN)* gene mapping to chromosome 7q22 (MIM #257320). *RELN* encodes an extracellular matrix-associated glycoprotein (reelin) that is secreted by Cajal-Retzius cells in the developing cerebral cortex and appears critical for the regulation of neuronal migration during cortical development (Hong et al. 2000). Affected children show severe neurological impairments frequently including hypotonia, ataxia, and generalized epilepsy beginning at an early age (Hong et al. 2000). MRI reveals predominant pachygyria with mild cortical thickening and anterior predominant gradient, hippocampal dysplasia, mild brainstem hypoplasia, and cerebellar hypoplasia ranging from midline hypoplasia to global cerebellar hypoplasia with disturbed foliation (Hong et al. 2000; Ross et al. 2001).

Lissencephaly with cerebellar hypoplasia is also correlated with mutations in the *VLDLR* gene on chromosome 9p24 coding for the very-low-density lipoprotein receptor (MIM #224050) (Boycott et al. 2005, 2009; Glass et al. 2005; Kolb et al. 2010). *VLDLR* binds to reelin and activates a downstream signaling cascade that is thought to influence cell migration (Boycott et al. 2005). *VLDLR*-associated cerebellar hypoplasia is characterized by nonprogressive congenital ataxia that is predominantly truncal and results in delayed ambulation (age >6 years), moderate-to-profound cognitive impairment, dysarthria, strabismus, and seizures (Glass et al. 2005; Boycott et al. 2009). Additional clinical findings are short stature and pes planus. MRI shows hypoplasia of the inferior portion of the cerebellar vermis and hemispheres, simplified gyration of the cerebral hemispheres with minimally thickened but uniform cortex and lack of clear anteroposterior gradient, and hypoplastic brainstem, particularly the pons (Glass et al. 2005; Boycott et al. 2009; Kolb et al. 2010).

The *α-tubulin 1a (TUBA1A)* gene on chromosome 12q12-q14 codes for a critical structural subunit of microtubules that is transiently expressed during neuronal development (Poirier et al. 2007). Mutations in this gene are associated with a wide phenotypic spectrum including (1) classic lissencephaly with posterior-anterior gradient, dysplastic hippocampi and corpus callosum, and a normal cerebellum, (2) classic lissencephaly with posterior-anterior gradient, dysplastic hippocampi and corpus callosum, and a hypoplasia of the cerebellar vermis, (3) diffuse pachygyria without agyria (most severe over the central convexity or the posterior pole), malformed hippocampi, absent corpus callosum, and moderate cerebellar hypoplasia with vermian predominance, and (4) lissencephaly with posterior-anterior gradient, agenesis of the corpus callosum, malformed hippocampi, severe global cerebellar hypoplasia, and pontine hypoplasia (MIM #611603) (Morris-Rosendahl et al. 2008; Kumar et al. 2010). Children with mutations in the *TUBA1A* gene present with microcephaly, severe to profound cognitive impairment, spastic quadriplegia, and epileptic seizures (Poirier et al. 2007).

Mutations in the *LIS1* gene on chromosome 17p13.3 are typically associated with classic lissencephaly with posterior-anterior gradient (MIM #607432) (Dobyns 2010). Uyanik et al. reported two patients with a mutation in exon 10 and additional mild cerebellar hypoplasia with vermian preponderance (Uyanik et al. 2007).

Mutations in the *doublecortin (DCX)* gene on chromosome Xq22.3 are known to cause classic lissencephaly with anterior-posterior gradient in males (MIM #300067), while heterozygous mutations in females are associated with subcortical band heterotopia (Dobyns 2010). Additionally, mutations in the *DCX* gene can be associated with isolated inferior vermis hypoplasia (Ross et al. 2001; Uyanik et al. 2007; Jissendi-Tchofo et al. 2009).

Mutations in the X-linked *ARX* gene cause a spectrum of abnormalities, including lissencephaly with posterior predominance, agenesis of the corpus callosum, and ambiguous genitalia (MIM #300215) (Dobyns 2010). Mild brainstem hypoplasia and moderate cerebellar hypoplasia have been reported in males with *ARX*-mutations (Kato et al. 2004).

Mutations in the *TUBB2B* gene on chromosome 6p25.2 cause a complex brain dysgenesis with bilateral, asymmetric and anteriorly predominant polymicrogyria, fusion of the caudate and putamen with internal capsule hypoplasia, corpus callosum agenesis or dysgenesis and, in most cases, hypoplasia of pons and cerebellum (MIM #610031) (Jaglin et al. 2009).

Mutations in the *TUBB3* gene on chromosome 16q24.3 may lead to malformations of cortical development (perisylvian polymicrogyria and frontoparietal gyral disorganization), hypoplasia of the corpus callosum, fusion or hypertrophy of the caudate nucleus and putamen, brainstem hypoplasia and hypoplasia/dysplasia of the cerebellum, mostly of the vermis (Poirier et al. 2010).

Mutations in the *human filamin A (FLNA)* gene on chromosome Xq28 are mostly associated with classic X-linked bilateral periventricular nodular heterotopia (MIM #300049) (Parrini et al. 2006). In rare cases, *FLNA* mutations can also cause temporo-occipital periventricular nodular heterotopias with hippocampal malformation and cerebellar hypoplasia (Parrini et al. 2006). Cerebellar abnormalities including cerebellar hypoplasia, cerebellar dysplasia, and cerebellar heterotopias have been reported also in *FLNA*-not-related nodular heterotopias (Srour et al. 2011).

Global cerebellar hypoplasia in genetic disorders

Global cerebellar hypoplasia has been reported in some genetic disorders (see Chapters 25 and 26) including:

- Cayman nonprogressive cerebellar ataxia (MIM #601238);
- Mutations in the *oligophrenin-1* gene (MIM #300486);
- X-linked nonprogressive ataxia mapping to chromosome Xp11.21-q21.3 (MIM %302500);
- X-linked nonprogressive ataxia mapping to chromosome Xq25-q27.1 (MIM %300703);
- Autosomal-recessive nonprogressive cerebellar ataxia mapping to chromosome 9q34-qter (MIM %213200);
- Cerebellar ataxia with mental retardation, optic atrophy, and skin abnormalities (CAMOS) due to mutations in the *ZNF592* gene on chromosome 15q24-q26 (MIM #606937);
- Nonprogressive ataxia with generalized tonic-clonic epilepsy and cognitive impairment, mapping to chromosome 16q21-q23;
- Nonprogressive cerebellar ataxia with cognitive and speech impairment, coarse face, hirsutism, and short stature, mapping to chromosome 17p (MIM %610185);
- Nonprogressive cerebellar ataxia associated with short stature, but without cognitive impairment, mapping to chromosome 20q11-q13;
- Nonprogressive cerebellar ataxia, neonatal diabetes mellitus, deafness, myopia, and developmental delay, due to mutations in the *NEUROD1* gene on chromosome 2q31;
- Several familial nonprogressive cerebellar ataxia with unknown gene locus.

Global cerebellar hypoplasia in syndromic disorders

In many syndromic disorders cerebellar hypoplasia has been reported as a typical, occasional, or rare neuroimaging finding.

Ritscher-Schinzel or *3C (cranio-cerebello-cardiac) syndrome* (MIM %220210) was first described in two sisters with similar craniofacial anomalies, malformations of the posterior fossa, and a congenital heart defect (Ritscher et al. 1987). Typical craniofacial anomalies include low-set ears, hypertelorism, down-slanting palpebral fissures, depressed nasal bridge, prominent occiput, cleft palate, micrognathia, and ocular coloboma (Leonardi et al. 2001). The most common cerebellar malformation is the Dandy-Walker malformation (present in about two-thirds of cases) (Leonardi et al. 2001). Cerebellar hypoplasia has been reported in about 20–25% of the patients. Cardiac malformations include mostly septal defects, while valvular defects and conotruncal anomalies are less frequent (Leonardi et al. 2001). Occasional features observed were unilateral hearing loss and growth hormone deficiency (Wheeler et al. 1999). One of the sisters in the initial description was subsequently found to have a secondary immunodeficiency (Zankl et al. 2003).

Hoyeraal-Hreidarsson syndrome (MIM #300240) is an X-linked multisystem disorder caused by mutations in the *DKC1* gene at Xq28 (Knight et al. 1999). Mutations in the same gene are associated with dyskeratosis congenita (Sznajer et al. 2003). This syndrome is characterized by prenatal onset of growth failure, secondary microcephaly, developmental delay, ataxia, immunodeficiency, and progressive bone marrow failure with aplastic anemia (Sznajer et al. 2003). Life expectancy of these children is markedly reduced (Sznajer et al. 2003). Cerebellar hypoplasia is one of the most characteristic abnormalities of this syndrome and is consistently reported (Sznajer et al. 2003; Kuwashima 2009). Additional neuroimaging findings include delayed myelination of cerebral white matter and hypoplastic corpus callosum (Akaboshi et al. 2000).

CHARGE syndrome (MIM #214800) is an autosomal dominant disorder characterized by colobomas, heart malformations, atresia of choanae, retarded mental development, genital anomalies, and ear anomalies with or without deafness (Sanlaville and Verloes 2007). About two-thirds of the patients have a truncating mutation in the *CHD7* gene on chromosome 8q12 (Lalani et al. 2006). Mutations in the *SEMA3E* gene can cause CHARGE syndrome as well (Lalani et al. 2004). Additional frequent findings include several dysmorphic features (square-shaped face with narrow bifrontal diameter, broad nasal bridge, small mouth, and inverted V-shaped upper lip), congenital facial paralysis, feeding and swallowing difficulties, and cleft palate (Sanlaville and Verloes 2007). Brain abnormalities have been found in 55–85% of the patients (Lin et al. 1990; Pinto et al. 2005). The most common brain anomalies are arrhinencephaly or hypoplastic olfactory bulbs and holoprosencephaly (Sanlaville and Verloes 2007). Dandy-Walker malformation and cerebellar hypoplasia as well as abnormalities in the forebrain (e.g., dysgenesis of the frontal lobe, agenesis of the septum pellucidum, nodular heterotopias, lissencephaly) have occasionally been found (Sanlaville and Verloes 2007).

Velocardiofacial syndrome (MIM #192430) is an autosomal dominant syndrome caused by a 1.5–3.0Mb hemizygous deletion of chromosome 22q11.2 (Fernandez et al. 2009). The most common clinical features include conotruncal congenital heart defects, velopharyngeal insufficiency, hypocalcemia (due to hypoparathyroidism), thymic aplasia or hypoplasia, and a characteristic craniofacial dysmorphism (Fernandez et al. 2009). Less frequent features included microcephaly, short stature, slender hands and digits, minor auricular anomalies, and inguinal hernia. In 25–40% of the patients, cognitive functions are impaired (mostly mild and particularly affecting visuospatial memory and arithmetic) (Gothelf et al. 2009). Children with this syndrome often show psychiatric disorders such as attention-deficit hyperactivity disorder (the most common), oppositional defiant disorder, specific and social phobias, generalized

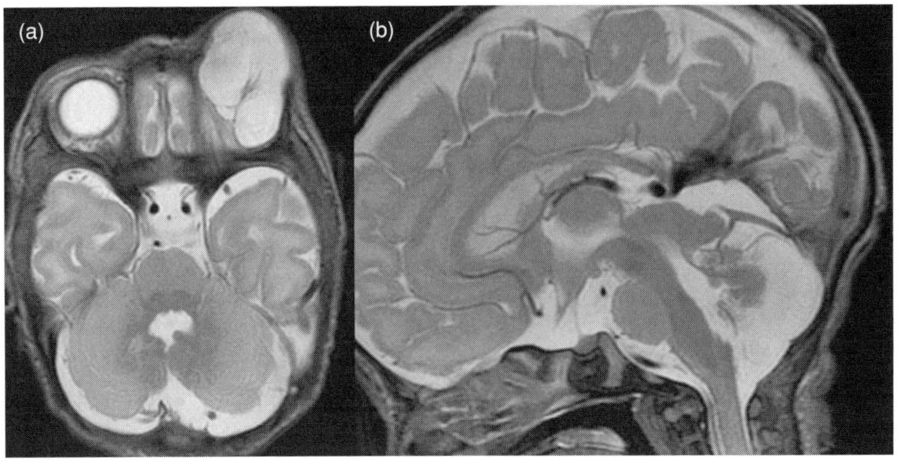

Fig. 8.6. Infant aged 6 days with oculo-cerebrocutaneous syndrome. **(a)** Axial T2-weighted MRI showing a cystic malformation of the left eye and cerebellar hypoplasia with vermian predominance; **(b)** sagittal T2-weighted images revealing enlarged and dysplastic tectum and vermian hypoplasia.

anxiety disorder, separation anxiety disorder, and obsessive-compulsive disorder (Gothelf et al. 2009). Neuroimaging findings in velocardiofacial syndrome include white matter reduction in brainstem, cerebellum, and occipitotemporal lobes, gray matter reduction in the cerebellum and the ventromedial occipital and posterior cingulated cortex, and reduced gyral pattern at the parieto-temporo-occipital junction (Campbell et al. 2006; Schaer et al. 2009; Tan et al. 2009).

Endosteal sclerosis is characterized by increased radiosensivity of bones and seems to be associated with cerebellar hypoplasia (MIM #213002) (Charrow et al. 1991; Ozgen et al. 2005). Clinical findings are ataxia, tremor, nystagmus, microcephaly, short stature, tooth eruption disturbances, optic atrophy, and congenital hip disclocation (Charrow et al. 1991; Ozgen et al. 2005). Additionally, neuroimaging may show delayed myelination (Ozgen et al. 2005).

Cerebellar hypoplasia is a possible neuroimaging pattern in *PHACE(S) syndrome* (MIM #606519) (Metry et al. 2009). Other cerebellar abnormalities include Dandy-Walker malformation, UCH, vermis hypoplasia, and cerebellar dysplasia (see Chapter 29) (Rossi et al. 2001; Bhattacharya et al. 2004; Church and Lowe 2006).

Oculocerebrocutaneous syndrome (OCCS) or Delleman syndrome (MIM #164180) is a rare (X-linked?) syndrome probably caused by abnormalities of the midbrain-rhombomere 1 boundary (Barkovich et al. 2009). It is characterized by the triad of eye, brain, and skin malformations, sometimes associated with other features such as craniofacial clefts, skull or rib defects, and urogenital anomalies (Moog et al. 1997; Hunter 2006). The eye malformations consist mainly of cystic anophthalmia or microphthalmia and colobomata, while the skin abnormalities consist of skin appendages and focal aplasia or hypoplasia (Moog et al. 1997). Giant and dysplastic midbrain tectum is a distinct neuroimaging finding in OCCS (Fig. 8.6) (Naafs et al. 1999; Pascual-Castroviejo et al. 2005; Moog et al. 2007). Other abnormalities of the posterior fossa include absence of the cerebellar vermis, hypoplastic and dysplastic cerebellar hemispheres, and a large posterior fossa fluid collection (Naafs et al. 1999; Pascual-Castroviejo et al. 2005; Moog et al. 2007). Other typical neuroimaging findings are frontal predominant polymicrogyria, periventricular nodular heterotopia always located beneath the polymicrogyria, complete or partial agenesis of the corpus callosum, sometimes associated with interhemispheric cysts, and enlarged third and lateral ventricles (Naafs et al. 1999; Pascual-Castroviejo et al. 2005; Moog et al. 2007).

Recently, Lamonica et al. reported two brothers with non-progressive congenital ataxia, iris heterochromia, cognitive impairment, language disorder (particularly affecting expressive language), and some dysmorphic features (long face, telecanthus) (Lamonica et al. 2010). In both children, MRI showed marked global cerebellar hypoplasia.

In *neurofibromatosis type 1* cerebellar hypoplasia has occasionally been reported and we have seen a few patients with this association.

Additionally, cerebellar hypoplasia has been reported in pseudo-TORCH syndrome (Abdel-Salam et al. 2008) and occasionally in oculodentodigital dysplasia (Amador et al. 2008), cri-du-chat syndrome (or distal 5p deletion) (Chen et al. 2004), Pallister-Killian syndrome (Saito et al. 2006), Galloway-Mowat syndrome (Steiss et al. 2005), Sengers syndrome (Perry and Sladky 2008), Cohen syndrome (Waite et al. 2010), and in two patients with postnatal growth failure, microcephaly, mental retardation, cataracts, large joint contractures, osteoporosis, and cortical dysplasia (Shotelersuk et al. 2003).

Pontocerebellar hypoplasias

In clinical practice the use of the term pontocerebellar hypoplasia (PCH) is not uniform. It is often used in a descriptive manner to imply that the volume of the cerebellum and the pons are reduced, generally in a nonspecific way. On the other hand it is used in the context of the so-called pontocerebellar hypoplasias, as previously conceptualized by Peter Barth (see Chapter 23) (Barth 1993, 2000). However, in the latter sense, PCH are not 'static' malformations, but early (prenatal)-onset degenerative disorders.

Similar MRI findings can be observed in several other conditions described below (Fig. 8.7).

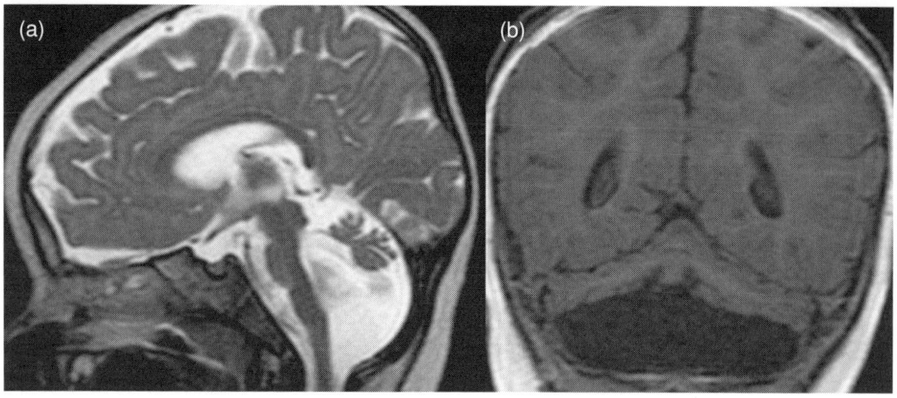

Fig. 8.7. Cerebellar hypoplasia in a 9-month-old infant with microcephaly, muscular hypotonia, and developmental delay, but without extrapyramidal movement disorders or epileptic seizures. **(a)** Sagittal T2-weighted and **(b)** coronal T1-weighted images show highly reduced cerebellar volume affecting the cerebellar hemispheres more than the vermis (pontocerebellar hypoplasia type 2 excluded).

Congenital disorders of glycosylation (CDG) are a rapidly growing family of diseases of protein glycosylation mostly due to defects in the *N*-glycosylation pathway, but also affecting the *O*-glycosylation pathway or combined *N*- and *O*-glycosylation pathways (Grunewald et al. 2002; Jaeken et al. 2008, 2009). The most common type is type 1a or PMM2-CDG due to defects in the phosphomannomutase-2 gene (MIM #601785) (Sparks 2006). Infants with PMM2-CDG generally present with muscular hypotonia, while older children have ataxia, progressive peripheral neuropathy, and mild to moderate non-progressive cognitive impairment (Miossec-Chauvet et al. 2003). Typical additional neurological findings are progressive microcephaly, stroke-like episodes, epileptic seizures, and progressive retinopathy (Drouin-Garraud et al. 2001; Miossec-Chauvet et al. 2003; Perez-Duenas et al. 2009). Non-neurological symptoms or findings are failure to thrive, inverted nipples, abnormal distribution of subcutaneous fat, hepatomegaly, episodes of ascites, and pericardial effusion (Miossec-Chauvet et al. 2003). Neuroimaging studies show marked cerebellar hypoplasia with super-imposed atrophy that may progress in infancy (Antoun et al. 1999; Mader et al. 2002; Miossec-Chauvet et al. 2003). The anterior vermis is most severely affected (Antoun et al. 1999; Mader et al. 2002). Associated neuroimaging findings include pontine hypoplasia, and supratentorial white matter hypoplasia or atrophy (Antoun et al. 1999; Drouin-Garraud et al. 2001; Mader et al. 2002; Miossec-Chauvet et al. 2003). Recently, in patients with abnormal glycosylation due to abnormalities in dolichol metabolism and mutation in the *SRD5A3* gene, different degrees of cerebellar hypoplasia have been reported (Morava et al. 2010).

CASK is a multi-domain scaffolding protein that interacts with the transcription factor TBR1 and regulates expression of genes involved in cortical development such as *RELN* (Najm et al. 2008; Bailey and Aldinger 2009). Mutations in the *CASK* gene on chromosome Xp11.4 (MIM #300749) cause ataxia, nystagmus, postnatal microcephaly, severe cognitive impairment, sensorineural hearing loss, and inconsistently cataract (Najm et al. 2008; Hackett et al. 2010). The neuroimaging correlates includes severe global cerebellar hypoplasia and pontine hypoplasia as well as reduced gyral pattern and unmyelinated corpus callosum (Najm et al. 2008; Takanashi et al. 2010). (See Chapter 25.)

Primary merosin-deficient congenital muscular dystrophies (MDC1A) as well as *dystroglycanopathies* are associated with cerebellar hypoplasia (mostly with vermian predominance) and pontine hypoplasia (see Chapter 15) (Clement et al. 2008).

In some forms of *migrational disorders* such as mutations in the *RELN*, *TUBA1A*, *VLDLR*, *TUBB2B*, and *TUBB3* genes cerebellar hypoplasia is associated with pontine hypoplasia (see 'Global cerebellar hypoplasia in migrational disorders' in this chapter) (Jissendi-Tchofo et al. 2009).

MRI findings similar to pontocerebellar hypoplasia can be found in children with *cerebellar agenesis* (see Chapter 7) (Poretti et al. 2009d) as well as in *extremely preterm infants with cerebellar disruption* (see Chapter 31) (Messerschmidt et al. 2005).

Diagnostic work-up

Cerebellar hypoplasia is a nonspecific neuroimaging finding, which can result from several aetiologies. Type of cerebellar hypoplasia (UCH, global cerebellar hypoplasia, pontocerebellar hypoplasia, or cerebellar hypoplasia with predominant involvement of the vermis), other neuroimaging findings, and clinical findings may offer some clues for the differential diagnosis. Serum creatine kinase is performed to rule out congenital muscular dystrophies. Isoelectric focusing of serum transferrin should be performed if CDG is suspected. Normal 7-dehydrocholesterol rules out Smith-Lemli-Opitz syndrome. Electrophysiological studies are not helpful unless migrational disorders are evident and seizures are present. Genetic studies including karyotype, fluorensce in situ hybridization (FISH), and array comparative genomic hybridization (CGH) may be indicated if dysmorphic signs or other features suggest a particular chromosomal or genetic disorder.

REFERENCES

Aarsen FK, Paquier PF, Arts WF, Van Veelen ML, Michiels E, Lequin M, Catsman-Berrevoets CE (2009) Cognitive deficits and predictors 3 years after diagnosis of a pilocytic astrocytoma in childhood. J Clin Oncol 27: 3526–3532.

Abdel-Salam GM, Zaki MS, Saleem SN, Gaber KR (2008) Microcephaly, malformation of brain development and intracranial calcification in sibs: pseudo-TORCH or a new syndrome. Am J Med Genet A 146A: 2929–2936.

Aeffner F, Ulrich R, Schulze-Ruckamp L, Beineke A (2006) Cerebellar hypoplasia in three sibling cats after intrauterine or early postnatal parvovirus infection. Dtsch Tierärztl Wochenschr 113: 403–406.

Akaboshi S, Yoshimura M, Hara T, Kageyama H, Nishikwa K, Kawakami T, Ieshima A, Takeshita K (2000) A case of Hoyeraal-Hreidarsson syndrome: delayed myelination and hypoplasia of corpus callosum are other important signs. Neuropediatrics 31: 141–144.

Aldinger KA, Lehmann OJ, Hudgins L, Chizhikov VV, Bassuk AG, Ades LC, et al. (2009) FOXC1 is required for normal cerebellar development and is a major contributor to chromosome 6p25.3 Dandy-Walker malformation. Nat Genet 41: 1037–1042.

Amador C, Mathews AM, Del Carmen Montoya M, Laughridge ME, Everman DB, Holden KR (2008) Expanding the neurologic phenotype of oculodentodigital dysplasia in a 4-generation Hispanic family. J Child Neurol 23: 901–905.

Amaral DG, Schumann CM, Nordahl CW (2008) Neuroanatomy of autism. Trends Neurosci 31: 137–145.

Andrieux J, Devisme L, Valat AS, Robert Y, Frnka C, Savary JB (2005) Prenatal diagnosis of ring chromosome 6 in a fetus with cerebellar hypoplasia and partial agenesis of corpus callosum: case report and review of the literature. Eur J Med Genet 48: 199–206.

Antoun H, Villeneuve N, Gelot A, Panisset S, Adamsbaum C (1999) Cerebellar atrophy: an important feature of carbohydrate deficient glycoprotein syndrome type 1. Pediatr Radiol 29: 194–198.

Applegarth DA, Toone JR (2004) Glycine encephalopathy (nonketotic hyperglycinaemia): review and update. J Inherit Metab Dis 27: 417–422.

Bailey KA, Aldinger KA (2009) An X-linked microcephaly syndrome caused by disruptions of CASK implicates the CASK-TBR1-RELN pathway in human brain development. Clin Genet 75: 424–425.

Barkovich AJ, Lindan CE (1994) Congenital cytomegalovirus infection of the brain: imaging analysis and embryologic considerations. AJNR Am J Neuroradiol 15: 703–715.

Barkovich AJ, Millen KJ, Dobyns WB (2009) A developmental and genetic classification for midbrain-hindbrain malformations. Brain 132: 3199–3230.

Barth PG (1993) Pontocerebellar hypoplasias. An overview of a group of inherited neurodegenerative disorders with fetal onset. Brain Dev 15: 411–422.

Barth PG (2000) Pontocerebellar hypoplasia – how many types? Eur J Paediatr Neurol 4: 161–162.

Baumgartner MR, Saudubray JM (2002) Peroxisomal disorders. Semin Neonatol 7: 85–94.

Bellini C, Massocco D, Serra G (2000) Prenatal cocaine exposure and the expanding spectrum of brain malformations. Arch Intern Med 160: 2393.

Bhattacharya JJ, Luo CB, Alvarez H, Rodesch G, Pongpech S, Lasjaunias PL (2004) PHACES syndrome: a review of eight previously unreported cases with late arterial occlusions. Neuroradiology 46: 227–233.

Bolduc ME, Limperopoulos C (2009) Neurodevelopmental outcomes in children with cerebellar malformations: a systematic review. Dev Med Child Neurol 51: 256–267.

Boltshauser E, Steinlin M, Martin E, Deonna T (1996) Unilateral cerebellar aplasia. Neuropediatrics 27: 50–53.

Boltshauser E (2004) Cerebellum-small brain but large confusion: a review of selected cerebellar malformations and disruptions. Am J Med Genet A 126A: 376–385.

Bookstein FL, Streissguth AP, Connor PD, Sampson PD (2006) Damage to the human cerebellum from prenatal alcohol exposure: the anatomy of a simple biometrical explanation. Anat Rec B New Anat 289: 195–209.

Boycott KM, Flavelle S, Bureau A, Glass HC, Fujiwara TM, Wirrell E, et al. (2005) Homozygous deletion of the very low density lipoprotein receptor gene causes autosomal recessive cerebellar hypoplasia with cerebral gyral simplification. Am J Hum Genet 77: 477–483.

Boycott KM, Bonnemann C, Herz J, Neuert S, Beaulieu C, Scott JN, et al. (2009) Mutations in VLDLR as a cause for autosomal recessive cerebellar ataxia with mental retardation (dysequilibrium syndrome). J Child Neurol 24: 1310–1315.

Campbell LE, Daly E, Toal F, Stevens A, Azuma R, Catani M, et al. (2006) Brain and behaviour in children with 22q11.2 deletion syndrome: a volumetric and voxel-based morphometry MRI study. Brain 129: 1218–1228.

Campeau PM, Ah Mew N, Cartier L, Mackay KL, Shaffer LG, Der Kaloustian VM, Thomas MA (2008) Prenatal diagnosis of monosomy 1p36: a focus on brain abnormalities and a review of the literature. Am J Med Genet A 146A: 3062–3069.

Carmi-Nawi N, Malinger G, Mandel H, Ichida K, Lerman-Sagie T, Lev D (2011) Prenatal brain disruption in molybdenum cofactor deficiency. J Child Neurol 26: 460–464.

Caruso PA, Poussaint TY, Tzika AA, Zurakowski D, Astrakas LG, Elias ER, et al. (2004) MRI and 1H MRS findings in Smith-Lemli-Opitz syndrome. Neuroradiology 46: 3–14.

Charrow J, Poznanski AK, Unger FM, Robinow M (1991) Autosomal recessive cerebellar hypoplasia and endosteal sclerosis: a newly recognized syndrome. Am J Med Genet 41: 464–468.

Chen CP, Lee CC, Chang TY, Town DD, Wang W (2004) Prenatal diagnosis of mosaic distal 5p deletion and review of the literature. Prenat Diagn 24: 50–57.

Chen CP, Chern SR, Lin CC, Wang TH, Li YC, Hsieh LJ, Leet al. (2006) Prenatal findings and molecular cytogenetic analyses of partial trisomy 12q (12q24.32 – >qter) and partial monosomy 21q (21q22.2 – >qter). Prenat Diagn 26: 313–320.

Chen WJ, McAlhany RE, Jr., Maier SE, West JR (1996) Cocaine exposure during the brain growth spurt failed to produce cerebellar Purkinje cell loss in rat pups. Teratology 53: 145–151.

Church DG, Lowe LH (2006) Case 103: PHACE syndrome. Radiology 241: 939–942.

Clement E, Mercuri E, Godfrey C, Smith J, Robb S, Kinali M, et al. (2008) Brain involvement in muscular dystrophies with defective dystroglycan glycosylation. Ann Neurol 64: 573–582.

Courchesne E, Saitoh O, Townsend JP, Yeung-Courchesne R, Press GA, Lincoln AJ, et al. (1994) Cerebellar hypoplasia and hyperplasia in infantile autism. Lancet 343: 63–64.

De Smet HJ, Baillieux H, Wackenier P, De Praeter M, Engelborghs S, Paquier PF, et al. (2009) Long-term cognitive deficits following posterior fossa tumor resection: a neuropsychological and functional neuroimaging follow-up study. Neuropsychology 23: 694–704.

de Vries LS, Gunardi H, Barth PG, Bok LA, Verboon-Maciolek MA, Groenendaal F (2004) The spectrum of cranial ultrasound and magnetic resonance imaging abnormalities in congenital cytomegalovirus infection. Neuropediatrics 35: 113–119.

Dobyns WB (2010) The clinical patterns and molecular genetics of lissencephaly and subcortical band heterotopia. Epilepsia 51 Suppl 1: 5–9.

Donald KA, Grotte R, Crutchley AC, Wilmshurst JM (2006) Gillespie syndrome: two further cases. J Child Neurol 21: 337–340.

Drouin-Garraud V, Belgrand M, Grunewald S, Seta N, Dacher JN, Henocq A, et al. (2001) Neurological presentation of a congenital disorder of glycosylation CDG-Ia: implications for diagnosis and genetic counseling. Am J Med Genet 101: 46–49.

Edery P, Chabrier S, Ceballos-Picot I, Marie S, Vincent MF, Tardieu M (2003) Intrafamilial variability in the phenotypic expression of adenylosuccinate lyase deficiency: a report on three patients. Am J Med Genet A 120A: 185–190.

Elson E, Perveen R, Donnai D, Wall S, Black GC (2002) De novo GLI3 mutation in acrocallosal syndrome: broadening the phenotypic spectrum of GLI3 defects and overlap with murine models. J Med Genet 39: 804–806.

Fernandez C, Soulier M, Coulibaly B, Liprandi A, Benoit B, Giuliano F, et al. (2008) Acrocallosal syndrome in fetus: focus on additional brain abnormalities. Acta Neuropathol 115: 151–156.

Fernandez L, Nevado J, Santos F, Heine-Suner D, Martinez-Glez V, Garcia-Minaur S, et al. (2009) A deletion and a duplication in distal 22q11.2 deletion syndrome region. Clinical implications and review. BMC Med Genet 10: 48.

Fink KR, Thapa MM, Ishak GE, Pruthi S (2010) Neuroimaging of pediatric central nervous system cytomegalovirus infection. Radiographics 30: 1779–1796.

Gabrielli O, Salvolini U, Maricotti M, Mariani MG, Coppa GV, Giorgi PL (1992) Cerebral MRI in two brothers with mucopolysaccharidosis type I and different clinical phenotypes. Neuroradiology 34: 313–315.

Glass HC, Boycott KM, Adams C, Barlow K, Scott JN, Chudley AE, et al. (2005) Autosomal recessive cerebellar hypoplasia in the Hutterite population. Dev Med Child Neurol 47: 691–695.

Gothelf D, Frisch A, Michaelovsky E, Weizman A, Shprintzen RJ (2009) Velo-Cardio-Facial Syndrome. J Ment Health Res Intellect Disabil 2: 149–167.

Graziano C, D'Elia AV, Mazzanti L, Moscano F, Guidelli Guidi S, Scarano E, et al. (2007) A de novo nonsense mutation of PAX6 gene in a patient with aniridia, ataxia, and mental retardation. Am J Med Genet A 143A: 1802–1805.

Grunewald S, Matthijs G, Jaeken J (2002) Congenital disorders of glycosylation: a review. Pediatr Res 52: 618–624.

Guerrini R, Dobyns WB, Barkovich AJ (2008) Abnormal development of the human cerebral cortex: genetics, functional consequences and treatment options. Trends Neurosci 31: 154–162.

Hackett A, Tarpey PS, Licata A, Cox J, Whibley A, Boyle J, et al. (2010) CASK mutations are frequent in males and cause X-linked nystagmus and variable XLMR phenotypes. Eur J Hum Genet 18: 544–552.

Hallahan B, Daly EM, McAlonan G, Loth E, Toal F, O'Brien F, et al. (2009) Brain morphometry volume in autistic spectrum disorder: a magnetic resonance imaging study of adults. Psychol Med 39: 337–346.

Hoffmann C, Ben-Zeev B, Anikster Y, Nissenkorn A, Brand N, Kuint J, Kushnir T (2007) Magnetic resonance imaging and magnetic resonance spectroscopy in isolated sulfite oxidase deficiency. J Child Neurol 22: 1214–1221.

Hong SE, Shugart YY, Huang DT, Shahwan SA, Grant PE, Hourihane JO, et al. (2000) Autosomal recessive lissencephaly with cerebellar hypoplasia is associated with human RELN mutations. Nat Genet 26: 93–96.

Hunter AG (2006) Oculocerebrocutaneous and encephalocraniocutaneous lipomatosis syndromes: blind men and an elephant or separate syndromes? Am J Med Genet A 140: 709–726.

Jaeken J, Hennet T, Freeze HH, Matthijs G (2008) On the nomenclature of congenital disorders of glycosylation (CDG). J Inherit Metab Dis 31: 669–672.

Jaeken J, Hennet T, Matthijs G, Freeze HH (2009) CDG nomenclature: time for a change! Biochim Biophys Acta 1792: 825–826.

Jaglin XH, Poirier K, Saillour Y, Buhler E, Tian G, Bahi-Buisson N, et al. (2009) Mutations in the beta-tubulin gene TUBB2B result in asymmetrical polymicrogyria. Nat Genet 41: 746–752.

Janecke AR, Muller T, Gassner I, Kreczy A, Schmid E, Kronenberg F, et al. (2004) Joubert-like syndrome unlinked to known candidate loci. J Pediatr 144: 264–269.

Jissendi-Tchofo P, Kara S, Barkovich AJ (2009) Midbrain-hindbrain involvement in lissencephalies. Neurology 72: 410–418.

Kato M, Das S, Petras K, Kitamura K, Morohashi K, Abuelo DN, et al. (2004) Mutations of ARX are associated with striking pleiotropy and consistent genotype-phenotype correlation. Hum Mutat 23: 147–159.

Kaufmann WE, Cooper KL, Mostofsky SH, Capone GT, Kates WR, Newschaffer CJ, et al. (2003) Specificity of cerebellar vermian abnormalities in autism: a quantitative magnetic resonance imaging study. J Child Neurol 18: 463–470.

Kelley RI, Hennekam RC (2000) The Smith-Lemli-Opitz syndrome. J Med Genet 37: 321–335.

Knight SW, Heiss NS, Vulliamy TJ, Aalfs CM, McMahon C, Richmond P, et al. (1999) Unexplained aplastic anaemia, immunodeficiency, and cerebellar hypoplasia (Hoyeraal-Hreidarsson syndrome) due to mutations in the dyskeratosis congenita gene, DKC1. Br J Haematol 107: 335–339.

Koenig R, Bach A, Woelki U, Grzeschik KH, Fuchs S (2002) Spectrum of the acrocallosal syndrome. Am J Med Genet 108: 7–11.

Kolb LE, Arlier Z, Yalcinkaya C, Ozturk AK, Moliterno JA, Erturk O, et al. (2010) Novel VLDLR microdeletion identified in two Turkish siblings with pachygyria and pontocerebellar atrophy. Neurogenetics 11: 319–325.

Kondo A, Saito Y, Floricel F, Maegaki Y, Ohno K (2007) Congenital ocular motor apraxia: clinical and neuroradiological findings, and long-term intellectual prognosis. Brain Dev 29: 431–438.

Kroes HY, Nievelstein RJ, Barth PG, Nikkels PG, Bergmann C, Gooskens RH, et al. (2005) Cerebral, cerebellar, and colobomatous anomalies in three related males: Sex-linked inheritance in a newly recognized syndrome with features overlapping with Joubert syndrome. Am J Med Genet A 135: 297–301.

Kumar RA, Pilz DT, Babatz TD, Cushion TD, Harvey K, Topf M, et al. (2010) TUBA1A mutations cause wide spectrum lissencephaly (smooth brain) and suggest that multiple neuronal migration pathways converge on alpha tubulins. Hum Mol Genet 19: 2817.2827.

Kuwashima S (2009) Hoyeraal-Hreidarsson syndrome: magnetic resonance imaging findings. Jpn J Radiol 27: 324–327.

Lalani SR, Safiullah AM, Molinari LM, Fernbach SD, Martin DM, Belmont JW (2004) SEMA3E mutation in a patient with CHARGE syndrome. J Med Genet 41: e94.

Lalani SR, Safiullah AM, Fernbach SD, Harutyunyan KG, Thaller C, Peterson LE, et al. (2006) Spectrum of CHD7 mutations in 110 individuals with CHARGE syndrome and genotype-phenotype correlation. Am J Hum Genet 78: 303–314.

Lamonica DA, Maximino LP, Abramides DV, Souza DH, Richieri-Costa A (2010) Nonprogressive congenital cerebellar ataxia, iris heterochromia, mental retardation and language impairment in two brothers. Clin Dysmorphol 19: 76–78.

Leonardi ML, Pai GS, Wilkes B, Lebel RR (2001) Ritscher-Schinzel cranio-cerebello-cardiac (3C) syndrome: report of four new cases and review. Am J Med Genet 102: 237–242.

Levisohn L, Cronin-Golomb A, Schmahmann JD (2000) Neuropsychological consequences of cerebellar tumour resection in children: cerebellar cognitive affective syndrome in a paediatric population. Brain 123: 1041–1050.

Lin AE, Siebert JR, Graham JM, Jr (1990) Central nervous system malformations in the CHARGE association. Am J Med Genet 37: 304–310.

Lin HY, Lin SP, Chen YJ, Hung HY, Kao HA, Hsu CH, et al. (2006) Clinical characteristics and survival of trisomy 18 in a medical center in Taipei, 1988–2004. Am J Med Genet A 140: 945–951.

Lincke CR, van den Bogert C, Nijtmans LG, Wanders RJ, Tamminga P, Barth PG (1996) Cerebellar hypoplasia in respiratory chain dysfunction. Neuropediatrics 27: 216–218.

Lindhard A, Graem N, Skovby F, Jeppesen D (1993) Postmortem findings and prenatal diagnosis of Zellweger syndrome. Case report. APMIS 101: 226–228.

Mader I, Dobler-Neumann M, Kuker W, Stibler H, Krageloh-Mann I (2002) Congenital disorder of glycosylation type Ia: benign clinical course in a new genetic variant. Childs Nerv Syst 18: 77–80.

Margari L, Ventura P, Presicci A, Buttiglione M, Perniola T (2004) Congenital ataxia and mental retardation in three brothers. Pediatr Neurol 31: 59–63.

Marien P, Brouns R, Engelborghs S, Wackenier P, Verhoeven J, Ceulemans B, De Deyn PP (2008) Cerebellar cognitive affective syndrome without global mental retardation in two relatives with Gillespie syndrome. Cortex 44: 54–67.

Marr JE, Green SH, Willshaw HE (2005) Neurodevelopmental implications of ocular motor apraxia. Dev Med Child Neurol 47: 815–819.

Messerschmidt A, Brugger PC, Boltshauser E, Zoder G, Sterniste W, Birnbacher R, Prayer D (2005) Disruption of cerebellar development: potential complication of extreme prematurity. AJNR Am J Neuroradiol 26: 1659–1667.

Metry D, Heyer G, Hess C, Garzon M, Haggstrom A, Frommelt P, et al. (2009) Consensus statement on diagnostic criteria for PHACE syndrome. Pediatrics 124: 1447–1456.

Miossec-Chauvet E, Mikaeloff Y, Heron D, Merzoug V, Cormier-Daire V, de Lonlay P, et al. (2003) Neurological presentation in pediatric patients with congenital disorders of glycosylation type Ia. Neuropediatrics 34: 1–6.

Moog U, de Die-Smulders C, Systermans JM, Cobben JM (1997) Oculocerebrocutaneous syndrome: report of three additional cases and aetiological considerations. Clin Genet 52: 219–225.

Moog U, Jones MC, Viskochil DH, Verloes A, Van Allen MI, Dobyns WB (2007) Brain anomalies in encephalocraniocutaneous lipomatosis. Am J Med Genet A 143A: 2963–2972.

Morava E, Wevers RA, Cantagrel V, Hoefsloot LH, Al-Gazali L, Schoots J, et al. (2010) A novel cerebello-ocular syndrome with abnormal glycosylation due to abnormalities in dolichol metabolism. Brain 133: 3210–3220.

Morris-Rosendahl DJ, Najm J, Lachmeijer AM, Sztriha L, Martins M, Kuechler A, et al. (2008) Refining the phenotype of alpha-1a Tubulin (TUBA1A) mutation in patients with classical lissencephaly. Clin Genet 74: 425–433.

Naafs GG, van der Vliet AM, Hew JM (1999) The oculocerebrocutaneous (Delleman-Oorthuys) syndrome. Neuroradiology 41: 55–59.

Najm J, Horn D, Wimplinger I, Golden JA, Chizhikov VV, Sudi J, et al. (2008) Mutations of CASK cause an X-linked brain malformation phenotype with microcephaly and hypoplasia of the brainstem and cerebellum. Nat Genet 40: 1065–1067.

Norman AL, Crocker N, Mattson SN, Riley EP (2009) Neuroimaging and fetal alcohol spectrum disorders. Dev Disabil Res Rev 15: 209–217.

Orssaud C, Ingster-Moati I, Roche O, Bui Quoc E, Dufier JL (2009) Familial congenital oculomotor apraxia: clinical and electro-oculographic features. Eur J Paediatr Neurol 13: 370–372.

Ozgen HM, Overweg-Plandsoen WC, Blees-Pelk J, Besselaar PP, Hennekam RC (2005) Cerebellar hypoplasia-endosteal sclerosis: a long term follow-up. Am J Med Genet A 134A: 215–219.

Parrini E, Ramazzotti A, Dobyns WB, Mei D, Moro F, Veggiotti P, et al. (2006) Periventricular heterotopia: phenotypic heterogeneity and correlation with Filamin A mutations. Brain 28: 34–38.

Pascual-Castroviejo I, Pascual-Pascual SI, Velazquez-Fragua R, Lapunzina P (2005) Oculocerebrocutaneous (Delleman) syndrome: report of two cases. Neuropediatrics 36: 50–54.

Perez-Duenas B, Garcia-Cazorla A, Pineda M, Poo P, Campistol J, Cusi V, et al. (2009) Long-term evolution of eight Spanish patients with CDG type Ia: typical and atypical manifestations. Eur J Paediatr Neurol 13: 444–451.

Perry MS, Sladky JT (2008) Neuroradiologic findings in Sengers syndrome. Pediatr Neurol 39: 113–115.

Pinto G, Abadie V, Mesnage R, Blustajn J, Cabrol S, Amiel J, et al. (2005) CHARGE syndrome includes hypogonadotropic hypogonadism and abnormal olfactory bulb development. J Clin Endocrinol Metab 90: 5621–5626.

Poirier K, Keays DA, Francis F, Saillour Y, Bahi N, Manouvrier S, et al. (2007) Large spectrum of lissencephaly and pachygyria phenotypes resulting from de novo missense mutations in tubulin alpha 1A (TUBA1A). Hum Mutat 28: 1055–1064.

Poirier K, Saillour Y, Bahi-Buisson N, Jaglin XH, Fallet-Bianco C, Nabbout R, et al. (2010) Mutations in the neuronal β-tubulin subunit TUBB3 result in malformation of cortical development and neuronal migration defects. Hum Mol Genet 19: 4462–4473.

Poretti A, Leventer RJ, Cowan FM, Rutherford MA, Steinlin M, Klein A, et al. (2008a) Cerebellar cleft: a form of prenatal cerebellar disruption. Neuropediatrics 39: 106–112.

Poretti A, Wolf NI, Boltshauser E (2008b) Differential diagnosis of cerebellar atrophy in childhood. Eur J Paediatr Neurol 12: 155–167.

Poretti A, Alber FD, Burki S, Toelle SP, Boltshauser E (2009a) Cognitive outcome in children with rhombencephalosynapsis. Eur J Paediatr Neurol 13: 28–33.

Poretti A, Dietrich Alber F, Brancati F, Dallapiccola B, Valente EM, Boltshauser E (2009b) Normal cognitive functions in Joubert sindrome. Neuropediatrics 40: 287–290.

Poretti A, Huisman TA, Cowan FM, Del Giudice E, Jeannet PY, Prayer D, et al. (2009c) Cerebellar cleft: confirmation of the neuroimaging pattern. Neuropediatrics 40: 228–233.

Poretti A, Prayer D, Boltshauser E (2009d) Morphological spectrum of prenatal cerebellar disruptions. Eur J Paediatr Neurol 13: 397–407.

Poretti A, Limperopoulos C, Roulet-Perez E, Wolf NI, Rauscher C, Prayer D, et al. (2010) Outcome of severe unilateral cerebellar hypoplasia. Dev Med Child Neurol 52: 718–724.

Ritscher D, Schinzel A, Boltshauser E, Briner J, Arbenz U, Sigg P (1987) Dandy-Walker(like) malformation, atrio-ventricular septal defect and a similar pattern of minor anomalies in 2 sisters: a new syndrome? Am J Med Genet 26: 481–491.

Riva D, Giorgi C (2000) The cerebellum contributes to higher functions during development: evidence from a series of children surgically treated for posterior fossa tumours. Brain 123: 1051–1061.

Rosati P, Guariglia L (1999) Cerebellar hypoplasia: could it be a sonographic finding of abnormal fetal karyotype in early pregnancy? Fetal Diagn Ther 14: 365–367.

Ross ME, Swanson K, Dobyns WB (2001) Lissencephaly with cerebellar hypoplasia (LCH): a heterogeneous group of cortical malformations. Neuropediatrics 32: 256–263.

Rossi A, Bava GL, Biancheri R, Tortori-Donati P (2001) Posterior fossa and arterial abnormalities in patients with facial capillary haemangioma: presumed incomplete phenotypic expression of PHACES syndrome. Neuroradiology 43: 934–940.

Saito Y, Masuko K, Kaneko K, Chikumaru Y, Saito K, Iwamoto H, et al. (2006) Brain MRI findings of older patients with Pallister-Killian syndrome. Brain Dev 28: 34–38.

Saneto RP, Friedman SD, Shaw DW (2008) Neuroimaging of mitochondrial disease. Mitochondrion 8: 396–413.

Sanlaville D, Verloes A (2007) CHARGE syndrome: an update. Eur J Hum Genet 15: 389–399.

Sargent MA, Poskitt KJ, Jan JE (1997) Congenital ocular motor apraxia: imaging findings. AJNR Am J Neuroradiol 18: 1915–1922.

Sass JO, Gunduz A, Araujo Rodrigues Funayama C, Korkmaz B, Dantas Pinto KG, Tuysuz B, et al. (2010) Functional deficiencies of sulphite oxidase: differential diagnoses in neonates presenting with intractable seizures and cystic encephalomalacia. Brain Dev 32: 544–549.

Schaer M, Glaser B, Cuadra MB, Debbane M, Thiran JP, Eliez S (2009) Congenital heart disease affects local gyrification in 22q11.2 deletion syndrome. Dev Med Child Neurol 51: 746–753.

Schmahmann JD, Sherman JC (1998) The cerebellar cognitive affective syndrome. Brain 121: 561–579.

Shah DK, Tingay DG, Fink AM, Hunt RW, Dargaville PA (2005) Magnetic resonance imaging in neonatal nonketotic hyperglycinemia. Pediatr Neurol 33: 50–52.

Shotelersuk V, Desudchit T, Suwanwela N (2003) Postnatal growth failure, microcephaly, mental retardation, cataracts, large joint contractures, osteoporosis, cortical dysplasia, and cerebellar atrophy. Am J Med Genet A 116A: 164–169.

Sparks SE (2006) Inherited disorders of glycosylation. Mol Genet Metab 87: 1–7.

Spiegel EK, Colman RF, Patterson D (2006) Adenylosuccinate lyase deficiency. Mol Genet Metab 89: 19–31.

Squier W, Hope PL, Lindenbaum RH (1990) Neocerebellar hypoplasia in a neonate following intra-uterine exposure to anticonvulsants. Dev Med Child Neurol 32: 737–742.

Srour M, Rioux MF, Varga C, Lortie A, Major P, Robitaille Y, et al. (2011) The clinical spectrum of nodular heterotopias in children: report of 31 patients. Epilepsia epub February 14.

Steinlin M, Martin E, Largo R, Boesch C, Boltshauser E (1990) Congenital ocular motor apraxia: a neurodevelopmental and neuroradiological study. Neuro-ophthalmology 10: 27–32.

Steinlin M, Schmid M, Landau K, Boltshauser E (1997) Follow-up in children with Joubert syndrome. Neuropediatrics 28: 204–211.

Steinlin M, Blaser S, Boltshauser E (1998) Cerebellar involvement in metabolic disorders: a pattern-recognition approach. Neuroradiology 40: 347–354.

Steinlin M, Styger M, Boltshauser E (1999) Cognitive impairments in patients with congenital nonprogressive cerebellar ataxia. Neurology 53: 966–973.

Steinlin M, Imfeld S, Zulauf P, Boltshauser E, Lovblad KO, Ridolfi Luthy A, Perrig W, Kaufmann F (2003) Neuropsychological long-term sequelae after posterior fossa tumour resection during childhood. Brain 126: 1998–2008.

Steinlin M (2008) Cerebellar disorders in childhood: cognitive problems. Cerebellum 7: 607–610.

Steiss JO, Gross S, Neubauer BA, Hahn A (2005) Late-onset nephrotic syndrome and severe cerebellar atrophy in Galloway-Mowat syndrome. Neuropediatrics 36: 332–335.

Sznajer Y, Baumann C, David A, Journel H, Lacombe D, Perel Y, et al. (2003) Further delineation of the congenital form of X-linked dyskeratosis congenita (Hoyeraal-Hreidarsson syndrome). Eur J Pediatr 162: 863–867.

Takanashi J, Arai H, Nabatame S, Hirai S, Hayashi S, Inazawa J, et al. (2010) Neuroradiologic features of CASK mutations. AJNR Am J Neuroradiol 31: 1619–1622.

Tan GM, Arnone D, McIntosh AM, Ebmeier KP (2009) Meta-analysis of magnetic resonance imaging studies in chromosome 22q11.2 deletion syndrome (velocardiofacial syndrome). Schizophr Res 115: 173–181.

Tavano A, Grasso R, Gagliardi C, Triulzi F, Bresolin N, Fabbro F, Borgatti R (2007) Disorders of cognitive and affective development in cerebellar malformations. Brain 130: 2646–2660.

Terhal P, Sakkers R, Hochstenbach R, Madan K, Rabelink G, Sinke R, Giltay J (2004) Cerebellar hypoplasia, zonular cataract, and peripheral neuropathy in trisomy 17 mosaicism. Am J Med Genet A 130A: 410–414.

Tsuda T, Yoshida K, Ohashi S, Yanase T, Sueyoshi M, Kamimura S, et al. (2004) Arthrogryposis, hydranencephaly and cerebellar hypoplasia syndrome in neonatal calves resulting from intrauterine infection with Aino virus. Vet Res 35: 531–538.

Turkmen S, Demirhan O, Hoffmann K, Diers A, Zimmer C, Sperling K, Mundlos S (2006) Cerebellar hypoplasia and quadrupedal locomotion in humans as a recessive trait mapping to chromosome 17p. J Med Genet 43: 461–464.

Uyanik G, Morris-Rosendahl DJ, Stiegler J, Klapecki J, Gross C, Berman Y, Martin P, et al. (2007) Location and type of mutation in the LIS1 gene do not predict phenotypic severity. Neurology 69: 442–447.

van der Knaap MS, Vermeulen G, Barkhof F, Hart AA, Loeber JG, Weel JF (2004) Pattern of white matter abnormalities at MR imaging: use of polymerase chain reaction testing of Guthrie cards to link pattern with congenital cytomegalovirus infection. Radiology 230: 529–536.

Ventura P, Presicci A, Perniola T, Campa MG, Margari L (2006) Mental retardation and epilepsy in patients with isolated cerebellar hypoplasia. J Child Neurol 21: 776–781.

Verrotti A, Spalice A, Ursitti F, Papetti L, Mariani R, Castronovo A, et al. (2010) New trends in neuronal migration disorders. Eur J Paediatr Neurol 14: 1–12.

Waite A, Somer M, O'Driscoll M, Millen K, Manson FD, Chandler KE (2010) Cerebellar hypoplasia and Cohen syndrome: a confirmed association. Am J Med Genet A 152A: 2390–2393.

Wassmer E, Davies P, Whitehouse WP, Green SH (2003) Clinical spectrum associated with cerebellar hypoplasia. Pediatr Neurol 28: 347–351.

Weller S, Rosewich H, Gartner J (2008) Cerebral MRI as a valuable diagnostic tool in Zellweger spectrum patients. J Inherit Metab Dis 31: 270–280.

Wheeler PG, Sadeghi-Nejad A, Elias ER (1999) The 3C syndrome: evolution of the phenotype and growth hormone deficiency. Am J Med Genet 87: 61–64.

Whitsel EA, Castillo M, D'Cruz O (1995) Cerebellar vermis and midbrain dysgenesis in oculomotor apraxia: MR findings. AJNR Am J Neuroradiol 16 (4 Suppl): 831–834.

Yapici Z, Eraksoy M (2005) Non-progressive congenital ataxia with cerebellar hypoplasia in three families. Acta Paediatr 94: 248–253.

Zankl A, Gungor T, Schinzel A (2003) Cranio-cerebello-cardiac (3C) syndrome: follow-up study of the original patient. Am J Med Genet A 118A: 55–59.

9 Nonprogressive Congenital Ataxia

Eugen Boltshauser and Andrea Poretti

Definition

The term nonprogressive cerebellar ataxia (NPCA) refers to children with early evidence of cerebellar ataxia, without progression on follow-up. The first obvious features of ataxia are preceded by muscle hypotonia and delayed motor (and often language) milestones. Ataxia is thus not 'congenital' in the strict sense. We do not use the term NPCA for children with evidence of prenatal infection, perinatal illness, brain malformation other than cerebellar hypoplasia, defined syndromal disorders associated with ataxia, and postnatally acquired neurological diseases (Steinlin et al. 1998). Although NPCA represents a heterogeneous group of patients, both clinically and genetically, it is a useful diagnostic 'label' in practice. We avoid the term 'ataxic cerebral palsy'.

The prevalence of NPCA is not recorded. In our clinical experience it is more common than any defined cerebellar malformation. It is likely that it is underdiagnosed.

Aetiology and genetics

Familial occurrence has been observed repeatedly, occasionally in successive generations, but more often among siblings. A genetic basis is likely. There is marked genetic heterogeneity: X-linked and autosomal dominant and recessive inheritances are now established, the latter being the most prevalent.

X-LINKED ATAXIAS

The X-linked ataxias are discussed in Chapter 25.

DOMINANTLY INHERITED NONPROGRESSIVE CEREBELLAR ATAXIA

Observations in a few families have been recorded (Kornberg and Shield 1991; Imamura et al. 1993; Dudding et al. 2004; Jen et al. 2006). As in recessive forms, typical findings were initial floppiness and delayed motor milestones preceding early-onset ataxia, nonprogressive clinical course, and normal or mildly impaired cognition. Neuroimaging revealed cerebellar hypoplasia, often more pronounced of the vermis, or a normal-appearing cerebellum. So far no gene has been identified. We have no personal experience with dominant NPCA.

AUTOSOMAL RECESSIVE NONPROGRESSIVE CONGENITAL ATAXIA

Table 9.1 lists the genes and gene loci found in NPCA with autosomal recessive inheritance. Occurrence of NPCA in siblings has been observed frequently, suggesting autosomal recessive inheritance (Guzzetta et al. 1993; Steinlin et al. 1998; Yapici and Eraksoy 2005).

Only in exceptional families (all consanguineous) a gene locus has been identified by homozygosity mapping to date (Delague et al. 2001; Tranebjaerg et al. 2003; Turkmen et al. 2006; Gribaa et al. 2007).

In Cayman island ataxia (MIM #601238) the gene (*caytaxin*) has been elucidated (Bomar et al. 2003).

In a 'dysequilibrium syndrome' initially observed in the Hutterite community, mutations in the *VLDLR* gene were found (MIM #224050) (Boycott et al. 2005). Subsequently *VLDLR* mutations were found in patients of Turkish, Iranian, and European descent (Boycott et al. 2009). *VLDLR* is part of the reelin pathway. Reelin mutations have a severe effect on cortical (lissencephaly) and cerebellar organization (pronounced cerebellar hypoplasia).

CA8 gene mutations (MIM #613227) have been identified in a consanguineous Iraqi family. *CA8* (carbonic anhydrase related protein 8) is highly expressed in Purkinje cells (Turkmen et al. 2009).

Mutations in the *ZNF592* gene have been found in a large Lebanese family with the CAMOS syndrome (cerebellar ataxia with mental retardation (UK: learning disability) optic atrophy, and skin abnormalities, MIM #606937) (Delague et al. 2002; Nicolas et al. 2010).

In Gillespie syndrome (aniridia, cerebellar ataxia, and mental retardation; MIM #206700) variable degrees of cognitive impairment as well as of cerebellar hypoplasia (affecting predominantly the vermis) have been reported (Marien et al. 2008). In some patients a mutation in the *PAX6* gene was found.

KCNJ10 mutations were identified in a multisystem channelopathy disorder consisting of early-onset epilepsy, ataxia, sensorineural deafness, and tubulopathy (MIM #612780) (Bockenhauer et al. 2009; Scholl et al. 2009). Brain MRI showed normal cerebral and cerebellar structures.

In clinical practice the diagnosis of NPCA is mostly considered as a sporadic observation, i.e., without positive family history. At this point we inform the parents of an increased recurrence risk. For these families genetic mutation analyses are not yet available.

Clinical features

As mentioned, signs of ataxia are always preceded by muscular hypotonia and delayed motor milestones. Obvious signs of truncal and/or limb ataxia are usually not seen before the second or third year. Truncal ataxia manifests as broad-based gait, occasional to frequent falls, inability or great difficulties in tandem gait and standing on one leg. Upper limb ataxia is

TABLE 9.1
Genes and gene loci in nonprogressive congenital ataxia with autosomal recessive inheritance

Gene locus	Gene	Disease	OMIM	Additional findings	Reference
9q34-qter	unknown		213200	Cognitive impairment, short stature, albinism (inconsistent)	Delague et al. 2001
20q11-q13	unknown		606937	Normal cognition, mild spasticity, short stature	Tranebjaerg et al. 2003
17p	unknown		610185	Cognitive impairment (may be severe), speech impairment (dysarthria-absent speech), short stature, hirsutism, coarse face	Turkmen et al. 2006
16q21–23	unknown			Epilepsy, cognitive impairment, reduced tendon reflexes	Gribaa et al. 2007
19p13.3	Caytaxin	Cayman ataxia	601238	Marked cognitive impairment	Bomar et al. 2003
9p24	VLDLR	Cerebellar hypoplasia with cerebral gyral simplification	224050	Moderate cognitive impairment, pes planus, strabismus, seizures (inconsistent), short stature (inconsistent), gyral simplification	Boycott et al. 2009
8q11-q12	Carbonic anhydrase VIII	Ataxia, cognitive impairment, and mild quadrupedal locomotion	613227	Cognitive impairment, quadrupedal gait (inconsistent)	Turkmen et al. 2009
15q24-q26	ZNF592	Cerebellar ataxia with mental retardation, optic atrophy, and skin abnormalities (CAMOS)	606937	Cognitive impairment, spasticity, speech disorder, severe microcephaly, short stature, optic atrophy, osmophilic skin vessels	Delague et al. 2002; Nicolas et al. 2010
11p13	PAX6	Gillespie syndrome	206700	Aniridia, ataxia, cognitive impairment	Marien et al. 2008
1q23.2	KCNJ10	Epilepsy, ataxia, sensorineural deafness, tubulopathy, and KCNJ10 mutations	612780	Early onset epilepsy, ataxia, sensorineural deafness, tubulopathy	Bockenhauer et al. 2009
2q31.1-q36.1	NEUROD1	Neonatal diabetes mellitus, ataxia, deafness, myopia		Cerebellar hypoplasia	Rubio-Cabezas et al. 2010
3q28-qter	KIAA0226	Salih ataxia		Epilepsy, cognitive impairment	Assoum et al. 2010

variable, but often interferes with normal play activities because of marked dysmetria (building a tower, peg boards, puzzle, drawing, and writing). Quadrupedal gait has been reported in some families (but not in all affected siblings) with a form of NPCA, with cerebellar hypoplasia as a neuro-imaging correlate. Quadrupedal gait was attributed mainly to environmental factors (Turkmen et al. 2009). Nystagmus is not consistently found. Delayed acquisition of expressive language is common, followed by variable degree of dysarthria. Areflexia, ocular motor apraxia, and visual and hearing impairment are not features of NPCA.

Patients with NPCA have an increased prevalence of epilepsy, autistic features, and microcephaly (Steinlin et al. 1998; Parmeggiani et al. 2003; Wassmer et al. 2003; Ventura et al. 2006). Seizure control is usually achieved with medication.

In addition to neurological deficits, cognitive impairment is a common finding in NPCA (Steinlin et al. 1998, 1999; Margari et al. 2004; Lamonica et al. 2010). Based on observations in adults with acquired lesions, Schmahmann and Sherman defined the 'cerebellar cognitive and affective syndrome' (Schmahmann and Sherman 1998). This concept was later confirmed in children with acquired (benign cerebellar tumours) lesions (Steinlin 2007). Clinical experience in children with congenital ataxia and cerebellar malformations supports the role of the cerebellum in nonmotor development. We found cognitive impairment in 22 of 34 children with NPCA (Steinlin et al. 1998). Detailed testing of 11 patients confirmed significant cognitive deficits and better verbal than nonverbal performance (Steinlin et al. 1999). Recent studies by Tavano and coworkers confirmed the role of the cerebellum in the acquisition of higher order cognitive and affective skills (Tavano et al. 2007; Tavano and Borgatti 2010).

Short- and long-term outcome

Infancy and preschool age are usually dominated by motor impairments. With increasing age, ataxia persists, but becomes less significant and tends not to be the primary difficulty in daily life. On the contrary, limitations in language and cognition become more evident as children get older, often resulting in significant impairments of scholastic and professional achievements. Many patients are incapable of a proper vocational training. A minority of affected patients have normal cognition.

On long-term follow-up of our cohort of 34 patients with NPCA, two individuals developed spasticity, and three a focal dystonia (Steinlin et al. 1998). Dystonic movements were also observed in a family with dominant NPCA (Dudding et al. 2004).

Neuroimaging

Neuroimaging in NPCA is variable and there is inter- and intra-familial variability. In a large proportion of affected children MRI is normal (Fig. 9.1). This fact is likely to be responsible for the fact that many paediatricians, neuroradiologists, and even paediatric neurologists dismiss a diagnosis of NPCA. Normal imaging raises the question whether inclusion of NPCA in a section on cerebellar malformations is meaningful. Our justification for doing so lies in the occurrence of cerebellar hypoplasia in some patients.

In some children with NPCA, neuroimaging shows cerebellar hypoplasia, i.e. reduced cerebellar volume with basically normal architecture, in a normal-sized or small posterior fossa. Occasionally unilateral or markedly asymmetric cerebellar hemispheres can be seen (Poretti et al. 2008).

In a further subgroup, neuroimaging reveals a small cerebellum with widened interfolial spaces, giving the impression of cerebellar atrophy (Fig. 9.2) (Steinlin et al. 1998; Yapici and Eraksoy 2005; Turkmen et al. 2006; Lamonica et al. 2010; and personal observations). In view of the static clinical course we consider this cerebellar appearance to be a form of cerebellar hypoplasia. This observation implies that a single neuroimaging study may not be able to distinguish progressive cerebellar atrophy from static cerebellar hypoplasia (Poretti et al. 2008).

Neuroimaging rarely points to a specific diagnosis. In patients with *VLDLR* mutations, MRI reveals an almost afoliar small cerebellum, a flattened pons, and a reduced cerebral gyral pattern (Barkovich et al. 2009; Boycott et al. 2009).

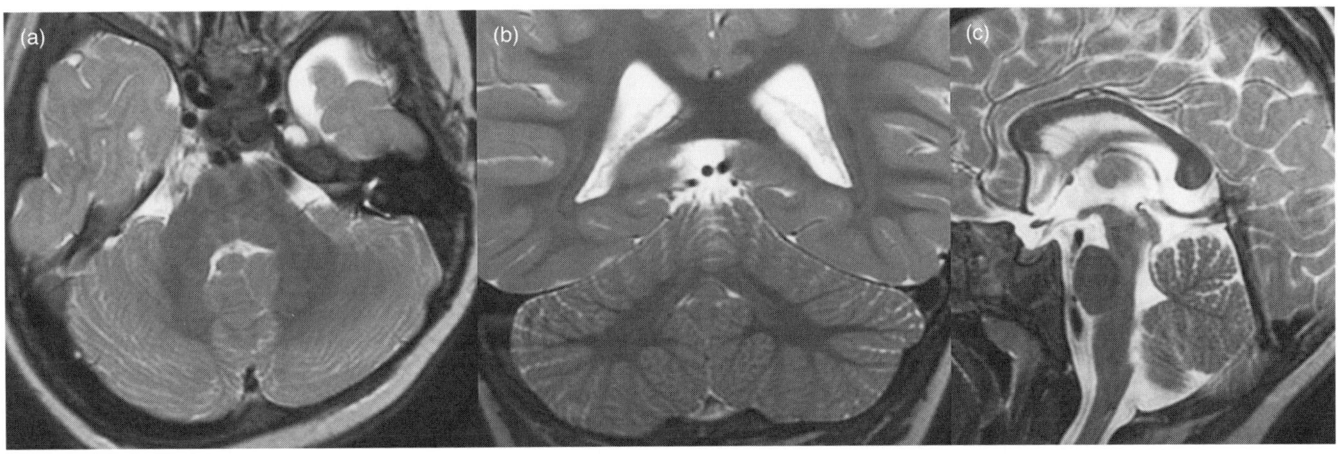

Fig. 9.1. Normal MRI of a 3 year old boy with a diagnosis of nonprogressive cerebellar ataxia. **(a)** Axial, **(b)** coronal, and **(c)** midsagittal T2-weighted MRI showing normal cerebellar structure.

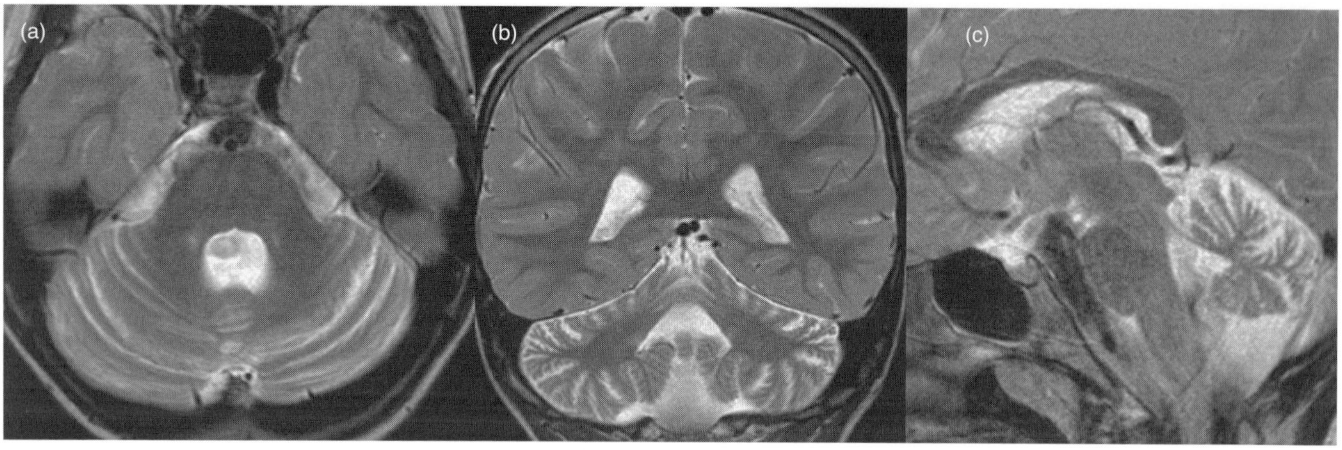

Fig. 9.2. Girl aged 8 years with nonprogressive cerebellar ataxia. **(a)** Axial, **(b)** coronal, and **(c)** midsagittal T2-weighted MRI demonstrating normal size of the cerebellum, but enlarged interfolial spaces mimicking cerebellar atrophy.

Diagnosis

In the absence of a positive family history (which is generally the case) diagnosis depends primarily on the patient history and the clinical context, supported by neuroimaging (revealing a normal cerebellum or a cerebellar hypoplasia; excluding defined cerebellar malformations and the rare midline posterior fossa tumour; and not providing pattern recognition evidence of a rare metabolic disorder such as glutaric aciduria, L-2-hydoxyglutaric aciduria). Prolonged observation may be required to confirm a nonprogressive course.

Differential diagnosis

Refer to Checklists, Table 1. Particularly at a young age (infancy), a long list of disorders associated with hypotonia and delayed motor milestones can mimic NPCA.

Neuroimaging is the most important additional diagnostic investigation (see Neuroimaging and Diagnosis).

We have seen two infants with a clinical suspicion of NPCA in whom MRI revealed a cerebellar tumour (without space-occupying effect and no focal cerebellar signs) as an unexpected 'incidental' finding. Removal of the tumour was not followed by neurological improvement.

Areflexia is not a feature of NPCA. If areflexia is present, nerve conduction studies are recommended. Rarely, a hereditary sensory neuropathy resulting in sensory ataxia can mimic NPCA.

Ataxia telangectasia at an early stage can present as NPCA; telangiectasias as well as oculomotor apraxia (a constant finding on follow-up) are late findings. In the initial stage MRI may not yet reveal cerebellar atrophy. Therefore, in view of management and genetic counselling, we recommend measuring alpha-fetoprotein, a reliable screening for ataxia telangiectasia (consistently and markedly elevated values).

The 'treatable ataxias' including coenzyme Q10 deficiency (see Checklists, Table 6) do not present as NPCA. Thus, measurements of vitamin E, cholesterol, and phytanic acid are not indicated, in our view.

Rarely, inborn errors of metabolism can mimic NPCA (personal observations). In order to confirm or rule out glutaric aciduria type 1, L-2-hydoxyglutaric aciduria, and congenital disorders of glycosylation (CDG), appropriate additional investigations can be considered (organic acids in urine, tandem mass spectroscopy, and transferrin isoform analysis). The rare conditions of pyruvate dehydrogenase deficiency and other mitochondrial disorders cannot be easily diagnosed by simple screenings.

An infant with substituted congenital hypothyroidism was seen with a typical clinical constellation of NPCA. When reviewed as a teenager he had only mild signs, compatible with benign hereditary chorea. This diagnosis was confirmed by mutation analysis (*NKX2-1* mutation encoding thyroid transcription factor 1). Benign hereditary chorea can behave as a 'chameleon'; hypothyroidism is not a consistent feature.

Summary

In our experience NPCA is more prevalent than any defined cerebellar malformation. It is under-recognized because of lack of awareness and frequently observed normal imaging. Neuroimaging is variable and may (inconsistently) reveal cerebellar hypoplasia or a small cerebellum with dilated interfolial spaces. NPCA is a congenital cerebellar malfunction, not always associated with a malformation. The motor deficits tend to improve with age, but a large proportion of affected children have permanent cognitive impairments. The assumed genetic basis is still largely unknown.

REFERENCES

Assoum M, Salih MA, Drouot N, H'Mida-Ben Brahim D, Lagier-Tourenne C, Al Drees A, et al. (2010) Rundataxin, a novel protein with RUN and diacylglycerol binding domains, is mutant in a new recessive ataxia. Brain 133: 2439–2447.

Barkovich AJ, Millen KJ, Dobyns WB (2009) A developmental and genetic classification for midbrain-hindbrain malformations. Brain 132: 3199–3230.

Bockenhauer D, Feather S, Stanescu HC, Bandulik S, Zdebik AA, Reichold M, et al. (2009) Epilepsy, ataxia, sensorineural deafness, tubulopathy, and KCNJ10 mutations. N Engl J Med 360: 1960–1970.

Bomar JM, Benke PJ, Slattery EL, Puttagunta R, Taylor LP, Seong E, et al. (2003) Mutations in a novel gene encoding a CRAL-TRIO domain cause human Cayman ataxia and ataxia/dystonia in the jittery mouse. Nat Genet 35: 264–269.

Boycott KM, Flavelle S, Bureau A, Glass HC, Fujiwara TM, Wirrell E, et al. (2005) Homozygous deletion of the very low density lipoprotein receptor gene causes autosomal recessive cerebellar hypoplasia with cerebral gyral simplification. Am J Hum Genet 77: 477–483.

Boycott KM, Bonnemann C, Herz J, Neuert S, Beaulieu C, Scott JN, et al. (2009) Mutations in VLDLR as a cause for autosomal recessive cerebellar ataxia with mental retardation (dysequilibrium syndrome). J Child Neurol 24: 1310–1315.

Delague V, Bareil C, Bouvagnet P, Salem N, Chouery E, Loiselet J, et al. (2001) Nonprogressive autosomal recessive ataxia maps to chromosome 9q34–9qter in a large consanguineous Lebanese family. Ann Neurol 50: 250–253.

Delague V, Bareil C, Bouvagnet P, Salem N, Chouery E, Loiselet J, et al. (2002) A new autosomal recessive non-progressive congenital cerebellar ataxia associated with mental retardation, optic atrophy, and skin abnormalities (CAMOS) maps to chromosome 15q24-q26 in a large consanguineous Lebanese Druze Family. Neurogenetics 4: 23–27.

Dudding TE, Friend K, Schofield PW, Lee S, Wilkinson IA, Richards RI (2004) Autosomal dominant congenital non-progressive ataxia overlaps with the SCA15 locus. Neurology 63: 2288–2292.

Gribaa M, Salih M, Anheim M, Lagier-Tourenne C, H'Mida D, Drouot N, et al. (2007) A new form of childhood onset, autosomal recessive spinocerebellar ataxia and epilepsy is localized at 16q21-q23. Brain 130: 1921–1928.

Guzzetta F, Mercuri E, Bonanno S, Longo M, Spano M (1993) Autosomal recessive congenital cerebellar atrophy. A clinical and neuropsychological study. Brain Dev 15: 439–445.

Imamura S, Tachi N, Oya K (1993) Dominantly inherited early-onset non-progressive cerebellar ataxia syndrome. Brain Dev 15: 372–376.

Jen JC, Lee H, Cha YH, Nelson SF, Baloh RW (2006) Genetic heterogeneity of autosomal dominant nonprogressive congenital ataxia. Neurology 67: 1704–1706.

Kornberg AJ, Shield LK (1991) An extended phenotype of an early-onset inherited nonprogressive cerebellar ataxia syndrome. J Child Neurol 6: 20–23.

Lamonica DA, Maximino LP, Abramides DV, Souza DH, Richieri-Costa, A (2010) Nonprogressive congenital cerebellar ataxia, iris heterochromia, mental retardation and language impairment in two brothers. Clin Dysmorphol 19: 76–78.

Margari L, Ventura P, Presicci A, Buttiglione M, Perniola T (2004) Congenital ataxia and mental retardation in three brothers. Pediatr Neurol 31: 59–63.

Marien P, Brouns R, Engelborghs S, Wackenier P, Verhoeven J, Ceulemans B, De Deyn PP (2008) Cerebellar cognitive affective syndrome without global mental retardation in two relatives with Gillespie syndrome. Cortex 44: 54–67.

Nicolas E, Poitelon Y, Chouery E, Salem N, Levy N, Megarbane A, Delague V (2010) CAMOS, a nonprogressive, autosomal recessive, congenital cerebellar ataxia, is caused by a mutant zinc-finger protein, ZNF592. Eur J Hum Genet 18: 1107–1113.

Parmeggiani A, Posar A, Scaduto MC, Chiodo S, Giovanardi-Rossi P (2003) Epilepsy, intelligence, and psychiatric disorders in patients with cerebellar hypoplasia. J Child Neurol 18: 1–4.

Poretti A, Wolf NI, Boltshauser E (2008) Differential diagnosis of cerebellar atrophy in childhood. Eur J Paediatr Neurol 12: 155–167.

Rubio-Cabezas O, Minton JA, Kantor I, Williams D, Ellard S, Hattersley AT (2010) Homozygous mutations in NEUROD1 are responsible for a novel syndrome of permanent neonatal diabetes and neurological abnormalities. Diabetes 59: 2326–2331.

Schmahmann JD, Sherman JC (1998) The cerebellar cognitive affective syndrome. Brain 121: 561–579.

Scholl UI, Choi M, Liu T, Ramaekers VT, Häusler MG, Grimmer J, et al. (2009) Seizures, sensorineural deafness, ataxia, mental retardation, and electrolyte imbalance (SeSAME syndrome) caused by mutations in KCNJ10. Proc Natl Acad Sci U S A 106: 5842–5847.

Steinlin M, Zangger B, Boltshauser E (1998) Non-progressive congenital ataxia with or without cerebellar hypoplasia: a review of 34 subjects. Dev Med Child Neurol 40: 148–154.

Steinlin M, Styger M, Boltshauser E (1999) Cognitive impairments in patients with congenital nonprogressive cerebellar ataxia. Neurology 53: 966–973.

Steinlin M (2007) The cerebellum in cognitive processes: supporting studies in children. Cerebellum 6: 237–241.

Tavano A, Borgatti R (2010) Evidence for a link among cognition, language and emotion in cerebellar malformations. Cortex 46: 907–918.

Tavano A, Grasso R, Gagliardi C, Triulzi F, Bresolin N, Fabbro F, Borgatti R (2007) Disorders of cognitive and affective development in cerebellar malformations. Brain 130: 2646–2660.

Tranebjaerg L, Teslovich TM, Jones M, Barmada MM, Fagerheim T, Dahl A, et al. (2003) Genome-wide homozygosity mapping localizes a gene for autosomal recessive non-progressive infantile ataxia to 20q11-q13. Hum Genet 113: 293–295.

Turkmen S, Demirhan O, Hoffmann K, Diers A, Zimmer C, Sperling K, Mundlos S (2006) Cerebellar hypoplasia and quadrupedal locomotion in humans as a recessive trait mapping to chromosome 17p. J Med Genet 43: 461–464.

Turkmen S, Guo G, Garshasbi M, Hoffmann K, Alshalah AJ, Mischung C, et al. (2009) CA8 mutations cause a novel syndrome characterized by ataxia and mild mental retardation with predisposition to quadrupedal gait. PLoS Genet 5: e1000487.

Ventura P, Presicci A, Perniola T, Campa MG, Margari L (2006) Mental retardation and epilepsy in patients with isolated cerebellar hypoplasia. J Child Neurol 21: 776–781.

Wassmer E, Davies P, Whitehouse WP, Green SH (2003) Clinical spectrum associated with cerebellar hypoplasia. Pediatr Neurol 28: 347–351.

Yapici Z, Eraksoy M (2005) Non-progressive congenital ataxia with cerebellar hypoplasia in three families. Acta Paediatr 94: 248–253.

10 Dandy-Walker Malformation

Andrea Poretti, Kathleen J. Millen, and Eugen Boltshauser

Historical note and nomenclature

Dandy-Walker malformation (DWM) is a cerebellar malformation first reported as the association of hydrocephalus, hypoplasia of the cerebellar vermis and posterior fossa cyst by Sutton in 1887 (Sutton 1887). This triad was later confirmed by Dandy and Blackfan in 1914 and subsequently studied in deeper detail by Taggart and Walker in 1942. In 1954, Benda coined the term 'Dandy-Walker syndrome' to describe this malformation. The DWM has been defined as an enlarged posterior fossa with high position of the tentorium, hypoplasia or agenesis of the cerebellar vermis, and a cystic dilatation of the fourth ventricle that fills nearly the entire posterior fossa. The observation of cases with hypoplasia and upward rotation of the cerebellar vermis as well as cystic enlargement of the fourth ventricle, but without enlargement of the posterior fossa, led some authors to introduce the term 'Dandy-Walker variant' (DWV). In 1989 Barkovich et al. introduced the terms 'Dandy-Walker complex' or 'Dandy-Walker continuum' including DWM, DWV, hypoplasia of the inferior cerebellar vermis, and mega cisterna magna, which could be part of the same spectrum of posterior fossa malformations (Barkovich et al. 1989). These different terms, particularly DWV, however, have been used with many different meanings. Some authors refer to the DWV as a hypoplastic inferior cerebellar vermis and a large cisterna magna without enlargement of the posterior fossa, while others use DVW to report a Dandy-Walker type malformation in which one or more of the fourth ventricular outflow foramina are patent. This leads to lack of specificity for the term DWV and confusion with the 'true' DWM. A detailed anatomic description (e.g., inferior cerebellar vermis or global cerebellar hypoplasia) is most sensible and preferable and the term DWV should be abandoned (Parisi and Dobyns 2003). The same should be applied to the terms 'Dandy-Walker complex' and 'Dandy-Walker continuum'.

For this chapter we will use only the term DWM. We define DWM based on its consistent neuroimaging features including (1) hypoplasia (or agenesis) of the cerebellar vermis, which is elevated and upwardly rotated and (2) a cystic dilatation of the fourth ventricle which extends posteriorly, filling nearly the entire posterior fossa (Parisi and Dobyns 2003). The elevation of the tentorium and torcula as well as hydrocephalus are not consistent and, therefore, are not diagnostic criteria. We wish to emphasize the importance of a consistent definition for DWM not only for clinical and diagnostic aims, but also for research purposes. We are aware of limitations of this definition because of its anatomic nature. A further understanding of the pathogenetic mechanisms of DWM might change the definition of this malformation in the future.

Finally we will discuss inferior cerebellar vermis hypoplasia. For posterior fossa cysts and cyst-like malformations, refer to Chapter 22.

Epidemiology

Dandy-Walker malformation is a relatively common malformation and the most prevalent human cerebellar malformation. The vast majority of patients with DWM are sporadic without familial recurrence or association with consanguinity. Consequently, the overall empiric recurrence risk has been estimated at between 1% and 5%. In a population-based survey of prenatal posterior fossa malformations the incidence of DWM has been estimated at about 1/11 000 (Long et al. 2006). This accounts for about 2–4% of all hydrocephalus cases in infants (Hirsch et al. 1984). The prevalence of isolated (not associated with another defined syndrome) DWM has been estimated at about 1/30 000 live births based on a neurosurgical cohort of patients (Osenbach and Menezes 1992). A mild female preponderance has been reported in some studies, particularly in patients with association between DWM and facial hemangioma (Hirsch et al. 1984; Osenbach and Menezes 1992).

Etiology

The etiology of DWM is poorly understood, probably multifactorial, and highly heterogeneous (Murray et al. 1985). Although environmental factors (such as exposure to teratogens) cannot be excluded, in the majority of patients DWM is due to a genetic etiology. DWM may occur as an isolated phenomenon or as part of a defined Mendelian disorder and with other syndromes such as *Aase-Smith syndrome* (MIM %147800; key features: hand abnormalities, joint contractures, and cleft palate) (Patton et al. 1985), *Aicardi syndrome* (MIM %304050; partial or complete absence of the corpus callosum, chorioretinal lacunae, and infantile spasms) (Jageerhussain et al. 2000), *Coffin-Siris syndrome* (MIM %135900; cognitive impairment, coarse face, hirsutism, and absent fifth fingernails/toenails/fifth distal phalanges) (Coulibaly et al. 2010), *cri-du-chat syndrome* (MIM #123450; characteristic cry, feeding problems, low birthweight, severe cognitive, speech, and motor impairment, and dysmorphic face) (Vialard et al. 2005), *Ellis-van Creveld syndrome* (MIM #225500; short limbs and ribs, postaxial polydactyly, dysplastic nails and teeth, and congenital cardiac defects) (Zangwill et al. 1988), *Fryns syndrome* (MIM %229850; diaphragmatic hernia, dysmorphic face, and distal limb hypoplasia) (Van Hove et al. 1995), *hydrolethalus syndrome* (MIM #236680; hydrocephalus, micrognathia, and polydactyly) (Morava et al. 1996), *Meckel syndrome* (different MIM numbers depending on the involved gene; occipital encephalocele, cystic kidneys, liver fibrosis, and polydactyly; there is significant overlap between Meckel syndrome and Joubert syndrome and related disorders and the molar tooth sign has been reported in several patients with Meckel syndrome) (Cincinnati et al. 2000), *Marden-Walker syndrome* (MIM %248700; blepharophimosis, microcephaly, micrognathia, multiple joint contractures, arachnodactyly, camptodactyly, kyphoscoliosis, and delayed motor development) (Ozkinay et al. 1995), *Ritscher-Schinzel or 3C syndrome* (MIM %220210; congenital cardiac and craniofacial anomalies) (Leonardi et al. 2001), *Rubinstein-Taybi syndrome* (MIM #180849 and #613684 for types 1 and 2, respectively; cognitive impairment, postnatal growth problems, microcephaly, broad thumbs and halluces, and dysmorphic face), and *PHACE(S)* syndrome (MIM 606519; posterior fossa malformations, hemangiomas of the face (large or complex), arterial anomalies, cardiac anomalies, eye abnormalities, and sternal clefting or supraumbilical raphe) (Rossi et al. 2001; Metry et al. 2009). Additionally, DWM has been associated with neurocutaneous melanosis (Berker et al. 2000; Marnet et al. 2009).

DWM has been also reported in association with various chromosomal anomalies including trisomy 9, 13, 18, triploidy, tetrasomy, and several partial duplications and deletions (Bordarier and Aicardi 1990; Altman et al. 1992; Ulm et al. 1997; Ecker et al. 2000; Parisi and Dobyns 2003; Poot et al. 2007; Jalali et al. 2008; Nakamura-Pereira et al. 2009). Karyotype abnormalities have been found in up to 32% of fetuses with DWM (Ecker et al. 2000).

Recently, mutations at three loci have been characterized in patients with DWM, as described below.

Pathogenesis

The sporadic nature and lack of large families segregating the DWM has made identification of the genetic basis of DWM difficult. Successful gene identification, however, has been possible due to the recognition of rare patients with chromosomal abnormalities and recent improvements in array-based methods to detect chromosomal copy number variants. To date, the genes associated with three rare DWM loci have been identified. Analysis of corresponding mouse models has allowed extensive embryonic analysis and delineation of the pathogenesis of DMW.

Analysis of nine patients with heterozygous deletions of chromosome 3q24 led to the identification of the linked *ZIC1* and *ZIC4* genes as the first DWM causative genes (Grinberg et al. 2004). These two linked genes encode two members of the five-member 'zinc finger in cerebellum' (zic) transcription factor family. They are widely expressed in developing mouse embryo and dynamically expressed in the developing cerebellum. Loss of *Zic1* and *Zic4* in mice causes disruption of multiple cerebellar developmental programs (Blank et al. 2011). Initially, there is a mispatterning of the cerebellar anlage during embryogenesis, leading to dysmorphic cerebellar foliation. Additionally, there is decreased proliferation of cerebellar granule cell progenitors in the external granule cell layer (EGL) of the developing cerebellum. The dramatic expansion of the size of the developing cerebellum is largely due to extensive proliferation of this population of cells, which also drives the elaboration of cerebellar foliation. Thus, decreased granule cell progenitor proliferation leads to considerable cerebellar hypoplasia and also contributes to aberrant foliation. The molecular pathways that the *Zic1* and *Zic4* genes regulate during cerebellar anlage patterning remain unknown. Loss of *Zic1* and *Zic4* function in granule cell progenitors, however, reduces reception in these cells to the Purkinje-cell derived sonic hedgehog (Shh) mitogenic signal required for their extensive expansion.

The second DWM locus to be delineated encompasses the *FOXC1* gene identified from a series of 21 patients with deletions and duplications of chromosome 6p25 and intragenic mutations of the *FOXC1* gene (Aldinger et al. 2009). *FOXC1* encodes a fork-head transcription factor which, intriguingly, is not expressed in the developing cerebellum, but rather is expressed in the adjacent posterior fossa mesenchyme – a complex mixture of head neural crest and mesoderm that gives rise to the meninges and skull. In mice, Foxc1 directs expression of a number of mesenchymal-derived growth factors, including members of the bone morphogenic (Bmp) and transforming growth factor beta (TGFβ) families. Foxc1-dependent expression of these growth factors is required to maintain organization of the adjacent rhombic lip and its major derivative, the EGL. One major molecular target in these cerebellar tissues is atonal homolog 1 (*Atoh1*), a gene essential for granule cell progenitor development in both the rhombic lip and EGL (Ben-Arie et al. 1997; Aldinger et al. 2009). Since granule cell progenitor proliferation is required for normal cerebellar growth and foliation, disruption of this developmental pathway is central to Foxc1-DWM pathogenesis. Notably, the rhombic lip also gives rise to the fourth ventricle roof plate, a precursor to the fourth ventricle choroid plexus epithelia (Chizhikov et al. 2010). In Foxc1 mouse mutants, the fourth ventricle is expanded because the roof plate and subsequent choroid plexus secondarily are expanded due to loss of Foxc1-dependent posterior fossa growth factors.

Most recently, fibroblast growth factor 17 (*FGF17*) has been implicated as a DWM gene based on the identification of a patient with a 2.3Mb deletion on chromosome 8p21 encompassing 19 genes (Zanni et al. 2011). Although it has not yet been directly established that these 19 genes have no role in DWM pathogenesis at this locus, notably, 1Mb proximal to the deletion lies the *FGF17* gene. Further, *Fgf17* expression is downregulated in the deletion patient's peripheral lymphocytes and skin fibroblasts. In mice *Fgf17* is expressed in the medial cerebellar anlage and loss of *Fgf17* causes vermis hypoplasia and foliation abnormalities due to very early proliferative defects in the vermis and aberrant vermis Purkinje cell differentiation (Xu et al. 2000).

Although the three characterized loci all appear to have considerably divergent mechanisms of pathogenesis, several important themes emerge. First, both the 3q24 and 6p25 DWM loci represent contiguous gene syndromes. Heterozygous deletion of either *Zic1* or *Zic4* alone is insufficient to model the DWM phenotype in mice. Both genes must be deleted (Grinberg et al. 2004). Similarly, mutation of *FOXC1* alone in humans causes a mild cerebellar phenotype. The full DWM phenotype is only apparent when additional adjacent genes are deleted (Aldinger et al. 2009). For the new 8p21 locus, there is insufficient data to yet determine whether *Fgf17* alone causes DWM, as most of the genes within the patient deletion have not been examined in detail (Zanni et al. 2011). It is likely that at least the two initial DWM loci were identified because the causative genes are adjacent to each other and the defining chromosomal abnormalities spanned all causative genes. However, since chromosomal abnormalities are rare in DWM and the genetics mostly non-Mendelian, 'true' DWM may more commonly be an oligogenic disorder involving at least two unlinked susceptibility alleles.

The 3q24 and 6p25 DWM loci are associated with a spectrum of cerebellar phenotypes; from mega cisterna magna to isolated vermis hypoplasia to 'true' DWM. Since deletion size does not easily correlate with phenotype severity (Grinberg et al. 2004; Aldinger et al. 2009), we speculate that stochastic events over the lengthy time period of cerebellar development can amplify early developmental disruptions, leading to a range of related developmental outcomes. Thus, DWM spectrum terminology may be appropriate for certain genetic loci. Notably however, there are several characterized inferior cerebellar vermis hypoplasia (IVH) loci that are never associated with DWM, including mutations of the *OPHN1* and *CASK* genes (Philip et al. 2003; Najm et al. 2008). Thus, until additional genes are identified for all posterior fossa malformations and their pathogenesis delineated, it will be extremely difficult to distinguish which patients merit a 'DWM spectrum' diagnosis versus diagnosis of a more specific malformation.

Based largely on analysis of *Foxc1* mutants, a working hypothesis is that DWM represents a complex disruption of the interaction of the developing posterior fossa and developing cerebellum. Further, the involvement of posterior fossa mesenchyme and its derivatives distinguish DWM loci from pure IVH loci (Aldinger et al. 2009). Notably, *Foxc1* mutation impacts all defining components of DWM. Specifically, it directly regulates posterior fossa size through its cell-autonomous regulation of meningeal and osteoblast development (Kume et al. 1998; Rice et al. 2003, 2005; Zarbalis et al. 2007; Vivatbutsiri et al. 2008) and indirectly controls both fourth ventricle and cerebellar size through its non-autonomous regulation of rhombic lip, roof plate, and EGL development (Aldinger et al. 2009). Although the roles of *Zic1* and *Zic4* have been characterized in cerebellar development, it has not yet been determined whether there is a posterior fossa phenotype in these mutants. Importantly however, both genes are expressed in posterior fossa mesenchyme (Blank et al. 2011) and *Zic1* is a known downstream target of *Foxc1* (Inoue et al. 2008). Finally, *Fgf17* is known to be expressed in the developing cerebellum (Xu et al. 2000); however, unpublished data (KJM) demonstrates that it is also highly expressed in the developing posterior fossa mesenchyme. It therefore remains to be determined whether all aspects of the *Fgf17* mouse cerebellar phenotype (and any potential posterior fossa phenotype) are attributable to this extracerebellar expression. Further phenotypic characterization of *Zic1/4* and *Fgf17* mutants is now imperative.

Clinical features

The vast majority of patients with DWM are asymptomatic during the neonatal period. The diagnosis of DWM is made before the age of 6 months in about 75% of patients and in more than 80% of patients by 1 year of age, mostly as a consequence of the symptoms of hydrocephalus (Hirsch et al. 1984; Pascual-Castroviejo et al. 1991). Macrocephaly, often with a dolichocephalic skull shape, is the most common manifestation in the first months of life, and is present in about 90–100% of affected children in this age group (Kumar et al. 2001; Yüceer et al. 2007; Alexiou et al. 2010). Bulging of the anterior fontanel and upward gaze palsy (both secondary to the hydrocephalus and found in 28% and 19% of the children, respectively, by Kumar et al. 2001), developmental delay, and muscular hypotonia are additional frequent signs in infants with DWM (Kumar et al. 2001). Atypical presentations in newborns or infants are apnea, seizures or cerebellar signs. Although all patients with DWM have hypoplasia of the cerebellar vermis, neurologic dysfunctions secondary to cerebellar abnormalities such as truncal and limb ataxia and nystagmus are present in about the half the patients and appear later in life (Gerszten and Albright 1995; Kumar et al. 2001). In older children symptoms of increased intracranial pressure include headaches, vomiting, and irritability, spasticity, hemiparesis, abnormal breathing pattern (e.g., apnea), cranial nerve dysfunction (e.g., seventh nerve palsy or trigeminal neuralgia), and strabismus (Hirsch et al. 1984; Gerszten and Albright 1995; Kumar et al. 2001; Ugur et al. 2005; Alexiou et al. 2010). Epileptic seizures have been reported in patients with DWM. In one series about a quarter of the patients present with seizures, while in our experience the frequency of seizures in patients with DWM is significantly lower (Gerszten and Albright 1995). Rarely patients come to clinical attention first as adults, or DWM may remain asymptomatic throughout life, particularly if hydrocephalus does not develop (Tal et al. 1980; Osenbach and Menezes 1992; Sato et al. 1996). These data are based mostly on previous neurosurgical studies and may be biased by patient selection. Our clinical experience (unpublished data), however, shows that the majority of patients are referred to a pediatric neurology centre shortly after birth because of a prenatal diagnosis of DWM, and most newborn infants have not yet developed hydrocephalus. Additionally, the number of patients presenting later (older children or adults) because of developmental delay, mild ataxia, or probably even as an incidental finding may be higher than was observed in the earlier neurosurgical reports.

The information about cognitive functions and the prevalence and degree of cognitive impairment in patients with DWM is conflicting. Several studies show different degrees of impairment of cognitive functions, whereas other reports present a more favorable cognitive outcome (Boddaert et al. 2003; Klein et al. 2003; Forzano et al. 2007; Bolduc et al. 2011). Overall, at least one-third of DWM patients have normal cognitive functions (Ecker et al. 2000; Has et al. 2004; Bolduc and Limperopoulos 2009; Bolduc et al. 2011). Normal lobulation of the cerebellar vermis and absence of associated brain abnormalities seem to be favorable prognostic indicators of normal cognitive functions (Bolduc and Limperopoulos 2009). Boddaert et al. (2003) assessed cognitive functions in 20 DWM patients and correlated them with neuroimaging findings. They found two groups with significant differences in cognitive outcome. While all patients with normal cognitive function had normal lobulation of the cerebellar vermis and no supratentorial anomalies, three of the six patients with cognitive impairment had an abnormal vermis as well as dysgenesis of the corpus callosum. A total of 82% of children with normal vermian lobulation had normal cognitive functions in contrast to none of the children with abnormal vermian lobulation. Similar results have been reported in a series including 26 patients with DWM (Klein et al. 2003). This point highlights the conclusion that cognitive impairment in DWM is primarily due to the cerebellar abnormality, not to increased intracranial pressure. Other studies compared DWM patients with and without additional brain anomalies such as agenesis or dysgenesis of the corpus callosum. Overall, these studies showed that all children with normal cognitive outcome did not have additional brain anomalies, while almost all children with cognitive impairment had associated brain malformations (Kölble et al. 2000; Kumar et al. 2001; Boddaert et al. 2003; Klein et al. 2003; Bolduc and Limperopoulos 2009). In a recent study of the spectrum of neurodevelopmental disabilities in children with cerebellar malformations, Bolduc et al. (2011) studied the cognitive outcome in five patients with DWM. They found impairments in fine motor functions in 40%, expressive language problems in 25%, and difficulties in receptive language, visual reception, and early learning in 20% of the patients. Additionally, they reported problems in externalizing and internalizing behaviors in 50% and 25% of patients, respectively.

Mostly as part of defined syndromes (see Etiology), DWM may be associated with systemic anomalies in 9–44% of affected patients (Kumar et al. 2001; Has et al. 2004). Various cardiovascular anomalies have been noted, including atrial and ventricular septal defects, patent ductus arteriosus, valvular aortic stenosis, tetralogy of Fallot, dextrocardia, or coarctation of the aorta (Ecker et al. 2000; Has et al. 2004; Yüceer et al. 2007). Other associated anomalies affect the urogenital system (e.g., vesico-ureteral reflux, hydronephrosis, multicystic dysplastic kidneys, horseshoe kidneys, undescended testes, hydrocele, and hypospadias), extremities (e.g., limb shortness, talipes, polydactyly, syndactyly, and overlapping fingers), and the face (e.g., micrognathia, cleft lip and/or palate, flat nasal bridge, hypertelorism, and facial hemangioma) (Ecker et al. 2000; Has et al. 2004; Yüceer et al. 2007). Finally, diaphragmatic hernia, tracheal atresia, hygroma, narrow thorax, omphalocele, duodenal atresia, cystic adenomatoid malformation of the lungs, and opaque lens have been reported in DWM (Ecker et al. 2000; Has et al. 2004; Yüceer et al. 2007).

Neuroimaging

Neuroimaging key features of DWM are hypoplasia (or rarely agenesis) of the cerebellar vermis and cystic dilatation of the fourth ventricle. Both are consistently present in all individuals with DWM and are required for the diagnosis.

The cerebellar vermis is elevated and upwardly rotated. Consequently it may be typically found behind the tectum and the quadrigeminal plate and may come in contact with the tentorium (Barkovich et al. 1989; Klein et al. 2003). Lobulation of the cerebellar vermis may be rudimentary (Boddaert et al. 2003; Klein et al. 2003). Mostly because of the enlargement of the fourth ventricle, the cerebellar hemispheres are typically displaced anterolaterally, and their size is usually reduced. The brainstem generally appears thin, mostly because of hypoplasia of the pons (Patel and Barkovich 2002; Klein et al. 2003; Abdel-Salam et al. 2006).

The fourth ventricle is consistently enlarged (Figs 10.1a, 10.2a, 10.3a) and may extend upwardly between the occipital lobes through a congenital dehiscence of the tentorium and inferiorly into the foramen magnum. Laterally, however, the extension of the fourth ventricle is limited by the cerebellar hemispheres. The fourth ventricle communicates widely with a retrocerebellar cystic compartment that may cause enlargement of the posterior fossa and elevation of the tentorium, torcula, and transverse sinuses (Figs 10.1a, 10.2a, 10.3a). Enlargement of the posterior fossa and upwards displacement of the tentorium are common, but are not consistent in all DWM cases (Parisi and Dobyns 2003). Therefore, they are not included in the diagnostic criteria of DWM. Lack of patency of the foramen of Magendie is usual, but not consistent, whereas the foramina of Luschka may be patent uni- or bilaterally. This variability in the foraminal patency may account for the different prevalence and degree of communicating hydrocephalus which is present in about 80–95% of patients in neurosurgical series (Fig. 10.2b) (Klein et al. 2003; Mohanty et al. 2006). The flow pattern of the cerebrospinal fluid (CSF) may be studied by CSF flow MR imaging (Yildiz et al. 2006). In DWM, aqueductal flow is present and typically directed into the posterior fossa cyst. In patients with hydrocephalus, the aqueductal flow is usually hyperdynamic (CSF flow through the Sylvian aqueduct into the cyst produces turbulent flow within the cyst and the turbulent flow is characterized by irregular movements of the fluid with high velocity), whereas in patients without hydrocephalus it may be hyperdynamic or diminished. A pulsatile signal of the CSF flow may be seen within the cyst.

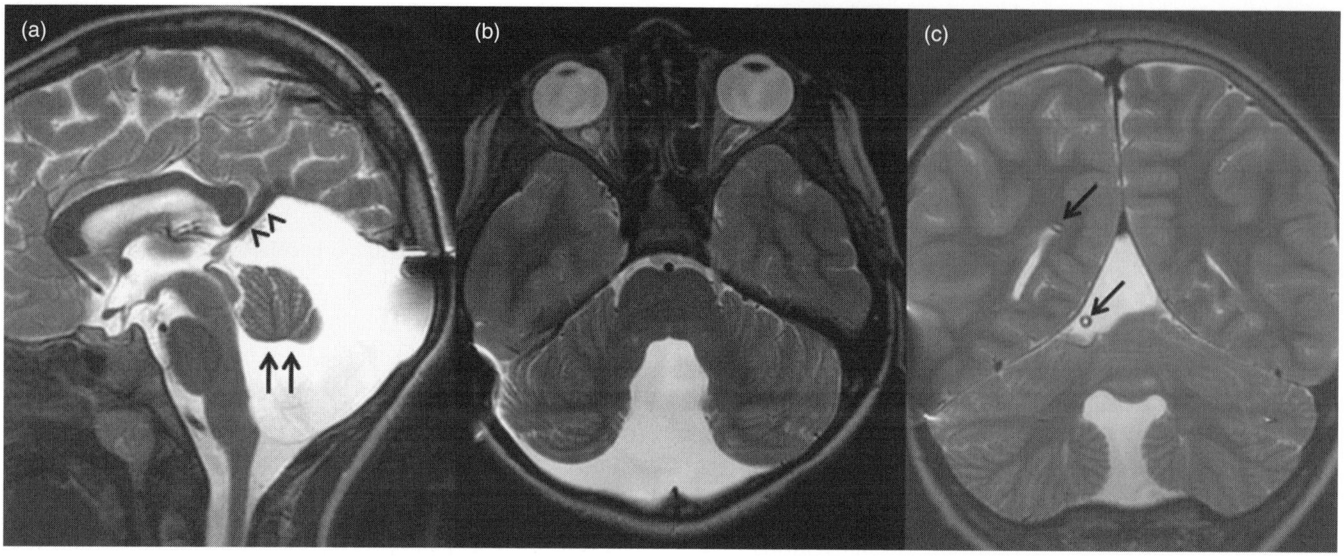

Fig. 10.1. Follow-up imaging in 10-year-old girl with Dandy-Walker malformation after shunting in the first year of life. **(a)** Sagittal, **(b)** axial, and **(c)** coronal T2-weighted MRI presenting a cystic dilatation of the fourth ventricle extending posteriorly and communicating with a retrocerebellar cystic compartment; the posterior fossa is enlarged; the cerebellar vermis is hypoplastic, elevated, and upwardly rotated (black arrows on (a)), the tentorium is elevated (black arrowheads on (a)). The cerebellar hemispheres are displaced anterolaterally. Notice the ventriculo- and the cysto-peritoneal shunts (black arrows on (c)).

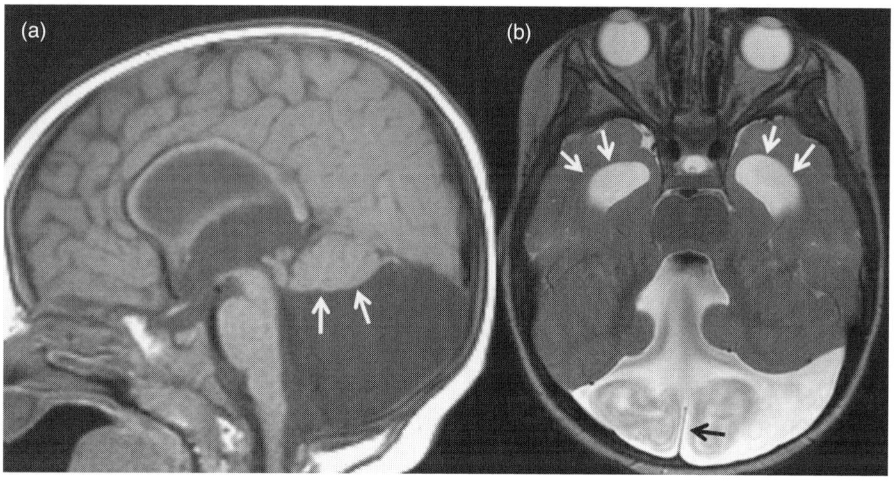

Fig. 10.2. Child aged 15 months with Dandy-Walker malformation before shunting. **(a)** Sagittal T1-weighted MRI and **(b)** axial T2-weighted MRI showing a hypoplastic cerebellar vermis which is counter-clockwise rotated (white arrows on (a)) and an enlargement of the posterior fossa which is filled with a retrocerebellar cystic compartment. The falx cerebelli is normal (black arrow on (b)). Notice the hydrocephalic dilatation of the temporal horns (white arrows on (b)).

Additional brain malformations are associated with DWM in about 30–50% of patients (Parisi and Dobyns 2003). Agenesis or dysgenesis of the corpus callosum has been reported in about 10–20% of DWM cases (Fig. 10.3a) (Parisi and Dobyns 2003; Has et al. 2004). Occipital encephaloceles, polymicrogyria, heterotopias, inferior olive malformation, aqueductal stenosis, and intracranial lipoma have also been described.

Recent advances in fetal imaging have significantly improved the prenatal diagnosis of DWM (Ecker et al. 2000; Has et al. 2004; Long et al. 2006; Forzano et al. 2007; Limperopoulos et al. 2008; Malinger et al. 2009; Prayer 2011). The neuroimaging criteria leading to a prenatal or a postnatal diagnosis are the same (Adamsbaum et al. 2005). In light of the prenatal diagnosis of DWM, it is important to know that an enlarged fourth ventricle may be a transient phenomenon between the 14th and 16th weeks of gestation. Therefore, a prenatal diagnosis of DWM is usually possible toward 20 weeks of gestation (Ecker et al. 2000). Additionally, the tentorium has its definitive orientation from the 20th gestational week. If the prenatal diagnosis of DWM is made or suspected, hydrocephalus and associated supratentorial malformations have to be carefully sought, as their presence represents a risk of poor cognitive outcome.

Diagnosis

Both the prenatal and the postnatal diagnosis of DWM are based on a detailed neuroimaging investigation, preferably MRI. The diagnostic criteria include hypoplasia of the cerebellar vermis, which is elevated and upwardly rotated, and cystic

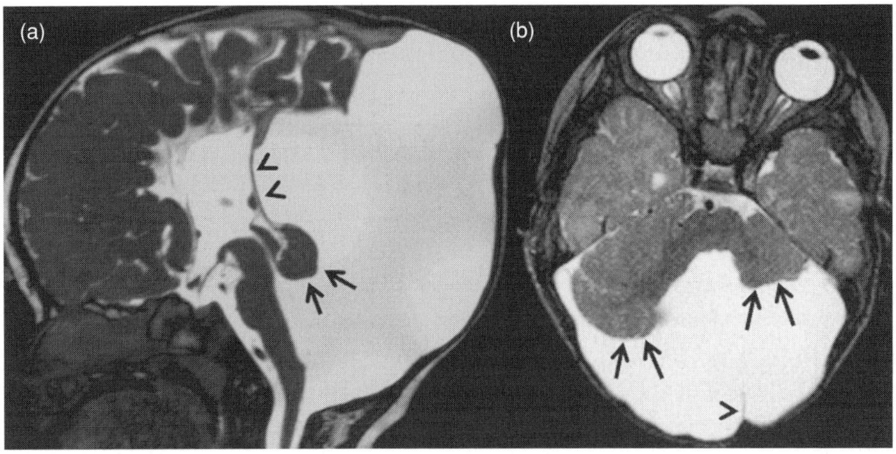

Fig. 10.3. Child aged 2 years with Dandy-Walker malformation. **(a)** Midsagittal constructive interference in steady-state (CISS) and **(b)** axial T2-weighted MRI demonstrating a severe hypoplasia, elevation, and upwardly rotation of the cerebellar vermis (black arrows on (a)), asymmetric hypoplasia of the cerebellar hemispheres (black arrows on (b)), marked elevation of the tentorium (black arrowheads on (a)), and marked enlargement of the posterior fossa. Notice associated agenesis of the corpus callosum, hypoplasia of the pons, and normal cerebellar falx (black arrowhead on (b)).

dilatation of the fourth ventricle which extends posteriorly filling nearly the entire posterior fossa. The lobulation of the cerebellar vermis should be carefully evaluated because of its prognostic relevance. Additional brain malformations have to be sought. A careful clinical investigation is mandatory for associated systemic abnormalities and/or dysmorphic features and to assess whether DWM is isolated or part of a defined syndrome. Chromosomal analysis is not indicated in isolated DWM.

Differential diagnosis

Based on the presence of associated systemic abnormalities and/or dysmorphic signs, isolated DWM should be differentiated from DWM as part of a defined syndrome. This is usually possible by a careful clinical investigation and, if necessary, additional targeted examinations.

DWM should be distinguished from other abnormalities of the posterior fossa such as mega cisterna magna, inferior cerebellar vermis hypoplasia, or Blake's pouch cyst. This is mostly not problematic if the diagnostic criteria for DWM are applied. The position of the choroid plexus in the fourth ventricle provides important clues to the nature of a posterior fossa cyst: normal in arachnoid cyst, absent in Dandy-Walker, displaced into the superior cyst wall in Blake's pouch (Nelson et al. 2004). CSF flow images may be useful in difficult cases. Exceptionally, DWM may mask recognition of the molar tooth sign in patients with Joubert syndrome (Sartori et al. 2010). Unfortunately, patients with clear-cut evidence of molar tooth sign are still misdiagnosed and reported as having DWM rather than Joubert syndrome (Sener 2007; Poretti and Boltshauser 2009; Shenoy and Kamath 2010). Finally, acquired cerebellar abnormalities such as disruption of cerebellar development in very preterm infants (Messerschmidt et al. 2005) and post-hemorrhagic cerebellar disruption (Limperopoulos et al. 2010) may mimic DWM.

Finally, hypoplasia of the inferior cerebellar vermis or inferior vermian hypoplasia (IVH) should be differentiated from DWM. IVH is defined by partial absence of the inferior portion of the cerebellar vermis with normal or near-normal shaped cerebellar hemispheres, a normal-sized posterior fossa without cystic lesions, and normal supratentorial structures (Limperopoulos et al. 2006). In the literature, however, the diagnostic entity of IVH remains inconsistently used. Some authors believe that IVH may represent a normal variant (Patel and Barkovich 2002). Other authors report this anatomic entity as 'Dandy-Walker variant', leading to confusion. The term IVH itself is not correct. 'Hypoplasia' means a small but complete anatomic structure with a congenital volume diminution. IVH, however, represents an arrested, incomplete downward growth of the cerebellar vermis and the term 'inferior vermian agenesis' seems to be more adequate (Malinger et al. 2009). 'Agenesis' is defined as either complete or partial absence of an anatomic structure. Because of the craniocaudal development of the vermis, partial agenesis involves its inferior (caudal) part, as occurs in IVH. Postnatally, the diagnosis of IVH is made best on midsagittal images and confirmed on axial and coronal imaging. Prenatally, IVH may be reliably diagnosed when caudal growth of the inferior vermis over the fourth ventricle remained incomplete after 18–20 weeks of gestation (Limperopoulos et al. 2006, 2008). The entire vermis is generally closed by the end of the 15th week of gestation, but Bromley et al. showed that its posterior-inferior aspect may remain open in about 4% of the fetuses until 17.5 weeks (Bromley et al. 1994).

The outcome of isolated IVH is mostly good. Limperopoulos et al. reported normal development in 77% of children with isolated IVH (Limperopoulos et al. 2006). In a recent study, the same group, however, presented mild functional deficits in fine motor activities and receptive language in 24%, early learning and visual reception in 18%, and expressive language in 12% of children with isolated IVH (Bolduc et al. 2011). Additionally, problems in internalizing and externalizing behavior have been found in 24% and 6% of such patients, respectively.

Management and treatment

Correction of hydrocephalus is the main treatment in DWM and the different possible technical procedures have been the subject of great controversy (Mohanty et al. 2006; Alexiou et al. 2010). Direct surgery on the posterior fossa involving excision of posterior fossa membranes to create unobstructed flow of CSF was reported in early series, but resulted in poor outcome and has been abandoned (Sawaya and McLaurin 1981; Asai et al. 1989). Currently, if progressive hydrocephalus is evident, the various treatment options include a shunt placement, either ventriculoperitoneal, cystoperitoneal, or combined ventriculoperitoneal and cystoperitoneal, or endoscopic procedures such as endoscopic third ventriculostomy (ETV) (Mohanty et al. 2006).

Shunt placement is currently considered the surgical procedure of choice, but there is considerable debate regarding the choice of shunt. Ventriculoperitoneal shunts are easier to place and have a lower incidence of malposition, migration, and overall complications than cystoperitoneal shunts and can be used in cases of significant hydrocephalus (Bindal et al. 1990; Gerszten and Albright 1995; Kalidasan et al. 1995; Mohanty et al. 2006). Nonetheless, ventriculoperitoneal shunts are not without complications. Permanent ventriculoperitoneal shunting is associated with general complications such as infection or shunt disconnection. Additionally, it has been suggested that, in DWM, ventriculoperitoneal shunt alone may lead to the development of acquired aqueductal stenosis necessitating the subsequent placement of a cystoperitoneal shunt as well in 29–77% of cases (Asai et al. 1989; Osenbach and Menezes 1992; Kumar et al. 2001). Moreover, an upward transtentorial herniation of the cyst after solitary ventriculoperitoneal shunt has been reported (Pillay et al. 1989). Cystoperitoneal shunt placement alone has been reported to drain both the cyst and the ventricles adequately, avoiding the risk of an entrapped fourth ventricle, and is considered by some to be the treatment of choice (Hirsch et al. 1984; Maria et al. 1987; Asai et al. 1989). Nevertheless, cystoperitoneal shunts may be associated with complications: difficult placement of the proximal end, frequent disconnection and migration, development of posterior fossa hematomas and brainstem tethering, need for frequent revisions, and an increased incidence of CSF leakage during the postoperative period (Bindal et al. 1990; Gerszten and Albright 1995; Kumar et al. 2001; Mohanty et al. 2006). Additionally, deaths of a few patients have been attributed to posterior fossa hematomas due to cystoperitoneal shunts (Bindal et al. 1990). Combined ventriculoperitoneal and cystoperitoneal shunt placement (with a common distal catheter) to equalize pressure across the tentorium has been advocated by other authors as the treatment of first choice (Pillay et al. 1989; Osenbach and Menezes 1992). Osenbach and Menezes reported a 92% success rate in alleviating hydrocephalus using combined shunts (Osenbach and Menezes 1992).

Recently, ETV has been proposed as an alternative method for the treatment of hydrocephalus in DWM (Mohanty et al. 2006). ETV is a less invasive procedure with lower morbidity and it obviates the need for placement of a shunt. In 21 patients with DWM treated with ETV, Mohanty et al. reported a success rate of 76%, which is comparable to the success rate of ETV treating obstructive hydrocephalus (Mohanty et al. 2006). Overall, the success rate of ETV ranges between 23% and 80%, with the lower success rates seen in infants and younger children (Mohanty et al. 2006). In cases of associated aqueductal stenosis, the placement of a cystoperitoneal shunt was combined with ETV to ensure patent communication between supratentorial and infratentorial compartments to prevent the development of a transtentorial upward herniation. In the series of Mohanty et al. (2006), the five ETV failures occurred between 1 and 6 months postoperatively and caused patient irritability and persistent increase in head circumference that required subsequent shunt insertion. Based on its high capacity to detect a flow defect through a ventriculostomy, Faggin et al. (2011) recently showed that performance of cine phase-contrast MRI during the follow-up of DWM patients treated with ETV may be useful in early detection of ETV failure.

In light of the frequently observed delayed milestones and cognitive impairment, careful neurodevelopmental evaluations help guide the need for supportive measures such as physical and occupational therapies.

Outcome and prognosis

The overall prognosis in DWM depends on several factors. Cognitive outcome seems to depend mostly on the lobulation of the vermis and the presence of additional supratentorial malformations. The presence of additional systemic abnormalities such as cardiac malformations may significantly affect prognosis. Mostly because of a higher frequency of associated findings and a higher prevalence of chromosomal aberrations, the prognosis in DWM was less favorable in a series of patients in whom the diagnoses was made *prenatally* (Ecker et al. 2000; Kölble et al. 2000). Additionally, complications related to the hydrocephalus and its treatment may significantly affect the prognosis. Even in centres with considerable expertise, the mortality of nontumoral infantile hydrocephalus during childhood is in the range of 10%. Moreover, sudden unexpected respiratory arrest and death in children with DWM have been reported (Tal et al. 1980; Elterman et al. 1995). Sudden death in DWM is not due to shunt problems, but may be related to pressure on the pontine respiratory centre by the posterior fossa cyst. Finally, in some cases the development of syringomyelia resulting from herniation of the Dandy-Walker cyst through the foramen magnum has been reported as an occasional late complication in DWM (Hammond et al. 2002; Richter and Pincus 2006).

REFERENCES

Abdel-Salam GM, Shehab M, Zaki MS (2006) Isolated Dandy-Walker malformation associated with brain stem dysgenesis in male sibs. Brain Dev 28: 529–533.

Adamsbaum C, Moutard ML, André C, Merzoug V, Ferey S, Quéré MP, et al. (2005) MRI of the fetal posterior fossa. Pediatr Radiol 35: 124–140.

Aldinger KA, Lehmann OJ, Chizhikov VV, Bassuk AG, Ades LC, Krantz ID, et al. (2009) FOXC1 is required for normal cerebellar development and is a major contributor to 6p25.3 Dandy-Walker malformation. Nat Genet 41: 1037–1042.

Alexiou GA, Sfakianos G, Prodromou N (2010) Dandy-Walker malformation: Analysis of 19 Cases. J Child Neurol 25: 188–191.

Altman NR, Naidich TP, Braffman BH (1992) Posterior fossa malformations. AJNR Am J Neuroradiol 13: 691–724.

Asai A, Hoffman HJ, Hendrick EB, Humphreys RP (1989) Dandy-Walker syndrome: experience at the Hospital for Sick Children, Toronto. Pediatr Neurosci 15: 66–73.

Barkovich AJ, Kjos BO, Norman D, Edwards MS (1989) Revised classification of posterior fossa cysts and cystlike malformations based on the results of multiplanar MR imaging. AJR Am J Roentgenol 153: 1289–1300.

Ben-Arie N, Bellen HJ, Armstrong DL, McCall AE, Gordadze PR, Guo Q, et al. (1997) Math1 is essential for genesis of cerebellar granule neurons. Nature 390: 169–172.

Benda CE (1954) The Dandy-Walker syndrome or the so-called atresia of the foramen Magendie. J Neuropathol Exp Neurol 13: 14–29.

Berker M, Oruckaptan HH, Oge HK, Benli K (2000) Neurocutaneous melanosis associated with Dandy-Walker malformation. Case report and review of the literature. Pediatr Neurosurg 33: 270–273.

Bindal AK, Storrs BB, McLone DG (1990) Management of the Dandy-Walker syndrome. Pediatr Neurosurg 16: 163–169.

Blank MC, Grinberg I, Aryee E, Laliberte C, Chizhikov VV, Henkelman RM, Millen KJ (2011) Multiple cerebellar developmental programs are altered by loss of Zic1 and Zic4 to cause Dandy-Walker malformation cerebellar pathogenesis. Development 138: 1207–1216.

Boddaert N, Klein O, Ferguson N, Sonigo P, Parisot D, Hertz-Pannier L, et al. (2003) Intellectual prognosis of the Dandy-Walker malformation in children: the importance of vermian lobulation. Neuroradiology 45: 320–324.

Bolduc ME, Limperopoulos C (2009) Neurodevelopmental outcomes in children with cerebellar malformations: a systematic review. Dev Med Child Neurol 51: 256–267.

Bolduc ME, Du Plessis AJ, Sullivan N, Khwaja OS, Zhang X, Barnes K, et al. (2011) Spectrum of neurodevelopmental disabilities in children with cerebellar malformations. Dev Med Child Neurol 53: 409–416.

Bordarier C, Aicardi J (1990) Dandy-Walker syndrome and agenesis of the cerebellar vermis: diagnostic problems and genetic counselling. Dev Med Child Neurol 32: 285–294.

Bromley B, Nadel AS, Pauker S, Estroff JA, Benacerraf BR (1994) Closure of the cerebellar vermis: evaluation with second trimester US. Radiology 193: 761–763.

Chizhikov VV, Lindgren AG, Mishima Y, Aldinger KA, Miesegaes GR, Currle DS, et al. (2010) Lmx1a regulates fates and location of cells in the cerebellar rhombic lip and telencephalic cortical hem. Proc Natl Acad Sci USA 107: 10725–10730.

Cincinnati P, Neri ME, Valentini A (2000) Dandy-Walker anomaly in Meckel-Gruber syndrome. Clin Dysmorphol 9: 35–38.

Coulibaly B, Sigaudy S, Girard N, Popovici C, Missirian C, Heckenroth H, et al. (2010) Coffin-Siris syndrome with multiple congenital malformations and intrauterine death: towards a better delineation of the severe end of the spectrum. Eur J Med Genet 53: 318–321.

Dandy WE, Blackfan KD (1914) Internal hydrocephalus: an experimental, clinical and pathological study. Am J Dis Child 8: 406–482.

Ecker JL, Shipp TD, Bromley B, Benacerraf B (2000) The sonographic diagnosis of Dandy-Walker and Dandy-Walker variant: associated findings and outcomes. Prenat Diagn 20: 328–332.

Elterman RD, Bodensteiner JB, Barnard JJ (1995) Sudden unexpected death in patients with Dandy-Walker malformation. J Child Neurol 10: 382–384.

Faggin R, Calderone M, Denaro L, Meneghini L, D'Avella D (2011) Long-term operative failure of endoscopic third ventriculostomy in pediatric patients: the role of cine phase-contrast MR imaging. Neurosurg Focus 30: E1.

Forzano F, Mansour S, Ierullo A, Homfray T, Thilaganathan B (2007) Posterior fossa malformation in fetuses: a report of 56 further cases and a review of the literature. Prenat Diagn 27: 495–501.

Gerszten PC, Albright AL (1995) Relationship between cerebellar appearance and function in children with Dandy-Walker syndrome. Pediatr Neurosurg 23: 320–324.

Grinberg I, Northrup H, Ardinger H, Prasad C, Dobyns WB, Millen KJ (2004) Heterozygous deletion of the linked genes ZIC1 and ZIC4 is involved in Dandy-Walker malformation. Nat Genet 36: 1053–1055.

Hammond CJ, Chitnavis B, Penny CC, Strong AJ (2002) Dandy-Walker complex and syringomyelia in an adult: case report and discussion. Neurosurgery 50: 191–194.

Has R, Ermis H, Yüksel A, Ibrahimoglu L, Yildrim A, Sezer HD, Basaran S (2004) Dandy-Walker Malformation: A Review of 78 Cases Diagnosed by Prenatal Sonography. Fetal Diagn Ther 19: 342–347.

Hirsch JF, Pierre-Kahn A, Renier D, Sainte-Rose C, Hoppe-Hirsch E (1984) The Dandy-Walker malformation. A review of 40 cases. J Neurosurg 61: 515–522.

Inoue T, Ogawa M, Mikoshiba K, Aruga J. (2008) Zic deficiency in the cortical marginal zone and meninges results in cortical lamination defects resembling those in type II lissencephaly. J Neurosci 28: 4712–4725.

Jageerhussain M, Dhinagar S, Nadaradjan S, Bhat BV (2000) Aicardi syndrome with Dandy-Walker malformation. Indian Pediatr 37: 673–676.

Jalali A, Aldinger KA, Chary A, McLone DG, Bowman RM, Le LC, et al. (2008) Linkage to chromosome 2q36.1 in autosomal dominant Dandy-Walker malformation with occipital cephalocele and evidence for genetic heterogeneity. Hum Genet 123: 237–245.

Kalidasan V, Carroll T, Allcutt D, Fitzgerald RJ (1995) The Dandy-Walker syndrome – a 10-year experience to its management and outcome. Eur J Pediatr Surg 5 Suppl 1: 16–18.

Klein O, Pierre-Kahn A, Boddaert N, Parisot D, Brunelle F (2003) Dandy-Walker malformation: prenatal diagnosis and prognosis. Childs Nerv Syst 19: 484–489.

Kölble N, Wisser J, Kurmanavicius J, Boltshauser E, Stallmach T, Huch A, Huch R (2000) Dandy-Walker malformation: prenatal diagnosis and outcome. Prenat Diagn 20: 318–327.

Kumar R, Jain MK, Chhabra DK (2001) Dandy-Walker syndrome: different modalities of treatment and outcome in 42 cases. Childs Nerv Syst 17: 348–352.

Kume T, Deng KY, Winfrey V, Gould DB, Walter MA, Hogan BL (1998). The forkhead/winged helix gene Mf1 is disrupted in the pleiotropic mouse mutation congenital hydrocephalus. Cell 93: 985–996.

Leonardi ML, Pai GS, Wilkes B, Lebel RR (2001) Ritscher-Schinzel cranio-cerebello-cardiac (3C) syndrome: report of four new cases and review. Am J Med Genet 102: 237–242.

Limperopoulos C, Robertson RL, Estroff JA, Barnewolt CE, Levine D, Bassan H, Du Plessis AJ (2006) Diagnosis of inferior vermian hypoplasia by fetal MRI: potential pitfalls and neurodevelopmental outcome. Am J Obstet Gynecol 194: 1070–1076.

Limperopoulos C, Robertson RL, Khwaja OS, Robson CD, Estroff JA, Barnwolt C, et al. (2008) How accurately does current fetal imaging identify posterior fossa anomalies? AJR Am J Roentgenol 190: 1637–1643.

Limperopoulos C, Folkerth R, Barnewolt CE, Connolly S, Du Plessis AJ (2010) Posthemorrhagic cerebellar disruption mimicking Dandy-Walker malformation: fetal imaging and neuropathology findings. Semin Pediatr Neurol 17: 75–81.

Long A, Moran P, Robson S (2006) Outcome of fetal cerebral posterior fossa anomalies. Prenat Diagn 26: 707–710.

Malinger G, Lev D, Lerman-Sagie T (2009) The fetal cerebellum. Pitfalls in diagnosis and management. Prenat Diagn 29: 372–380.

Maria BL, Zinreich SJ, Carson BC, Resenbaum AE, Freeman JM (1987) Dandy-Walker syndrome revised. Pediatr Neurosci 13: 45–51.

Marnet D, Vinchon M, Mostofi K, Catteau B, Kerdraon O, Dhellemmes P (2009) Neurocutaneous melanosis and the Dandy-Walker complex: an uncommon but not so insignificant association. Childs Nerv Syst 25: 1533–1539.

Messerschmidt A, Brugger PC, Boltshauser E, Zoder G, Sterniste W, Birnbacher R, Prayer D (2005) Disruption of cerebellar development: potential complication of extreme prematurity. AJNR Am J Neuroradiol 26: 1659–1667.

Metry D, Heyer G, Hess C, Garzon M, Haggstrom A, Frommelt P, et al. (2009) Consensus statement on diagnostic criteria for PHACE syndrome. Pediatrics 124: 1447–1456.

Mohanty A, Biswas A, Satish S, Shankar Praharaj S, Sastry KV (2006) Treatment options for Dandy-Walker malformation. J Neurosurg 105 (5 Suppl Pediatrics): 348–356.

Morava E, Adamovich K, Czeizel AE (1996) Dandy-Walker malformation and polydactyly: a possible expression of hydrolethalus syndrome. Clin Genet 49: 211–215.

Murray JC, Johnson JA, Bird TD (1985) Dandy-Walker malformation: etiologic heterogeneity and empiric recurrence risks. Clin Genet 28: 272–283.

Najm J, Horn D, Wimplinger I, Golden JA, Chizhikov VV, Sudi J, et al. (2008) Mutations of CASK cause an X-linked brain malformation phenotype with microcephaly and hypoplasia of the brainstem and cerebellum. Nat Genet 40: 1065–1067.

Nakamura-Pereira M, Cima LC, Llerena JC Guerra FA, Peixoto-Filho FM (2009) Sonographic findings in a case of tetrasomy 9p associated with increased nuchal translucency and Dandy-Walker malformation. J Clin Ultrasound 37: 471–474.

Nelson MD, Jr., Maher K, Gilles FH (2004) A different approach to cysts of the posterior fossa. Pediatr Radiol 34: 720–732.

Osenbach RK, Menezes AH (1992) Diagnosis and management of the Dandy-Walker malformation: 30 years of experience. Pediatr Neurosurg 18: 179–189.

Ozkinay F, Ozyürek AR, Bakiler AR, Narin N, Yüksel H, Ozkinay C, et al. (1995) A case of Marden-Walker syndrome with Dandy-Walker malformation. Clin Genet 47: 221–223.

Parisi MA, Dobyns WB (2003) Human malformations of the midbrain and hindbrain: review and proposal classification scheme. Mol Genet Metab 80: 36–53.

Pascual-Castroviejo I, Velez A, Pascual-Pascual SI, Roche MC, VIllarejo F (1991) Dandy-Walker malformation: analysis of 38 cases. Childs Nerv Syst 7: 88–97.

Patel S, Barkovich AJ (2002) Analysis and classification of cerebellar malformations. AJNR Am J Neuroradiol 23: 1074–1087.

Patton MA, Sharma A, Winter RM (1985) The Aase-Smith syndrome. Clin Genet 28: 521–525.

Philip N, Chabrol B, Lossi AM, Cardoso C, Guerrini R, Dobyns WB, et al. (2003) Mutations in the oligophrenin-1 gene (OPHN1) cause X linked congenital cerebellar hypoplasia. J Med Genet 40: 441–446.

Pillay PK, Barnett GH, Lanzeiri C, Cruse R (1989) Dandy-Walker cyst upward herniation: the role of magnetic resonance imaging and double shuntes. Pediatr Neurosci 15: 74–79.

Poot M, Kroes HY, v. d. Wijst SE, Eleveld MJ, Rooms L, Nievelstein RA, et al. (2007) Dandy-Walker complex in a boy with a 5 Mb deletion of region 1q44 due to a paternal t(1;20)(q44;q13.33). Am J Med Genet A 143A: 1038–1044.

Poretti A, Boltshauser E (2009) 'Rhombencephalosynapsis associated with Dandy-Walker malformation' is a molar tooth malformation. J Neuroimaging 19: 198.

Prayer D (2011) Fetal MRI, 1st edition. Berlin: Springer.

Rice R, Rice DP, Olsen BR, Thesleff I (2003) Progression of calvarial bone development requires Foxc1 regulation of Msx2 and Alx4. Dev Biol 262: 75–87.

Rice R, Rice DP, Thesleff I (2005) Foxc1 integrates Fgf and Bmp signalling independently of twist or noggin during calvarial bone development. Dev Dyn 233: 847–852.

Richter EO, Pincus DW (2006) Development of syringohydromyelia associated with Dandy-Walker malformation: treatment with cystoperitoneal shunt placement. Case report. J Neurosurg 104 (3 Suppl): 206–209.

Rossi A, Bava GL, Biancheri R, Tortori-Donati P (2001) Posterior fossa and arterial abnormalities in patients with facial capillary haemangioma: presumed incomplete phenotypic expression of PHACES syndrome. Neuroradiology 43: 934–940.

Sartori S, Ludwig K, Fortuna M, Marzocchi C, Calderone M, Toldo I, et al. (2010) Dandy-Walker malformation masking the molar tooth sign: an illustrative case with magnetic resonance imaging follow-up J Child Neurol 24: 1419–1422.

Sato K, Kubota T, Nakamura Y (1996) Adult onset of the Dandy-Walker syndrome. Br J Neurosurg 10: 109–112.

Sawaya R, McLaurin RL (1981) Dandy-Walker syndrome: clinical analysis of 23 cases. J Neurosurg 55: 89–98.

Sener RN (2007) Rhombencephalosynapsis associated with Dandy-Walker malformation. J Neuroimaging 17: 355–357.

Shenoy RD, Kamath N (2010) Dandy-Walker malformation, occipital meningoencephalocele, meso-axial polydactyly and bifid hallux. Clin Dysmorphol 19: 166–168.

Sutton JB (1887) The lateral recesses of the fourth ventricle: their relation to certain cysts and tumors of the cerebellum, and to occipital meningocele. Brain 9: 352.

Taggart JK, Walker AE (1942) Congenital atresia of the foramens of Luschka and Magendie. Arch Neurol Psychiatry 48: 583–612.

Tal Y, Freigang B, Dunn HG, Durity FA, Moyes PD (1980) Dandy-Walker syndrome: analysis of 21 cases. Dev Med Child Neurol 22: 189–201.

Ugur HC, Tortun F, Yilmaz E, Kanpolat Y (2005) Trigeminal neuralgia in a patient with Dandy Walker malformation. J Clin Neurosci 12: 815–817.

Ulm B, Ulm MR, Deutinger J, Bernaschek G (1997) Dandy-Walker malformation diagnosed before 21 weeks of gestation: associated malformations and chromosomal abnormalities. Ultrasound Obstet Gynecol 10: 167–170.

Van Hove JL, Spiridigliozzi GA, Heinz R, McConkie-Rosell A, Iafolla AK, Kahler SG (1995) Fryns syndrome survivors and neurologic outcome. Am J Med Genet 20: 334–340.

Vialard F, Robyr R, Hillion Y, Molina Gomes D, Selva J, Ville Y (2005) Dandy-Walker syndrome and corpus callosum agenesis in 5p deletion. Prenat Diagn 25: 311–313.

Vivatbutsiri P, Ichinose S, Hytönen M, Sainio K, Eto K, Iseki S (2008) Impaired meningeal development in association with apical expansion of calvarial bone osteogenesis in the Foxc1 mutant. J Anat 212: 603–611.

Xu J, Liu Z, Ornitz DM (2000) Temporal and spatial gradients of Fgf8 and Fgf17 regulate proliferation and differentiation of midline cerebellar structures. Development 127: 1833–1843.

Yildiz H, Yazici Z, Hakyemez B, Erdogan C, Parlak M (2006) Evaluation of CSF flow patterns of posterior fossa cystic malformations using CSF flow MR imaging. Neuroradiology 48: 595–605.

Yüceer N, Mertol T, Arda N (2007) Surgical treatment of 13 pediatric patients with Dandy-Walker syndrome. Pediatr Neurosurg 43: 358–363.

Zangwill KM, Boal DK, Ladda RL (1988) Dandy-Walker malformation in Ellis-van Creveld syndrome. Am J Med Genet 31: 123–129.

Zanni G, Barresi S, Travaglini L, Bernardini L, Rizza T, Digilio MC, et al. (2011) FGF17, a gene involved in cerebellar development, is downregulated in a patient with Dandy-Walker malformation carrying a de novo 8p deletion. Neurogenetics Apr 12, epub ahead of print.

Zarbalis K, Siegenthaler JA, Choe Y, May SR, Peterson AS, Pleasure SJ (2007) Cortical dysplasia and skull defects in mice with a Foxc1 allele reveal the role of meningeal differentiation in regulating cortical development. Proc Natl Acad Sci USA 104: 14002–14007.

11 Joubert Syndrome and Related Disorders

Enza Maria Valente, Francesco Brancati, and Bruno Dallapiccola

Joubert syndrome and related disorders (JSRD) are a group of highly heterogeneous conditions sharing a complex midbrain-hindbrain malformation known as the molar tooth sign (MTS). The main neurologic features include some or all of the following: hypotonia, ataxia, developmental delay, intellectual disability, altered breathing pattern in the neonatal period and abnormal eye movement. These are variably associated with multiorgan manifestations, mainly of the retina, kidneys, and liver. Such clinical variability requires a multidisciplinary approach for diagnosis and management.

JSRD are inherited in autosomal recessive fashion, with the exception of one form following X-linked inheritance. Ten causative genes have been identified to date, with relevant genotype-phenotype correlations. Notably, all genes encode for proteins of the primary cilium or the centrosome, making JSRD part of an expanding group of diseases known as ciliopathies.

Definition

The first report of Joubert syndrome (MIM #213300) dates back to 1969, when Dr Marie Joubert described a family with four siblings presenting agenesis of the cerebellar vermis, abnormal eye movements, breathing disturbances, ataxia, and intellectual disability (Joubert et al. 1969). In 1977, Boltshauser and Isler reported the same constellation of features in three additional patients from two families, and suggested this represented a distinct condition which they named Joubert syndrome (Boltshauser and Isler 1977). Several years later, a pathognomonic midbrain-hindbrain malformation, MTS, was recognized in patients with Joubert syndrome (Maria et al. 1997). The MTS was later identified in several other conditions previously considered as distinct entities, such as Dekaban-Arima syndrome (MIM %243910), COACH (Cerebellar vermis hypoplasia/aplasia, Oligophrenia, Ataxia, Coloboma, and Hepatic fibrosis) syndrome (MIM #216360), Varadi-Papp syndrome (or orofaciodigital type VI, MIM %277170), Malta syndrome and a minority of cases with Senior-Löken syndrome (SLS, MIM #266900) (Satran et al. 1999). Recently, the unifying term 'Joubert syndrome and related disorders' has been proposed to include all syndromes sharing the MTS (Gleeson et al. 2004), which represents the only mandatory criterion for diagnosis. This neuroradiological hallmark results from hypodysplasia of the cerebellar vermis, abnormally deep interpeduncular fossa at the level of the isthmus and upper pons, and horizontalized, thickened and elongated superior cerebellar peduncles (Maria et al. 1999b) (Fig. 11.1).

At the neuropathological level, the MTS corresponds to a picture of severe hypodysplasia of the cerebellar vermis with midline clefting, fragmentation of cerebellar nuclei, and heterotopia of Purkinje-like neurons, along with dysplasia of pontine and medullary structures such as the basis pontis, reticular formation, inferior olivary, dorsal column, and solitary tract nuclei. Moreover, there is lack of decussation both of the superior cerebellar peduncles and of the corticospinal tracts at the medullary pyramids (Friede and Boltshauser 1978; Yachnis and Rorke 1999) which is also evident from diffusion tensor imaging-tractography studies (Poretti et al. 2007).

Epidemiology

The reported incidence of JSRD ranges between 1/80 000 and 1/100 000 live births. However, these figures likely represent an underestimate, because of the limited awareness of the MTS, at least in the past (Parisi et al. 2007; Kroes et al. 2008). The higher incidence of JSRD in the Ashkenazi Jewish population may reflect a founder effect in this population, as all cases ascertained to date have a single recurrent mutation (p.R73L) in the *TMEM216* gene (Edvardson et al. 2010; Valente et al. 2010).

Genetics

Joubert syndrome and related disorders are characterized by marked genetic heterogeneity. Ten causative genes have been identified so far[1]: JBTS1/*INPP5E* (MIM *613037), JBTS2/*TMEM216* (MIM *613277), JBTS3/*AHI1* (MIM *608894), JBTS4/*NPHP1* (MIM *607100), JBTS5/*CEP290* (MIM *610142), JBTS6/*TMEM67* (MIM *609884), JBTS7/*RPGRIP1L* (MIM *610937), JBTS8/*ARL13B* (MIM *608922), JBTS9/*CC2D2A* (MIM *612013), JBTS10/*OFD1* (MIM *300170) (Table 11.1).

With the exception of *OFD1* associated with X-linked recessive inheritance (Coene et al. 2009), mutations in the other genes are transmitted in autosomal recessive manner, and the recurrence risk for a couple with an affected child is one in four. To date, published mutation screenings of known genes have allowed identification of mutations in fewer than half of patients with JSRD (Valente et al. 2008). Available genotype-phenotype correlates are discussed below.

[1] Since the submission of this chapter, three novel JSRD causative genes have been published (*KIF7* [MIM*611254], *TCTN2* [MIM*613846] and *TCTN1* [MIM*609863], the first two also causative of MS).

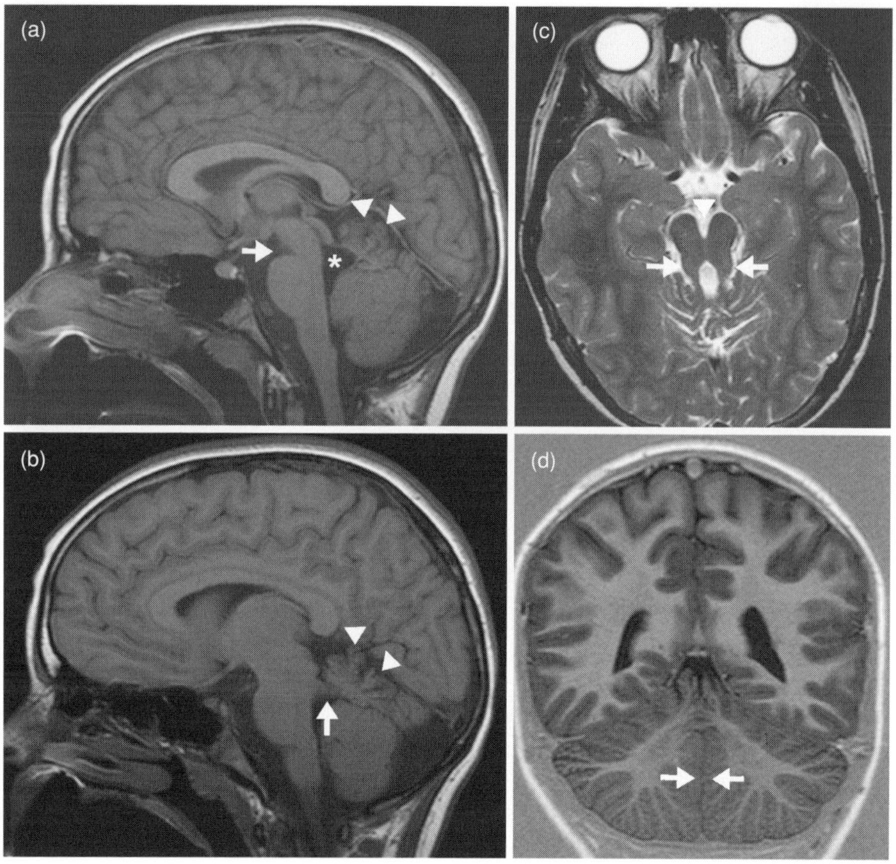

Fig. 11.1. Brain MRI sections in patients with Joubert syndrome and related disorders. **(a)** Mid-sagittal T1-weighted image shows deepening of the interpeduncular fossa (arrow), dysplastic cerebellar vermis (arrowheads), and abnormally high position of the fastigium of the fourth ventricle (asterisk); **(b)** parasagittal T1-weighted image shows thickened and maloriented superior cerebellar peduncle (arrow) and dysplastic vermis (arrowheads); **(c)** axial T2-weighted image at the pontomesencephalic junction confirms the deepened interpeduncular fossa (white arrowhead) and abnormal superior cerebellar peduncles (arrows), shaping the 'molar tooth sign'; **(d)** coronal inversion recovery image shows midline cerebellar cleft (arrows) indicating agenesis of the inferior vermis (the so-called 'buttock sign').

TABLE 11.1
Genes and loci causative of Joubert syndrome and related disorders and allelism with other ciliopathies

Gene	JSRD	MS	NPH	SLS	BBS
INPP5E	JBTS1				
TMEM216	JBTS2	MKS2			
AHI1	JBTS3				
NPHP1	JBTS4		NPHP1	SLSN1	
CEP290	JBTS5	MKS4	NPHP6	SLSN6	BBS14
TMEM67	JBTS6	MKS3			
RPGRIP1L	JBTS7	MKS5	NPHP8		
ARL13B	JBTS8				
CC2D2A	JBTS9	MKS6			
OFD1	JBTS10				

JSRD, Joubert syndrome and related disorders; MS, Meckel syndrome; NPH, nephronophthisis; SLS, Senior-Löken syndrome; BBS, Bardet-Biedl syndrome.

Clinical features and classification

A recently proposed clinical-genetic classification defines six JSRD subgroups based on the main organ(s) involvement and the established genotype-phenotype correlates (Brancati et al. 2010). These subgroups are described here, along with their characterizing clinical features and genetic correlates (Table 11.2).

Pure Joubert syndrome

This subgroup is dominated by the neurological symptoms of hypotonia evolving into ataxia and developmental delay, often associated with intellectual disability, altered respiratory pattern in the neonatal period, and abnormal eye movements (Joubert et al. 1968; Boltshauser and Isler 1977; Saraiva and Baraitser 1992; Maria et al. 1999a).

Early hypotonia is observed in the neonatal period or in infancy in most patients. Although this represents a nonspecific finding common to many disorders, its association with other peculiar features such as breathing abnormalities and altered eye movements should prompt the clinician to request a brain MRI. Patients often develop gait ataxia in the first years of independent ambulation (Maria et al. 1997), while tremor has only been occasionally reported (Maria et al. 1999a).

Respiratory abnormalities occur in about 40–50% of patients, with short alternate episodes of apnea and hyperpnea, or with episodic hyperpnea alone. These abnormalities present shortly after birth, intensify with emotional stress, and progressively resolve with age. Their severity can range from occasional short-lasting episodes manifesting every few days to extremely frequent (up to several per day) and prolonged attacks of apnea, requiring intensive care management and assisted ventilation (Joubert et al. 1968; Boltshauser et al. 1981).

Oculomotor apraxia is a common feature, which manifests with the inability to follow objects visually with compensatory head movements, decreased smooth pursuit, and abolition of the vestibulo-ocular reflex. Nystagmus, strabismus, and ptosis are also observed in a subset of patients. Such manifestations relate to the underlying midbrain-hindbrain malformation, and

TABLE 11.2
Classification of JSRD based on associated clinical features

	Pure Joubert syndrome	Joubert syndrome with ocular defect (JS-O)	Joubert syndrome with renal defect (JS-R)	Joubert syndrome with oculorenal defects (JS-OR)	Joubert syndrome with hepatic defect (JS-H)	Joubert syndrome with orofaciodigital defects (JS-OFD)
CNS:						
• MTS	+	+	+	+	+	+
• hypotonia, ataxia, psychomotor delay	+	+	+	+	+	+
• abnormal breathing, intellectual impairment, abnormal ocular movements	+/–	+/–	+/–	+/–	+/–	+/–
LCA/RD	—	+	—	+	n.r.	n.r.
NPH	—	—	+	+	+/–	+/–
CHF	—	—	—	—	+	—
Other:						
• polydactyly	+/–	+/–	+/–	+/–	+/–	+
• oral defects	—	—	—	—	—	+
• colobomas	+/–	+/–	+/–	+/–	+/– (common)	n.r.
Major gene(s)	mutations in many genes	*AHI1*	*NPHP1*, *RPGRIP1L*	*CEP290*	*TMEM67*	*TMEM216* (2 patients)

CHF, congenital hepatic fibrosis; CNS, central nervous system; JSRD, Joubert syndrome and related disorders; LCA, Leber congenital amaurosis; MTS, molar tooth sign; NPH, nephronophthisis; n.r., not reported; RD, retinal dystrophy.

are present independently from the specific ocular defects (see below) (Boltshauser et al. 1981; Maria et al. 1997; Braddock et al. 2006; Weiss et al. 2009).

Developmental delay of variable severity is present, particularly affecting language and motor skills (Deonna and Ziegler 1993; Gitten et al. 1998; Fennell et al. 1999; Braddock et al. 2006). Mild to severe intellectual disability is also common, although exceptional cases have been reported with borderline or even normal intellect (Poretti et al. 2009). Many patients have to attend special schools, but are able to learn specific job skills and even work in protected conditions (Steinlin et al. 1997). It has been suggested that developmental outcome in Joubert syndrome patients can be divided into (1) children who died young; (2) survivors who are severely developmentally delayed; and (3) survivors with mildly delayed development (Fennell et al. 1999). Behavioral problems reported in children include hyperactivity, aggressiveness, and dependency (Fennell et al. 1999). In an adult patient with Joubert syndrome a progressive movement disorder has been reported with rigidity, bradykinesia, tremor, ataxia, and masked facies (Gunzler et al. 2007).

Mutations in several genes have been reported to cause pure Joubert syndrome, including *INPP5E*, *TMEM216*, *AHI1*, *TMEM67*, *ARL13B*, *CC2D2A*, and *OFD1*, but none of these represents a major gene for this phenotype (Valente et al. 2006a; Baala et al. 2007; Cantagrel et al. 2008; Gorden et al. 2008; Bielas et al. 2009; Coene et al. 2009; Mougou-Zerelli et al. 2009; Edvardson et al. 2010; Valente et al. 2010).

Joubert syndrome with ocular defect

Joubert syndrome with ocular defect (JS-O) is a subgroup characterized by the association of the neurological features described above with retinal abnormalities, with variable age at onset, progression and severity. Retinal involvement can present with congenital retinal blindness (also known as Leber congenital amaurosis; LCA), or progressive retinal dystrophy with variably conserved vision (Lambert et al. 1989; Maria et al. 1997; Tusa and Hove 1999; Khan et al. 2008; Sturm et al. 2010). The diagnosis is made upon detection of reduced visual acuity, abnormal *fundus oculi* and/or electroretinogram (Satran et al. 1999). The most frequently mutated gene in patients with Joubert syndrome and retinal dystrophy is *AHI1*, which accounts for about 20% of cases; rarer mutations have been reported in the *INPP5E*, *CC2D2A*, and *OFD1* genes (Dixon-Salazar et al. 2004; Ferland et al. 2004; Parisi et al. 2006; Valente et al. 2006a; Gorden et al. 2008; Bielas et al. 2009; Coene et al. 2009).

Unilateral or bilateral chorioretinal colobomas do not characterize this specific subgroup as they can be variably found in all subgroups, with increased frequency in patient with Joubert syndrome congenital hepatic fibrosis (see below) (Gregory-Evans et al. 2004). Iris colobomas and other eye malformations are much rarer (Satran et al. 1999).

Joubert syndrome with renal defect

Joubert syndrome with renal defect (JS-R) is a subgroup in which neurological signs are associated with renal disease, typically nephronophthisis (NPH). This is a structural tubule-interstitial disorder characterized by irregular, thickened basal membrane of the tubular epithelium and progressive interstitial fibrosis, associated with small cysts at the corticomedullary junction. Juvenile NPH may remain asymptomatic for several years or present with subtle and often unrecognized signs such as polyuria and polydipsia, until acute or chronic renal insufficiency manifests in the late first or early second decade. End-stage renal failure is usually reached by the end of the second decade, requiring dialysis or kidney transplantation. A rarer infantile variant of NPH manifests within the first years of life, with a more rapid and severe course (Salomon et al. 2009). Interestingly, the renal disease in Dekaban-Arima syndrome, initially described as cystic dysplastic kidney (Dekaban 1969; Matsuzaka et al. 1986; Saraiva and Baraitser 1992), was recently reappraised as NPH, suggesting that all JSRD present the same renal phenotype (Kumada et al. 2004).

The two genes most commonly mutated in this rare phenotype are *NPHP1* and *RPGRIP1L*, while the *CEP290* G1890X mutation was detected in few cases (Parisi et al. 2004; Castori et al. 2005; Arts et al. 2007; Delous et al. 2007; Wolf et al. 2007; Brancati et al. 2007, 2008).

Joubert syndrome with oculorenal defects

Joubert syndrome with oculorenal defects (JS-OR) is a subgroup characterized by the association of neurological signs of Joubert syndrome with both retinal dystrophy and NPH. This phenotype comprises the subset of patients with SLS that also display the MTS (Satran et al. 1999; Brancati et al. 2007). About 50% of patients carry mutations in the *CEP290* gene (Sayer et al. 2006; Valente et al. 2006b; Brancati et al. 2007; Helou et al. 2007), and only a few patients display *AHI1* mutations (Parisi et al. 2006).

Joubert syndrome with hepatic defect

Joubert syndrome with hepatic defect (JS-H) is a subgroup characterized by the association of neurological signs with congenital hepatic fibrosis (CHF). This results from an embryonic malformation of the ductal plate, with cystic dilatation of primitive biliary structures and fibrous enlargement of the portal tracts (Desmet 1992). Liver disease may present with raised serum liver enzymes at least twice the normal values, early-onset hepato(spleno)megaly or more severe manifestations including portal hypertension and esophageal varices (Lewis et al. 1994; Brancati et al. 2009). Chorioretinal or optic nerve colobomas and NPH are frequently detected in JS-H patients. This subgroup encompasses both the condition known by the acronym COACH (cerebellar vermis hypoplasia, oligophrenia, ataxia, coloboma, and hepatic fibrosis) (Verloes and Lambotte 1989; Lewis et al. 1994), and so-called 'Gentile syndrome', characterized by the association of Joubert syndrome with CHF, in the absence of other clinical features.

The major causative gene in this subgroup is *TMEM67*, which accounts for over 70% of cases (Baala et al. 2007; Brancati et al. 2009; Otto et al. 2009; Doherty et al. 2010; Iannicelli et al. 2010), while *CC2D2A* and *RPGRIP1L* are occasionally mutated (Mougou-Zerelli et al. 2009; Doherty et al. 2010).

Joubert syndrome with orofaciodigital defects

In the subgroup Joubert syndrome with orofaciodigital defects (JS-OFD), neurological features are associated with bifid or lobulated tongue (often described as soft-tissue nodules or multiple hamartomas), multiple oral frenulae and polydactyly, usually mesaxial, with Y-shaped metacarpals (Varadi et al. 1980; Munke et al. 1990; Gleeson et al. 2004; Chodirker et al. 2005). This association was previously termed orofaciodigital syndrome type VI or Varadi-Papp syndrome (Varadi et al. 1980). Hypothalamic hamartoma and congenital absence of the pituitary gland may be part of this spectrum (Munke et al. 1990; Stephan et al. 1994; Al-Gazali et al. 1999).

To date, the only gene associated with this phenotype is *TMEM216*, mutations of which have been found in two patients (Valente et al. 2010). However, mutations in this gene were not detected in several other cases, suggesting that *TMEM216* is not the major causative gene in JS-OFD.

Additional features variably found in all subgroups

Many patients with JSRD present characteristic facial features that tend to change with age. These include long face, frontal prominence, bitemporal narrowing, ptosis, prominent nasal bridge and tip, prognathism, eyebrow abnormalities, trapezoid-shaped mouth, lower lip eversion, and thick ear lobes (Maria et al. 1999a; Braddock et al. 2007). Adult patients often present with midface hypoplasia ('flat cheeks').

Features occasionally reported by parents of an affected child include an abnormal sensitivity to noise, and swallowing impairment.

Polydactyly, most frequently postaxial and variably affecting hands and feet, is found in about 8–16% of patients (Joubert et al. 1968; Saraiva and Baraitser 1992; Pellegrino et al. 1997; Chance et al. 1999). Mild to severe scoliosis and structural anomalies of the vertebrae are rare findings. Interestingly, scoliosis has been reported in some patients carrying *RPGRIP1L* mutations, although the number of cases is still too limited to draw definite conclusions (Hodgkins et al. 2004; Brancati et al. 2008).

Occipital (meningo)encephalocele of variable severity can be present (Joubert et al. 1968; Shian et al. 1993; Wang et al. 1999). Other central nervous system (CNS) malformations occasionally found in JSRD patients include hydrocephalus, cystic enlargement of the posterior fossa, abnormalities of the corpus callosum, white matter cysts, hypomyelination, hypothalamic hamartoma, and absence of the pituitary gland (Kendall et al. 1990; van Dorp et al. 1991; Shian et al. 1993; Al-Gazali et al. 1999; Haug et al. 2000; Maria et al. 2001; Zamponi et al. 2002; Genel et al. 2004). Other rare structural malformations have been reported (Senocak et al. 2010), and abnormal migration defects, mainly periventricular nodular heterotopia, and cortical organization defects such as polymicrogyria (Dixon-Salazar et al. 2004; Giordano et al. 2009). Patients with these malformations present a higher incidence of epilepsy, which is otherwise a rare feature of JSRD (Haug et al. 2000; Dixon-Salazar et al. 2004).

Congenital heart defects and complete *situs inversus* have been occasionally reported in JSRD (Elmali et al. 2007; Aydinoz et al. 2007). Hirschsprung's disease has been described in two patients (Ozyurek et al. 2008).

Pathophysiology

The finding that all known JSRD genes encode for proteins expressed in the primary cilium or in the centrosome have linked these disorders to the fast-growing, fascinating field of ciliopathies.

Primary cilia are sophisticated organelles found in an extremely large number of tissues, including epithelium of renal tubules and bile ducts, retinal photoreceptors and neuronal cells in the fetal and adult brain. Many different proteins interact to form complexes that are necessary for cilia formation and multiple functions in different organs and tissues. For instance, in renal tubular epithelium, primary cilia have been shown to serve as cellular sensors transducing external signals (such as urinary osmolarity) to the nucleus and regulating cell cycle, proliferation and cell polarity. The impairment of these functions due to ciliary malfunctioning leads to cyst formation (a peculiar finding in all renal ciliopathies), which is variably associated with interstitial degeneration and fibrosis (Hildebrandt and Otto 2005; Hildebrandt et al. 2009). In the biliary epithelium, an early malfunctioning of primary cilia results in the arrest of the embryonic development of intrahepatic bile ducts at the stage of bilaminar plate formation ('ductal plate malformation'), with consequent cystic degeneration and congenital fibrosis (Johnson et al. 2003; Clotman et al. 2008). In the developing brain, primary cilia regulate some of the most powerful embryonic pathways, such as those of Wnt, sonic hedgehog and planar cell polarity. These molecular pathways are implicated in nearly every major developmental process, including the correct establishment of body plan, left-right axis determination, development and closure of the neural tube, and limb formation (Eggenschwiler and Anderson 2007; Smith et al. 2008; Spassky et al. 2008; Willaredt et al. 2008).

The multiple and distinct roles of primary cilia in different organs and tissues explain the marked pleiotropism observed in JSRD as well as in other autosomal recessive ciliopathies, such as Meckel syndrome (MIM #249000), isolated NPH (MIM #256100), SLS and Bardet-Biedl syndrome (BBS, MIM #209900). Meckel syndrome is a severe malformation that is often lethal in utero, presenting with encephalocele and other posterior fossa anomalies, ductal plate malformation of the liver, polycystic kidneys and polydactyly. Isolated NPH is a cystic renal disease characterized by progressive wasting of the filtering unit of the kidney and interstitial fibrosis, which represents the most common cause of end-stage renal failure in childhood. SLS is defined by the association of NPH with progressive retinal dystrophy, usually LCA. Typical features of BBS are obesity, retinal degeneration, polydactyly, renal and gonadal malformation, and behavioral and developmental problems.

The clinical overlap among these distinct ciliopathies is mirrored by an increasing genetic overlap, with mutations in one and the same gene causing different ciliopathies of variable severity (Table 11.1). For instance, mutations in the *CEP290* gene can cause many distinct ciliopathies, including isolated LCA or NPH, SLS, BBS, JSRD, and Meckel syndrome.

In particular, JSRD and Meckel syndrome seem to represent the two ends of a continuum of phenotypes, being allelic in at least seven genes. Preliminary genotype-phenotype correlates have emerged, with distinct mutation types correlating with the phenotypic severity: Meckel syndrome fetuses nearly invariably harbor truncating mutations, while at least one hypomorphic (e.g., missense) mutation is found in almost all JSRD cases (Brancati et al. 2007; Delous et al. 2007; Tallila et al. 2009; Mougou-Zerelli et al. 2009; Iannicelli et al. 2010; Valente et al. 2010).

However, these correlates do not entirely explain the phenotypic variability associated with mutations in one and the same ciliary gene. As an example, isolated NPH, SLS, and variable JSRD phenotypes can all be caused by the same homozygous deletion of the *NPHP1* gene, supporting the existence of additional genetic factors. A possible explanation has come from the genetics of BBS, for which up to 12 genes have been identified to date. In this condition, an oligogenic/triallelic mode of transmission has been demonstrated in some families, with mutations at different BBS loci genetically interacting to cause and/or modify the phenotype (Katsanis 2004; Badano et al. 2006). Interestingly, a similar mechanism was recently implicated in other ciliopathies. Two distinct studies showed that the p.R830W variant in the *AHI1* gene was associated with an increased risk of developing neurological or retinal involvement in a cohort of patients with NPH carrying the *NPHP1* homozygous deletion (Tory et al. 2007; Louie et al. 2010). Similarly, the p.A229T variant in the *RPGRIP1L* gene was found to increase the risk of developing retinal degeneration in patients with ciliopathies caused by mutations in other genes (Khanna et al. 2009). These data suggest that discrete heterozygous nucleotide changes in ciliary genes may act as modifier factors of the ciliary phenotype.

Diagnosis and management

Clinical investigations and follow-up

A diagnosis of JSRD should be suspected in all infants presenting with hypotonia, abnormal eye movements (in particular, oculomotor apraxia) and developmental delay. Abnormalities in the respiratory pattern, if present, reinforce the clinical suspicion of the disease. A brain MRI is necessary to confirm or exclude the diagnosis, based on the detection of the MTS. In neonates and children, particular care should be posed in managing respiratory and feeding problems related to either breathing abnormalities or hypotonia. Children should enter a diagnostic protocol to assess the degree of intellectual disability. Cognitive, behavioral and language problems must be addressed with appropriate rehabilitation programs, including early physical therapy, which may help to develop communicative skills. Recommended supportive measures for oculomotor apraxia and other eye movement abnormalities include physical and occupational therapy. Also, orthopedic management is relevant in the prevention of scoliosis.

TABLE 11.3
Multiorgan features and management of Joubert syndrome and related disorders

Organ	Features	Diagnosis (–) and management (→)
	MTS (mandatory for diagnosis of JSRD)	
CNS	Hypotonia Abnormal breathing Oculomotor apraxia, strabismus, other eye movement abnormalities Psychomotor delay Intellectual disability Ataxia Other CNS malformations (e.g. encephalocele, polymicrogyria)	– Perform neuropsychological testing (according to age) – Assess eye movements – EEG in case of seizures → *Prevent respiratory and feeding complications* → *Plan rehabilitation strategies targeted to the specific motor, cognitive, language and behavioural problems* → *'Vision therapy' for eye movement abnormalities* → *Treatment of seizures as appropriate*
Eye	Congenital blindness (LCA) Retinal dystrophy (any age) Colobomas (mainly chorioretinal)	– Visual acuity – Fundoscopy – ERG and slit lamp examination (whenever possible) → *If abnormal, refer to specialist for adequate management*
Kidney	Nephronophthisis (infantile or juvenile)	– Renal function and kidney ultrasound (at least every 2 years in children) – If urinary specific gravity is low or in the lower normal range, plan urinary concentration test (after desmopressin or water restriction) → *If abnormal, refer to specialist for adequate management*
Liver	Congenital hepatic fibrosis	– Liver function and liver ultrasound (at least every 2 years in children) – If repeatedly abnormal, perform liver MRI and/or biopsy → *If CHF is diagnosed, refer to specialist for adequate management*
Other	Polydactyly, scoliosis Lobulated/bifid tongue Pituitary defects Hypothalamic hamartoma Rarer features: cleft palate, CHD, Hirschsprung disease, *situs inversus*	– Check once for possibly associated abnormalities → *If abnormalities are detected, refer to specialist for adequate management*

CHD, congenital heart defects; CHF, congenital hepatic fibrosis; CNS, central nervous system; EEG, electroencephalogram; ERG, electroretinogram; JSRD, Joubert syndrome and related disorders; LCA, Leber congenital amaurosis; MRI, magnetic resonance imaging; MTS, molar tooth sign.

A careful assessment of multiorgan involvement is mandatory to plan appropriate management and to assess prognosis (Table 11.3).

Ocular investigations include evaluation of visual acuity, *fundus oculi* and, whenever possible, electroretinogram. Slit lamp examination can disclose abnormalities of the anterior segment of the eye. Besides correction of the visual deficit whenever possible, rehabilitation strategies must be planned in order to improve the use of residual visual abilities in the frame of the child's global development.

Kidney function should be tested, with special attention to urine specific gravity. Should this value be abnormal or towards the lower normal range, a challenge test to assess urinary concentration ability is recommended. This is usually performed with water restriction or, even better, by evaluating urine specific gravity after desmopressin stimulation. The detection of decreased urinary concentration ability often represents the first clue to a diagnosis of NPH in otherwise asymptomatic patients. This requires close monitoring to recognize and treat early signs of renal failure, and to delay the onset of associated complications such as growth defect or bone disease. In some cases, ultrasonography of the kidney will detect small cysts and loss of corticomedullar differentiation, which are suggestive of NPH. However, it must be noted that ultrasonography may prove uninformative in the first stages of the disease.

Liver function must be monitored and regular ultrasonography examinations carried out. Hepatic involvement is suspected in patients with repeatedly elevated liver serum enzymes (alanine aminotransferase, aspartate aminotransferase, and gamma-glutamyl transpeptidase), hepato(spleno)megaly, and/or abnormal parenchymal echogenicity. In these patients, further liver imaging techniques (such as MRI) can support the diagnosis by demonstrating bile ducts proliferation or fibrotic nodules, while liver biopsy is needed to confirm CHF. In this case, a specific follow-up should be planned to prevent or manage possible complications, including portal hypertension and esophageal varices. Liver disease usually manifests in the first decade of life, but the individual may remain asymptomatic for years.

Additional features should be investigated that are more rarely observed in JSRD, such as pituitary defects, cleft palate (including soft palate and bifid uvula), lobulated tongue, congenital heart defects, *situs inversus*, and Hirschsprung disease. A careful assessment of brain MRI is also requested to detect associated CNS malformations.

Once the clinical diagnosis of JSRD is confirmed, genetic testing may be indicated to identify the underlying causative mutation and offer the family appropriate counselling. It is estimated that mutations in the known JSRD genes are overall responsible for less than half cases. Genetic testing is currently based on sequential mutation screening of coding exons and exon-intron junctions of known genes, that should be prioritized by taking into account the available genotype-phenotype correlates (Table 11.2).

Diagnostic molecular analysis is available only for few genes, while selected laboratories offer molecular testing of known genes on a research basis.

Prenatal diagnosis

Chorionic villous sampling at around 11 weeks' gestation allows prenatal diagnosis only in those families in which the molecular defect has previously been identified in the proband. Fetal ultrasound may be useful in at-risk pregnancies, allowing detection of hypodysplasia of the cerebellar vermis and, when present, occipital encephalocele. Another useful indicator in prenatal diagnosis is polydactyly, which may be associated with all JSRD subgroups (Aslan et al. 2002, 2007). Fetal MRI, when available, represents the method of choice to delineate posterior fossa malformations, in some cases allowing diagnosis of the disease before 24 weeks of gestation (Doherty et al. 2005; Fluss et al. 2006; Saleem and Zaki 2010).

Differential diagnosis

All conditions involving neurological symptoms (hypotonia, abnormal breathing, abnormal eye movements, and developmental delay) and/or multiorgan manifestations seen in JSRD (e.g. polydactyly, retinal dystrophy, NPH, CHF) should be considered in the differential diagnosis. These include in particular the other ciliopathies such as isolated NPH, SLS and BBS, as well as cerebro-oculo-renal syndromes (Adams et al. 2007; Barkovich et al. 2009; Salomon et al. 2009; Schurman and Scheinman 2009). Other conditions to be considered are those mainly characterized by cerebellar vermis hypoplasia or dysplasia, such as the Dandy-Walker malformation (MIM %220200), X-linked cerebellar hypoplasia and cognitive impairment (MIM #300486), and pontocerebellar hypoplasias (PCH; MIM #607596).

Prognosis

Soon after birth, prognosis is related to the extent and severity of breathing dysregulation. In particular, recurrent episodes of prolonged apneas can be life-threatening and require assisted ventilation. In most cases, these respiratory abnormalities resolve spontaneously in the first year of life. Feeding difficulties may also represent a relevant problem in some patients. Afterwards, prognosis depends mostly on the extent of visual loss and on the occurrence of renal and hepatic complications that, if not diagnosed and managed, represent the major causes of death in patients with JSRD.

REFERENCES

Adams NA, Awadein A, Toma HS (2007) The retinal ciliopathies. Ophthalmic Genet 28: 113–125.

Al-Gazali LI, Sztriha L, Punnose J, Shather W, Nork M (1999) Absent pituitary gland and hypoplasia of the cerebellar vermis associated with partial ophthalmoplegia and postaxial polydactyly: a variant of orofaciodigital syndrome VI or a new syndrome? J Med Genet 36: 161–166.

Arts HH, Doherty D, van Beersum SE, Parisi MA, Letteboer SJ, Gorden NT, et al. (2007) Mutations in the gene encoding the basal body protein RPGRIP1L, a nephrocystin-4 interactor, cause Joubert syndrome. Nat Genet 39: 882–888.

Aslan H, Ulker V, Gulcan EM, Numanoglu C, Gul A, Agar M, Ark HC (2002) Prenatal diagnosis of Joubert syndrome: a case report. Prenat Diagn 22: 13–16.

Aslan H, Yildirim G, Ongut C, Ceylan Y (2007) Termination of pregnancy for fetal anomaly. Int J Gynaecol Obstet 99: 221–224.

Aydinoz S, Ersen A, Karademir F, Suleymanoglu S, Ozkaya H, Gocmen I. (2007) A case of cerebello-oculo-renal syndrome with situs inversus totalis: a new phenotype. J Child Neurol 22: 204–207.

Baala L, Romano S, Khaddour R, Saunier S, Smith UM, Audollent S, et al. (2007) The Meckel-Gruber syndrome gene, MKS3, is mutated in Joubert syndrome. Am J Hum Genet 80: 186–194.

Badano JL, Leitch CC, Ansley SJ, May-Simera H, Lawson S, Lewis RA, et al. (2006) Dissection of epistasis in oligogenic Bardet-Biedl syndrome. Nature 439: 326–330.

Barkovich AJ, Millen KJ, Dobyns WB (2009) A developmental and genetic classification for midbrain-hindbrain malformations. Brain 132: 3199–3230.

Bielas SL, Silhavy JL, Brancati F, Kisseleva MV, Al-Gazali L, Sztriha L, et al. (2009) Mutations in INPP5E, encoding inositol polyphosphate-5-phosphatase E, link phosphatidyl inositol signaling to the ciliopathies. Nat Genet 41: 1032–1036.

Boltshauser E, Herdan M, Dumermuth G, Isler W (1981) Joubert syndrome: clinical and polygraphic observations in a further case. Neuropediatrics 12: 181–191.

Boltshauser E, Isler W (1977) Joubert syndrome: episodic hyperpnea, abnormal eye movements, retardation and ataxia, associated with dysplasia of the cerebellar vermis. Neuropadiatrie 8: 57–66.

Braddock BA, Farmer JE, Deidrick KM, Iverson JM, Maria BL (2006) Oromotor and communication findings in joubert syndrome: further evidence of multisystem apraxia. J Child Neurol 21: 160–163.

Braddock SR, Henley KM, Maria BL (2007) The face of Joubert syndrome: a study of dysmorphology and anthropometry. Am J Med Genet A 143: 3235–3242.

Brancati F, Barrano G, Silhavy JL, Marsh SE, Travaglini L, Bielas SL, et al. (2007) CEP290 mutations are frequently identified in the oculo-renal form of Joubert syndrome-related disorders. Am J Hum Genet 81: 104–113.

Brancati F, Dallapiccola B, Valente EM (2010) Joubert Syndrome and related disorders. Orphanet J Rare Dis 5: 20.

Brancati F, Iannicelli M, Travaglini L, Mazzotta A, Bertini E, Boltshauser E, et al. and the International JSRD Study Group (2009) MKS3/TMEM67 mutations are a major cause of COACH Syndrome, a Joubert Syndrome related disorder with liver involvement. Hum Mutat 30: E432–E442.

Brancati F, Travaglini L, Zablocka D, Boltshauser E, Accorsi P, Montagna G, et al. (2008) RPGRIP1L mutations are mainly associated with the cerebello-renal phenotype of Joubert syndrome-related disorders. Clin Genet 74: 164–170.

Cantagrel V, Silhavy JL, Bielas SL, Swistun D, Marsh SE, Bertrand JY, et al. (2008) Mutations in the cilia gene ARL13B lead to the classical form of Joubert syndrome. Am J Hum Genet 83: 170–179.

Castori M, Valente EM, Donati MA, Salvi S, Fazzi E, Procopio E, et al. (2005) NPHP1 gene deletion is a rare cause of Joubert syndrome related disorders. J Med Genet 42: e9.

Chance PF, Cavalier L, Satran D, Pellegrino JE, Koenig M, Dobyns WB (1999) Clinical nosologic and genetic aspects of Joubert and related syndromes. J Child Neurol 14: 660–666.

Chodirker BN, Shah NS, Bunge MK, Reed MH (2005) Another case of Varadi-Papp Syndrome with a molar tooth sign. Am J Med Genet A 136A: 416–417.

Clotman F, Libbrecht L, Killingsworth MC, Loo CC, Roskams T, Lemaigre FP (2008) Lack of cilia and differentiation defects in the liver of human foetuses with the Meckel syndrome. Liver Int 28: 377–384.

Coene KL, Roepman R, Doherty D, Afroze B, Kroes HY, Letteboer SJ, et al. (2009) OFD1 is mutated in X-linked Joubert syndrome and interacts with LCA5-encoded lebercilin. Am J Hum Genet 85: 465–481.

Dekaban AS (1969) Hereditary syndrome of congenital retinal blindness (Leber), polycystic kidneys and maldevelopment of the brain. Am J Ophthalmol 68: 1029–1037.

Delous M, Baala L, Salomon R, Laclef C, Vierkotten J, Tory K, et al. (2007) The ciliary gene RPGRIP1L is mutated in cerebello-oculo-renal syndrome (Joubert syndrome type B) and Meckel syndrome. Nat Genet 39: 875–881.

Deonna T, Ziegler AL (1993) Cognitive development and behavior in Joubert syndrome. Biol Psychiatry 33: 854–855.

Desmet VJ (1992) Congenital diseases of intrahepatic bile ducts: variations on the theme 'ductal plate malformation'. Hepatology 16: 1069–1083.

Dixon-Salazar T, Silhavy JL, Marsh SE, Louie CM, Scott LC, Gururaj A, et al. (2004) Mutations in the AHI1 gene, encoding jouberin, cause Joubert syndrome with cortical polymicrogyria. Am J Hum Genet 75: 979–987.

Doherty D, Glass IA, Siebert JR, Strouse PJ, Parisi MA, Shaw DW, et al. (2005) Prenatal diagnosis in pregnancies at risk for Joubert syndrome by ultrasound and MRI. Prenat Diagn 25: 442–447.

Doherty D, Parisi MA, Finn LS, Gunay-Aygun M, Al-Mateen M, Bates D, et al. (2010) Mutations in 3 genes (MKS3, CC2D2A and RPGRIP1L) cause COACH syndrome (Joubert syndrome with congenital hepatic fibrosis). J Med Genet 47: 8–21.

Edvardson S, Shaag A, Zenvirt S, Erlich Y, Hannon GJ, Shanske AL, et al. (2010) Joubert syndrome 2 (JBTS2) in Ashkenazi Jews is associated with a TMEM216 mutation. Am J Hum Genet 86: 93–97.

Eggenschwiler JT, Anderson KV (2007) Cilia and developmental signaling. Annu Rev Cell Dev Biol 23: 345–373.

Elmali M, Ozmen Z, Ceyhun M, Tokatlioglu O, Incesu L, Diren B (2007) Joubert syndrome with atrial septal defect and persistent left superior vena cava. Diagn Interv Radiol 13: 94–96.

Fennell EB, Gitten JC, Dede DE, Maria BL (1999) Cognition, behavior, and development in Joubert syndrome. J Child Neurol 14: 592–596.

Ferland RJ, Eyaid W, Collura RV, Tully LD, Hill RS, Al-Nouri D, et al. (2004) Abnormal cerebellar development and axonal decussation due to mutations in AHI1 in Joubert syndrome. Nat Genet 36: 1008–1013.

Fluss J, Blaser S, Chitayat D, Akoury H, Glanc P, Skidmore M, Raybaud C (2006) Molar tooth sign in fetal brain magnetic resonance imaging leading to the prenatal diagnosis of Joubert syndrome and related disorders. J Child Neurol 21: 320–324.

Friede RL, Boltshauser E (1978) Uncommon syndromes of cerebellar vermis aplasia. I: Joubert syndrome. Dev Med Child Neurol 20: 758–763.

Genel F, Atlihan F, Ozdemir D, Targan S (2004) Development of hydrocephalus in a patient with Joubert syndrome. J Postgrad Med 50: 153.

Giordano L, Vignoli A, Pinelli L, Brancati F, Accorsi P, Faravelli F, et al. (2009) Joubert syndrome with bilateral polymicrogyria: clinical and neuropathological findings in two brothers. Am J Med Genet A 149A: 1511–1515.

Gitten J, Dede D, Fennell E, Quisling R, Maria BL (1998) Neurobehavioral development in Joubert syndrome. J Child Neurol 13: 391–397.

Gleeson JG, Keeler LC, Parisi MA, Marsh SE, Chance PF, Glass IA, et al. (2004) Molar tooth sign of the midbrain-hindbrain junction: occurrence in multiple distinct syndromes. Am J Med Genet A 125: 125–134.

Gorden NT, Arts HH, Parisi MA, Coene KL, Letteboer SJ, van Beersum SE, et al. (2008) CC2D2A Is Mutated in Joubert Syndrome and Interacts with the Ciliopathy-Associated Basal Body Protein CEP290. Am J Hum Genet 83: 559–571.

Gregory-Evans CY, Williams MJ, Halford S, Gregory-Evans K (2004) Ocular coloboma: a reassessment in the age of molecular neuroscience. J Med Genet 41: 881–891.

Gunzler SA, Stoessl AJ, Egan RA, Weleber RG, Wang P, Nutt JG (2007) Joubert syndrome surviving to adulthood associated with a progressive movement disorder. Mov Disord 22: 262–265.

Haug K, Khan S, Fuchs S, Konig R (2000) OFD II, OFD VI, and Joubert syndrome manifestations in 2 sibs. Am J Med Genet 91: 135–137.

Helou J, Otto EA, Attanasio M, Allen SJ, Parisi M, Glass I, et al. (2007) Mutation analysis of NPHP6/CEP290 in patients with Joubert-Syndrome and Senior-Loken-Syndrome. J Med Genet 44: 657–663.

Hildebrandt F, Attanasio M, Otto E (2009) Nephronophthisis: disease mechanisms of a ciliopathy. J Am Soc Nephrol 20: 23–35.

Hildebrandt F, Otto E (2005) Cilia and centrosomes: a unifying pathogenic concept for cystic kidney disease? Nat Rev Genet 6: 928–940.

Hodgkins PR, Harris CM, Shawkat FS, Thompson DA, Chong K, Timms C, et al. (2004) Joubert syndrome: long-term follow-up. Dev Med Child Neurol 46: 694–699.

Iannicelli M, Brancati F, Mougou-Zerelli S, Mazzotta A, Thomas S, Elkhartoufi N, et al. (2010) Novel TMEM67 mutations and genotype-phenotype correlates in meckelin-related ciliopathies. Hum Mutat 31: E1319–E1331.

Johnson CA, Gissen P, Sergi C (2003) Molecular pathology and genetics of congenital hepatorenal fibrocystic syndromes. J Med Genet 40: 311–319.

Joubert M, Eisenring JJ, Andermann F (1968) Familial dysgenesis of the vermis: a syndrome of hyperventilation, abnormal eye movements and retardation. Neurology 18: 302–303.

Joubert M, Eisenring JJ, Robb JP, Andermann F (1969) Familial agenesis of the cerebellar vermis. A syndrome of episodic hyperpnea, abnormal eye movements, ataxia, and retardation. Neurology 19: 813–825.

Katsanis N (2004) The oligogenic properties of Bardet-Biedl syndrome. Hum Mol Genet 13 Spec No 1: R65–R71.

Kendall B, Kingsley D, Lambert SR, Taylor D, Finn P (1990) Joubert syndrome: a clinico-radiological study. Neuroradiology 31: 502–506.

Khan AO, Oystreck DT, Seidahmed MZ, AlDrees A, Elmalik SA, Alorainy IA, Salih MA (2008) Ophthalmic features of Joubert syndrome. Ophthalmology 115: 2286–2289.

Khanna H, Davis EE, Murga-Zamalloa CA, Estrada-Cuzcano A, Lopez I, den Hollander AI, et al. (2009) A common allele in RPGRIP1L is a modifier of retinal degeneration in ciliopathies. Nat Genet 41: 739–745.

Kroes HY, van Zon PH, van de Putte DF, Nelen MR, Nievelstein RJ, Wittebol-Post D, et al. (2008) DNA analysis of AHI1, NPHP1 and CYCLIN D1 in Joubert syndrome patients from the Netherlands. Eur J Med Genet 51: 24–34.

Kumada S, Hayashi M, Arima K, Nakayama H, Sugai K, Sasaki M, et al. (2004) Renal disease in Arima syndrome is nephronophthisis as in other Joubert-related Cerebello-oculo-renal syndromes. Am J Med Genet A 131: 71–76.

Lambert SR, Kriss A, Gresty M, Benton S, Taylor D (1989) Joubert syndrome. Arch Ophthalmol 107: 709–713.

Lewis SM, Roberts EA, Marcon MA, Harvey E, Phillips MJ, Chuang SA, et al. (1994) Joubert syndrome with congenital hepatic fibrosis: an entity in the spectrum of oculo-encephalo-hepato-renal disorders. Am J Med Genet 52: 419–426.

Louie CM, Caridi G, Lopes VS, Brancati F, Kispert A, Lancaster MA, et al. (2010) AHI1 is required for photoreceptor outer segment development and is a modifier for retinal degeneration in nephronophthisis. Nat Genet 42: 175–180.

Maria BL, Boltshauser E, Palmer SC, Tran TX (1999a) Clinical features and revised diagnostic criteria in Joubert syndrome. J Child Neurol 14: 583–590.

Maria BL, Bozorgmanesh A, Kimmel KN, Theriaque D, Quisling RG (2001) Quantitative assessment of brainstem development in Joubert syndrome and Dandy-Walker syndrome. J Child Neurol 16: 751–758.

Maria BL, Hoang KB, Tusa RJ, Mancuso AA, Hamed LM, Quisling RG, et al. (1997) 'Joubert syndrome' revisited: key ocular motor signs with magnetic resonance imaging correlation. J Child Neurol 12: 423–430.

Maria BL, Quisling RG, Rosainz LC, Yachnis AT, Gitten J, Dede D, Fennell E (1999b) Molar tooth sign in Joubert syndrome: clinical, radiologic, and pathologic significance. J Child Neurol 14: 368–376.

Matsuzaka T, Sakuragawa N, Nakayama H, Sugai K, Kohno Y, Arima M (1986) Cerebro-oculo-hepato-renal syndrome (Arima' syndrome): a distinct clinicopathological entity. J Child Neurol 1: 338–346.

Mougou-Zerelli S, Thomas S, Szenker E, Audollent S, Elkhartoufi N, Babarit C, et al. (2009) CC2D2A mutations in Meckel and Joubert syndromes indicate a genotype-phenotype correlation. Hum Mutat 30: 1574–1582.

Munke M, McDonald DM, Cronister A, Stewart JM, Gorlin RJ, Zackai EH (1990) Oral-facial-digital syndrome type VI (Varadi syndrome): further clinical delineation. Am J Med Genet 35: 360–369.

Otto EA, Tory K, Attanasio M, Zhou W, Chaki M, Paruchuri Y, et al. (2009) Hypomorphic mutations in meckelin (MKS3/TMEM67) cause nephronophthisis with liver Fibrosis (NPHP11). J Med Genet 46: 663–670.

Ozyurek H, Kayacik OE, Gungor O, Karagoz F (2008) Rare association of Hirschsprung's disease and Joubert syndrome. Eur J Pediatr 167: 475–477.

Parisi MA, Bennett CL, Eckert ML, Dobyns WB, Gleeson JG, Shaw DW, et al. (2004) The NPHP1 gene deletion associated with juvenile nephronophthisis is present in a subset of individuals with Joubert syndrome. Am J Hum Genet 75: 82–91.

Parisi MA, Doherty D, Chance PF, Glass IA (2007) Joubert syndrome (and related disorders) (OMIM 213300). Eur J Hum Genet 15: 511–521.

Parisi MA, Doherty D, Eckert ML, Shaw DW, Ozyurek H, Aysun S, et al. (2006) AHI1 mutations cause both retinal dystrophy and renal cystic disease in Joubert syndrome. J Med Genet 43: 334–339.

Pellegrino JE, Lensch MW, Muenke M, Chance PF (1997) Clinical and molecular analysis in Joubert syndrome. Am J Med Genet 72: 59–62.

Poretti A, Boltshauser E, Loenneker T, Valente EM, Brancati F, Il'yasov K, Huisman TA (2007) Diffusion tensor imaging in Joubert syndrome. AJNR Am J Neuroradiol 28: 1929–1933.

Poretti A, Dietrich AF, Brancati F, Dallapiccola B, Valente EM, Boltshauser E (2009) Normal cognitive functions in joubert syndrome. Neuropediatrics 40: 287–290.

Saleem SN, Zaki MS (2010) Role of MR imaging in prenatal diagnosis of pregnancies at risk for Joubert syndrome and related cerebellar disorders. AJNR Am J Neuroradiol 31: 424–429.

Salomon R, Saunier S, Niaudet P (2009) Nephronophthisis. Pediatr Nephrol 24: 2333–2344.

Saraiva JM, Baraitser M (1992) Joubert syndrome: a review. Am J Med Genet 43: 726–731.

Satran D, Pierpont ME, Dobyns WB (1999) Cerebello-oculo-renal syndromes including Arima, Senior-Loken and COACH syndromes: more than just variants of Joubert syndrome. Am J Med Genet 86: 459–469.

Sayer JA, Otto EA, O'Toole JF, Nurnberg G, Kennedy MA, Becker C, et al. (2006) The centrosomal protein nephrocystin-6 is mutated in Joubert syndrome and activates transcription factor ATF4. Nat Genet 38: 674–681.

Schurman SJ, Scheinman SJ (2009) Inherited cerebrorenal syndromes. Nat Rev Nephrol 5: 529–538.

Senocak EU, Oguz KK, Haliloglu G, Topcu M, Cila A (2010) Structural abnormalities of the brain other than molar tooth sign in Joubert syndrome-related disorders. Diagn Interv Radiol 16: 3–6.

Shian WJ, Chi CS, Mak SC, Chen CH (1993) Joubert syndrome in Chinese infants and children: a report of four cases. Zhonghua Yi Xue Za Zhi (Taipei) 52: 342–345.

Smith DJ, Blake JR, Gaffney EA (2008) Fluid mechanics of nodal flow due to embryonic primary cilia. J R Soc Interface 5: 567–573.

Spassky N, Han YG, Aguilar A, Strehl L, Besse L, Laclef C, et al. (2008) Primary cilia are required for cerebellar development and Shh-dependent expansion of progenitor pool. Dev Biol 317: 246–259.

Steinlin M, Schmid M, Landau K, Boltshauser E (1997) Follow-up in children with Joubert syndrome. Neuropediatrics 28: 204–211.

Stephan MJ, Brooks KL, Moore DC, Coll EJ, Goho C (1994) Hypothalamic hamartoma in oral-facial-digital syndrome type VI (Varadi syndrome). Am J Med Genet 51: 131–136.

Sturm V, Leiba H, Menke MN, Valente EM, Poretti A, Landau K, Boltshauser E (2010) Ophthalmological findings in Joubert syndrome. Eye 24: 222–225.

Tallila J, Salonen R, Kohlschmidt N, Peltonen L, Kestila M (2009) Mutation spectrum of Meckel syndrome genes: one group of syndromes or several distinct groups? Hum Mutat 30: E813–E830.

Tory K, Lacoste T, Burglen L, Moriniere V, Boddaert N, Macher MA, et al. (2007) High NPHP1 and NPHP6 mutation rate in patients with Joubert syndrome and nephronophthisis: potential epistatic effect of NPHP6 and AHI1 mutations in patients with NPHP1 mutations. J Am Soc Nephrol 18: 1566–1575.

Tusa RJ, Hove MT (1999) Ocular and oculomotor signs in Joubert syndrome. J Child Neurol 14: 621–627.

Valente EM, Brancati F, Dallapiccola B (2008) Genotypes and phenotypes of Joubert syndrome and related disorders. Eur J Med Genet 51: 1–23.

Valente EM, Brancati F, Silhavy JL, Castori M, Marsh SE, Barrano G, et al. (2006a) AHI1 gene mutations cause specific forms of Joubert syndrome-related disorders. Ann Neurol 59: 527–534.

Valente EM, Logan CV, Mougou-Zerelli S, Lee JH, Silhavy JL, Brancati F, et al. (2010) Mutations in TMEM216 perturb ciliogenesis and cause Joubert, Meckel and related syndromes. Nat Genet 42: 619–625.

Valente EM, Silhavy JL, Brancati F, Barrano G, Krishnaswami SR, Castori M, et al. (2006b) Mutations in CEP290, which encodes a centrosomal protein, cause pleiotropic forms of Joubert syndrome. Nat Genet 38: 623–625.

van Dorp DB, Palan A, Kwee ML, Barth PG, van der Harten JJ (1991) Joubert syndrome: a clinical and pathological description of an affected male and a female fetus from the same sibship. Am J Med Genet 40: 100–104.

Varadi V, Szabo L, Papp Z (1980) Syndrome of polydactyly, cleft lip/palate or lingual lump, and psychomotor retardation in endogamic gypsies. J Med Genet 17: 119–122.

Verloes A, Lambotte C (1989) Further delineation of a syndrome of cerebellar vermis hypo/aplasia, oligophrenia, congenital ataxia, coloboma, and hepatic fibrosis. Am J Med Genet 32: 227–232.

Wang P, Chang FM, Chang CH, Yu CH, Jung YC, Huang CC (1999) Prenatal diagnosis of Joubert syndrome complicated with encephalocele using two-dimensional and three-dimensional ultrasound. Ultrasound Obstet Gynecol 14: 360–362.

Weiss AH, Doherty D, Parisi M, Shaw D, Glass I, Phillips JO (2009) Eye movement Abnormalities in Joubert Syndrome. Invest Ophthalmol Vis Sci 50: 4669–4677.

Willaredt MA, Hasenpusch-Theil K, Gardner HA, Kitanovic I, Hirschfeld-Warneken VC, Gojak CP, et al. (2008) A crucial role for primary cilia in cortical morphogenesis. J Neurosci 28: 12887–12900.

Wolf MT, Saunier S, O'Toole JF, Wanner N, Groshong T, Attanasio M, et al. (2007) Mutational analysis of the RPGRIP1L gene in patients with Joubert syndrome and nephronophthisis. Kidney Int 72: 1520–1526.

Yachnis AT, Rorke LB (1999) Neuropathology of Joubert syndrome. J Child Neurol 14: 655–659.

Zamponi N, Rossi B, Messori A, Polonara G, Regnicolo L, Cardinali C (2002) Joubert syndrome with associated corpus callosum agenesis. Eur J Paediatr Neurol 6: 63–66.

12 Chiari Type I Malformation

Michael S. Salman

Chiari type I malformation (CM1) is an anomaly in which the cerebellar tonsils are displaced more than 5mm below the foramen magnum (Aboulezz et al. 1985). The posterior fossa is usually small in CM1 and its contents are crowded. Other associated features include syringomyelia (the term most consistently used in medical literature) and cranial and vertebral abnormalities (Elster and Chen 1992).

In this chapter, historic aspects, nomenclature, and the frequency of CM1 are highlighted, then theories, characteristic features, and the clinical presentation of CM1 are discussed. The following sections deals with investigations, management, and prognosis of CM1.

Historic perspective

Hans Chiari (1851–1916) described three grades of hindbrain herniation in patients with chronic hydrocephalus in 1891 (Chiari 1891; Pearce 2000; Arnett 2003). In CM1, there is abnormal cerebellar tonsil elongation and herniation below the foramen magnum. Most patients with typical CM1 do not have associated hydrocephalus.

Nomenclature

Tonsillar ectopia or Chiari type I anomaly have been suggested as better names to describe CM1, since the cerebellum is not truly malformed and the tonsillar herniation is only a secondary event caused by a small posterior fossa size (Boltshauser 2004; Novegno et al. 2008; Rekate 2008). Others contend that the term 'malformation' is justified since there is increasing evidence for paraxial mesoderm disorder that leads to basioccipital hypoplasia, i.e., the malformation is that of the basal skull bones and not the cerebellum (Noudel et al. 2009).

If caudal descent of the brainstem accompanies tonsillar herniation, the term 'Chiari 1.5 malformation' has been used (Tubbs et al. 2004). However, the clinical presentation of 'Chiari 1.5 malformation' is similar to CM1, raising doubts as to whether it should be considered a separate disease entity from CM1, though a higher proportion of these patients require repeated operation for persistent syringomyelia (Tubbs et al. 2004).

Epidemiology

The true prevalence or incidence of CM1 is unknown. The National Institute of Neurological Disorders and Stroke estimate is 1 per 1000 births. This figure is likely to be higher since the widespread use of MRI has uncovered asymptomatic people with tonsillar ectopia (Voelker 2009). In a 2-year study between 1997 and 1998 of a pediatric population under the age of 20 years living in Northern California in the USA, the frequency of CM1 was 1% ($N = 51$) of all head and spine MRIs performed during that period ($N = 5248$). A third of the group was asymptomatic (Aitken et al. 2009). The figure is within the same frequency range (0.6–0.9%) reported in other similar radiological studies (Elster and Chen 1992; Wu et al. 1999).

Natural history, theories, and mechanisms

Cerebellar tonsils lying below the foramen magnum is not in itself a pathological finding, especially in children, where tonsillar displacement up to 6mm below the foramen magnum has been suggested to be a normal variant in the first decade of life (Mikulis et al. 1992). The same study reported that tonsillar ascent occurs with age. Other studies suggested 2mm caudal displacement below foramen magnum to be the upper limits of normal, 3–5mm to be a gray zone area that may be pathological in the presence of relevant symptoms and signs, and greater than 5mm tonsillar caudal displacement below foramen magnum to be pathological (Aboulezz et al. 1985; Barkovich et al. 1986).

With increasing use of brain and spinal MRI, more incidental cases of CM1 have been uncovered. Many were found to remain asymptomatic or to resolve spontaneously (Novegno et al. 2008), even in the presence of significant tonsillar herniation (Waldau et al. 2009) or syringomyelia (Guillen and Costa 2004).

CM1 is a multifactorial disorder with some evidence of familial clustering in a small percentage of patients, perhaps suggesting a genetic component to its pathogenesis (Milhorat et al. 1999; Szewka et al. 2006). The size of the posterior fossa is small in the majority of patients with the typical 'classic' nonacquired form of this disorder while brain volume is normal (Milhorat et al. 1999; Trigylidas et al. 2008; Furtado et al. 2009). One report suggested that the posterior fossa volume is small only if CM1 is associated with syringomyelia (Sgouros et al. 2006). Another study reported a normal posterior fossa size in a multigenerational family with CM1 (Tubbs et al. 2008). The cerebellar volume was reported to be normal in adolescents and adults with CM1 (Nishikawa et al. 1997). The classic form of the disorder has been referred to as congenital. This author and others (Furtado et al. 2010) disagree with this term as there is no evidence that the disorder is present at birth.

The small posterior fossa size usually associated with CM1 is postulated to result from a defect in paraxial mesoderm development with consequent occipital bone hypoplasia (Marín-Padilla 1991; also reviewed by Tubbs et al. 2007). One study reported that the entire skull base is morphologically different in children with CM1 with longer anterior fossa and a wider and steeper posterior fossa in comparison to children without CM1 (Sgouros et al. 2007).

Acquired CM1 may result from several factors including: (1) raised intracranial pressure which occurs in idiopathic intracranial hypertension or results from secondary causes, for example brain tumor or hydrocephalus; (2) a change in the cerebrospinal fluid (CSF) pressure gradient, for example CSF leak, ventriculo- or lumboperitonial shunting; and (3) cranial and vertebral bony abnormalities, for example skeletal dysplasia, osteopetrosis, acromegaly, hypophosphotemic rickets, various forms of craniosynostosis such as Crouzon, Carpenter, and rarely Apert syndromes (Wu et al. 1999; Tubbs et al. 2007; Caldarelli et al. 2009).

The mechanism by which syringomyelia is formed is unknown. Current theories suggest that it is caused by cranial-spinal pressure dissociation caused by foramen magnum obstruction by the tonsils (reviewed in Schijman 2004 and Tubbs et al. 2007).

Characteristic features

The main anatomic features of classical CM1 are characteristic (Aboulezz et al. 1985; Elster and Chen 1992; Milhorat et al. 1999) and consist of (1) a small posterior fossa; (2) herniation of at least one cerebellar tonsil 5mm or more below foramen magnum (Figs 12.1 and 12.2) or herniation of both cerebellar tonsils 3–5mm below foramen magnum accompanied by other features consistent with CM1, for example a syringomyelia; (3) no evidence of myelomeningocele; and (4) no secondary cause for the tonsillar displacement, for example brain tumor.

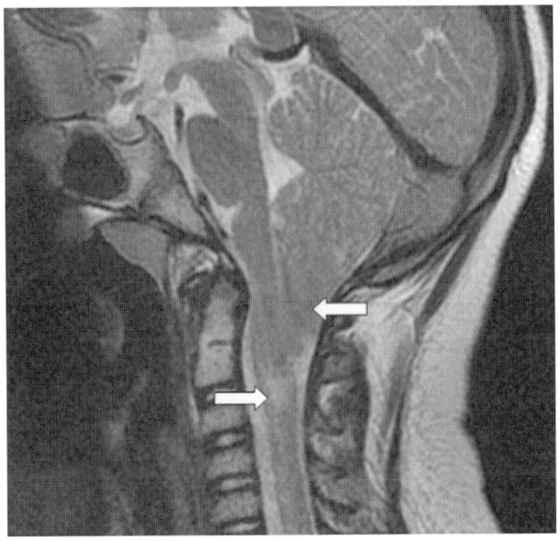

Fig. 12.1. T2-weighted midsagittal MRI of the lower brain and upper cervical spine (TR 2416.7ms, TE 102.2ms) in an 8-year-old girl who presented with frequent and prolonged episodes of nocturnal apnea. The figure illustrates several features of Chiari type I malformation including tonsillar herniation 25mm below foramen magnum (leftward pointing arrow), lack of the retrocerebellar CSF space, and hyperintense T2 signal within the upper cervical spinal cord at the level of C2-C3 (rightward pointing arrow) suggesting a myelopathy.

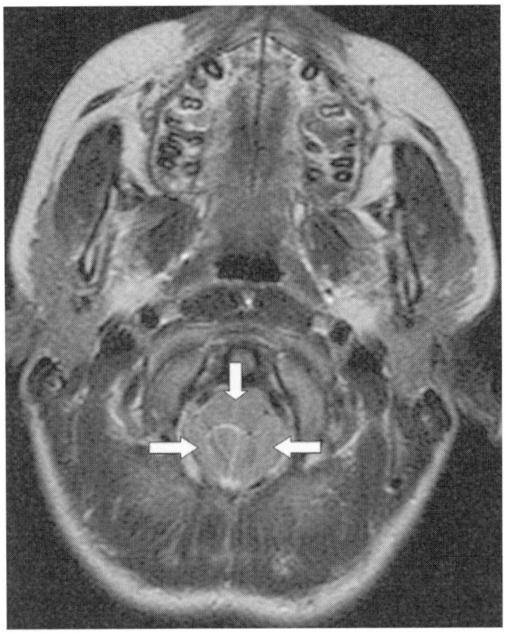

Fig. 12.2. T2-weighted axial MRI at the level of foramen magnum (TR 2650.0ms, TE 104.6ms) in a 12-year-old boy who presented with occipital headaches. The figure illustrates crowding of the foramen magnum caused by tonsillar tissue (horizontal arrows), displacing the medulla anteriorly (vertical arrow). His tonsils were displaced 20mm below the foramen magnum (not shown).

Pointed or 'peg-like' rather than round-shaped tonsils, stretching of the fourth ventricle (Aboulezz et al. 1985), and compression of the retrocerebellar CSF space (Fig. 12.1) suggest tissue crowding (Barkovich et al. 1986; Milhorat et al. 1999) but their presence is not necessarily associated with the more severe phenotype (Aitken et al. 2009). Other reported abnormalities include syringomyelia (Fig. 12.3) and bony deformities of the craniocervical junction (Elster and Chen 1992; Milhorat et al. 1999; Wu et al. 1999) (Table 12.1). Less common associations include hydrocephalus and cervico-medullary kinking (Amer and el-Shmam 1997). Other probably unrelated and uncommon associations include developmental disabilities and seizures (Brill et al. 1997; Wu et al. 1999).

Clinical presentation

Occipital or suboccipital headaches, made worse by the Valsalva maneuver, sudden postural change or physical exertion, and neck pain are the most common presenting features occurring in the majority of symptomatic patients with CM1 followed by visual disturbance, vertigo, and dizziness (Milhorat et al. 1999; Taylor and Larkins 2002). Other frequent presentations include limbs weakness, numbness and tingling, back or limb pain, tinnitus, ataxia, dysarthria, and scoliosis (Aitken et al. 2009). Oropharyngeal symptoms including dysphagia, choking, aspiration, and chronic cough are a more common mode of presentation in children under 3 years of age (Greenlee et al. 2002). Other symptoms suggestive of brainstem compression include sleep apnea, nystagmus (mostly horizontal and downbeat), vocal cord dysfunction or paralysis, and torticollis. Blurred

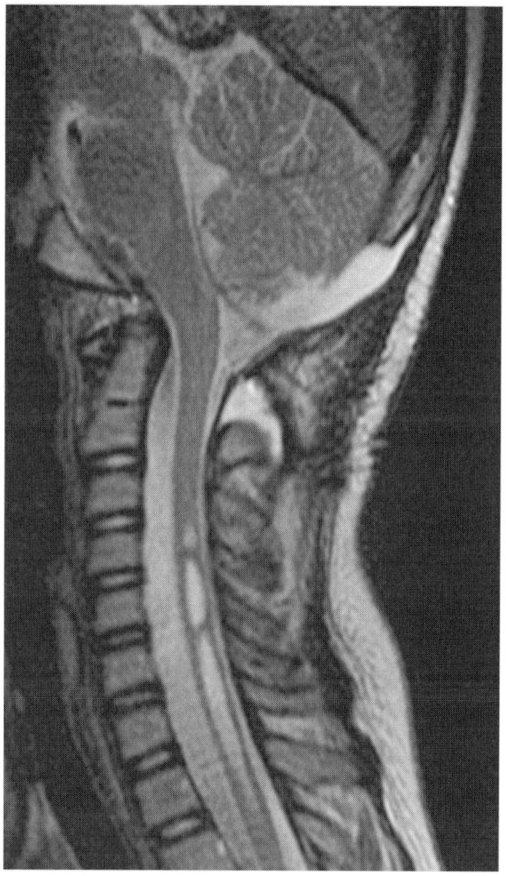

Fig. 12.3. T2-weighted midsagittal MRI of the lower posterior fossa and upper spinal cord (TR 3016.7ms, TE 113.6ms) in a 10-year-old girl with Chiari type I malformation following posterior fossa decompression showing syringomyelia of the cervical and thoracic spinal cord.

TABLE 12.1
Characteristic features and associated anomalies in Chiari type I malformation

A) Posterior fossa contents
1. Pathological tonsillar herniation below foramen magnum (usually >5mm)
2. Pointed tonsils
3. Anterior displacement of the cerebellum
4. Small posterior fossa size
5. Absence of the retrocerebellar fluid space
6. Inferior displacement of a small and stretched fourth ventricle
7. Increased slope of the tentorium
8. Medullary-cervical kink
9. Syringobulbia

B) Spinal cord, spine, and cranium
1. Syringomyelia
2. Myelopathy
3. Scoliosis or kyphosis
4. Atlanto-occipital assimilation
5. Platybasia
6. Basilar invagination
7. Klippel-Feil anomaly
8. Fused cervical vertebrae
9. Reduced height of the supraocciput and reduced length of the clivus
10. Hydrocephalus

TABLE 12.2
Summary of symptoms and signs associated with Chiari type I malformation

1. Headache, usually occipital and worse with Valsalva
2. Neck pain
3. Vertigo, dizziness, dysphagia, regurgitation, aspiration, apnoea, stridor, bradycardia, torticollis, facial pain, and nystagmus related to brainstem compression or syringobulbia (rarely)
4. Impaired saccadic smooth pursuit, saccadic dysmetria, strabismus, dysarthria, oscillopsia, nystagmus, and ataxia related to cerebellar compression
5. Sleep problems and snoring
6. Scoliosis
7. Limbs or back pain, sensory loss in a cape distribution, weakness, muscle atrophy, and spasticity related to the syringomyelia

vision, diplopia, syncope, hypertension, and urinary incontinence have also been described in patients with CM1 (Milhorat et al. 1999; Wu et al. 1999; Straus et al. 2009).

Physical findings include nystagmus, abnormal gag reflex, scoliosis, spasticity, weakness, muscle atrophy, ataxia, abnormal tendon reflexes, Babinski's sign, impaired temperature sensation and position sense (Milhorat et al. 1999; Greenlee et al. 2002; Tubbs et al. 2007). Table 12.2 summarizes the main symptoms and signs of CM1.

Some investigators have grouped the symptoms and signs of CM1 into those caused by: (1) brainstem compression, (2) cerebellar compression, and (3) the associated syringomyelia (Tubbs et al. 2007).

Syringomyelia occurs commonly in CM1 (Tubbs et al. 2007). Various estimates have been reported ranging from 12 to 65% or more (Milhorat et al. 1999; Wu et al. 1999; Greenlee et al. 2002; Aitken et al. 2009). Syringobulbia, presenting with cranial nerve palsies, is a rare association of CM1 and syringomyelia (Greenlee et al. 2005). The mechanism of syringobulbia formation is unknown and appears unrelated to specific morphometric changes in CM1 (Tubbs et al. 2009).

The degree of tonsillar ectopia does not correlate reliably with the symptoms of CM1 (Trigylidas et al. 2008; Aitken et al. 2009). Herniation of 9–14mm is associated most commonly with syringomyelia (Stovner and Rinck 1992); however, not all studies agree (Milhorat et al. 1999).

CSF fluid disturbance and direct neural tissue compression have been suggested as the cause of the symptoms and signs in CM1 (Milhorat et al. 1999). Some authors suggested that arachnoid adhesions and scarring at the foramen magnum cause the symptoms through obstruction of CSF flow (Barkovich et al. 1986). A histological study of 43 patients, aged 4 months to 20 years, who had cerebellar tonsillectomy as part of their posterior fossa decompression for CM1, revealed histological alteration in 38 patients. Purkinje cell loss and gliosis were the most frequent findings, likely to be secondary to injury from local trauma and possibly ischemia (Pueyrredon et al. 2007).

As more 'incidental' CM1 on MRI is being diagnosed, patients with vague symptoms or symptoms seemingly unrelated to CM1 present the clinician with a dilemma. Care should be exercised before attributing patients' symptoms to CM1 as it could lead to the wrong management plan.

Investigations

MRI of the brain and spinal cord is the investigation of choice in children suspected of having CM1 because the posterior fossa, its contents, and the syringomyelia can be seen in detail. In addition, myelopathy of the spinal cord may be detected on MRI and can be readily seen as an area of abnormal signal intensity on T2-weighted images. CSF flow studies using MRI imaging may be useful but its clinical role awaits future studies as the sensitivity and specificity in delineating patients with symptomatic CM1 from asymptomatic tonsillar ectopia is relatively low at 76% and 62%, respectively (Armonda et al. 1994; Hofkes et al. 2007; Trigylidas et al. 2008).

The vestibulocerebellum function may be impaired in CM1 since the tonsils and/or the brainstem are compressed. Vestibular function can be investigated by studying eye movements in response to different stimuli, for example, postural changes and caloric stimuli. These tests may aid surgical decisions in patients with mild to moderate symptoms with soft or non-specific neurological findings (Kumar et al. 2002). Hearing loss has been reported in these patients (Milhorat et al. 1999; Kumar et al. 2002), and audiometric testing may be useful in patients with CM1 and hearing loss.

Management

There are no widely accepted standards or guidelines for the management of CM1 because studies published on the treatment of this malformation are retrospective and generally limited by the small number of patients (Tubbs et al. 2007).

MEDICAL MANAGEMENT

Conservative management is advocated for asymptomatic and minimally symptomatic patients (Novegno et al. 2008). These patients usually have mild tonsillar ectopia and subtle neurological findings, and their lifestyle is not significantly affected by the symptoms. If pain is present, it is usually treated with simple analgesia (Tubbs et al. 2007). Routine follow-up looking for evidence of clinical progression associated with the development of brainstem or cerebellar compression, secondary hydrocephalus, syringobulbia, or syringomyelia is important.

SURGICAL MANAGEMENT

Posterior fossa decompression is the treatment of choice for patients with symptomatic CM1 (Fig. 12.4), especially when the symptoms are moderate to severe and are progressive. The operation is safe and results in improvements in the majority of patients in general (Tubbs et al. 2007). Headache, neck pain, sleep apnea, and scoliosis improve the most among all symptoms of CM1 (Tubbs et al. 2003). The operation is also effective in relieving the disabling ocular motor and vestibulo-ocular symptoms of CM1 (Liebenberg et al. 2005). Variations on the operative procedure exist, where decompression may involve one or more of the following options: limited suboccipital

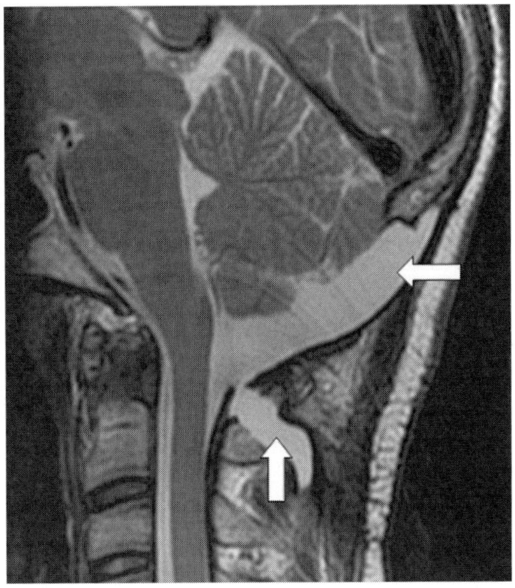

Fig. 12.4. T2-weighted midsagittal MRI of the lower brain and upper cervical spine (TR 2466.7ms, TE 111.9ms) in a 16-year-old patient with Chiari type I malformation illustrating postoperative changes following posterior fossa decompression. There is a pseudomeningocele (vertical arrow) and abundant retrocerebellar CSF space (horizontal arrow) following suboccipital craniectomy.

craniectomy, intradural dissection of adhesions, duraplasty, cervical laminectomy, or tonsillar resection (Alden et al. 2001; Tubbs et al. 2003; Durham and Fjeld-Olenec 2008). A minimalist surgical approach appears to produce satisfactory results (Caldarelli et al. 2007). Surgical complications are uncommon and include hemorrhage, CSF leakage, meningitis, and recurrence of CM1 (Alden et al. 2001).

Symptom recurrence has been reported in about 20% of pediatric patients with CM1 (McGirt et al. 2008). A third of these patients had recurrent hindbrain crowding or increased syringomyelia size and required further surgery.

Decompressive surgery is also recommended if there is clinical and radiographic evidence of progressive syringomyelia, which tends to resolve in 55–80% of pediatric patients following surgery (Depreitere et al. 2000; Attenello et al. 2008). Motor symptoms caused by the syringomyelia are more likely to resolve than sensory symptoms. Radiographic improvement of the syringomyelia lags behind clinical improvement by several months (Attenello et al. 2008).

SUPPORTIVE MANAGEMENT

Patient and family education and support should be part of the management plan.

Prognosis

Prognosis is very good for most patients with CM1. Some patients remain asymptomatic but others become symptomatic as their disease progresses. Most do well following decompressive surgery. Even in the minority of patients with symptom recurrence following the decompression surgery, their symptoms tend to be mild and rarely require further surgery (Caldarelli et al. 2007; McGirt et al. 2008). Self-perceived quality of life of adolescents older than 17 years and adults with CM1 is significantly improved after decompression surgery (Mueller and Oro' 2005). Similar studies in children have not been carried out.

The future

Systematic longitudinal clinical and neuroradiological studies in children and adolescents with CM1 are needed to better understand the natural history of this disorder. Multicenter trials investigating the best surgical options, timing of surgery, and extent of surgery should be undertaken in the future.

Summary

Chiari type I malformation is associated with pathological cerebellar tonsils displacement below foramen magnum. Other associated features include syringomyelia, scoliosis, and craniovertebral anomalies. Acquired causes of pathological tonsillar herniation include secondary causes of raised intracranial pressure and CSF shunts. Patients with CM1 present with headache, neck pain, and brainstem, cerebellar, motor, and sensory symptoms. The management of patients with CM1 includes conservative management in asymptomatic or mildly affected patients and decompression of the posterior fossa for the more severely affected patients. Surgery is safe and effective in the majority of patients.

REFERENCES

Aboulezz AO, Sartor K, Geyer CA, Gado MH (1985) Position of cerebellar tonsils in the normal population and in patients with Chiari malformation: a quantitative approach with MR imaging. J Comput Assist Tomogr 9: 1033–1036.

Aitken LA, Lindan CE, Sidney S, Gupta N, Barkovich AJ, Sorel M, Wu YW (2009) Chiari type I malformation in a pediatric population. Pediatr Neurol 40: 449–454.

Alden TD, Ojemann JG, Park TS (2001) Surgical treatment of Chiari I malformation: indications and approaches. Neurosurg Focus 11: E2.

Amer TA, el-Shmam OM (1997) Chiari malformation type I: a new MRI classification. Magn Reson Imaging 15: 397–403.

Armonda RA, Citrin CM, Foley KT, Ellenbogen RG (1994) Quantitative cine-mode magnetic resonance imaging of Chiari I malformations: an analysis of cerebrospinal fluid dynamics. Neurosurgery 35: 214–223.

Arnett B. (2003) Arnold-Chiari malformation. Arch Neurol 60: 898–900.

Attenello FJ, McGirt MJ, Gathinji M, Datoo G, Atiba A, Weingart J, et al. (2008) Outcome of Chiari-associated syringomyelia after hindbrain decompression in children: analysis of 49 consecutive cases. Neurosurgery 62: 1307–1313.

Barkovich AJ, Wippold FJ, Sherman JL, Citrin CM (1986) Significance of cerebellar tonsillar position on MR. AJNR Am J Neuroradiol 7: 795–799.

Boltshauser E (2004) Cerebellum-small brain but large confusion: a review of selected cerebellar malformations and disruptions. Am J Med Genet A 126A: 376–385.

Brill CB, Gutierrez J, Mishkin MM (1997) Chiari I malformation: association with seizures and developmental disabilities. J Child Neurol 12: 101–106.

Caldarelli M, Novegno F, Vassimi L, Romani R, Tamburrini G, Di Rocco C (2007) The role of limited posterior fossa craniectomy in the surgical treatment of Chiari malformation Type I: experience with a pediatric series. J Neurosurg 106(3 Suppl): 187–195.

Caldarelli M, Novegno F, Di Rocco C (2009) A late complication of CSF shunting: acquired Chiari I malformation. Childs Nerv Syst 25: 443–452.

Chiari H (1891) Ueber Veranderungen des Kleinhirns infolge von Hydrocephalie des Grosshirns. Dtsch Med Wochenschr 17: 1172–1175.

Depreitere B, Van Calenbergh F, van Loon J, Goffin J, Plets C (2000) Posterior fossa decompression in syringomyelia associated with a Chiari malformation: a retrospective analysis of 22 patients. Clin Neurol Neurosurg 102: 91–96.

Durham SR, Fjeld-Olenec K (2008) Comparison of posterior fossa decompression with and without duraplasty for the surgical treatment of Chiari malformation Type I in pediatric patients: a meta-analysis. J Neurosurg Pediatr 2: 42–49.

Elster AD, Chen MY (1992) Chiari I malformations: clinical and radiologic reappraisal. Radiology 183: 347–353.

Furtado SV, Reddy K, Hegde AS (2009) Posterior fossa morphometry in symptomatic pediatric and adult Chiari I malformation. J Clin Neurosci 16: 1449–1454.

Furtado SV, Thakre DJ, Venkatesh PK, Reddy K, Hegde AS (2010) Morphometric analysis of foramen magnum dimensions and intracranial volume in pediatric Chiari I malformation. Acta Neurochir (Wien) 152(2): 221–227.

Greenlee JD, Donovan KA, Hasan DM, Menezes AH (2002) Chiari I malformation in the very young child: the spectrum of presentations and experience in 31 children under age 6 years. Pediatrics 110: 1212–1219.

Greenlee JD, Menezes AH, Bertoglio BA, Donovan KA (2005) Syringobulbia in a pediatric population. Neurosurgery 57: 1147–1153.

Guillen A, Costa JM (2004) Spontaneous resolution of a Chiari I malformation associated syringomyelia in one child. Acta Neurochir (Wien) 146: 187–191.

Hofkes SK, Iskandar BJ, Turski PA, Gentry LR, McCue JB, Haughton VM (2007) Differentiation between symptomatic Chiari I malformation and asymptomatic tonsilar ectopia by using cerebrospinal fluid flow imaging: initial estimate of imaging accuracy. Radiology 245: 532–540.

Kumar A, Patni AH, Charbel F (2002) The Chiari I malformation and the neurotologist. Otol Neurotol 23: 727–735.

Liebenberg WA, Georges H, Demetriades AK, Hardwidge C (2005) Does posterior fossa decompression improve oculomotor and vestibulo-ocular manifestations in Chiari 1 malformation? Acta Neurochir (Wien) 147: 1239–1240.

Marín-Padilla M (1991) Cephalic axial skeletal-neural dysraphic disorders: embryology and pathology. Can J Neurol Sci 18: 153–169.

McGirt MJ, Attenello FJ, Atiba A, Garces-Ambrossi G, Datoo G, Weingart JD, et al. (2008) Symptom recurrence after suboccipital decompression for pediatric Chiari I malformation: analysis of 256 consecutive cases. Childs Nerv Syst 24: 1333–1339.

Mikulis DJ, Diaz O, Egglin TK, Sanchez R (1992) Variance of the position of the cerebellar tonsils with age: preliminary report. Radiology 183: 725–728.

Milhorat TH, Chou MW, Trinidad EM, Kula RW, Mandell M, Wolpert C, Speer MC (1999) Chiari I malformation redefined: clinical and radiographic findings for 364 symptomatic patients. Neurosurgery 44: 1005–1017.

Mueller D, Oro' JJ (2005) Prospective analysis of self-perceived quality of life before and after posterior fossa decompression in 112 patients with Chiari malformation with or without syringomyelia. Neurosurg Focus 18: ECP2.

Nishikawa M, Sakamoto H, Hakuba A, Nakanishi N, Inoue Y (1997) Pathogenesis of Chiari malformation: a morphometric study of the posterior cranial fossa. J Neurosurg 86: 40–47.

Noudel R, Jovenin N, Eap C, Scherpereel B, Pierot L, Rousseaux P (2009) Incidence of basioccipital hypoplasia in Chiari malformation type I: comparative morphometric study of the posterior cranial fossa. Clinical article. J Neurosurg 111: 1046–1052.

Novegno F, Caldarelli M, Massa A, Chieffo D, Massimi L, Pettorini B, et al. (2008) The natural history of the Chiari Type I anomaly. J Neurosurg Pediatr 2: 179–187.

Pearce JMS (2000) Arnold Chiari, or 'Cruveilhier Cleland Chiari' malformation. J Neurol Neurosurg Psychiatry 68: 13–16.

Pueyrredon F, Spaho N, Arroyave I, Vinters H, Lazareff J (2007) Histological findings in cerebellar tonsils of patients with Chiari type I malformation. Childs Nerv Syst 23: 427–429.

Rekate HL (2008) Natural history of the Chiari Type I anomaly. J Neurosurg Pediatr 2: 177–178.

Schijman E (2004) History, anatomic forms, and pathogenesis of Chiari I malformations. Childs Nerv Syst 20: 323–328.

Sgouros S, Kountouri M, Natarajan K (2006) Posterior fossa volume in children with Chiari malformation Type I. J Neurosurg 105(2 Suppl): 101–106.

Sgouros S, Kountouri M, Natarajan K (2007) Skull base growth in children with Chiari malformation Type I. J Neurosurg 107(3 Suppl): 188–192.

Stovner LJ, Rinck P (1992) Syringomyelia in Chiari malformation: relation to extent of cerebellar tissue herniation. Neurosurgery 31: 913–917.

Straus D, Foster K, Zimmerman F, Frim D (2009) Chiari drop attacks: surgical decompression and the role of tilt table testing. Pediatr Neurosurg 45: 384–389.

Szewka AJ, Walsh LE, Boaz JC, Carvalho KS, Golomb MR (2006) Chiari in the family: inheritance of the Chiari I malformation. Pediatr Neurol 34: 481–485.

Taylor FR, Larkins MV (2002) Headache and Chiari I malformation: clinical presentation, diagnosis, and controversies in management. Curr Pain Headache Rep 6: 331–337.

Trigylidas T, Baronia B, Vassilyadi M, Ventureyra EC (2008) Posterior fossa dimension and volume estimates in pediatric patients with Chiari I malformations. Childs Nerv Syst 24: 329–336.

Tubbs RS, McGirt MJ, Oakes WJ (2003) Surgical experience in 130 pediatric patients with Chiari I malformations. J Neurosurg 99: 291–296.

Tubbs RS, Iskandar BJ, Bartolucci AA, Oakes WJ (2004) A critical analysis of the Chiari 1.5 malformation. J Neurosurg 101(2 Suppl): 179–183.

Tubbs RS, Lyerly MJ, Loukas M, Shoja MM, Oakes WJ (2007) The pediatric Chiari I malformation: a review. Childs Nerv Syst 23: 1239–1250.

Tubbs RS, Hill M, Loukas M, Shoja MM, Oakes WJ (2008) Volumetric analysis of the posterior cranial fossa in a family with four generations of the Chiari malformation Type I. J Neurosurg Pediatr 1: 21–24.

Tubbs RS, Bailey M, Barrow WC, Loukas M, Shoja MM, Oakes W. (2009) Morphometric analysis of the craniocervical juncture in children with Chiari I malformation and concomitant syringobulbia. Childs Nerv Syst 25: 689–692.

Waldau B, Domeshek LF, Leigh FA, Lum KC, Fuchs HE, Marcus JR, et al. (2009) Spontaneous resolution of a 13-mm Chiari malformation Type I in relation to differential growth of the posterior fossa volume. J Neurosurg Pediatr 3: 110–114.

Wu YW, Chin CT, Chan KM, Barkovich AJ, Ferriero DM (1999) Pediatric Chiari I malformations: do clinical and radiologic features correlate? Neurology 53: 1271–1276.

Voelker R (2009) Chiari conundrum: researchers tackle a brain puzzle for the 21st century. JAMA 301: 147–149.

13
Chiari Type II Malformation

Michael S. Salman

Chiari type II malformation (CM2) occurs almost universally in neonates born with myelomeningocele (MMC), the most common and severe type of spina bifida (Wagner et al. 2002; Bowman et al. 2009). CM2 is a congenital anomaly that involves the cervical spinal cord, midbrain, and hindbrain (i.e., pons, medulla, and cerebellum) (Harding and Copp 2002; Barkovich 2005). In CM2, the posterior fossa is small and its contents are crowded and distorted. The cerebellar vermis herniates upward through the tentorial incisura and downward through foramen magnum. The lower brainstem is displaced downwards. Hydrocephalus and several supratentorial anomalies also occur in CM2.

In this chapter, historic aspects and the epidemiology of CM2 are highlighted, then the theories, characteristic features, and the clinical presentation of CM2 are discussed. The following sections deal with investigations, management, and prognosis of CM2. Issues related to the spinal cord lesion in MMC and its effects on lower limbs, tethered cord, renal and bowel functions are beyond the scope of this chapter.

Historic perspective

Hindbrain malformations were described in patients with spina bifida and hydrocephalus in an atlas by a professor of descriptive anatomy from Paris, Jean Cruveilhier (1791–1874), (Cruveilhier 1829; Pearce 2000). Hans Chiari (1851–1916), an Austrian-born professor of pathological anatomy in Prague's German University, described three grades of hindbrain herniation in patients with chronic hydrocephalus in a report in 1891 (Chiari 1891; Pearce 2000; Arnett 2003). In Chiari type I malformation, there is cerebellar tonsil elongation and herniation down the spinal canal. In CM2, there is cerebellar vermis and brainstem herniation down the spinal canal. In Chiari type III malformation, there is cerebellar-cervical encephalocele. A fourth grade, which was later called Chiari type IV malformation, was described in 1896 (Chiari 1896). It refers to cerebellar hypoplasia (Pearce 2000; Harding and Copp 2002; Barkovich 2005). The term Chiari type IV malformation is now obsolete.

John Cleland, a Scottish physician, described a hydrocephalic infant with spina bifida and distorted hindbrain in 1883. His work was acknowledged by Chiari (Cleland 1883; Gardner et al. 1975; Pearce 2000; Arnett 2003).

Julius Arnold (1835–1915), a German professor of pathological anatomy, reported herniation of the cerebellum into the spinal canal in spina bifida in 1894. His paper described the spinal myelomeningocele and theories of its cause (Arnold 1894; Arnett 2003).

Epidemiology

Since CM2 is an almost constant feature of MMC, the epidemiology of CM2 is reflected in the epidemiology of MMC, though fetal surgical repair of the MMC may alter that in the future if or when it becomes the first treatment of choice (Danzer et al. 2007).

The incidence of neural tube defects, of which MMC is the most common type, has been declining for three decades prior to the use of folic acid. Further reduction in incidence was reported following folic acid supplementation during pregnancy, food fortification with folic acid, and termination of pregnancy following prenatal diagnosis of MMC (Mills and Signore 2004; Bowman et al. 2009). The incidence of neural tube defects ranges between 0.17/1000 live births in non-Hispanic blacks in the USA to 6.39/1000 live births in northern China (Bowman et al. 2009). In the UK and North America, the incidence of neural tube defects is about 0.2–2/1000 live births. The incidence of MMC is about 0.2–0.5/1000 live births. The prevalence of MMC in 15- to 18-year-old teenagers in Sweden is 0.38/1000 (Olsson et al. 2007), suggesting a high survival rate in patients with MMC born after the mid-1980s.

Theories and mechanisms

Several theories have been proposed to explain the features of CM2 (Gardner et al. 1975; Gilbert et al. 1986; McLone and Knepper 1989; Harding and Copp 2002), including the following.

1. The traction theory suggests that hindbrain herniation into the spinal canal is due to downward pull of the lower spinal cord in MMC.
2. The dysgenesis theory proposes abnormal hindbrain tissue development.
3. The overgrowth theory postulates neural tissue overgrowth in the posterior fossa.
4. The hydrodynamic theory suggests that raised intracranial pressure from the hydrocephalus causes downward herniation of the hindbrain.
5. The molecular genetic theory states that abnormal rhombomere formation and ectopic expression of homeobox genes of the rostrocaudal axis of the neural tube may explain CM2 features (Sarnat 2000).

   None of these theories fully explain all the features described in CM2 (Marín-Padilla 1991; Stevenson 2004; Tubbs et al. 2008).
6. The popular unified theory proposes that normal distension of the embryonic ventricular system, through the pressure

generated from CSF build-up, does not occur in MMC because of cerebrospinal fluid (CSF) leakage through the spinal defect. Lack of ventricular distension in utero limits normal growth of the bony elements of the posterior fossa and results in a small posterior fossa (McLone and Knepper 1989; McLone and Dias 2003). The contents of the posterior fossa, which develop later, have to fit within a small posterior fossa (Griffiths et al. 2004). Crowding of hindbrain structures within a small posterior fossa is responsible for CM2 features (McLone and Knepper 1989; Marín-Padilla 1991). Consistent with this theory is the reduction in prevalence or prenatal resolution of hindbrain herniation following primary repair of the spinal defect in utero (Bruner et al. 1999; Sutton et al. 1999; Danzer et al. 2007) and a decrease in the incidence of brainstem compression in infancy and early childhood (Danzer et al. 2008).

7. Another theory states that genetic and environmental factors play a primary role in the causation of posterior fossa hypoplasia in CM2, which together with low spinal pressure, contributes to the development of CM2 (Williams 2008).
8. A recent paper reported the loss of ventricular lining (neuroepithelial/ependymal denudation) in the telencephalon and aqueduct during the early part of the second trimester prior to the development of CM2 or hydrocephalus in fetuses with MMC (de Wit et al. 2008). This resulted in permanent loss of cell function, which the authors postulated could lead to 'permanent cerebral pathology'.

Characteristic features

The small posterior fossa size usually associated with CM2 is detectable in fetuses with spina bifida as early as 16 weeks' gestation (Brocklehurst 1969; Hori 2002). CM2 can be identified during or after the second trimester using fetal ultrasonography (Fujisawa et al. 2006), and has been reported in about 54% of fetuses with spina bifida (Hori 2002). The anatomic deformity of CM2 is characteristic (McLone and Dias 2003) and involves the brainstem, cerebellum, supratentorial structures, spinal cord, and cranium (Table 13.1).

The brainstem

The brainstem is stretched down to the level of foramen magnum or cervical spine and narrowed in the anteroposterior diameter. A cervico-medullary kink may be seen (Barkovich 2005). The mesencephalic tectum is often distorted and is described on sagittal CT and MRI as 'beaking' of the tectum (Fig. 13.1). It occurs in 75% of CM2 patients, being more prominent as the age of the affected children increases and with more extensive MMC (Fletcher et al. 2004).

The cerebellum

The inferior vermis often herniates down to the upper cervical vertebrae (Fig. 13.1). The cerebellum wraps around the brainstem (Fig. 13.2). The superior part of the cerebellar vermis is displaced upwards. Other anomalies include dysplasia and low insertion of the tentorium cerebelli, cerebellar dysplasia, and agenesis or hypoplasia of the lateral cerebellar hemispheres (Gilbert et al. 1986; Harding and Copp 2002; Barkovich 2005; Juranek and Salman 2010).

TABLE 13.1
Characteristic features of Chiari type II malformation

A) Brainstem and cerebellum

1. Tectal beaking
2. Inferior displacement of the lower brainstem
3. Medullary-cervical kink
4. Aqueduct compression or stenosis
5. Inferior displacement of a small fourth ventricle
6. Enlargement of foramen magnum
7. Small posterior fossa size
8. Decreased cerebellar weight
9. Reduced cerebellar volume, especially the cerebellar hemispheres
10. Wrapping of the cerebellar hemispheres around the brainstem
11. Expanded midsagittal vermis area, including lobules I–V and VI–VII areas due to compression
12. Vermis (and tonsils) herniation below foramen magnum
13. Upward displacement of the superior vermis
14. Enlarged tentorium incisura
15. Dysplastic tentorium cerebelli and low insertion

B) Supratentorial structures, spinal cord, and cranium

1. Dilated lateral ventricles/hydrocephalus
2. Agenesis or hypoplasia of the corpus callosum
3. Thickening of the frontal cortical regions
4. Thinning of the posterior cortical regions
5. Disorganized white matter tracts in the long association pathways linking the posterior brain regions to the anterior brain regions
6. Abnormal gyration and interdigitation of the neocortex
7. Neuronal heterotopias
8. Enlarged massa intermedia
9. Total or partial absence of the septum pellucidum
10. Fenestration of the falx
11. Hydromyelia
12. Tethered spinal cord
13. Lower or upper spinal cord lesion as part of the myelomeningocele
14. Lacunar fenestrated skull (Luckenschadel)

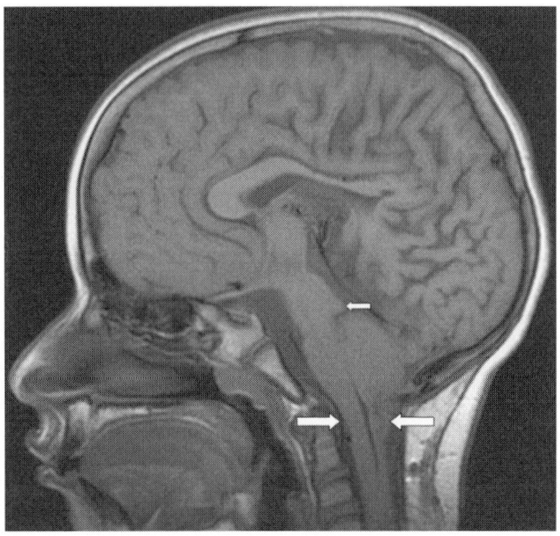

Fig. 13.1. T1-weighted midsagittal MRI (TR 410.0ms, TE 14.0ms) in a patient with Chiari type II malformation illustrating herniation of the inferior vermis and lower brainstem (large arrows), tectal beaking (small arrow), small posterior fossa, and abnormal posterior corpus callosum.

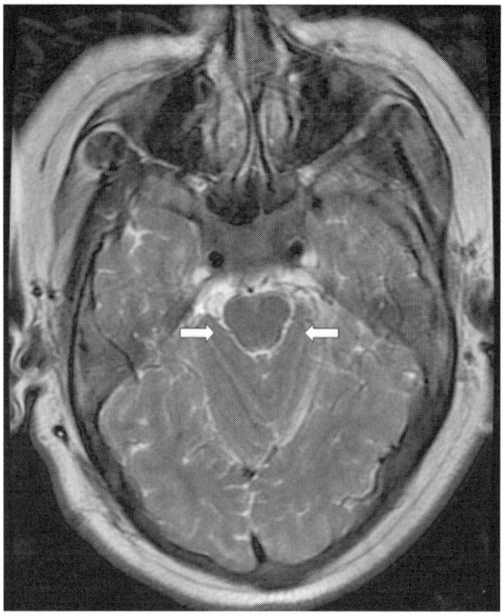

Fig. 13.2. T2-weighted axial MRI (TR 2500.0ms, TE 112.3ms) in a patient with Chiari type II malformation at the junction of the pons and midbrain illustrating wrapping of the cerebellum around the brainstem (arrows).

A study reported a reduction in the number of cells and DNA content involving the inferior more than the central vermis lobules in children with spina bifida (Emery and Gadsdon 1975). The herniated cerebellar tissue shows granule and Purkinje cell loss, reduction and gliosis of the folia, and myelin depletion (Harding and Copp 2002).

Reduced cerebellar size in CM2 has been reported in several studies. This reduction in size may occur earlier during pregnancy (Brocklehurst 1969; Hori 2002). Significant reduction in cerebellar weight was found in children with spina bifida who died within 4 weeks of birth (Variend and Emery 1973). Subsequent degeneration of the whole cerebellum, also referred to as 'vanishing cerebellum', and asymmetric reduction in cerebellar hemispheres on MRI have also been reported in children with CM2 (Sener 1995; Boltshauser et al. 2002).

Smaller cerebellar volumes were reported in children with MMC using MRI volumetric analysis (Dennis et al. 2004). The study also reported that the cerebellar gray and white matter volumes were reduced, especially in children with high spinal lesion levels. Similar findings were reported subsequently and correlated with neurobehavioral outcomes in 268 children with MMC (Fletcher et al. 2005). Upper spinal lesions in MMC are a marker of more severe brain dysmorphology, and are associated with poorer cognitive and behavioral outcomes (Fletcher et al. 2005). A recent MRI study on CM2 using cerebellar parcellation reported a smaller absolute volume and volume fraction of the inferior posterior cerebellar lobes and a larger absolute volume and volume fraction of the anterior lobes in CM2 in comparison with normal controls, despite an overall reduction in cerebellar size in CM2 patients (Dennis et al. 2009a; Juranek et al. 2010). The small cerebellar size has been blamed on tissue crowding and compression leading to parenchymal cerebellar loss. Compression may be exacerbated by the effects of hydrocephalus.

Wide variation in CM2 deformity has been reported on shape analyses (Tsai et al. 2002). Genetic and environmental factors may contribute to this variation including spinal lesion level, posterior fossa size, hydrocephalus severity, and subsequent need for shunt revisions. Age, sex, and head size do not appear to be important contributors to the cerebellar shape or size variability in CM2 (Tsai et al. 2002; Salman et al. 2006a).

Linear measurements and planimetry (area measurements) of the posterior fossa and its contents have been reported in CM2 to quantify abnormalities and predict function or prognosis. Longitudinal and transverse distances across the midsagittal vermis showed expansion, not reduction, in length in CM2 in comparison to age-matched controls (Salman et al. 2006a). Furthermore, a significant increase in midsagittal vermis area in CM2 compared to the normal vermis has been reported on MRI (Salman et al. 2006a). Midsagittal anterior, posterior, and inferior vermis lobules areas were each larger in patients with CM2 than in age-matched controls. The 25% increase in mean vermis area occurred despite a 9% reduction in posterior fossa area on midsagittal MRI (Salman et al. 2006a). The most likely explanation is vermis compression caused by tissue crowding (Salman et al. 2006a; Salman 2008). Expansion of the anterior vermis lobules is likely to be related to the larger size of the anterior cerebellar lobes reported recently in CM2 (Juranek et al. 2010).

Therefore, the reduction in cerebellar volume in CM2 is not uniform and involves the cerebellar hemispheres more because they have no place for expansion and growth within the confines of small posterior fossa, whereas the vermis is displaced upwards, downwards, and in a ventral-dorsal direction, thus preserving some of its functions (Salman 2008; Salman et al. 2009).

Supratentorial structures, spinal cord, and cranium

Brainstem and cerebellar herniation obstructs cerebrospinal fluid (CSF) outflow from the fourth ventricle and causes hydrocephalus in MMC (Sutton et al. 1999). Hydrocephalus may also occur, secondary to aqueduct compression or stenosis (Gilbert et al. 1986; Wagner et al. 2002). Hydrocephalus requiring CSF shunting occurs in 80–90% of neonates with MMC. However, more recent studies reported a shunt placement rate of 65% (Bowman et al. 2009). The reduced rate of shunting likely reflects the use of more stringent criteria for shunting because of the associated high rate of shunt-related complication (Bowman et al. 2009).

Other spinal cord and supratentorial anomalies associated with CM2 include hydromyelia (Fig. 13.3), tethered spinal cord, corpus callosum absence or hypogenesis (Fig. 13.1), cortical neuronal migration defects (heterotopias), interdigitation of the cortical gyri (Fig. 13.4), thalamic deformation, elongated cranial nerves, hypoplasia or aplasia of the cranial nerve nuclei, and septum pellucidum (Gilbert et al. 1986; Harding and Copp 2002; Barkovich 2005). More recently, abnormalities in the

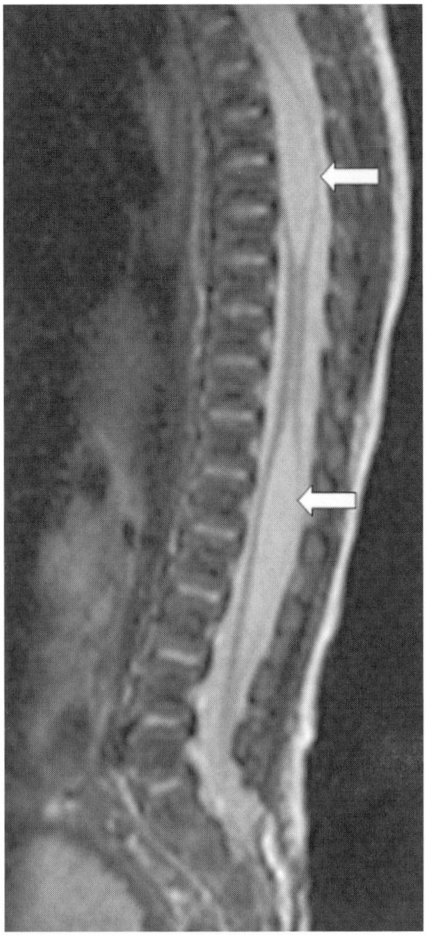

Fig. 13.3. T2-weighted sagittal MRI (TR 2350.0ms, TE 96.0ms) in a patient with Chiari type II malformation illustrating hydromyelia of the spinal cord (arrows).

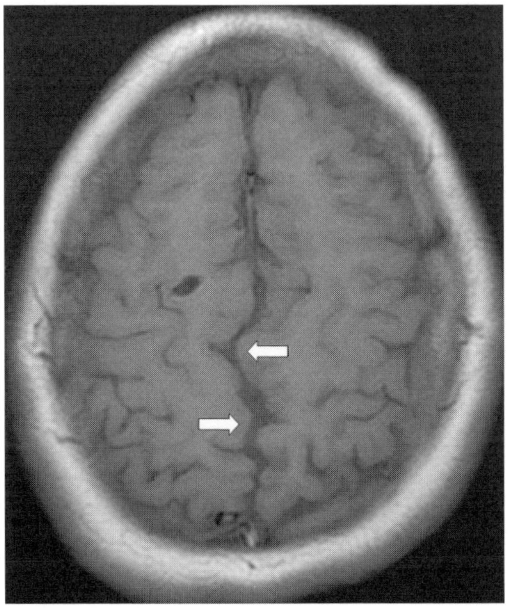

Fig. 13.4. T1-weighted axial MRI (TR 466.7ms, TE 14.0ms) in a patient with Chiari type II malformation at a level superior to the centrum semiovale illustrating fenestration of the interhemispheric falx and interdigitation of the parasagittal gyri (arrows).

cerebral hemispheres were reported on diffusion tensor tractography with thickening of the frontal cortical regions, thinning of the posterior cortical regions, abnormal gyrification, disruption of myelination, reduction in the total white matter volume, microstructural white matter abnormalities in the association pathways, and increased thickness of the anterior commissure (Hasan et al. 2008a, 2008b; Juranek et al. 2008; Herweh et al. 2009; Juranek and Salman 2010).

Secondary dysmorphologies also occur in CM2, some related to increased intracranial pressure (Fletcher et al. 2004; Barkovich 2005). These include secondary atrophy of the corpus callosum, compression of the diencephalon, and defects of the optic pathways. Luckenschadel (lacunar skull deformity) is associated with CM2 and MMC, where the fetal skull appears fenestrated (Vigliani 2008).

Clinical presentation

Ventricular dilatation occurs in the majority of neonates with CM2 and many develop hydrocephalus requiring shunting soon after birth. Therefore, an abnormally dilated fontanel accompanied by a rapid increase in head size should be looked for in neonates with MMC. The same signs may be present when shunt obstruction occurs in infancy prior to closure of the fontanels.

Intrinsic brainstem abnormalities, pressure on the brainstem from a crowded posterior fossa, and hydrocephalus cause diverse findings such as headaches, apnea, bradycardia, dysphagia, torticollis, and spasticity (Tubbs and Oakes 2004). Brainstem compression may occur in up to a third of patients with CM2, and may be fatal in a small proportion (Stevenson 2004).

Attention-deficit-hyperactivity disorder and seizures occur more commonly in patients with CM2 due to the multiple brain anomalies (McLone and Dias 2003; Fletcher et al. 2005). Upper limb motor dysfunction usually appears in late infancy or childhood (Jewell et al. 2009) and persists in young adults with MMC (Dennis et al. 2009b). Ataxia, weakness, and pyramidal tract dysfunction of the upper limbs occur to varying degrees (Wallace, 1973; Dennis et al. 2009b). Abnormal motor function of the lower limbs and impaired ambulation is mainly influenced by the spinal cord lesion rather than CM2.

Motor speech deficits, dysfunction in the speed and accuracy of rhythm perception, cognitive dysfunction, perceptual and motor timing deficits have been reported in children with MMC (Huber-Okrainec et al. 2002; Dennis et al. 2004, 2009a; Dennis and Barnes 2010). Several of these abnormalities were postulated to be the result of the cerebellar deformity of CM2, based on the increasing evidence for the role of the cerebellum in timing motor and cognitive functions (Salman 2002).

Ophthalmological problems occur commonly in patients with MMC and many are related to the hydrocephalus. Severe visual acuity impairment, cortical blindness, and optic atrophy are rarely seen nowadays because of improvement in the management of hydrocephalus (Biglan 1990; Caines et al. 2007). The visual and neuro-ophthalmological abnormalities include refractive errors, strabismus, and eye movement abnormalities, for example, impaired smooth ocular pursuit, saccadic dysmetria, impaired performance of the vestibular-ocular reflex, several types of pathological nystagmus such as gaze-evoked nystagmus and downbeat nystagmus, and internuclear ophthalmoplegia (Biglan 1990; Lennerstrand et al. 1990; Leigh and Zee 2006; Caines et al. 2007). Midsagittal vermis expansion, including the significant expansion of vermis lobules VI–VII area and preserved medial cerebellar volume corresponded to sparing of eye movements processed by the vermis, namely saccadic amplitude accuracy and smooth ocular pursuit (Salman et al. 2005, 2007) despite the overall reduction in cerebellar size in CM2. There is evidence for functional ocular motor circuits in many patients with CM2. For example, saccadic adaptation, a form of cerebellar ocular motor learning, still occurs in CM2 despite the cerebellar abnormalities (Salman et al. 2006b, 2009). Furthermore, other types of cerebellar motor learning have also been reported to be normal in patients with CM2, including adaptation on reaching or ballistic movements, mirror drawing performance, and weight judgments (Colvin et al. 2003; Edelstein et al. 2004; Dennis et al. 2006). Table 13.2 summarizes the clinical presentation of CM2.

Several factors need to be considered when clinical progression occurs in children with MMC, for example, shunt malfunction, the development of spinal or bulbar hydromyelia, tethered spinal cord or the presence of an unrelated neurological disorder. Neuroradiological progression can occur in CM2 in the absence of any obvious cause, as suggested by the 'vanishing cerebellum' described on MRI (Boltshauser et al. 2002) and anatomic changes in CM2 and the skull base as measured on MRI (Ruge et al. 1992).

Investigations

Elevated maternal serum alpha-fetoprotein between 15 and 20 weeks' gestation is usually indicative of open neural tube defects such as MMC. Antenatal fetal ultrasonography and MRI can be reliably used to diagnose CM2 (Fujisawa et al. 2006; Papadias et al. 2008). They may also reveal the spinal abnormality.

TABLE 13.2
Summary of symptoms and signs associated with Chiari type II malformation

1.	Apnea, stridor, bradycardia, dysphagia, torticollis, and nystagmus caused by brainstem dysfunction
2.	Enlarged head size in infancy, headache, nausea, vomiting, blurred vision, and reduced level of consciousness related to raised intracranial pressure from hydrocephalus or CSF shunt malfunction
3.	Cognitive deficits within some domains including perception, language, literacy, and numeracy
4.	Speech abnormalities
5.	Saccadic smooth pursuit, saccadic dysmetria, several types of nystagmus, strabismus, internuclear ophthalmoplegia, and rarely abnormalities of the visual pathways
6.	Attention-deficit hyperactivity disorder
7.	Seizures
8.	Sleep problems
9.	Spasticity, weakness, and ataxia of the upper limbs
10.	Limbs pain, sensory loss, weakness, or spasticity related to hydromyelia
11.	Scoliosis
12.	Lower limbs weakness and absent sensation, neuropathic bowel and bladder, and skin sores related to the myelomeningocele

Postnatal head ultrasound is used to assess and follow up the ventriculomegaly. Brain and spinal MRI are usually performed in the neonatal period to evaluate the hydrocephalus, features of CM2, assess the extent and level of the spinal lesion, and look for evidence of other abnormalities including a lipoma and tethered spinal cord. Brain and spinal MRI is also useful in infancy and childhood to look for causes of clinical progression such as tethered spinal cord and bulbar or spinal hydromyelia.

Auditory evoked potentials may be useful for the evaluation of brainstem function in patients with CM2 (Henriques-Filho and Pratesi 2006). Sleep studies should be considered if sleep difficulties, snoring, and apnea occur.

Management

Management of CM2 should take place in a multidisciplinary setting because the medical, surgical, and psychological needs of the patients and their families are complex due to the chronic and multiple disabilities (Olsson et al. 2007). There are no widely accepted standards or guidelines for the management of CM2 because studies published on the treatment of this malformation are retrospective and limited by the small number of patients (Tubbs and Oakes 2004).

Prevention

Prevention of CM2 has been achieved indirectly by the prevention of MMC. Food fortification with folic acid and folic acid supplementation during pregnancy led to further reduction in the incidence of MMC in the 1990s (Mills and Signore 2004; Bowman et al. 2009). Antenatal diagnosis of MMC and termination of pregnancy has also reduced the incidence of MMC (Bowman et al. 2009). Fetal surgery to repair the MMC has decreased the prevalence of hindbrain herniation on follow-up (Sutton et al. 1999).

Surgical management

Fetal surgical repair of the MMC has been shown to normalize the reduced subarachnoid extra-axial supratentorial and posterior fossa CSF spaces on postnatal MRI (Danzer et al. 2007). However, the authors also reported the persistence of an abnormally reduced brain thickness and cerebellar width on postnatal MRI in all neonates with MMC irrespective of whether the surgery to close their spinal defect was performed in utero or soon after birth (Danzer et al. 2007). It appears that the brain abnormalities in MMC occur early in utero (and prior to fetal surgical repair) and persist in the neonatal period. However, fetal surgery for MMC may reduce the incidence and severity of brainstem dysfunction (Danzer et al. 2008).

CSF shunting is usually performed during the neonatal period to reduce the adverse effects of hydrocephalus on the developing brain. Surgical decompression of the posterior fossa for neonates and infants with MMC who develop symptoms and signs of brainstem compression is required in 8–17% (Wagner et al. 2002). The surgery is effective and can be life saving (Pollack et al. 1992). Symptomatic and progressive hydromyelia is also treated surgically (La Marca et al. 1997) as is symptomatic tethered spinal cord, which usually present with pain, spasticity, and worsening lower limb function. Orthopedic surgery is helpful in certain circumstances, for example, in symptomatic or progressive scoliosis, tendon release for spasticity, or for hip dislocation. Strabismus surgery may be considered for significant ocular misalignment.

Medical management

This mainly involves the treatment of associated conditions such as seizures with anti-seizure medication and severe spasticity with baclofen or diazepam. Routine follow-up to look for evidence of clinical progression involving the brain (for example, disc edema from subacute shunt malfunction or torticollis from brainstem compression) or the spine (for example, upper limb weakness) is important.

Supportive management

This revolves around the patient and family education and ongoing psychological support. Physical therapy, occupational therapy, speech therapy and orthotist assessments form an integral part of managing patients with MMC and CM2. Arrangements should be made for educational support at school and vocational training for these patients.

Prognosis

Survival of patients with MMC and CM2 has improved markedly since the introduction of CSF shunting procedures in the 1960s. Before that time most patients died during childhood. Further improvement in survival and quality of life has followed due to advances in shunting technology over the last 50 years. Posterior fossa decompression has also contributed to improved survival beyond infancy.

The survival rate is 39% in patients born between 1963 and 1971 in the UK (Oakeshott et al. 2009), and 74% in patients born between 1975 and 1979 in the USA (Bowman et al. 2009). Causes of mortality nowadays are mostly related to renal failure or sepsis, shunt malfunction, epilepsy, and pulmonary embolus (Bowman et al. 2009).

Survivors appear to have a better quality of life in general; however, they have multiple and complex medical needs. Permanent motor impairment leading to compromised motor independence and cognitive dysfunction are two important causes of chronic disability in patients with MMC and CM2 that can impact negatively on their social functioning, employment opportunities, and quality of life in society (Fletcher et al. 2004).

The future

More longitudinal clinical and neuroradiological studies in patients with CM2 are needed to better understand the natural history of MMC and CM2, as prognosis continues to improve. The short- and long-term impact of fetal MMC repair requires continued evaluation. Multicenter trials investigating the best treatment options and their timing for dilated ventricles/hydrocephalus, posterior fossa decompression, and hydromyelia should be undertaken (Tubbs and Oakes 2004). Further research in CM2 using functional MRI, diffusion tensor imaging, and magnetoencephalographic imaging will also further our knowledge of this intriguing brain malformation.

Since patients with CM2 have multiple chronic medical issues, better transition to adult medical and surgical specialists needs to be planned and organized by health authorities (Tubbs and Oakes 2004), especially as most of these patients are surviving into adulthood (Bowman et al. 2009).

Summary

Chiari type II malformation is a congenital deformity of the brainstem, cerebellum, and cervical spine that occurs in people with myelomeningocele. There is reduction in cerebellar size likely resulting from crowding of tissue within the small posterior fossa and subsequent atrophy. Hydrocephalus and several supratentorial anomalies occur commonly in CM2. Brainstem, cognitive, speech, eye movement, and upper limb motor functions may be impaired in CM2. The management of patients with MMC and CM2 should be undertaken in a multidisciplinary setting and includes supportive, medical, and surgical treatments for the spinal cord defect and associated abnormalities.

REFERENCES

Arnett B (2003) Arnold-Chiari malformation. Arch Neurol 60: 898–900.

Arnold J (1894) Myelocyste, Transposition von Gewebskeimen und Sympodie. Beitr Pathol Anat 16: 1–28.

Barkovich J (2005) Pediatric Neuroimaging. Philadelphia, PA: Lippincott, Williams & Wilkins.

Biglan AW (1990) Ophthalmological Complications of Meningomyelocele: A longitudinal study. Trans Am Ophthalmol Soc 88: 389–462.

Boltshauser E, Schneider J, Kollias S, Waibel P, Weissert M (2002) Vanishing cerebellum in myelomeningocoele. Eur J Paediatr Neurol 6: 109–113.

Bowman RM, Boshnjaku V, McLone DG (2009) The changing incidence of myelomeningocele and its impact on pediatric neurosurgery: a review from the Children's Memorial Hospital. Childs Nerv Syst 25: 801–806.

Brocklehurst G (1969) A quantitative study of a spina bifida foetus. J Pathol 99: 205–211.

Bruner JP, Tulipan N, Paschall RL, Boehm FH, Walsh WF, Silva SR, et al. (1999) Fetal surgery for myelomeningocele and the incidence of shunt-dependent hydrocephalus. JAMA 282: 1819–1825.

Caines E, Dahl M, Holmström G (2007) Longterm oculomotor and visual function in spina bifida cystica: a population-based study. Acta Ophthalmol Scand 85(6): 662–666.

Chiari H (1891) Ueber Veranderungen des Kleinhirns infolge von Hydrocephalie des Grosshirns. Dtsch Med Wochenschr 17: 1172–1175.

Chiari H (1896) Uber Veranderungen des Kleinhirns, des pons und der Medulla oblongata infolge von congenitaler Hydrocephalie des Grosshirns. Denkschr der kais Akad Wiss Wien mathnaturw 63: 71–116.

Cleland J (1883) Contributions to the study of spina bifida, encephalocoele, and anencephalus. J Anat Physiol 17: 257–291.

Colvin AN, Yeates KO, Enrile BG, Coury DL (2003) Motor adaptation in children with myelomeningocele: Comparison to children with ADHD and healthy siblings. J Int Neuropsychol Soc 9: 642–652.

Cruveilhier LJB (1829–1842) L'Anatomie pathologique du corps humain, ou description, avec figures lithographi'ees et colori'ees, des diverses alterations morbides dont le corps humain est susceptible. 2 vol. Paris: JB Baillière.

Danzer E, Johnson MP, Bebbington M, Simon EM, Wilson RD, Bilaniuk LT, et al. (2007) Fetal head biometry assessed by fetal magnetic resonance imaging following in utero myelomeningocele repair. Fetal Diagn Ther 22: 1–6.

Danzer E, Finkel RS, Rintoul NE, Bebbington MW, Schwartz ES, Zarnow DM, et al. (2008) Reversal of hindbrain herniation after maternal-fetal surgery for myelomeningocele subsequently impacts on brain stem function. Neuropediatr 39: 359–362.

de Wit OA, den Dunnen WF, Sollie KM, Muñoz RI, Meiners LC, Brouwer OF, et al. (2008) Pathogenesis of cerebral malformations in human fetuses with meningomyelocele. Cerebrospinal Fluid Res 5: 4.

Dennis M, Edelstein K, Hetherington R, Copeland K, Frederick J, Blaser SE, et al. (2004) Neurobiology of perceptual and motor timing in children with spina bifida in relation to cerebellar volume. Brain 127: 1–10.

Dennis M, Jewell D, Edelstein K, Brandt ME, Hetherington R, Blaser SE, Fletcher JM (2006) Motor learning in children with spina bifida: Intact learning and performance on a ballistic task. J Int Neuropsychol Soc 12: 598–608.

Dennis M, Hopyan T, Juranek J, Cirino PT, Hasan KM, Fletcher J (2009a) Strong-meter and weak-meter rhythm identification in spina bifida meningomyelocele and volumetric parcellation of rhythm-relevant cerebellar regions. Ann N Y Acad Sci 1169: 84–88.

Dennis M, Salman MS, Jewell D, Hetherington R, Spiegler BJ, MacGregor DL, et al. (2009b) Upper limb motor function in young adults with spina bifida and hydrocephalus. Childs Nerv Syst 25: 1447–1453.

Dennis M, Barnes MA (2010) The cognitive phenotype of spina bifida meningomyelocele. Dev Disabil Res Rev 16: 31–39.

Edelstein K, Dennis M, Copeland K, Frederick J, Francis D, Hetherington R, et al. (2004) Motor learning in children with spina bifida: Dissociation between performance level and acquisition rate. J Int Neuropsychol Soc 10: 877–887.

Emery JL, Gadsdon DR (1975) A quantitative study of the cell population of the cerebellum in children with myelomeningocele. Dev Med Child Neurol 15 (Suppl 29): 20–25.

Fletcher JM, Dennis M, Northrup H, Barnes MA, Hannay HJ, Landry S, et al. (2004) Spina bifida: Genes, brain, and development. Int Rev Res Ment Retard 29: 63–117.

Fletcher JM, Copeland K, Frederick JA, Blaser SE, Kramer LA, Northrup H, et al. (2005) Spinal lesion level in spina bifida: a source of neural and cognitive heterogeneity. J Neurosurg Pediatrics 102 (3 suppl): 268–279.

Fujisawa H, Kitawaki J, Iwasa K, Honjo H (2006) New ultrasonographic criteria for the prenatal diagnosis of Chiari type 2 malformation. Acta Obstetricia et Gynecologica 85: 1426–1429.

Gardner E, O'Rahilly R, Prolo D (1975) The Dandy-Walker and Arnold-Chiari malformations. Clinical, developmental, and teratological considerations. Arch Neurol 32: 393–407.

Gilbert JN, Jones KL, Rorke LB, Chernoff GF, James HE (1986) Central nervous system anomalies associated with meningomyelocele, hydrocephalus, and the Arnold-Chiari malformation: reappraisal of theories regarding the pathogenesis of posterior neural tube closure defects. Neurosurgery 18: 559–564.

Griffiths PD, Wilkinson ID, Variend S, Jones A, Paley MN, Whitby E (2004) Differential growth rates of the cerebellum and posterior fossa assessed by post mortem magnetic resonance imaging of the fetus: Implications for the pathogenesis of the Chiari 2 deformity. Acta Radiol 45: 236–242.

Harding BN, Copp AJ (2002) Malformations. In: Greenfield's Neuropathology (eds DI Graham, PL Lantos). London: Edward Arnold; 376–386.

Hasan K, Eluvathingal T, Kramer LA, Ewing-Cobbs L, Dennis M, Fletcher JM (2008a) White matter microstructural abnormalities in children with spina bifida myelomeningocele and hydrocephalus: a diffusion tensor tractography study of the association pathways. J Magn Reson Imaging 27: 700–709.

Hasan KM, Sankar A, Halphen C, Kramer LA, Ewing-Cobbs L, Dennis M, Fletcher JM (2008b) Quantitative diffusion tensor imaging and intellectual outcomes in spina bifida: laboratory investigation. J Neurosurg Pediatr 2: 75–82.

Henriques Filho PS, Pratesi R (2006) Abnormalities in auditory evoked potentials of 75 patients with Arnold-Chiari malformations types I and II. Arq Neuropsiquiatr 64(3A): 619–623.

Herweh C, Akbar M, Wengenroth M, Blatow M, Mair-Walther J, Rehbein N, et al. (2009) DTI of commissural fibers in patients with Chiari II-malformation. Neuroimage 44: 306–311.

Hori A (2002) Chiari anomaly type II without cerebellar herniation. Acta Neuropathologica 105: 193–194.

Huber-Okrainec J, Dennis M, Brettschneider J, Spiegler BJ (2002) Neuromotor speech deficits in children and adults with spina bifida and hydrocephalus. Brain Lang 80: 592–602.

Jewell D, Fletcher J, Mahy CE, Hetherington R, MacGregor D, Drake JM, et al. (2009) Upper limb cerebellar motor function in children with spina bifida. Childs Nerv Syst 26: 67–73.

Juranek J, Fletcher JM, Hasan KM, Breier JI, Cirino PT, Pazo-Alvarez P, et al. (2008) Neocortical reorganization in spina bifida. Neuroimage 40: 1516–1522.

Juranek J, Dennis M, Cirino PT, El-Messidi L, Fletcher JM (2010) The cerebellum in children with spina bifida and Chiari II malformation: quantitative volumetrics by region. Cerebellum 9: 240–248.

Juranek J, Salman MS (2010) Anomalous development of brain structure and function in spina bifida myelomeningocele. Dev Disabil Res Rev 16: 23–30.

La Marca F, Herman M, Grant JA, McLone DG (1997) Presentation and management of hydromyelia in children with Chiari type-II malformation. Pediatr Neurosurg 26: 57–67.

Leigh RJ, Zee DS (2006) The neurology of eye movements, 4th edition. New York: Oxford University Press.

Lennerstrand G, Gallo JE, Samuelsson L (1990) Neuro-ophthalmological findings in relation to CNS lesions in patients with myelomeningocele. Dev Med Child Neurol 32: 423–431.

Marín-Padilla M (1991) Cephalic axial skeletal-neural dysraphic disorders: embryology and pathology. Can J Neurol Sci 18(2): 153–169.

McLone DG, Knepper PA (1989) The cause of Chiari II malformation: a unified theory. Pediatr Neurosci 15: 1–12.

McLone DG, Dias MS (2003) The Chiari II malformation: cause and impact. Childs Nerv Syst 19: 540–550.

Mills JL, Signore C (2004) Neural tube defect rates before and after food fortification with folic acid. Birth Defects Res A Clin Mol Teratol 70: 844–845.

Oakeshott P, Hunt GM, Poulton A, Reid F (2009) Expectation of life and unexpected death in open spina bifida: a 40-year complete, non-selective, longitudinal cohort study. Dev Med Child Neurol 2009 52: 749–753.

Olsson I, Dahl M, Mattsson S, Wendelius M, Aström E, Westbom L (2007) Medical problems in adolescents with myelomeningocele (MMC): an inventory of the Swedish MMC population born during 1986–1989. Acta Paediatr 96: 446–449.

Papadias A, Miller C, Martin WL, Kilby MD, Sgouros S (2008) Comparison of prenatal and postnatal MRI findings in the evaluation of intrauterine CNS anomalies requiring postnatal neurosurgical treatment. Childs Nerv Syst 24: 185–192.

Pearce JMS (2000) Arnold Chiari, or 'Cruveilhier Cleland Chiari' malformation. J Neurol Neurosurg Psychiatry 68: 13–16.

Pollack IF, Pang D, Albright AL, Krieger D (1992) Outcome following hindbrain decompression of symptomatic Chiari malformations in children previously treated with myelomeningocele closure and shunts. J Neurosurg 77: 881–888.

Ruge JR, Masciopinto J, Storrs BB, McLone DG (1992) Anatomical progression of the Chiari II malformation. Childs Nerv Syst 8: 86–91.

Salman MS (2002) The cerebellum: it's about time! But timing is not everything: New insights into the role of the cerebellum in timing motor and cognitive tasks. J Child Neurol 17: 1–9.

Salman MS, Sharpe JA, Eizenman M, Lillakas L, To T, Westall C, et al. (2005) Saccades in children with spina bifida and Chiari type II malformation. Neurology 64: 2098–2101.

Salman MS, Blaser SE, Sharpe JA, Dennis M (2006a) Cerebellar vermis morphology in children with spina bifida and Chiari type II malformation. Childs Nerv Syst 22: 385–393.

Salman MS, Sharpe JA, Eizenman M, Lillakas L, To T, Westall C, et al. (2006b) Saccadic adaptation in Chiari type II malformation. Can J Neurol Sci 33: 372–378.

Salman MS, Sharpe JA, Lillakas L, Steinbach MJ, Dennis M (2007) Smooth ocular pursuit in Chiari type II malformation. Dev Med Child Neurol 49: 289–293.

Salman MS (2008) The cerebellum in Chiari type II malformation. Neuroembryol Aging 5: 14–22.

Salman MS, Dennis M, Sharpe JA (2009) The cerebellar dysplasia of Chiari II malformation as revealed by eye movements. Can J Neurol Sci 36: 713–724.

Sarnat HB (2000) Molecular genetic classification of central nervous system malformations. J Child Neurol 15: 675–687.

Sener RN (1995) Cerebellar agenesis versus vanishing cerebellum in Chiari II malformation. Comput Med Imaging Graph 19: 491–494.

Stevenson KL (2004) Chiari Type II malformation: Past, present, and future. Neurosurg Focus 16(2): E5.

Sutton LN, Adzick NS, Bilaniuk LT, Johnson MP, Crombleholme TM, Flake AW (1999) Improvement in hindbrain herniation demonstrated by serial fetal magnetic resonance imaging following fetal surgery for myelomeningocele. JAMA 282: 1826–1831.

Tsai T, Bookstein FL, Levey E, Kinsman SL (2002) Chiari-II malformation: a biometric analysis. Eur J Pediatr Surg 12 (Suppl 1): S12–8.

Tubbs RS, Oakes WJ (2004) Treatment and management of the Chiari II malformation: an evidence-based review of the literature. Childs Nerv Syst 20: 375–381.

Tubbs RS, Shoja MM, Ardalan MR, Shokouhi G, Loukas M (2008) Hindbrain herniation: A review of embryological theories. Ital J Anat Embryol 113: 37–46.

Wagner W, Schwarz M, Perneczky A (2002) Primary myelomeningocele closure and consequences. Curr Opin Urol 12: 465–468.

Wallace SJ (1973) The effect of upper-limb function on mobility of children with myelomeningocele. Dev Med Child Neurol 15 (Supp 29): 84–91.

Williams H (2008) A unifying hypothesis for hydrocephalus, Chiari malformation, syringomyelia, anencephaly and spina bifida. Cerebrospinal Fluid Res 5: 7.

Variend S, Emery JL (1973) The weight of the cerebellum in children with myelomeningocele. Dev Med Child Neurol 15 (Suppl 29): 77–83.

Vigliani MB (2008) Luckenschadel skull: a forgotten entity. Obstet Gynecol 111(2 Pt 2): 562–565.

14 Cerebellar Dysplasia

Andrea Poretti and Eugen Boltshauser

The nomenclature of cerebellar dysplasia is inconsistent in the literature, and different terms have been used to describe this condition. Demaerel et al. (in their first reports) and Soto-Ares et al. used the term *cerebellar cortical dysplasia* (Demaerel et al. 1998, 1999; Soto-Ares et al. 2000, 2002). However, in his last review Demaerel changed the term to *abnormalities of cerebellar foliation and fissuration* (Demaerel 2002). Patel and Barkovich distinguished between diffuse cerebellar dysplasia as *diffuse dysplasia of the cerebellar cortex* (a descriptive term in contrast to known etiologies such as cerebellar dysplasia in lissencephalies, congenital muscular dystrophies, or prenatal cytomegalovirus infection) and focal dysplasia as *other focal dysplasias* (in contrast to well-known syndromes such as rhombencephalosynapsis or Joubert syndrome) (Patel and Barkovich 2002). In a recently published study Boddaert et al. referred to *hemispheric cerebellar dysgenesis* (Boddaert et al. 2010). The terms *cerebellar polymicrogyria* and *cerebellar polymicrophyllia* have also been proposed (Sasaki et al. 1997). However, because the cerebellum consists of folia and fissures instead of gyri and sulci, the term polymicrogyria is not semantically correct (Demaerel et al. 1999). The term polymicrophyllia is semantically correct, but not common and possibly ambiguous, and therefore should also be avoided (Barkovich 1997).

We prefer the term *cerebellar dysplasia*, implying a deranged development of the cerebellar tissue resulting in abnormal cerebellar foliation and fissuration (Demaerel 2002; Patel and Barkovich 2002). However, the abnormalities affect not only the cerebellar cortex (therefore we do not use *cerebellar cortical dysplasia*), but also the architecture of the cerebellar white matter as abnormal arborization of the cerebellar white matter and/or irregular cerebellar gray-white matter junction.

Cerebellar dysplasia includes a heterogeneous spectrum of different neuroimaging findings, clinical presentations, and etiologies leading to a purely descriptive definition.

Etiology and pathogenesis

The etiology of cerebellar dysplasia is heterogeneous and different causes, both genetic and acquired, are known. In most cases the etiology remains unknown (Boddaert et al. 2010).

Regarding genetic causes, Barkovich et al. hypothesized a defect in rhombomere 1 as causative for cerebellar heterotopia and foliation anomalies (Barkovich et al. 2009). However, the genes responsible have not yet been identified. Cerebellar dysplasia has been reported in congenital muscular dystrophies with defective dystroglycan *O*-glycosylation (CMD) such as Fukuyama congenital muscular dystrophy, Walker-Warburg syndrome, and muscle-eye-brain disease. Typical neuroimaging findings are disorderly alignment of the cerebellar folia, particularly in the midportion and dorsal surface of the hemispheres, and intraparenchymal subcortical cysts near the disorganized folia (Aida et al. 1994; Barkovich 1998; Clement et al. 2008). Cerebellar dysplasias have been described in chromosomal abnormalities (especially trisomy 13 with cerebellar heterotopia) (Rorke et al. 1968; Balci et al. 2008), in neurocutaneous syndromes such as PHACES syndrome (posterior fossa malformations, haemangiomas of the face, arterial anomalies, cardiac anomalies, eye abnormalities, and sternal clefting or supraumbilical raphe) (Rossi et al. 2001) or epidermal nevus syndrome (Pereira et al. 2009), and cerebellar malformations such as Joubert syndrome (Alorainy et al. 2006; Senocak et al. 2010) and Dandy-Walker malformation (Altman et al. 1992; Soto-Ares et al. 2000).

Cerebellar dysplasia can result from a prenatal cerebellar disruption. Prenatal infections (particularly congenital cytomegalovirus infection showing dysplastic cerebellar hemispheres with thin cerebellar cortex and shallow sulci, severe vermis hypoplasia, and not consistently cerebellar cortical calcifications) (Patel and Barkovich 2002), and exposure to gamma radiation (Inouye et al. 1992) and ethanol (Sakata-Haga et al. 2001; Soto-Ares et al. 2002) can cause generalized dysplasia of the cerebellar cortex. However, uni- or bilateral focal cerebellar dysplasia associated with a cerebellar cleft in one or both hemispheres may be the result of a prenatally acquired local event, mostly a haemorrhage (Poretti et al. 2008, 2009).

Cerebellar dysplasias are believed to arise from a genetic or environmental process affecting migration of Purkinje and granule cells, function of cellular and interstitial signaling that guide developing cells and axons, or both (Patel and Barkovich 2002). Migration and foliation occur at least in part simultaneously, and migration with an increase of cells represents the trigger for foliation (Demaerel 2002). Both Purkinje and external granular cells are involved in the foliation process (Voogd and Glickstein 1998). For example, aberrant migration and misorientation of the Purkinje cells in rats leads to an abnormal aggregation of granular cells and subsequently to abnormal cerebellar foliation (Demaerel 2002). Foliation is followed by fissuration. This explains why abnormal fissuration can be an isolated finding, while abnormalities of foliation are often associated with abnormal fissuration (Demaerel 2002). An important role in the foliation and lamination of the cerebellar cortex is also played by the meningeal cells: selective destruction of the leptomeninges has been shown to result in defective foliation, granule cell ectopia, and reduction in cerebellar size (Neumann et al. 1993).

Vermian and hemisphere dysplasia are closely related. The vermian and hemispheric parts of the anterior lobe develop together and the vermian foliation is in lateral continuity with the folia of the anterior lobe and of the first division of the posterior lobe (lobule VI) of both cerebellar hemispheres (Sasaki et al. 2001; Demaerel 2002). Therefore, dysplasia affecting the anterior vermian lobe extends to the cerebellar hemispheres (Demaerel et al. 1999). However, dysplasia in the posterior vermian lobe (caudal to the first division) occurs in isolation as well as dysplasia in the part of the posterior lobe of the cerebellar hemispheres, which are located caudally to lobule VI (the first division of the posterior lobe) (Sasaki et al. 2001). This is due to the noncontinuity of both vermian and hemispheric parts of the posterior lobes located caudally to the first division.

Clinical features

The clinical presentation of cerebellar dysplasia is highly variable, ranging from incidental finding without clinical relevance to multiple severe neurological impairments (Sekiguchi et al. 1998; Demaerel 2002). Frequent neurological findings include cognitive and motor developmental delay, cognitive impairment, speech and language disorders, muscular hypotonia, epileptic seizures, abnormal eye movements, and ataxia (Demaerel et al. 1999; Soto-Ares et al. 2000; Demaerel 2002). Cerebellar signs are associated with involvement of the cerebellar vermis, whereas patients with intact vermis do not show ataxia or ocular movement disorders (Demaerel et al. 1998, 1999; Demaerel 2002). The severity of the clinical symptoms seems to correlate with the degree of involvement of the cerebellum (Demaerel 2002). Mostly, isolated vermian abnormalities limited to malorientation of the fissures in the anterior lobe have been found as an incidental finding (for example, in children examined because of partial seizures or headaches) and are without clinical relevance (Demaerel 2002). All other abnormalities of foliation and fissuration are clinically significant to a variable degree. When present, supratentorial abnormalities typically dominate the clinical picture and the neurological disturbances are typically more severe. However, using positron emission tomography (PET) studies in two children with isolated cerebellar dysplasia, Jissendi Tchofo et al. demonstrated hypoperfusion and hypometabolism within the vermis, thalamus, and right striatum in one case, and hypometabolism in the basal ganglia and cerebellar deep gray nuclei in another case (Jissendi Tchofo et al. 2004). They hypothesized that these findings could explain the neurological symptoms, suggesting a pathological functional significance of cerebellar dysplasia.

Neuroimaging

The neuroimaging presentation of cerebellar dysplasia is highly variable. A classification of cerebellar dysplasia into subtypes from a neuroimaging point of view has been attempted by Demaerel (2002). Basically, this author distinguishes two types: type 1 involves the vermis (type 1a with abnormal fissuration only, or type 1b, associated with abnormal foliation); and type 2 involves the cerebellar hemispheres. They are variably associated with supratentorial abnormalities and have different clinical manifestations with more or less severe neurological impairments. Common sites of dysplasia are the vermis, nodulus, flocculus, and tonsils, but any portion of the cerebellar cortex may be affected (Demaerel et al. 1998). Abnormalities of foliation and fissuration are best seen on coronal T2-weighted images.

Abnormal foliation and fissuration including defective, enlarged, or vertical fissures represents the most common neuroimaging finding in cerebellar dysplasia (Figs 14.1b, 14.2a, 14.3b). Because foliation is embryologically followed by fissuration, abnormal fissuration can be an isolated finding, while irregular foliation is often associated with abnormal fissuration (Demaerel 2002). Localized fissural malorientation in the anterior lobe of the vermis can be isolated (corresponding to the type 1a in the classification of Demaerel) or associated with irregular foliation of the anterior and part of the posterior vermian lobe (type 1b) (Fig. 14.1b) (Demaerel 2002). Abnormalities of the cerebellar hemispheres (type 2) include irregular cerebellar gray-white matter junction, abnormal architecture of the cerebellar white matter, cortical thickening, aberrant orientation of the folia, and small cysts (Figs 14.1, 14.2, 14.3, 14.4) (Demaerel et al. 1998; Demaerel 2002). Type 1b changes in the vermis can be seen in more than 60% of hemispheric abnormalities. Cortical thickening results in an irregularly smooth cerebellar surface and can be focal or may diffusely involve both hemispheres (Demaerel et al. 1998; Demaerel 2002). The latter is frequent in prenatal infection and may be associated with subcortical calcification. Multiple, variably sized intra- or subcortical cysts can be present (Demaerel et al. 1998; Demaerel 2002). These are isointense with cerebraspinal fluid in all MRI sequences, preferentially involve the posterior portions of the cerebellar hemispheres and the upper part of the vermis, and are associated with absence of normal folia and fissures (Demaerel et al. 1998; Demaerel 2002). They likely represent remnants or sequelae of the migration of neurons forming the external granular layer of the cerebellar cortex at 11–13 weeks of gestation or remnants of daughter cells migrating inward to form part of the outer molecular layer and inner granular layer at 16 weeks (Demaerel et al. 1998). In cerebellar clefts, a form of prenatal cerebellar disruption, focal unilateral (or bilateral) cerebellar dysplasia including malorientation of the cerebellar folia, irregular gray-white matter junction, and abnormal architecture of the cerebellar white matter is confined only to the region adjacent to the cleft (Poretti et al. 2008, 2009).

Associated supratentorial abnormalities can be seen in more than 50% of the patients with cerebellar hemispheric abnormalities and occasionally in type 1b (Demaerel 2002). Supratentorial involvement is mostly bilateral and includes cerebral cortical dysplasia with irregular gray-white matter junction, polymicrogyria, subependymal nodular heterotopia, and agenesis or hypoplasia of the corpus callosum (Demaerel et al. 1998, 1999; Soto-Ares et al. 2000; Demaerel 2002; Srour

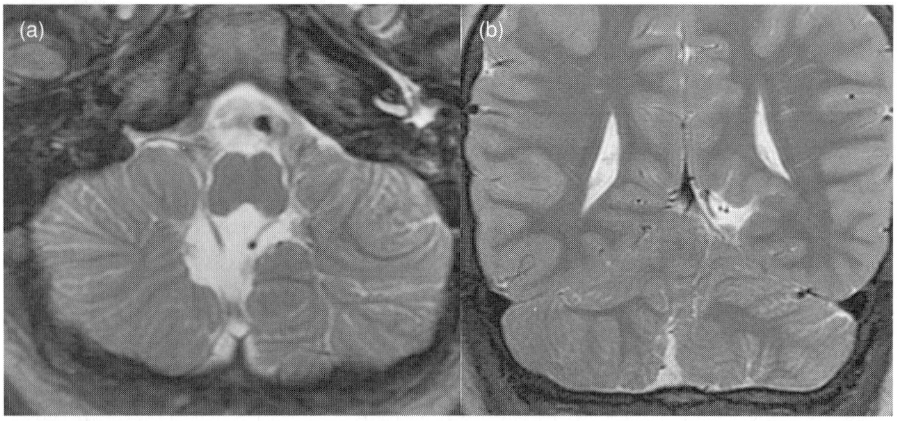

Fig. 14.1. Bilateral cerebellar dysplasia in an 11-year-old girl with severe congenital non-progressive ataxia, cognitive impairment, and bilateral periventricular nodular heterotopias (not shown) as well as temporal cortical dysplasia. **(a)** Axial T2-weighted MRI showing abnormal orientation of the cerebellar folia, irregular gray-white matter junction, abnormal cerebellar white-matter structure, and cortical thickening particularly in the left cerebellar hemisphere; **(b)** coronal T2-weighted MRI additionally demonstrating maloriented fissures and irregular foliation of the vermis as well as temporal cortical dysplasia.

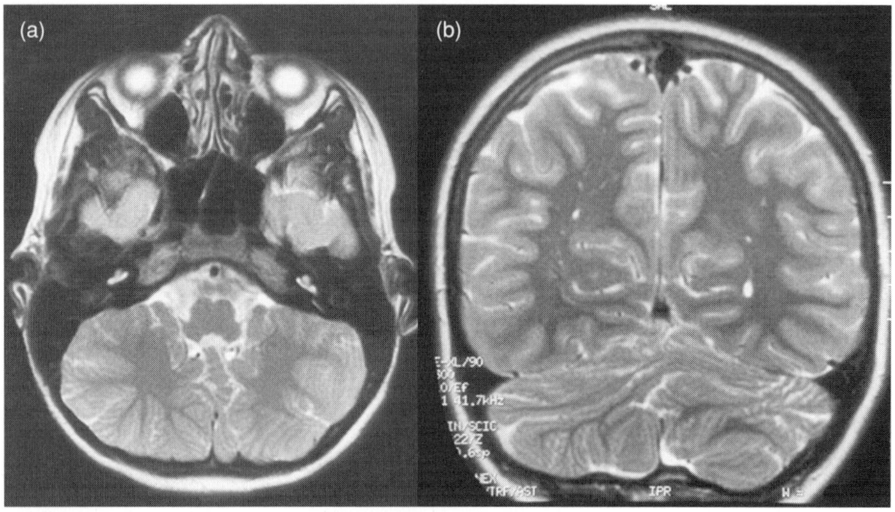

Fig. 14.2. Incidental finding of bilateral cerebellar dysplasia in a 9-year-old girl with benign paroxysmal vertigo and normal neurological examination. **(a)** Axial and **(b)** coronal T2-weighted MRI presenting abnormal orientation of the cerebellar folia, irregular gray-white matter junction, abnormal cerebellar white-matter structure, and cortical thickening particularly in the left cerebellar hemisphere and maloriented fissures of the vermis.

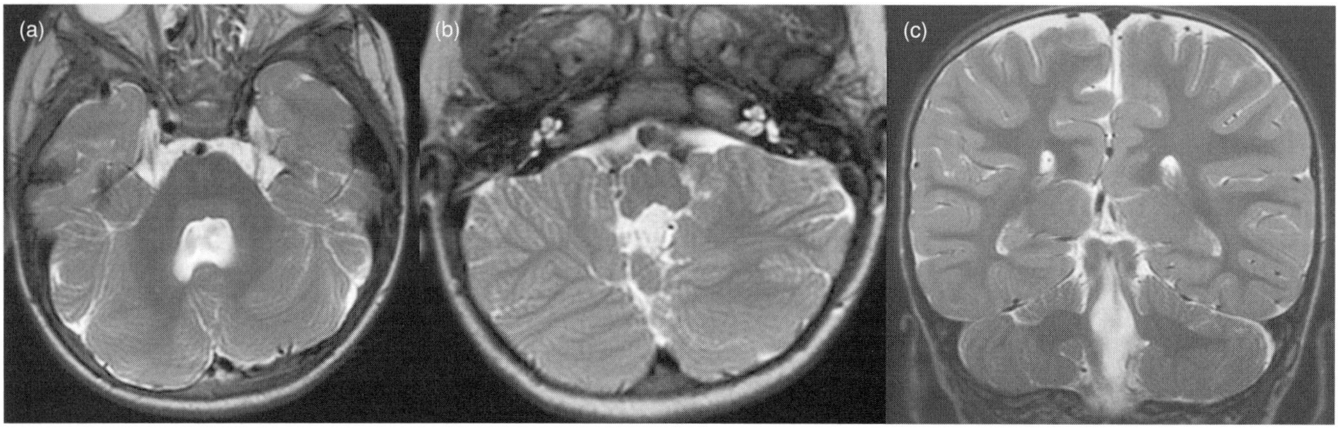

Fig. 14.3. Bilateral cerebellar dysplasia in a 2-year-old girl with craniofrontonasal dysplasia due to a mutation in the *EFNB1* gene and cognitive functions in the low normal range. **(a, b)** Axial and **(c)** coronal T2-weighted MRI revealing abnormal orientation of the cerebellar folia, irregular gray-white matter junction, abnormal cerebellar white-matter structure, and cortical thickening particularly in the left cerebellar hemisphere and maloriented fissures of the vermis.

et al. 2011). Ectopic neurohypophysis has been reported in a patient with unilateral cerebellar dysplasia and bilateral perisylvian polymicrogyria (Toldo et al. 2011).

Diagnosis

The diagnosis of cerebellar dysplasia depends on the neuroimaging appearance. If the diagnosis is suggestive, because of clinical presentation and additional neuroimaging findings, the underlying etiology, such as congenital muscular dystrophy or a congenital cytomegalovirus infection, has to be carefully sought.

Differential diagnosis

Vertical orientation of the cerebellar folia is occasionally associated with disorders characterized by severe vermian

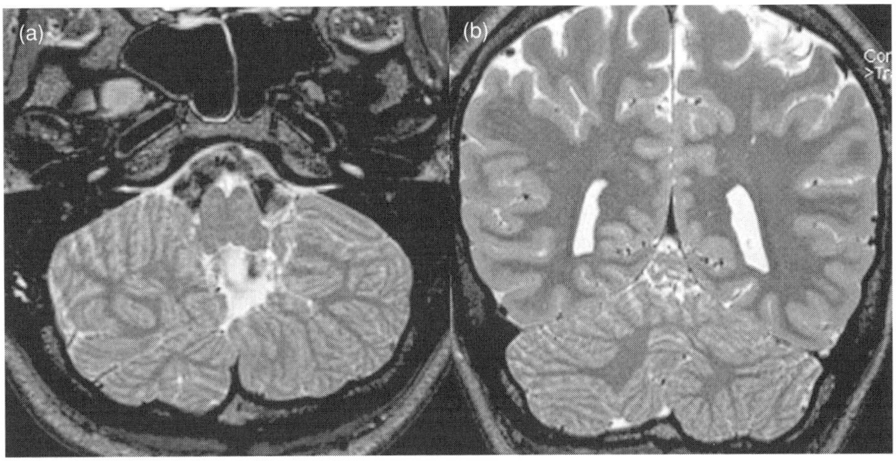

Fig. 14.4. Bilateral cerebellar cortical dysplasia in a 15-year-old girl with focal epileptic seizures **(a)** Axial and **(b)** coronal T2-weighted MRI showing abnormal orientation of the cerebellar folia, irregular gray-white matter junction, and abnormal cerebellar white-matter structure.

hypoplasia or agenesis, such as Joubert syndrome (Alorainy et al. 2006; Senocak et al. 2010), Dandy-Walker malformation (Altman et al. 1992; Soto-Ares et al. 2000), and congenital ocular motor apraxia (Cogan disease) (Sargent et al. 1997). Takanashi et al. reported vertically oriented cerebellar folia in the cerebellar hemispheres, hypoplastic cerebellar vermis, fusion of the inferior posterior cerebellum, and small cerebellar cysts in the superior cerebellar hemispheres in a child with hypotonia, nystagmus, ataxia, and cognitive impairment (Takanashi et al. 1999). Bilateral abnormal vertical orientation of the cerebellar folia seems to be a secondary change due to the absence of the vermis (Sasaki et al. 2001). However, vertically oriented folia and fissures at their posterior ends confined to one cerebellar hemisphere have been reported by Sasaki et al. in two patients without cerebellar clinical findings and normal vermis (Sasaki et al. 2001).

Management and treatment

If necessary, treatment of cerebellar cortical dysplasia is symptomatic.

Outcome

Because of the heterogeneous clinical manifestation ranging from incidental findings without clinical relevance to multiple severe neurological impairments, the outcome of cerebellar dysplasia is also extremely variable. Generally, a high degree of cerebellar involvement and associated supratentorial abnormalities correlate with a poor neurological outcome.

REFERENCES

Aida N, Yagishita A, Takada K, Katsumata Y (1994) Cerebellar MR in Fukuyama congenital muscular dystrophy: polymicrogyria with cystic lesions. AJNR Am J Neuroradiol 15: 1755–1759.

Alorainy IA, Sabir S, Seidahmed MZ, Farooqu HA, Salih MA (2006) Brain stem and cerebellar findings in Joubert syndrome. J Comput Assist Tomogr 30: 116–121.

Altman NR, Naidich TP, Braffman BH (1992) Posterior fossa malformations. AJNR Am J Neuroradiol 13: 691–724.

Balci S, Gucer S, Orhan D, Karagoz T (2008) A well-documented trisomy 13 case presenting with a number of common and uncommon features of the syndrome. Turk J Pediatr 50: 595–599.

Barkovich AJ (1997) Cerebellar polymicrogyria (editor's note). AJNR Am J Neuroradiol 18: 395–396.

Barkovich AJ (1998) Neuroimaging manifestations and classification of congenital muscular dystrophies. AJNR Am J Neuroradiol 19: 1389–1396.

Barkovich AJ, Millen KJ, Dobyns WB (2009) A developmental and genetic classification for midbrain-hindbrain malformations. Brain 132: 3199–3230.

Boddaert N, Desguerre I, Bahi-Buisson N, Romano S, Valayannopoulos V, Saillour Y, et al. (2010) Posterior fossa imaging in 158 children with ataxia. J Neuroradiol 37: 220–230.

Clement E, Mercuri E, Godfrey C, Smith J, Robb S, Kinali M, et al. (2008) Brain involvement in muscular dystrophies with defective dystroglycan glycosylation. Ann Neurol 64: 573–582.

Demaerel P (2002) Abnormalities of cerebellar foliation and fissuration: classification, neurogenetics and clinicoradiological correlations. Neuroradiology 44: 639–646.

Demaerel P, Lagae L, Casaer P, Baert AL (1998) MR of cerebellar cortical dysplasia. AJNR Am J Neuroradiol 19: 984–986.

Demaerel P, Wilms G, Marchal G (1999) Rostral vermian cortical dysplasia: MRI. Neuroradiology 41: 190–194.

Inouye M, Hayasaka S, Funahashi A, Yamamura H (1992) Gamma-radiation produces abnormal Bergmann fibers and ectopic granule cells in mouse cerebellar cortex. J Radiat Res (Tokyo) 33: 275–281.

Jissendi Tchofo P, De Tiege X, Goldman S, Van Bogaert P, David PH, Pruvo JP, Soto Ares G (2004) Supratentorial functional disturbances in two children with cerebellar cortical dysplasia. J Neuroradiol 31: 399–405.

Neumann PE, Garretson JD, Skabardonis GP, Mueller GG (1993) Genetic analysis of cerebellar folial pattern in crosses of C57BL/6J and DBA/2J inbred mice. Brain Res 619: 81–88.

Patel S, Barkovich AJ (2002) Analysis and classification of cerebellar malformations. AJNR Am J Neuroradiol 23: 1074–1087.

Pereira S, Serra D, Freitas PM, Santiago B, Brito O (2009) Epidermal nevus syndrome: an unusual cerebellar involvement. J Neuroradiol 36: 237–239.

Poretti A, Leventer RJ, Cowan FM, Rutherford MA, Steinlin M, Klein A, et al. (2008) Cerebellar cleft: a form of prenatal cerebellar disruption. Neuropediatrics 39: 106–112.

Poretti A, Huisman TA, Cowan FM, Del Giudice E, Jeannet PY, Prayer D, et al. (2009) Cerebellar cleft: confirmation of the neuroimaging pattern. Neuropediatrics 40: 228–233.

Rorke LB, Fogelson MH, Riggs HE (1968) Cerebellar heterotopia in infancy. Dev Med Child Neurol 10: 644–650.

Rossi A, Bava GL, Biancheri R, Tortori-Donati P (2001) Posterior fossa and arterial abnormalities in patients with facial capillary haemangiomas: presumed incomplete phenotypic expression of PHACES syndrome. Neuroradiology 43: 934–940.

Sakata-Haga H, Sawada K, Hisano S, Fukui Y (2001) Abnormalities of cerebellar foliation in rats prenatally exposed to ethanol. Acta Neuropathol 102: 36–40.

Sargent MA, Poskitt KJ, Jan JE (1997) Congenital ocular motor apraxia: imaging findings. AJNR Am J Neuroradiol 18: 1915–1922.

Sasaki M, Ehara S, Watabe T (1997) Cerebellar polymicrogyria. AJNR Am J Neuroradiol 18: 394–396.

Sasaki M, Oikawa H, Ehara S, Tamakawa Y, Takahashi S, Tohgi H (2001) Disorganised unilateral cerebellar folia: a mild form of cerebellar cortical dysplasia? Neuroradiology 43: 151–155.

Sekiguchi M, Abe H, Moriya M, Tanaka O, Nowakowski RS (1998) Cerebellar microfolia and other abnormalities of neuronal growth, migration, and lamination in the Pit1dw-J homozygote mutant mouse. J Comp Neurol 400: 363–374.

Senocak EU, Oguz KK, Haliloglu G, Topcu M, Cila A (2010) Structural abnormalities of the brain other than molar tooth sign in Joubert syndrome-related disorders. Diagn Interv Radiol 16: 3–6.

Soto-Ares G, Delmaire C, Deries B, Vallee L, Pruvo JP (2000) Cerebellar cortical dysplasia: MR findings in a complex entity. AJNR Am J Neuroradiol 21: 1511–1519.

Soto-Ares G, Devisme L, Jorriot S, Deries B, Pruvo JP, Ruchoux MM (2002) Neuropathologic and MR imaging correlation in a neonatal case of cerebellar cortical dysplasia. AJNR Am J Neuroradiol 23: 1101–1104.

Srour M, Rioux MF, Varga C, Lortie A, Major P, Robitaille Y, et al. (2011) The clinical spectrum of nodular heterotopias in children: report of 31 patients. Epilepsia 52: 728–737.

Takanashi J, Sugita K, Barkovich AJ, Takano H, Kohno Y (1999) Partial midline fusion of the cerebellar hemispheres with vertical folia: a new cerebellar malformation? AJNR Am J Neuroradiol 20: 1151–1153.

Toldo I, Calderone M, Sartori S, Mardari R, Gatta M, Boniver C, et al. (2011) Bilateral perisylvian polymicrogyria with cerebellar dysplasia and ectopic neurohypophysis. J Child Neurol 26: 361–365.

Voogd J, Glickstein M (1998) The anatomy of the cerebellum. Trends Neurosci 21: 370–375.

15
Cerebellar Cysts and Neuroimaging in Congenital Muscular Dystrophies

Andrea Poretti, Andrea Klein, and Eugen Boltshauser

Cerebellar cysts are rare, typically small and multiple, and located preferentially in involving the posterior portions of the cerebellar hemispheres and the upper part of the vermis. They are relatively specific for some forms of congenital muscular dystrophies (CMD), but have recently been reported in other disorders too, such as Aicardi syndrome and polymicrogyria. In this chapter we discuss the differential diagnosis of cerebellar cysts and also describe other cerebellar neuroimaging findings encountered in patients with CMD.

Congenital muscular dystrophies

Congenital muscular dystrophies are a heterogeneous group of rare autosomal recessive disorders characterized by onset of muscle weakness in the first 6 months of life, and muscle biopsy changes that range from myopathic to overtly dystrophic depending on the muscle biopsied and the age at biopsy (Muntoni and Voit 2004; Klein et al. 2008). The different genetically defined forms of CMD can be classified into three groups on the basis of the affected proteins: extracellular matrix proteins including laminin α2 and collagen VI, different glycosyltransferases necessary for *O*-glycosylation of α-dystroglycan (ADG), and selenoprotein N1 as a protein of the endoplasmic reticulum (Muntoni and Voit 2004; Peat et al. 2008). Collagen VI abnormalities and selenoproteinopathies do not affect the central nervous system, and the brain MRI in these patients is normal.

Primary merosin-deficient congenital muscular dystrophies

In patients with laminin α2 abnormalities or primary merosin-deficient CMD (MDC1A) the prominent neuroimaging findings are white matter changes (Caro et al. 1999; Philpot et al. 1999; Leite et al. 2005). Typically, in the first months of life white matter is near normal and the white matter abnormalities become evident after the first 6 months of life and progress only minimally over time (Philpot et al. 1999; Fujii et al. 2011). The abnormalities have a fronto-temporal predominance (Leite et al. 2005). The subcortical U fibres are initially spared and become involved only in the course of the disease (Philpot et al. 1999). Corpus callosum, internal capsule, optic radiation, brainstem, and cerebellar white matter are very rarely affected (Leite et al. 2005). Some patients with MDC1A also show cortical malformations, particularly bilateral (and sometimes asymmetric) occipital cortical dysplasia with agyria (Philpot et al. 1999; Leite et al. 2005). However, the gyral pattern of the rest of the cerebral hemispheres is typically normal. Pons and cerebellum can be hypoplastic (Philpot et al. 1999; Leite et al. 2005). Cerebellar cysts have not been reported in primary merosin-deficient CMD (Talim et al. 2000; Triki et al. 2003).

Congenital muscular dystrophies with defective dystroglycan *O*-glycosylation

This group includes CMD due to defective *O*-glycosylation of ADG, also termed dystroglycanopathies (Godfrey et al. 2007; Muntoni et al. 2007; Mercuri et al. 2009). These forms include a wide phenotypical spectrum of disorders: Walker-Warburg syndrome (WWS), Fukuyama CMD (FCMD), muscle-eye-brain disease (MEB), and CMD type 1C (MDC1C) and 1D (MDC1D) with mutations in six known glycosyltransferase genes: protein-O-mannosyl transferase 1 (*POMT1*; MIM 607423); protein-*O*-mannosyl transferase 2 (*POMT2*; MIM 607439); protein-*O*-mannose 1,2-N-acetylglucosaminyltransferase 1 (*POMGnT1*; MIM 606822); *Fukutin* (*FKTN*, MIM 607440); *Fukutin-related protein* (*FKRP*; MIM 606596); and *LARGE* (MIM 603590) (Mercuri et al. 2009). In the sections below we will briefly describe the main neuroimaging findings of the different phenotypes which reflect a smooth spectrum without clear borders.

Walker-Warburg syndrome

Typical neuroimaging findings in WWS are congenital hydrocephalus, always abnormal organization of the cerebral cortex with combination of agyria, pachygyria, and polymicrogyria and a pebbled surface corresponding to the cobblestone lissencephaly (Barkovich 1998; Clement et al. 2008). Severe hydrocephalus and the very thin cerebral mantle make it difficult to recognize the cortical abnormalities in an early stage or before shunting. The cerebral white matter shows a hyperintensity on T2-weighted images due to lack of myelination and multiple cysts may be present. The corpus callosum is often very thin or can be absent. The septum is absent too (Cormand et al. 2001). The cerebellum is highly hypoplastic involving both vermis and hemispheres and the vermis may also be absent. The cerebellar cortex is smooth, the cerebellar foliae are absent or very irregular, and multiple, small, subcortical isointense cysts are present involving the posterior portions of the cerebellar hemispheres (Barkovich 1998; Clement et al. 2008). The cerebellar white matter is not myelinated. The pons is extremely hypoplastic, the colliculi are fused, and the brainstem is kinked posteriorly at the ponto-mesencephalic junction (Barkovich 1998). The posterior fossa is often small.

Fukuyama congenital muscular dystrophy
In *FCMD* the cerebral cortex appears dysplastic typically with polymicrogyria in the frontotemporal and pachygyria in the occipital lobes (Barkovich 1998). The cerebral white matter appears normal at birth, but on repeated MRI the progress of myelination is sparse, resulting in hypomyelination. However, the cerebellar white matter usually has a normal appearance. The cerebellum and particularly the vermis are hypoplastic, the cerebellar cortex dysplastic with polymicrogyria, irregularly distorted folia, and multiple, small, subcortical cysts preferentially involving the posterior portions of the cerebellar hemispheres (Barkovich 1998). The pons appears flat; the colliculi can be fused. The ventricles are often mildly enlarged.

Muscle-eye-brain disease
In MEB the abnormalities of the cerebral cortex are variable (Barkovich 1998). The cortex presents mostly polymicrogyria with a fronto-occipital gradient (Figs 15.2c,d and 15.3c,d). The signal of the cerebral white matter is often abnormal (Fig. 15.3c,d). The corpus callosum can be dysplastic and thin. The cerebellum and in particular the vermis are hypoplastic (Figs 15.1a, 15.2a,b, 15.3a,b) and the cerebellar cortex shows polymicrogyria with small subcortical isointense cysts preferentially involving the posterior portions of the cerebellar hemispheres (Fig. 15.3b,d). In our patient these cysts were not visible on either the fetal MRI or the first postnatal MRI at the age of 4 days, but only on the second MRI at the age of 5 months (Fig. 15.3b,d). Barkovich and Longman et al. reported cerebellar cysts in MEB during the course of the disorder (several months postnatally) (Barkovich 1998; Longman et al. 2004). These observations suggest postnatal cerebellar migration disorder as a possible pathomechanism for cerebellar cysts. The pons is hypoplastic (Figs 15.1a, 15.2a, 15.3a) and presents a cleft in the ventral part most likely due to the absence of the ventral transverse pontine fibres (Fig. 15.3b) (Clement et al. 2008). The inferior colliculi are fused. In contrast to WWS, the septum is always present and the corpus callosum can be normal or at most thin, but not absent (Cormand et al. 2001).

Other dystroglycanopathies
Patients with MDC1C and mutations in the *FKRP* gene can have normal brain MRI (Mercuri et al. 2006a). Some patients may display cerebral abnormalities such as focal unilateral periventricular nodular heterotopia, and white matter changes which may regress with time (Louhichi et al. 2004; Mercuri et al. 2006a). However, in these patients the cerebellum can be particularly affected (Mercuri et al. 2006a). Several patients with MDC1C show hypoplasia of the vermis and cerebellar cysts (Topaloglu et al. 2003; Louhichi et al. 2004; Mercuri et al. 2006a). Additionally, in these patients the pons can be hypoplastic (Mercuri et al. 2006a).

MDC1D is a rare form of CMD characterized by white matter changes, hypoplastic brainstem, and mild pachygria with fronto-occipital gradient (Longman et al. 2003).

Neuroimaging-genotype correlation
Although involvement of different genes was originally reported in patients with distinct phenotypes, mutations in individual genes have subsequently been associated with a phenotypic spectrum (Table 15.1) (Mercuri et al. 2009; Waite et al. 2009). Therefore, Clement et al. searched for correlations between neuroimaging findings and genotype in 27 patients with CMD (Clement et al. 2008). Clement et al. and Godfrey et al. reported normal MRI or only minimal ventricular dilatation and/or minimal periventricular white matter changes in patients with *Fukutin* mutations (Godfrey et al. 2006; Clement et al. 2008). This is in contrast to patients with *Fukutin* mutations and phenotypically classic FCMD with cerebellar polymicrogyria and cysts (Aida et al. 1994), or MEB-like changes (Takada et al. 1984) reported in Japan. Therefore, the spectrum of

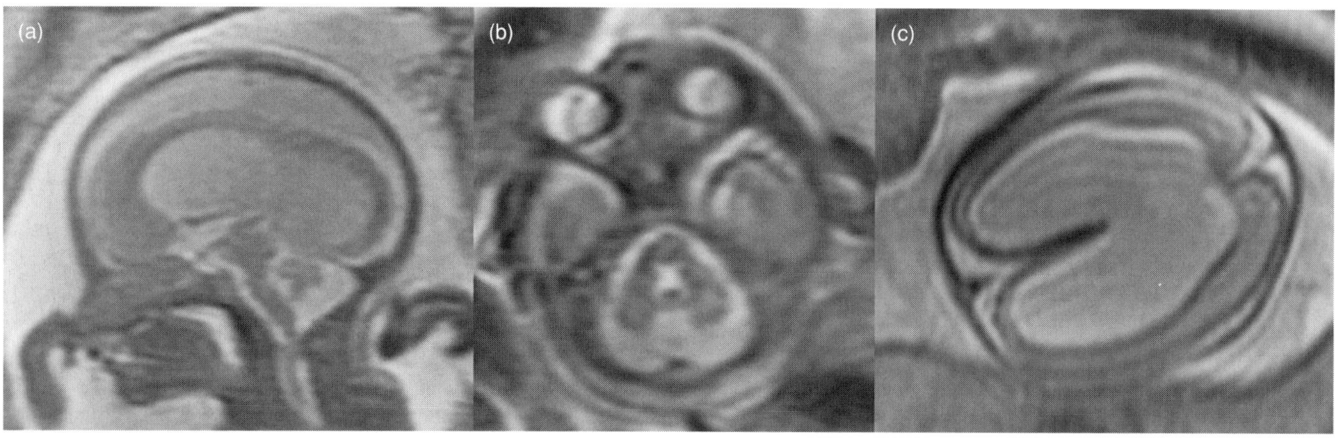

Fig. 15.1. Prenatal MRI at 25 weeks of gestation in a fetus with postnatal diagnosis of muscle-eye-brain disease (*POMGnT1* mutation). **(a)** Sagittal T2-weighted MRI showing severe ventriculomegaly, cerebellar hypoplasia, and flattened pons; **(b)** infratentorial axial T2-weighted MRI demonstrating cerebellar hypoplasia and dilatation of the fourth ventricle; **(c)** supratentorial T2-weighted MRI revealing bilateral ventriculomegaly and absence of the septum pellucidum.

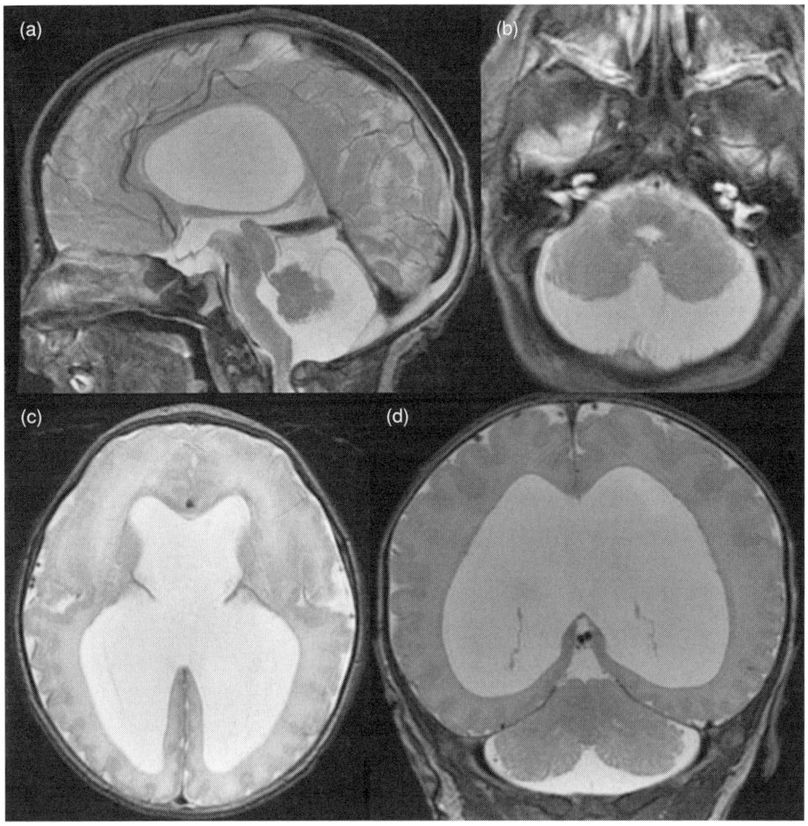

Fig. 15.2. MRI of the infant shown in Fig. 15.1, at the age of 4 days. **(a)** Sagittal T2-weighted MRI showing ventriculomegaly, thin corpus callosum, hypoplasia of the inferior vermis, flattened pons with a concave posterior border, and enlarged tectum; **(b)** infratentorial axial T2-weighted MRI demonstrating hypoplasia of both cerebellar vermis and hemispheres; **(c)** supratentorial T2-weighted MRI revealing bilateral ventriculomegaly and polymicrogyria with fronto-occipital gradient; **(d)** coronal T2-weighted MRI presenting ventriculomegaly, absence of the septum pellucidum, and cerebellar hypoplasia.

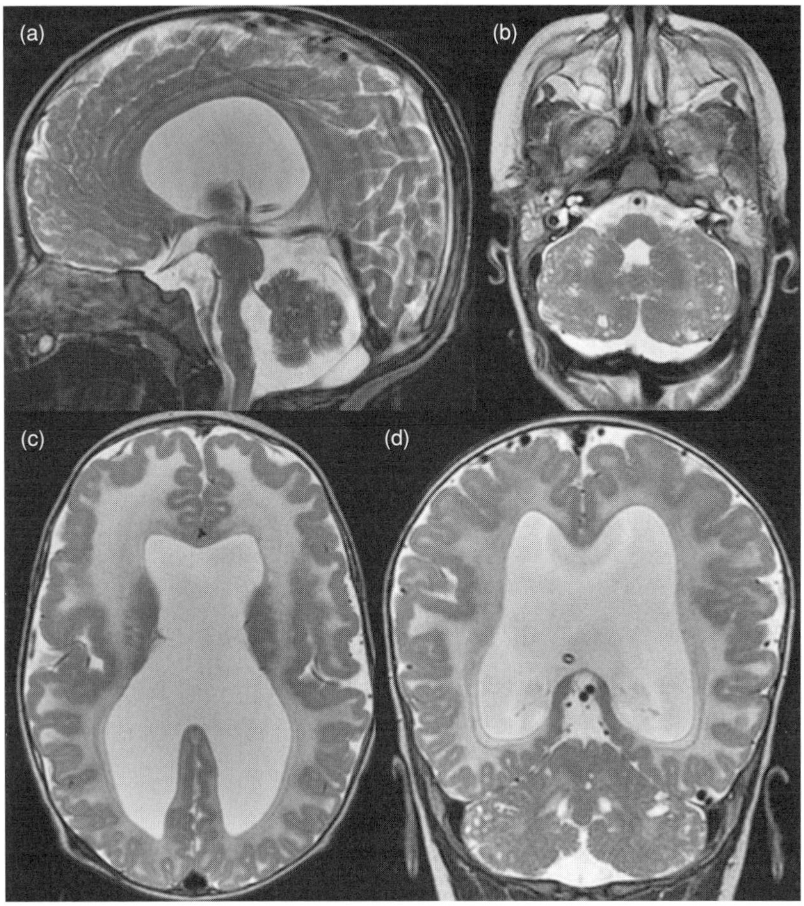

Fig. 15.3. MRI of the infant shown in Figs 15.1 and 5.2, at the age of 5 months. **(a)** Sagittal T2-weighted MRI showing ventriculomegaly, thin corpus callosum, hypoplasia of the inferior vermis, flattened pons with a concave posterior border, and enlarged tectum; **(b)** infratentorial axial T2-weighted MRI demonstrating cerebellar hypoplasia, multiple, subcortical cysts in both cerebellar hemispheres, and clefts in the dorsal and ventral pons; **(c)** supratentorial T2-weighted MRI revealing bilateral ventriculomegaly, polymicrogyria with fronto-occipital gradient, and abnormal high signal intensity of the white matter; **(d)** coronal T2-weighted MRI presenting ventriculomegaly, polymicrogyria, absence of the septum pellucidum, cerebellar hypoplasia, and multiple, subcortical cysts in both cerebellar hemispheres. (Parts (a–c) reprinted with permission from Clement E et al. Ann Neurol 2008; 64: 573–582.)

TABLE 15.1
Phenotype-genotype correlation in congenital muscular dystrophies

	FUKUTIN	*POMT1*	*POMT2*	*POMGnT1*	*LARGE*	*FKRP*
Normal MRI	+	+	—	—	—	+
WWS	+	+	+	+	—	+
FCMD	+	—	—	—	—	—
MEB	—	—	—	+	—	+
MDC1C	—	—	—	—	—	+
MDC1D	—	—	—	—	+	—

+, phenotype reported; —, phenotype not reported.
Cerebellar cysts have been reported in WWS, FCMD, MEB, and MDC1C. Walker-Warburg syndrome (WWS); Fukuyama congenital muscular dystrophy (FCMD); muscle-eye-brain disease (MEB); congenital muscular dystrophy type 1C (MDC1C); congenital muscular dystrophy type 1D (MDC1D). Modified from Topaloglu and Talim (2008).

neuroimaging findings in patients with *Fukutin* mutations ranges from normal MRI to WWS-like changes (Clement et al. 2008; Waite et al. 2009). This resembles the spectrum also reported in *FKRP* mutations by Mercuri et al. (2006a). Additionally, in *FKRP* mutations the cerebral cortex can be predominantly affected in the posterior areas, or cerebellar cysts can represent the predominant abnormalities. Most patients with *POMGnT1* mutations show changes consistent with MEB (Yoshida et al. 2001; Taniguchi et al. 2003; Diesen et al. 2004; Clement et al. 2008). However in *POMGnT1* mutations cerebellar cysts can be an isolated finding (Clement et al. 2008). Therefore, if cerebellar cysts are the predominant abnormality and/or a ventral pontine cleft is present, a targeted screening of *POMGnT1* and *FKRP* mutations should be considered (Clement et al. 2008). In patients with *POMT1* mutations, normal brain MRI has been reported (Balci et al. 2005; D'Amico et al. 2006; Liu et al. 2006; van Reeuwijk et al. 2006). However, the spectrum can also include minimal periventricular white matter changes (Clement et al. 2008), isolated cerebellar hypoplasia (Liu et al. 2006; van Reeuwijk et al. 2006), cortical and cerebellar abnormalities but normal pons (Clement et al. 2008), MEB-like phenotype (Liu et al. 2006), and WWS-like changes (Beltran-Valero de Bernabe et al. 2002; Liu et al. 2006). The spectrum of neuroimaging abnormalities in *POMT2* mutations is wide and includes mild ventricular dilatation (Clement et al. 2008), isolated cerebellar hypoplasia (Mercuri et al. 2006b; Yanagisawa et al. 2007; Clement et al. 2008), cerebellar hypoplasia with cysts, but without supratentorial changes (Clement et al. 2008), abnormalities of white matter and cortex, but normal cerebellum (Clement et al. 2008), cerebellar and cortical changes but normal pons (Clement et al. 2008), MEB-like phenotype (Clement et al. 2008), and WWS-like changes (van Reeuwijk et al. 2005, Clement et al. 2008). Patients with *LARGE* mutations can have white matter and cortical changes but normal cerebellum (Longman et al. 2003; Clement et al. 2008), MEB-like phenotype (Clement et al. 2008), and WWS-like changes (van Reeuwijk et al. 2007; Clement et al. 2008).

Prenatal diagnosis

The prenatal diagnosis of dystroglycanopathies (Fig. 15.1) remains difficult without a positive family history. Cortical migration disorders such as lissencephaly are typical findings in these CMD. However, the normal fetal brain is agyric and smooth until 24–25 weeks of gestation. Only thereafter does the absence of gyration raise the possibility of lissencephaly. Furthermore, the genotype of lissencephaly does not include only CMD (Dobyns 2010). Ventriculomegaly is often found in CMD, but prenatal finding of ventriculomegaly has other, far more common, causes (D'Addario et al. 2007). Vermian and pontine hypoplasia are also not specific (Malinger et al. 2009). Cerebellar cysts, which are highly suggestive of CMD, are reported to develop only postnatally (Barkovich 1998; Longman et al. 2004).

Pathogenesis

The role of ADG in brain development is not fully understood. Moore et al. showed that an appropriate *O*-glycosylation of ADG is crucial for its functions because it regulates its binding to extracellular matrix proteins such as laminin, neurexin, perlecan, and agrin (Moore et al. 2002). In particular, the interaction between ADG and laminin is important for stabilizing the basal lamina, and normal basal lamina formation is essential for neuronal migration. During brain development cells migrate from the ventricular zone to the cortical plate via radial glia, which are attached to the basal lamina. Because of the high expression of ADG in the basal lamina it is very likely that abnormal ADG-*O*-glycosylation causes reduced integrity of the basal lamina. It has been proposed that the resulting instability in the glial-guide interaction with the pial surface may be a mechanism by which defective ADG causes neuronal migration disorders (Moore et al. 2002). However, the regulated expression of ADG during development (Henion et al. 2003) and the expression of additional ADG ligands such as agrin and neurexin in the central nervous system (Sugita et al. 2001) suggest additional mechanisms of disturbed migration in CMD. Qu and Smith demonstrated that interactions involving ADG influence the strength of attachment of granule neurons to the ADG-expressing Bergmann glial cells that guide granule neuron migration in the cerebellum (Qu and Smith 2004).

Additional disorders with cerebellar cysts

Cerebellar cysts have also been reported in other disorders. We saw multiple cortical-subcortical cerebellar cysts of different

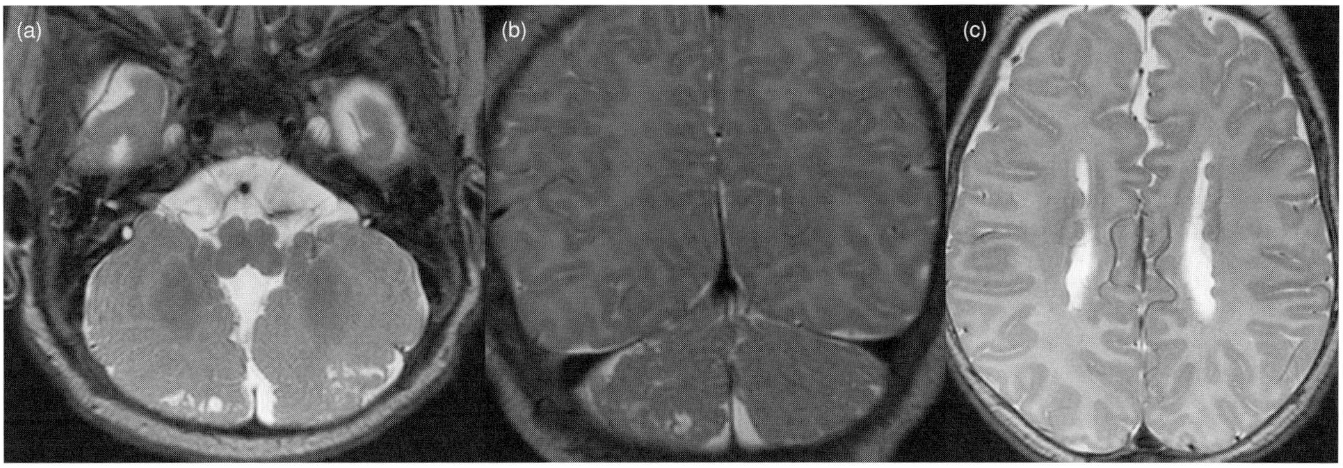

Fig. 15.4. MRI of a 4-month-old infant with poor visual fixation. **(a)** Infratentorial axial T2-weighted MRI showing multiple, subcortical cysts in both cerebellar hemispheres; **(b)** coronal T2-weighted MRI presenting multiple, subcortical cysts in both cerebellar hemispheres; **(c)** supratentorial axial T2-weighted MRI revealing multiple bilateral subependymal periventricular nodular heterotopia.

size (small as typically occurs in CMD, but also larger) and location (not only in the posterior portions of the cerebellar hemispheres, but also in the other parts of the hemispheres and in the vermis) in six children with developmental delay, ataxia, ocular motor apraxia, or ptosis as well as in one case additional complex brain malformation with multiple subependymal periventricular nodular heterotopia, hypoplasia of the corpus callosum, aplasia of the olfactory bulbs, and hypoplasia of the oculomotor nerve, but no obvious clinical or laboratory findings suggesting CMD (however, muscle biopsy has not been performed in all patients) (Fig. 15.4). The diagnostic categorization of these children is not yet clear.

Aicardi syndrome

Aicardi syndrome is a rare sporadic neurodevelopmental disorder affecting females and is characterized by a triad of infantile spasms, callosal dysgenesis (mostly callosal agenesis), and distinctive chorioretinal lacunae (Aicardi et al. 1965; Aicardi 2005). Typical additional structural brain abnormalities include polymicrogyria (predominantly frontal and perisylvian), periventricular or subcortical nodular heterotopia, underopercularization, intracranial cysts, sometimes papillomas of the choroid plexus, enlargement of the tectum in about the half of the patients, and cerebellar anomalies (Donnenfeld et al. 1989; Yamagata et al. 1990; Smith et al. 1996; Barkovich et al. 2001; Aicardi 2005; Palmer et al. 2006; Hopkins et al. 2008).

Posterior fossa abnormalities were reported in 95% of the patients studied by Hopkins et al. (2008). They included superior prominence of the vermis, inferior vermis hypoplasia, and dysplastic or hypoplastic cerebellar hemispheres in 65% of the patients. Cerebellar subcortical and/or periventricular heterotopia were noted in 27%, mega cisterna magna in 55%, and cerebellar cysts in 20%. In contrast to CMD, the cerebellar cysts in Aicardi syndrome seem to be larger in volume and not only subcortically located. Hopkins et al. speculated that superior foliar prominence and hypoplasia of the cerebellar vermis may be related to decreased cell proliferation as well as atrophy due to exposure to antiepileptic medication (Hopkins et al. 2008). However, cerebellar heterotopia and cerebellar cysts may indicate a neuronal migration defect (Steffensen et al. 2009).

Polymicrogyria

Polymicrogyria is a malformation of cortical development in which the process of normal cerebral cortical development is disturbed late in the stage of neuronal migration or early in the stage of cortical organization (Barkovich et al. 2005). Causes of polymicrogyria include prenatal infections, intrauterine localized or diffuse ischaemias, or mutations in some genes such as *GPR56* (Barkovich 2010b). It affects variable portions of the cerebral cortex, most commonly the Sylvian fissure, and can be isolated or associated with other brain malformations such as in specific syndromes. The neuroimaging appearance of polymicrogyria is variable. The cortical surface can have multiple small gyri or appear thick and irregular bumpy (Barkovich 2010b). Irregularities of the gray-white matter junction are often the most convincing evidence of dysplastic brain (Barkovich 2010a).

Recently, the neuroimaging pattern of *GPR56*-related polymicrogyria has been characterized (Bahi-Buisson et al. 2010). The polymicrogyria is commonly bilateral and frontoparietally located, or generalized with anterior to posterior gradient. Additional neuroimaging findings include cerebellar hypoplasia, moderate to severe cerebellar dysplasia with cortical or subpial cysts mainly affecting the superior vermis, pontine hypoplasia, thin corpus callosum, and patchy to diffuse white matter abnormalities (Bahi-Buisson et al. 2010). The white matter abnormalities showed a peculiar evolution from severe hypomyelination at 4 months to patchy lesions later in childhood. Children with *GPR56*-related polymicrogyria present with a clinical course characterized by severe mental and motor retardation and epileptic seizures (Bahi-Buisson et al.

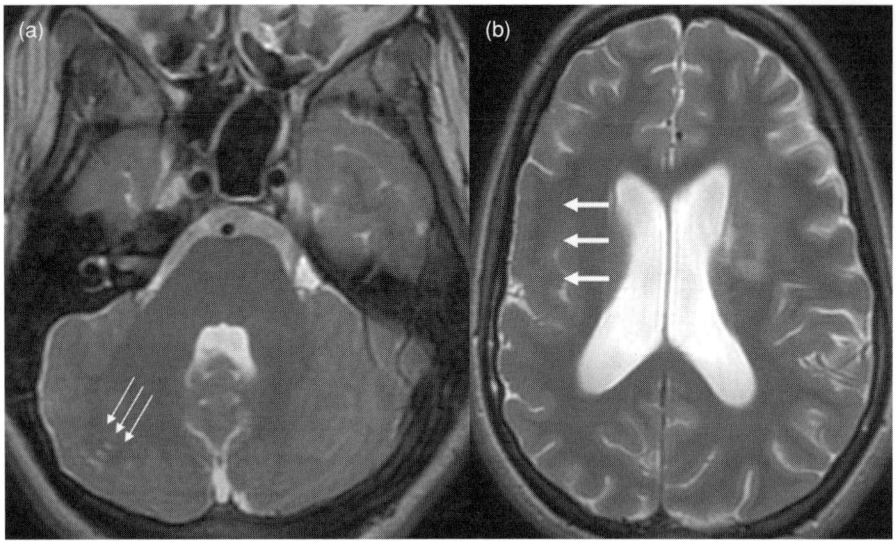

Fig. 15.5. MRI of a 23-year-old woman with left-sided congenital hemiparesis from ischaemic stroke in the left frontoparietal lobe, basal ganglia, and anterior part of the internal capsule due to an occlusion of the superior part of the left middle cerebral artery. **(a)** Infratentorial axial T2-weighted MRI showing multiple, subcortical cysts in the right cerebellar hemisphere (thin arrows); **(b)** supratentorial axial T2-weighted MRI presenting polymicrogyria in the right temporal lobe (thick arrows) and periventricular hyperintensity on the left side due to the subacute ischaemia. (Courtesy of Prof. A. Valavanis, Institute of Neuroradiology, University Hospital Zurich.

2010). Electroencephalographic changes are consistently characterized by predominantly anterior bursts of low amplitude α-like activity. Interestingly, loss of *GPR56* leads to a dysregulation of the maintenance of the pial basement membrane integrity in the forebrain and the rostral cerebellum (Li et al. 2008, Koirala et al. 2009). Both the neuroimaging pattern and the pathomechanism of *GPR56*-related polymicrogyria are very similar to those of the cobblestone malformation in dystroglycanopathies (Moore et al. 2002; Bahi-Buisson et al. 2010).

We are aware of an unreported case of a woman with unilateral perisylvian polymicrogyria and ipsilateral subcortical cerebellar cysts (Fig. 15.5). The unilaterality and perisylvian location of the polymicrogyria in this patient is not suggested to result from a mutation in the *GPR56* gene.

Other causes of cerebellar cysts

Typical MRI findings in multiple carboxylase deficiency are diffuse supratentorial white matter abnormalities, cortical atrophy, basal ganglia calcifications, and periventricular subependymal cystic lesions (Desai et al. 2008). Large subcortical cysts in the periphery of the both cerebellar hemispheres have been reported by Tsutsumi et al. (Y. Tsutsumi et al., personal communication at the Fetal MRI congress, Vienna, May 2010).

Takanashi et al. reported multifocal small cysts in the superior cerebellar hemispheres in a child with muscular hypotonia, nystagmus, ataxia, cognitive impairment, and severely impaired visual acuity due to 'retinal degeneration' (Takanashi et al. 1999). Additional neuroimaging findings were vertically oriented cerebellar folia, fusion of the inferior cerebellum, and hypoplasia of the cerebellar vermis. At the age of 4 years 6 months, muscle strength and serum creatinine kinase were normal.

The differential diagnosis of cerebellar cystic lesions also includes hydatid cysts (Is et al. 2009). These cysts can be very large, are well circumscribed, and typically unilateral. The cysts appear hypointense on T1-weighted images and hyperintense on T2-weighted images. Postcontrast T1-weighted images show enhancement of the rim of the cyst.

REFERENCES

Aida N, Yagishita A, Takada K, Katsumata Y (1994) Cerebellar MR in Fukuyama congenital muscular dystrophy: polymicrogyria with cystic lesions. AJNR Am J Neuroradiol 15: 1755–1759.

Aicardi J, Lefebvre J, Lerique-Koechlin A (1965) A new syndrome: spasm in flexion, callosal agenesis, ocular abnormalities. Electroencephalogr Clin Neurophysiol 19: 609–610.

Aicardi J (2005) Aicardi syndrome. Brain Dev 27: 164–171.

Bahi-Buisson N, Poirier K, Boddaert N, Fallet-Bianco C, Specchio N, Bertini E, et al. (2010) GPR56-related bilateral frontoparietal polymicrogyria: further evidence for an overlap with the cobblestone complex. Brain 133: 3194–3209.

Balci B, Uyanik G, Dincer P, Gross C, Willer T, Talim B, et al. (2005) An autosomal recessive limb girdle muscular dystrophy (LGMD2) with mild mental retardation is allelic to Walker-Warburg syndrome (WWS) caused by a mutation in the POMT1 gene. Neuromuscul Disord 15: 271–275.

Barkovich AJ (1998) Neuroimaging manifestations and classification of congenital muscular dystrophies. AJNR Am J Neuroradiol 19: 1389–1396.

Barkovich AJ, Simon EM, Walsh CA (2001) Callosal agenesis with cyst: a better understanding and new classification. Neurology 56: 220–227.

Barkovich AJ, Kuzniecky RI, Jackson GD, Guerrini R, Dobyns WB (2005) A developmental and genetic classification for malformations of cortical development. Neurology 65: 1873–1887.

Barkovich AJ (2010a) MRI analysis of sulcation morphology in polymicrogyria. Epilepsia 51 Suppl 1: 17–22.

Barkovich AJ (2010b) Current concepts of polymicrogyria. Neuroradiology 52: 479–487.

Beltran-Valero de Bernabe D, Currier S, Steinbrecher A, Celli J, van Beusekom E, van der Zwaag B, et al. (2002) Mutations in the O-mannosyltransferase gene POMT1 give rise to the severe neuronal migration disorder Walker-Warburg syndrome. Am J Hum Genet 71: 1033–1043.

Caro PA, Scavina M, Hoffman E, Pegoraro E, Marks HG (1999) MR imaging findings in children with merosin-deficient congenital muscular dystrophy. AJNR Am J Neuroradiol 20: 324–326.

Clement E, Mercuri E, Godfrey C, Smith J, Robb S, Kinali M, et al. (2008) Brain involvement in muscular dystrophies with defective dystroglycan glycosylation. Ann Neurol 64: 573–582.

Cormand B, Pihko H, Bayes M, Valanne L, Santavuori P, Talim B, et al. (2001) Clinical and genetic distinction between Walker-Warburg syndrome and muscle-eye-brain disease. Neurology 56: 1059–1069.

D'Addario V, Pinto V, Di Cagno L, Pintucci A (2007) Sonographic diagnosis of fetal cerebral ventriculomegaly: an update. J Matern Fetal Neonatal Med 20: 7–14.

D'Amico A, Tessa A, Bruno C, Petrini S, Biancheri R, Pane M, et al. (2006) Expanding the clinical spectrum of POMT1 phenotype. Neurology 66: 1564–1567.

Desai S, Ganesan K, Hedge A (2008) Biotinidase deficiency: a reversible metabolic encephalopathy. Neuroimaging and MR spectroscopic findings in a series of four patients. Pediatr Radiol 38: 848–856.

Diesen C, Saarinen A, Pihko H, Rosenlew C, Cormand B, Dobyns WB, et al. (2004) POMGnT1 mutation and phenotypic spectrum in muscle-eye-brain disease. J Med Genet 41: e115.

Dobyns WB (2010) The clinical patterns and molecular genetics of lissencephaly and subcortical band heterotopia. Epilepsia 51 Suppl 1: 5–9.

Donnenfeld AE, Packer RJ, Zackai EH, Chee CM, Sellinger B, Emanuel BS (1989) Clinical, cytogenetic, and pedigree findings in 18 cases of Aicardi syndrome. Am J Med Genet 32: 461–467.

Fujii Y, Sugiura C, Fukuda C, Maegaki Y, Ohno K (2011) Sequential neuroradiological and neurophysiological studies in a Japanese girl with merosin-deficient congenital muscular dystrophy. Brain Dev 33: 140–144.

Godfrey C, Escolar D, Brockington M, Clement EM, Mein R, Jimenez-Mallebrera C, et al. (2006) Fukutin gene mutations in steroid-responsive limb girdle muscular dystrophy. Ann Neurol 60: 603–610.

Godfrey C, Clement E, Mein R, Brockington M, Smith J, Talim B, et al. (2007) Refining genotype phenotype correlations in muscular dystrophies with defective glycosylation of dystroglycan. Brain 130: 2725–2735.

Henion TR, Qu Q, Smith FI (2003) Expression of dystroglycan, fukutin and POMGnT1 during mouse cerebellar development. Brain Res Mol Brain Res 112: 177–181.

Hopkins B, Sutton VR, Lewis RA, Van den Veyver I, Clark G (2008) Neuroimaging aspects of Aicardi syndrome. Am J Med Genet A 146A: 2871–2878.

Is M, Gezen F, Akyuz F, Aytekin H, Dosoglu M (2009) A 13-year-old girl with a cystic cerebellar lesion: consider the hydatid cyst. J Clin Neurosci 16: 712–713.

Klein A, Clement E, Mercuri E, Muntoni F (2008) Differential diagnosis of congenital muscular dystrophies. Eur J Paediatr Neurol 12: 371–377.

Koirala S, Jin Z, Piao X, Corfas G (2009) GPR56-regulated granule cell adhesion is essential for rostral cerebellar development. J Neurosci 29: 7439–7449.

Leite CC, Lucato LT, Martin MG, Ferreira LG, Resende MB, Carvalho MS, et al. (2005) Merosin-deficient congenital muscular dystrophy (CMD): a study of 25 Brazilian patients using MRI. Pediatr Radiol 35: 572–579.

Li S, Jin Z, Koirala S, Bu L, Xu L, Hynes RO, et al. (2008) GPR56 regulates pial basement membrane integrity and cortical lamination. J Neurosci 28: 5817–5826.

Liu J, Ball SL, Yang Y, Mei P, Zhang L, Shi H, et al. (2006) A genetic model for muscle-eye-brain disease in mice lacking protein O-mannose 1,2-N-acetylglucosaminyltransferase (POMGnT1). Mech Dev 123: 228–240.

Longman C, Brockington M, Torelli S, Jimenez-Mallebrera C, Kennedy C, Khalil N, et al. (2003) Mutations in the human LARGE gene cause MDC1D, a novel form of congenital muscular dystrophy with severe mental retardation and abnormal glycosylation of alpha-dystroglycan. Hum Mol Genet 12: 2853–2861.

Longman C, Mercuri E, Cowan F, Allsop J, Brockington M, Jimenez-Mallebrera C, et al. (2004) Antenatal and postnatal brain magnetic resonance imaging in muscle-eye-brain disease. Arch Neurol 61: 1301–1306.

Louhichi N, Triki C, Quijano-Roy S, Richard P, Makri S, Meziou M, et al. (2004) New FKRP mutations causing congenital muscular dystrophy associated with mental retardation and central nervous system abnormalities. Identification of a founder mutation in Tunisian families. Neurogenetics 5: 27–34.

Malinger G, Lev D, Lerman-Sagie T (2009) The fetal cerebellum. Pitfalls in diagnosis and management. Prenat Diagn 29: 372–380.

Mercuri E, Topaloglu H, Brockington M, Berardinelli A, Pichiecchio A, Santorelli F, et al. (2006a) Spectrum of brain changes in patients with congenital muscular dystrophy and FKRP gene mutations. Arch Neurol 63: 251–257.

Mercuri E, D'Amico A, Tessa A, Berardinelli A, Pane M, Messina S, et al. (2006b) POMT2 mutation in a patient with 'MEB-like' phenotype. Neuromuscul Disord 16: 446–448.

Mercuri E, Messina S, Bruno C, Mora M, Pegoraro E, Comi GP, et al. (2009) Congenital muscular dystrophies with defective glycosylation of dystroglycan: a population study. Neurology 72: 1802–1809.

Moore SA, Saito F, Chen J, Michele DE, Henry MD, Messing A, et al. (2002) Deletion of brain dystroglycan recapitulates aspects of congenital muscular dystrophy. Nature 418: 422–425.

Muntoni F, Voit T (2004) The congenital muscular dystrophies in 2004: a century of exciting progress. Neuromuscul Disord 14: 635–649.

Muntoni F, Brockington M, Godfrey C, Ackroyd M, Robb S, Manzur A, et al. (2007) Muscular dystrophies due to defective glycosylation of dystroglycan. Acta Myol 26: 129–135.

Palmer L, Zetterlund B, Hard AL, Steneryd K, Kyllerman M (2006) Aicardi syndrome: presentation at onset in Swedish children born in 1975–2002. Neuropediatrics 37: 154–158.

Peat RA, Smith JM, Compton AG, Baker NL, Pace RA, Burkin DJ, et al. (2008) Diagnosis and etiology of congenital muscular dystrophy. Neurology 71: 312–321.

Philpot J, Cowan F, Pennock J, Sewry C, Dubowitz V, Bydder G, Muntoni F (1999) Merosin-deficient congenital muscular dystrophy: the spectrum of brain involvement on magnetic resonance imaging. Neuromuscul Disord 9: 81–85.

Qu Q, Smith FI (2004) Alpha-dystroglycan interactions affect cerebellar granule neuron migration. J Neurosci Res 76: 771–782.

Smith CD, Ryan SJ, Hoover SL, Baumann RJ (1996) Magnetic resonance imaging of the brain in Aicardi's syndrome. Report of 20 patients. J Neuroimaging 6: 214–221.

Steffensen TS, Gilbert-Barness E, Lacson A, Margo CE (2009) Cerebellar migration defects in Aicardi syndrome: an extension of the neuropathological spectrum. Fetal Pediatr Pathol 28: 24–38.

Sugita S, Saito F, Tang J, Satz J, Campbell K, Sudhof TC (2001) A stoichiometric complex of neurexins and dystroglycan in brain. J Cell Biol 154: 435–445.

Takada K, Nakamura H, Tanaka J (1984) Cortical dysplasia in congenital muscular dystrophy with central nervous system involvement (Fukuyama type). J Neuropathol Exp Neurol 43: 395–407.

Takanashi J, Sugita K, Barkovich AJ, Takano H, Kohno Y (1999) Partial midline fusion of the cerebellar hemispheres with vertical folia: a new cerebellar malformation? AJNR Am J Neuroradiol 20: 1151–1153.

Talim B, Ferreiro A, Cormand B, Vignier N, Oto A, Gogus S, et al. (2000) Merosin-deficient congenital muscular dystrophy with mental retardation and cerebellar cysts unlinked to the LAMA2, FCMD and MEB loci. Neuromuscul Disord 10: 548–552.

Taniguchi K, Kobayashi K, Saito K, Yamanouchi H, Ohnuma A, Hayashi YK, et al. (2003) Worldwide distribution and broader clinical spectrum of muscle-eye-brain disease. Hum Mol Genet 12: 527–534.

Topaloglu H, Brockington M, Yuva Y, Talim B, Haliloglu G, Blake D, et al. (2003) FKRP gene mutations cause congenital muscular dystrophy, mental retardation, and cerebellar cysts. Neurology 60: 988–992.

Topaloglu H, Talim B (2008) Lissencephaly type II. In: Sarnat HB, Curatolo P, editors. Malformations of the Nervous System. New York: Elsevier; 219–234.

Triki C, Louhichi N, Meziou M, Choyakh F, Kechaou MS, Jlidi R, et al. (2003) Merosin-deficient congenital muscular dystrophy with mental retardation and cerebellar cysts, unlinked to the LAMA2, FCMD, MEB and CMD1B loci, in three Tunisian patients. Neuromuscul Disord 13: 4–12.

van Reeuwijk J, Janssen M, van den Elzen C, Beltran-Valero de Bernabe D, Sabatelli P, Merlini L, et al. (2005) POMT2 mutations cause alpha-dystroglycan hypoglycosylation and Walker-Warburg syndrome. J Med Genet 42: 907–912.

van Reeuwijk J, Maugenre S, van den Elzen C, Verrips A, Bertini E, Muntoni F, et al. (2006) The expanding phenotype of POMT1 mutations: from Walker-Warburg syndrome to congenital muscular dystrophy, microcephaly, and mental retardation. Hum Mutat 27: 453–459.

van Reeuwijk J, Grewal PK, Salih MA, Beltrán-Valero de Bernabé D, McLaughlan JM, Michielse CB, et al. (2007) Intragenic deletion in the LARGE gene causes Walker-Warburg syndrome. Hum Genet 121: 685–690.

Waite A, Tinsley CL, Locke M, Blake DJ (2009) The neurobiology of the dystrophin-associated glycoprotein complex. Ann Med 41: 344–359.

Yamagata T, Momoi M, Miyamoto S, Kobayashi S, Kamoshita S (1990) Multi-institutional survey of the Aicardi syndrome in Japan. Brain Dev 12: 760–765.

Yanagisawa A, Bouchet C, Van den Bergh PY, Cuisset JM, Viollet L, Leturcq F, et al. (2007) New POMT2 mutations causing congenital muscular dystrophy: identification of a founder mutation. Neurology 69: 1254–1260.

Yoshida A, Kobayashi K, Manya H, Taniguchi K, Kano H, Mizuno M, et al. (2001) Muscular dystrophy and neuronal migration disorder caused by mutations in a glycosyltransferase, POMGnT1. Dev Cell 1: 717–724.

16
Rhombencephalosynapsis and Gómez-López-Hernández Syndrome

Andrea Poretti and Eugen Boltshauser

Rhombencephalosynapsis is a rare, sporadic cerebellar malformation characterized by absence of the cerebellar vermis including its lobules, the fastigial nuclei, and efferent and afferent connections, fusion of the cerebellar hemispheres across the midsagittal plane, dentate nuclei appearing as an almost single structure consisting of contributions by left and right hemispheres, and fusion of the superior cerebellar peduncles leading to the characteristic keyhole-shaped appearance of the fourth ventricle (Toelle et al. 2002; Barth 2008; Poretti et al. 2009). This condition was first described by Obersteiner in 1916 in a 28-year-old man, who was employed as a clerical assistant and who committed suicide (Obersteiner 1916). With the advent of magnetic resonance imaging (MRI), rhombencephalosynapsis is being increasingly recognized including prenatally (Toelle et al. 2002; Dill et al. 2009; Poretti et al. 2009).

As of March 2011 about 142 cases had been reported, with 87 cases diagnosed by MRI (8 prenatally). The majority of the reported patients have nonsyndromic rhombencephalosynapsis. Rhombencephalosynapsis can be associated with other central nervous system anomalies (Toelle et al. 2002) or may occur in isolation. Nevertheless, in a minority of patients rhombencephalosynapsis is a key feature of Gómez-López-Hernández syndrome (GLHS) or cerebello-trigeminal-dermal dysplasia (OMIM 601853), whereof to date only 27 cases have been published (Gomez 1979; López-Hernández 1982; Truwit et al. 1991; Munoz et al. 1997; Brocks et al. 2000; Tan et al. 2005; Whetsell et al. 2006; Bowdin et al. 2007; Purvis et al. 2007; Gomy et al. 2008; Poretti et al. 2008; Schell-Apacik et al. 2008; Fernandez-Jaen et al. 2009; Sukhudyan et al. 2010). However, we are aware of additional, unreported cases. GLHS was first described in 1979 by Gómez and in 1982 by López-Hernández and is characterized by rhombencephalosynapsis, parietal alopecia, and trigeminal anesthesia as well as craniofacial dysmorphic signs (Poretti et al. 2008).

As GLHS may represent a syndromic form of rhombencephalosynapsis, they are included in the same chapter.

Etiology and pathogenesis

The etiology of rhombencephalosynapsis remains unclear. Cytogenetic studies usually show normal karyotype. An unbalanced subtelomeric translocation t(2p;10q) was found in a fetus (Lespinasse et al. 2004), and di Vera et al. reported rhombencephalosynapsis in a fetus with nonmosaic tetrasomy 9p and additional malformations (truncus arteriosus, atrioventricular septal defect, horseshoe kidney, micromelia, brachydactyly, bilateral cleft lip and palate, rocker-bottom feet, hypertelorism, preauricular tag, cupped ears) in a pregnancy achieved through intracytoplasmic sperm injection (di Vera et al. 2008). We are aware of unpublished cases with normal karyotype and array CGH results. All cases are sporadic.

The pathogenesis of rhombencephalosynapsis also remains unknown. Patel and Barkovich reported that rhombencephalosynapsis probably results from failure of induction of midline structures, rather than failure of fusion (Patel and Barkovich 2002). A defect in the dorsoventral patterning has been hypothesized (Barkovich et al. 2009). *LMX1a* acting at the mesencephalic-metencephalic junction of the early neural tube has been proposed as a candidate gene (Jellinger 2002; Yachnis 2002). Owing to a homozygous mutation of *Lmx1a*, the mutant mouse dreher has agenesis of the vermis with fusion of the cerebellar hemispheres and inferior colliculi (Manzanares et al. 2000; Millonig et al. 2000). Barkovich et al. proposed the human homolog *LBX1* as a candidate gene for rhombencephalosynapsis (Barkovich et al. 2009). LBX1 is a transcription factor that determines neuronal cell fate and identity in the developing brainstem and spinal cord (Gross et al. 2002; Sieber et al. 2007). Defective expression of other genes at the mesencephalic-metencephalic junction such as *WNT1*, *EN1*, or *EN2* represents a very unlikely pathomechanism for rhombencephalosynapsis, because mutations of these genes can cause brainstem disconnection, but not rhombencephalosynapsis (Sarnat et al. 2002).

In GLHS there is an association between rhombencephalosynapsis and developmental failure of the trigeminal placodes. Several transcription factors have been associated with development of the trigeminal placode. For example, the homeobox genes *Tlx-1* and *Tlx-3* are both expressed early in placode-derived cranial neurons, including the trigeminal placodes, and in the hindbrain in chicken (Logan et al. 1998; Baker and Bronner-Fraser 2001). However, the involvement of these genes in GLHS remains to be demonstrated. It has been speculated that the nax mouse, in which a novel recessive mutation of the lysosomal monoesterase *Acp2* gene induces disturbed cerebellar cortical architecture, ataxia and delayed hair appearance, might constitute an animal model for GLHS (Mannan et al. 2004). However, the involvement of the human homolog, *ACP2*, in GLHS could not be demonstrated (Gomy et al. 2008).

Gomy et al. speculated that some genes such as *FGF8*, *FGF17*, and *FGF20*, which are crucial for cerebellar and epithelial development, and *FGF22*, which plays a role in hair follicle development, might be studied as possible candidates for GLHS (Gomy et al. 2008).

Clinical features

Rhombencephalosynapsis

Clinical presentation in rhombencephalosynapsis is variable. Clinical information has been reported in 48 nonsyndromic cases. In these patients the first symptoms of rhombencephalosynapsis appeared at the mean age of 3.7 years (median: 1 year, range: a few days to 54 years). The first symptoms included delayed motor development (n=11), truncal ataxia (n=10), hydrocephalus/ventriculomegaly (n=10), neuro-ophthalmological findings (strabismus or nystagmus; n=6), dysmorphic signs (n=4), behavioural disorders (mostly depression; n=3), epileptic seizure (n=2), spasticity (n=1), and extrapyramidal movement disorder (n=1). Hydrocephalus/ventriculomegaly and dysmorphic signs are usually present at birth or in the first few days or weeks, oculomotor abnormalities and delayed motor development become evident in the first 4–10 months, truncal ataxia is recognized at the earliest at the age of 1.5–2 years, and behavioural disorders are manifest in adolescence. On average, the diagnosis of rhombencephalosynapsis was made about 5 years after the appearance of the first symptoms (mean age at diagnosis 8.6 years; median 3.5; range: a few days to 55 years). In 42 of 48 patients the diagnosis of rhombencephalosynapsis was made in infancy or childhood. At the last reported follow-up the mean age of these patients was 9.6 years (median 5 years, range 6 months to 55 years).

The most common manifestation of rhombencephalosynapsis includes truncal (n=28) and/or limb (n=6) ataxia and muscular hypotonia (n=9). These symptoms can vary considerably in severity, but are mostly mild. Indeed, only a few patients are restricted in activities of daily living (Demaerel et al. 1995; Guyot et al. 2000; Toelle et al. 2002; Poretti et al. 2009).

Muscular hypertonia has been reported in seven cases, as generalized (n=3), accentuated (n=2), and affecting only the lower extremities (n=2) (Romanengo et al. 1997; Scroop et al. 2000; Toelle et al. 2002; Pavone et al. 2005; Lespinasse et al. 2004; Chemli et al. 2007; Kalra et al. 2008). In four of the seven patients there was associated hyperreflexia. Supratentorial abnormalities were present in only one patient (Romanengo et al. 1997).

Strabismus has been reported in 16 patients with rhombencephalosynapsis, mostly as a convergent strabismus. Canturk et al. hypothesized an excess of convergence tone or defective horizontal phoria adaptation in rhombencephalosynapsis causing strabismus (Canturk et al. 2008). The dorsal vermis is suggested to be one area in the cerebellum controlling vergence and eye alignment (Gulyas and Roland 1994; Takagi et al. 2003). Other ocular motor abnormalities reported in rhombencephalosynapsis include nystagmus in eight cases and one case each with mild limitation of abduction bilaterally, dysconjugate gaze, and abnormal vertical eye movements (Phillips et al. 2008). In one patient with hypoplastic optic nerves, visual acuity was decreased and both optic disks were small (Subash and Minasian 2008).

Eight patients presented with rhythmical, regular, intermittent head stereotypies from the first years of life, described as a side-to-side head movement in seven cases and a backward head nodding in one (Demaerel et al. 1995; Toelle et al. 2002; Canturk et al. 2008; Poretti et al. 2009). In all cases, the frequency and intensity of head movements improved over the course of several years, but always persisted to some extent, causing impaired social interaction with peers. Head stereotypies were also reported in other cerebellar malformations (Hottinger-Blanc et al. 2002; Poretti et al. 2010).

Other reported findings are epileptic seizures in five patients (Toelle et al. 2002; Pavone et al. 2005 Poretti et al. 2009 Striano et al. 2011), choreo-athetoid movements of head and extremities (Toelle et al. 2002), and scoliosis in one (Chemli et al. 2007). Twelve patients exhibited dysmorphic signs such as low-set ears (n=9), hypertelorism (n=6), finger anomalies (n=3), long philtrum (n=2), thin lips (n=2), and broad and depressed nasal ridge (n=2) (Aydingoz et al. 1997; Romanengo et al. 1997; Montull et al. 2000; Verri et al. 2000; Odemis et al. 2003; Lespinasse et al. 2004; Pavone et al. 2005; Chemli et al. 2007; Canturk et al. 2008; Kalra et al. 2008; Koljonen et al. 2009; Poretti et al. 2009; Striano et al. 2011).

Speech and language impairments were present in nine patients and were characterized by dysarthria (n=4), expressive speech impairment (n=2), absence of speech with only nonverbal communication (n=2), and delay of speech development (n=1) (Truwit et al. 1991; Romanengo et al. 1997; Utsunomiya et al. 1998; Toelle et al. 2002; Bell et al. 2005).

Disorders of cognitive function and delayed cognitive development are reported present in the majority of cases of rhombencephalosynapsis (Demaerel et al. 1995; Montull et al. 2000; Verri et al. 2000; Toelle et al. 2002). In the literature we found data on the cognitive function of 23 patients with rhombencephalosynapsis. Remarkably, this was reported as normal in 11 cases. However, full-scale IQ measurement has only been reported in 4 cases, ranging between 90 and 114 (Bell et al. 2005; Michael et al. 2009; Poretti et al. 2009). Therefore, rhombencephalosynapsis is compatible with a favourable cognitive outcome and this is of particular importance in counselling parents when there is a prenatal diagnosis of rhombencephalosynapsis. We found full-scale IQ score lower than 50 in only one individual, who had complex additional brain malformation (Pavone et al. 2005). Toelle et al. hypothesized that additional supratentorial abnormalities and hydrocephalus may be crucial for the long-term cognitive outcome (Toelle et al. 2002). However, in view of all reports in the literature, this correlation appears uncertain. It is possible that a marked prenatal hydrocephalus is an unfavourable prognostic factor (Poretti et al. 2009). Verbal and performance IQ were reported in six cases (Verri et al. 2000; Bell et al. 2005; Michael et al. 2009; Poretti et al. 2009): verbal IQ ranged between 67 and 138 and performance IQ between 74 and 120. Both verbal and performance functions were normal in three patients and impaired in one, whereas in the other two patients either verbal function alone or performance function alone was affected. Because of this discrepancy a typical cognitive profile for rhombencephalosynapsis could not be detected.

Attention problems are the most frequent behavioural disturbance in rhombencephalosynapsis (n=4) (Michael et al. 2009; Poretti et al. 2009). Michael et al. reported that one patient with rhombencephalosynapsis exhibited greater reactivity to warning signals and difficulties interrupting attentive processing, whereas distraction was not increased (Michael et al. 2009). They concluded that the cerebellum modulates responsiveness and commands attentional and exploratory flexibility in response to sensory signals. Three patients had internalizing behavioural problems presenting as an obsessive-compulsive personality disorder with self-mutilation (n=2) (Verri et al. 2000; Toelle et al. 2002), and withdrawn, somatic complaints, and thought problems (n=1) (Poretti et al. 2009). These abnormalities appear to be consistent with the cerebellar cognitive affective syndrome described by Schmahmann and Sherman (1998). Indeed, in particular, dysregulation of affect as part of the cerebellar cognitive affective syndrome occurs when the lesions involve the 'limbic cerebellum' (vermis and fastigial nucleus) as in rhombencephalosynapsis (Schmahmann et al. 2007).

Gómez-López-Hernández syndrome

The clinical findings of GLHS can vary considerably in severity and are sometimes not easy to detect. Truncal (n=19) and limb (n=10) ataxia as well as muscular hypotonia (n=10) can be very mild and not restricting. Ten patients presented with rhythmical, regular, intermittent head stereotypies from the first years of life corresponding to an infinity sign (or a horizontally positioned number 8), backward head nodding, and side-to-side head movement (Brocks et al. 2000; Tan et al. 2005; Whetsell et al. 2006; Poretti et al. 2008; Sukhudyan et al. 2010). In all cases, these movements improved over the course of several years in frequency and intensity, but always persisted. Other neurological findings are strabismus (n=10), epileptic seizures (n=3), and spastic paraplegia and microcephaly (n=1).

Scalp alopecia (n=26) too may be only moderate and easily hidden. The typical alopecia in GLHS is bilateral (n=24), involving the parietal regions in a band-like pattern, and is present from the neonatal period (Munoz et al. 1997; Purvis et al. 2007). However, in rare cases it can be asymmetric (Poretti et al. 2008; Fernandez-Jaen et al. 2009; Sukhudyan et al. 2010).

Trigeminal anesthesia (n=15) most often affects the ophthalmic branch with abnormal sensation of forehead and cornea and can lead to repetitive microtrauma and subsequent corneal opacities (n=13) (Munoz et al. 1997; Poretti et al. 2008). Absent corneal reflexes due to lack of corneal sensation is an early and sensitive sign of abnormal trigeminal function and can even occur with normal sensation on the forehead (n=1) (Poretti et al. 2008). However, several cases without trigeminal anesthesia have also been reported (Bowdin et al. 2007; Purvis et al. 2007; Gomy et al. 2008; Sukhudyan et al. 2010) and we are aware of similar unreported cases.

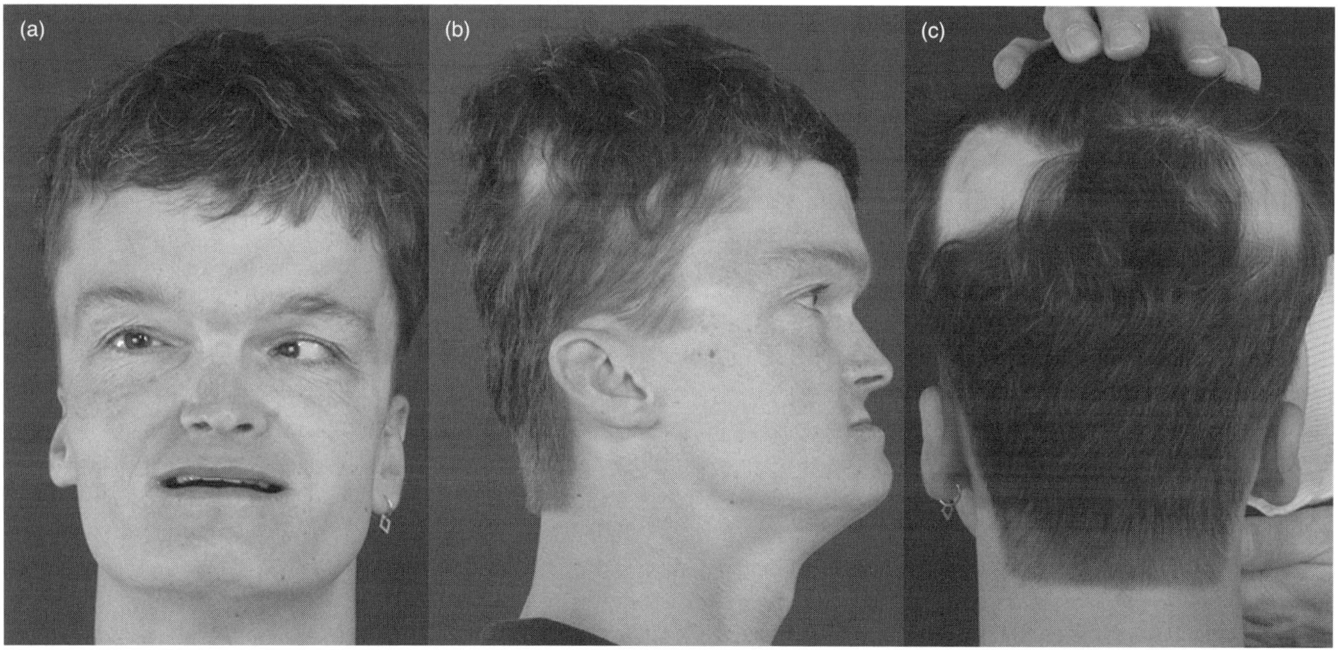

Fig. 16.1. Gómez-López-Hernández syndrome in a 34-year-old patient. **(a)** Front view showing broad, high forehead, hypertelorism, strabismus, small nose, and short and flat philtrum. Note the premature aging and scars on the forehead. **(b)** Right side view demonstrating pronounced brachyturricephaly, low-set, posteriorly rotated ears, prognathism, midface hypoplasia, and parietal alopecia. **(c)** Posterior view revealing bilateral parietal alopecia. (Reprinted with permission from Poretti A et al. Eur J Med Genet 2008; 51(3): 197–208.) (See color plate 24).

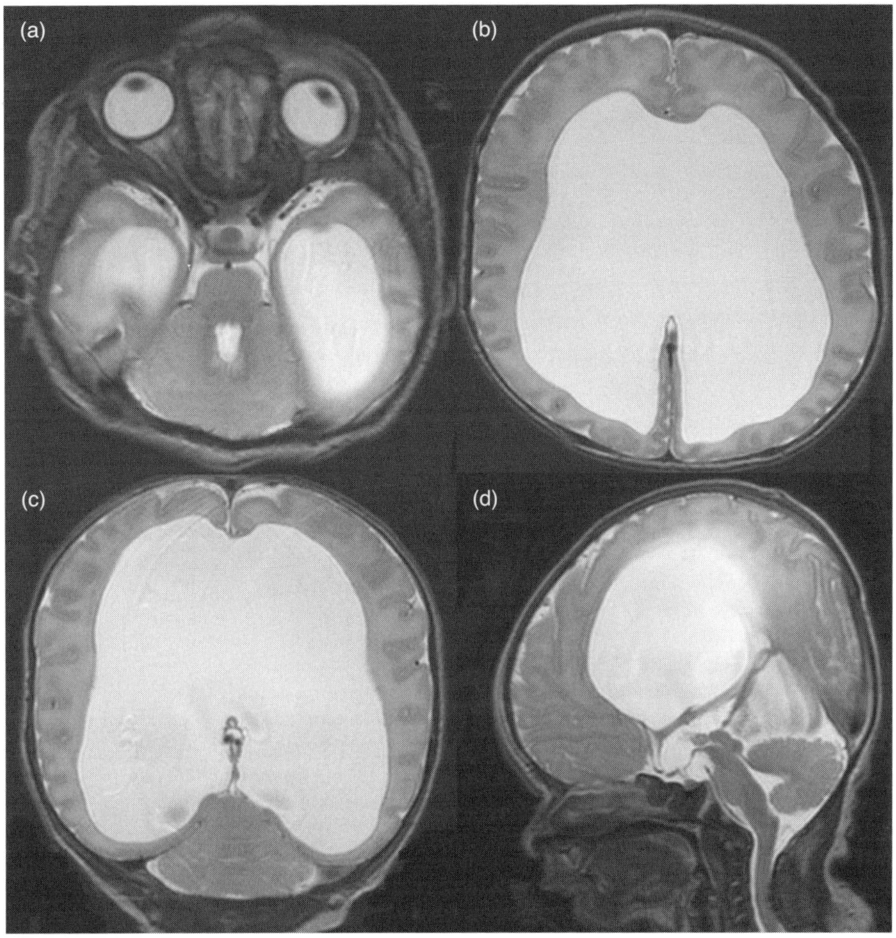

Fig. 16.2. Rhombencephalosynapsis in a 3-day-old patient investigated for macrocephaly. **(a)** Infratentorial axial T2-weighted image showing a small posterior fossa and midline fusion of the cerebellar peduncles, dentate nuclei, and cerebellar hemispheres without intervening vermis; **(b)** supratentorial axial T2-weighted MRI demonstrating hydrocephalus and absence of the septum pellucidum; **(c)** coronal T2-weighted MRI reveals hydrocephalus, absence of the septum pellucidum, and midline fusion of the cerebellar hemispheres without intervening vermis; **(d)** midsagittal T2-weighted MRI with abnormal configuration of the fourth ventricle and cerebellum due to the absence of the vermis. Aqueductal stenosis is noted.

Several dysmorphic signs are also typical of GLHS including midface hypoplasia and low-set, posteriorly rotated ears (n=23), brachycephaly (n=21), hypertelorism (n=15), clinodactyly (n=5), and mild ptosis (n=2) (Fig. 16.1) (Poretti et al. 2008; Sukhudyan et al. 2010).

Mental retardation (UK: learning disability) has been reported in the majority of patients with GLHS. However, six patients with normal cognition have also been reported (in three cases, full-scale IQ has been reported ranging from 90 to 114) (Truwit et al. 1991; Munoz et al. 1997; Purvis et al. 2007; Poretti et al. 2008; Sukhudyan et al. 2010). Ten patients had short stature, in two cases due to growth hormone deficiency (Brocks et al. 2000; Gomy et al. 2008). Most reported cases of GLHS are not associated with other diseases. One patient also suffered from neurogenic bladder dysfunction, one from esophageal atresia, and one from unilateral renal agenesis (Poretti et al. 2008; Sukhudyan et al. 2010).

Neuroimaging

The key neuroimaging features of rhombencephalosynapsis are agenesis of the cerebelli vermis and fusion of the cerebellar hemispheres, the superior and middle cerebellar peduncles, and the dentate nuclei, which arch in a horseshoe shape across the midline, resulting in a misshapen fourth ventricle mostly described as being keyhole-shaped on axial MRI images (Figs 16.2, 16.3) (Truwit et al. 1991; Danon et al. 2000; Montull et al. 2000; Toelle et al. 2002; Poretti et al. 2009). Additional neuroimaging findings include fusion of the colliculi (n=2) (Danon et al. 2000; Bell et al. 2005), which were closed in an additional case (Utsunomiya et al. 1998), fusion of the quadrigeminal plate (n=2) (Demaerel et al. 1995), hypoplastic olivary nuclei (n=1) (Demaerel et al. 1995), fused and posteriorly pointed tectum (n=1) (Utsunomiya et al. 1998), and in two patients with GLHS, lipoma of the quadrigeminal plate (n=1) and unilateral cleft in the brainstem-cerebellar junction (n=1) (Gomy et al. 2008; Sukhudyan et al. 2010). However, the nodulus appeared to be formed in three cases and the flocculi were also observed in one case (Utsunomiya et al. 1998; Mendonca et al. 2004). Neuropathological studies confirmed that in rhombencephalosynapsis the nodulus and flocculi are spared (Obersteiner 1916; Gross 1959; Gross and Hoff 1959; Yachnis 2002; Pasquier et al. 2009).

Hydrocephalus (Fig. 16.2) is the most common abnormality associated with rhombencephalosynapsis (Toelle et al. 2002). In 76 reported non-neuropathological cases the size of the lateral ventricles was increased in 44: in 18 cases it represented probable obstructive hydrocephalus, in the remaining 26 cases a mild ventriculomegaly (13 patients with GLHS). In

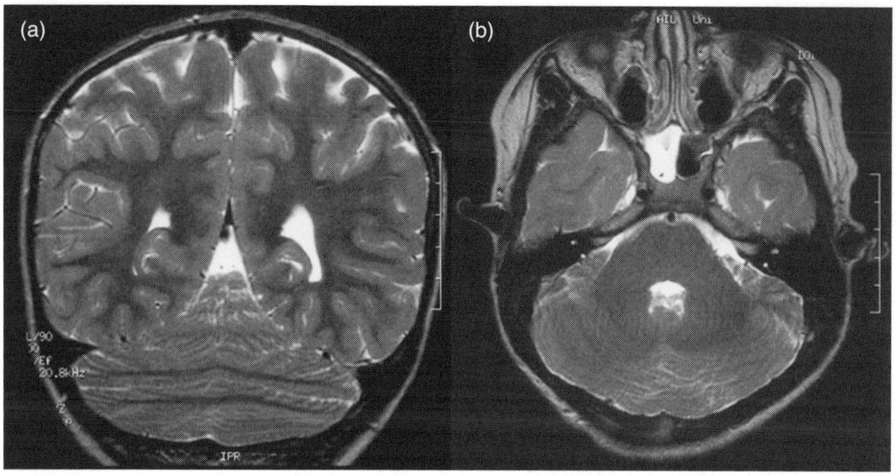

Fig. 16.3. Rhombencephalosynapsis in a patient aged 8 years 11 months. **(a)** Coronal T2-weighted MRI showing fused cerebellar hemispheres and abnormal, transverse orientation of cerebellar folia; **(b)** axial T2-weighted image demonstrating fusion of the cerebellar hemispheres without intervening vermis. (Reprinted with permission from Poretti A et al. Eur J Paediatr Neurol 2009; 13: 397–407.)

nine patients the hydrocephalus was treated by ventricular shunting. In rhombencephalosynapsis hydrocephalus is mostly caused by stenosis of the Sylvian aqueduct. In their neuropathological study, Pasquier et al. reported stenosis of the aqueduct in 5 of 36 cases (13%) (Pasquier et al. 2009). Evidence of aqueductal stenosis in rhombencephalosynapsis has been described as absence of the aqueductal flow void on MRI in five patients (GLHS, n=1) (Truwit et al. 1991; Utsunomiya et al. 1998; Gomy et al. 2008; Phillips et al. 2008; Poretti et al. 2009). Alternatively, obstruction of flow can be due to midline fusion of the thalami (Simmons et al. 1993), and obstruction or compression of the fourth ventricle by cerebellar tissue (Yachnis 2002) or retrocerebellar arachnoidal cyst (Toelle et al. 2002).

Aplasia of the septum pellucidum is often associated with rhombencephalosynapsis (n=29, in 7 cases GLHS) (Truwit et al. 1991; Brocks et al. 2000; Toelle et al. 2002; Bowdin et al. 2007; Gomy et al. 2008; Poretti et al. 2008, 2009). In 19 cases absence of the septum pellucidum was associated with hydrocephalus or ventriculomegaly (Fig. 16.2). In these cases, aplasia of the septum pellucidum can be secondary. In eight patients fusion of the fornices was specifically mentioned (Truwit et al. 1991; Boltenstern et al. 1995; Demaerel et al. 1995; Utsunomiya et al. 1998; Montull et al. 2000; Oei et al. 2001; McAuliffe et al. 2008; Poretti et al. 2009). Fusion of the fornices cannot be explained as a secondary phenomenon and may be regarded as evidence of a true midline defect (Barth 2008). Hypoplastic optic tract, which is typical of septo-optic-dysplasia, was reported in two cases of rhombencephalosynapsis (Truwit et al. 1991; Subash and Minasian 2008).

Hypoplasia of the corpus callosum was found in 18 cases of rhombencephalosynapsis (4 cases of GLHS) (Fig. 16.2) (Truwit et al. 1991; Demaerel et al. 1995; Utsunomiya et al. 1998; Danon et al. 2000; Guyot et al. 2000; Montull et al. 2000; Toelle et al. 2002; Mendonca et al. 2004; Chemli et al. 2007; Gomy et al. 2008; Kalra et al. 2008; Poretti et al. 2008, 2009). Because of the association of severe hydrocephalus (n=5), in some cases a thin corpus callosum can be a secondary phenomenon. However, hypoplastic corpus callosum has been also reported with mild ventriculomegaly (n=12) or without hydrocephalus or ventriculomegaly (n=1). In these cases it can be part of a midline defect. Hypoplasia of the anterior commissure was reported in two cases (Utsunomiya et al. 1998; Montull et al. 2000) and hippocampal abnormalities in eight: as malrotated hippocampi (n=4, in 3 cases GLHS) (Poretti et al. 2008, 2009), parahippocampal hypoplasia (Boltenstern et al. 1995), and vertically oriented (Mendonca et al. 2004), abnormal and globular (Bell et al. 2005), or hippocampal atrophy (Brocks et al. 2000).

The association between rhombencephalosynapsis and lobar holoprosencephaly was reported in vivo (McAuliffe et al. 2008) and postmortem (Siebert et al. 2005, Pasquier et al. 2009). In two cases (in one case of GLHS) fused thalami, a typical finding of alobar holoprosencephaly, were reported in association with rhombencephalosynapsis (Simmons et al. 1993; Poretti et al. 2008). Garfinkle reported the association between rhombencephalosynapsis, aventriculy, polymicrogyria, fused thalami, and absence of Sylvian fissures and both precentral and central sulci (Garfinkle 1996). Sergi et al. described a male fetus with rhombencephalosynapsis and telencephalosynapsis (Sergi et al. 1997). Pavone et al. presented a 15-year-old boy with rhombencephalosynapsis, distorted gyral patterns with deeply infolded mantle in the parietal-lateral and posterior-temporal lobes, fused thalami, thin white matter, collapsed ventricles, partial frontal corpus callosum agenesis, and closely apposed superior and middle cerebral peduncles (Pavone et al. 2005). Takano et al. demonstrated the association of rhombencephalosynapsis with aprosencephaly and hamartomatous midbrain dysplasia (Takano et al. 2010). Hypoplasia of the temporal lobes was present in two patients (Truwit et al. 1991; Montull et al. 2000). Other cortical abnormalities have been described in seven patients: cortical dysplasia of the right Sylvian fissure (Simmons et al. 1993), left parietal cleft (Simmons et al. 1993), focal dysplasia of the left temporal cortex (Mendonca et al. 2004), parietal cortical dysplasia and schizencephalic cleft (Phillips et al. 2008), temporal open-lip schizencephaly (McAuliffe et al. 2008), periventricular heterotopia (Toelle et al. 2002), and a thin gyrus cinguli (Poretti et al. 2009).

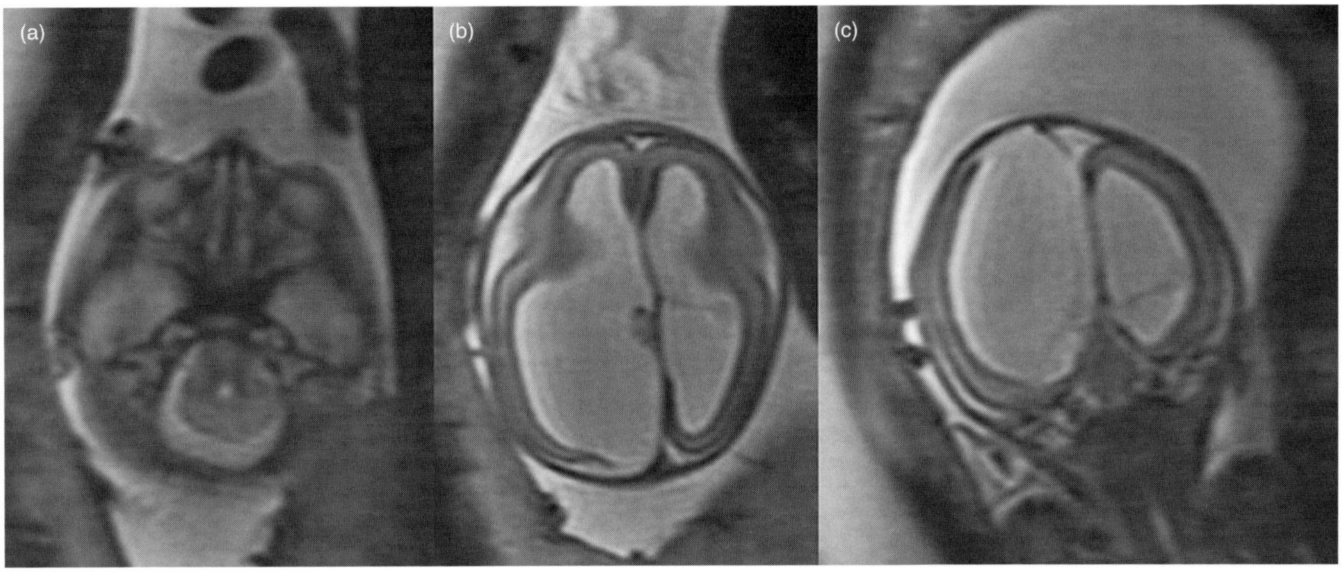

Fig. 16.4. Prenatal MRI at 22 weeks of gestation because of ventriculomegaly on routine ultrasound. **(a)** Axial infratentorial T2-weighted MRI showing a compact, small, single-lobed cerebellum suggesting rhombencephalosynapsis; **(b)** axial supratentorial T2-weighted MRI demonstrating an enlargement of both lateral ventricles; **(c)** coronal T2-weighted MRI presenting a compact, small, single-lobed cerebellum and enlarged lateral ventricles (RS was confirmed by postnatal MRI).

The association between rhombencephalosynapsis and encephalocele has been reported in two cases in vivo (one frontal and one occipital) (Simmons et al. 1993; Toelle et al. 2002), and postmortem (n=1) (Pasquier et al. 2009).

Diffusion tensor imaging (DTI) confirmed the absence of the transversely oriented fibres in the midsection of the cerebellum, demonstrated the vertical direction of the fibres in the midportion of the fused cerebellum, and showed that the deep cerebellar nuclei appeared more closely approximated (Widjaja et al. 2006).

Prenatal diagnosis of rhombencephalosynapsis (Fig. 16.4) has been reported in eight cases, the earliest at 21 weeks of gestation (Napolitano et al. 2004; Tan et al. 2005; McAuliffe et al. 2008; Dill et al. 2009). In all cases, fetal MRI has been performed because of bilateral ventriculomegaly on ultrasound screening.

In one patient with nonsyndromic rhombencephalosynapsis, single-voxel magnetic resonance spectroscopy revealed a reduced *N*-acetyl-aspartate to creatine ratio in the cerebellum compared with the control spectra (Striano et al. 2011).

Diagnosis

The diagnosis of rhombencephalosynapsis is made by the typical MRI findings and can be best confirmed on coronal MRI revealing an abnormal horizontal orientation of the cerebellar folia. Because neuroimaging findings in isolated rhombencephalosynapsis patients and patients with GLHS are identical, the typical clinical findings of GLHS must be accurately sought in all patients with rhombencephalosynapsis, otherwise the diagnosis can easily be missed (Poretti et al. 2008). Rhombencephalosynapsis is the only sign of GLHS that can be diagnosed in utero (Napolitano et al. 2004; Tan et al. 2005; McAuliffe et al. 2008; Dill et al. 2009). Therefore, prenatally it is not possible to distinguish between nonsyndromic rhombencephalosynapsis and GLHS (Poretti et al. 2008).

Differential diagnosis

Chiari II malformation is characterized by a small posterior fossa with herniation of the cerebellar vermis, caudal displacement of pons and medulla, kinking of the brainstem, loss of the pontine flexure, and beaking of the tectum (McLone and Dias 2003; Juranek and Salman 2010; see Chapter 13). Because of the small posterior fossa and herniation of the cerebellar vermis, on both coronal and axial MRI the vermis appears small and the cerebellar folia extend almost across the midline mimicking (partial) fusion of the cerebellar hemispheres and (partial) rhombencephalosynapsis (Guntur Ramkumar et al. 2010). Therefore, some authors have reported the association of rhombencephalosynapsis and Chiari II (Sener and Dzelzite 2003; Wang et al. 2005; Sandalcioglu et al. 2006). However, in our opinion a 'pseudo-fusion' of the cerebellar hemispheres is a typical neuroimaging finding in Chiari II without any association with rhombencephalosynapsis.

Fusion of the cerebellar hemispheres in the inferior posterior cerebellum was reported by Takanashi et al. in a child with muscular hypotonia, nystagmus, ataxia, and cognitive impairment (Takanashi et al. 1999). However, the additional neuroimaging findings (vertically oriented cerebellar folia, fusion of the inferior cerebellum, and hypoplasia of the cerebellar vermis) were clearly different than in rhombencephalosynapsis.

Management and treatment

In rhombencephalosynapsis and GLHS the treatment should be focused on symptoms to improve motor (particularly gait) and cognitive development and quality of life. Therefore, supporting therapies such as physical therapy (with emphasis on gait training) and occupational therapy as well as several aids can be utilized if necessary.

Because of corneal anesthesia in GLHS, prevention of repetitive microtrauma causing subsequent corneal opacities is mandatory.

Outcome

As extensively discussed in the clinical features section, ataxia is a frequent and persistent symptom, but is mostly mild and not restrictive of activities of daily living. However, a leading sign is mental retardation, which occurs in about half of the cases and is usually mild or moderate.

REFERENCES

Aydingoz U, Cila A, Aktan G (1997) Rhombencephalosynapsis associated with hand anomalies. Br J Radiol 70: 764–766.

Baker CV, Bronner-Fraser M (2001) Vertebrate cranial placodes I. Embryonic induction. Dev Biol 232: 1–61.

Barkovich AJ, Millen KJ, Dobyns WB (2009) A developmental and genetic classification for midbrain-hindbrain malformations. Brain 132: 3199–3230.

Barth PG (2008) Rhombencephalosynapsis. In: Sarnat HB, Curatolo P, editors. Malformations of the Nervous System. New York: Elsevier; 53–65.

Bell BD, Stanko HA, Levine RL (2005) Normal IQ in a 55-year-old with newly diagnosed rhombencephalosynapsis. Arch Clin Neuropsychol 20: 613–621.

Boltenstern M, Konrad A, Jost W, Uder M, Kujat C (1995) Rhombencephalosynapsis. Rofo 163: 91–93.

Bowdin S, Phelan E, Watson R, McCreery KM, Reardon W (2007) Rhombencephalosynapsis presenting antenatally with ventriculomegaly/hydrocephalus in a likely case of Gomez-Lopez-Hernandez syndrome. Clin Dysmorphol 16: 21–25.

Brocks D, Irons M, Sadeghi-Najad A, McCauley R, Wheeler P (2000) Gomez-Lopez-Hernandez syndrome: expansion of the phenotype. Am J Med Genet 94: 405–408.

Canturk S, Oto S, Kizilkilic O, Karaca S, Akova YA (2008) Rhombencephalosynapsis associated with infantile strabismus. Strabismus 16: 23–27.

Chemli J, Abroug M, Tlili K, Harbi A (2007) Rhombencephalosynapsis diagnosed in childhood: clinical and MRI findings. Eur J Paediatr Neurol 11: 35–38.

Danon O, Elmaleh M, Boukobza B, Fohlen M, Hadjnacer K, Hassan M (2000) Rhombencephalosynapsis diagnosed in childhood: clinical and MRI findings. Magn Reson Imaging 18: 99–101.

Demaerel P, Kendall BE, Wilms G, Halpin SF, Casaer P, Baert AL (1995) Uncommon posterior cranial fossa anomalies: MRI with clinical correlation. Neuroradiology 37: 72–76.

di Vera E, Liberati M, Celentano C, Calabrese G, Guanciali-Franchi PE, Morizio E, Rotmensch S (2008) Rhombencephalosynapsis in a severely polymalformed fetus with non-mosaic tetrasomy 9p, in intracytoplasmic-sperm-injection pregnancy. J Assist Reprod Genet 25: 577–580.

Dill P, Poretti A, Boltshauser E, Huisman TA (2009) Fetal magnetic resonance imaging in midline malformations of the central nervous system and review of the literature. J Neuroradiol 36: 138–146.

Fernandez-Jaen A, Fernandez-Mayoralas DM, Calleja-Perez B, Munoz-Jareno N, Moreno N (2009) Gomez-Lopez-Hernandez syndrome: two new cases and review of the literature. Pediatr Neurol 40: 58–62.

Garfinkle WB (1996) Aventriculy: a new entity? AJNR Am J Neuroradiol 17: 1649–1650.

Gomez MR (1979) Cerebellotrigeminal and focal dermal dysplasia: a newly recognized neurocutaneous syndrome. Brain Dev 1: 253–256.

Gomy I, Heck B, Santos AC, Figueiredo MS, Martinelli CE, Jr., Nogueira MP, Pina-Neto JM (2008) Two new Brazilian patients with Gomez-Lopez-Hernandez syndrome: reviewing the expanded phenotype with molecular insights. Am J Med Genet A 146A: 649–657.

Gross H (1959) Die Rhombencephalosynapsis, eine systemisierte Kleinhirnfehlbildung. Arch Psychiatr Nervenkr 199: 537–552.

Gross H, Hoff H (1959) Sur les dysraphies cranio-encéphaliques. In: Heuyer G, Feld M, Gruner J, editors. Malformations congénitales du cerveau. Paris: Masson; 287–296.

Gross MK, Dottori M, Goulding M (2002) Lbx1 specifies somatosensory association interneurons in the dorsal spinal cord. Neuron 34: 535–549.

Gulyas B, Roland PE (1994) Binocular disparity discrimination in human cerebral cortex: functional anatomy by positron emission tomography. Proc Natl Acad Sci U S A 91: 1239–1243.

Guntur Ramkumar P, Kanodia AK, Ananthakrishnan G, Roberts R (2010) Chiari II malformation mimicking partial rhombencephalosynapsis? A case report. Cerebellum 9: 111–114.

Guyot LL, Kazmierczak CD, Michael DB (2000) Adult rhombencephalosynapsis. Case report. J Neurosurg 93: 323–325.

Hottinger-Blanc PM, Ziegler AL, Deonna T (2002) A special type of head stereotypies in children with developmental (? cerebellar) disorder: description of 8 cases and literature review. Eur J Paediatr Neurol 6: 143–152.

Jellinger KA (2002) Rhombencephalosynapsis. Acta Neuropathol 103: 305–306.

Juranek J, Salman MS (2010) Anomalous development of brain structure and function in spina bifida myelomeningocele. Dev Disabil Res Rev 16: 23–30.

Kalra V, Sharma S, Garg A (2008) Rhombencephalosynapsis: association with single umbilical artery. Indian J Pediatr 75: 1175–1177.

Koljonen V, Leikola J, Valanne L, Hukki J (2009) Atypical craniosynostosis with torticollis and neurological symptoms: a rhombencephalosynapsis sequence. Case Report Med 2009: 919463.

Lespinasse J, Testard H, Nugues F, Till M, Cordier MP, Althuser M, et al. (2004) A submicroscopic unbalanced subtelomeric translocation t(2p;10q) identified by fluorescence in situ hybridization: fetus with increased nuchal translucency and normal standard karyotype with later growth and developmental delay, rhombencephalosynapsis (RES). Ann Genet 47: 405–417.

Logan C, Wingate RJ, McKay IJ, Lumsden A (1998) Tlx-1 and Tlx-3 homeobox gene expression in cranial sensory ganglia and hindbrain of the chick embryo: markers of patterned connectivity. J Neurosci 18: 5389–5402.

López-Hernández A (1982) Craniosynostosis, ataxia, trigeminal anaesthesia and parietal alopecia with pons-vermis fusion anomaly (atresia of the fourth ventricle). Report of two cases. Neuropediatrics 13: 99–102.

Mannan AU, Roussa E, Kraus C, Rickmann M, Maenner J, Nayernia K, et al. (2004) Mutation in the gene encoding lysosomal acid phosphatase (Acp2) causes cerebellum and skin malformation in mouse. Neurogenetics 5: 229–238.

Manzanares M, Trainor PA, Ariza-McNaughton L, Nonchev S, Krumlauf R (2000) Dorsal patterning defects in the hindbrain, roof plate and skeleton in the dreher (dr(J)) mouse mutant. Mech Dev 94: 147–156.

McAuliffe F, Chitayat D, Halliday W, Keating S, Shah V, Fink M, et al. (2008) Rhombencephalosynapsis: prenatal imaging and autopsy findings. Ultrasound Obstet Gynecol 31: 542–548.

McLone DG, Dias MS (2003) The Chiari II malformation: cause and impact. Childs Nerv Syst 19: 540–550.

Mendonca JL, Natal MR, Viana SL, Coimbra PP, Viana MA, Matsumine M (2004) Rhombencephalosynapsis: CT and MRI findings. Neurol India 52: 118–120.

Michael GA, Garcia S, Bussy G, Lion-Francois L, Guibaud L (2009) Reactivity to visual signals and the cerebellar vermis: Evidence from a rare case with rhombencephalosynapsis. Behav Neurosci 123: 86–96.

Millonig JH, Millen KJ, Hatten ME (2000) The mouse Dreher gene Lmx1a controls formation of the roof plate in the vertebrate CNS. Nature 403: 764–769.

Montull C, Mercader JM, Peri J, Martinez Ferri M, Bonaventura I (2000) Neuroradiological and clinical findings in rhombencephalosynapsis. Neuroradiology 42: 272–274.

Munoz RMv, Santos AC, Graziadio C, Pinta-Neto JM (1997) Cerebello-trigeminal-dermal dysplasia (Gomez-Lopez-Hernandez syndrome): description of three new cases and review. Am J Med Genet 72: 34–39.

Napolitano M, Righini A, Zirpoli S, Rustico M, Nicolini U, Triulzi F (2004) Prenatal magnetic resonance imaging of rhombencephalosynapsis and associated brain anomalies: report of 3 cases. J Comput Assist Tomogr 28: 762–765.

Obersteiner H (1916) Ein Kleinhirn ohne Wurm. Arb Neurol Inst Wien Univ 21: 124–136.

Odemis E, Cakir M, Aynaci FM (2003) Rhombencephalosynapsis associated with cutaneous pretibial hemangioma in an infant. J Child Neurol 18: 225–228.

Oei AS, Vanzieleghem BD, Kunnen MF (2001) Diagnostic imaging and clinical findings in rhombencephalosynapsis: case report and literature review. JBR-BTR 84: 197–200.

Pasquier L, Marcorelles P, Loget P, Pelluard F, Carles D, Perez MJ, et al. (2009) Rhombencephalosynapsis and related anomalies: a neuropathological study of 40 fetal cases. Acta Neuropathol 117: 185–200.

Patel S, Barkovich AJ (2002) Analysis and classification of cerebellar malformations. AJNR Am J Neuroradiol 23: 1074–1087.

Pavone P, Incorpora G, Ruggieri M (2005) A complex brain malformation syndrome with rhombencephalosynapsis, preaxial hexadactyly plus facial and skull anomalies. Neuropediatrics 36: 279–283.

Phillips PH, Glasier CM, Brodsky MC (2008) Neuro-ophthalmologic findings in patients with rhombencephalosynapsis. J AAPOS 12: 97–99.

Poretti A, Bartholdi D, Gobara S, Alber FD, Boltshauser E (2008) Gomez-Lopez-Hernandez syndrome: an easily missed diagnosis. Eur J Med Genet 51: 197–208.

Poretti A, Alber FD, Burki S, Toelle SP, Boltshauser E (2009) Cognitive outcome in children with rhombencephalosynapsis. Eur J Paediatr Neurol 13: 28–33.

Poretti A, Limperopoulos C, Roulet-Perez E, Wolf NI, Rauscher C, Prayer D, et al. (2010) Outcome of severe unilateral cerebellar hypoplasia. Dev Med Child Neurol 52: 718–724.

Purvis DJ, Ramirez A, Roberts N, Harper JI (2007) Gomez-Lopez-Hernandez syndrome: another consideration in focal congenital alopecia. Br J Dermatol 157: 196–198.

Romanengo M, Tortori-Donati P, Di Rocco M (1997) Rhombencephalosynapsis with facial anomalies and probable autosomal recessive inheritance: a case report. Clin Genet 52: 184–186.

Sandalcioglu IE, Gasser T, van de Nes JA, Menken U, Stolke D, Wiedemayer H (2006) Fusion of the cerebellar hemispheres ventral to the brainstem: a rare hindbrain-related malformation. Childs Nerv Syst 22: 73–77.

Sarnat HB, Benjamin DR, Siebert JR, Kletter GB, Cheyette SR (2002) Agenesis of the mesencephalon and metencephalon with cerebellar hypoplasia: putative mutation in the EN2 gene – report of 2 cases in early infancy. Pediatr Dev Pathol 5: 54–68.

Schell-Apacik CC, Cohen M, Vojta S, Ertl-Wagner B, Klopocki E, Heinrich U, von Voss H (2008) Gomez-Lopez-Hernandez syndrome (cerebello-trigeminal-dermal dysplasia): description of an additional case and review of the literature. Eur J Pediatr 167: 123–126.

Schmahmann JD, Sherman JC (1998) The cerebellar cognitive affective syndrome. Brain 121: 561–579.

Schmahmann JD, Weilburg JB, Sherman JC (2007) The neuropsychiatry of the cerebellum – insights from the clinic. Cerebellum 6: 254–267.

Scroop R, Sage M, Voyvodic F (2000) Rhombencephalosynapsis. Australas Radiol 44: 225–227.

Sener RN, Dzelzite S (2003) Rhombencephalosynapsis and a Chiari II malformation. J Comput Assist Tomogr 27: 257–259.

Sergi C, Hentze S, Sohn C, Voigtlander T, Jung C, Schmitt HP (1997) Telencephalosynapsis (synencephaly) and rhombencephalosynapsis with posterior fossa ventriculocele ('Dandy-Walker cyst'): an unusual aberrant syngenetic complex. Brain Dev 19: 426–432.

Sieber MA, Storm R, Martinez-de-la-Torre M, Muller T, Wende H, Reuter K, et al. (2007) Lbx1 acts as a selector gene in the fate determination of somatosensory and viscerosensory relay neurons in the hindbrain. J Neurosci 7: 4902–4909.

Siebert JR, Schoenecker KA, Resta RG, Kapur RP (2005) Holoprosencephaly and limb reduction defects: a consideration of Steinfeld syndrome and related conditions. Am J Med Genet A 134: 381–392.

Simmons G, Damiano TR, Truwit CL (1993) MRI and clinical findings in rhombencephalosynapsis. J Comput Assist Tomogr 17: 211–214.

Striano P, Morana G, Pezzella M, Beini T, Rossi A (2011) Rhombencephalosynapsis in a patient with mental retardation, epilepsy, and dysmorphisms. Neurol Sci 32: 193–194.

Subash M, Minasian M (2008) Reduced vision as a presenting feature of rhombencephalosynapsis. J AAPOS 12: 614–615.

Sukhudyan B, Jaladyan V, Melikyan G, Schlump JU, Boltshauser E, Poretti A (2010) Gómez–López-Hernández syndrome: reappraisal of the diagnostic criteria. Eur J Pediatr 169: 1523–1528.

Takagi M, Tamargo R, Zee DS (2003) Effects of lesions of the cerebellar oculomotor vermis on eye movements in primate: binocular control. Prog Brain Res 142: 19–33.

Takanashi J, Sugita K, Barkovich AJ, Takano H, Kohno Y (1999) Partial midline fusion of the cerebellar hemispheres with vertical folia: a new cerebellar malformation? AJNR Am J Neuroradiol 20: 1151–1153.

Takano T, Kinoshita N, Narumiya S, Takeuchi Y (2010) Aprosencephaly with rhombencephalosynapsis and hamartomatous midbrain dysplasia. Neuropathol Appl Neurobiol 36: 353–355.

Tan TY, McGillivray G, Goergen SK, White SM (2005) Prenatal magnetic resonance imaging in Gomez-Lopez-Hernandez syndrome and review of the literature. Am J Med Genet A 138: 369–373.

Toelle SP, Yalcinkaya C, Kocer N, Deonna T, Overweg-Plandsoen WC, Bast T, et al. (2002) Rhombencephalosynapsis: clinical findings and neuroimaging in 9 children. Neuropediatrics 33: 209–214.

Truwit CL, Barkovich AJ, Shanahan R, Maroldo TV (1991) MR imaging of rhombencephalosynapsis: report of three cases and review of the literature. AJNR Am J Neuroradiol 12: 957–965.

Utsunomiya H, Takano K, Ogasawara T, Hashimoto T, Fukushima T, Okazaki M (1998) Rhombencephalosynapsis: cerebellar embryogenesis. AJNR Am J Neuroradiol 19: 547–549.

Verri A, Uggetti C, Vallero E, Ceroni M, Federico A (2000) Oral self-mutilation in a patient with rhombencephalosynapsys. J Intellect Disabil Res 44: 86–90.

Wang SM, Khong PL, Ip P, Ooi GC (2005) Partial rhombencephalosynapsis and Chiari II malformation. Hong Kong Med J 11: 299–302.

Whetsell W, Saigal G, Godinho S (2006) Gomez-Lopez-Hernandez syndrome. Pediatr Radiol 36: 552–554.

Widjaja E, Blaser S, Raybaud C (2006) Diffusion tensor imaging of midline posterior fossa malformations. Pediatr Radiol 36: 510–517.

Yachnis AT (2002) Rhombencephalosynapsis with massive hydrocephalus: case report and pathogenetic considerations. Acta Neuropathol 103: 301–304.

17
Macrocerebellum

Andrea Poretti and Eugen Boltshauser

Macrocerebellum is an extremely rare condition characterized by abnormally large cerebellum with preservation of the overall shape. It may be a key feature of some syndromes (see Checklists, Table 25). Bodensteiner and colleagues published a report of four patients with isolated (nonsyndromal) macrocerebellum (Bodensteiner et al. 1997). We are aware of additional unreported patients.

Aetiology

Macrocerebellum can be caused by increased proliferation of cells, which usually occurs as part of a more widespread syndrome (Barkovich et al. 2009). It has been reported in the macrocephaly-capillary malformation syndrome which is associated with overgrowth of cerebral and cerebellar hemispheres, often resulting in cerebellar tonsillar herniation (Conway et al. 2007).

Macrocerebellum has been described in two patients with Sotos syndrome (Schaefer et al. 1997) as well as in Williams syndrome (enlarged cerebellum relative to a small cerebrum) (Jones et al. 2002). In both syndromes the presence of macrocerebellum is not an isolated phenomenon. In Sotos syndrome other neuroimaging findings include ventricular abnormalities, increased extracerebral fluid spaces, midline abnormalities, and migration anomalies. Furthermore, patients with Sotos syndrome have typical clinical findings such as macrocephaly, somatic overgrowth, characteristic facial dysmorphic signs, and mental retardation (UK: learning disability). Patients with Williams syndrome have a typical phenotype including characteristic 'elfin' facies, cardiac and pulmonary abnormalities, growth delays, hypercalcemia, and anxiety.

In Costello syndrome (severe failure to thrive, cardiac abnormalities, neurological abnormalities including developmental delay, mental retardation, nystagmus, and hypotonia, and susceptibility to papillomata and malignant tumour) Gripp et al. reported macrocerebellum with cerebellar tonsillar herniation in 96% of their patients (Gripp et al. 2010). In 59% the enlargement of the cerebellum was progressive on serial neuroimaging studies and caused several sequelae such as hydrocephalus requiring shunt or ventriculostomy (25%), Chiari I malformation (32%), and syrinx formation (25%). This process of evolving megalencephaly and cerebellar enlargement is in keeping with mouse model data, delineating abnormal genesis of neurons and glia, resulting in an increased number of astrocytes and enlarged brain volume (Gripp et al. 2010).

The aetiology of nonsyndromic macrocerebellum remains unknown. The association with delayed myelination of the supratentorial white matter (and not manifest in the cerebellum) leads to the hypothesis that in these patients the cerebellum is more mature from the standpoint of growth and the cerebellar tissue is responding to the elaboration of growth factors intended to augment the slow development of the cerebral structures (Bodensteiner et al. 1997).

Clinical features

Patients with nonsyndromic macrocerebellum were investigated because of delayed motor and cognitive development in all cases (motor delay mild to severe, cognitive delay moderate to severe), abnormal ocular movements (ocular motor apraxia in three cases and torsional nystagmus in one), slightly decreased coordination in three cases, and abnormalities of muscle tone (decreased in three, variable in one, and increased in the limbs and decreased in the trunk in the other patient) (Bodensteiner et al. 1997). Mild dysmorphic signs were present in three cases.

Neuroimaging

The 'typical' neuroimaging finding is the disproportionately large cerebellum with apparently normal architecture (Fig. 17.1). In the nonsyndromic form the neuroimaging features also include deficient or delayed myelination of the cerebral white matter in all cases, and subcortical band heterotopia in the frontal regions as described in one patient. In some cases of macrocephaly-capillary malformation syndrome, noticeable overgrowth of the cerebellum was observed during the first few months of life with progressive crowding of the posterior fossa and eventual herniation of the cerebellar tonsils (Conway et al. 2007).

Diagnosis

The diagnosis of macrocerebellum is made by the 'typical' MRI findings. Dysmorphic signs characteristic of Sotos, Williams, and Costello syndrome as well as of macrocephaly-capillary malformation have to be carefully sought because macrocerebellum can be part of these syndromes.

Differential diagnosis

Increased size of the cerebellum has been reported in rare instances of Alexander disease (van der Knaap et al. 2005). In these few patients the cerebellar as well as the periventricular

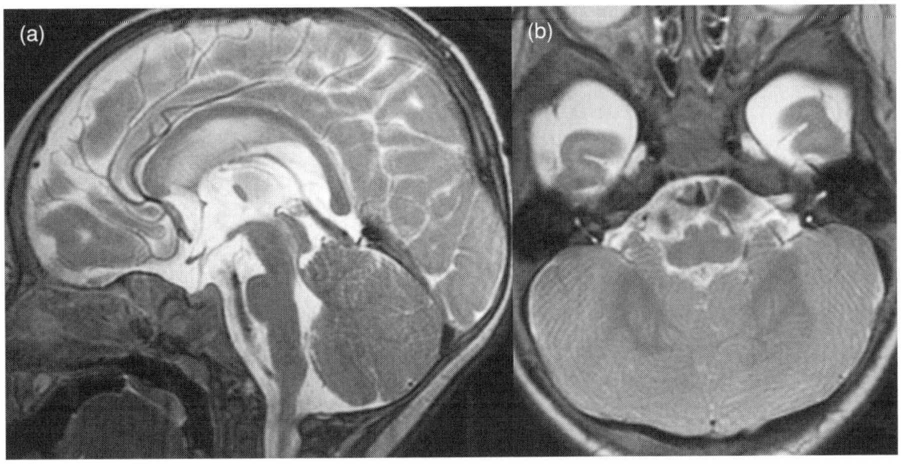

Fig. 17.1. MRI of a patient with macrocerebellum at the age of 7 months. **(a)** Midsagittal T2-weighted and **(b)** axial T2-weighted images showing marked increase in the size of the whole cerebellum without evidence of focal cortical dysplasia and with normal sized posterior fossa.

white matter was also abnormal and over time the size of the cerebellum decreased.

A significant global increase of the cerebellar volume has recently been reported in five patients with fucosidosis (Kau et al. 2011).

Enlargement of the cerebellum has been also reported in Lhermitte-Duclos syndrome (see Chapter 23) (Nowak and Trost 2002; Perez-Nunez et al. 2004). In this disease the cerebellar involvement is usually focal, although diffuse enlargement of the cerebellum has also been reported (Milbouw et al. 1988). The other neuroimaging findings of Lhermitte-Duclos disease (non-enhancing gyriform pattern corresponding to the enlargement of the cerebellar cortical folia, hypointensity on T1-weighted images, striated pattern with isointense bands in the area of hyperintensity on T2-weighted images) as well as the clinical features are distinct from those shared by children with macrocerebellum.

Enlargement of one half (ipsilateral) of the cerebellum is recognized in 'total hemimegalencephaly' (see Chapter 26) (Sener 1997). Hemimegalencephaly can occur as an isolated feature or associated with partial or total hemigigantism and/or several neurocutaneous syndromes (systemic form) such as Klippel-Trénaunay-Weber syndrome, epidermal nevus syndrome, or Ito's hypomelanosis (Flores-Sarnat 2002). Because of the supratentorial neuroimaging findings, the unilateral cerebellar enlargement, and the clinical findings (in the systemic form) the differentiation between macrocerebellum and total hemimegalencephaly is usually not problematic.

Management and treatment

Treatment of macrocerebellum is symptomatic and includes supporting therapies such as physical and occupational therapies.

REFERENCES

Barkovich AJ, Millen KJ, Dobyns WB (2009) A developmental and genetic classification for midbrain-hindbrain malformations. Brain 132: 3199–3230.

Bodensteiner JB, Schaefer GB, Keller GM, Thompson JN, Bowen MK (1997) Macrocerebellum: neuroimaging and clinical features of a newly recognized condition. J Child Neurol 12: 365–368.

Conway RL, Pressman BD, Dobyns WB, Danielpour M, Lee J, Sanchez-Lara PA, et al. (2007) Neuroimaging findings in macrocephaly-capillary malformation: a longitudinal study of 17 patients. Am J Med Genet A 143A: 2981–3008.

Flores-Sarnat L (2002) Hemimegalencephaly: part 1. Genetic, clinical, and imaging aspects. J Child Neurol 17: 373–384.

Gripp KW, Hopkins E, Doyle D, Dobyns WB (2010) High incidence of progressive postnatal cerebellar enlargement in Costello syndrome: brain overgrowth associated with HRAS mutations as the likely cause of structural brain and spinal cord abnormalities. Am J Med Genet A 152A: 1161–1168.

Jones W, Hesselink J, Courchesne E, Duncan T, Matsuda K, Bellugi U (2002) Cerebellar abnormalities in infants and toddlers with Williams syndrome. Dev Med Child Neurol 44: 688–694.

Kau T, Karlo C, Güngor T, Prietsch V, Kellenberger CJ, Scheer I, Boltshauser E (2011) Increased cerebellar volume in the early stage of fucosidosis: a case control study. Neuroradiology 53: 509–516.

Milbouw G, Born JD, Martin D, Collignon J, Hans P, Reznik M, Bonnal J (1988) Clinical and radiological aspects of dysplastic gangliocytoma (Lhermitte-Duclos disease): a report of two cases with review of the literature. Neurosurgery 22: 124–128.

Nowak DA, Trost HA (2002) Lhermitte-Duclos disease (dysplastic cerebellar gangliocytoma): a malformation, hamartoma or neoplasm? Acta Neurol Scand 105: 137–145.

Perez-Nunez A, Lagares A, Benitez J, Urioste M, Lobato RD, Ricoy JR, et al. (2004) Lhermitte-Duclos disease and Cowden disease: clinical and genetic study in five patients with Lhermitte-Duclos disease and literature review. Acta Neurochir (Wien) 146: 679–690.

Schaefer GB, Bodensteiner JB, Buehler BA, Lin A, Cole TR (1997) The neuroimaging findings in Sotos syndrome. Am J Med Genet 68: 462–465.

Sener RN (1997) MR demonstration of cerebral hemimegalencephaly associated with cerebellar involvement (total hemimegalencephaly). Comput Med Imaging Graph 21: 201–204.

van der Knaap MS, Salomons GS, Li R, Franzoni E, Gutierrez-Solana LG, Smit LM, et al. (2005) Unusual variants of Alexander's disease. Ann Neurol 57: 327–338.

18
Hemicerebellar Megalencephaly

Andrea Poretti and Eugen Boltshauser

Hemimegalencephaly (HME) is a rare malformation characterized by hamartomatous overgrowth limited to one cerebral hemisphere (Flores-Sarnat 2008). Its real frequency is unknown. Most reports consist of single cases and all patients are sporadic. Three forms of HME have been suggested. *Isolated HME* is not associated with hemicorporal hypertrophy, cutaneous or systemic involvement. *Associated HME* is accompanied by other conditions, mainly neurocutaneous syndromes, particularly the epidermal nevus syndrome (ENS) (Sugarman 2007; Menascu and Donner 2008), but also Klippel-Trenaunay-Weber (KTW) (Cohen 2002; Oduber et al. 2008), neurofibromatosis type 1 (NF1) (Balestri et al. 2003; Jett and Friedman 2010; Payne et al. 2010), encephalocraniocutaneous lipomatosis (Cruz et al. 2002; Moog et al. 2007; Moog 2009), Proteus syndrome (Dietrich et al. 1998; DeLone et al. 1999; Biesecker 2006), hypomelanosis of Ito (Ruggieri and Pavone 2000; Chapman and Cardenas 2008), and tuberous sclerosis (Galluzzi et al. 2002; Curatolo et al. 2008). Rarely HME occurs associated with Aicardi syndrome, Hirschsprung disease, Adams-Olivier syndrome, frontonasal dysplasia, giant congenital melanocytic nevi, cutis marmorata telangiectatica congenita or macrocephaly-capillary malformation (MCM) (Conway et al. 2007), and Gorlin syndrome. In a few cases the cerebellar hemisphere and the brainstem ipsilateral to the side of the cerebral enlargement are also enlarged and show abnormal foliation. This form is named *total HME* (THME) and was first described by Hallervorden (1923). To our knowledge, only 19 cases have been reported (Calzolari et al. 1996; Sener 1997; Di Rocco et al. 2001; Abdelhalim et al. 2003; Sato et al. 2007; Maruyama et al. 2010). We briefly mention two additional patients seen in our clinic.

Aetiology and pathogenesis

The aetiology of HME and THME is poorly understood. It was speculated that abnormalities of neuronal differentiation and cell migration in the affected cerebral hemisphere are involved. However, Flores-Sarnat proposed an early genetically programmed developmental disorder of symmetry and cellular lineage occurring at about the third week of gestation (Flores-Sarnat 2002; Flores-Sarnat et al. 2003). The neuroblast migratory abnormalities in HME are then secondary to both abnormal radial glial cells and abnormal neuroblasts occurring after the 8th gestational week. Additionally, the overgrowth suggests a disturbance in proliferation, which occurs early and continues beyond the normal proliferation period (Flores-Sarnat 2008). Because of the association between HME and some neurocutaneous syndromes a relationship between epidermal growth factor and excessive proliferation has been also considered (Takashima et al. 1991; Kato et al. 1996).

Clinical features

Patients with isolated HME usually manifest the first symptoms in infancy, often as soon as the neonatal period. The first neurological manifestation is usually macrocephaly which can progress in the first months of life, but without signs of intracranial hypertension (Hung and Wang 2005). The cranium can be asymmetric due to greater volume of the affected side. Global developmental delay is noted early and leads to cognitive impairment of varying severity. Mild cases with normal cognitive function are infrequent. Different degrees of contralateral hemiparesis are seen. Ipsilateral to the HME, hemianopsia can also be present (Vigevano et al. 1989; Rintahaka et al. 1993). Epilepsy has an early onset and can be of different types including generalized clonic and tonic-clonic, partial motor or partial complex, partial with secondary generalization, myoclonic, tonic, atonic, infantile spasms, and epilepsia partialis continua. Seizures are often intractable and correlate with poor outcome.

In associated HME the different skin lesions can be overlapping in the neurocutaneous syndromes. They include hyper- and hypopigmented lesions such as café-au-lait spots in NF1 and Proteus syndrome; white maculae in tuberous sclerosis, ENS, and Proteus syndrome; hypo- or hyperpigmented whorls in hypomelanosis of Ito and incontinentia pigmenti; cutaneous, subcutaneous, and internal vascular lesions in KTW, MCM, and Proteus syndrome; and lipomas in ENS, Proteus syndrome, and KTW (Flores-Sarnat 2008). Additionally, hemicorporal hypertrophy can be found in Proteus syndrome, KTW, ENS, MCM, and hypomelanosis of Ito, overgrowth of hands and feet in Proteus syndrome and KTW, intracranial calcifications in ENS, Proteus syndrome, and tuberous sclerosis, systemic involvement in tuberous sclerosis, ENS, MCM, and Proteus syndrome, and tumors in ENS, MCM, tuberous sclerosis, and NF1 (Flores-Sarnat 2008).

Detailed clinical information about THME is available for only four patients (Calzolari et al. 1996; Sener 1997; Abdelhalim et al. 2003). Sener reported a 1 year old boy with intractable seizures and an asymmetric cranium (Sener 1997). The patient presented by Abdelhalim et al. was 1 year old, started having myoclonic, tonic, and generalized tonic-clonic seizures at 8 weeks of age, which were poorly controlled despite several drugs (Abdelhalim et al. 2003). Additionally, he had pinpoint, flesh-colored papules linearly arranged along the

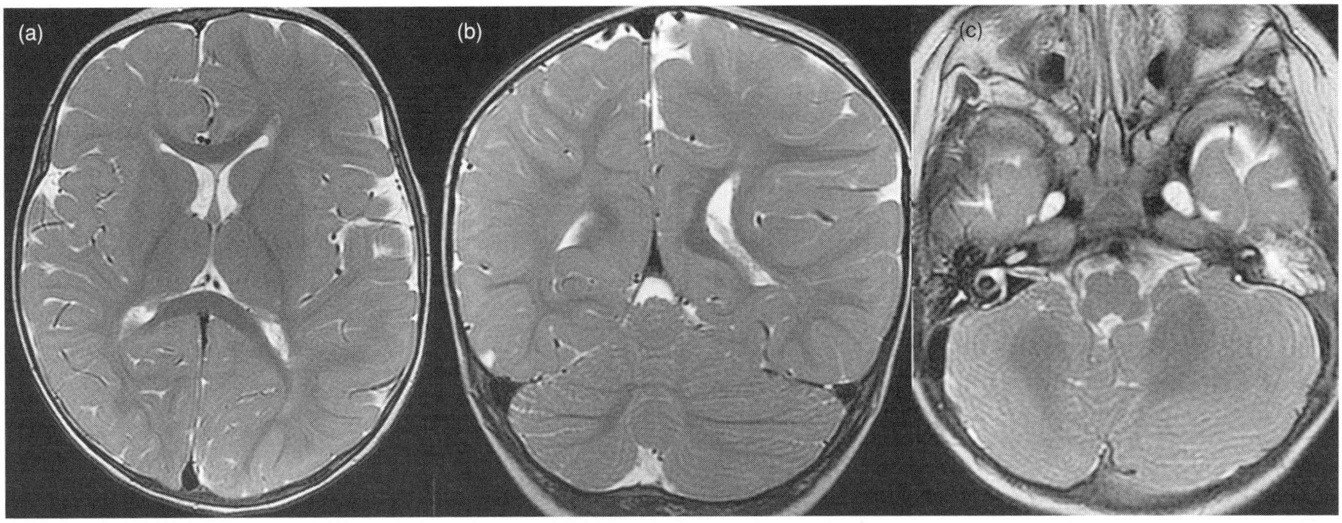

Fig. 18.1. Total hemimegalencephaly in a 13-month-old child with cutis marmorata teleangiectatica congenita and hemihypertrophy of the left face and arm. **(a)** Supratentorial axial T2-weighted MRI showing a moderate asymmetry of the cerebral hemispheres with enlargement of the left cortical hemisphere, mild occipital sign, cortical dysplasia, and increase in the white matter on the left side; **(b)** coronal T2-weighted MRI demonstrating asymmetry of the cerebral and cerebellar hemispheres with moderate enlargement of the left hemispheres, mild asymmetry of the lateral ventricles, and mild cortical dysplasia of the left cerebral hemisphere; **(c)** infratentorial T2-weighted MRI revealing asymmetry of the cerebellar hemisphere with mild enlargement of the left hemisphere.

left nasal bridge and keratotic plaques along the upper lip, suggesting ENS. One other patient presented with macrocephaly, asymmetric cranium, muscular hypotonia, generalized seizures, and hemihypertrophy of the face, trunk and limbs, and malformation of the feet (Calzolari et al. 1996). The fourth patient had generalized tonic seizures, a large, elastic subcutaneous mass in his right cheek, and a hemihypertrophy on the right side of the tongue (Maruyama et al. 2010). The first of our patients presented at birth with facial asymmetry with hypertrophy of the left hemiface and pinkish blue, reticular and patchy skin changes on the left trunk and right axilla suggesting cutis marmorata telangiectatica congenita. Brain MRI at the age of 13 months revealed a TMHE on the left side (Fig. 18.1). At the age of 16 months he also showed a very mild enlargement of the left arm causing minimal impairment in the function of the left hand. Otherwise the neurological examination and the development at the age of 16 months were normal. The second patient had a capillary malformation of the left forearm and hand as well as overgrowth of both hands at birth. At the age of 12 months he developed hydrocephalus; brain MRI showed TMHE on the left side and hydrocephalus due to Chiari I malformation, and shunting was placed. Additionally, this patient developed partial hypopituitarism and nephrotic syndrome.

Neuroimaging

The typical appearance of HME shows a moderate to marked enlargement of the affected cerebral hemisphere (Figs 18.1a,b, 18.2a,b). The cortex appears dysplastic with broad gyri, shallow sulci, blurring of the cortical-white matter junction, and cortical thickening (Figs 18.1a,b, 18.2a,b). The affected occipital lobe can be displaced to the contralateral side (the 'occipital sign') (Figs 18.1a, 18.2a). The white matter usually shows an increase in volume and abnormally high signal (Figs 18.1a, 18.2a) (Hoffmann et al. 2000; Herman and Siegel 2001; Flores-Sarnat 2002). The lateral ventricle frequently appears enlarged with straightening of the frontal horn and/or unilateral colpocephaly (Fig. 18.1b). The corpus callosum is almost always asymmetric with enlargement and dysplasia of the affected side (Griffiths et al. 1994).

In THME the cerebellar hemisphere and the brainstem ipsilateral to the affected cerebral hemisphere are enlarged and the architecture of the ipsilateral cerebellar folia can be abnormal (Figs 18.1b,c, 18.2b) (Sato et al. 2007; Flores-Sarnat et al. 2003). However, in some cases the ipsilateral enlarged cerebellar hemisphere can crowd the posterior fossa and is displaced downward, resulting in unilateral tonsillar herniation (Calzolari et al. 1996; Battaglia et al. 1999). In rare cases the cerebellar hemisphere ipsilateral to the HME can be hypoplastic (Ahmed et al. 2002). Other possible neuroimaging findings are ipsilateral enlargement of the olfactory and optic nerves and asymmetric vascular dilatations in the ipsilateral cerebral hemisphere and in both deep and superficial cerebral vessels (Sato et al. 2007).

Proton MR spectroscopy (n=1) shows marked reduction of glutamate and *N*-acetylaspartate in the white matter. In the affected hemispheres positron emission tomography (PET) demonstrates markedly reduced glucose uptake, suggesting little function in these patients save for acting as a seizure focus (Hoffmann et al. 2000).

Electroencephalography

Electroencephalography (EEG) is always abnormal in HME, both isolated and associated. EEG shows typically asymmetric

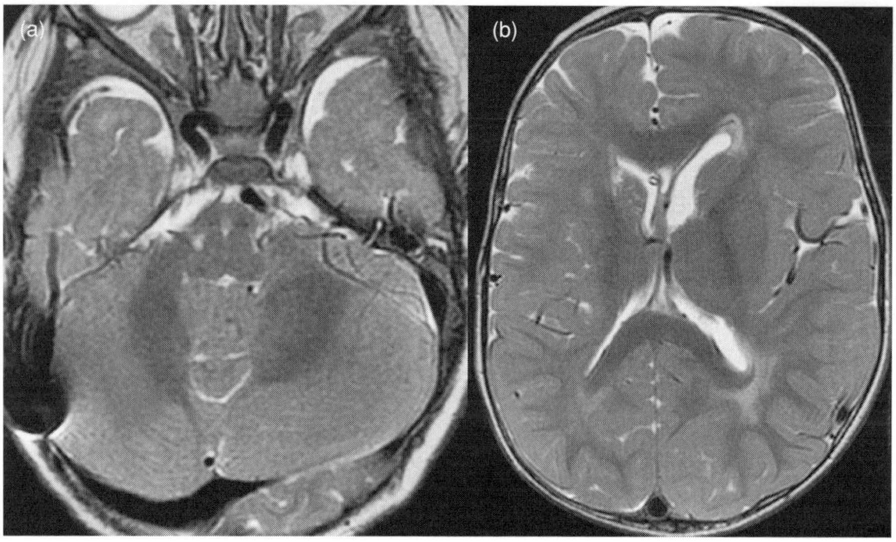

Fig. 18.2. Total hemimegalencephaly in a 15-month-old child with macrocephaly-capillary malformation. **(a)** Infratentorial T2-weighted MRI revealing asymmetry of the cerebellar hemisphere with mild enlargement of the left hemisphere; **(b)** supratentorial axial T2-weighted MRI showing a moderate asymmetry of the cerebral hemispheres with enlargement of the left cortical hemisphere, mild occipital sign, cortical dysplasia, and increase in the white matter on the left side with periventricular white matter hyperintensity.

continuous paroxysmal activity. This can include triphasic complexes of very large amplitude, predominating on the affected side, asymmetric suppression-burst pattern present at birth or after a few months, and asymmetric alpha-like activity with high amplitude and little modified in the waking phase (Paladin et al. 1989).

Diagnosis

HME and THME are almost always symptomatic at young age and can be suspected from the clinical presentation, but always require confirmation by neuroimaging.

Differential diagnosis

The neuroimaging findings are typical for HME and THME. However, enlargement of one cerebellar hemisphere can also be found in other disorders. In particular, HME should be differentiated from hemihypertrophy which is characterized by a simple increase in the volume of the white matter in the hypertrophied side of the cerebrum, but without cortical malformations, and seems to be associated with KTW (Torregrosa et al. 2000).

Focal enlargement of the cerebellum has also been reported in Lhermitte-Duclos syndrome (Nowak and Trost 2002; Perez-Nunez et al. 2004). Additional typical neuroimaging findings in this syndrome are non-enhancing gyriform patterns corresponding to enlargement of the cerebellar cortical folia, hypointensity on T1-weighted images, and striated pattern with isointense bands in the area of hyperintensity on T2-weighted images.

Jackson et al. reported a 10-year-old boy with duplication of the internal, middle, and external ear with an enlarged and duplicated right cerebellar hemisphere and proposed an aberrant notochordal split as the possible embryological pathomechanism (Jackson et al. 1990).

Management and treatment

Seizure control is the principal goal in the therapy of HME. Depending on the type of seizure, many antiepileptic drugs can be used. Usually, multiple antiepileptic drugs are required because of intractable seizures. For patients with frequent, intractable seizures, hemispherectomy should be evaluated (Di Rocco et al. 2006).

Surgical excision of lipomas is recommended, mainly for cosmetic reasons, with generally good results (Egan et al. 2001).

Supporting therapies such as physical and occupational therapies may be helpful for patients with spastic hemiparesis.

REFERENCES

Abdelhalim AN, Moritani T, Richfield E, Ekholm SE, Westesson PL (2003) Epidermal nevus syndrome: megalencephaly with bihemispheric and cerebellar involvement: imaging and neuropathologic correlation. J Comput Assist Tomogr 27: 534–537.

Ahmed I, Tope WD, Young TL, Miller DM, Bloom KE (2002) Neurocutaneous melanosis in association with encephalocraniocutaneous lipomatosis. J Am Acad Dermatol 47: S196–200.

Balestri P, Vivarelli R, Grosso S, Santori L, Farnetani MA, Galluzzi P, et al. (2003) Malformations of cortical development in neurofibromatosis type 1. Neurology 61: 1799–1801.

Battaglia D, Di Rocco C, Iuvone L, Acquafondata C, Iannelli A, Lettori D, Guzzetta F (1999) Neuro-cognitive development and epilepsy outcome in children with surgically treated hemimegalencephaly. Neuropediatrics 30: 307–313.

Biesecker L (2006) The challenges of Proteus syndrome: diagnosis and management. Eur J Hum Genet 14: 1151–1157.

Calzolari F, Chirico M, Tamisari L, Di Rocco C (1996) Hemimegalencephaly associated with somatic hemihypertrophy and a malformation of the feet: case report. Neuroradiology 38: 367–370.

Chapman K, Cardenas JF (2008) Hemimegalencephaly in a patient with a neurocutaneous syndrome. Semin Pediatr Neurol 15: 190–193.

Cohen MM (2002) More on vascular malformations. Plast Reconstr Surg 109: 2591–2594.

Conway RL, Pressman BD, Dobyns WB, Danielpour M, Lee J, Sanchez-Lara PA, et al. (2007) Neuroimaging findings in macrocephaly-capillary malformation: a longitudinal study of 17 patients. Am J Med Genet A 143A: 2981–3008.

Cruz AA, Schirmbeck T, Pina-Neto JM, Funayama CA (2002) Cicatricial upper eyelid retraction in encephalocraniocutaneous lipomatosis: a report of two cases and review of literature. Ophthal Plast Reconstr Surg 18: 151–155.

Curatolo P, Bombardieri R, Jozwiak S (2008) Tuberous sclerosis. Lancet 372: 657–668.

DeLone DR, Brown WD, Gentry LR (1999) Proteus syndrome: craniofacial and cerebral MRI. Neuroradiology 41: 840–843.

Dietrich RB, Glidden DE, Roth GM, Martin RA, Demo DS (1998) The Proteus syndrome: CNS manifestations. AJNR Am J Neuroradiol 19: 987–990.

Di Rocco F, Novegno F, Tamburrini G, Iannelli A (2001) Hemimegalencephaly involving the cerebellum. Pediatr Neurosurg 35: 274–276.

Di Rocco C, Battaglia D, Pietrini D, Piastra M, Massimi L (2006) Hemimegalencephaly: clinical implications and surgical treatment. Childs Nerv Syst 22: 852–866.

Egan CA, Meadows KP, Van Orman CB, Vanderhooft SL (2001) Neurologic variant of epidermal nevus syndrome with a facial lipoma. Int J Dermatol 40: 189–190.

Flores-Sarnat L (2002) Hemimegalencephaly: part 1. Genetic, clinical, and imaging aspects. J Child Neurol 17: 373–384.

Flores-Sarnat L, Sarnat HB, Davila-Gutierrez G, Alvarez A (2003) Hemimegalencephaly: part 2. Neuropathology suggests a disorder of cellular lineage. J Child Neurol 18: 776–785.

Flores-Sarnat L (2008) Hemimegalencephaly syndrome. In: Sarnat HB, Curatolo P, editors. Malformations of the nervous system. New York: Elsevier; pp. 153–176.

Galluzzi P, Cerase A, Strambi M, Buoni S, Fois A, Venturi C (2002) Hemimegalencephaly in tuberous sclerosis complex. J Child Neurol 17: 677–680.

Griffiths PD, Welch RJ, Gardner-Medwin D, Gholkar A, McAllister V (1994) The radiological features of hemimegalencephaly including three cases associated with Proteus syndrome. Neuropediatrics 25: 140–144.

Hallervorden J (1923) Angeborene Hemihypertrophie der linken Körperhälfte einschliesslich des Gehirns. Zentralbl Neurol Psychiatr 33: 518–519.

Herman TE, Siegel MJ (2001) Hemimegalencephaly and linear nevus sebaceous syndrome. J Perinatol 21: 336–338.

Hoffmann KT, Amthauer H, Liebig T, Hosten N, Etou A, Lehmann TN, et al. (2000) MRI and 18F-fluorodeoxyglucose positron emission tomography in hemimegalencephaly. Neuroradiology 42: 749–752.

Hung PC, Wang HS (2005) Hemimegalencephaly: cranial sonographic findings in neonates. J Clin Ultrasound 33: 243–247.

Jackson JM, Sadove AM, Weaver DD, Edwards MK, Bull MJ (1990) Unilateral duplication of the cerebellar hemisphere and internal, middle, and external ear: a clinical case study. Plast Reconstr Surg 86: 550–553.

Jett K, Friedman JM (2010) Clinical and genetic aspects of neurofibromatosis 1. Genet Med 12: 1–11.

Kato M, Mizuguchi M, Sakuta R, Takashima S (1996) Hypertrophy of the cerebral white matter in hemimegalencephaly. Pediatr Neurol 14: 335–338.

Maruyama K, Okumura A, Negoro T, Watanabe K (2010) Congenital infiltrating lipomatosis of the face with ipsilateral hemimegalencephaly, band heterotopia, and hypertrophy of brainstem and cerebellum. Neuropediatrics 41: 147–150.

Menascu S, Donner EJ (2008) Linear nevus sebaceous syndrome: case reports and review of the literature. Pediatr Neurol 38: 207–210.

Moog U, Jones MC, Viskochil DH, Verloes A, Van Allen MI, Dobyns WB (2007) Brain anomalies in encephalocraniocutaneous lipomatosis. Am J Med Genet A 143A: 2963–2972.

Moog U (2009) Encephalocraniocutaneous lipomatosis. J Med Genet 46: 721–729.

Nowak DA, Trost HA (2002) Lhermitte-Duclos disease (dysplastic cerebellar gangliocytoma): a malformation, hamartoma or neoplasm? Acta Neurol Scand 105: 137–145.

Oduber CE, van der Horst CM, Hennekam RC (2008) Klippel-Trenaunay syndrome: diagnostic criteria and hypothesis on etiology. Ann Plast Surg 60: 217–223.

Paladin F, Chiron C, Dulac O, Plouin P, Ponsot G (1989) Electroencephalographic aspects of hemimegalencephaly. Dev Med Child Neurol 31: 377–383.

Payne JM, Moharir MD, Webster R, North KN (2010) Brain structure and function in neurofibromatosis type 1: current concepts and future directions. J Neurol Neurosurg Psychiatry 81: 304–309.

Perez-Nunez A, Lagares A, Benitez J, Urioste M, Lobato RD, Ricoy JR, et al. (2004) Lhermitte-Duclos disease and Cowden disease: clinical and genetic study in five patients with Lhermitte-Duclos disease and literature review. Acta Neurochir (Wien) 146: 679–690.

Rintahaka PJ, Chugani HT, Messa C, Phelps ME (1993) Hemimegalencephaly: evaluation with positron emission tomography. Pediatr Neurol 9: 21–28.

Ruggieri M, Pavone L (2000) Hypomelanosis of Ito: clinical syndrome or just phenotype? J Child Neurol 15: 635–644.

Sato N, Yagishita A, Oba H, Miki Y, Nakata Y, Yamashita F, et al. (2007) Hemimegalencephaly: a study of abnormalities occurring outside the involved hemisphere. AJNR Am J Neuroradiol 28: 678–682.

Sener RN (1997) MR demonstration of cerebral hemimegalencephaly associated with cerebellar involvement (total hemimegalencephaly). Comput Med Imaging Graph 21: 201–204.

Sugarman JL (2007) Epidermal nevus syndromes. Semin Cutan Med Surg 26: 221–230.

Takashima S, Chan F, Becker LE, Kuruta H (1991) Aberrant neuronal development in hemimegalencephaly: immunohistochemical and Golgi studies. Pediatr Neurol 7: 275–280.

Torregrosa A, Marti-Bonmati L, Higueras V, Poyatos C, Sanchis A (2000) Klippel-Trenaunay syndrome: frequency of cerebral and cerebellar hemihypertrophy on MRI. Neuroradiology 42: 420–423.

Vigevano F, Bertini E, Boldrini R, Bosman C, Claps D, di Capua M, et al. (1989) Hemimegalencephaly and intractable epilepsy: benefits of hemispherectomy. Epilepsia 30: 833–843.

19 Brainstem Disconnection

Andrea Poretti and Eugen Boltshauser

Brainstem disconnection is a rare disorder characterized by brainstem dysfunction due to a discontinuation of the brainstem because of almost complete absence of a segment of the midbrain or pons, with the more rostral and caudal portions of the brainstem being connected by only a thin strand of white matter (Barkovich et al. 2007). Depending on the location of the disconnection, three different types of brainstem disconnection are distinguishable: *ponto-mesencephalic*, *ponto-medullary*, and *ponto-cervical* disconnection (Okumura et al. 2009). As of May 2010 only 12 cases had been reported (Robinson et al. 1993; Mamourian and Miller 1994; Sarnat et al. 2002; Bednarek et al. 2005; McCann et al. 2005; Poretti et al. 2007; Barth et al. 2008; Duffield et al. 2009; Govaert 2009; Jurkiewicz et al. 2009; Okumura et al. 2009). The absent segment typically includes the pons and can variably extend rostrally to the midbrain or caudally to the medulla oblongata.

Aetiology and pathogenesis

The pathogenesis of brainstem disconnection remains unknown and both genetic and disruptive causes have been suggested (Barkovich et al. 2007). It is also unclear whether different types of brainstem disconnection have the same pathogenesis.

Sarnat et al. hypothesized a malformation resulting from defective expression of the homeobox gene Engrailed-2 (*EN2*) (Sarnat et al. 2002). They extrapolate their hypothesis from experimental models. Homozygous deletion of this gene in murines results in agenesis of the mesencephalon and metencephalon (McMahon et al. 1992; Wurst et al. 1994; Joyner 1996; Mastick et al. 1996; Saint-Jeannet et al. 1997; Wassef and Joyner 1997). Mice with *En-2* deletions showed cerebellar hypoplasia with abnormal foliation (Millen et al. 1994; Kuemerle et al. 1997; Goldowitz and Hamre 1998). The abnormal rostral displacement of the cerebellum is consistent with a rostral shift of the mesencephalic boundary (Sarnat et al. 2002). Indeed, Engrailed defines the position of the dorsal dimesencephalic boundary by directly repressing the diencephalic fate (Araki and Nakamura 1999). Hypoplasia of the dentate and inferior olivary nuclei suggests an additional involvement of rhombomere 2 (Sarnat et al. 2002). The ectopic expression of *En-2* in mice Purkinje cells may also interfere with late-onset sagittal banding patterns, which might explain the imperfect lamination of the cerebellar cortex in humans (Sarnat et al. 2002; Baader et al. 1999). One patient also had ectopic and dysplastic thyroid tissue (Sarnat et al. 2002). Some studies suggest an antagonistic relation of Engrailed homeodomains to thyroid transcription factor 1 (Damante et al. 1996; Bruno et al. 2000). However, mutations in the *EN2* gene could not be demonstrated (Sarnat et al. 2002; Okumura et al. 2009). Additionally, vascular anomalies ranging from anomalous basilar and posterior cerebral arteries such as absence of the cervical portions of the vertebral arteries and the basilar artery, and intracranial portions of the vertebral arteries being supplied by bilateral persistent proatlantal intersegmental arteries, to absence of the basilar artery have been found in several patients (Mamourian and Miller 1994; Sarnat et al. 2002; Poretti et al. 2007; Barth et al. 2008; Okumura et al. 2009). Okumura et al. reported periventricular nodular heterotopia which are considered a disorder of neuronal migration caused mainly by gene mutations (Barkovich et al. 2005; Okumura et al. 2009). However, mutations in the *FLNA* gene could not be found in brainstem disconnection (Okumura et al. 2009). Finally, Sarnat et al. concluded that the absence of the midbrain and upper pons with cerebellar hypoplasia cannot be due to ischaemia from a vascular anomaly because the territory does not correspond to any single vessel and basilar artery occlusion would certainly have caused extensive infarction both in the brainstem and in the occipital cortex, but neither the brainstem caudal to the lesion nor the occipital lobes showed gliotic lesions suggesting hypoxia or ischaemia (Sarnat et al. 2002). This was interpreted as an additional point in favour of a malformation.

However, Aldinger et al. reported that in all experimental models the remaining transformed hindbrain segments always remain contiguous with each other (Sarnat 2004; Aldinger et al. 2009). This difference between models and human cases would favour an early disruptive vascular accident causing brainstem disconnection. Additionally nodular heterotopia have been reported after early-acquired prenatal insults in the germinative neuroepithelium (Battaglia et al. 2003a, 2003b). Barth et al. hypothesized a disruptive cause due to progressively insufficient perfusion through a hypoplastic basilar artery, and obstructed venous drainage through an abnormal glial barrier surrounding the posterior brainstem (Barth et al. 2008). They found central cavitation that they interpreted rather as a syrinx, as known occurs in disorders in which brainstem or spinal cord are damaged by a combination of mechanical and circulatory factors (Milhorat et al. 1995). Considering the maturity of the remaining parts of the pons, they estimated the onset of structural decline to be close to the time of birth (Barth et al. 2008). Finally, Okumura et al. proposed that the vascular aberration may result from disruption of the development of the brainstem (Okumura et al. 2009).

Clinical features

All children with brainstem disconnection were symptomatic at birth. In three cases symptoms of brainstem disconnection began prenatally and presented as polyhydramnios. The clinical manifestation of brainstem disconnection is characterized by brainstem dysfunction. At birth, in all patients suck was absent or weak, requiring nasogastric tube feeding. In one patient, a cyanotic episode had been described while feeding, demonstrating that not only suck, but also swallowing, is abnormal in patients with brainstem disconnection. Breathing was normal only in two patients. Five infants had been intubated in the first few minutes of life because of absent or markedly insufficient breathing. In one child, nasal continuous positive airway pressure was used to prevent respiratory failure because of tachypnea. In two other children, breathing was abnormal, but no mechanical assistance was necessary. In two unventilated patients, recurrent apneas occurred. Additionally, laryngeal stridor has been reported in two newborn infants.

At birth, in two patients spontaneous movements were absent and in one they were excessively jerky. Muscle tone of limbs and trunk has been reported in ten newborn infants and was increased in six and decreased in four. Facial innervation was normal in four children, but weak and hypertonic with trismus in one. Deep tendon reflexes were exaggerated in four patients (with limb clonus in two), and absent in one.

Visual fixation was studied in four children and was absent in all. When reported, pupillary response was normal, whereas the vestibulo-ocular reflex (VOR) and the corneal reflex were absent in all patients. Ocular movements were normal in one, but minimal in another child.

Clinical seizures have been reported in five of nine children (focal in one patient and myoclonic in another child). One newborn was microcephalic and in the other cases the head circumference was normal for gestational age. In three patients instability of temperature regulation was reported, and one lacked sleep- and wake-cycles.

Dysmorphic signs have been reported in four patients: microretrognathia, hypertelorism, and low-set ears in two; unusual hair patterning with frontal upsweep, unilateral anophthalmia, asymmetrically smaller right face with elevated nasal bridge and thin downturned upper lip in one; and bilateral anotia in one.

Extracerebral anomalies had been described in five patients. Four patients had congenital cardiac abnormalities (ventricular septal defect in two, atrial septal defect in one, and patent foramen ovale in one); two patients had hydronephrosis; and the following abnormalities occurred in at least one patient each: ectopic lingual thyroid gland with hypothyroidism, ectopic parathyroid glands, cleft palate, multiple thoracic spine segmentation anomalies, hypoplasia of the distal sacrum, uterus bicornute, scoliosis, ribs and vertebral anomalies as butterfly thoracic vertebra, hemivertebra, and posteriorly fused vertebra, congenital defects of middle ears, and abnormal epiglottis with short trachea and narrow spaces of the middle and inferior pharynx.

Neuroimaging

Discontinuation of the brainstem with absence of the pons (best evaluated on sagittal sections, Fig. 19.1) represents the neuroimaging hallmark of brainstem disconnection. The absent segment of the brainstem can variably extend rostrally to the midbrain or caudally to the medulla oblongata. Depending on the location of the disconnection, three different types of brainstem disconnection can be distinguished in the cases described: *ponto-mesencephalic* (Sarnat et al. 2002; Bednarek et al. 2005), *ponto-medullary* (Mamourian and Miller 1994; McCann et al. 2005; Poretti et al. 2007; Barth et al. 2008; Duffield et al. 2009; Govaert 2009), and *ponto-cervical* disconnection (Okumura et al. 2009). In *ponto-mesencephalic* disconnection the midbrain is almost absent and the disconnection is between the midbrain's remnant and the lower pons. However, in *ponto-medullary* as well as *ponto-cervical* disconnection the midbrain is normal, while the disconnection is located lower in the brainstem. In *ponto-medullary* disconnection, the disconnection is between upper pons and medulla oblongata. In *ponto-cervical* disconnection, the medulla oblongata is almost completely

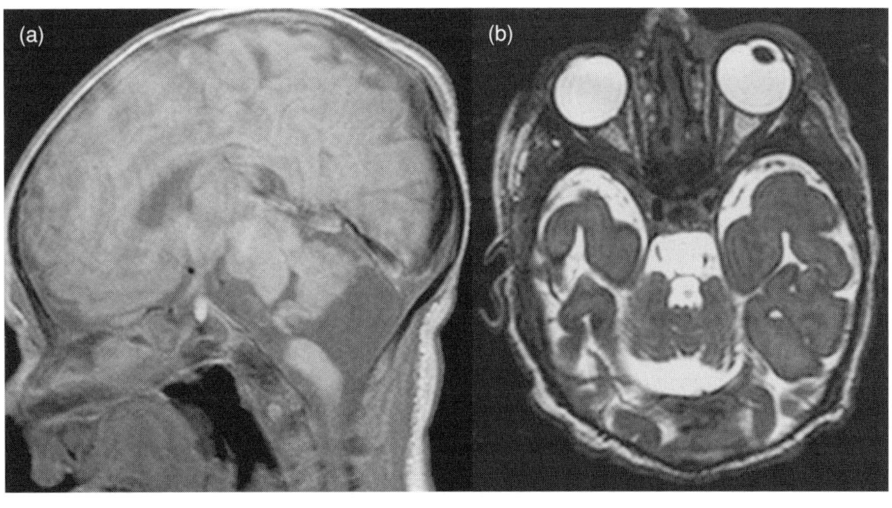

Fig. 19.1. Brainstem disconnection in an 11-day-old infant. **(a)** Midsagittal T1-weighted MRI showing absence of the lower pons and no apparent connection between the upper pons and the medulla oblongata. The cerebellum is hypoplastic. The basilar artery is not visible. Normal size of pituitary gland and optic chiasm as well as normal location of the cerebellar tentorium are apparent; **(b)** axial T2-weighted MRI showing only a thin strand of tissue at the level of the lower pons/upper medulla oblongata. The cerebellar hemispheres and the vermis are hypoplastic. The basilar artery is not visible. (Reprinted with permission from Poretti A et al. Neuropediatrics 2007; 38: 210–212.)

absent and the disconnection is between upper pons and cervical spinal cord. A thin strand of tissue connects the rostral and caudal potions of the brainstem. In all cases, brainstem disconnection is associated with cerebellar hypoplasia affecting both vermis and hemispheres. Because of the reduced volume, the cerebellar structures do not fill the normally configured posterior fossa. In one case, the middle and inferior cerebellar peduncles were absent.

Supratentorial abnormalities are rarely associated with brainstem disconnection. In three cases ventriculomegaly has been reported, with MRI showing a hypoplastic corpus callosum, small hypothalamus, and anophthalmia on the right side (Duffield et al. 2009), a large hamartoma of the tuber cinereum (Jurkiewicz et al. 2009), and several periventricular nodular heterotopia (Okumura et al. 2009), respectively.

A report of magnetic resonance spectroscopy in one case showed normal N-acetylaspartate/choline ratio and no lactate peak at the level of the basal ganglia (Barth et al. 2008).

Magnetic resonance angiography (MRA) was performed in three cases. In one case MRA failed to show a basilar artery (Barth et al. 2008) and in one only small vertebral arteries joining to form a very tiny proximal basilar artery were seen (Duffield et al. 2009). In the third case, MRA demonstrated absence of the cervical portions of the vertebral arteries; the basilar artery was supplied through proatlantal intersegmental arteries originating from the external carotid arteries. In four other cases, MRA has not been performed, but in the MRI sequences no normal signal void in the region of the basilar artery and the distal vertebral arteries was seen.

Additional examinations

Electrophysiological investigations have been performed in only a few patients. Brainstem auditory evoked potentials (BAER) showed no reproducible responses in one patient (Mamourian and Miller 1994) and abnormal responses in another (Okumura et al. 2009). Visual evoked potentials (VEP) demonstrated a delayed response in only one patient (Robinson et al. 1993). Somatosensory evoked potentials (SSEP) in one patient showed normal response at the cervical level, but no reproducible cortical response (Mamourian and Miller 1994). All these results confirm brainstem dysfunction. Electroencephalography (EEG) has been performed in four patients and was normal in three (Sarnat et al. 2002, Jurkiewicz et al. 2009, Okumura et al. 2009) but showed permanent discontinuous activity in another child. None of these four children had clinical seizures.

Diagnosis

The diagnosis of brainstem disconnection is made by the distinct neuroimaging pattern.

Differential diagnosis

Because of the typical neuroimaging findings the diagnosis of brainstem disconnection is not difficult. Homozygous mutations of the *HOXA1* gene which cause both the Bosley-Salih-Alorainy syndrome (BSAS) and the Athabascan brainstem dysgenesis syndrome (ABDS) also affect the brainstem, but clinical and neuroimaging findings as well as the course of the diseases are quite different (Tischfield et al. 2005; Bosley et al. 2008), with the brainstem showing normal structure in BSAS and ABDS.

Management and treatment

Most newborn infants with brainstem disconnection present with respiratory insufficiency or absent breathing at birth and require intubation and mechanical ventilation. Otherwise intubation and ventilation may be necessary because of frequent apneas. All reported patients with brainstem disconnection required intubation and mechanical ventilation at least temporarily. In most patients weaning was not possible. Only one patient was alive at the age of 5 months without any breathing support (Jurkiewicz et al. 2009). The condition and the very poor prognosis for these children need to be explained accurately to the parents; the care team and parents have to decide whether continuation of life-prolonging measures is in the best interests of the child.

Outcome

The outcome is very poor. In 2009 the two oldest of 12 patients were alive at the age of 5 months and 4 years, respectively (Jurkiewicz et al. 2009; Okumura et al. 2009). Both children remained hospitalized at the last follow-up and nutrition was maintained by feeding through a gastrostomy tube. One child required mechanical ventilation. The 4-year-old could lift her arms and legs slightly against gravity when crying or frustrated (probably unintentional movements). Spontaneous movements of the limbs were rarely observed. She could distinguish the faces of her parents and responded to verbal stimuli appropriately. Blood pressure, heart rate, and body temperature had been maintained appropriately. No epileptic seizures had been observed (Okumura et al. 2009).

REFERENCES

Aldinger KA, Elsen GE, Prince VE, Millen KJ (2009) Model organisms inform the search for the genes and developmental pathology underlying malformations of the human hindbrain. Semin Pediatr Neurol 16: 155–163.

Araki I, Nakamura H (1999) Engrailed defines the position of dorsal di-mesencephalic boundary by repressing diencephalic fate. Development 126: 5127–5135.

Baader SL, Vogel MW, Sanlioglu S, Zhang X, Oberdick J (1999) Selective disruption of ‘late onset’ sagittal banding patterns by ectopic expression of engrailed-2 in cerebellar Purkinje cells. J Neurosci 19: 5370–5379.

Barkovich AJ, Kuzniecky RI, Jackson GD, Guerrini R, Dobyns WB (2005) A developmental and genetic classification for malformations of cortical development. Neurology 65: 1873–1887.

Barkovich AJ, Millen KJ, Dobyns WB (2007) A developmental classification of malformations of the brainstem. Ann Neurol 62: 625–639.

Barth PG, de Vries LS, Nikkels PG, Troost D (2008) Congenital brainstem disconnection associated with a syrinx of the brainstem. Neuropediatrics 39: 1–7.

Battaglia G, Pagliardini S, Saglietti L, Cattabeni F, Di Luca M, Bassanini S, Setola V (2003a) Neurogenesis in cerebral heterotopia induced in rats by prenatal methylazoxymethanol treatment. Cereb Cortex 13: 736–748.

Battaglia G, Bassanini S, Granata T, Setola V, Giavazzi A, Pagliardini S (2003b) The genesis of epileptogenic cerebral heterotopia: clues from experimental models. Epileptic Disord 5 Suppl 2: S51–58.

Bednarek N, Scavarda D, Mesmin F, Sabouraud P, Motte J, Morville P (2005) Midbrain disconnection: an aetiology of severe central neonatal hypotonia. Eur J Paediatr Neurol 9: 419–422.

Bosley TM, Alorainy IA, Salih MA, Aldhalaan HM, Abu-Amero KK, Oystreck DT, et al. (2008) The clinical spectrum of homozygous HOXA1 mutations. Am J Med Genet A 146A: 1235–1240.

Bruno MD, Korfhagen TR, Liu C, Morrisey EE, Whitsett JA (2000) GATA-6 activates transcription of surfactant protein A. J Biol Chem 275: 1043–1049.

Damante G, Pellizzari L, Esposito G, Fogolari F, Viglino P, Fabbro D, et al. (1996) A molecular code dictates sequence-specific DNA recognition by homeodomains. EMBO J 15: 4992–5000.

Duffield C, Jocson J, Wootton-Gorges SL (2009) Brainstem disconnection. Pediatr Radiol 39: 1357–1360.

Goldowitz D, Hamre K (1998) The cells and molecules that make a cerebellum. Trends Neurosci 21: 375–382.

Govaert P (2009) Prenatal stroke. Semin Fetal Neonatal Med 14: 250–266.

Joyner AL (1996) Engrailed, Wnt and Pax genes regulate midbrain – hindbrain development. Trends Genet 12: 15–20.

Jurkiewicz E, Dobrzanska A, Nowak K, Pleskaczynska A (2009) MRI findings in the young infant with brainstem disconnection and extracerebral features. Report of one case and review of the literature. Brain Dev 32: 495–498.

Kuemerle B, Zanjani H, Joyner A, Herrup K (1997) Pattern deformities and cell loss in Engrailed-2 mutant mice suggest two separate patterning events during cerebellar development. J Neurosci 17: 7881–7889.

Mamourian AC, Miller G (1994) Neonatal pontomedullary disconnection with aplasia or destruction of the lower brain stem: a case of pontoneocerebellar hypoplasia? AJNR Am J Neuroradiol 15: 1483–1485.

Mastick GS, Fan CM, Tessier-Lavigne M, Serbedzija GN, McMahon AP, Easter SS, Jr (1996) Early deletion of neuromeres in Wnt-1-/-mutant mice: evaluation by morphological and molecular markers. J Comp Neurol 374: 246–258.

McCann E, Pilling D, Hesseling M, Roberts D, Subhedar N, Sweeney E (2005) Pontomedullary disconnection: fetal and neonatal considerations. Pediatr Radiol 35: 812–814.

McMahon AP, Joyner AL, Bradley A, McMahon JA (1992) The midbrain-hindbrain phenotype of Wnt-1-/Wnt-1- mice results from stepwise deletion of engrailed-expressing cells by 9.5 days postcoitum. Cell 69: 581–595.

Milhorat TH, Capocelli AL, Jr., Anzil AP, Kotzen RM, Milhorat RH (1995) Pathological basis of spinal cord cavitation in syringomyelia: analysis of 105 autopsy cases. J Neurosurg 82: 802–812.

Millen KJ, Wurst W, Herrup K, Joyner AL (1994) Abnormal embryonic cerebellar development and patterning of postnatal foliation in two mouse Engrailed-2 mutants. Development 120: 695–706.

Okumura A, Lee T, Shimojima K, Hisata K, Shoji H, Takanashi J, et al. (2009) Brainstem disconnection associated with nodular heterotopia and proatlantal arteries. Am J Med Genet A 149A: 2479–2483.

Poretti A, Boltshauser E, Plecko B (2007) Brainstem disconnection: case report and review of the literature. Neuropediatrics 38: 210–212.

Robinson RO, Trounce JQ, Janota I, Cox T (1993) Late fetal pontine destruction. Pediatr Neurol 9: 213–215.

Saint-Jeannet JP, He X, Varmus HE, Dawid IB (1997) Regulation of dorsal fate in the neuraxis by Wnt-1 and Wnt-3a. Proc Natl Acad Sci U S A 94: 13713–13718.

Sarnat HB (2004) Watershed infarcts in the fetal and neonatal brainstem. An aetiology of central hypoventilation, dysphagia, Möbius syndrome and micrognathia. Eur J Paediatr Neurol 8: 71–87.

Sarnat HB, Benjamin DR, Siebert JR, Kletter GB, Cheyette SR (2002) Agenesis of the mesencephalon and metencephalon with cerebellar hypoplasia: putative mutation in the EN2 gene – report of 2 cases in early infancy. Pediatr Dev Pathol 5: 54–68.

Tischfield MA, Bosley TM, Salih MA, Alorainy IA, Sener EC, Nester MJ, et al. (2005) Homozygous HOXA1 mutations disrupt human brainstem, inner ear, cardiovascular and cognitive development. Nat Genet 37: 1035–1037.

Wassef M, Joyner AL (1997) Early mesencephalon/metencephalon patterning and development of the cerebellum. Perspect Dev Neurobiol 5: 3–16.

Wurst W, Auerbach AB, Joyner AL (1994) Multiple developmental defects in Engrailed-1 mutant mice: an early mid-hindbrain deletion and patterning defects in forelimbs and sternum. Development 120: 2065–2075.

20 Pontine Tegmental Cap Dysplasia

Andrea Poretti and Eugen Boltshauser

Pontine tegmental cap dysplasia (PTCD) is characterized by distinct neuroimaging findings including vermal hypoplasia, subtotal absence of middle cerebellar peduncles, flattened ventral pons, vaulted pontine tegmentum, molar tooth aspect of the pontomesencephalic junction, and absent inferior olivary prominence (Barth et al. 2007). These neuroimaging findings are mandatory for the diagnosis.

As of July 2010 only 18 cases had been reported (Barth et al. 2007; Jissendi-Tchofo et al. 2009; Rauscher et al. 2009; Bacciu et al. 2010; Macferran et al. 2010; Szczaluba et al. 2010; and KRM Martin et al., personal communication, 2009). We saw another child in our clinic for a total of 19 patients reported in this chapter, but we are aware of two additional, unreported children with PTCD. All cases were sporadic.

Pathogenesis

Absence of normal decussating superior cerebellar peduncles (SCP), middle cerebellar peduncles (MCP), and axons of the pontine nuclei as well as vermian hypoplasia, elongated and laterally misplaced SCP, and an ectopic transverse fibre tract occupying the region of the dorsal vault are highly suggestive of PTCD, being a primary disorder of axon guidance (Engle 2010). Additionally, PTCD shares features with other disorders of axon guidance such as Joubert syndrome (Doherty 2009; Parisi 2009), horizontal gaze palsy with progressive scoliosis (HGPPS) (Jen et al. 2004; Bosley et al. 2005), and congenital cranial dysinnervation disorders (CCDD) (Gutowski et al. 2003; Engle 2007). Human genetic disorders resulting from defective axon guidance are caused by genetic mutations that alter axon growth cone ligands and receptors, downstream signalling molecules, and axon transport (Engle 2010).

Axonal guidance molecules such as netrins, slits, ephrins, semaphorins, and their receptors can be considered as candidate causative molecules (Dickson 2002; Finger et al. 2002; Barallobre et al. 2005; Bhat et al. 2007; Mann and Rougon 2007; Sibbe et al. 2007).

Netrins are extracellular proteins acting as a bifunctional signal: chemoattractive for some neurons and chemorepellent for others (Culotti and Merz 1998; Barallobre et al. 2005; Keleman and Dickson 2001). One of the clear functions of Netrin-1, the most studied member of the family, is the demarcation of the midline, where it acts as a guide for distinct axon populations inducing them to grow toward the midline. In this way, Netrin-1* stimulates the outgrowth of commissural axons at several levels of the central nervous system such as commissural axons leaving the cerebellum to cross the floor plate and inferior olivary axons (Shirasaki et al. 1996; Alcantara et al. 2000). Furthermore, in the midline Netrin-1 may act as a barrier for those axons that must not cross the midline (Colamarino and Tessier-Lavigne 1995; Guthrie and Pini 1995). In addition to its functions in axonal guidance, there is some evidence on the involvement of Netrin-1 in migration of distinct populations of neurons such as inferior olive and pontine neurons (Alcantara et al. 2000). Mice deficient in *Ntn1*, the gene producing Netrin-1, exhibit multiple commissural defects with ectopic fibre tracts and loss of pontine neurons (Serafini et al. 1996). Therefore, Barth et al. tested the human homolog *NTN1* as candidate gene for PTCD, but no mutations were detected within the coding regions of this gene (Barth et al. 2007).

To carry out their function, Netrins interact with specific receptors that belong to two protein families: Deleted in Colorectal Cancer (DCC) and UNC-5 (Barallobre et al. 2005). The DCC receptors mainly mediate attraction, but also participate in repulsion (Culotti and Merz 1998). In contrast, UNC-5 receptors appear to act only in repulsion (Keleman and Dickson 2001). Mice deficient in *Dcc* show a phenotype similar to *Ntn1*-deficient mice (Fazeli et al. 1997). DCC was initially isolated as a tumour suppressor gene and unless it is engaged by its ligand, Netrin-1, DCC induces apoptosis (Fearon et al. 1990). Indeed, in the absence of Netrin-1 massive neuronal death occurs in the inferior olivary nuclei which are absent or hypoplastic in PTCD (Llambi et al. 2001). Therefore, Barth et al. considered the human homolog *DCC* as candidate gene for PTCD, but no mutations were detected within the coding regions of this gene (Barth et al. 2007).

Another Netrin-1 receptor, UNC-5H3, is also involved in neuronal-migration guidance and its loss may result both in abnormal neuronal migration and axonal guidance impairment (Finger et al. 2002); additionally, like DCC, it induces apoptosis in the absence of Netrin-1 (Llambi et al. 2001). Therefore, UNC-5H3 may be another candidate gene for PTCD.

Axon guidance by netrins needs to be regulated in mice by a signaling system from the midline mediated by slit and its receptors of the Roundabout (Robo) family (Dickson 2002; Jen et al. 2004; Woods 2004; Devine and Key 2008). When bound to each other, Slit and Robo act as a chemorepellent, inducing growth of axon tips away from the midline (Wong

* Nomenclature in this chapter: protein designation in roman; human genes italic, all upper case; mice genes italic, first letter upper case.

et al. 2001; Bulow and Hobert 2004; Woods 2004; Bhat et al. 2007). The interaction between the midline pairs Slit/Robo and Netrin/DCC occurs through the inhibition of the midline attractant Netrin by Robo1 and Robo2 which block the DCC's response to Netrin (Stein et al. 2001; Tamada et al. 2008). In this way the Slit repellent signal presumably overcomes the attraction of Netrin and blocks the neurons from crossing the midline. The effects of Robo1 are antagonized by Robo3, which differs from the other Robo proteins in two crucial respects: it is a chemoattractant (and not a repellent to axons trying to cross the midline) and, if it is expressed in the hindbrain, axons cross the midline (Jen et al. 2004; Sabatier et al. 2004; Tamada et al. 2008). Indeed, a mutation in the *ROBO3* gene causes the human disorder, horizontal gaze palsy with progressive scoliosis (HGPPS) (Bosley et al. 2005). Typical structural abnormalities are absent midline crossing at the pontine and mesencephalic levels. However, ectopic fibre bundles have not been identified (Sicotte et al. 2006; Otaduy et al. 2009; Avadhani et al. 2010). In HGPPS somatosensory evoked responses (SSEP) are dominant ipsilateral to the stimulation side (Haller et al. 2008), whereas in one patient with PTCD SSEPs showed a normal crossed cortical response (Barth et al. 2007). Therefore, *ROBO3* is an unlikely candidate gene for PTCD.

An additional signaling system for *Netrin (Net)* uses the receptor *Frazzled (Fra)* functioning as a midline attractant for the tracts at the point of midline crossing (Devine and Key 2008). Jissendi et al. hypothesized that a loss of *Net-Fra* or overexpression of *Sli-Robo* function could explain the absence of SCP decussation, the molar-tooth-like appearance, and the dorsal transverse axon band in PTCD (Jissendi-Tchofo et al. 2009).

Some neuroimaging findings such as vermis hypoplasia, molar tooth sign (MTS), and absent decussation of the SCPs are reminiscent of Joubert syndrome (Poretti et al. 2007). Furthermore, in a patient with PTCD Macferran et al. reported a 96.6-kb deletion at 2q13 involving the target gene *NPHP1* which is a gene reported to be the cause of Joubert syndrome in 1–2% of cases (Castori et al. 2005; Macferran et al. 2010). However, some clinical (involvement of kidneys, liver, and retina) as well as neuroimaging (ventral pontine hypoplasia, near absence of the MCPs, absence of transverse pontine fibres) findings are quite different (Doherty 2009; Parisi 2009).

A combination of hindbrain anomalies, cranial nerve dysfunction, and vertebral anomalies may suggest changes in the function of the *Hox* genes, whose expression results in both the segmental formation of somites (from which the vertebrae derive) and rhombomeres (from which pons, medulla, and cerebellum develop) (Gavalas et al. 2003; Wellik 2007). Thus, abnormalities of *Hox* genes could be another pathomechanism of PTCD.

Clinical features

The clinical findings are dominated by the involvement of several cranial nerves (Barth et al. 2007; Jissendi-Tchofo et al. 2009; Rauscher et al. 2009; Bacciu et al. 2010; Macferran et al. 2010; Szczaluba et al. 2010; and KRM Martin et al., personal communication, 2009).

In all 19 cases the cochlear nerves were involved, causing bilateral sensory deafness in 17 and a moderate hearing loss on the left side in one patient. The vestibular ocular reflex was absent in both patients who were tested.

The facial nerve was involved in 14 cases: bilaterally in 11 cases (symmetrically in 7 cases); in 2 children only the left side was affected.

The trigeminal sensory nerve was involved in 11 patients (bilaterally in 7) causing corneal anesthesia and absent corneal reflex and resulting in corneal ulcers in 5 children. Two patients presented as newborn infants with impaired mouth opening, probably resulting from reduced mouth movements because of a trigeminal motor nerve palsy.

The glossopharyngeal nerve was involved in 11 cases causing swallowing disorders and feeding difficulties necessitating gastrostomy in six cases and nasogastric tube in one. In one child feeding difficulties improved with age.

Ocular movement disorders affected 15 patients: nystagmus (8: vertical in 4 cases, 1 with downbeat nystagmus), ocular motor apraxia (OMA) (2 cases), impaired smooth pursuit (2 cases), impaired horizontal gaze (2 cases), and near-absent voluntary eye movements (1). In one case trochlear paresis has been reported.

Speech was impaired in eight children: five were mute and three had indistinct language. Four children communicated by sign language. Epileptic seizures have been reported in one patient.

Cerebellar signs were present in all patients who could be tested: truncal and limb ataxia in eight and three, respectively, uncoordinated movements in four, and head titubation in three patients. Two children reported by Barth et al. could walk at 4 and 6 years, respectively, but both were clearly ataxic (Barth et al. 2007). Another child walks with assistance of a walker at 10 years. Two children could not walk, but were able to sit at the age of 2 years 2 months and 2 years 3 months, respectively. Three other patients had poor head control and were unable to sit. Pyramidal tract signs present in four cases included brisk reflexes (three children) and bilateral ankle clonus (one).

Developmental delay was present in 12 of 13 patients tested, and was severe in 7. One child had an overall IQ of 94 (Barth et al. 2007), but one child had normal cognitive abilities at the age of 6 years (Bacciu et al. 2010).

One patient had flat affect and developed self-injurious behaviours such as digging at his eyes and biting his lips and tongue.

Ten patients had vertebral segmentation anomalies such as butterfly-shaped vertebral bodies (4), hemivertebrae (4), split vertebral body (1), fused vertebral bodies (2), and wedge-shaped vertebral body (1) (Fig. 20.1). Rib malformations were present in five cases as an increased or decreased number of ribs or fusion of part of a rib. Five patients had a congenital heart defect (atrial septal defect in two cases, ventricular

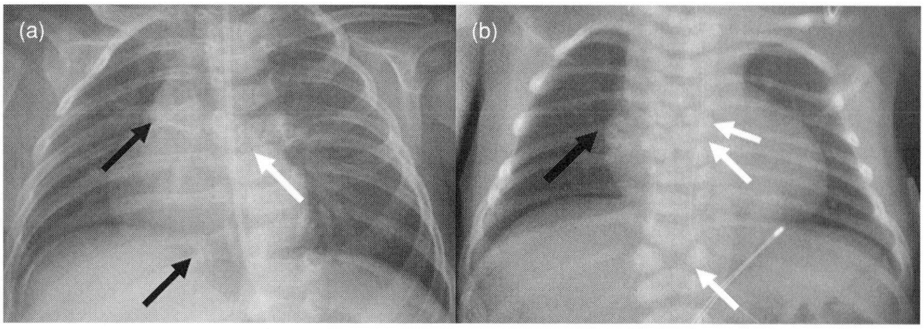

Fig. 20.1. **(a)** Chest radiograph of one patient showing on the right side only 11 ribs and partial fusion of the dorsal part of both pairs of ribs 5/6 and 9/10 (black arrows), butterfly shape of the vertebral body T5, wedge-shaped vertebral body T6 (white arrow), and nasogastric tube. **(b)** Chest radiograph of another patient showing on the right side fusion of ribs 4/5 (black arrows), butterfly shape of vertebral bodies T4, T5, and T9 (white arrows), and nasogastric tube. (Reprinted with permission from Rauscher C et al. Neuropediatrics 2009; 40: 43–46.)

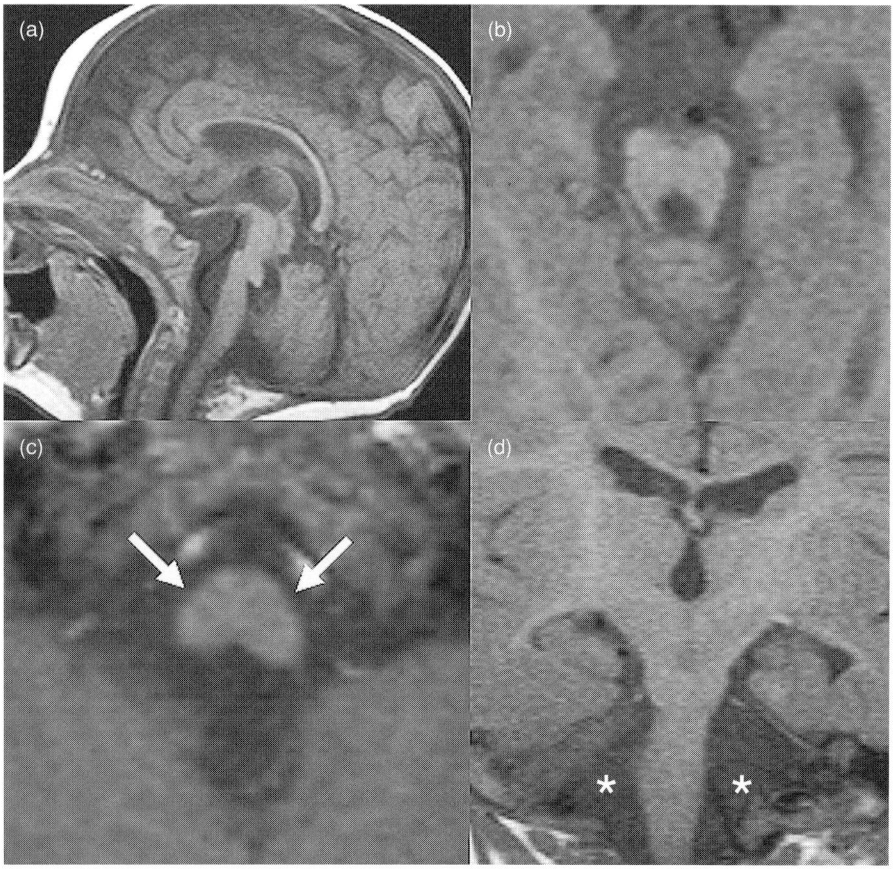

Fig. 20.2. MRI of a patient at 6 months of age. **(a)** Midsagittal T1-weighted MRI showing the flat profile of the ventral side of the pons, the vaulted structure protruding into the fourth ventricle, shortening of the mesencephalic isthmus, hypoplastic and dysplastic superior vermis, and slightly enlarged fourth ventricle partially occupied by the cap; **(b)** axial T1-weighted MRI revealing abnormal shape of the superior cerebellar peduncles reminiscent of a 'molar tooth' appearance; **(c)** axial T1-weighted MRI at the level of the medulla oblongata demonstrating absence of the contours of the inferior olivary nuclei (arrows); **(d)** coronal T1-weighted MRI showing absence of both middle cerebellar peduncles (asterisks), slightly enlarged lateral ventricles, and hippocampal malrotation. (Reprinted with permission from Rauscher C et al. Neuropediatrics 2009; 40: 43–46.)

septal defect in two, variant right subclavian artery in one), two had bilateral vesico-ureteral reflux, and one had a submucous cleft palate and bilateral inguinal hernias, horseshoe kidneys, partial duplication of the left kidney, bilateral coxa valga and left acetabular dysplasia with hip subluxation, external rotation of the right leg, deformity of the right third toe, pectus excavatum and broad chest, inguinal hernia on the right side, haemangioma in the popliteal fossa, esophageal atresia, and anal atresia.

Mild, nonspecific dysmorphic features were described in three patients (retrognathia in two individuals, relative macrocephaly, cranial frontal bossing and parietal prominence, low frontal hairline, long eyelashes, low-set ears, soft ear cartilage, prominent ears, broad nasal root, small upturned nose, flattened nasal bridge, long smooth upper lip, high arched and narrow palate, large tongue that was frequently protruding from the mouth during infancy, and tendency to have an open-mouthed appearance).

Neuroimaging

PTCD has a distinct neuroimaging pattern (Fig. 20.2). In our opinion, the MRI in the case reported by Macferran et al. is not absolutely convincing (Macferran et al. 2010). The typical pattern includes: a flat profile of the ventral pons; an abnormal curved structure ('cap') covering the middle third of the pontine tegmentum and projecting into the fourth ventricle; quite small MCPs; short ponto-mesencephalic isthmus; lateralized course of the SCPs in 10 cases; slightly elongated shape of the SCPs in axial images with almost horizontal orientation and convergent course are remotely reminiscent of a MTS (but this 'atypical MTS' is quite different from a classic MTS in Joubert syndrome where the superior cerebellar peduncles are thickened and elongated and their orientation is more horizontal) (Maria et al. 1999; Gleeson et al. 2004; Poretti et al. 2007); hypoplasia and dysplasia of the vermis in 14 and 11 cases respectively; normal cerebellar hemispheres in all but 3 patients (slightly hypoplastic); small or not identifiable inferior cerebellar peduncles (ICP); a slightly enlarged fourth ventricle in 12 patients; and altered shape of the medulla oblongata on axial sections due to hypoplasia or aplasia of the inferior olivary nuclei.

In six patients the 7th and 8th cranial nerves were severely reduced in width. Supratentorial findings were hypoplastic or dysplastic corpus callosum in four and two patients, respectively, mild lateral ventricular dilatation in four, hippocampal malrotation in two, and unilateral closed lip schizencephaly in one.

Fractional anisotropy (FA) color maps and fibre tractography have been obtained for two patients (Barth et al. 2007; Jissendi-Tchofo et al. 2009). In one case decussation of MCPs as well as the fibres to the pontine nuclei were absent at the level of the upper pons, a likely explanation of the decreased size of the ventral pons (Jissendi-Tchofo et al. 2009). At the same level, an abnormal bundle of transverse directed ectopic fibres crossed the midline in the dorsal pons directly beneath the fourth ventricle, extending from one MCP to the other to form the pontine 'cap' (Barth et al. 2007; Jissendi-Tchofo et al. 2009). These fibres appeared to terminate at the sites of crossing of the SCPs projecting to the cerebellar hemispheres. The SCPs appeared elongated and running laterally in both cases. In one case the decussation was not visible in its normal midbrain location (Jissendi-Tchofo et al. 2009). However, in the other patient a transverse band across the midline indicated decussation of the SCPs (Barth et al. 2007). Two tracts of longitudinal axons were located in the anterior pons, at the sites normally occupied by the corticospinal and corticopontine tracts. However, they were smaller than in healthy individuals.

Additional examinations

Electrophysiological investigations have been performed in some patients. Brainstem auditory evoked potentials (BAER) were sought in eight patients and were absent in all.

Electroencephalography (EEG) has been performed in seven patients and was normal in five. EEG showed multifocal sharp waves without clinical seizures and seizures with clonic upper limb movements and facial twitching in the other cases.

SSEP in one patient showed normal crossed cortical response (Barth et al. 2007).

Diagnosis

The diagnosis of PTCD is made by the distinct neuroimaging pattern.

Differential diagnosis

Because of the typical neuroimaging findings the diagnosis of PTCD is straightforward.

Involvement of cranial nerves has also been reported in Moebius syndrome (Verzijl et al. 2003), swallowing difficulties and retrognathia in Pierre Robin syndrome (Benko et al. 2009), and OMA in congenital OMA of type Cogan (Kondo et al. 2007). However, the extent of brainstem involvement and the neuroimaging findings distinguish PTCD clearly from these syndromes.

Roig et al. reported five patients with muscular hypotonia, facial diplegia, jaw ankylosis, velopharyngeal incoordination with feeding difficulties, pyramidal tract signs, and OMA, and named this syndrome 'brainstem dysgenesis' (Roig et al. 2003). All these clinical signs are present in PTCD too. However, in all the patients with brainstem dysgenesis, MRI recorded normal brainstem structures.

Management and treatment

In PTCD the treatment should be focused on symptoms to improve motor and cognitive development (including visual and auditory perception and communication) and quality of life.

For sensorineural hearing loss (SNHL) a trial with hearing aids or a frequency-modulation device is appropriate, although for those with severe to profound SNHL, as is typical in PTCD, the approach is more complex. For these children, the earliest decision may be focused on the choice of communication: auditory-oral, which includes auditory verbal training, oral training, lip reading, and cued speech; visual, gestural, and manual training, which include variously recognized sign languages; and a combination of speech and sign, referred to as total communication. Additionally, cochlear implantation has become standard treatment when there is lack of progress with well-fitted hearing aids and intensive auditory training (Smith et al. 2005). To our knowledge, to date cochlear implantation has only been performed in two patients with PTCD. In one child, perception, cognition, and communication did not improve after cochlear implantation (personal observation). Bacciu et al. reported some improvements in speech perceptions, but overall poor results in a girl implanted at the advanced age of 6 years (Bacciu et al. 2010).

For paediatric corneal opacities, keratoplasty remains the management of choice. However, it is associated with several complications such as a high risk of graft failure or failure of amblyopia therapy in clear grafts (Vanathi et al. 2009). Therefore, careful preoperative evaluation is required. To our knowledge, to date keratoplasty has not been performed in children with PTCD.

For swallowing and feeding difficulties a nasogastric tube and gastrostomy are helpful. Additionally, supporting therapies such as physical and occupational therapies as well as several aids can be utilized if necessary.

Outcome

Four children died: two from pneumonia at the ages of 2 years 8 months and 6 months, respectively; one at 2 years from unknown cause; and one at 1 year 4 months from recurrent respiratory infections. The other patients are alive at the last follow-up at a mean age of 6 years 11 months (median 5 years 6 months, range: 5 months to 19 years).

Developmental delay was present in 11 of 12 tested patients, and was severe in 7. One child had an overall IQ of 94 (Barth et al. 2007). Two children reported by Barth et al. could walk at 4 and 6 years, respectively, but both were clearly ataxic (Barth et al. 2007). Two children walk with support of a walker at 10 and 16 years, respectively. Two children could not walk, but sat at the age of 2 years 2 months and 2 years 3 months, respectively. Three other patients had poor head control and were unable to sit. Speech was impaired in 8 children: five were mute and three produced indistinct language. Four children learned sign language.

REFERENCES

Alcantara S, Ruiz M, De Castro F, Soriano E, Sotelo C (2000) Netrin 1 acts as an attractive or as a repulsive cue for distinct migrating neurons during the development of the cerebellar system. Development 127: 1359–1372.

Avadhani A, Ilayaraja V, Shetty AP, Rajasekaran S (2010) Diffusion tensor imaging in horizontal gaze palsy with progressive scoliosis. Magn Reson Imaging 28: 212–216.

Bacciu A, Ormitti F, Pasanisi E, Vincenti V, Zanetti D, Bacciu S (2010) Cochlear implantation in pontine tegmental cap displasia. Int J Pediatr Otorhinolaryngol 74: 962–966.

Barallobre MJ, Pascual M, Del Rio JA, Soriano E (2005) The Netrin family of guidance factors: emphasis on Netrin-1 signalling. Brain Res Rev 49: 22–47.

Barth PG, Majoie CB, Caan MW, Weterman MA, Kyllerman M, Smit LM, et al. (2007) Pontine tegmental cap dysplasia: a novel brain malformation with a defect in axonal guidance. Brain 130: 2258–2266.

Benko S, Fantes JA, Amiel J, Kleinjan DJ, Thomas S, Ramsay J, et al. (2009) Highly conserved non-coding elements on either side of SOX9 associated with Pierre Robin sequence. Nat Genet 41: 359–364.

Bhat KM, Gaziova I, Krishnan S (2007) Regulation of axon guidance by slit and netrin signaling in the Drosophila ventral nerve cord. Genetics 176: 2235–2246.

Bosley TM, Salih MA, Jen JC, Lin DD, Oystreck D, Abu-Amero KK, et al. (2005) Neurologic features of horizontal gaze palsy and progressive scoliosis with mutations in ROBO3. Neurology 64: 1196–1203.

Bulow HE, Hobert O (2004) Differential sulfations and epimerization define heparan sulfate specificity in nervous system development. Neuron 41: 723–736.

Castori M, Valente EM, Donati MA, Salvi S, Fazzi E, Procopio E, et al.; Italian MTS Study Group (2005) NPHP1 gene deletion is a rare cause of Joubert syndrome related disorders. J Med Genet 42: e9.

Colamarino SA, Tessier-Lavigne M (1995) The axonal chemoattractant netrin-1 is also a chemorepellent for trochlear motor axons. Cell 81: 621–629.

Culotti JG, Merz DC (1998) DCC and netrins. Curr Opin Cell Biol 10: 609–613.

Devine CA, Key B (2008) Robo-Slit interactions regulate longitudinal axon pathfinding in the embryonic vertebrate brain. Dev Biol 313: 371–383.

Dickson BJ (2002) Molecular mechanisms of axon guidance. Science 298: 1959–1964.

Doherty D (2009) Joubert syndrome: insights into brain development, cilium biology, and complex disease. Semin Pediatr Neurol 16: 143–154.

Engle EC (2007) Oculomotility disorders arising from disruptions in brainstem motor neuron development. Arch Neurol 64: 633–637.

Engle EC (2010) Human genetic disorders of axon guidance. Cold Spring Harb Perspect Biol 2: a001784.

Fazeli A, Dickinson SL, Hermiston ML, Tighe RV, Steen RG, Small CG, et al. (1997) Phenotype of mice lacking functional Deleted in colorectal cancer (Dcc) gene. Nature 386: 796–804.

Fearon ER, Cho KR, Nigro JM, Kern SE, Simons JW, Ruppert JM, et al. (1990) Identification of a chromosome 18q gene that is altered in colorectal cancers. Science 247: 49–56.

Finger JH, Bronson RT, Harris B, Johnson K, Przyborski SA, Ackerman SL (2002) The netrin 1 receptors Unc5h3 and Dcc are necessary at multiple choice points for the guidance of corticospinal tract axons. J Neurosci 22: 10346–10356.

Gavalas A, Ruhrberg C, Livet J, Henderson CE, Krumlauf R (2003) Neuronal defects in the hindbrain of Hoxa1, Hoxb1 and Hoxb2 mutants reflect regulatory interactions among these Hox genes. Development 130: 5663–5679.

Gleeson JG, Keeler LC, Parisi MA, Marsh SE, Chance PF, Glass IA, et al. (2004) Molar tooth sign of the midbrain-hindbrain junction: occurrence in multiple distinct syndromes. Am J Med Genet A 125A: 125–134.

Guthrie S, Pini A (1995) Chemorepulsion of developing motor axons by the floor plate. Neuron 14: 1117–1130.

Gutowski NJ, Bosley TM, Engle EC (2003) 110th ENMC International Workshop: the congenital cranial dysinnervation disorders (CCDDs). Naarden, The Netherlands, 25–27 October, 2002. Neuromuscul Disord 13: 573–578.

Haller S, Wetzel SG, Lutschg J (2008) Functional MRI, DTI and neurophysiology in horizontal gaze palsy with progressive scoliosis. Neuroradiology 50: 453–459.

Jen JC, Chan WM, Bosley TM, Wan J, Carr JR, Rub U, et al. (2004) Mutations in a human ROBO gene disrupt hindbrain axon pathway crossing and morphogenesis. Science 304: 1509–1513.

Jissendi-Tchofo P, Doherty D, McGillivray G, Hevner R, Shaw D, Ishak G, et al. (2009) Pontine tegmental cap dysplasia: MR imaging and diffusion tensor imaging features of impaired axonal navigation. AJNR Am J Neuroradiol 30: 113–119.

Keleman K, Dickson BJ (2001) Short- and long-range repulsion by the Drosophila Unc5 netrin receptor. Neuron 32: 605–617.

Kondo A, Saito Y, Floricel F, Maegaki Y, Ohno K (2007) Congenital ocular motor apraxia: clinical and neuroradiological findings, and long-term intellectual prognosis. Brain Dev 29: 431–438.

Llambi F, Causeret F, Bloch-Gallego E, Mehlen P (2001) Netrin-1 acts as a survival factor via its receptors UNC5H and DCC. EMBO J 20: 2715–2722.

Macferran KM, Buchmann RF, Ramakrishnaiah R, Griebel ML, Sanger WG, Saronwala A, Schaefer GB (2010) Pontine tegmental cap dysplasia with a 2q13 microdeletion involving the NPHP1 gene: insights into malformations of the mid-hindbrain. Semin Pediatr Neurol 17: 69–74.

Mann F, Rougon G (2007) Mechanisms of axon guidance: membrane dynamics and axonal transport in semaphorin signalling. J Neurochem 102: 316–323.

Maria BL, Quisling RG, Rosainz LC, Yachnis AT, Gitten J, Dede D, Fennell E (1999) Molar tooth sign in Joubert syndrome: clinical, radiologic, and pathologic significance. J Child Neurol 14: 368–376.

Otaduy MC, Leite Cda C, Nagae LM, Pinho Mda C, Bueno C, Reed UC, Kok F (2009) Further diffusion tensor imaging contribution in horizontal gaze palsy and progressive scoliosis. Arq Neuropsiquiatr 67: 1054–1056.

Parisi MA (2009) Clinical and molecular features of Joubert syndrome and related disorders. Am J Med Genet C 151C: 326–340.

Poretti A, Boltshauser E, Loenneker T, Valente EM, Brancati F, Il'yasov K, Huisman TA (2007) Diffusion tensor imaging in Joubert syndrome. AJNR Am J Neuroradiol 28: 1929–1933.

Rauscher C, Poretti A, Neuhann TM, Forstner R, Hahn G, Koch J, et al. (2009) Pontine tegmental cap dysplasia: the severe end of the clinical spectrum. Neuropediatrics 40: 43–46.

Roig M, Gratacos M, Vazquez E, Del Toro M, Foguet A, Ferrer I, Macaya A (2003) Brainstem dysgenesis: report of five patients with congenital hypotonia, multiple cranial nerve involvement, and ocular motor apraxia. Dev Med Child Neurol 45: 489–493.

Sabatier C, Plump AS, Le M, Brose K, Tamada A, Murakami F, et al. (2004) The divergent Robo family protein rig-1/Robo3 is a negative regulator of slit responsiveness required for midline crossing by commissural axons. Cell 117: 157–169.

Serafini T, Colamarino SA, Leonardo ED, Wang H, Beddington R, Skarnes WC, Tessier-Lavigne M (1996) Netrin-1 is required for commissural axon guidance in the developing vertebrate nervous system. Cell 87: 1001–1014.

Shirasaki R, Mirzayan C, Tessier-Lavigne M, Murakami F (1996) Guidance of circumferentially growing axons by netrin-dependent and -independent floor plate chemotropism in the vertebrate brain. Neuron 17: 1079–1088.

Sibbe M, Taniguchi M, Schachner M, Bartsch U (2007) Development of the corticospinal tract in Semaphorin3A- and CD24-deficient mice. Neuroscience 150: 898–904.

Sicotte NL, Salamon G, Shattuck DW, Hageman N, Rub U, Salamon N, et al. (2006) Diffusion tensor MRI shows abnormal brainstem crossing fibers associated with ROBO3 mutations. Neurology 67: 519–521.

Smith RJ, Bale JF, Jr., White KR (2005) Sensorineural hearing loss in children. Lancet 365: 879–890.

Stein E, Zou Y, Poo M, Tessier-Lavigne M (2001) Binding of DCC by netrin-1 to mediate axon guidance independent of adenosine A2B receptor activation. Science 291: 1976–1982.

Szczaluba K, Szymanska K, Bekiesinka-Figatowska M, Jurkiewicz E, Madzik J, Obersztyn E, Mazurczak T (2010) Pontine tegmental cap dysplasia: A hindbrain malformation caused by defective neuronal migration. Neurology 74: 1835.

Tamada A, Kumada T, Zhu Y, Matsumoto T, Hatanaka Y, Muguruma K, et al. (2008) Crucial roles of Robo proteins in midline crossing of cerebellofugal axons and lack of their up-regulation after midline crossing. Neural Dev 3: 29.

Vanathi M, Panda A, Vengayil S, Chaudhuri Z, Dada T (2009) Pediatric keratoplasty. Surv Ophthalmol 54: 245–271.

Verzijl HT, van der Zwaag B, Cruysberg JR, Padberg GW (2003) Mobius syndrome redefined: a syndrome of rhombencephalic maldevelopment. Neurology 61: 327–333.

Wellik DM (2007) Hox patterning of the vertebrate axial skeleton. Dev Dyn 236: 2454–2463.

Wong K, Ren XR, Huang YZ, Xie Y, Liu G, Saito H, Tang H, Wen L, Brady-Kalnay SM, Mei L, Wu JY, Xiong WC, Rao Y (2001) Signal transduction in neuronal migration: roles of GTPase activating proteins and the small GTPase Cdc42 in the Slit-Robo pathway. Cell 107: 209–221.

Woods CG (2004) Neuroscience. Crossing the midline. Science 304: 1455–1456.

21
Brainstem Malformations Associated with Cerebellar Abnormalities

Andrea Poretti and Eugen Boltshauser

Because of the same embryological origin (hindbrain), abnormalities of the brainstem (particularly of the pons and medulla oblongata) are almost always associated with cerebellar anomalies. Malformations of the brainstem and cerebellum can occur as the only recognized brain anomaly, such as in pontine tegmental cap dysplasia (see Chapter 20), but they have also been increasingly recognized in patients with supratentorial anomalies such as some forms of lissencephaly (Fig. 21.1) (see Chapter 8, section on migrational disorders), congenital muscular dystrophies (see Chapter 15), or callosal anomalies, and in patients with additional developmental disorders in other organ systems such as kidneys or eyes, for example, Joubert syndrome and related disorders (see Chapter 11) or oculocerebrocutaneous syndrome (see Chapter 8, Barkovich et al. 2009). Additionally, the pons is involved (mostly as hypoplasia) in several genetic disorders (e.g., the group of the pontocerebellar hypoplasia reported by Peter Barth; see Chapter 23), *CASK* mutation (see Chapter 8), or *PTF1A* mutation (see Chapter 7) or metabolic diseases (mostly the group of congenital disorders of glycosylation, see Chapter 27) with prenatal onset (see Checklists, Table 24).

Recently, Barkovich et al. classified the malformations that primarily affect the brainstem on the basis of the possible embryological pathomechanisms (Barkovich et al. 2007, 2009). In their classification, they reported in part largely unrecognized anomalies, but also well-known disorders such as some forms of congenital muscular dystrophies (Clement et al. 2008), brainstem disconnection (Poretti et al. 2007a), and the oculocerebrocutaneous syndrome (OCC) (Moog et al. 2005). The authors proposed two embryological pathomechanisms: (1) *abnormal brainstem segmentation* and (2) *abnormal cell migration, cell proliferation, or axon navigation* (Barkovich et al. 2007, 2009).

Abnormal brainstem segmentation

Malformations secondary to abnormal brainstem segmentation are defects of early brainstem patterning that affect the anteroposterior or dorsoventral mid-hindbrain segmentation.

Disorders of anteroposterior segmentation are due to gain, loss, or transformation of segments at boundaries between sections of the neural tube (diencephalon and midbrain, midbrain and rhombomere 1, and lower hindbrain structures) (Barkovich et al. 2009). If gain, loss, or transformation affect the diencephalon and midbrain, the midbrain can be enlarged, short, or elongated, but the cerebellum is normal (e.g., midbrain enlargement with dorsoventral midline hyperintensity; Fig. 21.2) (Barkovich et al. 2007, 2009). Loss of midbrain and rhombomere 1 causes deletion of posterior midbrain, pons, vermis, and most of the cerebellar hemispheres such as in pontomesencephalic brainstem disconnection (Poretti et al. 2007a). However, gain of midbrain and loss of rhombomere 1 results in elongated midbrain, enlarged tectum, absent cerebellar vermis, and hypoplasia of the cerebellar hemispheres such as in OCC (see Fig. 6, Chapter 8; Moog et al. 2005). Loss of midbrain combined with gain of rhombomere 1 leads to a short midbrain with long pons and large cerebellum involving both vermis (particularly the anterior lobes) and hemispheres (Barkovich et al. 2007). Gain, loss, or transformation can affect also the lower hindbrain structures. Loss of pons or medulla results in the pontomedullary brainstem disconnection (Poretti et al. 2007a), mixed gains and losses of pons or medulla in anomalies characterized by short pons and long medulla, sometimes with associated ventral and/or dorsal midline clefts (Fig. 21.1) (Barkovich et al. 2007), and segmental shifts of pons or medulla in defects of some hindbrain segments such as mutations in the *HOXA1* gene resulting in Athabaskan brainstem dysgenesis syndrome and Bosley-Salih-Alorainy syndrome (Bosley et al. 2007, 2008). Four of five patients with 6q terminal deletion syndrome had an abnormal brainstem with elongated midbrain and relatively small pons (Elia et al. 2006). Additionally, pontine hypoplasia has been reported in cri-du-chat syndrome or partial deletion of the short arm of chromosome 5 (Ninchoji and Takanashi 2010).

Mid-hindbrain dorsoventral patterning defects are postulated to result in abnormal development or function of specific mid-hindbrain ventricular zones and structures including abnormal formation of brainstem nuclei, cranial nerves, and any cerebellar structures (Barkovich et al. 2009). These defects can involve the alar or basal ventricular zone. Alar defects result in rhombencephalosynapsis (if more than one dorsoventral subregion is involved, see Chapter 16), in diffuse granule cell hypoplasia (if roof plate and rhombic lip derivates are affected), and cerebellar agenesis due to mutations in the *PTF1A* gene (if the defects involve the cerebellar ventricular zone, particularly the GABAergic neurons, see Chapter 7). Basal ventricular zone defects result in defects of specific cranial nerve nuclei leading to Duane retraction syndrome (Engle 2010) or Moebius syndrome (Verzijl et al. 2003).

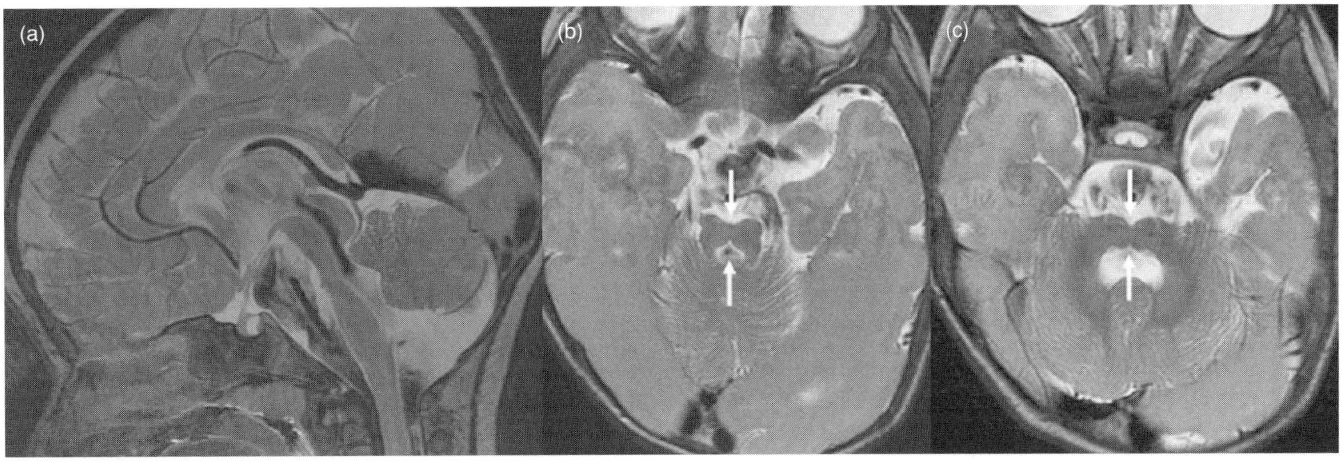

Fig. 21.1. A 5-month-old girl with infantile spasms and lissencephaly as well as supratentorial T2-hyperintensity of the white matter (not shown). **(a)** Midsagittal T2-weighted MRI showing a long midbrain with proportionally long tectum, practically absent pons, long medulla, and slightly hypoplastic cerebellum. **(b, c)** Axial T2-weighted MRI presenting ventral and dorsal clefts in the pons (arrows).

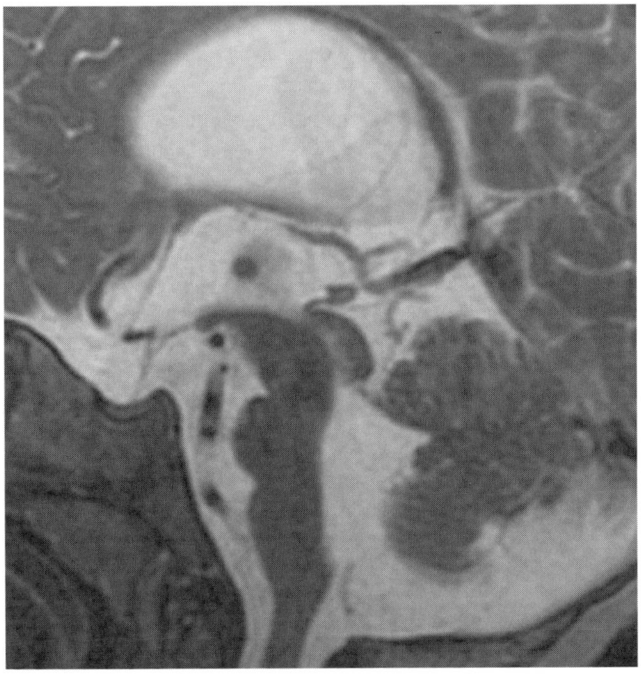

Fig. 21.2. A 10-month-old infant with ocular motor abnormalities, severe global developmental delay, and hemiparesis on the left side. Midsagittal T2-weighted MRI demonstrating enlarged and long midbrain, small pons, long medulla, and mild cerebellar hypoplasia.

Abnormal cell migration or proliferation

These disorders can affect the entire brain, but the involvement of mid- and hindbrain is often prominent. They affect cell proliferation, cell migration, and probably axon navigation (Barkovich et al. 2009). Barkovich et al. distinguish five groups: (1) developmental encephalopathies associated with mid-hindbrain malformations; (2) mesenchymal-neurepithelial signalling defects associated with mid-hindbrain malformations; (3) malformations of neuronal and glial proliferation that prominently affect the brainstem and cerebellum; (4) malformation of neuronal migration that prominently affect the brainstem and cerebellum; and (5) Joubert syndrome and related disorders characterized by the molar tooth sign and associated with defects in ciliary proteins (Barkovich et al. 2009).

Developmental encephalopathies associated with mid-hindbrain malformations include disorders characterized by cognitive impairment, autism, and global cerebellar hypoplasia or vermian hypoplasia, for example, cognitive impairment with cerebellar vermis hypoplasia due to mutations in the *OPHN1* gene (Bergmann et al. 2003; Zanni et al. 2005) or X-linked nonprogressive cerebellar hypoplasia mapping to chromosome Xp11.21.q24 (Illarioshkin et al. 1996).

Mesenchymal-neurepithelial signalling defects associated with mid-hindbrain malformations include a wide range of anomalies in the posterior fossa ranging from Dandy-Walker malformation to vermis hypoplasia or mega cisterna magna (Barkovich et al. 2009). This range of posterior fossa abnormalities can be caused by mutations in the *FOXC1* gene (Aldinger et al. 2009), loss of *ZIC1-ZIC4* because of deletion of 3q24 (Grinberg and Millen 2005), neurocutaneous melanosis (Marnet et al. 2009), and PHACES (Posterior fossa malformations, Hemangiomas, Arterial anomalies, Coarctation of the aorta and cardiac defects, Eye abnomalities); syndrome (Metry et al. 2009).

Abnormal cell proliferation seems to cause a number of brainstem malformations (Barkovich et al. 2009). Proliferation of abnormal cells results in focal areas of overgrowth containing dysplastic cells. Cerebellar dysplastic gangliocytoma (Lhermitte Duclos disease, see Chapter 33; Nowak and Trost 2002), cortical hamartoma in the cerebellum in children with tuberous sclerosis (see Chapter 29; Eluvathingal et al. 2006; Ertan et al. 2010), and hemicerebellar hemimegalencephaly (see Chapter 18; Flores-Sarnat, 2008) are part of this group. Increased proliferation is very uncommon and can result in macrocerebellum (see Chapter 17). It has been reported in the macrocephaly-capillary malformation syndrome resulting in overgrowth of cerebral and cerebellar hemispheres, often leading to cerebellar tonsillar herniation (Conway et al. 2007) and in the Costello syndrome which is mostly also characterized by macrocerebellum (which can be progressive) with cerebellar tonsillar herniation (Gripp et al. 2010). However, decreased proliferation results in microcephaly with severe and disproportionate brainstem and cerebellar hypoplasia such as in mutations in the *CASK* gene (see Chapter 8; Najm et al. 2008).

Malformations of cortical development may be associated with midbrain-hindbrain involvement (Jissendi-Tchofo et al. 2009). These include lissencephalies (e.g., lissencephaly with mild cerebellar hypoplasia such as in mutations of the *LIS1* or *DCX* gene and lissencephaly with nearly afoliar cerebellum and hypoplastic pons such as in mutations of the *RELN* or *VLDLR* gene; see Chapter 8), polymicrogyria, nodular heterotopias (periventricular such in mutations of the *FLNA* gene, or subcortical; see Chapter 8), and dystroglycanopathies with cobblestone malformations (see Chapter 15 on cerebellar cysts and neuroimaging in congenital muscular dystrophies; Clement et al. 2008).

Joubert syndrome and related disorders or molar tooth malformations are characterized by abnormalities of the white matter tracts in the brainstem, abnormal superior cerebellar peduncles, and dysplastic-hypoplastic cerebellar vermis (see Chapter 11; Gleeson et al. 2004; Alorainy et al. 2006; Poretti et al. 2007b; Zaki et al. 2008; Senocak et al. 2010).

Tectocerebellar dysraphism with occipital encephalocele (TCD-OE) was defined by Friede as a cerebellar malformation characterized by agenesis of the cerebellar vermis (in some cases with exception of small anterior/superior remnants), an occipital encephalocele, and a deformation of the tectum (mostly an exaggeration of the beaking seen in the Chiari II malformation) (Friede 1978). The cases reported so far in the literature and fulfilling the three diagnostic criteria present additional heterogeneous findings (Demaerel et al. 1995; Dehdashti et al. 2004; Anik et al. 2010). Elongated, horizontally orientated, and thickened superior cerebellar peduncles reminiscent of the molar tooth sign in Joubert syndrome and related disorders have also been found in some patients with TCD-OE (Demaerel et al. 1995; Dehdashti et al. 2004). In our opinion it is doubtful whether TCD-OE represents an entity.

There are some additional localized brain malformations that significantly affect brainstem and cerebellum whose pathogenesis may include defects in local proliferation, cell specification, cell migration, and axonal guidance (Barkovich et al. 2009).

In this group are included so-called *developmental clefts* (see Checklists, Table 29), which may be seen in the dorsal and/or ventral midline surface of the pons and are mostly, but not consistently, associated with cerebellar hypoplasia or dysplasia (Barkovich et al. 2007). The most common clefts are localized ventrally and longitudinally in the midline and involve the pons. They are likely to result from the absence of the decussation of the middle cerebellar peduncles and the transverse pontine axons migrating from the cerebellar cortex to the pontine nuclei (Barkovich et al. 2009).

However, midline dorsal clefts seem to originate from abnormal development of the median longitudinal fasciculus and the tectospinal tract (Barkovich et al. 2007). The best example is horizontal gaze palsy with progressive scoliosis (HGPPS) due to mutations in the *ROBO3* gene (Jen et al. 2004; Bosley et al. 2005). It is characterized by absent midline crossing of the major pontine axons and the superior cerebellar peduncles resulting in brainstem hypoplasia with absence of the facial colliculi, presence of a deep midline dorsal pontine cleft, and a butterfly configuration of the medulla (Rossi et al. 2004; Sicotte et al. 2006). Other brainstem malformations probably resulting from abnormal axonal guidance are PTCD (see Chapter 20) and L1 syndrome with X-linked hydrocephalus (Kanemura et al. 2006).

L1 syndrome is a highly variable X-linked neurological disorder resulting from mutations in the *L1CAM* gene on chromosome Xq28 and originally recognized as four distinct entities: X-linked hydrocephalus; MASA (cognitive impairment, aphasia, shuffling gait, adducted thumbs, MIM #303350); X-linked complicated spastic paraplegia type 1; and X-linked corpus callosum agenesis (Weller and Gärtner 2001). The L1 cell adhesion molecule is a transmembrane neural adhesion glycoprotein and acts as a short-range axon guidance molecule (Kenwrick et al. 2000). It is highly expressed in developing and migrating axons such as in the corpus callosum and corticospinal tract. Binding several extra- and intracellular molecules, L1 may potentiate cell adhesion and enhance neuronal migration and neurite outgrowth or may induce growth cone collapse and axon repulsion, respectively, depending on the binding partner molecules (Kenwrick et al. 2000). The clinical presentation includes a combination of macrocephaly due to severe hydrocephalus, cognitive impairment, aphasia, spastic paraparesis, and thumb adduction deformities (Vos et al. 2010). An association with Hirschsprung disease has been reported. The neuroimaging criteria suggesting L1 syndrome include severe congenital hydrocephalus, rippled ventricular wall after shunt placement, hypoplasia of the corpus callosum, large massa intermedia, enlarged quadrigeminal plate, and hypoplasia of the cerebellar vermis (Kanemura et al. 2006).

Localized abnormalities of cell specification caused Duane retraction syndrome (due to mutation in the *CHN1* gene; Al-Baradie et al. 2002), Okihiro syndrome including Duane syndrome, radial ray anomalies, and deafness (caused by mutations in the *SALL4* gene; Kohlhase et al. 2005), and congenital fibrosis of the extraocular muscles (because of mutations in the *PHOX2A* gene; Bosley et al. 2006).

REFERENCES

Al-Baradie R, Yamada K, St Hilaire C, Chan WM, Andrews C, McIntosh N, et al. (2002) Duane radial ray syndrome (Okihiro syndrome) maps to 20q13 and results from mutations in SALL4, a new member of the SAL family. Am J Hum Genet 71: 1195–1199.

Aldinger KA, Lehmann OJ, Hudgins L, Chizhikov VV, Bassuk AG, Ades LC, et al. (2009) FOXC1 is required for normal cerebellar development and is a major contributor to chromosome 6p25.3 Dandy-Walker malformation. Nat Genet 41: 1037–1042.

Alorainy IA, Sabir S, Seidahmed MZ, Farooqu HA, Salih MA (2006) Brain stem and cerebellar findings in Joubert syndrome. J Comput Assist Tomogr 30: 116–121.

Anik I, Koc K, Anik Y, Yildiz DK, Ceylan S (2010) Tetocerebellar dysraphism with vermian encephalocele. J Child Neurol 25: 1411–1414.

Barkovich AJ, Millen KJ, Dobyns WB (2007) A developmental classification of malformations of the brainstem. Ann Neurol 62: 625–639.

Barkovich AJ, Millen KJ, Dobyns WB (2009) A developmental and genetic classification for midbrain-hindbrain malformations. Brain 132: 3199–3230.

Bergmann C, Zerres K, Senderek J, Rudnik-Schoneborn S, Eggermann T, Hausler M, et al. (2003) Oligophrenin 1 (OPHN1) gene mutation causes syndromic X-linked mental retardation with epilepsy, rostral ventricular enlargement and cerebellar hypoplasia. Brain 126: 1537–1544.

Bosley TM, Salih MA, Jen JC, Lin DD, Oystreck D, Abu-Amero KK, et al. (2005) Neurologic features of horizontal gaze palsy and progressive scoliosis with mutations in ROBO3. Neurology 64: 1196–1203.

Bosley TM, Oystreck DT, Robertson RL, al Awad A, Abu-Amero K, Engle EC (2006) Neurological features of congenital fibrosis of the extraocular muscles type 2 with mutations in PHOX2A. Brain 129: 2363–2374.

Bosley TM, Salih MA, Alorainy IA, Oystreck DT, Nester M, Abu-Amero KK, et al. (2007) Clinical characterization of the HOXA1 syndrome BSAS variant. Neurology 69: 1245–1253.

Bosley TM, Alorainy IA, Salih MA, Aldhalaan HM, Abu-Amero KK, Oystreck DT, et al. (2008) The clinical spectrum of homozygous HOXA1 mutations. Am J Med Genet A 146A: 1235–1240.

Clement E, Mercuri E, Godfrey C, Smith J, Robb S, Kinali M, et al. (2008) Brain involvement in muscular dystrophies with defective dystroglycan glycosylation. Ann Neurol 64: 573–582.

Conway RL, Pressman BD, Dobyns WB, Danielpour M, Lee J, Sanchez-Lara PA, et al. (2007) Neuroimaging findings in macrocephaly-capillary malformation: a longitudinal study of 17 patients. Am J Med Genet A 143A: 2981–3008.

Dehdashti AR, Abouzeid H, Momjian S, Delavelle J, Rilliet B (2004) Occipital extra- and intracranial lipoencephalocele associated with tectocerebellar dysraphia. Childs Nerv Syst 20: 225–228.

Demaerel P, Kendall BE, Wilms G, Halpin SFS, Casaer P, Baert AL (1995) Uncommon posterior cranial fossa anomalies: MRI with clinical correlation. Neuroradiology 37: 72–76.

Elia M, Striano P, Fichera M, Gaggero R, Castiglia L, Galesi O, et al. (2006) 6q terminal deletion syndrome associated with a distinctive EEG and clinical pattern: a report of five cases. Epilepsia 47: 830–838.

Eluvathingal TJ, Behen ME, Chugani HT, Janisse J, Bernardi B, Chakraborty P, et al. (2006) Cerebellar lesions in tuberous sclerosis complex: neurobehavioral and neuroimaging correlates. J Child Neurol 21: 846–851.

Engle EC (2010) Human genetic disorders of axon guidance. Cold Spring Harb Perspect Biol 2: a001784.

Ertan G, Arulrajah S, Tekes A, Jordan L, Huisman TA (2010) Cerebellar abnormality in children and young adults with tuberous sclerosis complex: MR and diffusion weighted imaging findings. J Neuroradiol 37: 231–238.

Flores-Sarnat L (2008) Hemimegalencephaly syndrome. In: Sarnat HB, Curatolo P, editors. Malformations of the nervous system. New York: Elsevier. p. 153–176.

Friede RL (1978) Uncommon syndromes of cerebellar vermis aplasia. II: Tcto-cerebellar dysraphism with occipital encephalocele. Dev Med Child Neurol 20: 764–772.

Gleeson JG, Keeler LC, Parisi MA, Marsh SE, Chance PF, Glass IA, et al. (2004) Molar tooth sign of the midbrain-hindbrain junction: occurrence in multiple distinct syndromes. Am J Med Genet A 125A: 125–134.

Grinberg I, Millen KJ (2005) The ZIC gene family in development and disease. Clin Genet 67: 290–296.

Gripp KW, Hopkins E, Doyle D, Dobyns WB (2010) High incidence of progressive postnatal cerebellar enlargement in Costello syndrome: brain overgrowth associated with HRAS mutations as the likely cause of structural brain and spinal cord abnormalities. Am J Med Genet A 152A: 1161–1168.

Illarioshkin SN, Tanaka H, Markova ED, Nikolskaya NN, Ivanova-Smolenskaya IA, Tsuji S (1996) X-linked nonprogressive congenital cerebellar hypoplasia: clinical description and mapping to chromosome Xq. Ann Neurol 40: 75–83.

Jen JC, Chan WM, Bosley TM, Wan J, Carr JR, Rub U, et al. (2004) Mutations in a human ROBO gene disrupt hindbrain axon pathway crossing and morphogenesis. Science 304: 1509–1513.

Jissendi-Tchofo P, Kara S, Barkovich AJ (2009) Midbrain-hindbrain involvement in lissencephalies. Neurology 72: 410–418.

Kanemura Y, Okamoto N, Sakamoto H, Shofuda T, Kamiguchi H, Yamasaki M (2006) Molecular mechanisms and neuroimaging criteria for severe L1 syndrome with X-linked hydrocephalus. J Neurosurg (5 Suppl Pediatrics) 105: 403–412.

Kenwrick S, Watkins A, De Angelis E (2000) Neural cell recognition molecule L1: relating biological complexity to human disease mutations. Hum Molec Genet 9: 879–886.

Kohlhase J, Chitayat D, Kotzot D, Ceylaner S, Froster UG, Fuchs S, et al. (2005) SALL4 mutations in Okihiro syndrome (Duane-radial ray syndrome), acro-renal-ocular syndrome, and related disorders. Hum Mutat 26: 176–183.

Marnet D, Vinchon M, Mostofi K, Catteau B, Kerdraon O, Dhellemmes P (2009) Neurocutaneous melanosis and the Dandy-Walker complex: an uncommon but not so insignificant association. Childs Nerv Syst 25: 1533–1539.

Metry D, Heyer G, Hess C, Garzon M, Haggstrom A, Frommelt P, et al. (2009) Consensus statement on diagnostic criteria for PHACE syndrome. Pediatrics 124: 1447–1456.

Moog U, Jones MC, Bird LM, Dobyns WB (2005) Oculocerebrocutaneous syndrome: the brain malformation defines a core phenotype. J Med Genet 42: 913–921.

Najm J, Horn D, Wimplinger I, Golden JA, Chizhikov VV, Sudi J, et al. (2008) Mutations of CASK cause an X-linked brain malformation phenotype with microcephaly and hypoplasia of the brainstem and cerebellum. Nat Genet 40: 1065–1067.

Ninchoji T, Takanashi J (2010) Pontine hypoplasia in 5p-syndrome: a key MRI finding for a diagnosis. Brain Dev 32: 571–573.

Nowak DA, Trost HA (2002) Lhermitte-Duclos disease (dysplastic cerebellar gangliocytoma): a malformation, hamartoma or neoplasm? Acta Neurol Scand 105: 137–145.

Poretti A, Boltshauser E, Plecko B (2007a) Brainstem disconnection: case report and review of the literature. Neuropediatrics 38: 210–212.

Poretti A, Boltshauser E, Loenneker T, Valente EM, Brancati F, Il'yasov K, Huisman TA (2007b) Diffusion tensor imaging in Joubert syndrome. AJNR Am J Neuroradiol 28: 1929–1933.

Rossi A, Catala M, Biancheri R, Di Comite R, Tortori-Donati P (2004) MR imaging of brain-stem hypoplasia in horizontal gaze palsy with progressive scoliosis. AJNR Am J Neuroradiol 25: 1046–1048.

Senocak EU, Oguz KK, Haliloglu G, Topcu M, Cila A (2010) Structural abnormalities of the brain other than molar tooth sign in Joubert syndrome-related disorders. Diagn Interv Radiol 16: 3–6.

Sicotte NL, Salamon G, Shattuck DW, Hageman N, Rub U, Salamon N, et al. (2006) Diffusion tensor MRI shows abnormal brainstem crossing fibers associated with ROBO3 mutations. Neurology 67: 519–521.

Verzijl HT, van der Zwaag B, Cruysberg JR, Padberg GW (2003) Mobius syndrome redefined: a syndrome of rhombencephalic maldevelopment. Neurology 61: 327–333.

Vos YJ, Vos YJ, de Walle HE, Bos KK, Stegeman JA, Ten Berge AM, et al. (2010) Genotype-phenotype correlations in L1 syndrome: a guide for genetic counselling and mutation analysis. J Med Genet 47: 169–175.

Weller S, Gärtner J (2001) Genetic and clinical aspects of X-linked hydrocephalus (L1 disease): mutations in the LICAM gene. Hum Mutat 18: 1–12.

Zanni G, Saillour Y, Nagara M, Billuart P, Castelnau L, Moraine C, et al. (2005) Oligophrenin 1 mutations frequently cause X-linked mental retardation with cerebellar hypoplasia. Neurology 65: 1364–1369.

Zaki MS, Abdel-Aleem A, Abdel-Salam G, Marsh SE, Silhavy JL, Barkovich AJ, et al. (2008) The molar tooth sign: a new Joubert syndrome and related cerebellar disorders classification system tested in Egyptian families. Neurology 70: 556–565.

22

Posterior Fossa Cysts and Cyst-like Malformations (Blake's Pouch Cyst, Arachnoid Cysts, and Mega Cisterna Magna)

Andrea Poretti, Ianina Scheer, and Eugen Boltshauser

In this chapter we focus on posterior fossa cysts and cyst-like malformations, although – in a strict sense – they do not represent cerebellar malformations. This is a challenging topic in view of difficulties and controversies in terminology (often changing with time) and pathogenetic concepts. We will not solve these controversies nor do we suggest that the distinction (although theoretically possible) is always straightforward in clinical practice. Our emphasis here is on clinical relevance. We focus on persistent Blake's pouch cyst (BPC), arachnoid cysts, and mega cisterna magna (MCM) (Nelson et al. 2004; Yildiz et al. 2006). Diagnosis and differential diagnosis of these cystic malformations is generally based on the morphology of the cyst, fourth ventricle, subarachnoid spaces, vermis, and cerebellar hemispheres, the size of the posterior fossa, the position of the torcular, and the presence of hydrocephalus. MR imaging studies of cerebrospinal fluid flow may be helpful in determining whether there is free communication between the cyst and the fourth ventricle (Yildiz et al. 2006). Nevertheless, as recently emphasized (Raybaud 2010), it is not always easy to distinguish between the different forms because of their overlapping features.

Blake's pouch cyst

Blake's pouch is a physiological, transient structure during the embryology of the posterior fossa (Nelson et al. 2004). It is a marked midline protrusion of the intact roof of the fourth ventricle. Blake's pouch extends posteriorly and inferiorly to the cerebellum and initially does not communicate with the surrounding subarachnoid space. The subsequent fenestration of Blake's pouch results in the foramen of Magendie. Failure of the perforation of Blake's pouch and its postnatal persistence result in the so-called Blake's pouch cyst (BPC) (Nelson et al. 2004). Therefore, the BPC is characterized by the absence of communication between the fourth ventricle and the subarachnoid spaces, usually resulting in hydrocephalus.

Clinical features

Hydrocephalus and macrocephaly are the most common presenting features in the neonatal or infant age range (Cornips et al. 2010). BPC may also present later in life without hydrocephalus. In these patients the normal function of the foramina of Luschka may help to maintain the CSF flow between the fourth ventricle and subarachnoid space, avoiding the development of hydrocephalus. Older patients may still present with hydrocephalus which may decompensate after an intercurrent event such as trauma or infection (Calabrò et al. 2000; Cornips et al. 2010). Other possible presentations later in life include acute or progressive ataxia, nystagmus, or vertigo that may develop also after an intercurrent event (typically after head trauma) (Calabrò et al. 2000; Cornips et al. 2010). Exceptionally, BPC may present with symptoms of syringomyelia (Conti et al. 2003).

Neuroimaging

The location of a BPC may be purely infracerebellar, or infraretrocerebellar (Tortori-Donati et al. 1996) (Figs 22.1, 22.2). The fourth ventricle is usually enlarged. The degree of the enlargement of the fourth ventricle is variable from marked (particularly when the BPC is purely infravermian) to mild (when there is retrocerebellar extension of the BPC with some degree of mass effect on the cerebellum and the fourth ventricle). If the BPC has a retrocerebellar extension, the posterior fossa may be enlarged and the tentorium displaced upwards. Secondary to the enlargement of the BP as a protrusion of the roof of the fourth ventricle, the choroid plexus may be displaced to the superior wall of the cyst inferiorly to the cerebellar vermis (Nelson et al. 2004). Mass effect often leads to caudal flattening or even impression of the lower vermis, but not to vermal rotation. The space-occupying effect also may lead to medial indentation of the cerebellar hemispheres. In practice the membranous outline of BPC is not consistently demonstrable by MRI. The appearance of the cerebellum, however, is consistently normal. Neuroimaging makes it possible to differentiate between BPC and mega cistern magna (there is consistent absence of hydrocephalus in mega cisterna magna because the communication between the fourth ventricle and subarachnoid spaces is present) and between BPC and Dandy-Walker malformation (the cerebellum appears consistently normal in BPC). The differentiation between BPC and arachnoid cysts is more difficult (Raybaud 2010).

Treatment

The treatment of the BPC is surgical. The best procedure is the placement of a ventriculo-peritoneal shunt, but endoscopic

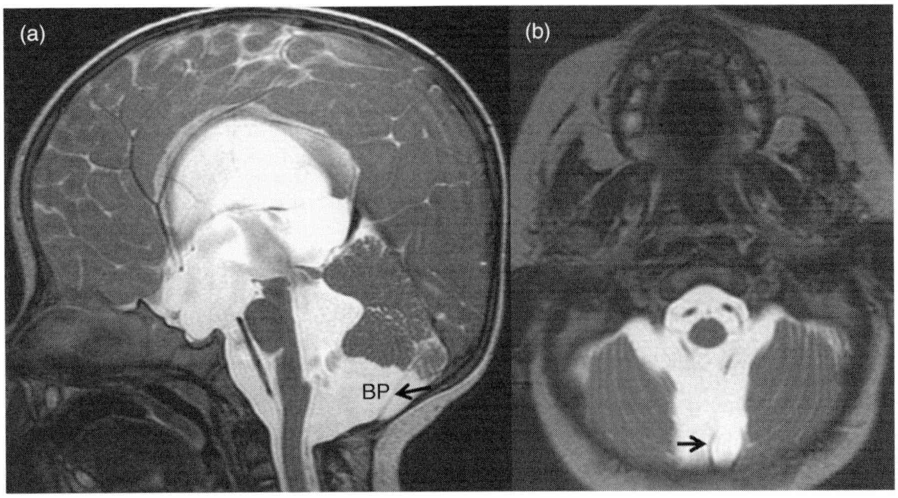

Fig. 22.1. A 7-month-old intant with Blake's pouch cyst. **(a)** Sagittal and **(b)** axial T2-weighted MRI reveals tetraventricular hydrocephalus, marked enlargement of the fourth ventricle that communicates with an infravermian cystic formation representing Blake's pouch cyst (BP). The cerebellar vermis is normally formed and not rotated; the size of the posterior fossa is normally. The medial parts of the cerebellar hemispheres are winged outwards by the cyst. Notice that the membrane (black arrow on (a) and (b)) represents the normal cerebellar falx, not the wall of the Blake's pouch cyst, which is not recognizable.

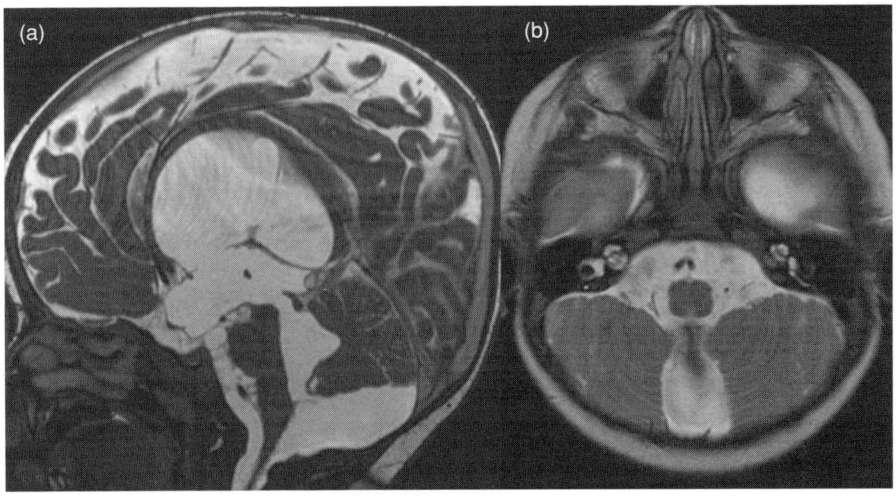

Fig. 22.2. An 8-month-old infant with Blake's pouch cyst demonstrate with progressive macrocephaly and signs of increased intracranial pressure. **(a)** Sagittal and **(b)** axial T2-weighted MRI presenting tetraventricular hydrocephalus. There is a marked enlargement of the fourth ventricle which communicates with an infravermian cystic compartment corresponding to the Blake's pouch cyst (BP). The cerebellar vermis is well formed, the size of the posterior fossa appears normal, and the medial part of the cerebellar hemispheres are laterally displaced by the cyst.

third ventriculostomy has been reported as an alternative, less invasive therapeutic option (Conti et al. 2003; Cornips et al. 2010).

Outcome and prognosis

We are not aware of studies on neurodevelopmental and cognitive outcome in chidlren with BPC. In our experience, the prognosis of these children depends mostly on complications related to the hydrocephalus and its treatment. In the absence of shunt-related complications, the prognosis seems to be favourable because of the normal cerebellar structure.

Arachnoid cysts

Arachnoid cysts are congenital CSF-filled lesions of the arachnoid membrane that do not communicate with the surrounding subarachnoid space and ventricular system. The temporal fossa is the most common location for arachnoid cysts, accounting for about 35–45% of such lesions (Sinha and Brown 2004; Al-Holou et al. 2010).

The posterior fossa represents the second most common location and accounts for about 10–25% (Samii et al. 1999). In the posterior fossa arachnoid cysts are usually large (>5cm) and may be located inferior or posterior to the vermis in a midsagittal location (retrocerebellar) (Fig. 22.3), cranial to the vermis in the tentorial hiatus (*supravermian*), lateral to the cerebellar hemispheres, anterior to the brainstem, or anterolaterally in the cerebellopontine angle cistern (Fig. 22.4) (Marin-Sanabria et al. 2007). On MRI, arachnoid cysts appear as well-defined non-enhancing intracranial masses that are isointense to CSF in all sequences, although a mild hyperintensity may be caused by a fluid content high in proteins.

Clinical features

Presenting signs and symptoms of arachnoid cysts are generally related to the size and the topography of the cyst. Most arachnoid cysts are considered to be congenital and become symptomatic in early infancy, particularly if CSF flow is obstructed (Fig. 22.3). Boltshauser et al. reported the outcome of 11 patients with

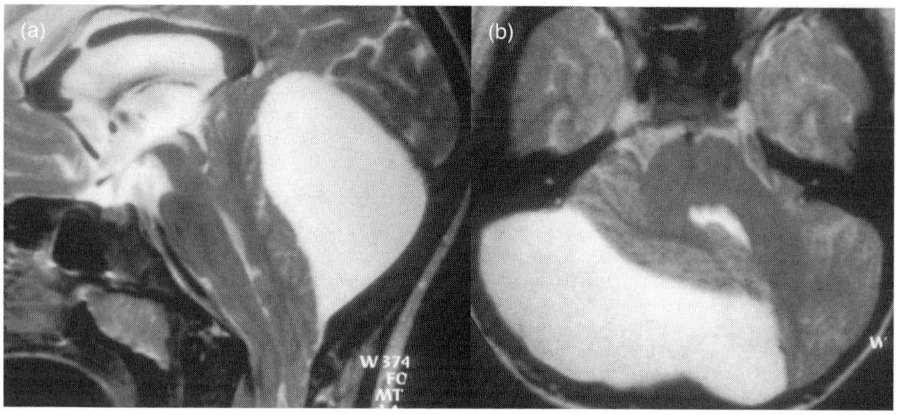

Fig. 22.3. A 10-year-old girl with a retrocerebellar asymmetric arachnoid cyst after ventriculo-peritoneal shunting in the first year of life (in view of excellent scholastic performance including violin playing and normal neurologic examination, the cyst was not fenestrated). **(a)** Sagittal T2-weighted MRI showing a retrocerebellar arachnoid cyst compressing and distorting the cerebellum and a defect of the corpus callosum after shunting; **(b)** axial T2-weighted MRI documents asymmetric retrocerebellar arachnoid cyst compressing the right cerebellar hemisphere. (Reprinted with permission from Boltshauser E et al. Neuropediatrics 2002; 33: 118–121.)

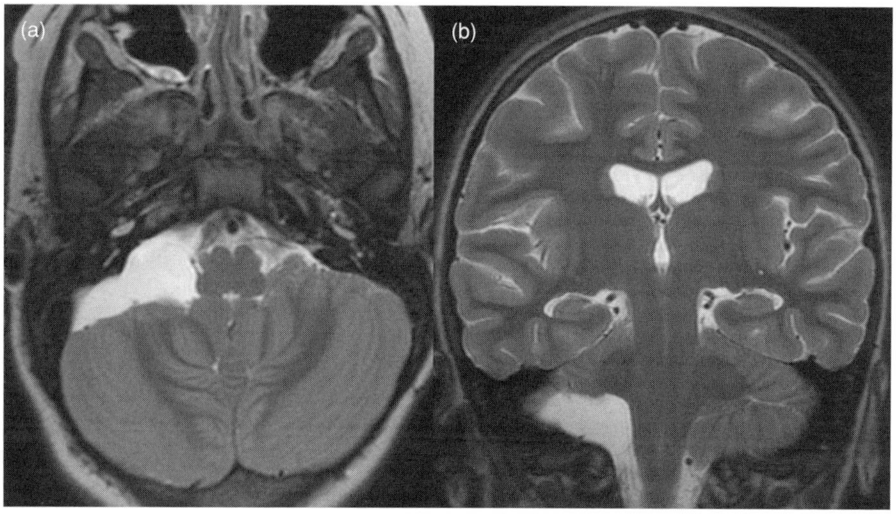

Fig. 22.4. An 8-year-old girl investigated for headaches. **(a)** Axial and **(b)** coronal T2-weighted MRI demonstrating an arachnoid cyst in the right cerebellopontine angle cistern. This was considered as an incidental finding not responsible for the headaches.

space-occupying arachnoid cysts resulting in obstructive hydrocephalus in the first year of life. These patients were identified over a 20-year period, showing that the prevalence of space-occupying arachnoid cysts in the posterior fossa seems to be very low (Boltshauser et al. 2002). However, some arachnoic cysts become symptomatic only later in life and others are an incidental finding. Marin-Sanabria et al. reported 23 patients with arachnoid cysts in the posterior fossa presenting at a mean age of 12.7 years (Marin-Sanabria et al. 2007). Macrocephaly, signs of increased intracranial pressure, and developmental delay were the initial clinical findings. Ataxia has not been found in this series too. In our experience, ataxia is not a feature of arachnoid cysts localized in the posterior fossa.

Treatment

Treatment for arachnoid cysts should be restricted to patients with raised intracranial pressure. There are different therapeutic methods including cyst fenestration, cyst marsupialization in the subarachnoid space, cyst-peritoneal shunting, and ventriculo-peritoneal shunting (Samii et al. 1999). In the series of Boltshauser et al. all but one patient were treated with ventriculo-peritoneal and/or cyst-peritoneal shunting (Boltshauser et al. 2002).

Outcome and prognosis

At the mean follow-up age of 10 years 8 months (range 2–22 years) truncal ataxia and cognitive impairment were present in only two patients (Boltshauser et al. 2002). Additionally, in one case neurological impairments were the result of neurosurgical complications following extensive intraventricular and intracerebral haemorrhage as well as several shunt complications. Because of the generally high incidence of shunt revisions, Marin et al. considered surgical procedures such as cyst marsupialization or fenestration as a first-line surgery and CSF shunting as the second-line procedure (Marin-Sanabria et al. 2007). In conclusion, the overall outcome is favourable in patients who were treated with both surgical procedures (with and without shunting) (Boltshauser et al. 2002; Marin-Sanabria et al. 2007). In contrast to children with cerebellar hypoplasia, even patients with persistent compression and distortion of the cerebellum or reduced cerebellar volume had generally normal neurological and cognitive functions (Boltshauser et al. 2002).

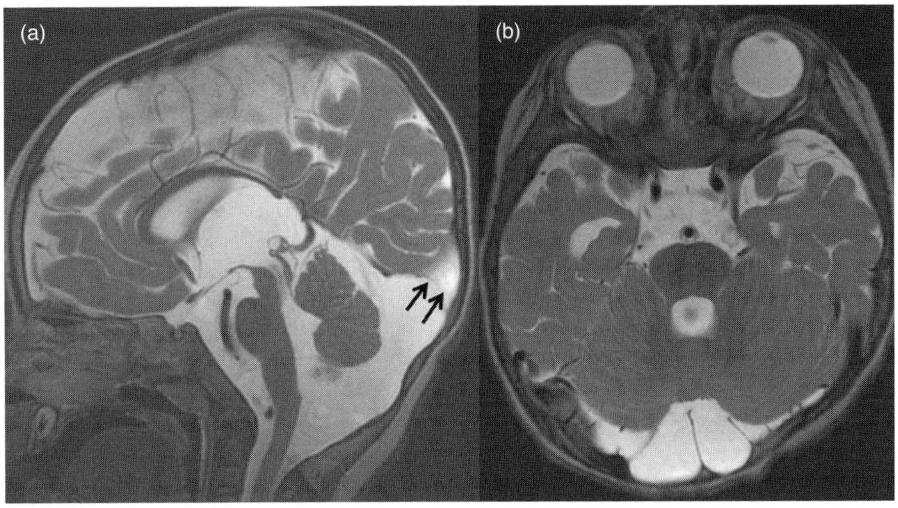

Fig. 22.5. Mega cisterna magna as an incidental finding in a 4-year-old child who has been investigated for focal seizures. **(a)** Sagittal and **(b)** axial T2-weighted MRI demonstrating retro- and supravermian extension of the mega cisterna magna (black arrows on (a)). Notice the normal size and shape of the cerebellar vermis and cerebellar hemispheres.

Mega cisterna magna

A mega cisterna magna (MCM) is defined as a cystic posterior fossa malformation characterized by an intact vermis, an enlarged cisterna magna (≥10mm on midsagittal images), and absence of hydrocephalus (Fig. 22.5) (Barkovich et al. 1989; Altman et al. 1992; Tortori-Donati et al. 1996). MCM is generally a very common finding, representing about 50% of all cystic posterior fossa abnormalities (Altman et al. 1992). In a recent study the prevalence of MCM has been reported as 2.5/1,000 (Zimmer et al. 2007). MCM is hypothesized to result from a late fenestration of Blake's pouch. The pouch persists and expands posterior to the cerebellum and the vermis resulting in an expanded posterior fossa with a free communication between the 'cyst' (MCM) and the fourth ventricle (Nelson et al. 2004; Robinson and Goldstein 2007; Zimmer et al. 2007). The free communication between MCM, fourth ventricle, and spinal subarachnoid spaces results in consistent absence of hydrocephalus in MCM. The extent of MCM is variable: it may be purely infravermian, it may extend laterally, posteriorly, and superiorly, and sometimes it reaches the quadrigeminal plate cistern or may extend into a focal dehiscence of the falcotentorial junction (Altman et al. 1992; Tortori-Donati et al. 1996). The posterior fossa is often enlarged and in about 12% of cases the torcular is displaced upwards (Tortori-Donati et al. 1996). The cerebellum (vermis and hemispheres) and the brainstem are, however, consistently normal. A normal cerebellum strongly favours the diagnosis of MCM versus an arachnoid cyst. The presence (or absence) of hydrocephalus helps to differentiate between MCM and Blake's pouch cyst (Tortori-Donati et al. 1996). MCM should be differentiated from inferior vermis hypoplasia (IVH). In MCM the size and shape of the vermis are normal and in IVH there is no cystic formation in the posterior fossa.

The neurodevelopmental outcome of children with isolated MCM is mostly good. The vast majority (90–95%) of children with isolated MCM develop normally (Limperopoulos et al. 2006; Long et al. 2006; Forzano et al. 2007; Bolduc and Limperopoulos 2009; Bolduc et al. 2011). Data from adults with MCM, however, show mild impairment in some cognitive functions and language, particularly verbal memory and fluency, executive functions, and semantic fluency (Zimmer et al. 2007). MCM is often an incidental finding in patients with brain or systemic anomalies such as dysgenesis of the corpus callosum or renal, cardiac and liver anomalies (Long et al. 2006; Forzano et al. 2007). In this group the proportion of neurological impairments such as cognitive, motor, or language problems is significantly higher than in children with isolated MCM (Long et al. 2006; Bolduc and Limperopoulos 2009).

Retrocerebellar fluid pouches

In clinical practice a quite common finding is an increased retrocerebellar fluid accumulation: (1) without mass effect on the cerebellum, and thus no hydrocephalus; (2) without indentation of cerebellar structures; (3) without obvious visible cyst membranes; and (4) without abnormal cerebellar structures and no apparent hypoplasia. A retrocerebellar fluid pouch should be differentiated from a retrocerebellar arachnoid cyst and a mega cisterna magna (MCM). While retrocerebellar arachnoid cysts may demonstrate mass effect with displacement of the cerebellum causing hydrocephalus, retrocerebellar fluid pouches do not have mass effect. The differentiation between retrocerebellar fluid pouches and retrocerebellar arachnoid cysts without mass effect is difficult and may be possible only with demonstration of the cystic membrane. Some authors used both terms interchangeably (Yildiz et al. 2006). The differentiation between retrocerebellar fluid pouches and MCM may be difficult too. The cisterna magna is a CSF-filled space at the base of the brain. In MCM a significant part of the cyst is located infravermian, while retrocerebellar fluid pouches are only retrovermian, not infravermian. Retrocerebellar fluid pouches are often an incidental finding in the diagnostic work-up of any neurological sign or symptom. In our experience it has no clinical significance, and follow-up neuroimaging is not indicated. Depending on the terminology, these pouches may be regarded as being within the mega cisterna magna spectrum.

REFERENCES

Al-Holou WN, Yew AY, Boomsaad ZE, Garton HJ, Muraszko KM, Maher CO (2010) Prevalence and natural history of arachnoid cysts in children. J Neurosurg Pediatr 5: 578–585.

Altman NR, Naidich TP, Braffman BH (1992) Posterior fossa malformations. AJNR Am J Neuroradiol 13: 691–724.

Barkovich AJ, Kjos BO, Norman D, Edwards MS (1989) Revised classification of posterior fossa cysts and cystlike malformations based on the results of multiplanar MR imaging. AJR Am J Roentgenol 153: 1289–1300.

Bolduc ME, Limperopoulos C (2009) Neurodevelopmental outcomes in children with cerebellar malformations: a systematic review. Dev Med Child Neurol 51: 256–267.

Bolduc ME, Du Plessis AJ, Sullivan N, Khwaja OS, Zhang X, Barnes K, et al. (2011) Spectrum of neurodevelopmental disabilities in children with cerebellar malformations. Dev Med Child Neurol 53: 409–416.

Boltshauser E, Martin F, Altermatt S (2002) Outcome in children with space-occupying posterior fossa arachnoid cysts. Neuropediatrics 33: 118–121.

Calabrò F, Arcuri T, Jinkins JR (2000) Blake's pouch cyst: an entity within the Dandy-Walker continuum. Neuroradiology 42: 290–295.

Conti C, Lunardi P, Bozzao A, Liccardo G, Fraioli B (2003) Syringomyelia associated with hydrocephalus and Blake's pouch cyst: case report. Spine 28: E279-E283.

Cornips EM, Overvliet GM, Weber JW, Postma AA, Hoeberigs CM, Baldewijns MM, Vles JS (2010) The clinical spectrum of Blake's pouch cyst: report of six illustrative cases. Childs Nerv Syst 26: 1757–1764.

Forzano F, Mansour S, Ierullo A, Homfray T, Thilaganathan B (2007) Posterior fossa malformation in fetuses: a report of 56 further cases and a review of the literature. Prenat Diagn 27: 495–501.

Limperopoulos C, Robertson RL, Estroff JA, Barnewolt CE, Levine D, Bassan H, Du Plessis AJ (2006) Diagnosis of inferior vermian hypoplasia by fetal MRI: potential pitfalls and neurodevelopmental outcome. Am J Obstet Gynecol 194: 1070–1076.

Long A, Moran P, Robson S (2006) Outcome of fetal cerebral posterior fossa anomalies. Prenat Diagn 26: 707–710.

Marin-Sanabria EA, Yamamoto H, Nagashima T, Kohmura E (2007) Evaluation of the management of arachnoid cyst of the posterior fossa in pediatric population: experience over 27 years. Childs Nerv Syst 23: 535–542.

Nelson MD, Jr., Maher K, Gilles FH (2004) A different approach to cysts of the posterior fossa. Pediatr Radiol 34: 720–732.

Raybaud C (2010) Comment to the paper (CNS-09–0420) 'The clinical spectrum of Blake's pouch cyst: report of 6 illustrative cases'. Childs Nerv Syst 26: 1065–1066.

Robinson AJ, Goldstein R (2007) The cisterna magna septa: vestigial remnants of Blake's pouch and a potential new marker for normal development of the rhombencephalon. J Ultrasound Med 26: 83–95.

Samii M, Carvalho GA, Schuhmann MU, Matthies C (1999) Arachnoid cysts of the posterior fossa. Surg Neurol 51: 376–382.

Sinha S, Brown JI (2004) Familial posterior fossa arachnoid cyst. Childs Nerv Syst 20: 100–103.

Tortori-Donati P, Fondelli MP, Rossi A, Carini S (1996) Cystic malformations of the posterior cranial fossa originating from a defect of the posterior membranous area. Mega cisterna magna and persisting Blake's pouch: two separate entities. Childs Nerv Syst 12: 303–308.

Yildiz H, Yazici Z, Hakyemez B, Erdogan C, Parlak M (2006) Evaluation of CSF flow patterns of posterior fossa cystic malformations using CSF flow MR imaging. Neuroradiology 48: 595–605.

Zimmer EZ, Lowenstein L, Bronshtein M, Goldsher D, Aharon-Peretz J (2007) Clinical significance of isolated mega cisterna magna. Arch Gynecol Obstet 276: 487–490.

Part 5
Genetic and Metabolic Disorders

23
Pontocerebellar Hypoplasias

Peter G. Barth

History

The first recorded case of pontocerebellar hypoplasia (PCH) is attributed to R. Brun (1917) at the Institute of Brain Anatomy in Zürich. His description is embedded in a treatise linking cerebral malformations to different stages of fetal brain development. Referring to cerebellar hypoplasia, he emphasized that the image of the fragmented cerebellar dentate in pontocerebellar hypoplasia was strikingly similar to a stage in normal development (Brun 1917). Subsequent reports (Brouwer 1924; Koster 1926; Krause 1929; Biemond 1955) established an entity defined by hypoplasia combined with atrophy of the cerebellum, with the hemispheres significantly more affected than the vermis, relative sparing of the flocculi, atrophy of the ventral pons due to loss of neurons, fragmentation of the cerebellar dentate nucleus and loss of neurons, loss of the arcuate nuclei and an immature aspect of the inferior olivary nuclei. The cerebral hemispheres were underweight, but showed relatively few abnormalities. Because of the clinical setting of the later authors some of the emphasis shifted from developmental neuroanatomy to clinical detail. The case study of Krause (1929) was probably the first that included such details: it featured a boy who lacked any motor or cognitive development from birth, and also had feeding difficulty and spastic tetraparesis. This may well have been the first report of pontocerebellar hypoplasia type 2 (PCH2). Peiffer and Pfeiffer (1977) described the neuropathology and added another important clinical detail: chorea. Later serial studies, combining clinical data with MR profiles, confirmed the phenotype of PCH2 (Barth et al. 1995; Goasdoue et al. 2001; Steinlin et al. 2007).

Another subtype of PCH showed the distinctive feature of spinal anterior horn involvement, strikingly similar to Werdnig-Hoffmann disease. It was first reported by Norman (1961), whose name has become linked to the later type 1 (PCH1). A case similar to Norman's was reported by Weinberg and Kirkpatrick (1975) and a very detailed description of a family with three affected siblings by Goutières et al. (1977) providing coverage of clinical, genetic as well as neuropathological aspects. It became clear that more than one type of PCH existed. A first proposal of classification defined two distinct autosomal recessive disease entities: PCH1 for the association of PCH with spinal anterior horn disease and PCH2 for the association of PCH with chorea/dystonia (Barth 1993). A third distinct phenotype was proposed by Rajab et al. (2003), featuring optic atrophy, not present in the other types. An updated classification by Patel et al. (2006) proposed a type 4, a clinically more severe entity with neonatal lethality, previously described as olivo-ponto-cerebellar hypoplasia (OPCH), and type 5 with predominant involvement of the vermis. Type 6, discovered in 2006, became the first subtype to be identified by its gene mutation (*RARS2*). It was followed by the discovery of pathogenic mutations in tRNA endonuclease subunit ('*TSEN*') genes as a major cause of PCH2 and PCH4 (Budde et al. 2008). The later study linked both PCH2 and PCH4 to the TSEN spectrum of gene mutations. Further, a homozygous founder mutation of *TSEN54* was found in the large majoritiy of PCH2 patients in families of European origin. The classified subtypes and their main characteristics are summarized in Table 23.1.

TABLE 23.1
Subtypes of pontocerebellar hypoplasia (PCH)

PCH subtype	Distinguishing aspect	Molecular genetic findings	Key references
PCH1	Spinal anterior horn involvement	*VRK1* mutation in single family with mild variant	Norman 1961; Goutières et al. 1977; Rudnik-Schöneborn et al. 2003
PCH2	Chorea/dystonia, rarely spasticity only	Subunit genes of tRNA endonuclease, mainly *TSEN54*, rarely *TSEN2* or *TSEN34*	Barth et al. 1995; Steinlin et al. 2007; Budde et al. 2008
PCH3 (CLAM)	Optic atrophy	Chr. 7q11-21	Rajab et al. 2003; Durmaz et al. 2009
PCH4 (OPCH)	Severe neonatal course due to hypoventilation; hypertonia and severe clonus; immature aspect inferior olivary nuclei on autopsy	Subunit genes of tRNA endonuclease, mostly heterozygosity for *TSEN54* mutation with stopcodon on one allele	Albrecht et al. 1993; Park et al. 1998; Chaves-Vischer et al. 2000; Budde et al. 2008
PCH5	Lethal course, neonatal death, vermis more affected than cerebellar hemispheres	unknown	Patel et al. 2006
PCH6	Lactic acidemia and/or lactic acid increase in CSF	*RARS2*	Edvardson et al. 2007

CLAM, cerebellar atrophy with progressive microcephaly; OPCH, olivo-ponto-cerebellar-hypoplasia.

Pontocerebellar hypoplasia type 1

Pontocerebellar hypoplasia type 1 (PCH1) has the synonym 'infantile olivo-ponto-cerebellar atrophy and anterior horn degeneration'.

Patients with this subtype have pontocerebellar hypoplasia combined with spinal anterior horn degeneration. The morphological similarity between the anterior horn degeneration in what we now call PCH1 and Werdnig-Hoffman was such that Norman considered his case to be a variant of Werdnig-Hoffmann disease with cerebellar hypoplasia (Norman 1961). Despite the morphological similarity of anterior horn degeneration in PCH1 to spinal muscular atrophy (SMA) type 1, mutations in the *SMN* gene are absent in PCH1 (Muntoni et al. 1999; Rudnik-Schöneborn et al. 1995), confirming that the two diseases are different, and not variants of the same gene defect. Beginning with the signal report of Norman (1961), 14 studies on PCH1 have been published that form the basis of the present review. These studies deal with the severe type with a lethal course in the first year and a less severe variant with longer survival, first proposed by Rudnik-Schöneborn et al. (2003).

Clinical findings in severe PCH1

Including the signal case report of Norman (1961), 14 patient studies on the common (severe type) have been published in English (Weinberg and Kirkpatrick 1975; Goutières et al. 1977; Steiman et al. 1980; De León et al. 1984; Moerman and Barth 1987; Chou et al. 1990; Kamoshita et al. 1990; Barth 1993; Rudnik-Schöneborn et al. 1995; Görgen-Pauly et al. 1999; Muntoni et al. 1999; Szabó et al. 2008; Okanishi et al. 2010). The number of reported cases is 32, and includes 7 families with more than one affected offspring. One is an aborted fetus. The male/female ratio is 13/19. None of the parents had signs of the disease. Parental consanguinity was present in two cases. All patients were born with severe hypotonia and peripheral paresis. Neurogenic loss of swallowing in utero caused polyhydramnios in a fourth (8/32) and congenital contractures, obviously caused by intrauterine paresis, in about half of the patients (17/32). Contractures affected proximal as well as distal joints. In a few cases they were absent at birth but developed soon afterwards. Sometimes hip dislocation was present. Peripheral paresis present at birth often necessitated prolonged mechanical ventilation. Paresis involved intercostal muscles and spared the diaphragm, resulting in paradoxic respiratory movements, similar to end-stage SMA type 1.

The severest affected patient was born with pulmonary hypoplasia (Moerman and Barth 1987). Involvement of cranial motor nerves was present leading to partial or total paralysis of the laryngeal muscles and stridor. Stridor or confirmed paralysis through laryngoscopy was present in 9/32. This may be an underestimate since many patients were permanently intubated from birth. Some patients had symmetric or asymmetric facial palsy. Tendon reflexes were mostly absent from the beginning or became negative shortly after birth. Patients who survived the neonatal period showed lack of visual contact. Nystagmoid eye movements were stated to be present in some cases but not interpreted. Frank epilepsy was reported in five cases, including two with infantile spasms. Several observations indicate a progressive character of the disease, such as worsening paresis. Two published observations are testimony of declining head growth which is similar to the much better-known situation in PCH2. Most patients die before their first birthday, or even in the neonatal period, the usual cause of death being respiratory failure or pulmonary infection. A patient who was alive at 6 years was on continuous mechanical ventilation (Okanishi et al. 2010).

Neurophysiological tests in PCH1

Motor nerve conduction velocities were measured in eight patients with results reported as normal (one), mild slowing (one), and moderate slowing (six). Decreased compound muscle action potential was found in another case. Denervation was present on electromyography in three patients and absent in one. The EEG may show epileptogenic activity. An EEG trace with suppression burst pattern was seen from the first day in one patient (Görgen-Pauly et al. 1999, case 3). Electroretinography carried out in one patient was normal (Muntoni et al. 1999, patient 3). Salman et al. (2003) reported subtle macular and electroretinographic abnormalities in one family.

Biochemical screening

No abnormalities have been reported in routine biochemical investigations aimed at inborn errors of metabolism. Congenital disorder of glycosylation, type 1A, known to cause cerebellar hypoplasia/atrophy, was specifically excluded in two patients (Görgen-Pauly et al. 1999; Muntoni et al. 1999). Results of testing for SMN and NAIP deletions were negative in PCH1 (Muntoni et al. 1999; Ryan et al. 2000; Rudnik-Schöneborn et al. 1995). Testing for *TSEN* mutations, associated with PCH2 and PCH4, was equally negative (Budde et al. 2008).

Neuroradiological findings in PCH1

Neuroradiological findings are characterized by a flat ventral aspect of the pons due to volume loss of the ventral pons, and severe cerebellar hypoplasia mainly affecting the cerebellar hemispheres with relative sparing of the vermis. Occasionally destruction cysts are seen in the vermis or hemispheres. Supratentorial findings may show a delay in development of the neocortex (Okanishi et al. 2010). No demyelination is seen. No malformations are seen above the tentorium. Neuroradiological and neuropathological findings in PCH1 and PCH2 are essentially similar, except for the presence of spinal anterior horn degeneration in the former. Typical findings in the brainstem and cerebellum, as illustrated in Fig. 23.4 for types 2 and 4, also apply to type 1.

Neuropathological findings in PCH1

Muscle biopsies and muscle specimens from autopsies show group atrophy as the most frequent finding, followed by nonspecific changes such as increased variation in fibre diameter. Autopsy findings of the brain are generally diminished weight, a tiny cerebellum with flattened hemispheres and relative sparing of the vermis, and a small, flattened pons. The cerebral hemispheres may show some ventriculomegaly and mild or moderate neocortical atrophy. The severest case (Moerman and Barth 1987) also had neocortical dysplasia present as patches of polymicrogyria. Microscopic examination of the cerebellum shows diminished folial branching and focal loss of Purkinje cells and internal and external granule cells. The distribution is variable, with relative sparing of the flocculi and vermis (especially the nodule) and predominant affection of the inferior parts of the hemispheres most often mentioned. The dentate nuclei are depleted and the remaining neurons clustered in islands, reminiscent of their fetal stage. The inferior olivary nuclei are always affected with lack of undulation (sometimes complete, giving the nucleus a horseshoe-like appearance), loss of neurons and loss of hilar fibres. Detailed descriptions are given by Norman (1961) and Chou et al. (1990).

Visceral abnormalities or malformations outside the nervous system were occasionally observed; no consistent pattern of extracerebral malformations can be distilled from the reported cases. Incidental findings include nonspecific cardiomegaly (Chou et al. 1990), renal microcysts (Chou et al. 1990), proteinuria, renal tubular hyaline casts (Ryan et al. 2000), dysplastic ovaries (Muntoni et al. 1999), cleft palate (Muntoni et al. 1999), and rib anomalies (Chou et al. 1990).

Clinical, laboratory, and radiological findings in mild PCH1

Rudnik-Schöneborn et al. (2003) reported an extension of the phenotype of PCH1 in nine patients from six sibships. Onset was before or after birth. Lifespan was 2–4 years in the mildest cases. Neuromuscular findings were similar to infantile spinal muscular atrophy, with typical findings of denervation in muscle biopsies, but also signs of peripheral neuropathy on electrophysiological testing. Symptomatology was dominated by severe peripheral paresis and also by absent cognitive development. In some patients suprasegmental motor involvement was obvious with some hypertonicity, and increased tendon reflexes. Radiological findings deviated from the classic pattern with the outline of the ventral pons preserved, and cerebellar hemispheres less affected by hypoplasia, and more compatible with postnatal atrophy, suggestive of a later onset of the process. The family reported by Salman et al. (2003) overlaps with the extended phenotype with a normal aspect of the pons on MRI and survival of 40 months in one sibling.

Molecular genetic studies in PCH1

Results of testing for SMN mutations are negative in both severe PCH1 (Rudnik-Schöneborn et al. 1995; Muntoni et al. 1999; Ryan et al. 2000) and extended PCH1 (Rudnik-Schöneborn et al. 2003). *TSEN* mutations have been excluded in a small number tested so far (Budde et al. 2008). A homozygous nonsense mutation in the *VRK1* (vaccinia related kinase 1) gene was present in the offspring of a single consanguineous family, with progressive microcephaly from birth, relatively mild course, and mild cerebellar hypoplasia on computed tomography (Renbaum et al. 2009). So far the finding has not been confirmed in other families. Phenotypic details in the *VRK1* mutated family deviate in several regards from the PCH1 spectrum as outlined above, including the extended phenotype: severe microcephaly at birth (–6.0 s.d. in the proband), a very mild course permitting assisted walking, and prolonged survival until 11.5 years. In a single case of severe neonatal PCH with lactic acid elevation in the cerebrospinal fluid and a clinical diagnosis of PCH6, bi-allelic mutations of the *RARS2* gene were found including a splice site mutation. Surprisingly autopsy revealed additional involvement of the spinal anterior horn cells similar to PCH1.

Pontocerebellar hypoplasia type 2

Pontocerebellar hypoplasia type 2 (PCH2) was probably first reported by Krause (1929). Its most common expression, i.e., with chorea, was first reported in 1977 by Peiffer and Pfeiffer. Serial studies (Barth et al. 1995; Steinlin et al. 2007) and case reports (Barbot et al. 1997; Iso et al. 1997; Coppola et al. 2000; Grellner et al. 2000; Grosso et al. 2002, case 1) present a consistent phenotype. Patients with PCH2 are usually born at full term. Head circumference in all cases is normal at birth, but always below the 50th centile. Head growth levels off progressively and is below –2 SD after the first birthday. The neonatal period is characterized by 'unrest', mainly the result of excessive clonus on arousal and handling. Feeding is difficult from the beginning, which is mainly due to inability to initiate and maintain a rapid succession of sucking and swallowing movements in the absence of overt weakness. Parents who had a previous child with the disease recorded that this inability was the first symptom by which they recognized their second baby with PCH2. Many patients have to be fed by gavage, and subsequently undergo gastrostomy. Retina and optic nerves are normal, but central visual information processing is severely abnormal. Visual tracking and visually guided social interaction fail in the large majority, but some patients manage to look intentionally or make visual tracking movements. Exceptionally patients make visual contact and smile. Postural control is completely lacking in the majority; a minority achieve head control. Control of manual movements is completely absent in the majority, but a small minority is able to reach for objects. Patients who are able to 'handle' objects are very rare. Muscle tone may be variable in the first months. Within the first half-year most patients develop chorea, often combined with spasticity. In rare cases pure spasticity is found without chorea. Contractures in the large joints and scoliosis may develop. About half of all patients develop seizures, which vary from febrile seizures to infantile spasms. Life expectancy used to be limited, mainly because of feeding difficulty and the ever present risk of aspiration of food. This risk has been reduced by gastrostomy. Specific risks are cot death in the first year and malignant hyperthermia. While most patients die before puberty, a few reach adulthood, and one patient known to the author is alive at 31 years. Two cases are on record with rhabdomyolysis (Barth et al. 2008), one with acute multisystem disorder (Sans-Fitó et al. 2002). Rhabdomyolysis appears to be related to a latent myopathy, since approximately half of all PCH2 patients have increased creatine kinase activity in blood. The large majority of reported patients are of European origin (Barth et al. 1995; Steinlin et al. 2007; Budde et al. 2008). Other reported families classified as PCH2 or fulfilling all requirements for that diagnosis are ethnically Turkish, Pakistani, Arab (Budde et al. 2008), and Japanese (Iso et al. 1997).

NEURORADIOLOGICAL AND NEUROPATHOLOGICAL FINDINGS

The key findings in pontocerebellar hypoplasia are a small cerebellum and a flattened ventral pons. The cerebellar anomaly is disproportionate in the sense that the cerebellar hemispheres are more affected than the vermis. These properties characterize PCH2 on MR images (Barth et al. 1995; Goasdoue et al. 2001) (Fig. 23.1). The supratentorial parts of the brain are also affected. Myelination is delayed, the corpus callosum is complete but too thin, and in most patients there is some degree of ventriculomegaly resulting from tissue loss. The cerebral cortex shows a variable degree of atrophy, which appears to be age related (Fig. 23.2). The growth of the cerebellum is impaired from its earliest stages resulting in shorter folia and diminished folial branching. This results in flattening of the cerebellar growth profile during pregnancy. A curve of transverse cerebellar growth in a fetus at risk for PCH2 illustrates the progressive nature of cerebellar involvement, as captured by ultrasonography (Fig. 23.3).

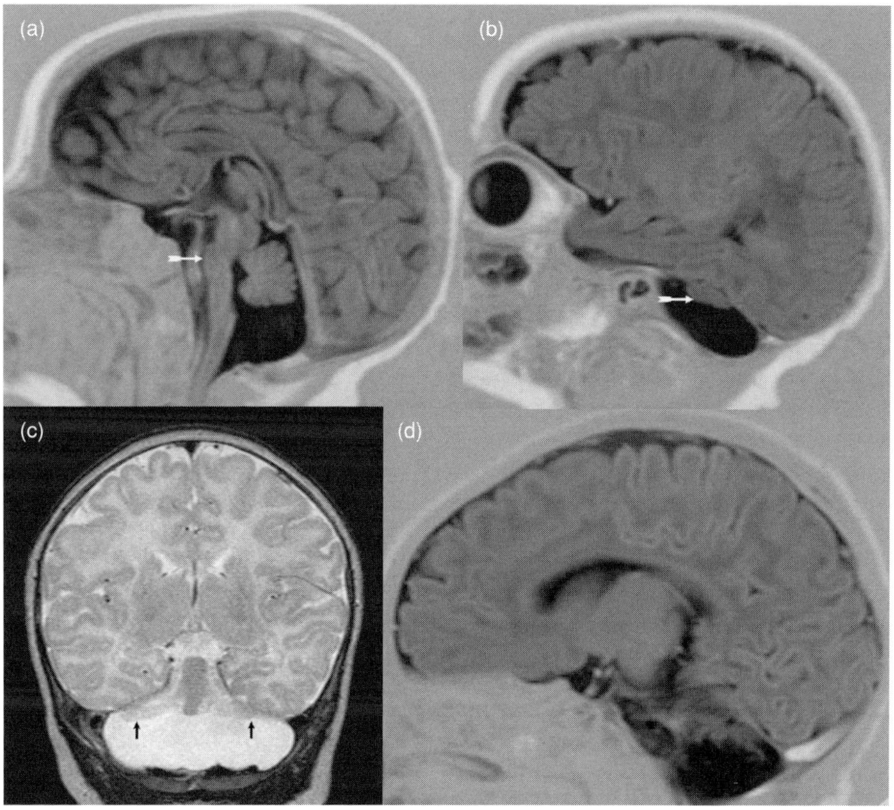

Fig. 23.1. MRI in PCH2. **(a)** Midsagittal IR section from a 2-month-old patient with PCH2 shows flattening of the ventral aspect of the pons (arrow) and an hypoplastic cerebellar vermis; above the tentorium the corpus callosum is thin but complete; **(b)** sagittal section from the same series shows hypoplasia of the cerebellar hemisphere (arrow) rendering a large part of the posterior fossa empty; **(c)** coronal T2-weighted image from same patient shows discrepancy between the short but relatively preserved vermis and severe hypoplasia of the cerebellar hemispheres (arrows); **(d)** lateral IR section from a 1-month-old patient shows cerebellar folial atrophy as well as hypoplasia. (Figs 23.1a and 23.1c are reproduced from Barth PG et al. Acta Neuropathol (Berl) 2007; 114: 373–386 with kind permission of Springer Science and Business Media.)

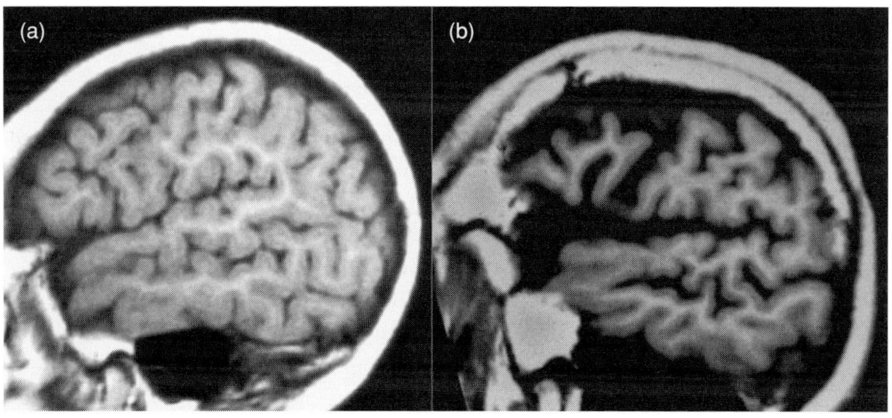

Fig. 23.2. Variable neocortical atrophy in PCH2. Lateral sagittal T1-weighted images from two patients. **(a)** Patient aged 23 months shows mild atrophy. **(b)** Patient aged 15 years shows severe atrophy. Subcortical myelin in both cases is unaffected.

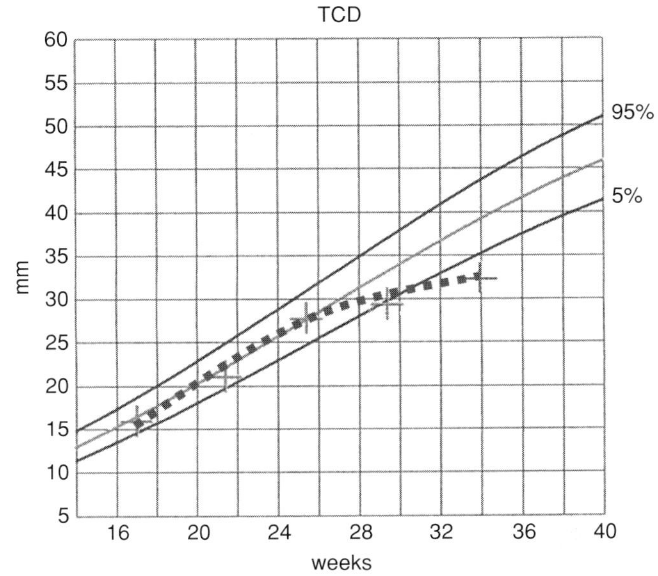

Fig. 23.3. Ultrasound follow-up of transverse cerebellar diameter (TCD) in a fetus at risk for PCH2, who eventually was diagnosed with the disease. A flattening of the curve can be seen from approximately 25 weeks, the probable time when folial growth started to level off. (Reproduced with kind permission of Prof. Catia Bilardo, Department of Obstetrics, Academic Medical Centre, Amsterdam.)

Reconstruction of events from neuropathological findings suggests that embryonic stages of cerebellar cortical development proceed normally until the start of foliation, but subsequent growth by the formation of folia stalls, resulting in short folia and diminished lateral branching. This is followed by a continuous process of cerebellar degeneration. Cerebellar cortical degeneration is partly diffuse with retained architecture. In part it takes the character of segmental loss of full-thickness segments of cortex leading to denudation. Examination of these areas of segmental degeneration reveals remaining cortical elements in a maze of glial tissue. The main focus of degeneration is found in the bottom region between folia (Fig. 23.4a,b) but the process is ubiquitous (Barth et al. 2007). Some regions, such as the flocculus and the vermis, are relatively spared. The most typical expression of cerebellar involvement in PCH2, however, is in the dentate nucleus which is broken up into small islands of neurons, easily seen in microscopic slides, but as yet inaccessible to routine MR imaging (Fig. 23.4c). The ventral pons is affected by severe neuronal loss. There may be a link between neuronal degeneration in the ventral pons and the cerebellar cortex because ventral pontine nuclei project to the contralateral cerebellar hemispheres. Therefore cerebellar cortical atrophy could result either from deafferentiation due to loss of pontine neurons or to an intrinsically driven process of degeneration – probably both. A similar process, resulting from loss of the inferior olivary nuclei, is also expected to affect the contralateral cerebellar cortex. On the other hand the flocculus, which receives its main afferents from the vestibular nuclei, is relatively spared. The inferior olivary nuclei are affected by diffuse and segmental degeneration. They are also less folded than normal, suggesting that the pathological process may begin during their formation (Fig. 23.4d,e).

Neurophysiological tests in PCH2

No systematic studies have been performed. Electroencephalography often shows epileptogenic activity, varying from bursts at wake or during sleep to hypsarrhythmia. Brainstem acoustic evoked responses may be normal, but in most recorded cases show increased latency of later peaks, consistent with anomalies within the brainstem (Barth et al. 1990; Coppola et al. 2000).

Biochemical tests in PCH2

No abnormalities are reported in routine biochemical investigations aimed at inborn errors of metabolism. Disialotransferrin electrophoresis is normal. No abnormalities in mitochondrial function studies have been reported in PCH2. Creatine kinase activity is elevated in blood in approximately half of the patients.

Molecular basis and genetic testing in PCH2

In the human nuclear genome, 32 of a total of 631 tRNA genes possess an intron positioned close to the anticodon. The removal of this intron is catalyzed by tRNA endonuclease. This protein is made up of four protein subunits encoded by four different genes: *TSEN2, TSEN15, TSEN34* and *TSEN54* (Fig. 23.5). The enzyme cleaves intron containing pre-tRNAs at both ends of the intron, after which ligation of the two halves of the tRNA takes place by a separate process. The finding of mutations in three of four *TSEN* genes by Budde et al. (2008) highlights their crucial role in fetal and postnatal brain growth. Most (>90%) of the patients clinically diagnosed with PCH2 have a homozygous mutation in *TSEN54*, causing the amino acid substitution p.Ala307Ser. A segment of 285 kbase surrounding the 8 kbase of the *TSEN54* gene is also shared by patients and healthy heterozygotes, strongly endorsing the finding as a founder mutation. Rare patients with PCH2 have different mutations affecting *TSEN54*, or mutations in *TSEN2* or *TSEN34*. Heterozygous double mutations in *TSEN54* causing stopcodons on one allele and the common p.Ala307Ser on the other allele were identified in patients with PCH4, endorsing a single spectrum of gene defects, encompassing PCH2 and PCH4. Almost all patients with PCH2 and the common *TSEN54* p.Ala307Ser are of European descent. In a multicentre study of 169 patients clinically and radiologically diagnosed with PCH (all kinds), 88 had the common *TSEN54* mutation in homozygous form, making this the most prevalent cause of PCH in Europe and probably also in North Americans of Western European origin (Namavar et al. 2011a).

Pontocerebellar hypoplasia type 3

The initial study was based on a single consanguineous family from Oman (Rajab et al. 2003). Patients with PCH3 are characterized by severe developmental delay, progressive microcephaly with brachycephaly, seizures, hypotonia with hyperreflexia, and appendicular spasticity in two of the three

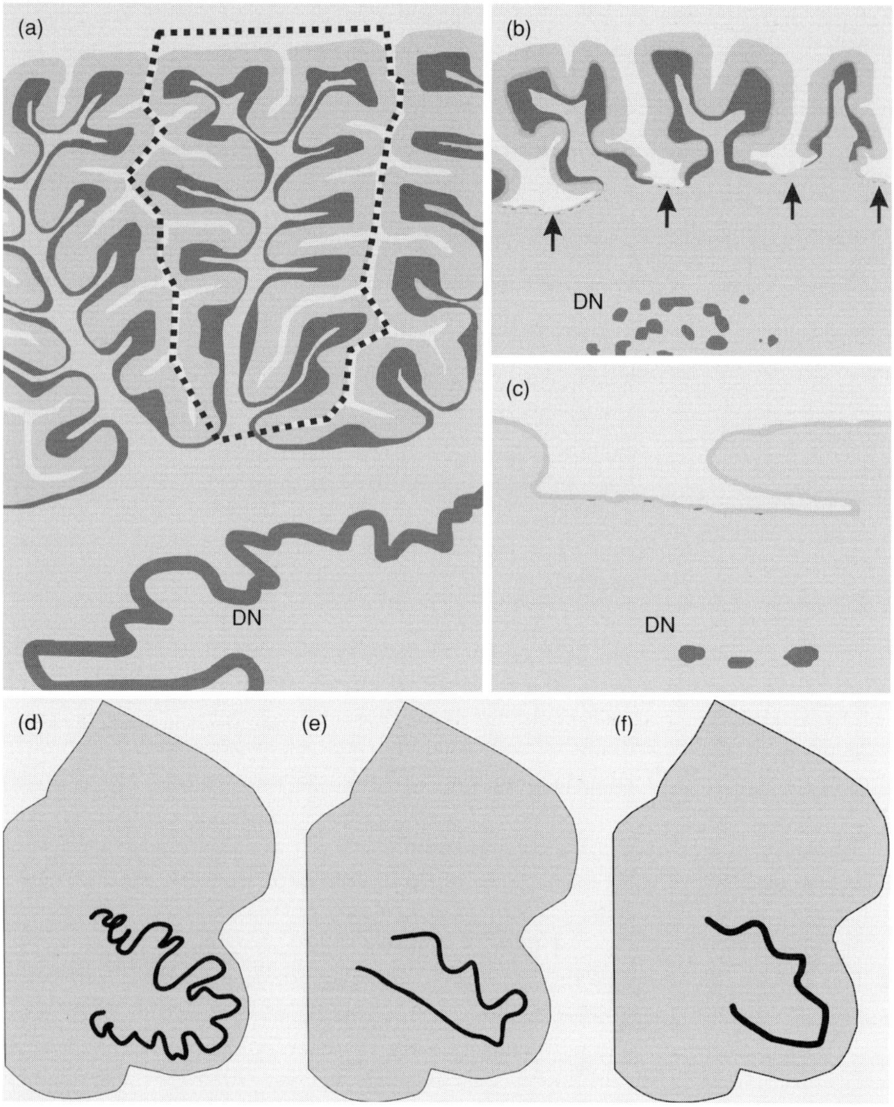

Fig. 23.4. (a–c) Cerebellum in pontocerebellar hypoplasia types 2 and 4. **(a)** Normal cerebellar folia with 8 to 15 branches. The confines of one folium are indicated by a broken line. The dentate nucleus (DN) is shown beneath the cerebellar cortex as an undulating unbroken line. **(b)** An example of pontocerebellar hypoplasia type 2 with short folia and limited branching. Cortex between the folia is depleted (arrows), with microsopic remnants of destroyed cortex. The dentate nucleus (DN) is broken up into small islands, possibly related to loss of segments of overlying cortex by antegrade degeneration. **(c)** Findings in cerebellar cortex and dentate nucleus (DN) in pontocerebellar hypoplasia type 4. The cortex is largely denuded, and a ghost folium can be recognized with its fine structure lost. Only minute islands of dentate nucleus (DN) remain. **(d–f)** The inferior olivary nucleus in pontocerebellar hypoplasia, types 2 and 4. **(d)** Normal undulation in control. **(e)** Pontocerebellar hypoplasia type 2 showing diminished undulation reflecting early fetal disruption. **(f)** Pontocerebellar hypoplasia type 4 with primitive shape of olivary nucleus and nearly absent undulation. (Reproduced from Barth PG. Pontocerebellar hypoplasia. In: Gilman S, editor. MedLink Neurology. San Diego: MedLink Corporation. www.medlink.com. By permission of MedLink Corporation.)

affected siblings, short stature, and optic atrophy. MRI shows a small atrophic cerebellum and brainstem, ventriculomegaly and cerebral atrophy. The gene was mapped to chromosome 7q11–21 and has not been identified yet, although further studies (Durmaz et al. 2009) in a family diagnosed with PCH3 showed homozygosity within the earlier defined interval, restricting the gene to an interval of 7Mb. The mechanism underlying the optic atrophy has not been clarified. Little is known about the pathomechanism underlying PCH3. Its inclusion in the group of pontocerebellar hypoplasias is therefore not uniformly supported.

Pontocerebellar hypoplasia type 4

Patients with PCH4, also known as olivo-ponto-cerebellar hypoplasia (OPCH) or congenital OPCA (olivo-ponto-cerebellar atrophy) are born with polyhydramnios and/or contractures due to fetal onset of neurological dysfunction. Neonatal behaviour is grossly abnormal with hypertonia and severe generalized clonus on passive movements or arousal. Life expectancy is severely shortened because of respiratory impairment, making continuous mechanical ventilation necessary for prolonged periods. Swallowing is impaired. Some patients can be weaned from the respirator only temporarily. All patients die in the first year, the majority in the neonatal period. Only single families have been reported. This suggests that the disease is very rare (Albrecht et al. 1993; Park et al. 1998; Hashimoto et al. 1998; Chaves-Vischer et al. 2000; Grosso et al. 2002, patient 2; Leroy et al. 2007). A detailed review of the literature on this subtype is included in the paper by Leroy et al. (2007). Neuropathological findings are similar to type 2 to some extent, but more severe. The vermis is less affected than the hemispheres. Hypoplastic development of cerebellar folia is more severe than in type 2, with parts of the hemispheres completely denuded. Flat parts of cerebellar cortex are gliotic and show remnants of neurons, a telling witness of regression following a period of stunted growth. The cerebellar dentate nuclei are grossly reduced in size, sometimes wholly absent on routine staining, and often reduced to tiny clusters instead of its typical folded structure. The inferior olivary nuclei are in their proper place, but gliotic with loss of neurons. Its mature folded structure is absent, with

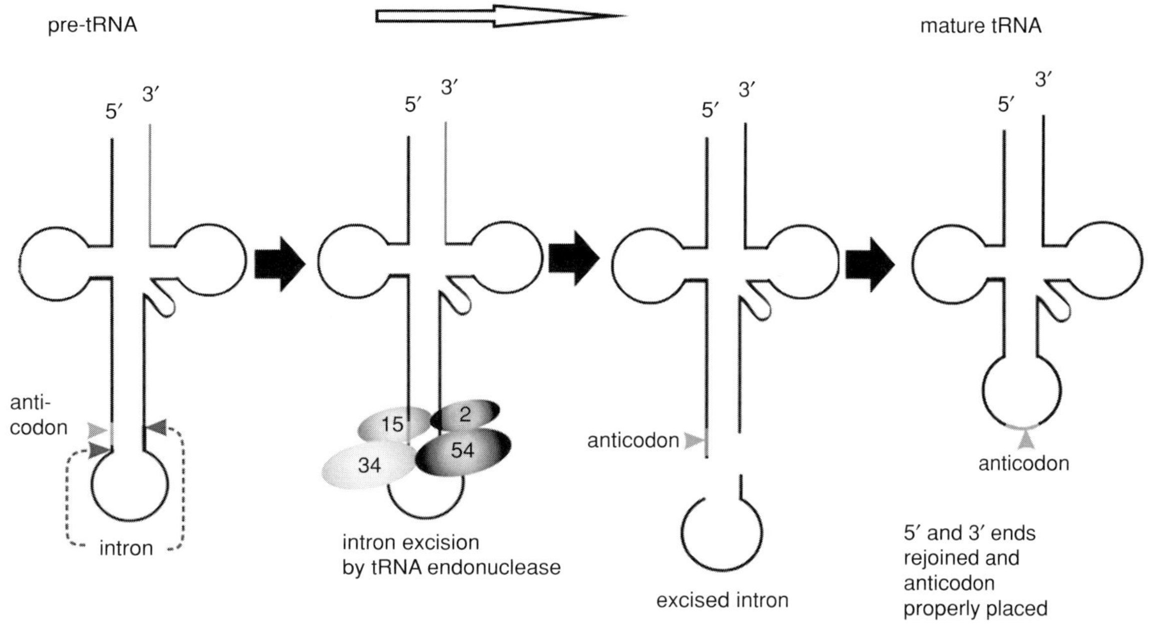

Fig. 23.5. Scheme to illustrate the process of tRNA maturation by the splicing of an intron from pre-tRNA (primary DNA transcript). The numbers (2, 15, 34, 54) in the second frame indicate the 4 TSEN subunits comprising the enzyme tRNA endonuclease. In the first and last frame, the change in position of the anticodon is indicated. The anticodon is a nucleotide triplet that specifies the amino acid that is added to the growing peptide chain. In the last frame, the anticodon is in the middle of the anticodon loop and prepared for its role in protein synthesis. (Reproduced from Barth PG. Pontocerebellar hypoplasia. In: Gilman S, editor. MedLink Neurology. San Diego: MedLink Corporation. www.medlink.com. By permission of MedLink Corporation.)

instead an unfolded, horseshoe-like structure, reminiscent of the embryonal stage, which clearly has persisted (Fig. 23.4f). From the neuropathological point of view this is the most specific difference between PCH4 and PCH2. Hypoplasia of the pons is found with almost total absence of neurons in the ventral part and loss of transverse pontocerebellar fibres, which normally connect to the contralateral cerebellar hemisphere. Changes in the basal ganglia, thalami, and neocortex are variable. Some degree of gliosis in the hemispheric white matter is reported in most cases, probably indicating another point of divergence from PCH2. A family with neocortical dysplasia, otherwise overlapping with PCH2 and PCH4, was reported by Leroy et al. (2007). Patients also had areas of denudation affecting the insular cortex and neocortical disorganization especially affecting layer 2, and absence of the claustrum. Lack of growth in the insular area resulted in wide open Sylvian fossae, visible on MRI, lending the brain a more immature aspect than its actual fetal age. The molecular genetic status of this family has still to be determined. From the clinical point there is some analogy between PCH4 and PCH1, because polyhydramnios, contractures, and respiratory impairment are shared symptoms. PCH4 and PCH1 differ in other regards with hypertonia and clonus in the former and hypotonia and areflexia in the latter. No systematic studies have yet been performed on neuroradiological findings in PCH4. Typical MRI findings of PCH4 appear from a small number of observations (Namavar et al. 2011a). Beside the pontocerebellar hypoplasia, there is increased pericerebral cerebrospinal fluid, broad persistent midline cava, and decreased gyral maturation. This indicates that the impact on supratentorial brain growth and maturation is more severe in PCH4 than in PCH2.

Molecular basis and genetic testing in PCH4

A small number of patients have been studied for *TSEN* gene mutation. In two individuals, *TSEN54* was heterozygously mutated with the common Ala307Ser on one allele and a stop-codon inducing mutation in the same gene on the other allele (Namavar et al. 2011a).

Pontocerebellar hypoplasia type 5

A family of European ancestry with three affected siblings, reported by Patel et al. (2006), was proposed as a new subtype on the basis of cell paucity in the vermis exceeding that in the cerebellar hemispheres. Other findings were poor development of neocortical layer 2. Otherwise the findings resemble PCH4 including arrested maturation of the inferior olivary nuclei and diffuse gliosis. Symptoms started in mid-pregnancy with seizure-like intrauterine movements. Lethargy, hypertonia, and apnea were present in the firstborn, the only one of the three who reached term and died of apnea. The status of PCH5, whether different from or just forming part of the PCH2-PCH4 spectrum, needs further analysis through gene studies. More recent evaluation of the index patient of this family showed compound heterozygosity for the common *TSEN54* mutation (p.A307S) and a novel splice site mutation of the same gene (Namavar et al. 2011b). The finding confirms that PCH5 and PCH4 are closely related, clinically and genetically. If allowance is made for gradual rather than absolute differences in involvement of the vermis in both phenotypes, their continued separation can only be supported for historic reasons.

Pontocerebellar hypoplasia type 6

A severe homozygous defect was found in the nuclear gene *RARS2* which encodes mitochondrial arginyl-transfer RNA synthetase (Edvardson et al. 2007). The defect was established in three members of a consanguineous family in Israel with rapidly fatal pontocerebellar hypoplasia, hypotonia, failing mental and motor development, severe epilepsy, progressive microcephaly, and cerebral atrophy. General screening for inborn errors of metabolism, including organic acids, was normal. Plasma lactate was normal in one and mildly elevated in the other two. Cerebrospinal fluid lactate was increased in one of the siblings. Respiratory chain complex activities in three patients were found variably decreased in muscle and fibroblasts. *RARS2* deficiency is the first discovered genetic deficiency of an amino-acyl-tRNA synthetase that causes PCH. Recently a second family was reported in the UK (Rankin et al. 2010).

Differential diagnosis

One particular group of inherited disorders that mimick pontocerebellar hypoplasias is made up of disorders of neuronal migration that, outside the cerebral cortex, involve neurons generated at the embryonic rhombic lip, destined to populate the ventral pons and parts of the cerebellum. Dystroglycanopathies (Walker-Warburg syndrome, muscle-eye-brain disease, and others) are expressed in this way and cause hypoplasia of the pons and cerebellum. Preliminary differentiation of these disorders from PCH by radiological means is possible because dystroglycanopathies cause neocortical and cerebellar malformation (Barkovich et al. 2009), whereas in PCH progressive and atrophic changes predominate, both above and below the tentorium. Cerebellar hypoplasia may also be encountered in congenital disorders of glycosylation, especially type 1A, excluded by sialotransferrin electrophoresis. Cerebellar abnormalities resembling pontocerebellar hypoplasia have been described in preterm infants born at 26 weeks' gestation or earlier. Three types of this abnormality have been detailed (Messerschmidt et al. 2005).

In one particular disorder, CLAM (cerebellar atrophy with progressive microcephaly); OPCH (olivo-ponto-cerebellar-hypoplasia deficiency), the differentiation from the PCH group by MRI appears difficult.

CASK DEFICIENCY

CASK is an X-linked gene on Xp11.4. It encodes regulatory protein that interacts with ion channels in synapses. It also translocates to the nucleus to interact with Tbr1, an important transcription factor during embryogenesis, which in turn interacts with Reelin (Bailey and Aldinger 2009). Loss of Reelin is known to result in cerebro-cerebellar lissencephaly in men. Najm et al. (2008) reported progressive microcephaly from birth, moderate to severe developmental delay, sensorineuronal hearing loss (2/5), and optic nerve anomalies (3/5) in five patients, four of whom were female. CASK was deleted in three and mutated in two patients including the single male. MRI abnormalities were pontocerebellar hypoplasia and subtle abnormalities in gyral development of the frontal cortex. Neuropathological examination in one patient showed a neocortical layering abnormality, especially affecting layers V and VI and a vague transition between layer VI and the subcortical white matter. In the hypoplastic cerebellum, decreased density of the internal granular layer was associated with a thickened external granular layer, strongly suggesting a migratory failure. Both the regulatory function of the gene and the neuropathological findings suggest that CASK deficiency has a purely developmental character, as opposed to the partly trophic effects of PCH.

REFERENCES

Albrecht S, Schneider MC, Belmont J, Armstrong DL (1993) Fatal infantile encephalopathy with olivopontocerebellar hypoplasia and micrencephaly. Acta Neuropathol 85: 394–399.

Bailey KA, Aldinger KA (2009) An X-linked microcephaly syndrome caused by disruptions of CASK implicates the CASK-TBR1-RELN pathway in human brain development. Clin Genet 75: 424–425.

Barbot C, Carneiro G, Melo J (1997) Pontocerebellar hypoplasia with microcephaly and dyskinesia: report of two cases. Dev Med Child Neurol 39: 554–557.

Barkovich AJ, Millen KJ, Dobyns WB (2009) A developmental and genetic classification for midbrain-hindbrain malformations. Brain 132: 3199–3230.

Barth PG, Vrensen GFJM, Uylings HBM, Oorthuys JWE, Stam FC (1990) Inherited syndrome of microcephaly, dyskinesia and pontocerebellar hypoplasia – a systemic atrophy with early onset. J Neurol Sci 97: 25–42.

Barth PG (1993) Pontocerebellar hypoplasias: An overview of a group of inherited neurodegenerative disorders with fetal onset. Brain Dev 15: 411–422.

Barth PG, Blennow G, Lenard H-G, Begeer JH, van der Kley JM, Hanefeld F, et al. (1995) The syndrome of autosomal recessive pontocerebellar hypoplasia, microcephaly and extrapyramidal dyskinesia (pontocerebellar hypoplasia type 2): compiled data from ten pedigrees. Neurology 45: 311–317.

Barth PG, Aronica E, de Vries L, Nikkels PG, Scheper W, Hoozemans JJ, et al. (2007) Pontocerebellar hypoplasia type 2: a neuropathological update. Acta Neuropathol (Berl) 114: 373–386.

Barth PG, Ryan MM, Webster RI, Aronica E, Kan A, Ramkema M, et al. (2008) Rhabdomyolysis in pontocerebellar hypoplasia type 2 (PCH-2). Neuromuscul Disord 18: 52–58.

Biemond A (1955) Hypoplasia ponto-neocerebellaris, with malformation of the dentate nucleus. Folia Psychiatr Neurol (Amst) 58: 2–7.

Brouwer B (1924) Hypoplasia ponto-neocerebellaris. Psychiatr Neurol (Amst) 6: 461–473.

Brun R (1917) Zur Kenntnis der Bildungsfehler des Kleinhirns. Epikritische Bemerkungen zur Entwicklungspathologie, Morphologie und Klinik der umschriebenen Entwicklungshemmungen des Neozerebellums. Schweiz Arch Neurol Psychiat 1: 61–123.

Budde BS, Namavar Y, Barth PG, Poll-The B, Nurnberg G, Becker C, et al. (2008) tRNA splicing endonuclease mutations cause pontocerebellar hypoplasia. Nat Genet 40: 1113–1118.

Chaves-Vischer V, Pizzolato GP, Hanquinet S, Maret A, Bottani A, Haenggeli CA (2000) Early fatal pontocerebellar hypoplasia in premature twin sisters. Eur J Paediatr Neurol 4: 171–176.

Chou SM, Gilbert EF, Chun RW, Laxova R, Tuffli GA, Sufit RL, Krassikot N. (1990) Infantile olivopontocerebellar atrophy with spinal muscular atrophy (infantile OPCH + SMA). Clin Neuropathol 9: 21–32.

Coppola G, Muras I, Pascotto A (2000) Pontocerebellar hypoplasia type 2 (PCH2): report of two siblings. Brain Dev 22: 188–192.

De León GA, Grover WE, D'Cruz CA (1984) Amyotrophic cerebellar hypoplasia: A specific form of infantile spinal atrophy. Acta Neuropathol (Berl) 63: 282–286.

Durmaz B, Wollnik B, Cogulu O, Li Y, Tekgul H, Hazan F, Ozkinay F (2009) Pontocerebellar hypoplasia type III (CLAM): Extended phenotype and novel molecular findings. J Neurol 256: 416–419.

Edvardson S, Shaag A, Kolesnikova O, Gomori JM, Tarassov I, Einbinder T, et al. (2007) Deleterious mutation in the mitochondrial arginyl-transfer RNA synthetase gene is associated with pontocerebellar hypoplasia. Am J Hum Genet 81: 857–862.

Goasdoue P, Rodriguez D, Moutard ML, Robain O, Lalande G, Adamsbaum C (2001) Pontoneocerebellar hypoplasia: definition of MR features. Pediatr Radiol 31: 613–618.

Görgen-Pauly U, Sperner J, Reiss I, Gehl H-B, Reusche E (1999) Familial pontocerebellar hypoplasia type I with anterior horn cell disease. Eur J Paediat Neurol 3: 33–38.

Goutières F, Aicardi J, Farkas E (1977) Anterior horn cell disease associated with pontocerebellar hypoplasia in infants. J Neurol Neurosurg Psychiat 40: 370–378.

Grellner W, Rohde K, Wilske J (2000) Fatal outcome in a case of pontocerebellar hypoplasia type 2. Forensic Sci Int 113: 165–172.

Grosso S, Mostadini R, Cioni M, Galluzzi P, Morgese G, Balestri P (2002) Pontocerebellar hypoplasia type 2: further clinical characterization and evidence of positive response of dyskinesia to levodopa. J Neurol 249: 596–600.

Hashimoto K, Takeuchi Y, Kida Y, Hasegawa H, Kantake M, Sasaki A, et al. (1998) Three siblings of fatal infantile encephalopathy with olivopontocerebellar hypoplasia and microcephaly. Brain & Development 20: 169–174.

Iso A, Ozawa H, Kurokawa T, Kubota M, Mori K, Takashima S (1997) Olivopontocerebellar atrophy of neonatal onset with muscle hypertonia in two siblings. Neuropathology 17: 225–229.

Kamoshita S, Takei Y, Miyao M, Yanagisawa M (1990) Pontocerebellar hypoplasia associated with infantile motor neuron disease (Norman's disease). Pediatr Pathol 10: 133–142.

Koster S (1926) Two cases of hypoplasia ponto-neocerebellaris. Acta Psychiatr (Copenhagen) 1926; 47–76.

Krause F (1929) Über einen Bildungsfehler des Kleinhirns und einige faseranatomische Beziehungen des Organs. Zeitschr Gesamt Neurol Psychiatr 119: 788–815.

Leroy JG, Lyon G, Fallet C, Amiel J, De Praeter C, Van den Broecke C, Vanhaesebrouck P (2007) Congenital pontocerebellar atrophy and telencephalic defects in three siblings: a new subtype. Acta Neuropathol 114: 387–399.

Messerschmidt A, Brugger PC, Boltshauser E, Zoder G, Sterniste W, Birnbacher R, Prayer D (2005) Disruption of cerebellar development: potential complication of extreme prematurity. Am J Neuroradiol 26: 1659–1667.

Moerman P, Barth PG (1987) Olivo-ponto-cerebellar atrophy with muscular atrophy, joint contractures and pulmonary hypoplasia of prenatal onset. Virchows Arch A 410: 339–345.

Muntoni F, Goodwin F, Sewry C, Cox P, Cowan F, Airaksinen E, et al. (1999) Clinical spectrum and diagnostic difficulties of infantile pontocerebellar hypoplasia type 1. Neuropediatrics 30: 243–248.

Najm J, Horn D, Wimplinger I, Golden JA, Chizhikov VV, Sudi J, et al. (2008) Mutations of CASK cause an X-linked brain malformation phenotype with microcephaly and hypoplasia of the brainstem and cerebellum. Nat Genet 40: 1065–1067.

Namavar Y, Barth PG, Kasher PR, van Ruissen F, Brockmann K, Bernert G, et al. (2011a) Clinical, neuroradiological and genetic findings in pontocerebellar hypoplasia. Brain 134: 143–156.

Namavar Y, Chitayat D, Barth PG, van Ruissen F, de Wissel MB, Poll-The BT, et al. (2011b) TSEN54 mutations cause pontocerebellar hypoplasia type 5. Eur J Hum Genet 19: 724–726.

Norman RM (1961) Cerebellar hypoplasia in Werdnig-Hoffmann disease. Arch Dis Child 36: 96–101.

Okanishi T, Mori Y, Shirai K, Kobayashi S, Nakashima H, Kibe T, et al. (2010) Delayed gyration with pontocerebellar hypoplasia type 1. Brain Dev 32: 258–262.

Park SH, Becker-Catania S, Gatti RA, Crandall BF, Emelin JK, Vinters HV (1998) Congenital olivopontocerebellar atrophy – report of two siblings with paleo- and neocerebellar atrophy. Acta Neuropathol 96: 315–321.

Patel MS, Becker LE, Toi A, Armstrong DL, Chitayat D (2006) Severe, fetal-onset form of olivopontocerebellar hypoplasia in three sibs: PCH type 5? Am J Med Genet A 140: 594–603.

Peiffer J, Pfeiffer RA (1977) Hypoplasia ponto-neocerebellaris. J Neurol 215: 241–251.

Rajab A, Mochida GH, Hill A, Ganesh V, Bodell A, Riaz A, et al. (2003) A novel form of pontocerebellar hypoplasia maps to chromosome 7q11–21. Neurology 60: 1664–1667.

Rankin J, Brown R, Dobyns WB, Harington J, Patel J, Quinn M, Brown G (2010) Pontocerebellar hypoplasia type 6: A British case with PEHO-like features. Am J Med Genet A 152A: 2079–2084.

Renbaum P, Kellerman E, Jaron R, Geiger D, Segel R, Lee M, et al. (2009) Spinal muscular atrophy with pontocerebellar hypoplasia is caused by a mutation in the VRK1 gene. Am J Hum Genet 85: 281–289.

Rudnik-Schöneborn S, Wirth B, Rohrig D, Saule H, Zerres K (1995) Exclusion of the gene locus for spinal muscular atrophy on chromosome 5q in a family with infantile olivopontocerebellar atrophy (OPCA) and anterior horncell degeneration Neuromuscul Disord 5: 19–23.

Rudnik-Schöneborn S, Sztriha L, Aithala GR, Houge G, Laegreid LM, Seeger J, et al. (2003) Extended phenotype of pontocerebellar hypoplasia with infantile spinal muscular atrophy. Am J Med Genet A 117A: 10–17.

Ryan MM, Cooke-Yarborough CM, Procopis PG, Ouvrier RA (2000) Anterior horn cell disease and olivopontocerebellar hypoplasia. Pediatr Neurol 23: 180–184.

Salman MS, Blaser S, Buncic JR, Westall CA, Heon E, Becker L (2003) Pontocerebellar hypoplasia type 1: New leads for an earlier diagnosis. J Child Neurol 18: 220–225.

Sans-Fitó A, Campistol-Plana J, Mas-Salguero MJ, Poo-Arguelles P, Fernandez-Alvarez E (2002) Pontocerebellar hypoplasia type 2 and Reye-like syndrome. J Child Neurol 17: 132–134.

Steiman GS, Rorke LB, Brown MJ (1980) Infantile neuronal degeneration masquerading as Werdnig-Hoffmann disease. Ann Neurol 8: 317–324.

Steinlin M, Klein A, Haas-Lude K, Zafeiriou D, Strozzi S, Muller T, et al. (2007) Pontocerebellar hypoplasia type 2: variability in clinical and imaging findings. Eur J Paediatr Neurol 11: 146–152.

Szabó N, Szabó H, Hortobágyi T, Túri S, Sztriha L (2008) Pontocerebellar hypoplasia type 1. Pediatr Neurol 39(4): 286–288.

Weinberg AG, Kirkpatrick JB (1975) Cerebellar hypoplasia in Werdnig-Hoffmann disease. Dev Med Child Neurol 17: 511–516.

24
Autosomal Dominant Spinocerebellar Ataxias

Andrea H. Nemeth

This chapter addresses dominant ataxias seen in children that are not covered in the sections on leukodystrophies and metabolic disorders. The common terminology of spinocerebellar ataxias (SCA's) is somewhat confusing: strictly speaking there should be evidence of impairment of the spinocerebellar tracts in addition to the cerebellum itself. Of course one of the most common types is Friedreich ataxia but we do not use the term SCA's for this condition; generally speaking, SCA's has come to be used for autosomal dominant ataxias, usually degenerative, irrespective of the underlying pathology.

In general terms the SCA's are thought to be uncommon causes of childhood ataxia, although there is actually very little epidemiological data on the prevalence of these conditions in children. Furthermore, only the SCA's caused by repeat expansions (SCA1, 2, 3, 6, 7, and 17) have easily available genetic tests because they are polymerase chain reaction (PCR) based; this may bias the limited prevalence data that is available. Recent advances in high-throughput sequencing mean that more genetic tests are likely to be available in the next few years and this may increase diagnostic rates and give better prevalence data on individual disorders.

Since autosomal dominant disorders are often seen in successive generations of a family, it might be supposed that the diagnosis is relatively straightforward, since an affected child should have an affected parent. However, there are many exceptions to this general rule and there are diagnostic pitfalls for the unwary. These will be highlighted in the relevant sections.

Genetic concepts in autosomal dominant ataxias

'Autosomal dominant' refers to a pattern of inheritance in which an affected individual has one copy of a mutant gene and one copy of a normal gene on opposite alleles of a pair of autosomal (non X-linked) chromosomes. This contrasts with autosomal recessive conditions which require that the individual have two copies of the mutant gene on opposite alleles. In autosomal dominant disorders there is a 50% (1:2) chance that an individual carrying a mutant dominant gene will pass this on to a child, whereas in autosomal recessive conditions both parents are usually unaffected carriers and there is a 25% (1:4) chance of passing the condition to a child.

Autosomal dominant inheritance can be readily identified in some human pedigrees by drawing a family tree. In the simplest and classic case approximately equal numbers of males and females are affected, and offspring of affected parents have a 50:50 chance of developing the disorder at some time in their life. Transmission can be from male to male (which is not seen in X-linked conditions) and there are affected individuals in successive generations.

Penetrance

Reduced penetrance (sometimes erroneously referred to as 'incomplete' penetrance) describes the situation when an unaffected individual carries a pathogenic gene change but does not appear to have the disorder. On inspection of a family tree an affected individual may not have an affected parent, although sometimes there may be other family members with the condition. This is colloquially referred to as 'skipping' a generation, an incorrect term since the intervening parent without the condition carries the genetic change. In some cases the unaffected parent may genuinely never develop any symptoms or signs of the disorder. However, there are other explanations. If there is *age-related penetrance* then the unaffected person may simply not yet have developed symptoms or signs of the disorder. There may be *variable expressivity*, a term that is used to describe the variability of clinical phenotype in different family members with the same mutation. Or the 'unaffected' person may simply have subtle features that have not previously been detected by the individual or by a physician. Close questioning, examination and other investigations such as imaging of such individuals, *with appropriate genetic counseling beforehand*, may reveal features of the condition.

However, even with extensive investigations some individuals who have one mutant gene and one normal gene, are able to pass the condition on to their children and yet do not develop the condition themselves. This true *reduced penetrance* is a well-recognized genetic phenomenon and illustrates the molecular complexities underlying autosomal dominant disorders. The phenomenon implies that although the gene mutation is a prerequisite for developing the condition, there are other genetic or environmental factors which are important in the ultimate development of a disease. In some cases these 'genetic modifiers' have been identified (for example the codon 129 polymorphism in the Prion gene), but in many cases we still have limited knowledge of them.

In the case of *trinucleotide repeat disorders* (Huntington disease and some of the dominant spinocerebellar ataxias, see below) the molecular basis of reduced penetrance can partly be attributed to the smaller repeat size in some individuals, leading some to develop the condition and others not. However, the variability of age at onset in different individuals carrying the same allele size suggests that other genetic or environmental factors are important. A recent hypothesis is that there is somatic mosaicism such that in some individuals the central nervous system neurons may have larger repeat sizes than in the peripheral blood lymphocytes which are the ones usually analysed in clinical diagnostics. The result may be a difference in the age at onset that might be predicted from measurement of the peripheral sample alone. A further complexity is the presence of *genetic anticipation* in which there is a reduction in age at onset in successive generations. This phenomenon has been noted for many years but the molecular basis only became apparent with the identification of pathogenic expanded trinucleotide repeats which are unstable in parental transmission. The size of the repeat sometimes inversely correlates with the age at onset, and as the repeat expands in successive generations the age at onset decreases.

In nucleotide repeat disorders, *reduced penetrance* alleles need to be distinguished from *non-disease-causing unstable alleles* (sometimes known as '*intermediate alleles*' or '*normal-sized mutable alleles*'). These alleles can increase in size during parental transmission but appear to confer little or no risk of developing the condition. Such alleles are well described in Huntington disease and occur in some of the SCA's as well. They create many complexities in interpretation and genetic counselling.

In cases where reduced penetrance is noted or reported in other families, the risk to offspring of developing the disease is less than 50% (as opposed to the risk of inheriting the mutant gene which remains at 50%). This can have profound consequences for genetic counselling regarding reproductive risks.

De novo dominant inheritance

Sometimes an affected child with a known mutation has two parents who do not have the mutation on routine testing of DNA extracted from a peripheral blood sample. This can be the result of non-paternity (or, more rarely, non-maternity) but a well-recognized genetic mechanism is a *de novo* mutation that has occurred in the germline of one of the parents. Such a parent will not have the condition themselves (unless there is also somatic mosaicism), but may have a small proportion of germline cells with the mutation ('*germline mosaicism*'), conferring a risk of the disease in subsequent children. The risk depends on the specific condition and is often not known with certainty. In these cases a 1–3% risk is generally quoted but referral for genetic counselling is advised. If the affected child grows up to reproductive potential then their children will be at 50% risk of developing the condition, as with any other autosomal dominant disorder, and therefore genetic counselling should also be offered to the affected child at an appropriate age.

Accurate genetic counselling therefore forms a significant part of the diagnostic process in investigating a child with ataxia. In some cases it is justified to delay investigation until the parents have had the opportunity to be reviewed by an experienced clinical geneticist.

Chromosomal rearrangements

Large-scale rearrangements of chromosomes also can result in autosomal dominant patterns of inheritance. For example, in SCA15 (see below), the pathogenic mutations are generally large deletions of the gene. Since standard sequencing does not detect large deletions, the disease-associated mutations in *ITPR1* (SCA15) took many years to identify. In some cases deletions may involve several genes (contiguous gene deletions) resulting in more complex phenotypes.

Another type of rearrangement is a chromosomal translocation. This is a common occurrence (~1/800) in the population and often does not result in any net gain or loss of genetic material, but may result in abnormal segregation products at meiosis resulting in loss or gain of genetic material in the offspring (also contiguous gene deletions). In addition, some translocations directly disrupt a gene (see SCA27) and can be associated with the disease. Duplications, insertions and inversions also may be associated with the disease.

The techniques used to identify chromosomal rearrangements currently are quite different from those used to screen for small nucleotide changes, and advice should always be sought from a molecular genetics and cytogenetics laboratory when embarking on testing.

Mechanisms of disease in autosomal dominant spinocerebellar ataxias

In the normal situation there are two copies of each autosomal gene. If one of the copies has a mutation then there are at least three different mechanisms to account for the occurrence of disease when a normal copy of the gene is also present.

Haploinsufficiency

In diploid organisms, including humans, there are two copies of autosomal genes. In some instances only one functioning copy of a gene is required for health (for example, in carriers of recessive mutations), but in some cases both copies of a gene are required, a situation known as *dosage dependence*. In *haploinsufficiency* there is an absence of one of the two copies of the gene, often as a result of a large deletion, truncating or nonsense mutation which results in absence of the protein product from one allele. Experimentally, an animal model with one of the two genes knocked out would be expected to show a similar phenotype to the human disease. An example of this is SCA15.

Dominant negative effect

A dominant negative describes a molecular mechanism in which the mutant protein interferes directly or indirectly with the function of the normal ('wild type') gene. Experimentally, knockout of one gene would not be expected to produce a phenotype and there would be evidence of interaction of the mutant protein with the wild-type protein in the pathogenic process. In some instances a single missense mutation can result in a more severe phenotype than deletion of the whole gene because of this mechanism. An example of this is SCA13.

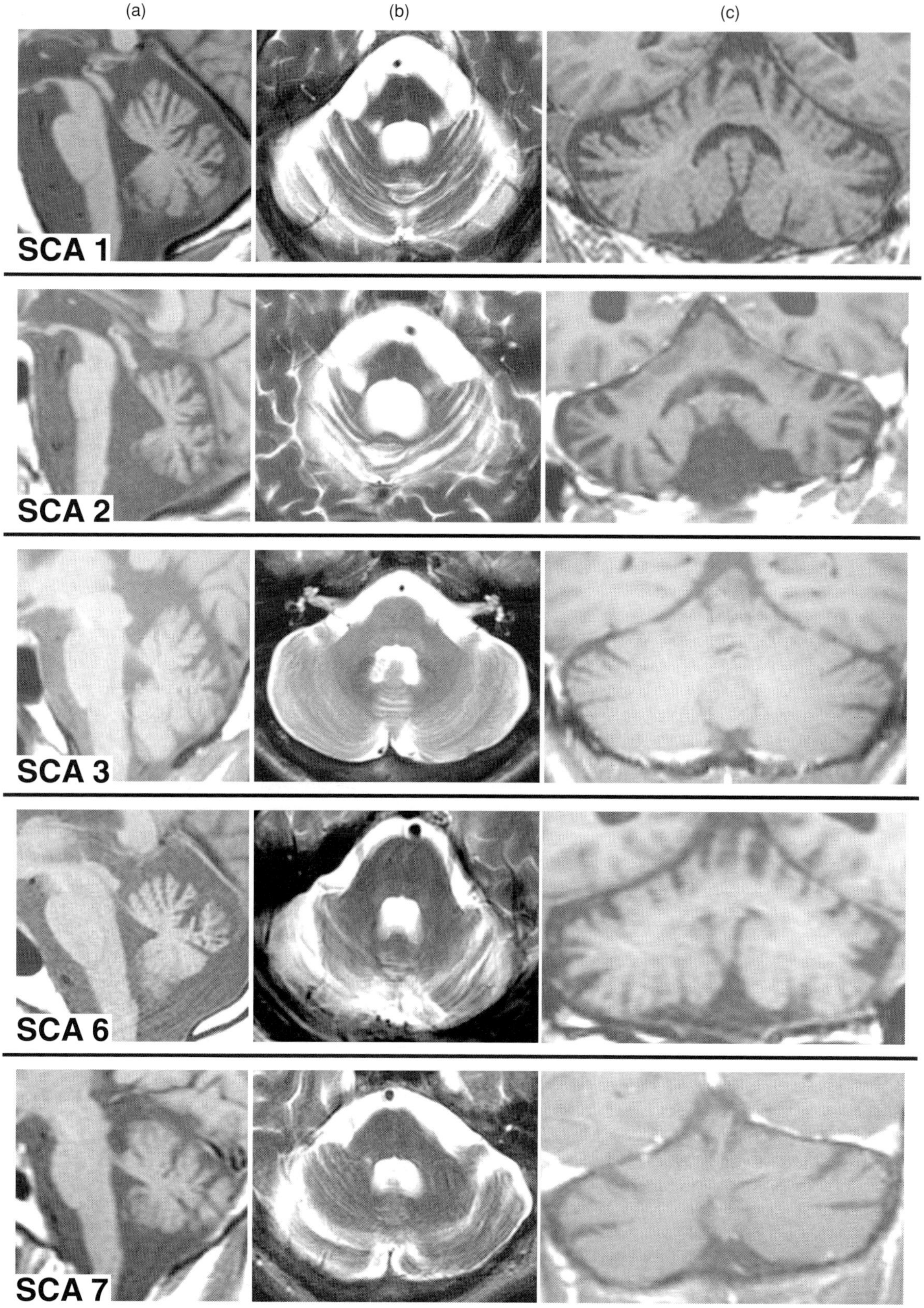

Fig. 24.1. Magnetic resonance brain images of adult patients with selected autosomal dominant spinocerebellar ataxias. **(a)** T1-weighted images in the mid-sagittal plane. **(b)** T2-weighted images, axial plane. **(c)** T1-weighted images, coronal plane. The higher-quality image in the SCA1 case is a magnetized prepared rapid acquisition gradient echo (MPRAGE) sequence. The patient with SCA1 is a 56-year-old man with 45 CAG repeats, 8 years into his illness, mildly affected with a Brief Ataxia Rating Scale (BARS) score of 7 (out of 30). The patient with SCA2 is 33 years of age, with a CAG expansion of 43 CAG repeats, and 11 years after disease onset is moderately impaired with a BARS score of 17/30. The SCA3 patient is 39 years of age, his CAG repeat length is 77, and at 12 years of disease progression his BARS score is 9/30, reflecting mild to moderate disability. The SCA6 gentleman is 69 years of age, CAG repeat length 24, with a BARS score of 14/30 reflecting mild to moderate disability now 23 years into the symptomatic phase of his illness. The patient with SCA7 is 56 years of age with 46 CAG repeats. At age 37 he developed retinitis pigmentosis, and at age 49 he developed gait instability. After 9 years of ataxia progression his BARS score is still relatively mild at 7/30. (Images courtesy of Jeremy D. Schmahmann, and Neuroradiology Department, Massachusetts General Hospital.)

Dominant positive effect or toxic gain of function

A toxic gain of function refers to the situation where the mutation confers a function not seen in the wild type and which causes toxicity to the cell. Experimentally the disease is only produced when the specific type of mutation is present and again will not be present when one or both genes are knocked out.

One of the best-studied dominant gain-of-function mechanisms in the dominant spinocerebellar ataxias is that of the trinucleotide repeat expansion disorders, examples of which include SCA1, 2, 3, 6, and 7. The clinical features and specific details are described below; in general terms these are often CAG repeat expansions in the coding region of genes, resulting in proteins containing polyglutamine repeats. Genetic testing is well established in most medical genetics laboratories because they are PCR based and therefore cheap and easy to set up. There is an inverse correlation between the size of the expansion such that the age at onset is earlier with larger expansions and the clinical features in children may be markedly different (see Fig. 24.2). The most common CAG trinucleotide repeat disorder is Huntington disease; although this only extremely rarely presents with a cerebellar syndrome it has molecular similarities with the dominant SCA's associated with CAG repeats. Thus it is hoped that disease-modifying therapies will be relevant for the entire group of disorders. A common feature of the CAG repeat disorders is the instability of the repeat in paternal and most frequently paternal transmission, which has been particularly noted in SCA1, SCA2, and SCA7 in addition to Huntington disease. This leads to the phenomenon of '*genetic anticipation*' as previously described. In some cases this may lead to the diagnosis being made in a child before a parent is symptomatic and thus testing for these conditions in children requires counselling of the parents first.

Therefore, understanding the existence of different types of mutations has important clinical consequences: different types of genetic tests must be requested by the clinician, the type of mutation will give important information about risks to other family members (for example, *reduced penetrance* or instability in parental transmission resulting in *anticipation*), and ultimately understanding the molecular mechanisms may result in the development of rational treatment strategies.

Laboratory testing in dominant ataxias

Currently, mutation testing for ataxias in many European Centres is limited to Spinocerebellar ataxias (SCA's) 1, 2, 3, 6, 7, 17, Dentato-rubro-pallido-luysian atrophy (DRPLA), Fragile X Associated Tremor Syndrome (FXTAS) and Friedreich Ataxia (FRDA), in addition to Episodic Ataxias (EA) 1–3. In the USA SCA 5, 8, 10, 13 and 14 are also available. The remainder are done in individual laboratories, sometimes on a research basis. It is likely that in the next few years much wider testing will become available as technological advances in next-generation sequencing are made which allow parallel sequencing of multiple genes. Several such projects are under way in Oxford and Newcastle in the UK and some European centres (Hoischen et al. 2010). The availability of sequence-based genetic testing clearly has a significant impact on diagnosis and genetic counselling. However, sequencing is not the only technology required for genetic testing. As noted above, PCR is used to detect mutations associated with repeats. Sequencing technology of any kind currently does not easily detect large deletions, so other methods are required, usually multiplex ligation probe amplification (MLPA), comparative genome hybridization single nucleotide polymorphism (SNP), array technology, or fluorescent in situ hybridization. Karyotyping remains necessary for detecting balanced translocations. Good liaison with local clinical genetics teams and molecular genetic laboratories will aid in the choice of genetic tests and technology. Table 24.1 summarizes the different spinocerebellar ataxias seen in children, the mutation mechanism, normal and pathogenic sizes in the repeat disorders, and the key clinical features.

Autosomal dominant spinocerebellar ataxias

Spinocerebellar ataxias caused by nucleotide repeat expansions

Spinocerebellar ataxia type 1

Spinocerebellar ataxia type 1 (SCA1) is caused by a CAG repeat expansion on chromosome 6p23 and was originally linked using markers near the HLA locus (Zoghbi et al. 1988). In 1993 the gene for SCA1 was identified and found to be a CAG trinucleotide repeat expansion. Two juvenile-onset cases were reported (Orr et al. 1993), one with onset at age 4 and the other at age 15. Five of the six children were born to affected fathers, and larger alleles (mutable normal-sized, reduced penetrance, and disease associated) were more unstable in paternal transmission. There is an inverse correlation between the age at onset and the repeat size. The prevalence of the disorder is thought to be in the region of 1–2 per 100 000 of the population, making it approximately ten times less common than Huntington disease. SCA1 appears to be found in many different ethnic groups including in Poland, Thailand, North America, Italy, India, and China (reviewed in Shibata-Hamaguchi et al. 2009).

In adults the most frequent presenting clinical features are progressive cerebellar ataxia with a gait and balance disturbance, dysmetria, dysarthria, nystagmus, mild dysphagia, and brisk reflexes. As the disease progresses they may develop ophthalmoparesis with impaired up-gaze, slow saccadic velocity, and proprioceptive loss. In the later stages patients develop muscle atrophy, chorea, dystonia, cognitive impairment, and more severe bulbar dysfunction. The age at onset is typically in the third or fourth decade. Almost one-quarter of affected patients in the pedigree presented by Zoghbi et al. (1988) were affected under the age of 15 and in the families reported by Orr et al. (1993) the youngest onset was 4 years of age. They had gait ataxia, dysdiadochokinesis, dysmetria, dysphagia, and impaired eye movements but in addition all had cognitive impairment and a more rapid progression than their relatives with adult onset. Cerebellar atrophy was noted on CT in this family and was also clearly visible on MRI (see Fig. 24.1).

TABLE 24.1
Summary of spinocerebellar ataxias seen in children with mutations, size of repeats, and key clinical features

Disease Name	HGNC gene symbol	Chromosomal locus	Protein name	Protein function	Type of mutation	Clinical features in children in addition to cerebellar ataxia
SCA1	*ATXN1*	6p23	ataxin 1	Transcriptional regulation	CAG expansion in exon 8 Normal size alleles 6–44 repeats Mutable normal size alleles 36–38 repeats Full penetrance disease associated alleles 39–91 repeats	Cognitive impairment, rapid progression Cerebellar atrophy on imaging
SCA2	*ATXN2*	12q23-q24.1	ataxin 2	RNA metabolism	CAG expansion in exon 1 Normal size alleles 31 and under Reduced penetrance alleles (later onset) 32 and 33 Full penetrance alleles 37–39 in adult cases, 100s in infantile cases	Neonatal hypotonia, developmental delay/cognitive impairment, retinitis pigmentosa, visual inattention, severe hypotonia and absent reflexes, cerebellar atrophy on imaging EEG: hypsarrhythmia, discharges of sharp and slow wave activity and slowing of the EEG background
SCA3	*ATXN3*	14q24.3-q31	ataxin 3	De-ubiquitination	CAG expansion in exon 10 Normal repeat sizes range 14–47 Reduced penetrance alleles 44–47 Full penetrance alleles 44–86	Abnormal eye movements, dysarthria upper motor neuron signs, a spastic and athetotic, twisting movements of hands, cerebellar and vermis atrophy on imaging
SCA5	*SPTBN2*	11q13.2	spectrin, beta, non-erythrocytic 2	Cytoskeleton	Missense and small in-frame deletions	Abnormal eye movements, dysarthria
SCA6	*CACNA1A*	19p13	Calcium channel, voltage gated P/Q type	Neuronal calcium regulation	CAG expansion in exon 47 Normal allele sizes 18 or less Mutable normal size 19 Full penetrance alleles 20–33	Brisk reflexes, muscle weakness, more rapid progression than adults
SCA7	*ATXN7*	3p21.2-p12	Ataxin 7	Transcriptional regulation	CAG expansion in exon 1 Normal alleles 4–18 repeats Reduced penetrance 28–35 Full penetrance alleles over 38, in infants over 300 described	Childhood: dysmetria, intention tremor, dysarthria, dysphagia and brisk reflexes Infancy: includes failure to thrive, weight loss, weakness and hypotonia patent ductus arteriosus, multiple organ failure, retinal dystrophy
SCA8	*ATXN8OS*	13q21	ATXN8OS/ATXN8	Unknown	CTG expansions (noncoding strand)/CAG expansions (coding strand)	Congenital ataxia, myoclonic epilepsy, developmental delay
SCA10	*ATXN10*	22q13	Ataxin 10	Cytoplasmic protein	ATTCT pentanucleotide repeat in intron 9	Scanning dysarthria, and dysphagia, cognitive dysfunction, behavioural disturbances, mood disorders, mild pyramidal signs, peripheral neuropathy

SCA11	*TTBK2*	15q14-q15.3	Tau-tubulin kinase 2	Tau phosphorylation	Frameshift mutations	abnormal eye movements, less commonly pyramidal features, hyper-reflexia, peripheral neuropathy, dystonia
SCA12	*PPP2R2B*	5q31-q33	Serine threonine protein phosphatase 2A 55kd regulatory subunit B beta isoform	Serine threonine protein phosphatase thought to be involved in numerous cellular processes	CAG expansion in noncoding region	action tremor, bradykinesia, hyper-reflexia, psychiatric symptoms, dystonia, dementia
SCA13	*KCNC3*	19q13.3-q13.4	Potassium voltage-gated channel subfamily C member 3	Voltage gated Potassium channel	Missense mutations	nystagmus, dysarthria, developmental delay, hyperreflexia, in some cases mild cognitive impairment and seizures
SCA14	*PRKCG*	19q13.4	Protein kinase C gamma type	Signal transduction	Missense, in-frame deletion, splice	nystagmus, dysarthria, brisk reflexes
SCA15	*ITPR1*	3p26.1	Inositol 1,4,5-triphosphate receptor type 1	Calcium signalling	Large deletions	nystagmus, dysarthria, titubation, tremor, mild hyperreflexia, impaired vestibulo-ocular reflex, dysphagia, oscillopsia
SCA16	Now known as *SCA15*					
SCA17	TBP	6q27	Tata box binding protein	Nuclear transcription factor	CAG expansion Normal allele sizes 25–44 Reduced penetrance alleles sizes 43–48 Full penetrance alleles sizes 43–63	abnormal eye movements, psychiatric disorders, learning difficulties or cognitive decline, basal ganglia dysfunction, seizures
SCA27	*FGF14*	13q34	Fibroblast Growth factor 14	Interacts with voltage gated Na channels	Missense, nonsense, translocation	abnormal eye movements, dysarthria, memory loss, depression, learning difficulties, tremor, orofacial dyskinesias, brisk knee reflexes, absent vibration sense, pes cavus, microcephaly
SCA28	*AFG3L2*	18p11.21	AFG3 ATPase family gene 3-like 2 (S. cerevisiae)	Component of m-AAA metalloprotease complex involved in maintenance of mitochondrial proteome	Missense mutations	abnormal eye movements, ptosis dysarthria, brisk reflexes, bilateral clonus and extensor plantars
DRPLA	*ATN1*	12p13.31	atrophin 1	Unknown (? transcriptional co-repressor)	CAG trinucleotide repeat expansion Normal repeat sizes are 7–34 Expanded in patients up to 88	severe myoclonic epilepsy and other seizures types, severe cognitive impairment, choreoathetosis, autistic spectrum disorder, obstructive sleep apnoea

Gene information from HGNC: http://www.genenames.org/aboutHGNC.html

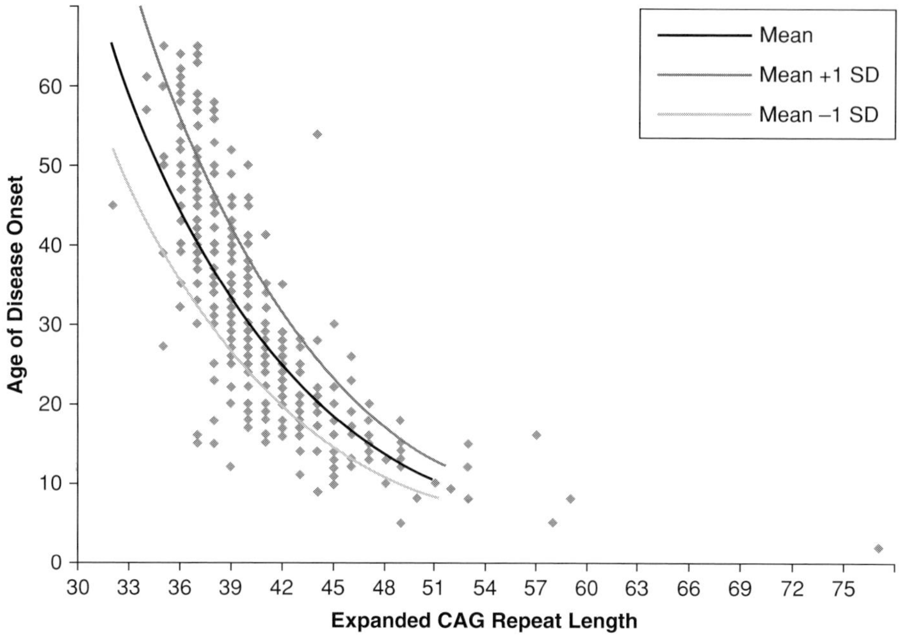

Fig. 24.2. Scatterplot of SCA2 CAG repeat length and age at onset in Cuban SCA2 patients: dashed and dotted red and yellow lines denote one standard deviation boundaries for age at onset. (Reproduced with permission from Pulst S et al. Brain 2005; 128: 2297–2303.) (See color plate 25).

Spinocerebellar ataxia type 2

Spinocerebellar ataxia type 2 (SCA2) is caused by an expansion of a CAG trinucleotide repeat near the 5′ coding region of the *ataxin 2* gene on chromosome 12q24. As in the other CAG repeat disorders there is an inverse correlation between the repeat size and the age at onset (Pulst et al. 2005; see Fig. 24.2). The condition has been described in many European populations, in a huge pedigree in Cuba, and in India. The prevalence is highly variable in different populations.

The condition was originally reported by several investigators as an autosomal dominant disorder characterized by gait ataxia, dysarthria, dysmetria, dysdiadochokinesis, cramps, tremor, hypotonia, abnormal reflexes, and slowed/limited eye movements. Although it is usually seen in adults the age at onset was reported to range from 2 to 65 years in the Cuban pedigree and 8 to 30 in the Indian pedigree (Orozco Diaz et al. 1990; Wadia and Swami 1971). Full penetrance alleles are usually 37–39 in adult cases but very large expansions of over 200 have been reported in infants with neonatal hypotonia, absent reflexes, developmental delay, retinitis pigmentosa, and visual inattention (Babovic-Vuksanovic et al. 1998; Mao et al. 2002). MRI findings include cerebellar atrophy and delayed myelination but in some patients the scan is reported to be normal (see Fig. 24.1). EEG findings in children included hypsarrhythmia, discharges of sharp and slow wave activity, and slowing of the EEG background. There is one report of polyphagia in affected children from an Egyptian family (Abdel-Aleem and Zaki 2008) and a strikingly different pattern of disease progression in two siblings from a Turkish family, one of whom deteriorated very quickly and one of whom remains at school with limited cognition. Interestingly, in the latter case the more severely affected child had a smaller repeat than the less severely affected child (70 versus 84), illustrating that other genetic modifiers are operating (Yiş et al. 2009).

Spinocerebellar ataxia type 3

Spinocerebellar ataxia type 3 (SCA3) is also known as Machado-Joseph disease (MJD) which is the variant first described in the Portuguese or those of Portuguese descent. The mutation is a CAG repeat in the *SCA3/MJD* gene on chromosome 14q32.1 (Kawaguchi et al. 1994). It was originally described in two families from the Azores (Machado family from San Miguel and Joseph family from Flores) and was subsequently found in patients from Europe, Japan, China, the United States, and worldwide in individuals of Portuguese descent. The repeat is unstable during paternal transmission and there is an overlap between normal reduced penetrance and full penetrance alleles (see Table 24.1).

The phenotypes are sometimes subdivided thus: type 1 early onset (<20 years of age with pronounced pyramidal and extrapyramidal signs and a more rapid course); type 2 in which there are pyramidal and cerebellar signs only and an age at onset in 20s–30s; type 3 in which there are more peripheral signs, a later age at onset, and slower progression; and type 4 with neuropathy, parkinsonism, and a variable age at onset (Rosenberg 1992). The patients with MJD of Portuguese descent sometimes have a slightly different phenotype from other SCA3 patients, with lid retraction giving a 'staring eyes' appearance, dystonia, rigidity, and facial myokymia.

The reported age at onset is in the range 5–75 years. Two patients with onset at age 5 and 11, respectively, were both heterozygous for an 83-repeat expansion (Zhou et al. 1997). The main presenting features were nystagmus, brisk tendon reflexes, and extensor plantars which progressed to spastic gait, abnormal saccadic eye movements, a spastic dysarthria, athetotic, twisting movements of hands, and cerebellar ataxia. One of the patients had lid retraction and facial myokymia.

There is only one published report of a patient who was homozygous for the repeat: this was the only child of a consanguineous couple both aged 22 at the birth of their child. She had normal early development, and was referred for regression of motor skills at the age of 4. She had an unsteady gait, slow speech, and difficulty in swallowing, and the clinical syndrome progressed to spasticity of limbs, dystonia, bradykinesia, brisk reflexes, extensor plantars, facial hypomimia, mild ataxia, and action tremor. By 8 she was no longer able to walk, had generalized dystonia, bulging eyes, and nystagmus and by 11 was bedridden, rigid, dystonic, and had pyramidal signs and cachexia. One repeat size of 67 was inherited from the mother and the other of 72 was inherited from the father (with three additional repeats). The mother had a normal neurological examination; the father (and several of his relatives with repeat sizes of 69 or 70) had minor signs of cerebellar ataxia. Therefore the child had similar repeat sizes to her parents but was homozygous and had a much more severe phenotype (Carvalho et al. 2008).

MRI of patients shows cerebellar hemisphere and vermis atrophy, pontine atrophy, and enlargement of the fourth ventricle (see Fig. 24.1). Volumetric analysis shows putamen and caudate atrophy. Postmortem analysis reveals depigmentation of the substantia nigra in addition to widespread involvement of the cerebellum, thalamus, midbrain, pons, medulla, and spinal cord (reviewed in Riess et al. 2008).

As in the other progressive disorders, treatment is supportive: parkinsonism may respond to L-dopa, amantadine has been reported to help dystonia and bradykinesia, and muscle cramps may respond to quinine, magnesium or mexilitene. Spasticity may be treated with baclofen, tizanidine or memantine. Patients should have assessments for gait support and physiotherapy.

Spinocerebellar ataxia type 6

Spinocerebellar ataxia type 6 (SCA6) is an autosomal dominant disorder caused by expansion of a CAG trinucleotide repeat in the last exon of the *CACNA1A* gene on chromosome 19p. Normal-size alleles are 18 repeats or less and full penetrance alleles over 20 repeats. Repeats of 19 are probably reduced penetrance alleles. This gene encodes a voltage-dependent, P/Q type calcium channel. Mutations in this gene can also cause familial hemiplegic migraine (FHM) and episodic ataxia type 2 (EA2). FHM tends to be caused by point mutations (although a large gene deletion has been associated with this phenotype) and EA2 associated with nonsense, frameshift or splice mutations. There is more phenotypic overlap between EA2 and SCA6 than FHM, in that EA2 patients may develop a progressive ataxia, and SCA6 patients may report migraine, but some FHM patients with point mutations have been reported to have ataxia. MRI in SCA6 reveals cerebellar atrophy (see Fig. 24.1).

SCA6 has almost always been reported as a late adult-onset disorder, and there is only one report of the condition in developing adolescence (Wang et al. 2010). There was a progressive cerebellar syndrome in two siblings with age at onset at 16 and 18 years with brisk reflexes and no evidence of dementia or neuropathy. The patients died 13–16 years after onset. Both patients had 25 repeats.

Spinocerebellar ataxia type 7

Spinocerebellar ataxia type 7 (SCA7) is an autosomal dominant disorder caused by expansion of a CAG trinucleotide repeat in the first coding exon of the gene located on chromosome 3p (Michalik et al. 2004). There is an inverse correlation between the size of the repeat and age at onset. Expanded repeats are among the most unstable described to date, resulting in marked anticipation and occasionally a presymptomatic diagnosis in a parent. There also are reports of repeats expanding during maternal transmission (Benton et al. 1998).

In typical adult-onset cases SCA7 causes a macular dystrophy with cone involvement first, which progresses to a cone-rod dystrophy. Clinically there is impairment of central and color vision first, leading eventually to total loss of vision. This is associated with a progressive ataxia that renders the patient wheelchair bound in early to mid-adult life and cerebellar atrophy is seen on MRI (see Fig. 24.1). Although typically described as presenting with visual loss, some patients develop ataxia first and visual onset later. In childhood the phenotype is similar with cerebellar ataxia, visual loss, dysmetria, intention tremor, dysarthria, dysphagia, and brisk reflexes, but may also include psychosis and behavioural disturbance as well as extrapyramidal signs (Benton et al. 1998). There may be visual disturbance. However, the phenotype in infancy is quite different from that in adolescent and adulthood and includes failure to thrive, weight loss, weakness, hypotonia, and acquired microcephaly. Patients may have a patent ductus arteriosus and evidence of multiple organ failure (Benton et al. 1998; van de Warrenburg et al. 2001; Whitney et al. 2007). The MRI may show cerebellar and cerebral atrophy and ventricular dilatation. The repeat sizes in infantile cases can be over 300. Neurological deterioration and a retinal dystrophy are present but, in the context of other features, a metabolic abnormality may be suspected. The retinal dystrophy may not be evident without investigation by an experienced ophthalmologist. Families reported in the literature have highly variable ages of onset, even in a single family, partly reflecting the repeat size.

Spinocerebellar ataxia type 8

Spinocerebellar ataxia type 8 (SCA8) is described as an autosomal dominant disorder caused by a trinucleotide repeat expansion in the *ATXN8OS* gene on chromosome 13q21. There is considerable debate about whether the trinucleotide repeat identified in the 3′ untranslated part of the gene is a polymorphism or is pathogenic (Koob et al. 1999; Day et al. 2000; Stevanin et al. 2000; Worth et al. 2000; Cellini et al. 2001; Brusco et al. 2002; Tazón et al. 2002; Schöls et al. 2003; Zeman et al. 2004).

The age at onset is generally described to be in early adult life but there are reports of symptoms and signs being present in a 1-year-old, a 3-year-old, and several teenagers (Koob et al. 1999; Day et al. 2000; Silveira et al. 2000; Felling and Baron 2005). The child with congenital ataxia had cerebellar signs from the age of 1, did not walk until aged 5, and had myoclonic epilepsy from age 3. A young girl with congenital ataxia within the first year of life had myoclonic epilepsy and was mentally retarded. She had 105 repeats. Adolescents are described with gait and limb ataxia and marked cerebellar atrophy with a slow disease progression. In summary, the childhood onset of SCA8 is very variable and should be considered in a child with unexplained ataxia *even without* a family history (see below). Several atypical phenotypes including parkinsonism in children have been reported but their relationship to the molecular mutation is unclear. Adults may have a more variable and complex neurological phenotype including dysarthria, oculomotor abnormalities, extensor plantars, migraine, sensory abnormalities, myoclonus, seizure-like episodes without EEG correlates, and cognitive impairment.

The molecular mechanisms underlying SCA8 remain unclear. The genetic abnormality was initially reported as a CTG expansion in the noncoding part of a novel gene in a large family with autosomal dominant ataxia. However, reduced penetrance of the condition was noted in the MN-A family (22/35 individuals were unaffected) and, in this family, the repeat length tended to be shorter in the unaffected individuals. In subsequent reports affected individuals sometimes do not have a family history or there are only a few affected individuals and the penetrance very low. Normal alleles have been defined as 15–50 repeats and repeat lengths most often associated with ataxia range from 80 to 250; however, repeat lengths ranging from 71 to more than 1300 have been found in some individuals with ataxia. Although reduced penetrance is observed for alleles of all repeat lengths, it is most often observed with alleles of fewer than 100 repeats. The repeat size varies from 70 to over 1000 and cannot be used to predict the age at onset. There is also no clear pathogenic range of repeat size in comparison to normal. The initial reports suggested that the noncoding CTG repeat gene (*ATXNOS8*) coded for an antisense RNA transcript that has a toxic gain-of-function effect by interfering with normal splicing of other genes. Subsequently, it was discovered that there is a second gene spanning the repeat in the CAG direction and that this gene is transcribed producing a polyglutamine-containing protein that is present in intranuclear inclusions in human autopsy SCA8 patient Purkinje cells (Moseley et al. 2006). The current hypotheses are that this complex gene is bidirectionally expressed and that both RNA gain of function and protein gain of function may be involved in its aetiology.

Genetic counselling of families is strongly advised before embarking on genetic testing for this condition; indeed, some authors suggest that genetic testing should not be performed on a clinical basis until more is understood about the relationship between the repeat and the disease (Munhoz et al. 2009). Genetic testing for SCA8 is not routinely performed in the UK for this reason.

Spinocerebellar ataxia type 10

Spinocerebellar ataxia type 10 (SCA10) is caused by a repeat expansion of an ATTCT pentanucleotide repeat in intron 9 of a gene originally known as E46L, now *ATXN10* on chromosome 22q13.3. Normal alleles range from 10 to 29 repeats and pathogenic alleles from 800 repeats (4kb) to 4500 repeats (22.5kb). The function of *ATXN10* and mechanism of pathogenicity of the repeat expansion remains unknown (Lin and Ashizawa 2005). To date, SCA10 has only been identified in individuals of Mexican and Brazilian descent.

The condition frequently presents as a combination of a cerebellar syndrome with epilepsy, but epilepsy has only been described in patients of Mexican descent (25–80% of the cases). In addition to poor balance and unsteady gait, followed by upper limb ataxia, there may be a scanning dysarthria, and dysphagia. Abnormal tracking eye movements are common. Patients of Mexican origin have also been described with cognitive dysfunction, behavioural disturbances, mood disorders, mild pyramidal signs, and peripheral neuropathy. The age at onset in the Mexican families was 14–44 and in Brazilian families 12–48 years. It is still unclear whether the condition affects other ethnic groups. Cerebellar atrophy is almost invariably present.

Spinocerebellar ataxia type 12

Spinocerebellar ataxia type 12 (SCA12) has only been identified in two families, one of German and one of Indian descent (Holmes et al. 1999; Fujigasaki et al. 2001; Srivastava et al. 2001). The most common features are an action tremor, bradykinesia, cerebellar signs, hyperreflexia, psychiatric symptoms, dystonia, and dementia. The age at onset is in the range 8–55 with most individuals presenting in their 30s. The MRI shows diffuse cerebral cortical and cerebellar atrophy in older patients and pathology shows loss of Purkinje cell and cortical atrophy with no evidence of tangles plaques, Lewy bodies or Pick bodies (O'Hearn, unpublished). The condition is thought to be caused by a CAG expansion just upstream of exon 7 in the brain-specific gene *PPP2R2B* (Holmes et al. 1999). This is a subunit of PP2A, a protein serine/threonine phosphatase involved in a wide range of cellular processes. The CAG expansion is thought to be located in the promoter region of the gene and segregates with the disease in both families. The normal range of alleles is 9–28 and in the two pedigrees described the pathogenic alleles are 66–78 repeats. There appears to be little correlation between the repeat size and age at onset. Several individuals in the pedigrees and in other series reported in the literature have repeat sizes in the pathogenic range. It is unclear whether this represents age-related penetrance or reduced penetrance. Further work is required to elucidate the pathogenic mechanisms responsible for SCA12.

Spinocerebellar ataxia type 17

Spinocerebellar ataxia type 17 (SCA17) is caused by an expanded complex CAG/CAA trinucleotide repeat coding for glutamine in exon 3 of the TATA-box binding protein, a general transcription initiation factor located on chromosome 6q27 (reviewed in Stevanin and Brice 2008). The glutamine coding repeat size in normal alleles ranges from 25 to 44 and in pathological alleles from 43 to 63. Repeat sizes from 43 to 48 are considered to be reduced penetrance alleles. Further work is still required to fully understand the nature of the repeats and their relation to clinical phenotype. There is intergenerational instability, as with the other CAG repeat disorders, and this seems more marked in paternal transmission. About half the cases appear to be sporadic, making diagnosis very challenging, although the genetic test is straightforward and available in many countries. SCA17 has been reported in those of European, Japanese, Chinese, Finnish, Brazilian, and Mexican descent and the overall prevalence has been estimated at 1–10/100 000.

SCA17 is most commonly reported in adults with a mean age at onset of 30 (range 4–55). Cerebellar symptoms and signs are sometimes the presenting feature with gait ataxia being the most common and other features such as dysarthria less common. There may be oculomotor abnormalities such as jerky pursuit, hypometric or slowed saccades, and gaze-evoked nystagmus. However, other presenting features include psychiatric disorders (personality change, depression, psychosis, hallucinations, aggressive behaviour, mutism), mental retardation (UK: learning disability) or cognitive decline; basal ganglia dysfunction (dystonia, chorea, rigidity, bradykinesia, tics, orofacial dyskinesia) may also occur as early features. Seizures are reported. These features may be present alone or in combination with ataxia. The EEG may be normal, show diffuse slowing or epileptic discharges. The MRI may show cerebellar, cortical, brainstem, and basal ganglia atrophy, but some patients are reported to have normal MRI appearances.

There are only rare reports of children affected with SCA17 and they do not seem to have clinical features that are different from adults although the progression appears to be faster. There may also be growth retardation and hypogonadotropic hypogonadism (Maltecca et al. 2003; Rasmussen et al. 2007).

Dentatorubropallidoluysian atrophy

Dentatorubropallidoluysian atrophy (DRPLA) is a complex autosomal dominant disorder which includes the clinical features of ataxia. However, there are always other neurological features and the brain pathology, as indicated by the name, is more widespread than just the cerebellum (Kanazawa 1998). The condition has been most frequently described in the Japanese population but is also rarely found in other ethnic groups.

The gene mutation is located on chromosome 12p13.31 and is a CAG trinucleotide repeat in exon 5 of the *Atrophin1* gene. The normal repeat size is 7–34 and in patients is up to 88. As with the other CAG repeat disorders, there is an inverse correlation between the repeat size and the age at onset. However, only 62% of the variation in age at onset is explained by the repeat size, suggesting that other factors are involved. There is anticipation with marked instability of the repeat with paternal transmission. Homozygous cases show a more severe clinical phenotype.

Some authors classify DRPLA into juvenile onset (under 20 years of age) and adult onset (over 20 years of age) (Komure et al. 1995). This is based on the difference in presentation of the two groups. In juvenile-onset cases there is usually severe myoclonic epilepsy and other types of seizures, severe cognitive impairment, and mild cerebellar ataxia. As the condition progresses myoclonus, choreoathetosis, and severe ataxia develop. Two patients have been reported who also had autistic spectrum disorder and obstructive sleep apnea in addition to the other features (Licht and Lynch 2002). In adult-onset cases there is usually cerebellar ataxia and choreoathetosis, behavioural and psychiatric disorders, while myoclonus, seizures, and dementia are less common. The condition progresses more quickly in the juvenile-onset cases. EEG abnormalities are common, especially in early-onset cases, with paroxysmal diffuse spike and wave abnormalities and a slow basic rhythm. Up to half of early-onset cases also have photosensitivity. CT and MRI shows cerebellar and cortical atrophy, dilatation of the lateral and fourth ventricles, tegmental atrophy of the midbrain, and in later-onset cases high signal lesions on T2-weighted MRI. Pathologically the cerebellum has been described as small but well formed, which raises the issue of whether it is hypoplastic to begin with. Microscopically, the neurons of the dentate nucleus are severely affected, with some gliosis. Those neurons that remain are atrophic or vacuolated. The Luys body (subthalamic nucleus) sometimes shows neuronal loss but this is milder than the pallidum, of which the external segments are usually more affected. The red nucleus neurons are the least affected. There is decreased staining for myelin in the cerebral white matter which is thought to be the pathological correlate of the high intensity lesions seen on MRI and is thought to be responsible for the dementia.

A variant of DRPLA is the Haw River syndrome described in a several African-American families. It is characterized by a lack of myoclonic epilepsy, extensive demyelination of the subcortical white matter, basal ganglia calcification, and neuroaxonal dystrophy. The genetic change is the same with 63–68 repeats of the CAG in the *Atrophin 1* gene (Burke et al. 1994). Haplotype analysis reveals a different founder origin from those of both Japanese and Caucasian background.

Spinocerebellar ataxias caused by mechanisms other than nucleotide repeat expansion

Spinocerebellar ataxia type 5

Spinocerebellar ataxia type 5 (SCA5) is an uncommon, relatively 'pure' cerebellar ataxia caused by mutations in the ß III spectrin gene (*SPTBN2*) located on chromosome 11q13. It is a well-known condition because an enormous family related to the US President Abraham Lincoln were affected, but otherwise appears to be very rare (Ranum et al. 1994). Other families from France and Germany have also been identified; all have different mutations, two are in-frame deletions, the third a missense mutation (Ikeda et al. 2006). The most common clinical features are gait and limb ataxia, dysarthria, abnormalities of saccadic eye movements, and nystagmus. The age at onset can be as early as 10 years old, although this only occurred in a very small fraction of the family members and most cases developed symptoms in the third or fourth decade. These patients also had pyramidal and bulbar dysfunction. MRI show cerebellar but no brainstem atrophy.

Spinocerebellar ataxia type 11

Spinocerebellar ataxia type 11 (SCA11) has only been described in two families, one from the UK and the other from Pakistan. The age at onset ranges from 15 to 43 and the predominant clinical features include progressive cerebellar ataxia of gait, limbs and trunk, and abnormal eye movements (jerky pursuit, horizontal and vertical nystagmus). Less commonly there are pyramidal features with hyperreflexia, a peripheral neuropathy, and dystonia. Two separate mutations in the two families have been found, both of which result in frameshifts in the tau-tubulin kinase 2 gene (*TTBK2*) resulting in nonsense-mediated decay (Houlden et al. 2007). The mechanism of action therefore appears to be haploinsufficiency of *TTBK2*. MRI shows atrophy of the cerebellar hemispheres. One case has come to postmortem examination and revealed loss of the Purkinje cell layer and proliferation of Bermann glial cells. No intranuclear inclusions such as those observed in the trinucleotide repeat disorders were seen (Johnson et al. 2008).

Spinocerebellar ataxia type 13

Spinocerebellar ataxia type 13 (SCA13) is a rare autosomal dominant ataxia resulting from mutations in the KCNV3 voltage-gated potassium channel located on chromosome 19q13 (Waters et al. 2006). A total of seven families have been reported. In three of these families the age at onset is in infancy to early childhood, with little or no progression throughout life. The condition is fully penetrant in the reported families. In the first family to be reported there was delay of developmental motor milestones, with independent walking achieved between 3 and 12 years. The patients had truncal and limb ataxia, dysarthria, nystagmus, and hyperreflexia. Mild cognitive impairment was present (IQ 62–76). Absence seizures were present in one patient. A Phe448Leu mutation was identified in the S5 transmembrane domain which is predicted to slow cerebellar neuron firing by reducing the closing rate of the channel. There were no seizures and in a single patient there was lower limb spasticity. In two other patients the phenotype was rather different, with no cognitive impairment and no seizures. CT was reported as normal in one of the affected children at age 3 but in older patients the MRI shows cerebellar atrophy. An Arg423His mutation was found and coexpression of mutant and wild-type subunits in a *Xenopus* oocyte system revealed a strong dominant negative effect.

The other four reported families have a late-onset, slowly progressive ataxia with gait and limb involvement, titubation, hypotonia, dysarthria, and occasional nystagmus and hyperreflexia. The mutation Arg420His also results in a nonfunctional subunit with dominant negative properties. Although specific mutations were associated with specific phenotypes it remains unclear why apparently similar functional effects give different phenotypes (Figueroa et al. 2010).

Spinocerebellar ataxia type 14

Spinocerebellar ataxia type 14 (SCA14) is caused by missense mutations in the protein kinase C gamma gene (*PRKCG*) located on chromosome 19q13.4 (Chen et al. 2003). The initial symptoms are usually a progressive gait ataxia, associated later on with dysarthria and nystagmus. There may be brisk reflexes. There is no peripheral neuropathy, seizures, parkinsonian features or cognitive decline. The age at onset ranges from 5 to 60 but is usually in early adult life. Most people remain ambulatory and have a normal lifespan. Some patients from Japan are reported to have myoclonus, vertigo, and dystonia. A Dutch family has been reported in which the age at onset was 3 years and clinical features included gait ataxia and action myoclonus (Vlak et al. 2006). Cerebellar atrophy was noted on MRI. *PRKCG*-null mice are neurologically normal, suggesting that the missense mutations result in a toxic gain of function.

Spinocerebellar ataxia type 15

Spinocerebellar ataxia type 15 (SCA15) was originally mapped to distal chromosome 3p and SCA16 to 3p26. Mutation screening of the *ITPR1* (inositol 1,4,5-trisphosphate receptor type 1) gene within the candidate initially did not reveal any pathogenic changes (Knight et al. 2003). Subsequently, a mouse model with ataxia revealed mutations in the *ITPR1* gene and this gene was retested in families with SCA15 and SCA16 mapping to this region (van de Leemput et al. 2007). Mutations were not identified by standard sequencing and were only found once alternative techniques were used which identify large gene deletions. The total loss of one functional copy of *ITPR1* suggests that this the disorder is caused by haploinsufficiency. Evaluation of an SCA16 family also demonstrated a large deletion in *ITPR1* which encompasses most of the gene (Iwaki et al. 2008). Therefore SCA15 and SCA16 are both caused by mutations in this gene and the term SCA16 is no longer used. One family has been described with a 'missense mutation' but the pathogenicity of this change has yet to be proven.

The clinical features of SCA15 include a slowly progressive gait and limb ataxia, dysarthria, titubation, upper limb postural tremor, mild hyperreflexia, gaze-evoked nystagmus, and an impaired vestibulo-ocular reflex. Onset is between ages 7 and 66 years, usually with gait ataxia but sometimes with tremor. Affected individuals remain ambulant for 10 to 54 years after onset. Mild dysphagia and movement-induced oscillopsia after several decades of symptoms have been observed in members of two of the seven families known to have SCA15. MRI showed prominent atrophy of the cerebellar vermis with minimal cerebellar hemisphere involvement and sparing of the brainstem. One patient in an Italian family also showed bilateral frontoparietal atrophy (Di Gregorio et al. 2010).

Spinocerebellar ataxia type 27

Spinocerebellar ataxia type 27 (SCA27) is caused by mutations of the gene for fibroblast growth factor 14 isoform b, located on chromosome 13q34. The first family described was of Dutch descent and the presenting clinical features were tremor or trembling exacerbated by stress or exercise in childhood followed by gait and upper limb ataxia in adolescence or early adulthood. There were aggressive outbursts and depression in some patients and several did not complete primary education. Neurological examination revealed abnormal pursuit and saccadic eye movements, dysarthria, a high-frequency low amplitude tremor of the hands, and in some a head tremor and orofacial dyskinesias. Some had brisk knee reflexes and absent vibration sense at the ankles. Moderate cerebellar atrophy was present on MRI in some but not all patients. The first mutation identified was a missense mutation, *F145S* (van Swieten et al. 2003).

A second case was reported with a frameshift mutation. This patient had an age at onset of 12 years with a progressive gait disturbance, memory loss, and depression. He had a mild mental retardation (IQ 70). On examination he had gait and trunk ataxia, tremor in both hands, nystagmus, and pes cavus. Nerve conduction studies revealed a mild sensory axonal neuropathy. His father was reported to have memory loss, gait disturbance, and pes cavus but had died of other causes and could not be examined (Dalski et al. 2005). A third family has been reported with a more severe phenotype caused by a translocation through the gene (Misceo et al. 2009). The mother and daughter had an identical translocation breakpoint through the *FGF14* gene. The clinical features in the daughter included developmental delay and microcephaly from birth, truncal ataxia, gait ataxia, an intention tremor, occasional dyskinetic jerky movements, and mild dysmorphic features including a short neck and fifth finger clinodactyly. MRI and nerve conduction studies were normal. The mother had mild learning difficulties and went to a special school. She was treated for seizures as a child and had a mild loss of balance.

Spinocerebellar ataxia type 28

Spinocerebellar ataxia type 28 (SCA28) is caused by missense mutations in *AFG3L2*, a mitochondrial metalloprotease on chromosome 18p11.21 (Di Bella et al. 2010). The mutations are reported to cause defective complex IV function in yeast cells. There is evidence for both haploinsufficiency (*AFG3L2* knockout mice have a cerebellar phenotype) and a dominant negative effect (replacement of wild-type gene does not correct some cellular models with missense mutations). Some prevalence data suggest that up to 3% of cases which are negative for triplet expansions may be caused by *AFG3L2* mutations (Cagnoli et al. 2010). The clinical features of SCA28 include a generally early onset (many in later childhood or adolescence, 12–36, mean 19.5 years), with gait and limb ataxia, nystagmus, mild ophthalmoparesis, dysarthria, brisk reflexes, bilateral clonus, and extensor plantars. As the disease progresses some individuals have a more severe ophthalmoparesis, very slow saccades, ptosis, and a wide-based gait. Most individuals have a normal lifespan. There is no cognitive impairment (Cagnoli et al. 2006). Another missense change has been reported in a German family but the pathogenicity remains unproven. The age at onset in this family was 10 years (Edener et al. 2010).

Conclusions

Genetic testing for cerebellar ataxias in children should be directed by the clinical presentation and the family history. However, the neurological features are highly variable and genetic testing may need to be extensive, in which case referral to a specialist centre for both neurological and clinical genetics assessments is advised. Genetic testing may expand in the future because of advances in technology but this will require expert interpretation to determine the pathogenicity of specific genetic changes. At the current time many patients will remain without a secure molecular diagnosis and further research is required in these cases.

REFERENCES

Abdel-Aleem A, Zaki MS (2008) Spinocerebellar ataxia type 2 (SCA2) in an Egyptian family presenting with polyphagia and marked CAG expansion in infancy. J Neurol 255: 413–419.

Babovic-Vuksanovic D, Snow K, Patterson MC, Michels VV (1998) Spinocerebellar ataxia type 2 (SCA 2) in an infant with extreme CAG repeat expansion. Am J Med Genet 79: 383–387.

Benton CS, de Silva R, Rutledge SL, Bohlega S, Ashizawa T, Zoghbi HY (1998) Molecular and clinical studies in SCA-7 define a broad clinical spectrum and the infantile phenotype. Neurology 51: 1081–1086.

Brusco A, Cagnoli C, Franco A, Dragone E, Nardacchione A, Grosso E, et al. (2002) Analysis of SCA8 and SCA12 loci in 134 Italian ataxic patients negative for SCA1-3, 6 and 7 CAG expansions. J Neurol 249: 923–929.

Burke JR, Wingfield MS, Lewis KE, Roses AD, Lee JE, Hulette C, et al. (1994) The Haw River syndrome: dentatorubropallidoluysian atrophy (DRPLA) in an African-American family. Nat Genet 7: 521–524.

Cagnoli C, Stevanin G, Brussino A, Barberis M, Mancini C, Margolis RL, et al. (2010) Missense mutations in the AFG3L2 proteolytic domain account for <1.5% of European autosomal dominant cerebellar ataxias. Hum Mutat 31: 1117–1124.

Cagnoli C, Mariotti C, Taroni F, Seri M, Brussino A, Michielotto C, et al. (2006) SCA28, a novel form of autosomal dominant cerebellar ataxia on chromosome 18p11.22-q11.2. Brain 129(Pt 1): 235–242.

Carvalho DR, La Rocque-Ferreira A, Rizzo IM, Imamura EU, Speck-Martins CE (2008) Homozygosity enhances severity in spinocerebellar ataxia type 3. Pediatr Neurol 38: 296–299.

Cellini E, Nacmias B, Forleo P, Piacentini S, Guarnieri BM, Serio A, et al. (2001) Genetic and clinical analysis of spinocerebellar ataxia type 8 repeat expansion in Italy. Arch Neurol 58: 1856–1859.

Chen DH, Brkanac Z, Verlinde CL, Tan XJ, Bylenok L, Nochlin D, et al. (2003) Missense mutations in the regulatory domain of PKC gamma: a new mechanism for dominant nonepisodic cerebellar ataxia. Am J Hum Genet 72: 839–849.

Dalski A, Atici J, Kreuz FR, Hellenbroich Y, Schwinger E, Zühlke C (2005) Mutation analysis in the fibroblast growth factor 14 gene: frameshift mutation and polymorphisms in patients with inherited ataxias. Eur J Hum Genet 13(1): 118–120.

Day JW, Schut LJ, Moseley ML, Durand AC, Ranum LP (2000) Spinocerebellar ataxiam type 8: clinical features in a large family. Neurology 55: 649–657.

Di Bella D, Lazzaro F, Brusco A, Plumari M, Battaglia G, Pastore A, et al. (2010) Mutations in the mitochondrial protease gene AFG3L2 cause dominant hereditary ataxia SCA28. Nat Genet 42: 313–321.

Di Gregorio E, Orsi L, Godani M, Vaula G, Jensen S, Salmon E, et al. (2010) Two Italian families with ITPR1 gene deletion presenting a broader phenotype of SCA15. Cerebellum 9: 115–123.

Edener U, Wöllner J, Hehr U, Kohl Z, Schilling S, Kreuz F, et al. (2010) Early onset and slow progression of SCA28, a rare dominant ataxia in a large four-generation family with a novel AFG3L2 mutation. Eur J Hum Genet 18: 965–968.

Felling RJ, Barron TF (2005) Early onset of ataxia in a child with a pathogenic SCA8 allele. Pediatr Neurol 33: 136–138. Review.

Figueroa KP, Minassian NA, Stevanin G, Waters M, Garibyan V, Forlani S, et al. (2010) KCNC3: phenotype, mutations, channel biophysics-a study of 260 familial ataxia patients. Hum Mutat 31: 191–196.

Fujigasaki H, Verma IC, Camuzat A, Margolis RL, Zander C, Lebre AS, et al. (2001) SCA12 is a rare locus for autosomal dominant cerebellar ataxia: a study of an Indian family. Ann Neurol 49: 117–121.

Hoischen A, Gilissen C, Arts P, Wieskamp N, van der Vliet W, Vermeer S, et al. (2010) Massively parallel sequencing of ataxia genes after array-based enrichment. Hum Mutat 31: 494–499.

Holmes SE, O'Hearn EE, McInnis MG, Gorelick-Feldman DA, Kleiderlein JJ, Callahan C, et al. (1999) Expansion of a novel CAG trinucleotide repeat in the 5′ region of PPP2R2B is associated with SCA12. Nat Genet 23: 391–392.

Houlden H, Johnson J, Gardner-Thorpe C, Lashley T, Hernandez D, Worth P, et al. (2007) Mutations in TTBK2, encoding a kinase implicated in tau phosphorylation, segregate with spinocerebellar ataxia type 11. Nat Genet 39: 1434–1436.

Ikeda Y, Dick KA, Weatherspoon MR, Gincel D, Armbrust KR, Dalton JC, et al. (2006) Spectrin mutations cause spinocerebellar ataxia type 5. Nat Genet 38: 184–190.

Iwaki A, Kawano Y, Miura S, Shibata H, Matsuse D, Li W, et al. (2008) Heterozygous deletion of ITPR1, but not SUMF1, in spinocerebellar ataxia type 16. J Med Genet 45: 32–35.

Johnson J, Wood N, Giunti P, Houlden H (2008) Clinical and genetic analysis of spinocerebellar ataxia type 11. Cerebellum 7: 159–164.

Kanazawa I (1998) Dentatorubral-pallidoluysian atrophy or Naito-Oyanagi disease. Neurogenetics 2: 1–17.

Kawaguchi Y, Okamoto T, Taniwaki M, Aizawa M, Inoue M, Katayama S, et al. (1994) CAG expansions in a novel gene for Machado-Joseph disease at chromosome 14q32.1. Nat Genet 8: 221–228.

Knight MA, Kennerson ML, Anney RJ, Matsuura T, Nicholson GA, Salimi-Tari P, et al. (2003) Spinocerebellar ataxia type 15 (sca15) maps to 3p24.2–3pter: exclusion of the ITPR1 gene, the human orthologue of an ataxic mouse mutant. Neurobiol Dis 13: 147–157.

Komure O, Sano A, Nishino N, Yamauchi N, Ueno S, Kondoh K, et al. (1995) DNA analysis in hereditary dentatorubral-pallidoluysian atrophy: correlation between CAG repeat length and phenotypic variation and the molecular basis of anticipation. Neurology 45: 143–149.

Koob MD, Moseley ML, Schut LJ, Benzow KA, Bird TD, Day JW, Ranum LP (1999) An untranslated CTG expansion causes a novel form of spinocerebellar ataxia (SCA8). Nat Genet 21: 379–384.

Licht DJ, Lynch DR (2002) Juvenile dentatorubral-pallidoluysian atrophy: new clinical features. Pediatr Neurol 26: 51–54.

Lin X, Ashizawa T (2005) Recent progress in spinocerebellar ataxia type-10 (SCA10). Cerebellum 4(1): 37–42.

Maltecca F, Filla A, Castaldo I, Coppola G, Fragassi NA, Carella M, et al. (2003) Intergenerational instability and marked anticipation in SCA-17. Neurology 61(10): 1441–1443.

Mao R, Aylsworth AS, Potter N, Wilson WG, Breningstall G, Wick MJ, et al. (2002) Childhood-onset ataxia: testing for large CAG-repeats in SCA2 and SCA7. Am J Med Genet 110: 338–345.

Michalik A, Martin JJ, Van Broeckhoven C (2004) Spinocerebellar ataxia type 7 associated with pigmentary retinal dystrophy. Eur J Hum Genet 12: 2–15.

Misceo D, Fannemel M, Barøy T, Roberto R, Tvedt B, Jaeger T, et al. (2009) SCA27 caused by a chromosome translocation: further delineation of the phenotype. Neurogenetics 10: 371–374.

Moseley ML, Zu T, Ikeda Y, Gao W, Mosemiller AK, Daughters RS, et al. (2006) Bidirectional expression of CUG and CAG expansion transcripts and intranuclear polyglutamine inclusions in spinocerebellar ataxia type 8. Nat Genet 38: 758–769.

Munhoz RP, Teive HA, Raskin S, Werneck LC (2009) CTA/CTG expansions at the SCA 8 locus in multiple system atrophy. Clin Neurol Neurosurg 111: 208–210.

Orozco Diaz G, Nodarse Fleites A, Cordovés Sagaz R, Auburger G (1990) Autosomal dominant cerebellar ataxia: clinical analysis of 263 patients from a homogeneous population in Holguín, Cuba. Neurology 40: 1369–1375.

Orr HT, Chung MY, Banfi S, Kwiatkowski TJ Jr, Servadio A, Beaudet AL, et al. (1993) Expansion of an unstable trinucleotide CAG repeat in spinocerebellar ataxia type 1. Nat Genet 4: 221–226.

Ranum LP, Schut LJ, Lundgren JK, Orr HT, Livingston DM (1994) Spinocerebellar ataxia type 5 in a family descended from the grandparents of President Lincoln maps to chromosome 11. Nat Genet 8: 280–284.

Rasmussen A, De Biase I, Fragoso-Benítez M, Macías-Flores MA, Yescas P, Ochoa A, et al. (2007) Anticipation and intergenerational repeat instability in spinocerebellar ataxia type 17. Ann Neurol 61: 607–610.

Riess O, Rüb U, Pastore A, Bauer P, Schöls L (2008) SCA3: neurological features, pathogenesis and animal models. Cerebellum 7: 125–137.

Rosenberg RN (1992) Machado-Joseph disease: an autosomal dominant motor system degeneration. Mov Disord 7: 193–203.

Schöls L, Bauer I, Zühlke C, Schulte T, Kölmel C, Bürk K, et al. (2003) Do CTG expansions at the SCA8 locus cause ataxia? Ann Neurol 54: 110–115.

Shibata-Hamaguchi A, Ishida C, Iwasa K, Yamada M (2009) Prevalence of spinocerebellar degenerations in the Hokuriku district in Japan. Neuroepidemiology 32: 176–183.

Silveira I, Alonso I, Guimarães L, Mendonça P, Santos C, Maciel P, et al. (2000) High germinal instability of the (CTG)n at the SCA8 locus of both expanded and normal alleles. Am J Hum Genet 66: 830–840.

Srivastava AK, Choudhry S, Gopinath MS, Roy S, Tripathi M, Brahmachari SK, Jain S (2001) Molecular and clinical correlation in five Indian families with spinocerebellar ataxia 12. Ann Neurol 50: 796–800.

Stevanin G, Brice A (2008) Spinocerebellar ataxia 17 (SCA17) and Huntington's disease-like 4 (HDL4). Cerebellum 7: 170–178.

Stevanin G, Herman A, Dürr A, Jodice C, Frontali M, Agid Y, Brice A (2000) Are (CTG)n expansions at the SCA8 locus rare polymorphisms? Nat Genet 24: 213.

Tazón B, Badenas C, Jiménez L, Muñoz E, Milà M (2002) SCA8 in the Spanish population including one homozygous patient Clin Genet 62: 404–409.

van de Leemput J, Chandran J, Knight MA, Holtzclaw LA, Scholz S, Cookson MR, et al. (2007) Deletion at ITPR1 underlies ataxia in mice and spinocerebellar ataxia 15 in humans. PLoS Genet 3: e108.

van de Warrenburg BP, Frenken CW, Ausems MG, Kleefstra T, Sinke RJ, Knoers NV, Kremer HP (2001) Striking anticipation in spinocerebellar ataxia type 7: the infantile phenotype. J Neurol 248: 911–914.

van Swieten JC, Brusse E, de Graaf BM, Krieger E, van de Graaf R, de Koning I, et al. (2003) A mutation in the fibroblast growth factor 14 gene is associated with autosomal dominant cerebellar ataxia [corrected]. Am J Hum Genet 72: 191–199.

Vlak MH, Sinke RJ, Rabelink GM, Kremer BP, van de Warrenburg BP (2006) Novel PRKCG/SCA14 mutation in a Dutch spinocerebellar ataxia family: expanding the phenotype. Mov Disord 21: 1025–1028.

Wadia NH, Swami RK (1971) A new form of heredo-familial spinocerebellar degeneration with slow eye movements (nine families). Brain 94: 359–374.

Wang X, Wang H, Xia Y, Jiang H, Shen L, Wang S, et al. (2010) A neuropathological study at autopsy of early onset spinocerebellar ataxia 6. J Clin Neurosci 17: 751–755.

Waters MF, Minassian NA, Stevanin G, Figueroa KP, Bannister JP, Nolte D, et al. (2006) Mutations in voltage-gated potassium channel KCNC3 cause degenerative and developmental central nervous system phenotypes. Nat Genet 38: 447–451.

Whitney A, Lim M, Kanabar D, Lin JP (2007) Massive SCA7 expansion detected in a 7-month-old male with hypotonia, cardiomegaly, and renal compromise. Dev Med Child Neurol 49: 140–143.

Worth PF, Houlden H, Giunti P, Davis MB, Wood NW (2000) Large, expanded repeats in SCA8 are not confined to patients with cerebellar ataxia. Nat Genet 24: 214–215.

Yiş U, Dirik E, Kurul SH, Eken AG, Başak AN (2009) Two young sisters with spinocerebellar ataxia type 2 showing different clinical progression of disease. Cerebellum 8: 127–129.

Zeman A, Stone J, Porteous M, Burns E, Barron L, Warner J (2004) Spinocerebellar ataxia type 8 in Scotland: genetic and clinical features in seven unrelated cases and a review of published reports. J Neurol Neurosurg Psychiatry 75: 459–465.

Zhou YX, Takiyama Y, Igarashi S, Li YF, Zhou BY, Gui DC, et al. (1997) Machado-Joseph disease in four Chinese pedigrees: molecular analysis of 15 patients including two juvenile cases and clinical correlations. Neurology 48: 482–485.

Zoghbi HY, Pollack MS, Lyons LA, Ferrell RE, Daiger SP, Beaudet AL (1988) Spinocerebellar ataxia: variable age of onset and linkage to human leukocyte antigen in a large kindred. Ann Neurol 23: 580–584.

25
X-linked Cerebellar Disorders

Ginevra Zanni and Enrico Bertini

X-linked cerebellar disorders (XLCD) are a genetically and clinically heterogeneous group of disorders in which the hallmark is cerebellar dysgenesis (hypoplasia, atrophy or dysplasia) visible on brain imaging, associated with gene mutations or genomic imbalances on the X chromosome. The neurological features of XLCD include hypotonia at birth, developmental delay, abnormal eye movements, ataxia and/or other cerebellar signs, intellectual disability or normal cognitive development. Cerebellar dysgenesis may be isolated or associated with other brain malformations or multiorgan involvement. To date, at least three genes (*OPHN1*, *CASK*, and *SLC9A6*) encoding for proteins involved in neuronal morphogenesis and synaptic plasticity have been consistently associated with X-linked forms of cerebellar disorders. In other X-linked syndromes, cerebellar defects are increasingly being recognized. A number of loci have been mapped on the X chromosome and several families with an X-linked cerebellar phenotype have been reported. The clinical, neuroradiological and molecular aspects of these rare conditions will be explored in detail.

X-linked cerebellar disorders with known genes

OPHN1 SYNDROME

Clinical and genetic aspects

OPHN1 syndrome (MIM 300486) was first described in a 12-year-old female, carrier of a de novo translocation t(X;12)(q11;q15) which was successively found to disrupt the Oligophrenin-1 (*OPHN1*) gene (Bienvenu et al. 1997; Billuart et al. 1998). The girl had congenital hypotonia, severe developmental delay, moderate cognitive impairment, early-onset complex partial seizures, and bilateral divergent strabismus and dysmetria. At a later reevaluation, brain MRI showed a posterior vermis dysplasia including a partial agenesis of lobules VI and VII associated with right vermian parasagittal cleft and mild hypoplasia of the cerebellar hemispheres. A consistent dilatation of the lateral cerebral ventricles and a mild cortical atrophy was also present. A similar clinico-radiological phenotype (Table 25.1, Fig. 25.1a–c) was found in the affected males

TABLE 25.1
Clinical and neuroimaging features of the main X-linked cerebellar disorders

	OPHN1	***CASK***	***SLC9A6***
Developmental delay/ hypotonia	Moderate	Moderate to severe	Severe
Intellectual disability	Moderate to severe	Normal to severe	Severe
Cerebellar ataxia/signs	+ (Ataxia is rare)	+	+
Seizures	+ (50%)	+ (50%)	+
Other neurological signs	—	Spasticity, tremor	Hyperkinetic movements, dystonia, hemiparesis
Ocular findings	Strabismus, nystagmus, ophthalmoplegia	Nystagmus, optic nerve hypoplasia, cataract, retinal coloboma	Strabismus, ophthalmoplegia
Behavior	Hyperactive anxious	nd	Angelman-like autistic behavior
Craniofacial features	Normal OFC/macrocephaly, long face, deep-set eyes, large ears, prominent jaw	Normal OFC/micro- or macrocephaly, hypertelorism, broad nasal bridge, large ears, micrognathia	Microcephaly, large ears, square jaw
Other associated findings	Hypogenitalism, tall stature	Hearing loss, short stature, scoliosis	Flexed arms, adducted thumbs, swallowing difficulties
MRI findings	Cerebellar hypoplasia (vermis lobules VI–VII), vermischisis, cystic dilatation of posterior fossa, ventriculomegaly, cortical atrophy, caudate nuclei hypoplasia	Cerebellar hypoplasia, flat pons, enlarged 4th ventricle, thin corpus callosum, simplified cortical gyri	Cerebellar atrophy, prominent cisterna magna, pontine atrophy, ↑ glutamate in the basal ganglia (MRS)

nd, not determined; OFC, occipito-frontal circumference; MRS, magnetic resonance spectroscopy.

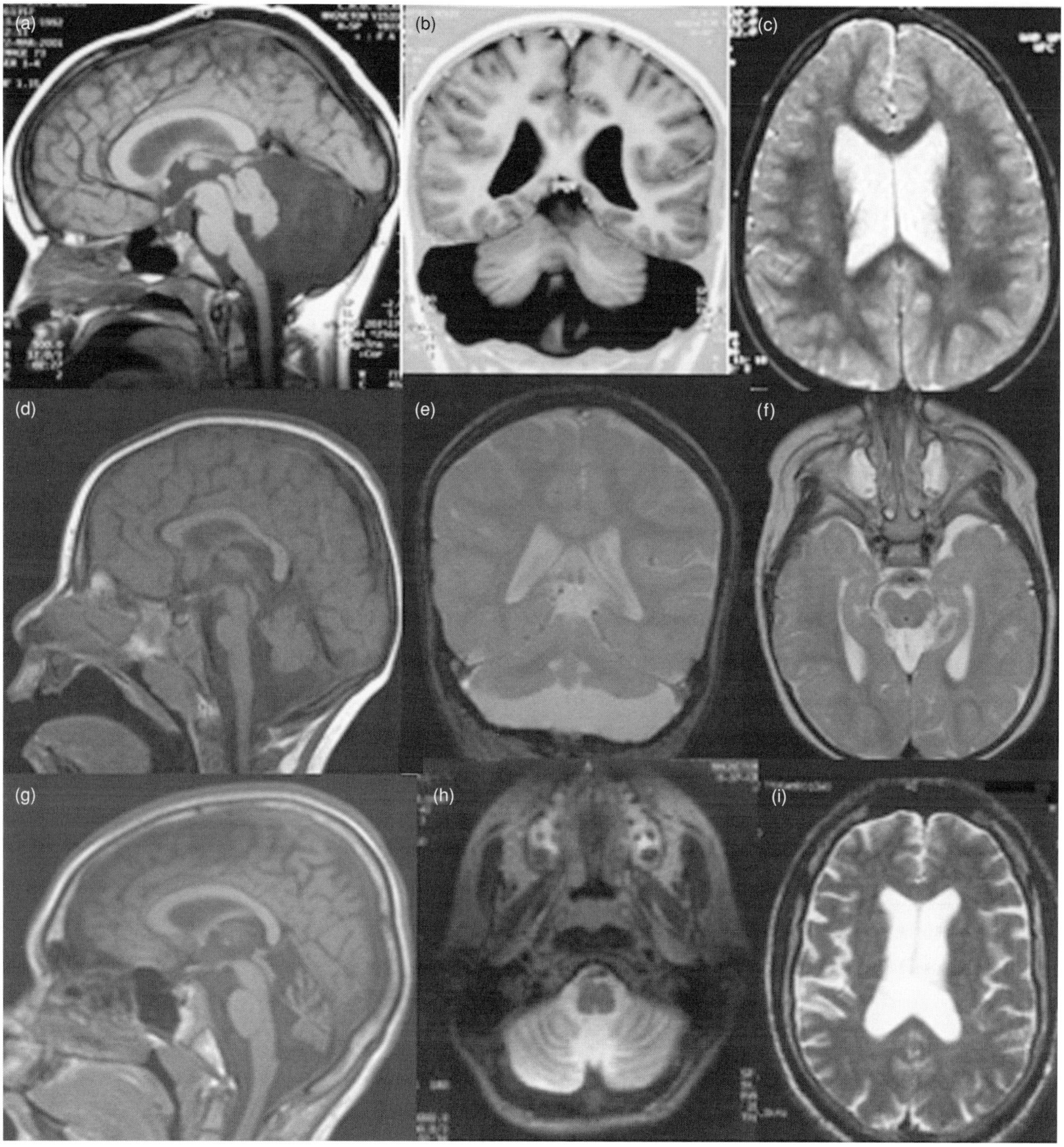

Fig. 25.1. Brain MRI studies of patients with *OPHN1, CASK* and *SLC9A6* mutations. 1a–c (*OPHN1*): midsagittal T1-weighted image showing hypoplastic cerebella vermis and enlarged cisterna magna **(a)** coronal Inversion Recovery image showing global cerebellar hypoplasia **(b)** axial T2-weighted image showing lateral ventricle dilatation **(c)**. 1d–f (*CASK*): midsagittal T1-weighted image showing moderate vermis hypoplasia and flat pons **(d)** coronal T2-weighted image showing global cerebellar hypoplasia and simplified cortical gyri **(e)** axial T2-weighted image showing simplified gyral pattern **(f)**. 1g–i (*SLC9A6*): midsagittal T1-weighted image **(g)** and axial T2-weighted image **(h)** showing cerebellar atrophy. Axial T2 weighted image showing moderate ventricular enlargement and sulcal widening **(i)**. Figures **(a)**, **(b)** and **(c)** reproduced with permission from Neurology 2005; 65(9): 1364–9. Figure **(g)** reproduced with permission from Am J Hum Genet 2008; 82(4): 1003–10. Figure **(h)** reproduced with permission from J Med Genet 1999; 36(10): 759–66. Figure **(i)** reproduced with permission from Brain 2010; (Pt 5): 1391–402.

of a family carrying a single nucleotide deletion in exon 19 of the *OPHN1*, initially diagnosed with nonsyndromic X-linked mental retardation (UK usage: learning disability) (Des Portes et al. 2004). Another deletion comprising exon 19 of the *OPHN1* gene was identified by Bergmann et al. (2003) in a family with five affected males showing moderate to severe mental retardation, infantile-onset epilepsy, hypotonia, strabismus, and ataxia. Cryptorchidism and genital hypoplasia were present in all affected males. Neuroradiological findings included cortical atrophy, enlargement of the cerebral ventricles, bilateral hypoplasia of the head of the caudate nucleus, lower vermis and cerebellar hemisphere hypoplasia. One carrier sister had mild learning disabilities and strabismus but her brain MRI was normal. Philip et al. (2003) found a stop mutation in exon 3 and an 8bp insertion in exon 9 of the *OPHN1* gene in two families with congenital hypotonia, moderate to severe cognitive and motor delay, macrocephaly, tall stature, and dysmorphic facial features: deep-set eyes, long nose, short philtrum, and prominent chin. One affected individual showed abnormal behaviour with stereotypies and tendency to self-mutilation.

At brain MRI studies, large pericerebral spaces, ventricular dilatation requiring ventriculoperitoneal shunt placement, cerebellar hypoplasia, and cystic dilatation of the posterior fossa were noted. Chabrol et al. (2005) reported a family with a 2bp deletion in exon 8 of *OPHN1* leading to a premature stop codon. The patients showed developmental and cognitive delay with IQ ranging from 46 to 54, strabismus, early-onset generalized tonico-clonic seizures, abnormal behaviour, and a characteristic facial phenotype with long face, prominent forehead, infraorbital creases, deep-set eyes, upturned philtrum, and large ears. The obligate carrier females showed only mild cognitive impairment and subtle facial changes. Brain MRI studies performed in the propositus at 3 months of age showed underdeveloped frontal lobes, loss of brain volumes with enlarged lateral ventricles, prominent subarachnoid spaces, and a particular square shape of the frontal horns. Cerebellar hypoplasia and dysplastic vermis with a large cisterna magna and a retrocerebellar cyst were also recognized.

A girl with mild mental retardation, early-onset ataxia, seizures started at 10 months, and tall stature was found to be a carrier of a de novo translocation t(X;9)(q12;p13.3) disrupting the *OPHN1* gene (Menten et al. 2007). Brain MRI showed moderately enlarged cerebral ventricles with the frontal horn of lateral ventricles most prominently enlarged, hypoplasia of the caudate nucleus, dilated fourth ventricle, and vermian hypoplasia. Intragenic deletions of *OPHN1*, detected by array-comparative genomic hybridization (CGH) were reported in a male patient and in two families in which affected males all showed the characteristic clinico-radiological phenotype associated with OPHN1 syndrome (Froyen et al. 2007; Madrigal et al. 2008; Al-Owain et al. 2010). Contiguous gene deletions and a duplication encompassing the *OPHN1* gene have also been reported (Tentler et al. 1999; Wieland et al. 2007; Bedeschi et al. 2008). Screening *OPHN1* in a large cohort of patients (Zanni et al. 2005) identified mutations in 12% of individuals with intellectual deficit and cerebellar hypoplasia, suggesting that the screening of this gene should be implemented in boys with vermis hypoplasia enlarged cerebral ventricles and developmental delay and that those families should be counseled for high risk of X-linked inheritance.

Molecular aspects

The *OPHN1* gene (MIM 300127) is located in Xq12 and contains 23 coding exons. It encodes for a RhoGTPase activating protein (RhoGAP). Dysfunction of OPHN1 results in the constitutive activation of Rho signaling pathways, involved in cellular processes such as cell migration, neuronal morphogenesis and synaptic function (Billuart et al. 1998). OPHN1 protein is expressed in multiple tissues with the highest expression in the developing CNS. Expression in the brain is enriched in the hippocampus, the olfactory bulb, and the PC layer of the cerebellum. In vivo and in vitro analysis of the hippocampi of mice mutants showed an increase of immature spines and a reduction of size and number of mature spines coupled with alterations of short-term synaptic plasticity (Govek et al. 2004; Khelfaoui et al. 2007). OPHN1 loss of function was found to reduce endocytosis both at the presynaptic (synaptic vesicle recycling) and at the postsynaptic level (glutamate receptors AMPAR internalization) through upregulation of the RhoA/ROCK pathway and possibly impaired interaction with proteins involved in clathrin mediated endocytosis (Khelfaoui et al. 2009; Nakano-Kobayashi et al. 2009).

CASK SYNDROME

Clinical and genetic aspects

Calcium/calmodulin dependent serine protein kinase (CASK) syndrome (MIM 300749) was first described by (Naijm et al. 2008) in a 4-year-old girl, carrier of an apparently de novo paracentric inversion 46X, inv(X)(p11.4p22.3) disrupting the *CASK* gene. The patient showed marked congenital and postnatal microcephaly, severe developmental delay, seizures, and sensorineural hearing loss. She had minor facial anomalies: low forehead, hypertelorism, broad nasal bridge, smooth philtrum, large ears, and micrognathia. She also had episodic hyperpnea and optic disc pallor with anisocoria. Brain MRI showed cerebellar hypoplasia predominant in the vermis, a small pons with flattened basis pontis, mildly enlarged fourth ventricle, and reduced number and complexity of cortical gyri. By screening a series of patients with microcephaly, developmental delay, and pontine and cerebellar hypoplasia, Najm et al. (2008) found, in three girls with a clinical and neuroradiological phenotype very similar to the first described patient (Table 25.1, Fig. 25.1d–f), de novo mutations of *CASK*: two heterozygous deletions (one 740kb deletion covering *CASK* and a double deletion in the 5′ and 3′ regions of the gene) identified by array-CGH and one missense mutation in exon 21 leading to a premature stop codon. A hemizygous mutation partially affecting the splice of exon 9 in a severely affected boy who died at 2 weeks was also found. Mid-hindbrain hypoplasia was more severe, the corpus callosum was thin and unmyelinated, and the cortex showed an area of pachygyria. Neuropathological examination of the cerebellum showed poorly formed and unbranched folia, a virtually absent internal granular layer, and an abnormally thick external granular layer. The molecular layer was hypercellular and disorganized.

Previous to *CASK* identification, two large deletions including the *CASK* gene had been identified by array-CGH in two girls with severe developmental delay, microcephaly, and multiple congenital anomalies partially overlapping the severe

CASK phenotype (Froyen et al. 2007; Hayashi et al. 2008). Piluso et al. (2009) found a missense mutation of *CASK* which partially disrupts the splicing of exon 2 in a family with three affected males diagnosed with FG syndrome (MIM 305450) who showed congenital hypotonia, chronic constipation, severe mental retardation, bilateral sensorineural deafness, seizures, and hyperactive aggressive behaviour. The mother of the proband showed mild intellectual impairment and suffered from absence attacks. In addition all mutated males had relative macrocephaly and minor facial anomalies: broad forehead, frontal upsweep of the hair, hypertelorism, saddled root of the nose, long philtrum, and micrognathia. Brain MRI of the proband was normal. Hackett et al. (2010) identified three novel missense mutations and one splice site mutation of *CASK* in four families with mild to moderate X-linked mental retardation and congenital nystagmus. Affected individuals had normal occipito-frontal circumference or relative macrocephaly. Brain imaging was only performed in two of the four families: in the proband of one family MRI showed pachygyria and cerebellar hypoplasia, while in the other family with half of the affected individuals having normal cognitive development, MRI was reported normal. Ocular findings included strabismus, cataracts, myopia or reduced visual acuity. Unsteady gait and seizures were present in some but not all affected individuals. In two additional families with apparently nonsyndromic XLMR, Hackett et al. (2010) found novel missense mutations in exon 8 and 27 of the *CASK* gene. The phenotypes associated with *CASK* mutations thus range from mild, apparently nonsyndromic MR with or without congenital nystagmus, to severe cognitive impairment associated with cerebellar and pontine hypoplasia and abormalities of cortical development.

Molecular aspects

The *CASK* gene (MIM 300749) is located at Xp11.4 and contains 27 coding exons. It encodes for a multidomain scaffolding protein that belongs to the membrane-associated guanylate kinase protein family of proteins which target to neuronal synapses and regulate trafficking, targeting, and signaling of ion channels. CASK is not a neural-specific protein but it is strongly expressed in fetal and adult brain (Stevenson et al. 2000). CASK controls synapse formation and function in many different ways.

1. At the nuclear level, CASK regulates the expression of genes such as *REELIN*, involved in cortical lamination and cerebellum development (Najm et al. 2008).
2. At the presynaptic level, CASK controls neurotransmitter release through its interaction with N-type calcium channels and protein complexes involved in synaptic vesicle recycling. CASK also regulates synaptic targeting of neurexin, a protein involved in transsynaptic adhesion.
3. At the postsynaptic level, CASK is involved in the stabilization of dendritic spines morphology and participates in the differential sorting and trafficking of glutamate receptors (Hsueh 2009). A specific role of CASK has been demonstrated in the biogenesis, transport, sorting, and recycling of glutamate receptors NMDA in a functionally distinct secretory pathway to dendritic Golgi outposts which bypasses the somatic Golgi for a more efficient synaptic delivery of these receptors (Jeyifous et al. 2009).

Christianson syndrome

Clinical and genetic aspects

Christianson syndrome (MIM 300243) was first described in a South African family of Norwegian descent in which 16 affected males suffered from profound mental retardation, absence of speech, early-onset generalized tonic-clonic epilepsy, bilateral ophthalmoplegia, and truncal/gait ataxia (Table 25.1). Three of the 10 obligate carrier females had mental retardation. In the patients, developmental milestones were severely retarded, with hypotonia progressing to spasticity, autistic features, microcephaly, and minor facial anomalies consisting of a long narrow face, prominent nose, square prognathic jaw, large ears, deep sunken eyes, and bushy eyebrows were noted. The chest was narrow, limb muscles were poorly developed, and joints were stiff and contractured. MRI showed a prominent cisterna magna, enlarged fourth ventricle, cerebellopontine and supracerebellar cisterna, atrophy of the cerebellum predominant in the vermis and of the pons (Fig. 25.1g–i). Most of the affected males in this family died prematurely, around 25–30 years of age. Neuropathological examination showed an atrophic cerebellum, especially of the vermis. The molecular layer dysplayed microcystic changes and there was widespread neuronal loss in the granular and Purkinje cell layers, in the pons and in the hippocampi. The condition was mapped by linkage analysis studies to Xq24-q27 (Christianson et al. 1999). In this family, a 2bp deletion within the coding sequence of the *Solute Carrier family 9 member 6* (*SLC9A6*) gene encoding for a Na+/H+ exchanger NHE6 was identified (Gilfillan et al. 2008).

Additional mutations – a 6pb deletion, a nonsense mutation R468X, a splice site mutation causing skipping of exon 3 – were identified in three other families with an Angelman-like phenotype characterized by developmental delay, postnatal microcephaly, and epilepsy occurring between 9 and 26 months of age. Patients exhibited ataxia, hyperkinetic movements, and frequent smiling with episodes of unprovoked laughter, open mouth, profuse drooling, and swallowing difficulties, gastroesophageal reflux, and thin body habitus. MRI studies performed at 3 years of age in an affected child, showed a mild progression of the cerebellar atrophy. Proton magnetic resonance spectroscopy (MRS) showed elevated glutamate/glutamine in the basal ganglia of affected individuals. An additional family with six affected males showing severe mental retardation, absent speech, autism spectrum disorder, epilepsy, late-onset ataxia, weakness, and dystonia with stereotyped hand movements was reported and an in-frame 9pb deletion in *SLC9A6* was identified. Brain MRI showed moderate ventricular enlargement and sulcal widening due to atrophy of the brain, thin corpus callosum but normal cerebellum and brainstem.

Postmortem examination of two affected males revealed widespread neuronal loss and deposits of the microtubule-binding protein tau in cortical and subcortical regions which are generally the defining neuropathological characteristics of a number of adult-onset neurodegenerative disorders but had been never associated before with early-onset mental retardation or autism (Garbern et al. 2010).

Molecular aspects

SLC9A6 (MIM 300231) is located at Xq26.3 and contains 16 coding exons. It encodes for a sodium/hydrogen exchanger protein 6 (NHE6) that belongs to the NHE family of proteins found in the membranes of intracellular organelles. In particular NHE6 is found in sorting/recycling endosomes where it regulates the endoluminal pH by exporting H+ out of the lumen (Bowers et al. 2000). Depletion of NHE6 leads to acidification of early endosomes disrupting the trafficking of proteins (e.g., AMPAR) essential for growth and maintenance of dendritic spines (Roxrud et al. 2009).

Other X-linked syndromes with cerebellar involvement

Table 25.2 presents the X-linked genes associated with cerebellar dysgenesis.

Hoyeraal-Hreidarsson syndrome

Hoyeraal-Hreidarsson syndrome (HHS; MIM 300240) is a rare X-linked recessive disorder, characterized by intrauterine growth retardation, microcephaly, intellectual disability, bone marrow failure, cancer predisposition, and cerebellar hypoplasia (Hoyeraal et al. 1970). It is caused by mutations of the *DCK1* gene located on Xq28, encoding the nucleolar protein dyskerin which interacts with the human telomerase RNA complex (Yaghmai et al. 2000). Detailed neuroimaging studies of a patient with HHS showed global cerebellar hypoplasia, a small brainstem, a thin corpus callosum, and intracranial cerebral calcifications (Kuwashima 2009).

X-linked sideroblastic anaemia with ataxia

X-linked sideroblastic anaemia with ataxia (XLSA/A; MIM 301310) is a rare X-linked disorder characterized by early-onset, slowly progressive ataxia associated with a sideroblastic anaemia due to mitochondrial iron accumulation. It is caused by mutation of the *ABC7* gene which maps to Xq13 and encodes for an ATP-binding mitochondrial iron transporter located in the inner mitochondrial membrane, involved in mitochondrial iron homeostasis as well as in the maturation of cytosolic iron-sulfur proteins (Allikmets et al. 1999). Neuroimaging studies showed a global cerebellar hypoplasia with signs of atrophy in affected individuals (Bekri et al. 2000).

Oral-facial digital type I/X-linked Joubert syndrome

Oral-facial digital type I (OFD1; MIM 311200) is a rare male lethal X-linked dominant syndrome characterized by malformations of the oral cavity, face, and digits in affected females. CNS anomalies have been found in 40% of OFD1 patients, in particular vermis hypoplasia, corpus callosum agenesis, hydrocephalus, and perventricular heterotopia (Thauvin-Robinet et al. 2006). *OFD1* maps to Xp22 and encodes for a ciliary protein.

TABLE 25.2
X-linked genes associated with cerebellar dysgenesis

Gene	Chromosomal localization	Syndrome (MIM #)	Cerebellar phenotype	References
DCK1	Xq28	Hoyeraal-Hreidarsson (MIM 300240)	Global cerebellar hypoplasia	Yaghmai et al. 2000; Kuwashima 2009
ABC7	Xq13	X-linked sideroblastic anemia/ataxia (MIM 301310)	Global cerebellar atrophy	Allikmets et al. 1999; Bekri et al. 2000
OFD1	Xp22	Oral-facial-digital I (MIM 311200)	Vermis hypoplasia, molar tooth sign	Thauvin-Robinet et al. 2006; Coene et al. 2009
MID1	Xp22	Opitz G/BBB (MIM 300000)	Anterior vermis hypoplasia	Pinson et al. 2004; Fontanella et al. 2008
FMR1	Xq27	Fragile X (MIM 300624)	Posterior vermis hypoplasia	Reiss 1991; Gothelf et al. 2008
MECP2	Xq28	Rett/Dup *MECP2* (MIM 312750/MIM 300260)	Cerebellar atrophy	Murakami et al. 1992; Reardon et al. 2010
ZIC3	Xq26	X-linked heterotaxy (MIM 306955)	Vermis hypoplasia	Grinberg & Millen 2005
L1CAM	Xq28	X-linked hydrocephalus (MIM 30700)	Global or anterior vermis hypoplasia	Kanemura et al. 2006
AP1S2	Xp22	Fried (MIM 300630)	Mild vermis hypoplasia	Saillour et al. 2007
ARX	Xp21	XLAG (MIM 300004)	Severe cerebellar hypoplasia	Kato et al. 2004
DCX	Xq22	X-linked lissencephaly (MIM 300067)	Mild cerebellar hypoplasia (vermis)	Ross et al. 2001; Bahi-Buisson et al. 2008
FLNA	Xq28	Oto-palato-digital II (MIM 300049)	Mild cerebellar hypoplasia	Parrini et al. 2006
—	Xq28	Xq28 duplication (MIM 300815)	Dandy-Walker malformation spectrum	Vandewalle et al. 2009; Martinez et al. 2010

OFD1 mutations have been identified in two families with retinitis pigmentosa and postaxial polydactyly in association with the molar tooth sign (Coene et al. 2009).

X-linked Opitz GBBB syndrome

Opitz GBBB syndromes (MIM 300000) are an X-linked recessive or autosomal dominant conditions characterized by developmental delay and midline malformations: hypertelorism, cleft lip/palate, esophagolaryngotracheal defects, imperforate anus and hypospadia, first described by Opitz et al. (1969). The X-linked form is caused by mutations in the *MID1* gene which maps to Xp22.3 and encodes for a microtubule-associated protein involved in microtubules and ribonucleoprotein complex stabilization (Quaderi et al. 1997; Aranda-Orgillés et al. 2008). Anterior vermis hypoplasia and corpus callosum abnormalities were found in more than one-third of patients with *MID1* mutations (Pinson et al. 2004; Fontanella et al. 2008) and lack of *Mid1* in the mouse causes abnormal development of the anterior cerebellar vermis (Lancioni et al. 2010).

Fragile X syndrome

The FRAXA syndrome (MIM 300624) is the most frequent cause of monogenic mental retardation in the male population. It is mainly caused by CGG triplet expansion in the first noncoding exon of the *FMR1* gene leading to a block of gene transcription (Verkerk et al. 1991). Loss of function of the FMRP protein leads to abnormalities of dendritic spine maturation associated with altered synaptic plasticity and cerebellar motor learning (eyeblink conditioning) also seen in FRAXA patients (Koekkoek et al. 2005). A comparative study of the posterior fossa of a group of patients with the mutation and a group of age-matched comparisons has revealed a significant reduction of the posterior vermis (lobules VI–VII) in the Fragile X population. These data were recently confirmed by three-dimensional MRI morphometric studies (Reiss et al. 1991; Lee et al. 2007; Gothelf et al. 2008).

X-linked heterotaxy

X-linked heterotaxy (MIM 306955) is caused by mutations of the Zinc finger transcription factor *ZIC3* located in Xq26 and coding for a transcription factor involved in the establishment of the left/right axis in early embryonic development (Gebbia et al. 1997). Vermis hypoplasia is found in association with X-linked heterotaxy and has been reported in males hemizygous for *ZIC3* mutations (Debrus et al. 1997; Grinberg and Millen 2005). Cerebellar dysgenesis predominant in the flocculonodular lobe has been described in *Zic3*-deficient mice (Aruga et al. 2004). Proteins belonging to the ZIC family have been implicated in the proliferation and differentiation of cerebellar granular cells and heterozygous deletions of the autosomal genes *ZIC1–4* have been shown in patients with Dandy-Walker malformation (Grinberg et al. 2004).

Rett syndrome/MECP2 duplication syndrome

Rett syndrome (MIM 312750) is an X-linked dominant neurodevelopmental disorder which represents the most important cause of severe mental retardation in the female population (1/10 000). It is due, in the majority of cases, to mutations of the *MECP2* gene in Xq28 which encodes for a Methyl-CpG DNA binding protein functioning as transcriptional repressor (Amir et al. 1999). MECP2 is highly expressed in the CNS, in particular in the cortex, hippocampus, and cerebellum. The psychomotor development of Rett patients is apparently normal, then regresses around 6–18 months with the appearance of stereotyped hand movements, breathing irregularities, seizures, epilepsy, loss of speech, hypotonia, ataxia, and hyperreflexia. MRI studies of young patients with Rett syndrome have demonstrated the presence of a mild cerebellar hypoplasia especially of lobules I–IV, whereas in adult patients a progressive cerebellar atrophy was detected and also confirmed by postmortem neuropathological studies of the cerebellum in older Rett patients (Murakami et al. 1992; Bauman et al. 1995). *Mecp2* mice mutants show cerebellar and hyppocampal-based learning deficits and develop gait incoordination (Pelka et al. 2006). Most recently, Reardon et al. (2010) reported neuroradiological evidence of progressive cerebellar atrophy, emerging in the second decade of life, in males of three families carrying duplications of the MECP2 region (MIM300260), which cause a syndrome characterized by infantile hypotonia, profound intellectual deficit, autistic features, and recurrent infections (Van Esch et al. 2005).

X-linked cortical dysgenesis

The gene *DCX* located in Xq22 and encoding for the doublecortin protein is mutated in 40% of patients with type 1 lissencephaly. The cortical dysgenesis is associated with severe mental retardation and seizures in affected males and subcortical laminal heterotopia in hemizygous females (Des Portes et al. 1998; Gleeson et al. 1998). Doublecortin is a microtubule-associated protein which participates in the assembling and stabilization of microtubules in migrating neuronal cells. It is reported that 25% of male patients with *DCX* mutations show a mild cerebellar hypoplasia, predominant in the vermis (Ross et al. 2001; Bahi-Buisson et al. 2008).

The *ARX* gene located in Xp21 encodes for an Aristaless-related homeobox transcription factor involved in multiple aspects of cortical development (Kitamura et al. 2002; Bienvenu et al. 2002). In a severe case of X-linked lissencephaly and abnormal genitalia (XLAG) due to *ARX* mutations, neuroimaging studies showed a hypoplastic vermis and enlarged fourth ventricle associated with agenesis of the corpus callosum and lissencephaly (Kato et al. 2004).

The gene *FLNA* maps to Xq28 and encodes for Filamin 1, a protein interacting with F-actin, involved in brain neurogenesis and neuronal migration (Fox et al. 1998). *FLNA* mutations cause several different syndromes with a predominant skeletal phenotype: oto-palato digital type I and II, Melnick Needles dysplasia, frontometaphyseal dysplasia, and FG-like syndrome (Robertson 2005). Mutations of *FLNA* have also been found in a high proportion of individuals with bilateral periventricular nodular heterotopia, mega cisterna magna, cardiovascular malformations, and epilepsy. Almost all patients with *FLNA* mutations had mild to moderate cerebellar hypoplasia (Parrini et al. 2006).

Xq28 microduplication syndrome

In four families with X-linked intellectual disability Vandewalle et al. (2009) identified a copy number gain of an identical 0.3Mb region on chromosome band Xq28 that included 19 annotated genes including *FLNA* and *GDI1* (a gene mutated in non-syndromic X-linked mental retardation) but not *MECP2*. These patients presented with hypotonia, severely delayed psychomotor development, mild ataxic gait, strabismus or nystagmus, but no other cerebellar signs. MRI of the brain showed a mildly enlarged fourth ventricle and ventricular dilatation in two unrelated patients and a classic Dandy-Walker malformation with cerebellar hypoplasia and agenesis of the corpus callosum in two other affected males. Mild dysmorphic features were present in all patients. A fifth family with three affected males carrying an identical Xq28 duplication and showing mild to moderate intellectual disability associated with Dandy-Walker malformation was reported by Martinez et al. (2010).

X-linked hydrocephalus

X-linked hydrocephalus with aqueductal stenosis (MIM 30700) is the most common form of hereditary hydrocephalus with an incidence of 1/30 000 in male neonates. Most cases of X-linked hydrocephalus are caused by mutations in the *L1CAM* gene, encoding for a cellular adhesion protein which has also been implicated in the regulation of vesicle cycling through its interaction with proteins of clathrin-mediated endocytosis (Thelen et al. 2002). In patients with loss-of-function mutations of *L1CAM*, a global vermis hypoplasia or anterior vermis hypoplasia has been observed (Kanemura et al. 2006).

In families with X-linked mental retardation and hydrocephalus, Tarpey et al. (2006) and Saillour et al. (2007) identified mutations of *AP1S2* (sigma subunit of the clathrin adaptor protein complex 1). Brain MRI imaging of affected males in one family showed ventricular dilatation without aqueductal stenosis, calcifications of the basal ganglia, and mild vermis hypoplasia. Loss of function of the clathrin adaptor AP1 determines defects in synaptic vesicle cycling with accumulation of large endosome-like vacuoles, defects which are paired with reduced motor coordination and long-term spatial memory in mutant mice (Glyvuk et al. 2010).

X-linked cerebellar disorders with mapped gene loci

X-linked nonprogressive congenital ataxia

This form was described for the first time in a large family of Eastern Russian descent with seven affected males over three generations, displaying X-linked recessive inheritance. All patients had markedly delayed early developmental milestones, cerebellar ataxia, external ophthalmoplegia, pyramidal signs, normal cognitive development, and nonprogressive course. Neuroimaging studies revealed marked hypoplasia/atrophy of the cerebellar vermis and hemispheres. Linkage studies mapped the gene to a large genetic interval on Xp11.21-Xq24 with a maximum logarithm of the odds (LOD) score (logarithm base 10 of odds) of 4.66 at DXS1059 (Illarioshkin et al. 1996; see Fig. 25.3). A second family with a similar phenotype, with the propositus and his maternal uncle suffering from severe hypotonia at birth, psychomotor delay, slow eye movements, nonprogressive ataxia, and normal intelligence was reported by Bertini et al. (2000). Neuroimaging studies revealed global cerebellar atrophy that was not evident in the first years of life (Fig. 25.2a,b). As is expected in congenital ataxias, the clinical situation was static with a tendency to improvement (Batten 1905), despite the progression of cerebellar changes. A genetic interval, partially overlapping with the first reported family, was identified by exclusion mapping. A large family of Norwegian descent with six affected males over three generations with nonprogressive X-linked congenital ataxia and normal cognitive development was reported by Zanni et al. 2008; see Fig. 25.3). Hypotonia and overall delay or motor development were noted since birth. Nystagmus, dysarthria, and truncal ataxia were present. Neuroimaging studies showed a global atrophy of the cerebellum, predominant in the vermis (Fig. 25.2c,d). The disease was mapped to a genetic interval of 12Mb at Xq25-q27.1 with a maximum LOD score of 3.44 at DXS1192 not overlapping with the previously identified locus, indicating that there are at least two genes responsible for this rare form of X-linked congenital ataxia.

Other X-linked syndromes

Pettigrew et al. (1991) reported a four-generation family of Dutch descent with nine affected males presenting with severe cognitive delay, early hypotonia with progression to spasticity and contractures, choreoathetosis, seizures, and a long narrow face with coarse features. Brain imaging studies revealed a cystic enlargement of the fourth ventricle with cerebellar hypoplasia and iron accumulation in the basal ganglia with neuroaxonal dystrophy. The disease was mapped to the long arm of the X chromosome with a maximum LOD score of 2.19 at DXS425 in Xq25-q27 (Huang et al. 1991) (see Fig. 25.3).

Bertini et al. (1991) reported a family of Italian descent with seven affected males. Two of them showed a severe congenital ataxia, generalized hypotonia, psychomotor delay, recurrent bronchopulmonary infections, and later developed myoclonic encephalopathy and macular degeneration. Serial neuroimaging studies showed cerebellar vermis and corpus callosum hypoplasia, a cyst of the septum pellucidum, and persistence of the cavum vergae. The other five affected males in the family had recurrent bronchopneumonia with severe congenital hypotonia and died within the first years of life. Immunological investigations only showed a reduced level of IgG2 subclass in one sib. Des Portes et al. (1996) mapped the condition to the short arm of the X chromosome with a maximum LOD score of 2.48 at DXS7099 in Xp22.33-pter (see Fig. 25.3).

Arena et al. (1992) described a family with a syndromic form of X-linked mental retardation characterized by absent

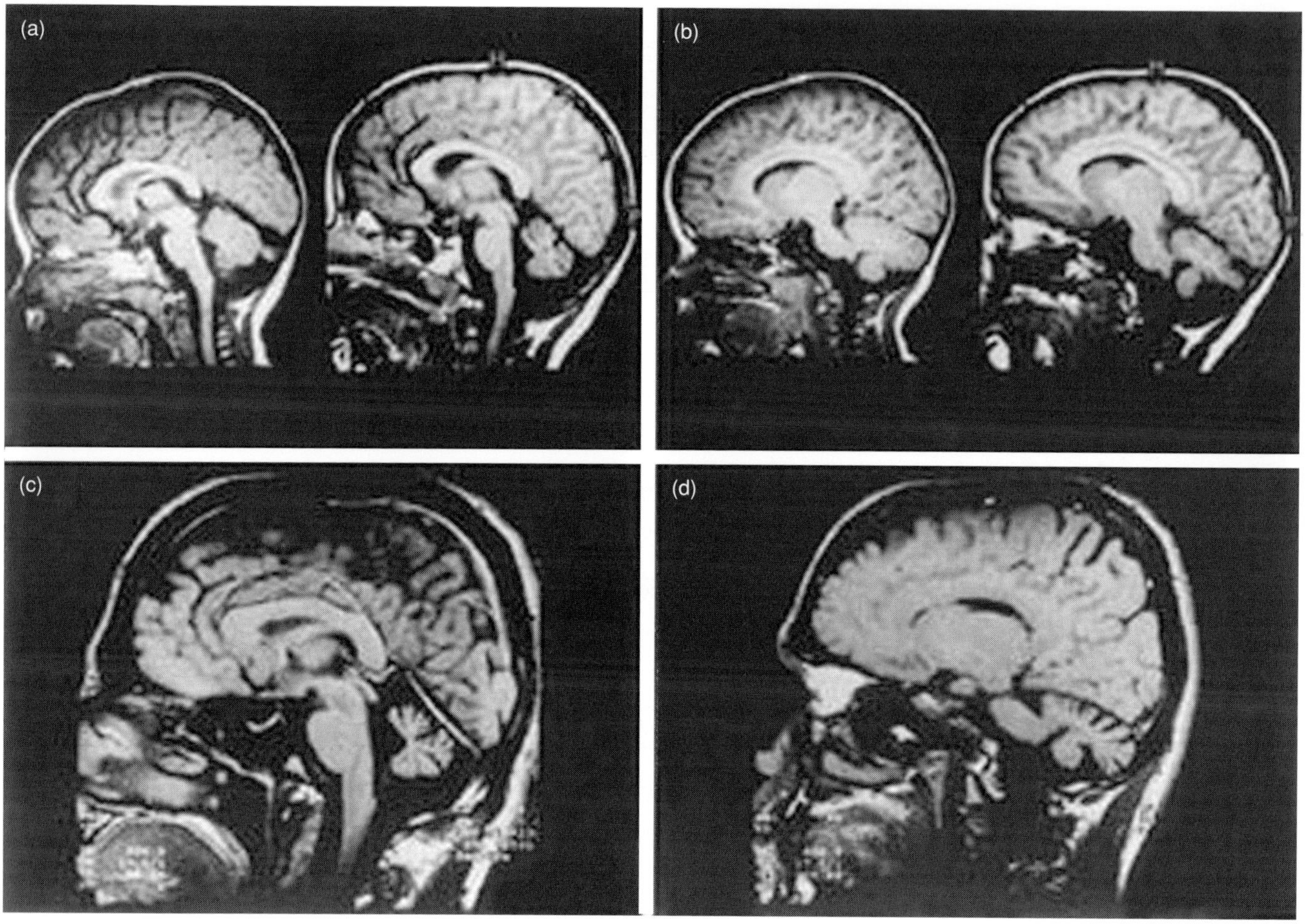

Fig. 25.2. Brain MRI studies of a family with non progressive X-linked congenital ataxia. 2a–b: midsagittal **(a)** and parasagittal **(b)** T1-weighted sections of the propositus. The left sides correspond to the propositus at age 2 years; the right sides correspond to 3 years of age. Notice theprogressive atrophy of the cerebellum with age. 2c–d: midsagittal **(c)** and parasagittal **(d)** T1-weighted image showing marked atrophy of cerebellar folia in the maternal uncle. Reproduced from Am J Med Genet A. 2008; 146(A): 593–600. With permission from John Wiley & Sons.

speech, truncal ataxia, contractures, and hypoplasia of the cerebellum and the brainstem revealed at neuroimaging studies. Only one of the affected males developed seizures and showed changes in the basal ganglia, suggesting iron deposits. The condition was mapped to Xq23-q24 (see Fig. 25.3).

Gustavson et al. (1993) described a family in which affected males showed congenital cerebellar hypoplasia, microcephaly, short stature, profound developmental delay, blindness, deafness, and seizures. Death occurred in infancy or early childhood. This syndrome has been mapped to Xq24-Xq27 (see Fig. 25.3).

Strømme et al. (1999) described a family with seven affected males presenting moderate to severe intellectual impairment and infantile spasms. Neuroimaging studies showed cerebellar atrophy or corpus callosum hypoplasia or both, in half of the affected individuals. The condition was mapped to Xp11.4-p22.11 (see Fig. 25.3).

Chudley et al. (1999) identified a family with three males in two generations affected with moderate intellectual deficit and dysmorphic features: prominent glabella, synophris, prognathism, generalized hirsutism, and bilateral single palmar creases. All patients developed seizures in childhood and two of them showed a progressive gait disturbance and prolonged nerve conduction velocity and hypogammaglobulinemia. Neuroimaging studies in one patient revealed cerebellar atrophy. The disease was mapped to Xq21.33-Xq23 (see Fig. 25.3).

Guo et al. (2006) reported a Chinese family in which six males were affected by early hypotonia, severe psychomotor delay, cerebellar ataxia, congenital cataracts, and short stature. Carrier females only showed cataracts. Neuroimaging studies were not performed. The disease gene was mapped to Xpter-Xq13.1 (see Fig. 25.3).

A description of the clinical features of unmapped X-linked conditions is summarized in Table 25.3.

A diagnostic approach to the patient with suspected X-linked cerebellar disorder

An X-linked cerebellar disorder should generally be suspected in a patient with a positive family history or in an affected male, if sporadic, presenting with early developmental or cognitive delay, hypotonia, and oculomotor signs: nystagmus, strabismus or ophthalmoplegia.

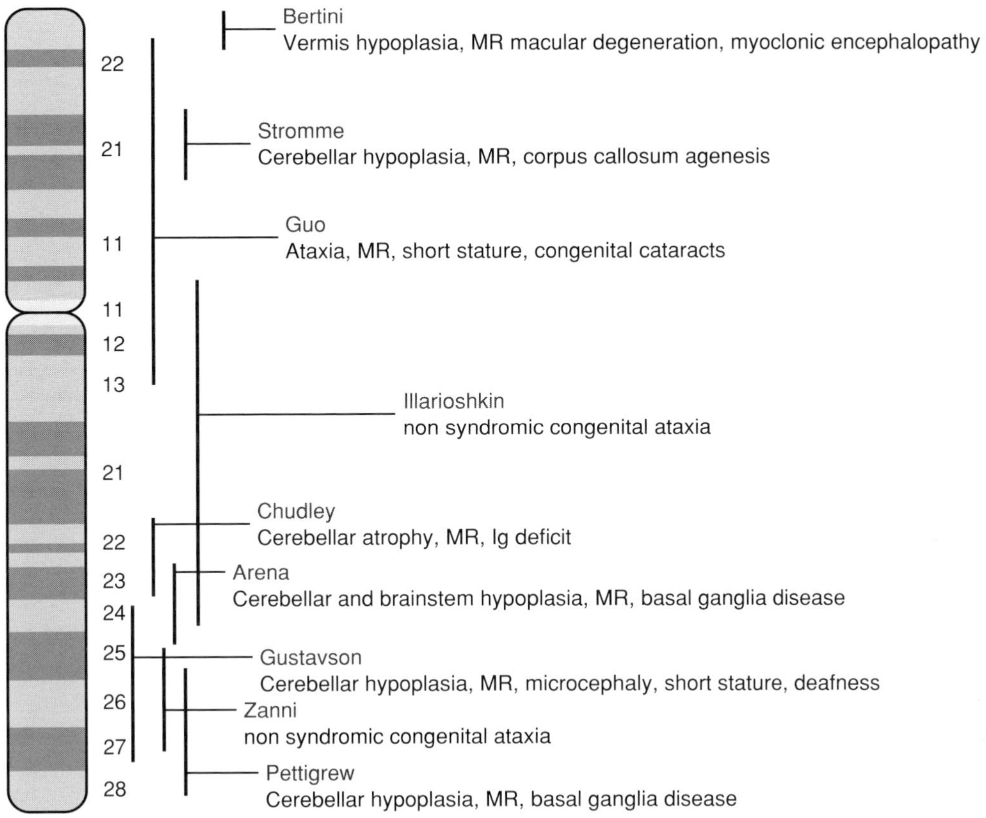

Fig. 25.3. Ideogram of the X-chromosome with linkage mapping limits of families with X-linked cerebellar disorders. (See color plate 26).

TABLE 25.3
X-linked cerebellar disorders for which no mapping data are available

	Turner & Roberts 1938	Malamud & Cohen 1958	Shokeir 1970	Spira et al. 1979	Lutz et al. 1989	Young et al. 1987	Margari et al. 2004	Kroes et al. 2005
Affected males	9	7	3	10	3	3	3	3
Age of onset	5y	Congenital	16–21y	6–16y	Congenital	Congenital	Congenital	Congenital
Developmental delay, hypotonia	+	—	+	+	+	+	+	+
Cerebellar ataxia/signs	+	+	+	+	+	+	+	–
Ocular findings	Nystagmus	Nystagmus, strabismus, OA	Nystagmus	—	Nystagmus	Nystagmus	Nystagmus	Retinal colobomas
Other neurological signs	—	Myoclonic seizures	Spasticity	Spasticity	—	—	Spasticity	Seizures, apnea/tachypnea
Intellectual deficit	+	—	—	—	+	+	+	
Progressive course	+	+	+	+	+	—	—	+
Other associated findings	Scoliosis	nd	nd	Scoliosis	nd	Scoliosis	df	df
Neuroradiological findings	CA/CH	CA/CH	CA/CH	CA/CH	CA/CH, brainstem hypoplasia	CA/CH	CA/CH	CH (vermis), callosal/cortical dysgenesis

CA, cerebellar atrophy; CH, cerebellar hypoplasia; OA, optic atrophy; df, dysmorphic features; nd, not determined.

The differential diagnosis with other (X-linked) diseases is not easy at birth, in particular because specific cerebellar signs may appear after the cerebellum has completed its development, around the second year of age.

Optimal management of these patients requires a multidisciplinary approach with particular attention to three-generation family history and personal prenatal and postnatal history to exclude infectious, toxic, or traumatic etiology.

A complete physical examination focused on the presence of minor anomalies, an assessment of multiorgan involvement and the search for associated problems – neurosensorial deficits, seizures, specific learning problems – is important because most of these conditions are syndromic. A cognitive and behavioural assessment (Wechsler scales, Vineland) is essential because X-linked cerebellar disorders are frequently associated with mild to severe developmental or cognitive delay.

A metabolic work-up (lactate/pyruvate ratio in blood and cerebrospinal fluid, lysosomal enzymes, isoelectro-focusing of transferrin, creatine kinase, very long chain fatty acids, plasmatic and urinary amino acids and urinary organic acids chromatography) together with nerve conduction studies should be performed to exclude metabolic or neuromuscular causes (X-linked adrenoleukodystrophy, X-linked dystrophinopathies). Neuroimaging studies of the cerebellum with particular attention to the brainstem and cerebral cortex can be fundamental for the differential diagnosis between different X-linked cerebellar syndromes and other noncerebellar X-linked disorders that can present with ataxic symptoms (e.g., Arts syndrome, characterized by ataxia, deafness, and neuropathy).

A clinical and neuroradiological follow-up is also necessary for the assessment of the evolution or nonprogressive course of the condition.

Rehabilitation and therapeutic strategies should be planned for motor, cognitive and behavioural difficulties as well as for specific manifestations such as visual impairment or seizures.

In the last few years molecular cytogenetic studies (array-CGH and high-resolution single nucleotide polymorphism (SNP) arrays) have proven that submicroscopic genomic imbalances are a major cause of developmental disorders due to copy number changes of dosage-sensitive genes. On the X chromosome, a high incidence of causal deletions and microduplications was found, demonstrating that dysregulated expression of tightly regulated genes can disturb normal brain and cognitive development. At least one-third of cases with OPHN1 or CASK syndrome were found to be carriers of a chromosomal or subchromosomal abnormality. It is therefore recommended, in patients with a documented (X-linked) cerebellar disorder, especially when two or more dysmorphic features are present, to perform standard karyotype followed by array-CGH studies.

Genetic testing (with the possible exception of FMRI) should be performed only in well-selected cases. The identification of the molecular defects in couples at risk allows early prenatal testing, whereas fetal brain neuroimaging may prove uninformative. Given the report of several forms of X-linked cerebellar disorders and the excess of males with ataxia (Lesny 1970; Neuhäuser 1975), families of children with congenital cerebellar hypoplasia, atrophy or Dandy-Walker malformation with or without intellectual deficit should be counseled for high risk of X-linked inheritance.

REFERENCES

Allikmets R, Raskind WH, Hutchinson A, Schueck ND, Dean M, Koeller DM (1999) Mutation of a putative mitochondrial iron transporter gene (ABC7) in Xlinked sideroblastic anemia and ataxia (XLSA/A). Hum Mol Genet 8: 743–749.

Al-Owain M, Kaya N, Al-Zaidan H, Al-Hashmi N, Al-Bakheet A, Al-Muhaizea M, et al. (2010) Novel intragenic deletion in OPHN1 in a family causing XLMR with cerebellar hypoplasia and distinctive facial appearance. Clin Genet 4: 1–8.

Amir RE, Van den Veyver IB, Wan M, Tran CQ, Francke U, Zoghbi HY (1999) Rett syndrome is caused by mutations in X-linked MECP2, encoding methyl-CpG-binding protein 2. Nat Genet 23: 185–188.

Aranda-Orgillés B, Trockenbacher A, Winter J, Aigner J, Köhler A, Jastrzebska E, et al. (2008) The Opitz syndrome gene product MID1 assembles a microtubule-associated ribonucleoprotein complex. Hum Genet 123: 163–176.

Arena JF, Schwartz C, Stevenson R, Lawrence L, Carpenter A, Duara R, et al. (1992) Spastic paraplegia with iron deposits in the basal ganglia:a new X-linked mental retardation syndrome. Am J Med Genet 43: 479–490.

Aruga J, Ogura H, Shutoh F, Ogawa M, Franke B, Nagao S, Mikoshiba K (2004) Locomotor and oculomotor impairment associated with cerebellar dysgenesis in Zic3-deficient (Bent tail) mutant mice. Eur J Neurosci 20: 2159–2167.

Bahi-Buisson N, Boddaert N, Saillour Y, Souville I, Poirier K, Léger PL, et al. (2008) [Epileptogenic brain malformations: radiological and clinical presentation and indications for genetic testing]. Rev Neurol (Paris) 164: 995–1009.

Batten FE (1905) Ataxia in childhood. Brain 28: 484.

Bauman ML, Kemper TL, Arin DM (1995) Microscopic observations of the brain in Rett syndrome. Neuropediatrics 26(2): 105–108.

Bedeschi MF, Novelli A, Bernardini L, Parazzini C, Bianchi V, Torres B, et al. (2008) Association of syndromic mental retardation with an Xq12q13.1 duplication encompassing the oligophrenin 1 gene. Am J Med Genet 146A: 1718–1724.

Bekri S, Kispal G, Lange H, Fitzsimons E, Tolmie J, Lill R, Bishop DF (2000) Human ABC7 transporter: gene structure and mutation causing X-linked sideroblastic anemia with ataxia with disruption of cytosolic iron-sulfur protein maturation. Blood 96: 3256–3264.

Bergmann C, Zerres K, Senderek J, Rudnik-Schoneborn S, Eggermann T, Häusler M, et al. (2003) Oligophrenin 1 (OPHN1) gene mutation causes syndromic X-linked mental retardation with epilepsy, rostral ventricular enlargement and cerebellar hypoplasia. Brain 126: 1537–1544.

Bertini E, Cusmai R, de Saint Basile G, Le Deist F, Di Capua M, Gaggero DR, et al. (1991) Congenital X-linked ataxia, progressive myoclonic encephalopathy, macular degeneration and recurrent infections. Am J Med Genet 43: 443–451.

Bertini E, des Portes V, Zanni G, Santorelli F, Dionisi-Vici C, Vicari S, et al. (2000) X-linked congenital ataxia: a clinical and genetic study. Am J Med Genet 92: 53–56.

Bienvenu T, Der-Sarkissian H, Billuart P, Tissot M, Des Portes V, Brulst T, et al. (1997) Mapping of the X-breakpoint involved in a balanced X;12 translocation in a female with mild mental retardation. Eur J Hum Genet 5: 105–109.

Bienvenu T, Poirier K, Friocourt G, Bahi N, Beaumont D, Fauchereau F, et al. (2002) ARX, a novel Prd-class-homeobox gene highly expressed in the telencephalon, is mutated in X-linked mental retardation. Hum Mol Genet 11: 981–991.

Billuart P, Bienvenu T, Ronce N, des Portes V, Vinet MC, Zemni R, et al. (1998) Oligophrenin-1 encodes a rhoGAP protein involved in X-linked mental retardation. Nature 392: 923–926.

Bowers K, Levi BP, Patel FI, Stevens TH (2000) The sodium/proton exchanger Nhx1p is required for endosomal protein trafficking in the yeast Saccharomyces cerevisiae. Mol Biol Cell 11: 4277–4294.

Chabrol B, Girard N, N'Guyen K, Gérard A, Carlier M, Villard L, Philip N (2005) Delineation of the clinical phenotype associated with OPHN1 mutations based on the clinical and neuropsychological evaluation of three families. Am J Med Genet 138: 314–317.

Christianson AL, Stevenson RE, van der Meyden CH, Pelser J, Theron FW, van Rensburg PL, et al. (1999) X linked severe mental retardation, craniofacial dysmorphology, epilepsy, ophthalmoplegia, and cerebellar atrophy in a large South African kindred is localised to Xq24-q27. Med Genet 36: 759–766.

Chudley AE, Tackels DC, Lubs HA, Arena JF, Stoeber WP, Kovnats S, et al. (1999) X-linked mental retardation syndrome with seizures, hypogammaglobulinemia, and progressive gait disturbance is regionally mapped between Xq21.33 and Xq23. Am J Med Genet 85: 255–262.

Coene KL, Roepman R, Doherty D, Afroze B, Kroes HY, Letteboer SJ, et al. (2009) OFD1 is mutated in X-linked Joubert syndrome and interacts with LCA5-encoded lebercilin. Am J Hum Genet 85: 465–481.

Debrus S, Sauer U, Gilgenkrantz S, Jost W, Jesberger H-J, Bouvagnet P (1997) Autosomal recessive lateralization and midline defects: Blastogenesis recessive 1. Am J Med Genet 68: 401–404.

Des Portes V, Bachner L, Bruls T, Beldjord C, Billuart P, Soufir N, et al. (1996) X-linked neurodegenerative syndrome with congenital ataxia, late-onset progressive myoclonic encephalopathy and selective macular degeneration, linked to Xp22.33-pter. Am J Med Genet 64: 69–72.

Des Portes V, Pinard JM, Billuart P, Vinet MC, Koulakoff A, Carrie A, et al. (1998) A novel CNS gene required for neuronal migration and involved in X-linked subcortical laminar heterotopia and lissencephaly syndrome. Cell 92: 51–61.

Des Portes V, Boddaert N, Sacco S, Briault S, Maincent K, Bahi N, et al. (2004) Specific clinical and brain MRI features in mentally retarded patients with mutations in the Oligophrenin-1 gene. Am J Med Genet 124A: 364–371.

Fontanella B, Russolillo G, Meroni G (2008) MID1 mutations in patients with X-linked Opitz G/BBB syndrome. Hum Mutat 29: 584–594.

Fox JW, Lamperti ED, Eksioglu YZ, Hong SE, Feng Y, Graham DA, et al. (1998). Mutations in filamin 1 prevent migration of cerebral cortical neurons in human periventricular heterotopia. Neuron 21: 1315–1325.

Froyen G, Van Esch H, Bauters M, Hollanders K, Frints SG, Vermeesch JR, et al. (2007) Detection of genomic copy number changes in patients with idiopathic mental retardation by high-resolution X-array-CGH: important role for increased gene dosage of XLMR genes. Hum Mutat 28: 1034–1042.

Garbern JY, Neumann M, Trojanowski JQ, Lee VM, Feldman G, Norris JW, et al. (2010) A mutation affecting the sodium/proton exchanger, SLC9A6, causes mental retardation with tau deposition. Brain 133(Pt 5): 1391–402.

Gebbia M, Ferrero GB, Pilia G, Bassi MT, Aylsworth A, Penman-Splitt M, et al. (1997) X-linked situs abnormalities result from mutations in ZIC3. Nat Genet 17: 305–308.

Gilfillan GD, Selmer KK, Roxrud I, Smith R, Kyllerman M, Eiklid K, et al. (2008) SLC9A6 mutations cause X-linked mental retardation, microcephaly, epilepsy, and ataxia, a phenotype mimicking Angelman syndrome. Am J Hum Genet 82: 1003–1010.

Gleeson JG, Allen KM, Fox JW, Lamperti ED, Berkovic S, Scheffer I, et al. (1998) Doublecortin, a brainspecific gene mutated in human X-linked lissencephaly and double cortex syndrome, encodes a putative signaling protein. Cell 92: 63–72.

Glyvuk N, Tsytsyura Y, Geumann C, D'Hooge R, Hüve J, Kratzke M, et al. (2010) AP-1/sigma1B-adaptin mediates endosomal synaptic vesicle recycling, learning and memory. EMBO J 29: 1318–1330.

Gothelf D, Furfaro JA, Hoeft F, Eckert MA, Hall SS, O'Hara R, et al. (2008) Neuroanatomy of fragile X syndrome is associated with aberrant behavior and the fragile X mental retardation protein (FMRP). Ann Neurol 63: 40–51.

Govek EE, Newey SE, Akerman CJ, Cross JR, Van der Veken L, Van Aelst L (2004) The X-linked mental retardation protein oligophrenin-1 is required for dendritic spine morphogenesis. Nat Neurosci 7: 364–372.

Grinberg I, Northrup H, Ardinger H, Prasad C, Dobyns WB, Millen KJ (2004) Heterozygous deletion of the linked genes ZIC1 and ZIC4 is involved in Dandy-Walker malformation. Nat Genet 36: 1053–1055.

Grinberg I, Millen KJ (2005) The ZIC gene family in development and disease. Clin Genet 67: 290–296.

Guo X, Shen H, Xiao X, Dai Q, Li S, Jia X, Hejtmancik JF, Zhang Q (2006) Cataracts, ataxia, short stature, and mental retardation in a Chinese family mapped to Xpter-q13.1. J Hum Genet 51: 695–700.

Gustavson KH, Anneren G, Malmgren H, Dahl N, Ljunggren CG, Backman H (1993) New X-linked syndrome with severe mental retardation, severely impaired vision, severe hearing defect, epileptic seizures, spasticity, restricted joint mobility, and early death. Am J Med Genet 45: 654–658.

Hackett A, Tarpey PS, Licata A, Cox J, Whibley A, Boyle J, et al. (2010) CASK mutations are frequent in males and cause X-linked nystagmus and variable XLMR phenotypes. Eur J Hum Genet 18: 544–552.

Hayashi S, Mizuno S, Migita O, Okuyama T, Makita Y, Hata A, et al. (2008) The CASK gene harbored in a deletion detected by array-CGH as a potential candidate for a gene causative of X-linked dominant mental retardation. Am J Med Genet 146A: 2145–2151.

Hoyeraal HM, Lamvik J, Moe PJ (1970) Congenital hypoplastic thrombocytopenia and cerebral malformations in two brothers. Acta Paediatr Scand 59: 185–191.

Hsueh YP (2009) Calcium/calmodulin-dependent serine protein kinase and mental retardation. Ann Neurol 66: 438–443.

Huang TH, Hejtmancik JF, Edwards A, Pettigrew AL, Herrera CA, Hammond HA, et al. (1991) Linkage of the gene for an X-linked mental retardation disorder to a hypervariable (AGAT)n repeat motif within the human hypoxanthine phosphoribosyltransferase (HPRT) locus (Xq26). Am J Hum Genet 49: 1312–1319.

Illarioshkin SN, Tanaka H, Markova ED, Nikolskaya NN, Ivanova-Smolenskaya IA, Tsuji S (1996) X-linked nonprogressive congenital cerebellar hypoplasia: clinical description and mapping to chromosome Xq. Ann Neurol 40: 75–83.

Jeyifous O, Waites CL, Specht CG, Fujisawa S, Schubert M, Lin EI, et al. (2009) SAP97 and CASK mediate sorting of NMDA receptors through a previously unknown secretory pathway. Nat Neurosci 12: 1011–1019.

Kanemura Y, Okamoto N, Sakamoto H, Shofuda T, Kamiguchi H, Yamasaki M (2006) Molecular mechanisms and neuroimaging criteria for severe L1 syndrome with X-linked hydrocephalus. J Neurosurg 105(5 Suppl): 403–412.

Kato M, Das S, Petras K, Kitamura K, Morohashi K, Abuelo DN, et al. (2004) Mutations of ARX are associated with striking pleiotropy and consistent genotype-phenotype correlation. Hum Mutat 23: 147–159.

Khelfaoui M, Denis C, van Galen E, de Bock F, Schmitt A, Houbron C, et al. (2007) Loss of X-linked mental retardation gene oligophrenin1 in mice impairs spatial memory and leads to ventricular enlargement and dendritic spine immaturity. J Neurosci 27: 9439–9450.

Khelfaoui M, Pavlowsky A, Powell AD, Valnegri P, Cheong KW, Blandin Y, et al. (2009) Inhibition of RhoA pathway rescues the endocytosis defects in Oligophrenin1 mouse model of mental retardation. Hum Mol Genet 18: 2575–2583.

Kitamura K, Yanazawa M, Sugiyama N, Miura H, Iizuka-Kogo A, Kusaka M, et al. (2002) Mutation of ARX causes abnormal development of forebrain and testes in mice and X-linked lissencephaly with abnormal genitalia in humans. Nat Genet 32: 359–369.

Koekkoek SK, Yamaguchi K, Milojkovic BA, Dortland BR, Ruigrok TJ, Maex R, et al. (2005) Deletion of FMR1 in Purkinje cells enhances parallel fiber LTD, enlarges spines, and attenuates cerebellar eyelid conditioning in Fragile X syndrome. Neuron 47: 339–352.

Kroes HY, Nievelstein RJ, Barth PG, Nikkels PG, Bergmann C, Gooskens RH, et al. (2005) Cerebral, cerebellar and colobomatous anomalies in three related males: Sex-Linked inheritance in a newly recognized syndrome with features overlapping with Joubert syndrome. Am J Med Genet 135A: 297–301.

Kuwashima S (2009) Hoyeraal-Hreidarsson syndrome: magnetic resonance imaging findings. Jpn J Radiol 27: 324–327.

Lancioni A, Pizzo M, Fontanella B, Ferrentino R, Napolitano LM, De Leonibus E, Meroni G (2010) Lack of Mid1, the mouse ortholog of the Opitz syndrome gene, causes abnormal development of the anterior cerebellar vermis. J Neurosci 30: 2880–2887.

Lee AD, Leow AD, Lu A, Reiss AL, Hall S, Chiang MC, et al. (2007) 3D pattern of brain abnormalities in Fragile X syndrome visualized using tensor-based morphometry. Neuroimage 34: 924–938.

Lesny I (1970) [Symmetric cerebellar hypogenesis (Study of chronic ataxias).] Cesk Pediatr 25:530–531.

Lutz R, Bodensteiner J, Schaefer B, Gay C (1989) X-linked olivopontocerebellar atrophy. Clin Genet 35: 417–422.

Madrigal I, Rodríguez-Revenga L, Badenas C, Sánchez A, Milà M (2008) Deletion of the OPHN1 gene detected by aCGH. J Intellect Disabil Res 52: 190–194.

Malamud N, Cohen P (1958) Unusual form of cerebellar ataxia with sex-linked inheritance Brain 19: 261–266.

Margari L, Ventura P, Presicci A, Buttiglione M, Perniola T (2004) Congenital ataxia and mental retardation in three brothers. Pediatr Neurol 31: 59–63.

Martinez F, Monfort S, Rosello MP, Oltra S, Quiroga R, Orellana C (2010) Association of Xq28 recurrent duplication with Dandy Walker Malformation: a putative role for filamin A as a predisposing factor.Eur J Hum Genet 18(S1): 274.

Menten B, Buysse K, Vermeulen S, Meersschaut V, Vandesompele J, Ng BL, et al. (2007) Report of a female patient with mental retardation and tall stature due to a chromosomal rearrangement disrupting the OPHN1 gene on Xq12. Eur J Med Genet 50: 446–454.

Murakami JW, Courchesne E, Haas RH, Press GA, Yeung-Courchesne R (1992) Cerebellar and cerebral abnormalities in Rett syndrome: a quantitative MR analysis. Am J Roentgenol 159: 177–183.

Najm J, Horn D, Wimplinger I, Golden JA, Chizhikov VV, Sudi J, et al. (2008) Mutations of CASK cause an X-linked brain malformation phenotype with microcephaly and hypoplasia of the brainstem and cerebellum. Nat Genet 40: 1065–1067.

Nakano-Kobayashi A, Kasri NN, Newey SE, Van Aelst L (2009) The Rho-linked mental retardation protein OPHN1 controls synaptic vesicle endocytosis via endophilin A1. Curr Biol 19: 1133–1139.

Neuhäuser G (1975) Differentialdiagnose von Koordinationsstörungen im Kindesalter. Med Mschr 29: 355–361.

Opitz J, Frias JL, Gutenberger JE, Pellett JR (1969) The G syndrome of multiple congenital anomalies. Birth Defects Orig Art Ser (2): 95–101.

Parrini E, Ramazzotti A, Dobyns WB, Mei D, Moro F, Veggiotti P, et al. (2006) Periventricular heterotopia: phenotypic heterogeneity and correlation with Filamin A mutations. Brain 129: 1892–906.

Pelka GJ, Watson CM, Radziewic T, Hayward M, Lahooti H, Christodoulou J, Tam PP (2006) Mecp2 deficiency is associated with learning and cognitive deficits and altered gene activity in the hippocampal region of mice. Brain 129: 887–898.

Pettigrew AL, Jackson LG, Ledbetter DH (1991) New X-linked mental retardation disorder with Dandy-Walker malformation, basal ganglia disease, and seizures. Am J Med Genet 38: 200–207.

Philip N, Chabrol B, Lossi AM, Cardoso C, Guerrini R, Dobyns WB, et al. (2003) Mutations in the oligophrenin-1 gene (OPHN1) cause X linked congenital cerebellar hypoplasia. J Med Genet 40: 441–446.

Piluso G, D'Amico F, Saccone V, Bismuto E, Rotundo IL, Di Domenico M, et al. (2009) A missense mutation in CASK causes FG syndrome in an Italian family. Am J Hum Genet 84): 162–77.

Pinson L, Auge J, Audollent S, Mattei G, Etchevers H, Gigarel N, et al. (2004) Embryonic expression of the human MID1 gene and its mutations in Opitz syndrome J Med Genet 41: 381–386.

Quaderi NA, Schweiger S, Gaudenz K, Franco B, Rugarli EI, Berger W, et al. (1997) Opitz G/BBB syndrome, a defect of midline development, is due to mutations in a new RING finger gene on Xp22. Nat Genet 17: 285–291.

Reardon W, Donoghue V, Murphy AM, King MD, Mayne PD, Horn N, Birk Moller L (2010) Progressive cerebellar degenerative changes in the severe mental retardation syndrome caused by duplication of MECP2 and adjacent loci on Xq28. Eur J Pediatr 169: 941–949.

Reiss AL, Freund L, Tseng JE, Joshi PK (1991) Neuroanatomy in fragile X females: the posterior fossa. Am J Hum Genet 49: 279–288.

Robertson SP (2005) Filamin A: Phenotypic diversity. Curr Opin Genet Dev 15: 301–307.

Ross ME, Swanson K, Dobyns WB (2001) Lissencephaly with cerebellar hypoplasia (LCH): a heterogeneous group of cortical malformations. Neuropediatrics 32: 256–263.

Roxrud I, Raiborg C, Gilfillan GD, Strømme P, Stenmark H (2009) Dual degradation mechanisms ensure disposal of NHE6 mutant protein associated with neurological disease. Exp Cell Res 315: 3014–3027.

Saillour Y, Zanni G, Des Portes V, Heron D, Guibaud L, Iba-Zizen MT, et al. (2007) Mutations in the AP1S2 gene encoding the sigma 2 subunit of the adaptor protein 1 complex AP1S2 are associated with syndromic X-linked mental retardation with hydrocephalus and calcifications in basal ganglia. J Med Genet 44: 739–744.

Shokeir MHK (1970) X-linked cerebellar ataxia. Clin Genet 1: 225–231.

Spira PJ, McLeod JG, Evans WA (1979) A spinocerebellar degeneration with X-linked inheritance. Brain 102: 27–41.

Stevenson D, Laverty HG, Wenwieser S, Douglas M, Wilson JB (2000) Mapping and expression analysis of the human CASK gene. Mamm Genome 11: 934–937.

Strømme P, Sundet K, Mørk C, Cassiman JJ, Fryns JP, Claes S (1999) X linked mental retardation and infantile spasms in a family: new clinical data and linkage to Xp11.4-Xp22.11. J Med Genet 36: 374–378.

Tarpey PS, Stevens C, Teague J, Edkins S, O'Meara S, Avis T, et al. (2006) Mutations in the gene encoding the Sigma 2 subunit of the adaptor protein 1 complex, AP1S2, cause X-linked mental retardation Am J Hum Genet 79: 1119–1124.

Tentler D, Gustavsson P, Leisti J, Schueler M, Chelly J, Timonen E, et al. (1999) Deletion including the oligophrenin-1 gene associated with enlarged cerebral ventricle, cerebellar hypoplasia, seizures and ataxia. Eur J Hum Genet 7: 541–548.

Thauvin-Robinet C, Cossee M, Cormier-Daire V, Van Maldergem L, Toutain A, Alembik Y, et al. (2006) Clinical, molecular, and genotype-phenotype correlation studies rom 25 cases of oral-facial-digital syndrome type 1: a French and Belgian collaborative study J Med Genet 43: 54–61.

Thelen K, Kedar V, Panicker AK, Schmid RS, Midkiff BR, Maness PF (2002) The neural cell adhesion molecule L1 potentiates integrin-dependent cell migration to extracellular matrix proteins. J Neurosci 22: 4918–4931.

Turner EV, Roberts E (1938) A family with a sex-linked hereditary ataxia. J Nerv Ment Dis 97: 74–80.

Vandewalle J, van Esch H, Govaerts K, Verbeeck J, Zweier C, Madrigal I, et al. (2009) Dosage-dependent severity of the phenotype in patients with Mental retardation due to a recurrent copy-number gain at Xq28 mediated by an unusual recombination. Am J Hum Genet 85: 809–822.

Van Esch H, Bauters M, Ignatius J, Jansen M, Raynaud M, Hollanders K, et al. (2005) Duplication of the MECP2 region is a frequent cause of severe mental retardation and progressive neurological symptoms in males. Am J Hum Genet 77: 442–453.

Verkerk AJ, Pieretti M, Sutcliffe JS, Fu YH, Kuhl DP, Pizzuti A, et al. (1991) Identification of a gene (FMR-1) containinga CGG repeat coincident with a breakpoint cluster region exhibiting lengthvariation in fragile X syndrome. Cell 65: 905–914.

Wieland I, Weidner C, Ciccone R, Lapi E, McDonald-McGinn D, Kress W, et al. (2007) Contiguous gene deletions involving EFNB1, OPHN1, PJA1 and EDA in patients with craniofrontonasal syndrome. Clin Genet 72: 506–516.

Yaghmai R, Kimyai-Asadi A, Rostamiani K, Heiss NS, Poustka A, Eyaid W, et al. (2000) Overlap of dyskeratosis congenita with the Hoyeraal-Hreidarsson syndrome. J Pediatr 136: 390–393.

Young ID, Moore JR, Tripp JH (1987) Sex-linked recessive congenital ataxia. J Neurol Neurosurg Psychiatr 50: 1230–1232.

Zanni G, Saillour Y, Nagara M, Billuart P, Castelnau L, Moraine C, et al. (2005) Mutations of Oligophrenin 1 frequently cause X-linked mental retardation with cerebellar hypoplasia. Neurology 65: 1364–1369.

Zanni G, Bertini E, Bellcross C, Nedelec B, Froyen G, Neuhäuser G, et al. (2008) X-linked congenital ataxia: a new locus maps to Xq25-q27.1. Am J Med Genet 146A: 593–600.

26
Recessive Ataxias

Alessandra Terracciano, Ginevra Zanni, and Enrico Bertini

Autosomal recessive cerebellar ataxias (ARCA) are neurological disorders characterized by abnormal development of the cerebellum alone or associated with neurodegeneration, peripheral neuropathy, and brainstem and spinal cord involvement. By definition these conditions have autosomal recessive inheritance and, in most cases, they have early onset occurring in infancy and childhood or, at the latest, before the age of 25 years. This group encompasses a large number of rare diseases. Peripheral neuropathy, ophthalmological abnormalities, and additional extra-neurological signs and symptoms may provide important clues for diagnosis. Thus a clinical classification has been proposed as follows:

1. ARCA with sensory involvement and spinocerebellar ataxias;
2. ARCA with sensory-motor polyneuropathy;
3. ARCA with purely cerebellar ataxias.

Examples of the first category include ataxia with isolated vitamin E deficiency, abetalipoproteinemia, Refsum disease, infantile-onset spinocerebellar ataxia, and ataxia with blindness and deafness. Examples of ataxia with sensorimotor polyneuropathy include ataxia with oculomotor apraxia 1 and 2, spinocerebellar ataxia with neuropathy, and autosomal recessive spastic ataxia of Charlevoix-Saguenay. Examples of purely cerebellar ataxia include most of the autosomal recessive congenital ataxias, and ataxia with hypogonadotropic hypogonadism (Koenig 2003).

Friedreich ataxia, the most common ARCA, was first described in 1863 and is seen worldwide (Palau and Espinós 2006; Fogel et al. 2007). In the last few years, several other conditions have also been recognized and their loci and genes identified.

On the basis of the underlying pathological mechanisms, ARCA can be classified into five main groups: (1) congenital; (2) metabolic; (3) DNA repair defects; (4) neurodegenerative; (5) unknown pathogenesis. Although congenital ataxia is not a pathogenetic subcategory we will keep it as a separate entity because it includes a complex group of heterogeneous disorders starting early in life and all with symptoms of hypotonia and delayed motor development.

Congenital ataxias

Congenital ataxia is defined and extensively discussed in Chapter 9. We will particularly focus on conditions with autosomal recessive inheritance.

Congenital ataxias, first described by Batten (in 1905) as 'cases in which ataxia has been noted early in life and in which there is a tendency to gradual improvement', are a heterogeneous group of disorders accounting for 10% of nonprogressive infantile encephalopathies (Sanner and Hagberg 1974; Esscher et al. 1996). Many of these conditions were first classified under the term 'dysequilibrium syndrome' first employed by Alajouanine et al. (1943) and subsequently by Hagberg et al. (1972) and Sanner (1973) to encompass what we now know as a spectrum of genetically heterogeneous conditions that combine autosomal recessive, nonprogressive cerebellar ataxia with mental retardation (UK: learning disability). They are characterized by severe hypotonia at birth and delayed motor development followed by the appearance of nonprogressive cerebellar ataxia and other typical signs of cerebellar dysfunction in the first years of life.

In two-thirds of cases there is neuroradiological evidence of structural cerebellar anomalies without any other gross abnormality of the central nervous system. Mild to moderate mental retardation is present in more than half of the patients (Steinlin et al. 1999). These conditions can be caused by autosomal recessive, autosomal dominant or X-linked traits.

Congenital ataxias are clinically classified into pure cerebellar and syndromic forms (Steinlin 1998) although neuroimaging is of pivotal importance for subclassification of congenital ataxia, dividing this group of disorders into (1) CA with cerebellar malformations or early-onset abnormalities, (2) CA with cerebellar hypoplasia, and (3) CA with nonprogressive cerebellar ataxia and cerebellar atrophy. Pure cerebellar congenital ataxias include all nonprogressive encephalopathies showing typical features of cerebellar dysfunction in the absence of pyramidal tract dysfunction or dysmorphic features.

The main conditions under the classification of CA with cerebellar malformations or early-onset abnormalities are Dandy-Walker malformation, Joubert syndrome, and pontocerebellar hypoplasia (PCH). Dandy-Walker malformation, Joubert syndrome, rhomboencephalosynapsis, and PCH are presented in chapters 10, 11, 16 and 23, respectively, of this volume.

CA with cerebellar hypoplasia can be distinguished from global cerebellar hypoplasia such as in X-linked OPHN1 (oligophrenin 1) deficiency (see Chapter 25) or in association with haploinsufficiency of *ZIC1* and *ZIC4* (Grinberg et al. 2004) and cerebellar hypoplasia limited to the vermis. Many conditions of CA with cerebellar hypoplasia are associated with dysmorphic syndromes and cognitive impairment with unknown underlying genetic cause. We will describe in more detail some conditions such as the very rare CA with cerebellar hypoplasia defined as Cayman ataxia where the molecular basis has been elucidated.

Finally, CA with nonprogressive cerebellar ataxia and cerebellar atrophy is a heterogeneous group of conditions with X-linked or autosomal recessive inheritance. Genetic causes of most of these conditions are unknown but some genetic loci have been recognized. Mutations in the *ADCK3/COQ8* gene (MIM *606980) associated with coenzyme Q10 deficiency have been characterized in the last years; however, the *ADCK3/COQ8* gene is not associated with a congenital ataxia but is responsible for ataxia starting later in childhood.

Congenital ataxia with cerebellar malformations or early-onset abnormalities

Joubert syndrome, Dandy-Walker malformation, and rhomboencephalosynapsis are covered elsewhere in this volume (see above).

Pontocerebellar hypoplasia

Pontocerebellar hypoplasia is discussed in Chapter 23.

Cerebellar agenesis and diabetes mellitus

Neonatal diabetes mellitus with cerebellar hypoplasia/agenesis (MIM #609069) was first described by Hoveyda et al. (1999) in three patients born from consanguineous parents. Patients had dysmorphic facial features consisting of beaked nose and low-set, dysplastic ears. Later another patient was described by Sellick et al. (2004) with an identical phenotype. No pancreas was present at autopsy, and detailed macroscopic and microscopic examination failed to detect any pancreatic tissue in the abdominal cavity. By using a positional cloning candidate gene approach, they found a mutation in the *PTF1A* gene (MIM *607194).

Congenital ataxia with cerebellar hypoplasia

Chapter 8 contains an extensive discussion on cerebellar hypoplasia.

Several dysmorphic and multiple malformation syndromes have been reported to be associated with cerebellar hypoplasia, but autosomal recessive conditions are very few. The best characterized form is Ritscher-Schinzel cranio-cerebello-cardiac (3C) syndrome (MIM %220210). Ritscher and Schinzel described the first two patients with 3C syndrome in 1987 (Herman and Siegel 2008). Current diagnostic criteria for this condition in a patient with normal chromosomes are the following: (1) congenital heart disease more complicated than simple patent ductus arteriosus; (2) Dandy-Walker malformation or vermian hypoplasia; and (3) craniofacial malformations: either cleft palate and ocular colobomas or four of the following: prominent occiput, prominent forehead, hypertelorism, micrognathia, depressed nasal bridge, downward slanting palpebral fissures, low-set ears, and depressed nasal bridge. The severity of the congenital heart disease determines the prognosis of patients with 3C syndrome.

Additional findings reported in 3C syndrome patients include rib anomalies (18%), hypospadias (14%), renal hypoplasia, anal anomalies, lymphedema, human growth hormone deficiency, single umbilical artery, and heterochromia iritidis.

Other well-known conditions associated with cerebellar hypoplasia are seen in some patients with 22q11 microdeletion (Bish 2006), hemizygous mutations in *MID1* (MIM *300552) in X-linked Opitz G/BBB syndrome (MIM #300000) (De Falco et al. 2003). Interestingly, cerebellar vermis hypoplasia has also been obtained in a mouse line carrying a nonfunctional ortholog of the human *MID1* gene, *Mid1*. *Mid1*-null mice show the brain anatomical defect observed in patients with X-linked Opitz G/BBB syndrome (i.e., hypoplasia of the anterior portion of the medial cerebellum, the vermis) (Lancioni et al. 2010). Moreover several conditions associated with lissencephaly are associated with isolated cerebellar hypoplasia (Ross et al. 2001) or cerebellar and brainstem hypoplasia (Jissendi-Tchofo et al. 2009). Lissencephaly syndromes in which cerebellar and/or brainstem hypoplasia are frequently associated and can be an important clue for diagnosis are the following:

1. X-linked conditions such as bilateral periventricular nodular heterotopia as a consequence of Filamin A (MIM *300017) mutations (Parrini et al. 2006), X-linked cerebral malformations associated with abnormal genitalia with mutations in ARX (MIM *300382) (Kato et al. 2004), or X-linked lissencephaly (MIM #300067) and mutations in *DCX* (MIM *300121) (Doublecortin) (Leger et al. 2008);
2. Recessive mutations in *Reelin* (MIM *600514) (Fatemi 2005), and *GPR56* (MIM *604110) (Koirala et al. 2009; see Fig. 26.1), defects of *O*-glycosylation (Clement et al. 2008), and other microlissencephaly syndromes with unknown genetic cause (Barkovich et al. 1998);
3. Dominant mutations in *alpha-tubulin 1a* gene (*TUBA1A*; MIM *602529) (Kumar et al. 2010) and *TUBB2B* (MIM *612850) (Jaglin et al. 2009).

Furthermore, two autosomal recessive conditions in which the genetic basis has been disclosed are cerebellar hypoplasia and mutations in VLDL receptor, and Cayman ataxia, which are discussed in Chapters 8 and 9.

Congenital ataxia with nonprogressive cerebellar ataxia and cerebellar atrophy

Evidence for autosomal recessive inheritance of nonprogressive cerebellar ataxia and cerebellar atrophy has been reported (Guzzetta et al. 1993). The MRI generally shows isolated atrophy of the cerebellum with visible sulci (Fig. 26.2). More recently, linkage to chromosomes 9q, 15q, and 20q has been described in recessively inherited syndromic (Delague et al. 2002) and nonsyndromic (Delague et al. 2001; Tranebjaerg et al. 2003) forms of CA with severe mental retardation. Some of these conditions may fall in the classification of Norman type of cerebellar atrophy, which is discussed in the section 'Ataxias with unknown pathogenesis', below.

The syndromic form, cerebellar ataxia with mental retardation, optic atrophy and skin abnormalities (CAMOS), (MIM #606937) is a rare autosomal recessive syndrome characterized

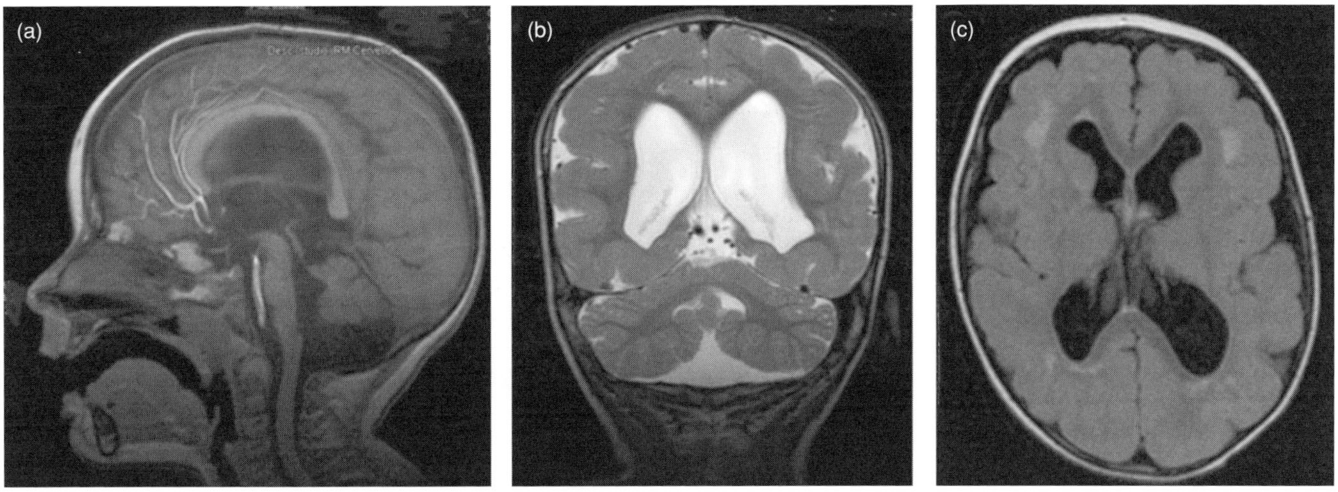

Fig. 26.1. (a–c) Patient affected by a homozygous mutation in the *GPR56* gene. **(a)** Sagittal T1-weighted image shows a flattened pons and cerebellar vermal hypoplasia. **(b)** Notice small multiple cerebellar cysts and simplified gyral sulci of the neocortex in the coronal T2-weighted section of (b). **(c)** Axial FLAIR image showing white matter periventricular abnormal signals.

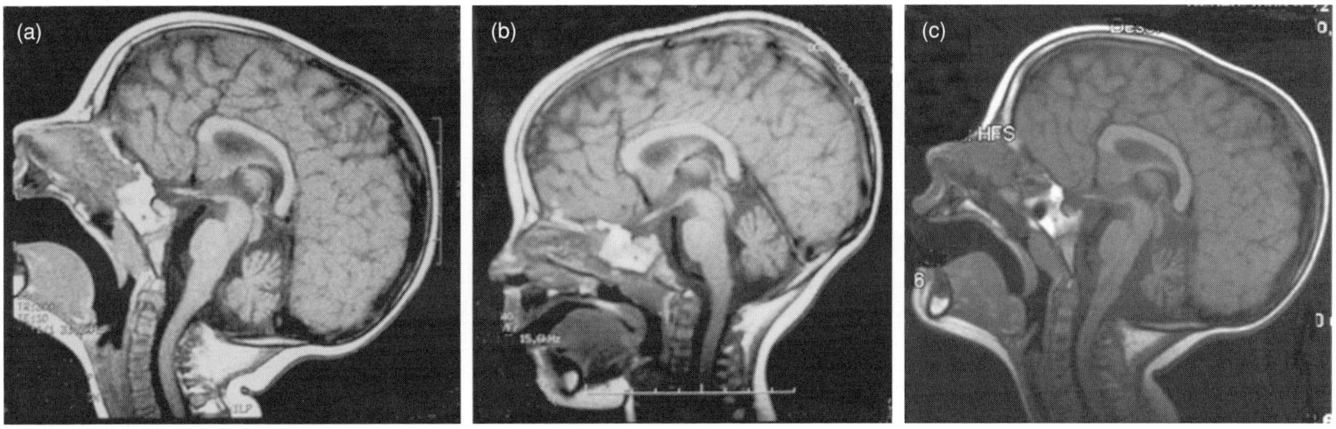

Fig. 26.2. (a–c) Serial Sagittal T1-weighted images of the same patient at different ages: **(a)** at 1 year old, **(b)** at around age 2 years, and **(c)** at around age 3 years. The serial images show a progressive global atrophy of the cerebellum, indicated, in the images, by the progressive atrophy of the vermis. The patient is now aged 4 years 6 months and is affected by a congenital ataxia of undefined genetic cause. Parents are not consanguineous. The child had hypotonia in the neonatal period and developed strabismus at age 3 months. He was able to walk with support from the age of 4 years and is slowly improving.

by a nonprogressive congenital cerebellar ataxia associated with mental retardation, optic atrophy, and skin abnormalities. Homozygosity mapping in a large inbred Lebanese Druze family, which was previously mapped to chromosome 15q24–q26, led to the identification of a homozygous p.Gly1046Arg missense mutation in *ZNF592*, in all five affected individuals of the family. *ZNF592* encodes a 1267-amino-acid zinc-finger (ZnF) protein and seems to be implicated in a complex developmental pathway, and it is likely that mutations disturb the highly orchestrated regulation of this gene during cerebellar development (Nicolas et al. 2010).

Metabolic ataxias

Metabolic ataxias can be treatable disorders, and it is particularly important to make an early and accurate diagnosis in this group of ARCA. In this section we summarize the following conditions: ataxia with vitamin E deficiency, abetalipoproteinemia, hypobetalipoproteinemia, Refsum disease, and cerebrotendinous xanthomatosis, avoiding most of the mitochondrial, lysosomal, and peroxisomal conditions that are reviewed in Chapter 27.

Friedreich ataxia

Friedreich ataxia (FRDA; MIM #229300) is the most common recessive ataxia worldwide, with an estimated prevalence in the Caucasian population of 1:30 000 to 1:50 000 (Pandolfo 2008), and a carrier frequency of 1:85 (Fogel and Perlman 2007). Its onset is usually in the second decade of life, but can vary from 2 to 25 years of age. Clinical manifestations are characterized by a combination of sensory and cerebellar symptoms, and gait instability is usually the first recognized abnormality. Diabetes is generally insulin dependent, and appears in about 10–15% of patients (Pandolfo 2008). Relentlessly progressive ataxia is characteristic, and 10–15 years after onset, patients are usually wheelchair bound. Dysarthria is also an early and incapacitating symptom, leading to almost incomprehensible speech. Vibratory and positional sense is affected, and Romberg sign is usually positive. Deep tendon reflexes are absent, but extensor plantar reflex (Babinski sign) is usually present. Abnormal eye movements and defective fixation are also observed. Cognitive function is preserved, but communication abilities can be affected, with changes in working and visuo-spatial memory (Mantovan et al. 2006). Systemic abnormalities such as hypertrophic cardiomyopathy, cardiac conduction defects, and diabetes can occur. As disease progresses, pes cavus and scoliosis are almost always present. Although there are significant variations in the onset and rate of disease progression, the mean age at death has been reported to be approximately 38 years, with a range as wide as 5 to 70 years. Death is usually secondary to progressive cardiomyopathy (Pandolfo 2008) but other patients may die from aspiration pneumonia. Brain MRI in Friedreich ataxia does not show cerebellar atrophy but may show a mild degree of cerebellar volume. Spinal cord MRI can disclose mild atrophy of its cervical segment, which is explained by the large loss of primary sensory neurons in the dorsal root ganglia, early in the course of the disease. Nerve conduction studies characteristically show axonal sensory neuropathy (Koeppen et al. 2007). Atypical forms of Friedreich ataxia, such as late onset or with maintained reflexes, have been proposed, but it is now clear that they are also caused by mutations in the same gene.

Friedreich ataxia is neuropathologically characterized by the presence of the most conspicuous neurodegeneration involving the spinal cord (posterior columns, spinocerebellar tracts, and corticospinal tracts) (Lamarche et al. 1984; Oppenheimer and Esiri 1992).

In about 98% of cases, the disease is associated with a triplet GAA expansion in the first intron of the *FRDA* gene on chromosome 9q13. This mutation causes the formation of a 'sticky' triplex DNA structure that interferes with the transcription of the gene and reduces the synthesis of frataxin, a mitochondrial protein of 210 amino acids, normally expressed at high levels in the human spinal cord (Campuzano et al. 1996; Koutnikova et al. 1997).

There is evidence that frataxin is closely involved in the early steps of the iron-sulfur cluster (ISC) biosynthesis and acts as an iron storage protein, maintaining iron in a nontoxic and bioavailable form (Gerber et al. 2003). Yeast strains disrupted for yeast frataxin homolog gene (*YFH1*) show a severe defect of mitochondrial respiration, intramitochondrial iron accumulation, and increased sensitivity to oxidative stress (Koutnikova et al. 1997; Lodi et al. 2006). Furthermore, findings from animal models demonstrate that the tissue-specific targeted disruption of the frataxin gene in the heart muscle causes decreased activity of mitochondrial complex II and late-stage iron accumulation (Puccio et al. 2001).

On the basis of previous studies, it has been supposed that an excess of unbound reactive iron in mitochondria, by virtue of its capacity to produce free oxygen radicals, via iron-catalyzed Fenton chemistry, may cause the oxidation of cellular components and the inactivation of mitochondrial enzymes (Schon and Manfredi 2003).

The key role of oxidative stress in the pathophysiology of the disease has been confirmed by studies showing elevated levels of oxidative stress markers in FRDA patients (Edmond et al. 2000; Schulz et al. 2000; Piemonte et al. 2001; Tozzi et al. 2002) and demonstrating the protective effect of antioxidants, such as idebenone and vitamin E, in animal or in vitro disease models (Jauslin et al. 2007). Moreover, we found decreased levels of free glutathione, a tissue sensor of oxidative stress, in blood and fibroblasts of patients with FRDA (Piemonte et al. 2001; Pastore et al. 2003).

Coenzyme Q10 and its synthetic analog idebenone, vitamin E, and, more recently, the iron chelator deferiprone have been used for treating Friedreich ataxia (Cooper et al. 2008; Gonçalves et al. 2008). Deferiprone, an atypical iron chelator, may decrease accumulation of toxic iron in the mitochondria in patients, but the recommended dose and the efficiency of this is controversial treatment. Recent preclinical studies delivering HDAC inhibitors in FRDA patient cells and a knock-in mouse model have demonstrated to reverse gene silencing for the FXN gene (Gonçalves et al. 2008).

Ataxia with coenzyme Q10 deficiency

Primary deficiency of coenzyme Q10 (MIM #607426) is a genetically heterogeneous disorder, with a highly variable clinical spectrum, which includes multisystemic manifestations as well as central nervous system (CNS) involvement. Five clinical subtypes have been recognized: (1) encephalomyopathic, with mitochondrial myopathy, recurrent myoglobinuria, and CNS symptoms and signs (Ogasahara et al. 1989); (2) early infantile multisystemic, with severe visceral and brain manifestations (Rotig et al. 2000); (3) Leigh syndrome (van Maldergem et al. 2002); (4) pure myopathic (Lalani et al. 2005); (5) ataxic (Quinzii et al. 2006).

The ataxic subtype is the most common presentation of CoQ10 deficiency. It is characterized by progressive ataxia, cerebellar atrophy, and reduced muscle CoQ10. Early symptoms may include developmental delay, hypotonia, and frequent falls. Global, progressive ataxia and dysarthria start before adolescence. Epileptic seizures, proximal or distal muscle weakness, dysphagia, ophthalmoparesis, nystagmus, peripheral axonal neuropathy, pyramidal signs, and scoliosis may also be present. Mental retardation or cognitive decline is also sometimes seen. The adult-onset form of ataxia and CoQ10 deficiency is usually associated with hypergonadotropic hypogonadism.

CoQ10 (also known as ubiquinone) is a lipophilic compound which is involved in electron transport from complex I and II to complex III of the mitochondrial respiratory chain. CoQ10 deficiency impairs proton transfer across the internal mitochondrial membrane and consequently leads to a reduction in ATP production (Duncan et al. 2009).

The main source of CoQ10 is endogenous synthesis, which involves a still-uncharacterized complex pathway. More than

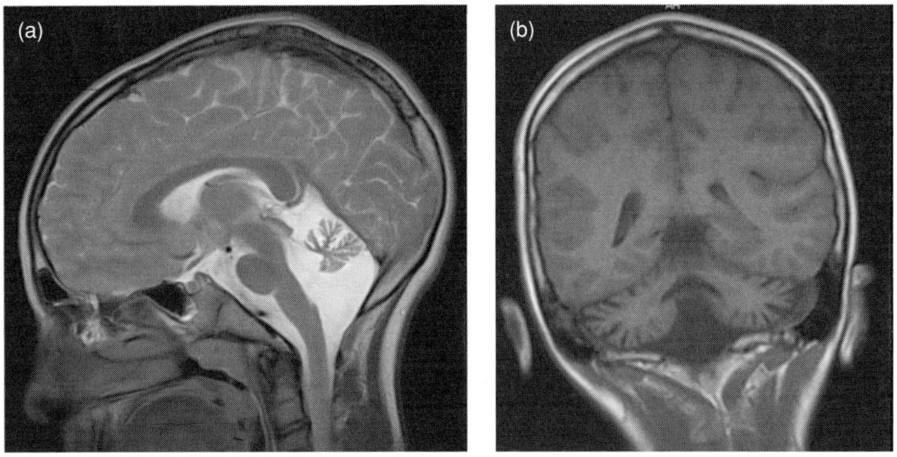

Fig. 26.3. **(a)** T2-weighted sagittal and **(b)** T1-weighted coronal images of a patient with coenzyme Q10 deficiency in the muscle biopsy, in which we did not find any mutations of the *ADCK3* gene, confiming the genetic heterogeneity of the pattern of congenital ataxia of later onset with coenzyme Q10 deficiency in skeletal muscle biopsy and cultured fibroblasts wih global cerebellar atrophy. Notice normal preservation of the supratentorial neocortical structures and of the brainstem. The patient is now 5 years old and is slowly improving with time but has a clear ataxia with clumsy gait and severe dysarthria. A pattern of global cerebellar atrophy is frequent in many ataxic syndromes of metabolic and DNA repair defects having several neurodegenerative causes.

ten genes are involved in the CoQ10 biosynthesis cascade, but up to now only five genes have been described as causative of pathogenic CoQ10 biosynthesis: *PDSS1* (MIM *607429) and *PDSS2* (MIM *607429) (subunits 1 and 2 of prenyldiphosphate synthase) (Mollet et al. 2007), *COQ2* (MIM *609825) (OH-benzoate polypreniltransferase) (Quinzii et al. 2006), *ADCK3/CABC1* (MIM *606980), which acts as a chaperone (Mollet et al. 2008), and *COQ9* (MIM *612837) (coenzyme Q9 homolog *S. cerevisiae*) (Duncan et al. 2009). Mutation in the *APTX* gene (MIM *606350) is associated with secondary CoQ10 deficiency (Quinzii et al. 2005).

Diagnosis is based on a reduced amount of CoQ10 in muscle, as plasma CoQ10 levels are usually normal. Muscle histopathology is essentially normal and brain MRI discloses global cerebellar atrophy (Fig. 26.3). Treatment with oral CoQ10 should be adjusted according to clinical results, with doses varying from 300 to 3000mg/day (Rotig et al. 2000). Treatment outcome is quite variable: in some patients disease stabilized while in others it progressed relentlessly. It is probable that treatment response is dependent on the underlying biochemical defect as well as stage of disease.

Ataxia with mutations in polymerase gamma

Polymerase gamma (*POLG*) (MIM *174763) is a nuclear encoded gene, whose product is responsible for maintaining the integrity of mitochondrial DNA (mtDNA) (Chan and Copeland 2009). Mutations in *POLG* are associated with a variety of clinical phenotypes, which includes Alpers disease, parkinsonism, and external progressive ophthalmoplegia. Two similar forms of ARCA are associated with mutations in *POLG*: mitochondrial recessive ataxic syndrome (MIRAS) and sensory ataxia, neuropathy, dysarthria, and ophthalmoplegia (SANDO) (Van Goethem et al. 2004; Milone et al. 2008).

MIRAS is the most frequent recessive ataxia in Finland (Winterhun et al. 2005). Clinical manifestations generally become apparent between 5 and 40 years of age, and are characterized by cerebellar ataxia, nystagmus, dysarthria, ophthalmoplegia, tremor, cognitive decline, and myoclonus. Loss of vibratory and position perception is commonly seen. Epilepsy is a frequent manifestation in MIRAS, but not in SANDO (MIM #607459), with both partial and generalized seizures, sometimes becoming refractory to antiepileptic drugs and evolving to status epilepticus (Van Goethem et al. 2004; Winterhun et al. 2005; Milone et al. 2008). Neuroimaging discloses cerebellar atrophy and T2-weighed hypersignal on thalamus, and dentate and inferior olivary nuclei. Nerve conduction studies also demonstrate axonal sensory neuropathy. Elevated protein may be detected in CSF. Muscle biopsy is not diagnostic, but Southern blotting analysis may detect multiple deletions in muscle mtDNA. Diagnosis is based on sequencing of the *POLG* gene, with two mutations (p.A467T and p.W748S) being responsible for most cases of this disorder in Caucasians (Van Goethem et al. 2004; Winterhun et al. 2005).

Infantile-onset spinocerebellar ataxia

Infantile-onset spinocerebellar ataxia (IOSCA) (MIM #271245) is currently identified only in Finland and is characterized by acute or subacute cerebellar signs triggered by an unspecific infection around the age of 1 year (Koskinen et al. 1995; Lönnqvist et al. 1998). The clinical features are similar to MIRAS (MIM #607459). Hypotonia, athetosis of hands and face, and ataxia with absent reflexes are the early symptoms of this disease. Later, at preschool age, ophthalmoplegia and neurosensorial deafness may be seen. Tactile, proprioceptive, and vibratory impairment, without pain or temperature compromise, are detected after the first decade. Adolescents are usually wheelchair bound with severe distal muscular atrophy, pes cavus, mild to moderate cognitive impairment, and optic atrophy without significant visual impairment. Refractory epilepsy and status epilepticus may contribute to rapid neurological deterioration and death. Further recognized abnormalities are autonomic dysfunction and, in females, primary hypogonadism (Koskinen et al. 1995; Lönnqvist et al. 1998).

There is no biochemical marker for IOSCA. Nerve conduction studies and nerve biopsy demonstrate a severe, mostly sensory, axonal neuropathy. Sensory ganglia are more severely affected than motor neurons (Koskinen et al. 1995; Lönnqvist et al. 1998). Neuroimaging studies at early stages of the disease demonstrate reduced size of cerebellar hemispheres which progress to a more widespread olivopontocerebellar atrophy.

Muscle biopsy is nondiagnostic but mtDNA depletion may be seen in this tissue. Pathological studies disclose spinal cord atrophy (more intense on the posterior funiculi), cerebellum, and brainstem; there is also marked loss of myelinated fibers on peripheral nerves (Lönnqvist et al. 1998).

IOSCA is caused by a mutation in the *C10ORF2* gene (MIM *606075), which codes for Twinkle, a specific mtDNA helicase, and one of its smaller isoforms, Twinky. Twinkle is important for maintenance and replication of mtDNA, and twinky function is currently unknown. The same founder mutation (p.Y508C) was detected in most Finnish patients with classic IOSCA. Mutations in *C10ORF2* may also be associated with different phenotypes, such as Alpers disease (early-onset encephalopathy with untreatable epilepsy, mtDNA depletion, and liver failure) and autosomal dominant progressive external ophthalmoplegia (Nikali et al. 2005).

Ataxia with vitamin E deficiency

Ataxia with vitamin E deficiency (AVED) (MIM #277460) is similar to Friedreich ataxia. Age at onset is usually between 4 and 20 years, with outliers ranging from 2 to 52 years. Clinical manifestations are characterized by progressive trunk and limb ataxia, dysarthria, disturbance of positional and vibratory lower limb senses, Babinski sign, and abolished deep tendon reflexes. Scoliosis and pes cavus are commonly seen (Cavalier et al. 1998; Mariotti et al. 2004; Marzouki et al. 2005), but retinopathy is less frequent. Dystonia (13%) and head titubation (28%) are more commonly seen in AVED than in Friedreich ataxia. Cardiomyopathy and an acute cardiac event may be associated with premature death among AVED cases (Mariotti et al. 2004; Marzouki et al. 2005).

AVED is caused by mutations in the α-tocopherol transfer protein gene (*TTPA*; MIM *600415), which codes a protein responsible for transferring α-tocopherol from chilomicrons to very-low-density lipoprotein (Marzouki et al. 2005; Mariotti et al. 2004). TTPA dysfunction causes very low levels of circulating α-tocopherol and tissue deficiency of this vitamin (Arita et al. 1995). Several different pathogenic mutations have been reported so far. Two mutations, associated with a severe phenotype, are particularly frequent in Europe, North Africa, and North America: c.744delA and c.486delT (Cavalier et al. 1998; Marzouki et al. 2005). On the other hand, the mutation p.H101G has only been detected in Japanese families and is associated with later onset and pigmentary retinopathy. Age at onset, clinical manifestations, and rate of progression are quite variable in AVED. It is usually stated that mutations causing profound TTPA protein depletion are responsible for a more severe phenotype, and mutations leading to amino acid substitution are associated with a milder form of the disease (Cavalier et al. 1998; Mariotti et al. 2004; Marzouki et al. 2005).

Diagnosis in a symptomatic individual is established with the determination of α-tocopherol (vitamin E) serum level, which is always below 2.5μg/mL (reference values: 5–15μg/mL) (Marzouki et al. 2005). Brain MRI is usually normal, but mild cerebellar atrophy may also be seen (Mariotti et al. 2004). A pattern of axonal sensitive neuropathy is often observed in nerve conduction studies (Cavalier et al. 1998).

AVED treatment consists of vitamin E oral administration at a dose of 600–2400mg/day. Serum levels may be used as guidance for oral dose adjustment (Cavalier et al. 1998; Mariotti et al. 2004; Marzouki et al. 2005). Differential diagnosis of α-tocopherol primary deficiency includes intestinal fat malabsorption and abetalipoproteinemia (Mariotti et al. 2004). As a rule, vitamin E serum levels should be checked in all patients with the Friedreich ataxia clinical phenotype without molecular confirmation for this condition.

Abetalipoproteinemia or Bassen-Kornzweig disease

Abetalipoproteinemia (ABL; MIM #200100), a multisystem disorder caused by a defect in lipoprotein metabolism, is characterized by acanthocytosis, atypical pigmentary retinopathy, and spinocerebellar degeneration (Berriot-Varoqueaux et al. 2000; Di Leo et al. 2008). In the first year of life, main clinical manifestations are chronic diarrhea and failure to thrive. Neurological features appear after the first decade of life, including absent deep tendon reflexes, superficial and deep sensory abnormalities, weakness and global ataxia (Di Leo et al. 2008). As the disease progresses, atypical pigmentary retinopathy characterized by small, irregularly distributed white spots, and night and color blindness is detected (Di Leo et al. 2008). Clinical manifestations of ABL are secondary to deficient absorption of the lipid-soluble vitamins A, D, E, and K (Berriot-Varoqueaux et al. 2000).

Apolipoprotein B (ApoB) is the main protein of both VLDL and LDL, and their assembly is dependent on microsomal triglyceride transfer protein (*MTP*; MIM *157147). Mutations in the gene coding for the large (88kD) subunit of MTP is responsible for ABL and determine very low levels of LDL and VLDL cholesterol. Decreased levels of vitamins A, K, and E, anemia, very low sedimentation rate, increased prothrombin time, and elevated creatine kinase are also observed. Deficient MTP can also lead to lipid infiltration of small bowel mucosa and hepatic steatosis (Berriot-Varoqueaux et al. 2000; Di Leo et al. 2008). Nerve conduction velocity usually discloses sensory axonal peripheral neuropathy (Di Leo et al. 2008).

ABL is treated with supplementation of vitamin A (100–400IU/kg/day), vitamin E (2400–14 400IU/day), and vitamin K (5mg/day). A low-fat diet combined with essential fatty acid supplementation is also recommended (Berriot-Varoqueaux et al. 2000; Di Leo et al. 2008). Coagulation tests are used to monitor vitamin K and serum levels of vitamin A and E to check for adequate vitamin supplementation (Berriot-Varoqueaux et al. 2000; Di Leo et al. 2008).

Refsum disease

Refsum disease (MIM #266500) is a peroxisomal disorder clinically characterized by pigmentary retinopathy, cerebellar ataxia, mixed motor-sensory neuropathy, and elevated CSF protein. Its onset usually occurs before 20 years of age, with night blindness secondary to retinopathy, followed by progressive constriction of visual field and optic atrophy, cataracts, vitreous opacities, and nystagmus. Other common clinical manifestations are anosmia, nerve deafness, ichthyosis, bone dysplasia, and cardiac conduction abnormalities (Wierzbicki et al. 2002; Jansen et al. 2004). Psychiatric disorders are uncommon. If not adequately treated, Refsum disease can cause premature cardiac death (Wierzbicki et al. 2002; Jansen et al. 2004).

Elevation of serum phytanic acid is very suggestive, but not specific for Refsum disease (Wierzbicki et al. 2002; Jansen et al. 2004) because it can be found in other peroxisomal disorders. Phytanic acid is a branched long-chain fatty acid present in dairy products and red meat (Wierzbicki et al. 2002). It is a byproduct of chlorophyll catabolism and is not endogenously synthesized (Wierzbicki et al. 2002; Jansen et al. 2004). Diagnostic confirmation can be obtained by measuring the activity of phytanoyl-CoA hydroxylase in fibroblasts or by molecular analysis of the responsible gene (Jansen et al. 2004).

Refsum disease is genetically heterogeneous. Most cases are caused by mutations in *PHYH* (encoding phytanoyl-CoA hydroxylase; MIM *602026), a peroxisomal matrix enzyme which catalyses oxidation of branched-chain fatty acids (Wanders et al. 2001). Deficiency in *PEX7* (encoding peroxin-7), a protein involved in peroxisomal import of some enzymes, including phytanoyl-CoA hydroxylase, also results in this phenotype. *PEX7* (MIM *601757) mutations may also cause a severe peroxisomal biogenesis disorder known as rhizomelic chondrodysplasia punctata (Wanders et al. 2001; Wierzbicki et al. 2002; Jansen et al. 2004).

Treatment is based on phytanic acid dietary restriction, combined, if necessary, with plasmapheresis. With reduction of phytanic acid serum levels, Refsum disease symptoms stabilize and there may be some improvement of ataxia and ichthyosis, albeit effects on pigmentary retinopathy are uncertain (Wierzbicki et al. 2002; Jansen et al. 2004).

Cerebrotendinous xanthomatosis

Cerebrotendinous xanthomatosis (CTX; MIM #213700) is a rare disorder of bile acid synthesis (Keren and Falik-Zaccai 2009). Its main clinical manifestations are juvenile cataracts, chronic diarrhea, and tendinous xanthomas (Barkhof et al. 2000; Gallus et al. 2006).

In the neonatal period, a potentially lethal cholestatic syndrome has been reported. After the second decade of life, progressive neurological deterioration may occur, characterized by cognitive decline, psychiatric manifestations, cerebellar ataxia, progressive spastic paraplegia, dysphagia, and less frequently, seizures and peripheral neuropathy (Barkhof et al. 2000; Gallus et al. 2006; Berginer et al. 2009; Keren and Falik-Zaccai 2009). Exceptionally, neurological manifestations are restricted to the spinal cord (Barkhof et al. 2000). There is a wide intra- and inter-familial clinical variability (Barkhof et al. 2000; Gallus et al. 2006; Berginer et al. 2009; Keren and Falik-Zaccai 2009). Coronary heart disease without elevated cholesterol is an important cause of morbidity and mortality in adults (Keren and Falik-Zaccai 2009).

CTX is caused by mutations in the *CYP27A1* gene (MIM *606530), which codes for sterol 27-hydroxylase, a protein expressed mostly in liver. This enzyme is essential for bile acids synthesis, including chenodeoxycholic acid. In the absence of sterol 27-hydroxylase, the substrate of this enzyme is converted to cholestanol by the action of 7α-hydroxylase. Elevated serum cholestanol is the biochemical hallmark of CTX (Barkhof et al. 2000; Gallus et al. 2006; Berginer et al. 2009; Keren and Falik-Zaccai 2009). Increased urinary excretion of bile alcohol glucuronides may also be present. This disorder can be treated by oral administration of chenodeoxycholic acid, which inhibits 7α-hydroxylase and consequentely cholestanol synthesis (Barkhof et al. 2000; Gallus et al. 2006; Berginer et al. 2009; Keren and Falik-Zaccai 2009). Liver transplant is another therapeutic alternative (Keren and Falik-Zaccai 2009). Cholestanol determination in asymptomatic siblings of CTX patients is recommended in order to improve clinical outcome (Barkhof et al. 2000; Gallus et al. 2006; Berginer et al. 2009).

On brain MRI the most distinctive abnormalities are detected on T2-weighed and FLAIR sequences, which demonstrate bilateral, heterogeneous, and hyperintense sign in dentate nuclei and adjacent cerebellar white matter (Barkhof et al. 2000; Gallus et al. 2006). Other less characteristic abnormalities which may be detected are brainstem, cerebellar and cerebral atrophy and diffuse hyperintense cerebral white matter lesions. MR spectroscopy of CTX patients discloses reduction of *N*-acetylaspartate and increase in lactate (Gallus et al. 2006).

Ataxias and DNA repair defects

A common pathogenic cause of this group of disorders is a defect in double-strand or single-strand DNA repair. Extrinsic ocular movements are frequently associated with ataxia. Ataxia-telangiectasia, ataxia-telangiectasia-like disorder, apraxia, and oculomotor apraxia types 1, 2 and 3, and spinocerebellar ataxia with axonal neuropathy type 1 can be classified in this group of disorders.

Ataxia-telangiectasia

Ataxia-telangiectasia (MIM #208900) has an estimated frequency in the USA of 1/40 000 individuals (Chun and Gatti 2004) but is considered approximately eight times less frequent than FRDA following other epidemiological studies (Anheim et al. 2010). Progressive ataxia with onset before 3 years of age is the main clinical characteristic. Telangiectasias are another hallmark of disease and appear in at least 90% of affected individuals and their age at onset ranges from 2 to 8 years; they are more easily seen in conjunctivas, ears, face, and neck (Farr et al. 2002; Perlman et al. 2003; Chun and Gatti 2004). A large range of ophthalmological abnormalities may also be detected, including: optokinetic nystagmus (present in 81% of cases), gaze-induced nystagmus (seen in 29%), hypometric or delayed saccades (76%), delayed eye tracking (63%), strabismus (38%), and oculomotor apraxia (30%). Dysarthria, dysphagia, facial hypomimia, generalized hypotonia, peripheral neuropathy, and movement disorder, as tremor or choreoathetosis, are seen after 5 years of age (Farr et al. 2002; Perlman et al. 2003; Chun and Gatti 2004). Cognitive level is usually normal, even though severe dysarthria and incoordination may leave an impression of mental retardation. Independent gait is lost by the end of first decade (Perlman et al. 2003; Chun and Gatti 2004). Immunodeficiency (mainly humoral) leading to chronic sinopulmonary infection and increased susceptibility to cancer are other important features in ataxia-telangiectasia. Risk of lymphoproliferative disorders such as leukemia and lymphoma are dramatically increased in ataxia-telangiectasia (Perlman et al. 2003; Chun and Gatti 2004). Treating cancer in ataxia-telangiectasia patients is particularly challenging, because of their increased radiosensitivity and the adverse side effects of chemotherapy (Perlman et al. 2003). Female carriers of one mutated copy of the gene have a three- to four-fold increased risk of breast cancer when compared to the general population. The *ATM* gene encodes for an ATM serine/threonine kinase, a large protein with 3056 amino acids which is part of the phosphatidyl-inositol-3-kinase (PI3-K) complex, responsible for DNA repair during the cell cycle, avoiding incorporation of deleterious mutations (Chun and Gatti 2004). The *ATM* gene containes 66 exons, and its sequencing with current technology is still a challenge. Most patients are compound heterozygotes for *ATM* mutations and a large variety of sequence variants have been recognized, thus making interpretation of results difficult. Pathogenic mutations are usually nonsense mutations (85%), and missense mutations are responsible for 10% of detected pathogenic changes (Farr et al. 2002; Perlman et al. 2003; Chun and Gatti 2004). Some laboratory tests may help in the investigation of ataxia-telangiectasia: serum alpha-fetoprotein is elevated in more than 95% of cases and low levels of IgA and IgE and reduced T-lymphocyte count, with normal or elevated B-lymphocytes, are usually detected. Karyotype may show translocation between chromosomes 7 and 14 (Farr et al. 2002; Perlman et al. 2003; Chun and Gatti 2004) and radiosensivity tests may be used to demonstrate a predisposition to chromosomal breakage.

Follow-up neuroimaging generally shows cerebellar atrophy, which is initially more evident on the hemispheres and superior vermis and later becomes diffuse (Chun and Gatti 2004). CT scan and plain radiography should be avoided because of increased X-ray sensitivity.

Affected individuals are very sensitive to the effects of radiation exposure, including medical radiographs. Although people with ataxia-telangiectasia usually live into adulthood, their life expectancy is reduced.

Ataxia-telangiectasia-like disorder

Ataxia-telangiectasia-like disorders (ATLD; MIM #604391) is a very rare clinical condition which is characterized by slowly progressive ataxia with onset between 1 and 7 years of age, associated with oculomotor apraxia and dysarthria (Fernet et al. 2005). No ocular or facial telangiectasias are detected and cognition is preserved. Reflexes may be initially brisk and become reduced. At advanced stages of disease, tongue and facial dyskinesia, choreoathetosis, and dystonia, suggesting basal ganglia compromise, may be seen. ATLD is progressive up to adolescence, when it stabilizes. There is no increased risk for infections or neoplasias, as is seen in ataxia-telangiectasia, but occasionally microcephaly is present (Delia et al. 2004; Fernet et al. 2005).

Brain MRI detects cerebellar atrophy, and laboratory tests are non-informative. Radiosensitivity test is usually present but in a lesser degree than in ataxia-telangiectasia (Delia et al. 2004; Taylor et al. 2004; Fernet et al. 2005).

ATL is caused by mutations in the *MRE11* gene, located in chromosome 11q21, near the *ATM* gene. Its product is part of the MRN complex, which recognizes DNA double-strand breakage. Both missense and null mutations have been reported. Severity varies according to the type of molecular defect. Most of the reported cases were originally from Saudi Arabia (Delia et al. 2004; Taylor et al. 2004; Fernet et al. 2005).

Ataxia with oculomotor apraxia type 1

Ataxia with oculomotor apraxia type 1 (AOA1; MIM #208920) is a condition characterized by involuntary movements (chorea and dystonia) and/or progressive global ataxia, with dysarthria associated with hands and head tremor. Onset can vary between 1 and 20 years of age and developmental delay may be seen before clinical symptoms become apparent. As the disease progresses, movement disorders are attenuated and peripheral neuropathy signs, such as distal atrophy, pes cavus, superficial and deep sensory impairment, hypo/arreflexia, become apparent. The most distinctive clinical signs in AOA1 are related to external eye movements: gaze-evoked nystagmus (found in all patients), oculomotor apraxia (seen in 86%), saccadic pursuit, hypometric saccades, fixation instability, and excessive blinking (Barbot et al. 2001; Le Ber et al. 2003; Ferrarini et al. 2007). In advanced stages, oculomotor apraxia may be masked by progressive external ophthalmoparesis, which starts with upward gaze paralysis. Optic atrophy and retinal exudative lesions have been occasionally reported (Barbot et al. 2001; Le Ber et al. 2003). Variable cognitive impairment may be seen and mental retardation is not uncommon (Barbot et al. 2001; Le Ber et al. 2003).

Laboratory findings include hypoalbuminemia and hypercholesterolemia (Le Ber et al. 2003; Ferrarini et al. 2007). Elevated creatine kinase is occasionally detected. Nerve conduction velocity studies disclose sensory-motor axonal neuropathy. MRI reveals marked cerebellar atrophy, mild brainstem atrophy and, in advanced cases, cortical atrophy (Barbot et al. 2001; Le Ber et al. 2003; Ferrarini et al. 2007). Loss of myelinated fibers with maintenance of amyelinic fibers is seen at the sural nerve (Barbot et al. 2001; Le Ber et al. 2003; Ferrarini et al. 2007).

AOA1 is caused by mutation in the *APTX* gene (MIM *606350), which encodes aprataxin, a nuclear protein involved in single-strand DNA repair, acting in the same pathway of the ATM protein (Le Ber et al. 2003). Several mutations have been reported so far, most of them in exons 5, 6, and 7 of the *APTX* gene (Ferrarini et al. 2007). This condition was originally reported in Japan (where it is the most common cause of ARA) but is found worldwide. In Portugal, AOA1 is the second most common cause of ARCA (Le Ber et al. 2003).

Ataxia with oculomotor apraxia type 2 or spinocerebellar ataxia type 1

Ataxia with oculomotor apraxia type 2 (AOA2 or SCAR1; MIM #606002) is characterized by global progressive ataxia with onset usually between 8 and 25 years of age (Le Ber et al. 2004; Tazir et al. 2009), dysarthria, axonal motor sensory neuropathy, and oculomotor apraxia, which is seen in less than 50% of cases (Le Ber et al. 2004; Duquette et al. 2005; Tazir et al. 2009). Saccadic pursuit is seen in all patients, gaze-evoked nystagmus in 89%, and bilateral limited abduction of the eyes with strabismus in 61% of the patients (Le Ber et al. 2004). Dystonia, head and postural tremor, chorea, dysphagia, pes cavus, and scoliosis are occasionally seen. Cognitive function is usually preserved, but executive dysfunction is sometimes observed (Le Ber et al. 2004; Duquette et al. 2005; Tazir et al. 2009). Premature ovarian failure was also reported in some patients (Le Ber et al. 2004). Progression is slow, and most patients are wheelchair bound 10 years after disease onset (Le Ber et al. 2004; Tazir et al. 2009).

Serum alpha-fetoprotein is mildly to moderately elevated in all patients with AOA2 (Le Ber et al. 2004; Duquette et al. 2005; Tazir et al. 2009). Increased serum creatine kinase, cholesterol, and immunoglobulin IgG and IgA, and reduced serum albumin are inconstantly seen (Le Ber et al. 2004; Duquette et al. 2005). Brain MRI discloses diffuse cerebellar atrophy, more intense in the vermis, occasionally associated with pontine atrophy (Duquette et al. 2005). Nerve conduction studies detect sensory-motor axonal neuropathy and nerve biopsy demonstrates that large myelinated fibers are more severely affected than thin fibers (Le Ber et al. 2004; Duquette et al. 2005).

AOA2 is caused by mutation in the *SETX* gene (encoding senataxin; MIM *608465), a protein with DNA and RNA helicase activity and which is involved in RNA processing and DNA repair (Le Ber et al. 2004; Duquette et al. 2005; Tazir et al. 2009). Amyotrophic lateral sclerosis type 4 (ALS4) is caused by dominant mutations in senataxin (Duquette et al. 2005).

Ataxia with oculomotor apraxia type 3

Ataxia with oculomotor apraxia type 3 (AOA3) is a recently described ARCA with a phenotype similar to ataxia-telangiectasia, but with onset after 8 years of age. Reported clinical features are ataxic gait, dysarthria, oculomotor apraxia, and cerebral atrophy. No telangiectasia, biochemical abnormalities, or nerve conduction impairment was detected. Studies performed in fibroblasts demonstrated a defect in repairing DNA, making these cells sensitive to agents that cause single-strand breaks in DNA. Nevertheless, a locus for AOA3 remains elusive (Gueven et al. 2007).

Spinocerebellar ataxia with axonal neuropathy type 1

Spinocerebellar ataxia with axonal neuropathy type 1 (SCAN1; MIM #607250) is a rare disorder recognized in 2002 in a large consanguineous family from Saudi Arabia (Takashima et al. 2002). Age at onset is around 14 years, characterized by moderate ataxia, dysarthria, muscular weakness, distal atrophy, pes cavus, and reduction of vibratory and postural sense. Epilepsy may occur, but there is no cognitive decline or oculomotor abnormality. Nerve conduction studies disclose motor-sensory axonal neuropathy and biochemical tests are nondiagnostic, but low serum albumin and elevated cholesterol are occasionally seen (Takashima et al. 2002). Mild cerebellar and cerebral atrophy may be present on MRI studies. SCAN1 is caused by mutation in the *TDP1* gene, which codes for tyrosil DNA phosphodiesterase 1 (MIM *607198), a protein involved in single-strand DNA repair. SCAN1 is an additional example of nervous system vulnerability to impaired DNA repair, as occurs in AOA1, AOA2, and ataxia-telangiectasia (Takashima et al. 2002; El-Khamisy and Caldecott 2006).

Degenerative ataxias

Degenerative ataxias have as a common feature the compromise of a protein that acts as a chaperone, helping protein folding. Two conditions belong to this group: autosomal recessive ataxia of Charlevoix-Saguenay and Marinesco-Sjögren syndrome. Another condition is related to the defect of a protein that is a component of the nuclear lamina.

Autosomal recessive ataxia of Charlevoix-Saguenay

In the Saguenay-Lac-St-Jean (SLSJ) region of Quebec, Bouchard et al. (1978) identified a distinctive form of early-onset spastic ataxia. They named this syndrome autosomal recessive spastic ataxia of Charlevoix-Saguenay (ARSACS; MIM #270550). None of the patients ever walked normally, and the disease had a long course with little progression after age 20 years. Ataxia, dysarthria, spasticity, distal muscle wasting, nystagmus, defect in conjugate pursuit ocular movements, and hypermyelination of retinal fibers constitute the most frequent progressive neurological signs; the frequent presence (57%) of mitral valve prolapse is reported. The disorder bore some similarity to Troyer syndrome. Deafness is reported in two independent patients segregating a deletion spanning the *SACS* gene, responsible for the disease (Breckpot et al. 2008; Terracciano et al. 2009); however, clinical presentation of patients harboring a deleted allele does not seem to differ significantly from typical individuals harboring loss-of-function mutations in *SACS*. Cognitive skills are preserved in the long term as individuals remain able to perform tasks of daily living late into adulthood. Death commonly occurs in the sixth decade. Brain MRI generally shows cerebellar atrophy that may be limited for many years to the cerebellar vermis (Fig. 26.4).

Although initially confined to Quebec, genetically confirmed ARSACS has now been reported in individuals from France, Tunisia, Italy, Spain, Japan, Turkey, and the Netherlands

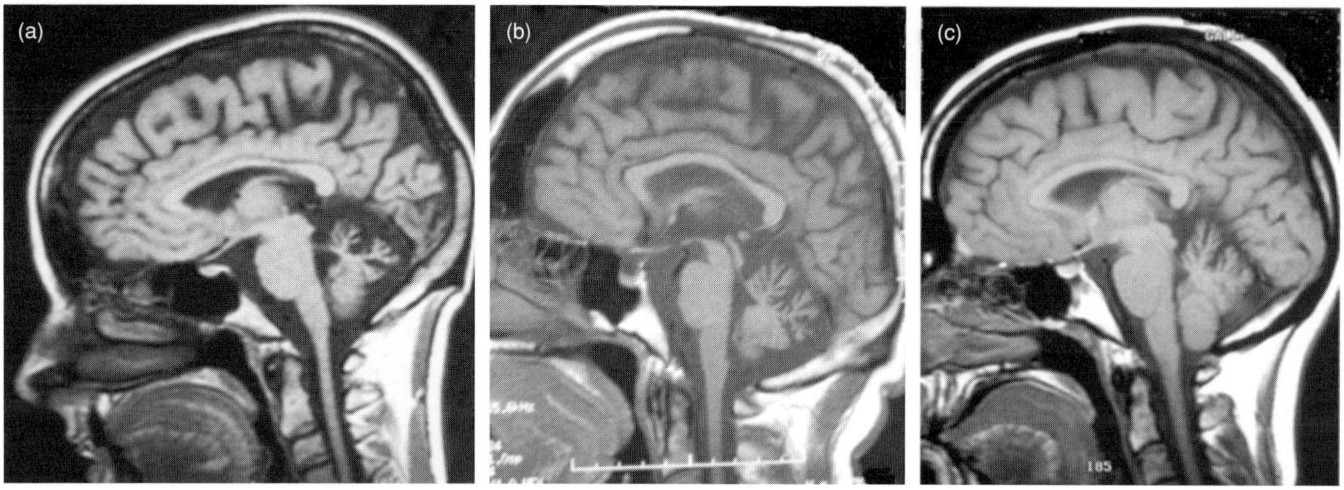

Fig. 26.4. (a–c) Sagittal T1-weighted images of three young adult patients with confirmed mutations in the *SACS* gene, showing a characteristic pattern mostly limited to the anterior and superior cerebellar lobuli. Notice mild hypoplasia of the corpus callosum. This pattern is generally evident during the first decade of life.

(Criscuolo et al. 2004, 2005; Grieco et al. 2004; Ogawa et al. 2004; Takiyama 2006; Vermeer et al. 2008). A probable founder effect accounts for an estimated ARSACS carrier frequency in the French Canadian population of 1:21, with a birth incidence of 1:1932; meanwhile the true worldwide incidence remains unknown as underdiagnosis is likely.

The *sacsin* (SACS; MIM *604490) gene, identified by linkage in the chromosome 13q12 region, was initially described as a unique large exon spanning 12 794bp with an 11 487bp open reading frame (Engert et al. 2000), then the gene structure was revised and eight new exons were discovered in addition to the first recognized gigantic exon (Ouyang et al. 2006). Despite the gene structure revision, the gigantic exon still segregates most of the pathological allelic variants, to date at least 21 mutations on the *SACS* gene have been found in Quebec and non-Quebec patients (reviewed by Takiyama 2006); in individuals with ARSACS born in Quebec the 6594delT mutation in homozygosity accounts for 92.6% of the mutated population, while 3.7% of individuals were compound heterozygotes for the common deletion and a missense 5254C>T mutation. Up till now, *SACS* is the only gene associated with ARSACS, although the existence of some patients, showing all strict diagnostic criteria but not harboring *SACS* gene mutations, suggests the presence of a second disease gene. In 2007 Bouslam et al. identified in an informative consanguineous Moroccan family a novel locus, named SAX2, to chromosome 17p13.

Recent implementation of quantitative approaches in routine diagnostic tests has led to the identification of a large deletion spanning the whole *SACS* gene in heterozygosity with a point mutation in Belgian, Italian, and English patients (Breckpot et al. 2008; Terracciano et al. 2009, 2010). One patient with the gene deletion is reported in a French Canadian population segregating *SACS* deletion in homozygosity (McMillan et al. 2009).

Sacsin is a 479kDa protein of yet unknown function. The carboxy-terminus domain harbors a 'DnaJ' motif that has the potential to interact with members of the HSP70 family of heat-shock proteins and stimulate its ATPase activity. The *N*-terminus has extensive homology for HSP90, a subtype of heat-shock protein that can act as a chaperone molecule important in the regulation of protein folding. Wild-type sacsin is expressed throughout the CNS, in skeletal muscles, and in skin fibroblasts (Parfitt et al. 2009). However, no knockout transgenic models of ARSACS are yet available to assess the potential lethality of mutated sacsin.

Marinesco-Sjögren syndrome

Marinesco-Sjögren syndrome (MSS; MIM #248800) is a rare, multisystem disorder, characterized by congenital or early-onset cataracts, developmental delay, cerebellar ataxia, and mild to severe mental retardation. Microcephaly, nystagmus, short stature, scoliosis, hypergonadotropic hypogonadism, and myopathy are common additional features (Lagier-Tourenne et al. 2003; Senderek et al. 2005). Peripheral neuropathy, deafness, optic atrophy, strabismus, spasticity, and seizures may be present. Disease progression is slow and long survival can be expected.

Brain MRI usually discloses a global cerebellar atrophy. Additional uncommon findings are cortical atrophy and leukoencephalopathy. Serum creatine kinase is usually elevated and muscle biopsy shows chronic myopathy with rimmed subsarcolemmal vacuoles (Lagier-Tourenne et al. 2003; Senderek et al. 2005).

MSS is caused by mutations in the *SIL1* gene (encoding a nucleotide exchange factor for heat-shock protein 70 family member, HSPA5 (MIM *608005). Heat-shock protein 70 family members are the highly conserved molecular chaperones that assist in stabilization and folding of newly synthesized polypeptides. Decrease of *SIL1* gene product leads to a reduction of protein synthesis in endoplasmic reticulum (Anttonen et al. 2005; Senderek et al. 2005).

ARCA1

Spinocerebellar ataxia, autosomal recessive 8 (ARCA1; MIM #610743) is a form identified by Gros-Louis et al. (2007) in a geographically defined group of 26 French Canadian families, including 53 affected family members, most of whom originated from the Beauce and Bas-St. Laurent regions of the province of Quebec, Canada. All of the affected family members had a similar phenotype, which consisted of adult-onset cerebellar ataxia with slow progression accompanied by dysarthria, with few associated features other than dysmetria, occasional brisk lower-extremity tendon reflexes, and minor abnormalities in saccades and smooth pursuit. None of the individuals showed optic atrophy, auditory loss, sensory abnormalities, autonomic disturbances, or extrapyramidal signs. Nerve conduction studies carried out in 18 affected individuals were all within normal limits. Imaging by CT or MRI invariably showed diffuse pure cerebellar atrophy. This disorder represents a 'pure' autosomal recessive cerebellar ataxia and is also known as recessive ataxia of Beauce. This disorder was mapped on chromosome 6q and the responsible gene identified was *SYNE1* (MIM *608441), which spans over 0.5Mb of genomic DNA. *SYNE1* or *Nesprin 1* gene is composed of two main transcripts, SYNE1A and SYNE1B. SYNE1A transcript is expressed in skeletal and cardiac muscle and a 10-kb SYNE1B transcript in multiple tissues, including heart, muscle, kidney, liver, and brain. Immunofluorescence on adult mouse tissues localized *Syne1* to nuclei in skeletal, smooth, and cardiac muscle cells. In skeletal muscle, high levels of expression were detected in nuclei associated with synaptic sites (Apel et al. 2000). *SYNE1* requires its C-terminal transmembrane domain to localize to the nuclear envelope (Zhang et al. 2001). Recently an Emery-Dreifuss muscular dystrophy phenotype has been related to heterozygous mutations in the *SYNE1* gene (Zhang et al. 2007).

Other rare forms of autosomal recessive cerebellar ataxia

One form of cerebellar ataxia has been characterized in one consanguineous family associating cerebellar atrophy with a peripheral neuropathy and was linked to 9q33–34, and in a second family there was associated hearing impairment and optic atrophy, and was linked to 6p21–23.

In the first family, the four affected Japanese siblings had spinocerebellar ataxia associated with elevated levels of serum creatine kinase, gamma-globulin, and alpha-fetoprotein. Homozygosity over a 20cM region allowed demonstration of linkage at 9q33.3–34.3 with a logarithm of odds (LOD) score of 3.0. Genotyping two unrelated Japanese patients from first-degree consanguineous parents revealed that one was homozygous for the same region but did not share the biochemical features.

In the second family, an Israeli uncle and a niece were affected by an early-onset recessive ataxia and subsequently developed hearing impairment and optic atrophy. Homozygosity over a 17cM region allowed demonstration of linkage at 6p21–23 with an LOD score of 3.25 (Bomont et al. 2000).

Another form of ARCA has been published recently in a large consanguineous family from Saudi Arabia with four affected children presenting with generalized tonic-clonic epilepsy, ataxia, and mental retardation, but neither myoclonus nor mental deterioration. MRI and muscle biopsy of one patient revealed, respectively, posterior white matter hyperintensities and vacuolization of the sarcotubular system. The defective gene was localized by homozygosity mapping to a 19Mb interval in 16q21–q23 between markers D16S3091 and D16S3050 (Gribaa et al. 2007). Linkage studies in this region will allow testing for homogeneity of this novel ataxia-epilepsy entity.

Ataxias with unknown pathogenesis

Cerebellar atrophy, Norman type

Cerebellar atrophy, Norman type (MIM %213200), was first described by Norman (1940) in three siblings in one family and two siblings in another who had cerebellar ataxia and mental retardation since early life. Postmortem examinations showed severe cerebellar granule cell loss. One child showed delayed motor development and mental retardation in infancy. Other features included small head, cataracts, increased knee jerks, and intention tremor. He died at age 20 years. Postmortem examination showed marked cerebellar atrophy with complete absence of granule cells in the lateral lobes of the cerebellum and the superior part of the vermis. There were heterotopic Purkinje cells and gliosis (Weiner and Konigsmark 1971). Other similar cases have been reported by Scherer (1933) and Jervis (1950) in three affected siblings and in monozygotic Italian twin sisters (Jervis 1954).

In an inbred Christian Maronite family originating from a village in the northeast of Lebanon, Megarbane et al. (1999) described hereditary congenital nonprogressive cerebellar ataxia. The authors believed that the 12 affected members had autosomal recessive Norman type of cerebellar atrophy, also known as primary granular cell atrophy of the cerebellum. The patients in the Lebanese family were of short stature, varying from 136cm in a 44-year-old female to 164cm in a 40-year-old male. Delague et al. (2001) found linkage to a 12.1cM interval on chromosome 9q34–qter between markers D9S67 and D9S312. This form can be included in the group of patients with congenital nonprogressive cerebellar ataxia defined above.

Aniridia, cerebellar ataxia, and mental retardation

The syndrome of aniridia, cerebellar ataxia, and mental retardation (Gillespie syndrome; MIM #206700) can be caused by heterozygous mutations in the *PAX6* gene (MIM *607108) (Ticho et al. 2006); however, an autosomal recessive condition has been reported by Gillespie (1965) who first described brothers and sisters with the combination of aniridia, cerebellar ataxia, and mental retardation. The karyotype of each patient was normal. Later Sarsfield (1971) reported a further example of the above syndrome complex with evidence of autosomal recessive transmission occurring in a male, the second child of normal parents. Bilateral partial aniridia was noted at birth and developmental milestones were subsequently delayed. Although muscle biopsies and nerve conduction times were normal, there was persistent hypotonia with normal tendon reflexes and sensation, but with gross uncoordination, attention tremor, and scanning speech. There was some improvement in motor performance with age, but mental retardation was evident. All laboratory investigations, including karyotype, were normal. Nelson et al. (1997) described two unrelated patients with Gillespie syndrome with the typical presentation of fixed dilated pupils in a hypotonic infant. In one patient, Nelson et al. (1997) found cerebral and cerebellar atrophy with white matter changes on MRI. Finally, Boughamoura et al. (2006) reported a sister and brother, born of consanguineous parents, who had congenital bilateral partial aniridia, cerebellar ataxia, and mental retardation. Brain MRI showed cerebellar atrophy in the girl and mild cortical and subcortical atrophy involving the subtentorial region and hypoplasia of the inferior vermis in the boy. Ophthalmological examination of the boy revealed bilateral partial aniridia with peripheral tufting, iris strands on the anterior lens, and dysgenesis of the iridocorneal angle. The karyotype was normal in both children.

Besides these reports, a heterozygous splice site mutation in the *PAX6* gene was reported in a 6-year-old Caucasian boy with atypical Gillespie syndrome, consisting of partial aniridia, mild balance disorder, hand tremor, and learning disability, by Ticho et al. (2006). In addition, in a girl aged 9 years 6 months with a phenotype suggestive of Gillespie syndrome, Graziano et al. (2007) identified heterozygosity for a nonsense mutation in the *PAX6* gene, suggesting that screening for *PAX6* in patients with suspected Gillespie syndrome should be performed with up-to-date methodology.

Cerebellar ataxia and hypogonadotropic hypogonadism

Holmes (1907) first described the association of cerebellar ataxia and hypogonadism (Gordon Holmes syndrome; MIM %212840). He reported three brothers and one sister who, in their mid-30s, developed cerebellar symptoms and signs of sex steroid deficiency. As gonadotropin assays were developed, both hypo- and hypergonadotropic forms were reported. The hypogonadism of most patients with Gordon Holmes syndrome is hypogonadotropic, with a defect in the production or release of gonadotropins by the pituitary gland. Neuhauser and Opitz (1975) described a kindred in which two brothers and two sisters born from second-cousin parents had the combination of ataxia and hypogonadotropic hypogonadism. In three siblings the onset of cerebellar ataxia was between 12 and 20 years and, in the fourth, in the 30s. Hypogonadotropism was reflected in failure of secondary sexual characteristics, eunuchoidism, absence of libido, and infertility. Limber et al. (1989) provided a follow-up on the family described by Neuhauser and Opitz (1975) and demonstrated that the affected members had a syndrome that includes, in addition to spinocerebellar ataxia and hypogonadotropic hypogonadism, chorioretinal dystrophy. Later, Berciano et al. (1982) described conclusive evidence of autosomal recessive inheritance of an ataxia associated with hypogonadotropic hypogonadism in an affected brother and sister from consanguineous parents. Furthermore they found that hypogonadotropism was due to deficiency of hypothalamic luteinizing hormone-releasing hormone (LHRH). Raised gonadotropin levels were found after repeated stimulation with exogenous LHRH. CT in one case showed cerebellar and brainstem atrophy. Abs et al. (1990) also described a 20-year-old male with longstanding, nonprogressive ataxia due to hypoplasia of the inferior cerebellar vermis. He also showed hypogonadism with low serum gonadotropin and prolactin levels, which were judged to be due to a primary deficiency of the gonadotroph and lactotroph cells, rather than a hypothalamic lesion, because of the response to administration of gonadotropin-releasing hormone. The patient was born from an incestuous relationship between a brother and sister. Seminara et al. (2002) described the largest kindred with Gordon Holmes syndrome. The parents of the three affected siblings were first cousins, suggesting that the disease was inherited as an autosomal recessive trait. The siblings' initial evaluation was notable for low serum levels of sex steroids and gonadotropins (consistent with hypogonadotropic hypogonadism), progressive ataxia, and dementia. Extended treatment with physiological doses of pulsatile GNRH (LNRH) failed to stimulate a gonadotropin response. Brain imaging revealed volume loss in the cerebellum, with extensive abnormalities in the cerebral white matter. Two years later, late-onset cerebellar ataxia was reported in a female patient with hypogonadism and muscle coenzyme Q10 deficiency (Gironi et al. 2004).

Conclusions

ARCA is a group of extremely heterogeneous disorders and a coherent methodology is required to approach the differential diagnosis of these disorders. Moreover ataxia can be the presenting symptom of leukodystrophies such as metachromatic leukodystrophy, vanishing white matter, or Paelizeus-Merzbacher disease, and of other metabolic and neurodegenerative disorders such as neuroaxonal dystrophy, neuronal lipofuscinosis ceroid or juvenile Tay-Sachs disease which can simulate ARCA, particularly at onset of symptoms. In addition it is important to highlight that autosomal dominant cerebellar ataxias generally appear in adulthood; however, some patients can have a very early onset because of the phenomenon of anticipation due to triplet nucleotide expansion that occurs in most of these conditions while segregating along the generations.

First of all it is important to distinguish between ARCA with or without the presence of a peripheral neuropathy. Thus electrophysiological examinations have to be performed systematically in ARCA and possibly repeated over time when dealing with unclassified forms in order to rule in or out the association of a peripheral neuropathy or other neuropathy (optic or auditory). Moreover it is important to detect any other associated symptoms indicating multisystem involvement.

Detailed neuroimaging studies, particularly brain MRI, are pivotal for subclassification of this group of disorders.

Other laboratory examinations can be useful such as serum creatine kinase, which may be slightly increased in AOA1, or the elevation of serum alpha-fetoprotein that is characteristic of ataxia-telangiectasia and AOA2, or hypoalbuminemia be found in AOA2, while hypercholesterolemia is characteristic for AOA1 or AOA2.

Additional biochemical tests can be useful in the diagnosis such as determination of vitamin E, phytanic acid, and serum cholestanol, and measurement of muscle CoQ10 levels.

REFERENCES

Abs R, Van Vleymen E, Parizel PM, Van Acker K, Martin M, Martin J-J (1990) Congenital cerebellar hypoplasia and hypogonadotropic hypogonadism J Neurol Sci 98: 259–265.

Anttonen AK, Mahjneh I, Hämäläinen RH, Lagier-Tourenne C, Kopra O, Waris L, et al. (2005) The gene disrupted in Marinesco-Sjögren syndrome encodes SIL1, an HSPA5 cochaperone. Nat Genet 37: 1309–1311.

Apel ED, Lewis RM, Grady RM, Sanes JR (2000) Syne-1, a dystrophin- and Klarsicht-related protein associated with synaptic nuclei at the neuromuscular junction. J Biol Chem 275: 31986–31995.

Alajouanine T, Aubrey M, Nehlil J (1943) Sur une affection familiale caractérisée par un syndrome de déséquilibration avec importantes pertubations vestibulaires centrales. Rev Neurol 75: 252–254.

Anheim M, Fleury M, Monga B, Laugel V, Chaigne D, Rodier G, et al. (2010) Epidemiological, clinical, paraclinical and molecular study of a cohort of 102 patients affected with autosomal recessive progressive cerebellar ataxia from Alsace, Eastern France: implications for clinical management. Neurogenetics 11(1): 1–12.

Arita M, Sato Y, Miyata A, Tanabe T, Takahashi E, Kayden HJ, et al. (1995) Human α-tocoferol transfer protein: cDNA cloning, expression and chromosomal localization. Biochem J 306: 437–443.

Barbot C, Coutinho P, Chorão R, Ferreira C, Barros J, Fineza I, et al. (2001) Recessive ataxia with ocular apraxia: review of 22 portuguese patients. Arch Neurl 58: 201–205.

Barkhof F, Verrips A, Wesseling P, van Der Knaap MS, van Engelen BG, Gabreëls FJ, et al. (2000) Cerebrotendinous xanthomatosis: the spectrum of imaging findings and the correlation with neuropathogic findings. Neuroradiology 217: 869–876.

Barkovich AJ, Ferriero DM, Barr RM, Gressens P, Dobyns WB, Truwit CL, Evrard P (1998) Microlissencephaly: a heterogeneous malformation of cortical development. Neuropediatrics 29: 113–119.

Batten FE (1905) Ataxia in childhood. Brain 28: 484.

Berciano J, Amado JA, Freijanes J, Rebollo M, Vaquero A (1982) Familial cerebellar ataxia and hypogonadotropic hypogonadism: evidence for hypothalamic LHRH deficiency J Neurol Neurosurg Psychiat 45: 747–751.

Berginer VM, Gross B, Morad K, Kfir N, Morkos S, Aaref S, Falik-Zaccai TC (2009) Chronic diarrhea and juvenile cataracts: think cerebrotendinous xanthomatosis and treatment. Pediatrics 123: 143–147.

Berriot-Varoqueaux N, Aggerbeck LP, Samson-Bouma ME, Wetterau JR (2000) The role of the microsomal triglyceride transfer protein in abetalipoproteinemia. Annu Rev Nutr 20: 663–697.

Bish JP, Pendyal A, Ding L, Ferrante H, Nguyen V, McDonald-McGinn D, et al. (2006) Specific cerebellar reductions in children with chromosome 22q11.2 deletion syndrome. Neurosci Lett 399: 245–248.

Bomont P, Watanabe M, Gershoni-Barush R, Shizuka M, Tanaka M, Sugano J, et al. (2000) Homozygosity mapping of spinocerebellar ataxia with cerebellar atrophy and peripheral neuropathy to 9q33–34, and with hearing impairment and optic atrophy to 6p21–23. Eur J Hum Genet 8: 986–990.

Bouchard JP, Barbeau A, Bouchard R, Bouchard RW (1978) Autosomal recessive spastic ataxia of Charlevoix-Saguenay. Can J Neurol Sci 5, 61–69.

Boughamoura L, Yacoub M, Abroug M, Chabchoub I, Bouguezzi R, Charfeddine L, et al. (2006) Le syndrome de Gillespie: a propos de 2 cas familiaux Gillespie syndrome: 2 familial cases. Arch Pediat 13: 1323–1325.

Bouslam N, Bouhouche A, Benomar A, Hanein S, Klebe S, Azzedine H, et al. (2007) A novel locus for autosomal recessive spastic ataxia on chromosome 17p. Hum Genet 121: 413–420.

Breckpot J, Takiyama Y, Thienpont B, Van Vooren S, Vermeesch JR, Ortibus E, Devriendt K (2008) A novel genomic disorder: a deletion of the SACS gene leading to spastic ataxia of Charlevoix-Saguenay. Eur J Hum Genet 16: 1050–1054.

Campuzano V, Montermini L, Moltò MD, Pianese L, Cossée M, Cavalcanti F, et al. (1996) Friedreich's ataxia: autosomal recessive disease caused by an intronic GAA triplet repeat expansion. Science 271: 1423–1427.

Cavalier L, Ouahchi K, Kayden HJ, Di Donato S, Reutenauer L, Mandel JL, Koenig M (1998) Ataxia with isolated vitamin E deficiency: heterogeneity of mutations and phenotypic variability in a large number of families. Am J Hum Genet 62: 301–310.

Chun HH, Gatti RA (2004) Ataxia-telangiectasia, an evolving phenotype. DNA Repair 3: 1187–1196.

Chan SS, Copeland WC (2009) DNA polymerase gamma and mitochondrial disease: understanding the consequence of POLG mutations. Biochim Biophys Acta 1787: 312–319. Review.

Cooper JM, Korlipara LVP, Korlipara PE, Hart PE, Bradley JL, Schapira AHV (2008) Coenzyme Q10 and vitamin E in Friedreich's ataxia: predictor of efficacy of vitamin E and coenzyme Q10 therapy. Eur J Neurol 15: 1371–1379.

Clement E, Mercuri E, Godfrey C, Smith J, Robb S, Kinali M, et al. (2008) Brain involvement in muscular dystrophies with defective dystroglycan glycosylation. Ann Neurol 64: 573–582.

Criscuolo C, Banfi S, Orio M, Gasparini P, Monticelli A, Scarano V, et al. (2004) A novel mutation in SACS gene in a family from southern Italy. Neurology 62: 100–102.

Criscuolo C, Saccà F, De Michele G, Mancini P, Combarros O, Infante J, et al. (2005) Novel mutation of SACS gene in a Spanish family with autosomal recessive spastic ataxia. Mov Disord 20: 1358–1361.

Delia D, Piane M, Buscemi G, Savio C, Palmeri S, Lulli P, et al. (2004) MRE11 mutations and impaired ATM-dependent responses in na Italian family with ataxia-telangiectasia-like disorder. Hum Mol Genet 13: 2155–2163.

De Falco F, Cainarca S, Andolfi G, Ferrentino R, Berti C, Rodríguez Criado G, et al. (2003) X-linked Opitz syndrome: novel mutations in the MID1 gene and redefinition of the clinical spectrum. Am J Med Genet A 120A: 222–228. Review.

Delague V, Bareil C, Bouvagnet P, Salem N, Chouery E, Loiselet J, et al. (2001) Nonprogressive autosomal recessive ataxia maps to chromosome 9q34–9qter in a large consanguineous Lebanese family. Ann Neurol 50: 250–253.

Delague V, Bareil C, Bouvagnet P, Salem N, Chouery E, Loiselet J, et al. (2002) A new autosomal recessive nonprogressive congenital cerebellar ataxia associated with mental retardation, optic atrophy, and skin abnormalities (CAMOS) maps to chromosome 15q24–q26 in a large consanguineous Lebanese Druze family. Neurogenetics 4: 23–27.

Di Leo E, Magnolo L, Bertolotti M, Bourbon M, Carmo Pereira S, Pirisi M, et al. (2008) Variable phenotypic expression of homozygous familial hypobetalipoproteinaemia due to novel APOB gene mutations. Clin Genet 74: 267–273.

Duncan AJ, Bitner-Glindzicz M, Meunier B, Costello H, Hargreaves IP, Lopez LC, et al. (2009) A nonsense mutation in COQ9 causes autosomal-recessive neonatal-onset primary coenzyme Q10 deficiency: a potentially treatable form of mitochondrial disease. Am J Hum Genet 84: 558–566.

Duquette A, Roddier K, McNabb-Baltar J, Gosselin I, St-Denis A, Dicaire MJ, et al. (2005) Muattions in senataxin responsible for Quebec cluster of ataxia with neuropathy. Ann Neurol 57: 408–414.

Edmond M, Lepage G, Vanasse M, Pandolfo M (2000) Increased levels of plasma malondialdehyde in Friedreich ataxia. Neurology 55: 1752–1753.

El-Khamisy SF, Caldecott KW (2006) TDP1-dependent DNA single-strand break repair and neurodegeneration. Mutagenesis 21: 219–224.

Engert JC, Berube P, Mercier J, Dore C, Lepage P, Ge B, Bouchard J-P, et al. (2000) ARSACS, a spastic ataxia common in northeastern Quebec, is caused by mutations in a new gene encoding an 11.5-kb ORF. Nature Genet 24: 120–125.

Esscher E, Flodmark O, Hagberg G, Hagberg B (1996) Nonprogressive ataxia: Origins, brain pathology and impairments in 78 Swedish children. Dev Med Child Neurol 38: 285–296.

Fatemi SH (2005) Reelin glycoprotein: structure, biology and roles in health and disease. Mol Psychiatry 10: 251–257. Review.

Farr AK, Shalev B, Crawford TO, Lederman HM, Winkelstein JA, Repka MX (2002) Ocular manifestations of ataxia-telangiectasia. Am J Ophthalmol 134: 891–896.

Fernet M, Gribaa M, Salih MAM, Seidahmed MZ, Hall J, Koenig M (2005) Identification and functional consequences of a novel MRE11 mutation affecting 10 Saudi Arabian patients with the ataxia telangiectasia-like disorder. Hum Mol Genet 14: 307–318.

Ferrarini M, Squintani G, Cavallaro T, Ferrari S, Rizzuto N, Fabrizi GM (2007) A novel mutation of aprataxin associated with ataxia ocular apraxia type 1: Phenotypical ang genotypical characterization. J Neurol Sci 260: 219–224.

Fogel BL, Perlman S (2007) Clinical features and molecular genetics of autosomal recessive cerebellat ataxias. Lancet Neurol 6: 245–257.

Gerber J, Muhlenhoff U, Lill R (2003) An interaction between frataxin and Isu1/Nfs1 that is crucial for Fe/S cluster synthesis on Isu1. Embo Rep 4: 906–911.

Gallus GN, Dotti MT, Federico A (2006) Clinical and molecular diagnosis of cerebrotendinous xanthomatosis with a review of the mutations in the CYP27A1 gene. Neurol Sci 27: 143–149.

Gillespie FD (1965) Aniridia, cerebellar ataxia, and oligophrenia in siblings. Arch Ophthal 73: 338–341.

Gironi M, Lamperti C, Nemni R, Moggio M, Comi G, Guerini FR, et al. (2004) Late-onset cerebellar ataxia with hypogonadism and muscle coenzyme Q10 deficiency. Neurology 62: 818–820.

Gonçalves S, Paupe V, Dassa EP, Rustin P (2008) Deferiprone targets aconitase: Implication for Friedreich's ataxia. BMC Neurol 8: 1–4.

Graziano C, D'Elia AV, Mazzanti L, Moscano F, Guidi SG, Scarano E, et al. (2007) A de novo nonsense mutation of PAX6 gene in a patient with aniridia, ataxia, and mental retardation. Am J Med Genet 143A: 1802–1805.

Gribaa M, Salih M, Anheim M, Lagier-Tourenne C, H'mida D, Drouot N, et al. (2007) A new form of childhood onset, autosomal recessive spinocerebellar ataxia and epilepsy is localized at 16q21–q23. Brain 130: 1921–1928.

Grieco GS, Malandrini A, Comanducci G, Leuzzi V, Valoppi M, Tessa A, et al. (2004) Novel SACS mutations in autosomal recessive spastic ataxia of Charlevoix-Saguenay type. Neurology 62: 103–106.

Grinberg I, Northrup H, Ardinger H, Prasad C, Dobyns WB, Millen KJ (2004) Heterozygous deletion of the linked genes ZIC1 and ZIC4 is involved in Dandy-Walker malformation. Nat Genet 36: 1053–1055.

Gros-Louis F, Dupre N, Dion P, Fox MA, Laurent S, Verreault S, et al. (2007) Mutations in SYNE1 lead to a newly discovered form of autosomal recessive cerebellar ataxia. Nature Genet 39: 80–85.

Gueven N, Chen P, Nakamura J, Becherel OJ, Kijas AW, Grattan-Smith P, Lavin MF (2007) A subgroup of spinocerebellar ataxias defective in DNA damage responses. Neuroscience 145: 1418–1425.

Guzzetta F, Mercuri E, Bonanno S, Longo M, Spano M (1993) Autosomal recessive congenital cerebellar atrophy: a clinical and neuropsychological study. Brain Dev 15: 439–445.

Hagberg B, Sanner G, Steen M (1972) The dysequilibrium syndrome in cerebral palsy: clinical aspects and treatment. Acta Paediat Scand 61: 1–63.

Herman TE, Siegel MJ (2008) Ritscher-Schinzel cranio-cerebello-cardiac syndrome. J Perinatol 28: 715–718.

Holmes G (1907) A form of familial degeneration of the cerebellum. Brain 30: 466–489 .

Hoveyda N, Shield JPH, Garrett C, Chong WK, Beardsall K, Bentsi-Enchill E, et al. (1999) Neonatal diabetes mellitus and cerebellar hypoplasia/agenesis: report of a new recessive syndrome. J Med Genet 36: 700–704.

Jaglin XH, Poirier K, Saillour Y, Buhler E, Tian G, Bahi-Buisson N, et al. (2009) Mutations in the beta-tubulin gene TUBB2B result in asymmetrical polymicrogyria. Nat Genet 41: 746–752.

Jansen GA, Waterham HR, Wanders RJA (2004) Molecular basis of Refsum disease: sequence variations in phytanoyl-CoA hydroxylase (PHYH) and the PTS2 receptor (PEX7). Hum Mutat 23: 209–218.

Jauslin ML, Vertuani S, Durini E, Buzzoni L, Ciliberti N, Verdecchia S, et al. (2007) Protective effects of Fe-Aox29, a novel antioxidant derived from a molecular combination od idebenone and vitamin E, in immortalized fibroblasts and fibroblasts from patients with Friedreich ataxia. Mol Cell Biochem 302: 79–85.

Jervis GA (1950) Early familial cerebellar degeneration (report of three cases in one family) J Nerv Ment Dis 111: 398–407.

Jervis GA (1954) Concordant primary atrophy of cerebellar granules in monozygotic twins. Acta Genet Med Gemellol 3: 153–162.

Jissendi-Tchofo P, Kara S, Barkovich AJ (2009) Midbrain-hindbrain involvement in lissencephalies. Neurology 72(5): 410–418.

Kato M, Das S, Petras K, Kitamura K, Morohashi K, Abuelo DN, et al. (2004) Mutations of ARX are associated with striking pleiotropy and consistent genotype-phenotype correlation. Hum Mutat 23: 147–159.

Keren Z, Falik-Zaccai TC (2009) Cerebrotendinous xanthomatosis (CTX): a treatable lipid storage disease. Pediatr Endocrinol Rev 7: 6–11. Review.

Koenig M (2003) Rare forms of autosomal recessive neurodegenerative ataxia. Semin Pediatr Neurol 3: 183–192. Review.

Koeppen AH, Michael SC, Knutson MD, Haile DJ, Qian J, Levi S, et al. (2007) The dentate nucleus in Friedreich's ataxia: the role of iron-responsive proteins. Acta Neuropathol 114: 163–173.

Koirala S, Jin Z, Piao X, Corfas G (2009) GPR56-regulated granule cell adhesion is essential for rostral cerebellar development. J Neurosci 29: 7439–7449.

Koskinen T, Valanne L, Ketonen LM, Pihko H (1995) Infantile-onset spinocerebellar ataxia: MR and CT findings. Am J Neuroradiol 16: 1427–1433.

Koutnikova H, Campuzano V, Foury F, Dolle P, Cazzalini O, Koenig M (1997) Studies of human, mouse and yeast homologues indicate a mitochondrial function for frataxin. Nat Genet 16: 345–351.

Kumar RA, Pilz DT, Babatz TD, Cushion TD, Harvey K, Topf M, et al. (2010) TUBA1A mutations cause wide spectrum lissencephaly (smooth brain) and suggest that multiple neuronal migration pathways converge on alpha tubulins. Hum Mol Genet 19: 2817–2827.

Lagier-Tourenne C, Tranebaerg L, Chaigne D, Gribaa M, Dollfus H, Silvestri G, et al. (2003) Homozygosity mapping of Marinesco-Sjögren syndrome to 5q31. Eur J Hum Genet 11: 770–778.

Lalani SR, Vladutiu GD, Plunkett K, Lotze TE, Adesina AM, Scaglia F (2005) Isolated mitochondrial myopathy associated with muscle coenzyme Q10 deficiency Arch Neurol 62: 317–320.

Lamarche JB, Lemieux B, Lieu HB (1984) The neuropathology of 'typical' Friedreich's ataxia in Quebec. Can J Neurol Sci 11(Suppl. 4): 592–600.

Lancioni A, Pizzo M, Fontanella B, Ferrentino R, Napolitano LM, De Leonibus E, Meroni G (2010) Lack of Mid1, the mouse ortholog of the Opitz syndrome gene, causes abnormal development of the anterior cerebellar vermis. J Neurosci 30: 2880–2887.

Le Ber I, Moreira MC, Rivaud-Péchoux S, Chamayou C, Ochsner F, Kuntzer T, et al. (2003) Cerebellar ataxia with oculomotor apraxia type 1: clinical and genetic studies. Brain 126: 2761–2772.

Le Ber I, Bouslam N, Rivaud-Péchoux S, Guimarães J, Benomar A, Chamayou C, et al. (2004) Frequency and phenotypic spectrum of ataxia with oculomotor apraxia 2: a clinical and genetic stydy in 18 patients. Brain 127: 759–767.

Leger PL, Souville I, Boddaert N, Elie C, Pinard JM, Plouin P, et al. (2008) The location of DCX mutations predicts malformation severity in X-linked lissencephaly. Neurogenetics 9: 277–285.

Limber ER, Bresnick GH, Lebovitz RM, Appen RE, Gilbert-Barness EF, Pauli RM (1989) Spinocerebellar ataxia, hypogonadotropic hypogonadism, and choroidal dystrophy (Boucher-Neuhauser syndrome) Am J Med Genet 33: 409–414.

Lodi R, Tonon C, Calabrese V, Shapira A (2006) Friedreich's ataxia: from disease mechanisms to therapeutic interventention. Antioxid Redox Signal 8: 438–443.

Lönnqvist T, Paetau A, Nikali K, von Boguslawski K, Pihko H (1998) Infantile onset spinocerebellar ataxia with sensory neuropathy (IOSCA): neuropathological features. J Neurol Sci 161: 57–65.

Mantovan MC, Martinuzzi A, Squarzanti F, Bolla A, Silvestri I, Liessi G, et al. (2006) Exploring mental status in Friedreich's ataxia: a combined neuropsychological, behavioral and neuroimaging study. Eur J Neurol. 13(8): 827–35.

Mariotti C, Gellera C, Rimoldi M, Mineri R, Uziel G, Zorzi G, et al. (2004) Ataxia with isolated vitamin E deficiency: neurological phenotype, clinical follow-up and novel mutations in TTPA gene in Italian families. Neurol Sci 25: 130–137.

Marzouki N, Benomar A, Yahyaoui M, Birouk N, Elouazzani M, Chkili T, Benlemlih M (2005) Vitamin E deficiency ataxia with (744del A) mutation on α-TTP gene: genetic and clinical peculiarities in Moroccan patients. Eur J Med Genet 48: 21–28.

McMillan HJ, Carter MT, Jacob PJ, Laffan EE, O'Connor MD, Boycott KM (2009) Homozygous contiguous gene deletion of 13q12 causing LGMD2C and ARSACS in the same patient. Muscle Nerve 39: 396–399.

Megarbane A, Delague V, Salem N, Loiselet J (1999) Autosomal recessive congenital cerebellar hypoplasia and short stature in a large inbred family. Am J Med Genet 87: 88–90.

Milone M, Brunetti-Pierri N, Tang LY, Kumar N, Mezei MM, Josephs K, et al. (2008) Sensory ataxic neuropathy with ophthalmoparesis caused by POLG mutations. Neuromuscul Disord 18: 626–632.

Mollet J, Giurgea I, Schlemmer D, Dallner G, Chretien D, Delahodde A, et al. (2007) Prenyldiphosphate synthase, subunit 1 (PDSS1) and OH-benzoate polyprenyltransferase (COQ2) mutations in ubiquinone deficiency and oxidative phosphorylation disorders. J Clin Invest 117: 765–772.

Mollet J, Delahodde A, Serre V, Chretien D, Schlemmer D, Lombes A, et al. (2008) CABC1 gene mutations cause ubiquinone deficiency with cerebellar ataxia and seizures. Am J Hum Genet 82: 623–630.

Nelson J, Flaherty M, Grattan-Smith P (1997) Gillespie syndrome: a report of two further cases. Am J Med Genet 71: 134–138.

Neuhauser G, Opitz JM (1975) Autosomal recessive syndrome of cerebellar ataxia and hypogonadotropic hypogonadism. Clin Genet 7: 426–434.

Nicolas E, Poitelon Y, Chouery E, Salem N, Levy N, Mégarbané A, Delague V (2010) CAMOS, a nonprogressive, autosomal recessive, congenital cerebellar ataxia, is caused by a mutant zinc-finger protein, ZNF592. Eur J Hum Genet 18: 1107–1113.

Nikali K, Suomalainen A, Saharinen J, Kuokkanen M, Spelbrink JN, Lönnqvist T, Peltonen L (2005) Infantile onset spinocerebellar ataxia is caused by recessive mutations in mitochondrial proteins Twinkle and Twinky. Hum Mol Genet 14: 2981–2990.

Norman RM (1940) Primary degeneration of the granular layer of the cerebellum: an unusual form of familial cerebellar atrophy occurring in early life. Brain 63: 365–379.

Ogasahara S, Engel AG, Frens D, Mack D (1989) Muscle coenzyme Q deficiency in familial mitochondrial encephalomyopathy. Proc Nat Acad Sci 86: 2379–2382.

Ogawa T, Takiyama Y, Sakoe K, Mori K, Namekawa M, Shimazaki H, et al. (2004) Identification of a SACS gene missense mutation in ARSACS. Neurology 62: 107–109.

Ouyang Y, Takiyama Y, Sakoe K, Shimazaki H, Ogawa T, Nagano S, et al. (2006) Sacsin-related ataxia (ARSACS): expanding the genotype upstream from the gigantic exon. Neurology 66: 1103–1104.

Palau F, Espinós C (2006) Autosomal recessive cerebellar ataxias. Orphanet J Rare Dis 1: 1–19.

Pandolfo M (2008) Friedreich ataxia. Arch Neurol 65: 1296–1303.

Parfitt DA, Michael GJ, Vermeulen EG, Prodromou NV, Webb TR, Gallo JM, et al. (2009) The ataxia protein sacsin is a functional co-chaperone that protects against polyglutamine-expanded ataxin-1. Hum Mol Genet 18: 1556–1565.

Parrini E, Ramazzotti A, Dobyns WB, Mei D, Moro F, Veggiotti P, et al. (2006) Periventricular heterotopia: phenotypic heterogeneity and correlation with Filamin A mutations. Brain 129: 1892–1906.

Pastore A, Tozzi G, Gaeta LM, Bertini E, Serafini V, Di Cesare S, et al. (2003) Actin glutathionylation increases in fibroblasts of patients with Friedreich's ataxia: a potential role in the pathogenesis of the disease. J Biol Chem 43: 42588–42595.

Perlman S, Becker-Catania S, Gatti RA (2003) Ataxia-telangiectasia: diagnosis and treatment. Semin Pediatr Neurol 10: 173–182.

Piemonte F, Pastore A, Tozzi G, Tagliacozzi D, Santorelli FM, Carrozzo R, et al. (2001) Glutathione in blood of patients with Friedreich's ataxia. Eur J Clin Invest 31: 1007–1011.

Puccio H, Simon D, Cossee M, Criqui-Filipe P, Tiziano F, Melki J, et al. (2001) Mouse models for Friedreich ataxia exhibit cardiomyopathy, sensory nerve defect and Fe-S enzyme deficiency followed by intramitochondrial iron deposits. Nat Genet 27: 181–186.

Oppenheimer D, Esiri M (1992) Disease of the basal ganglia, cerebellum and motor neurons. In: Greenfield's Neuropathology, 5th edition (eds Adams JH, Corsellis J, Duchen LW). London: Arnold; 988–1054.

Quinzii CM, Kattah AG, Naini A, Akman HO, Mootha VK, DiMauro S, Hirano M (2005) Coenzyme Q deficiency and cerebellar ataxia associated with an aprataxin mutation. Neurology 64: 539–541.

Quinzii C, Naini A, Salviati L, Trevisson E, Navas P, DiMauro S, Hirano M (2006) A mutation in para-hydroxybenzoate-polyprenyl transferase (COQ2) causes primary coenzyme Q10 deficiency. Am J Hum Genet 78: 345–349.

Ross ME, Swanson K, Dobyns WB (2001) Lissencephaly with cerebellar hypoplasia (LCH): a heterogeneous group of cortical malformations. Neuropediatrics 32: 256–263.

Rotig A, Appelkvist E-L, Geromel V, Chretien D, Kadhom N, Edery P, et al. (2000) Quinone-responsive multiple respiratory-chain dysfunction due to widespread coenzyme Q10 deficiency. Lancet 356: 391–395.

Sandi C, Pinto RM, Al-Mahdawi S, Ezzatizadeh V, Barnes G, Jones S, et al. (2011) Prolonged treatment with pimelic o-aminobenzamide HDAC inhibitors ameliorates the disease phenotype of a Friedreich ataxia mouse model. Neurobiol Dis. 42(3): 496–505.

Sanner G (1973) The dysequilibrium syndrome: a genetic study. Neuropädiatrie 4: 403–413.

Sanner G, Hagberg B (1974) 188 cases of nonprogressive ataxic syndromes in childhood: aspects of aetiology and classification. Neuropädiatrie 5: 224–235.

Sarsfield JK (1971) The syndrome of congenital cerebellar ataxia, aniridia and mental retardation. Dev Med Child Neurol 13: 508–511.

Seminara SB, Acierno JS, Abdulwahid NA, Crowley WF, Margolin DH (2002) Hypogonadotropic hypogonadism and cerebellar ataxia: detailed phenotypic characterization of a large, extended kindred. J Clin Endocr Metab 87: 1607–1612.

Sellick GS, Barker KT, Stolte-Dijkstra I, Fleischmann C, Coleman RJ, Garrett C, et al. (2004) Mutations in PTF1A cause pancreatic and cerebellar agenesis. Nature Genet 36: 1301–1305.

Senderek J, Krieger M, Stendel C, Bergmann C, Moser M, Breitbach-Faller N, et al. (2005) Mutations in SIL1 cause Marinesco-Sjögren syndrome, a cerebellar ataxia with cataract and myopathy. Nat Genet 37: 1312–1314.

Scherer HJ (1933) Beitraege zur pathologischen Anatomie des Kleinhirns: genuine Kleinhirnatrophien. Z Neurol Psychiat 145: 335–405.

Schon EA, Manfredi G (2003) Neuronal degeneration and mitochondrial dysfunction. J Clin Invest 111: 303–312.

Schulz JB, Dehmer T, Schols L, Mende H, Hardt C, Vorgerd M, et al. (2000) Oxidative stress in patients with Friedreich ataxia. Neurology 55: 719–721.

Steinlin M (1998) Nonprogressive congenital ataxias. Brain Dev 20: 199–208.

Steinlin M, Styger M, Boltshauser E (1999) Cognitive impairments in patients with congenital nonprogressive cerebellar ataxia. Neurology 53: 966–973.

Takashima H, Boerkoel CF, John J, Saifi GM, Salih MA, Armstrong D, et al. (2002) Mutation of TDP1, encoding a topoisomerase I-dependent DNA damage repair enzyme, in spinocerebellar ataxia with axonal neuropathy. Nat Genet 32: 267–272.

Takiyama Y (2006) Autosomal recessive spastic ataxia of Charlevoix-Saguenay. Neuropathology 26: 368–375.

Taylor AMR, Groom A, Byrd PJ (2004) Ataxia-telangiectasia-like disorder (ATLD) – its clinical presentation and molecular basis. DNA Repair 3: 1219–1225.

Tazir M, Ali-Pacha L, M'Zahem A, Delaunoy JP, Fritsch M, Nouioua S, et al. (2009) Ataxia with oculomotor apraxia type 2: a clinical and genetic study of 19 patients. J Neurol Sci 278: 77–81.

Terracciano A, Casali C, Grieco GS, Orteschi D, Di Giandomenico S, Seminara L, et al. (2009) An inherited large-scale rearrangement in SACS associated with spastic ataxia and hearing loss. Neurogenetics 10: 151–155.

Terracciano A, Foulds NC, Ditchfield A, Bunyan DJ, Crolla JA, Huang S, et al. (2010) Pseudodominant inheritance of spastic ataxia of Charlevoix-Saguenay. Neurology 74: 1152–1154.

Ticho BH, Hilchie-Schmidt C, Egel RT, Traboulsi EI, Howarth RJ, Robinson D (2006) Ocular findings in Gillepsie-like syndrome: association with a new PAX6 mutation. Ophthal Genet 27: 145–149.

Tozzi G, Nuccetelli M, Lo Bello M, Bernardini S, Bellincampi L, Ballerini S, et al. (2002) Antioxidant enzymes in blood of patients with Friedreich's ataxia. Arch Dis Child 86: 376–379.

Tranebjaerg L, Teslovich TM, Jones M, Barmada MM, Fagerheim T, Dahl A, et al. (2003) Genome-wide homozygosity mapping localizes a gene for autosomal recessive non-progressive infantile ataxia to 20q11–q13. Hum Genet 113: 293–295.

Van Goethem G, Luoma P, Rantamäki M, Al Memar A, Kaakkola S, Hackman P, et al. (2004) POLG mutations in neurodegenerative disorders with ataxia but no muscle involvement. Neurology 63: 1251–1257.

Van Maldergem L, Trijbels F, DiMauro S, Sindelar PJ, Musumeci O, Janssen A, et al. (2002) Coenzyme Q-responsive Leigh's encephalopathy in two sisters. Ann Neurol 52: 750–754.

Vermeer S, Meijer RP, Pijl BJ, Timmermans J, Cruysberg JRM, Bos MM, et al. (2008) ARSACS in the Dutch population: a frequent cause of early-onset cerebellar ataxia. Neurogenetics 9: 207–214.

Wanders RJA, Jansen GA, Skjeldal OH (2001) Refsum disease, Peroxisomes and phytanic acid oxidation: a review. J Neuropathol Exp Neurol 60: 1021–1031.

Weiner LP, Konigsmark BW (1971) Hereditary disease of the cerebellar parenchyma. Birth Defects Orig Art Ser VII(1): 192–196.

Wierzbicki AS, Lloyd MD, Schofield CJ, Feher MD, Gibberd FB (2002) Refsum's disease: a peroxisomal disorder affecting phytanic acid α-oxidation. J Neurochem 80: 727–735.

Winterhun S, Ferrari G, He L, Taylor RW, Zeviani M, Turnbull DM, et al. (2005) Autosomal recessive mitochondrial ataxic syndrome due to mitochondrial polymerase γ mutations. Neurology 64: 1204–1208.

Zhang Q, Skepper JN, Yang F, Davies JD, Hegyi L, Roberts RG, et al. (2001) Nesprins: a novel family of spectrin-repeat-containing proteins that localize to the nuclear membrane in multiple tissues. J Cell Sci 114: 4485–4498.

Zhang Q, Bethmann C, Worth NF, Davies JD, Wasner C, Feuer A, et al. (2007) Nesprin-1 and -2 are involved in the pathogenesis of Emery Dreifuss muscular dystrophy and are critical for nuclear envelope integrity. Hum Molec Genet 16: 2816–2833.

27
Ataxia in Metabolic and White Matter Disorders

Nicole I. Wolf

Ataxia is a frequent and, unfortunately, nonspecific sign in many metabolic disorders (Sedel et al. 2008; Garcia-Cazorla et al. 2009). It is also encountered in many white matter disorders. In some of these disorders, ataxia is slowly progressive. In others, especially in mitochondrial disorders, it may be exacerbated by minor infections and show a relapsing and partially remitting course. There may also be stable ataxia, resembling congenital ataxia, e.g. in the congenital disorders of glycosylation (CDG). It should be remembered that all kinds of intoxication can lead to cerebellar signs. Endogenous intoxication from high levels of ammonia or other toxic metabolites causes broad-based, unstable gait and other cerebellar signs, suggesting decompensation in children with urea cycle defects or certain organic acidurias. Intermittent ataxia is also a feature of a rare aminoaciduria, Hartnup disease. Exogenous intoxication with benzodiazepines, antiepileptic drugs or alcohol also causes disturbed cerebellar function.

Which investigations should be performed if a metabolic type of ataxia is suspected? As in other types of ataxia too, MRI is the most valuable tool in the differential diagnosis and should be the first step. Additional metabolic or genetic investigations have to be done taking into account age at onset, MRI findings and clinical course.

Leukoencephalopathies

Several white matter disorders present with ataxia. In some of these, ataxia may be the only neurological abnormality for several years. Cerebral MRI often suggests a diagnosis which can then be confirmed by demonstrating the underlying biochemical or genetic defect.

Metachromatic leukodystrophy (MLD; MIM 250100) is one of the most common inherited white matter disorders (Gieselmann and Krageloh-Mann 2010). Depending on the age at onset, MLD is classified as infantile (age at onset 6 months–3 years), juvenile (early-juvenile 3–6 years, late-juvenile 6–16 years) or adult (>16 years). In the infantile form, the first symptom is an unsteady gait, usually due to a combination of demyelinating peripheral neuropathy and ataxia. Tendon reflexes may be brisk or already lost. Children regress further and develop frank truncal ataxia, titubation, and dysarthria. Nystagmus may be present. Spastic tetraplegia develops later, as well as a combination of bulbar and pseudobulbar palsy leading to feeding problems and repeated aspirations. Epilepsy and status epilepticus are common. In the last stage of the disease, patients are in a decerebrate stage, unable to make contact. The early-juvenile form resembles the infantile form, but deterioration is slower. In the late-juvenile variant, children come to attention with deterioration of school performance, behavioral problems and, only later, gait problems due to a mixture of spasticity, cerebellar ataxia, and peripheral neuropathy. The adult form starts typically with slow dementia. Many patients develop psychiatric symptoms (psychosis, disinhibition, depression). Ataxia and later spastic paraparesis are late symptoms, and patients can remain ambulatory for a long time. Peripheral neuropathy is not always present. Cerebrospinal fluid protein is elevated. The gallbladder is also involved, and some patients develop acute cholecystitis or hemobilia.

MRI shows progressive changes of the white matter, sparing the subcortical fibers. T2 signal intensity is elevated, and in the infantile and juvenile form there is a tigroid pattern with stripes of more normal signal around blood vessels. The corpus callosum is always affected (Fig. 27.1). If onset is early, the signal abnormalities have an occipital preponderance, but can also start frontally. Atrophy is a late sign in patients with early onset, but is frequently seen in adults, including variable cerebellar atrophy (Eichler et al. 2009).

The disease is caused by deficiency of arylsulfatase A (ASA) leading to lysosomal storage of sulfatides. Sulfatides are also excreted in urine. The remaining enzyme activity correlates with disease severity, and homozygosity for null alleles leads to the infantile form. About 1–2% of Europeans have a low ASA activity of 5–15% without clinical symptoms and without increased excretion of sulfatides. This has been named 'pseudodeficiency' and is due to two different polymorphisms, one leading to the loss of one of the three oligosaccharide side chains, the other one to the loss of a polyadenylation signal. These polymorphisms also occur independently, and they have also been found in combination with disease-causing mutations. There is also a rare activator protein deficiency with normal in vitro ASA activity.

The prototype of a hypomyelinating disorder is **Pelizaeus-Merzbacher disease** (PMD; MIM 312080). Its clinical features were well described by Pelizaeus in a large German family in 1885. He noted that the disease was transmitted by asymptomatic females, and that only males were affected. These patients develop a pendular nystagmus at the age of several weeks, similar to infants with congenital nystagmus. Shortly thereafter, delayed psychomotor development becomes apparent. Infants show axial hypotonia with difficult head control and later titubation, scissoring, and exaggerated tendon reflexes and a combination of ataxia and extrapyramidal features. Nystagmus may lessen or even disappear over time. In later

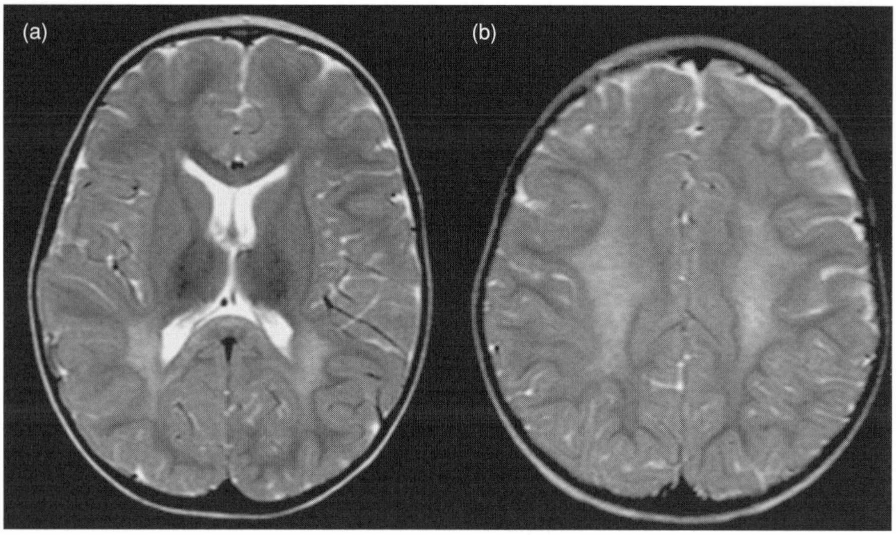

Fig. 27.1. T2 axial MR images of a 2-year-old child with the infantile form of metachromic leukodystrophy (MLD). Signal of the periventricular matter is high; the splenium of the corpus callosum is also affected. The thalami appear dark **(a)**. The subcortical fibers are spared. In **(b)**, a tigroid pattern with stripes of more normal signal is evident.

stages, optic atrophy is common. In the classic form of PMD, patients are not able to walk, and are often unable to sit without support. Many develop only poor active speech which is difficult to understand. Mental retardation (UK: learning disability) is common, although motor impairment is usually more pronounced than cognitive disability. In congenital PMD, symptoms are evident shortly after birth and often include congenital stridor, feeding difficulties, and profound hypotonia. Overt spasticity may never develop in these children. Development is much more impaired than in the classic form: patients with connatal PMD do not learn to talk or sit without support. Transitional PMD is intermediate in severity. These three subtypes form a continuous spectrum. Epilepsy is rare in PMD. A rare clinical variant is the null form caused by functional null mutations. Patients suffering from this form show only mild ataxia and spasticity in addition to peripheral neuropathy. Until late childhood or early adolescence, patients with all forms of the disease may improve and make slow developmental progress. From this age, however, slow deterioration begins, with insidious progression of neurological symptoms. While difficult to predict, life expectancy is reduced, and depends on severity of neurological deficits and additional complications (Garbern 2007).

PMD is caused by alterations of the proteolipid protein 1 (*PLP1*) gene which is located on Xq22.2 (Hudson et al. 1989; Ellis and Malcolm 1994). PLP1 constitutes about half of all myelin protein. Duplication of the entire gene is found in 60–70% of PMD cases and is associated with the classic form of the disease (Sistermans et al. 1998). Missense mutations account for 10–15% of cases. Deletions or null mutations are rare. Triplications are probably present in 1–2% of cases; even higher copy numbers have been described in one child (Wolf et al. 2005b). Complex chromosomal rearrangements involving PLP1 or its promotor region have been described in individual cases. In about 15% of cases, no mutations in *PLP1* can be identified. PMD is allelic with a much milder disorder, X-linked spastic paraplegia type 2 (SPG2), also caused by *PLP1* mutations. In its pure form, the sole symptom associated with SPG2 is slowly increasing spasticity, more of the legs than of the arms, which begins during childhood or adolescence. In the complicated forms, additional symptoms such as nystagmus, ataxia, dysarthria and mild mental retardation are present.

MRI in PMD shows hypomyelination, indicated by diffusely elevated T2 white matter signal (Fig. 27.2). Myelin is usually present in the brainstem and sometimes in the cerebellar hemispheric white matter; the cerebellar volume is normal. Generalized cerebral atrophy develops over time, usually in the second decade. Proton MR spectroscopy reveals low choline, due to reduced membrane turnover, and normal to elevated *N*-acetylaspartate (NAA).

Pelizaeus-Merzbacher-like disease (PMLD; MIM 608804) shows a similar clinical presentation, albeit its inheritance is autosomal recessive. The primary clinical features include early nystagmus, ataxia, and spasticity. The disorder is genetically heterogeneous. In most cases, the underlying genetic abnormality is not known. In a subset of patients with PMLD (fewer than 10%), mutations in *GJC2* (formerly called *GJA12*), coding for Connexin 46.6 (Cx47) located on chromosome 1q41–42, have been found (Uhlenberg et al. 2004; Henneke et al. 2008). Connexins (Cx) form intercellular gap junctions which are an essential component of the large glial syncytium of astrocytes and oligodendrocytes in the CNS. Patients with mutations in *GJC2* have a better initial development than PMD patients. Cerebellar signs are prominent, and some of the children had been classified as having spastic ataxia. There is however a much more pronounced decline, and the children become wheelchair-bound in adolescence. Epilepsy is common and may even be severe in some subject patients. Mild demyelinating peripheral neuropathy has been described in some patients. MRI shows hypomyelination; T2 hyperintensity of the brainstem pyramidal tract portion is frequently seen (Fig. 27.2).

The initial and most prominent neurological symptom of **4H syndrome** (MIM 612440) is ataxia. 4H stands for hypomyelination, hypodontia, and hypogonadotropic hypogonadism

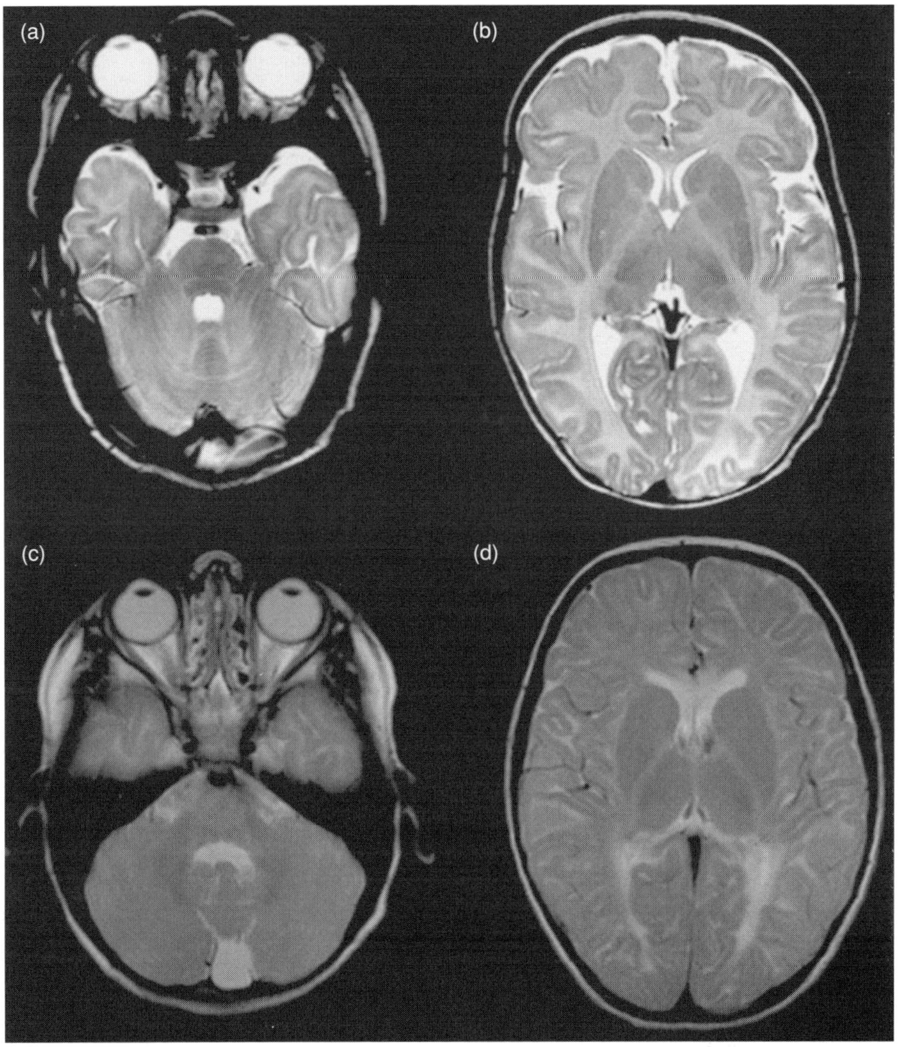

Fig. 27.2. **(a, b)** T2-weighted axial MR images of a 2-year-old child with Pelizaeus-Merzbacher disease (PMD) **(c, d)** and a 5-year-old child with Pelizaeus-Merzbacher-like disease (PMLD), demonstrating the diffuse high signal intensity of unmyelinated white matter. In the child with PMD, the cerebellar white matter is also affected **(a)**. In the child with PMLD, the signal intensity of the brainstem is abnormally high **(c)**.

(Wolf et al. 2005a; Timmons et al. 2006). This disease is rare; its genetic defect has not yet been elucidated. As affected siblings of both sexes are known, inheritance is probably autosomal recessive. Initial development is normal, and affected children often start to walk without support before 18 months. By the age of 2–3 years, parents note that gait remains clumsy and the children frequently fall. Neurological examination reveals ataxic gait, mild intention tremor, and dysmetria. There is also a prominent cerebellar eye movement disorder with saccadic pursuit and gaze-evoked nystagmus. During the first decade, clinical course is more or less stable although many parents describe episodic deterioration with infections and subsequent recovery. Ataxia progresses towards the end of the first decade, and pyramidal signs develop. Many children become wheelchair-bound in the second decade, and are ultimately almost unable to move, despite only mildly impaired cognitive function. As in many other disorders, there is a considerable spectrum of severity: about 10% of children are never able to walk without support; others show only minor ataxia even in early adulthood. Most children show mild to moderate learning disability. Many have a language disorder. Peripheral neuropathy is an inconstant finding. Hypodontia is distinctive and allows early diagnosis. Eruption of deciduous teeth is delayed, and its order disturbed. In children with 4H syndrome, the deciduous molars erupt first, followed by the mandibular incisors, and finally the upper median incisors. Despite this delayed and disorganized eruption, the deciduous teeth are usually complete, although the upper median incisors may never erupt, probably because of resorption. In the permanent dentition however, some teeth are missing in most patients. The incisors have an abnormal convex shape and often also a yellowish color. About 20% of patients have natal teeth, an otherwise very rare finding. Hypogonadotropic hypogonadism can only be diagnosed in adolescence when patients fail to enter puberty. Luteinizing hormone (LH) and follicle stimulating hormone (FSH) are low. Other symptoms found in the majority of patients include myopia and small stature.

MRI shows hypomyelinated white matter. T2 signal in the supratentorial white matter is diffusely elevated, with the exception of the optic radiation and a part of the posterior limb of the internal capsule. T1 white matter signal varies from hypointense to hyperintense, depending on the amount of myelin deposited.

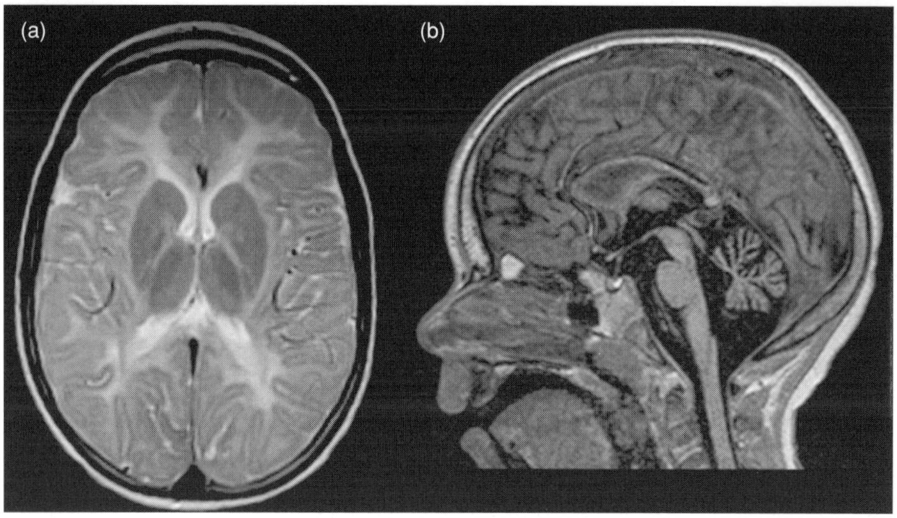

Fig. 27.3. **(a)** T2-weighted axial **(b)** and T1-weighted sagittal image of a 7-year-old child with 4H syndrome (hypomyelination, hypodontia, and hypogonadotropic hypogonadism). There is diffuse hypomyelination **(a)** and considerable cerebellar atrophy **(b)**.

There is cerebellar atrophy early in the disease, more so of the vermis than of the hemispheres (Fig. 27.3). Later on in the disease course, cortical atrophy and white matter loss develop, indicating ongoing myelin loss.

Vanishing white matter disease (VWM; MIM 306896), also called childhood ataxia with central hypomyelination (CACH) or myelinopathia centralis diffusa, is one of the more frequent white matter disorders (van der Knaap et al. 2006). In its classic form, development during infancy and early childhood is normal. Symptoms start between the age of 2 and 6 years. The children slowly develop progressive cerebellar ataxia and mild spasticity. Cognitive decline is mild. The disease is exacerbated by mild head traumas or febrile infections triggering rapid deterioration with loss of motor functions, profound hypotonia, seizures, and finally coma. Some children recover, but do not reach their previous level; others die. The mildest variant has its onset only in adulthood as the mildest form. Ovarian failure is common. The most severe form starts in utero with decreased fetal movements, microcephaly, and arthrogryposis multiplex congenita. Affected infants do not gain any milestones and die within the first months of life. This early and severe form of VWM is a multisystem disease including, for example, cataract, hepatosplenomegaly, and ovarian dysgenesis. There is no known cure for this disease. Care should be taken to prevent fever by using antipyretics or even cooling. Vaccinations should be kept up to date. In older patients with milder disease, contact sports are discouraged.

There are no specific laboratory abnormalities in patients with VWM. The diagnosis is made on MRI. In the classic form, the white matter signal, is diffusely elevated in T2-weighted images. In the course of the disease, white matter rarefies, which is best seen in FLAIR or proton density images demonstrating cystic degeneration, and radial stripes which are compatible with better preserved strands of white matter (Fig. 27.4). Subcortical fibers may be spared. In younger children, white matter appears swollen; in older patients, the brain may become atrophic. The cortex does not collapse, however, in spite of the white matter disappearance. Cerebellar atrophy is a late finding except in severely affected infants where it may be an early feature. MRI criteria for the diagnosis have been published (van der Knaap et al. 2006).

VWM is caused by recessive mutations in each one of the five genes (*EIF2B1–5*) coding for the subunits of eIF2B, a translation initiation factor important in the regulation of protein synthesis (Pronk et al. 2006). In two-thirds of all patients with VWM, mutations are found in *EIF2B5* coding for the largest eIF2B subunit. There seems to be a certain genotype-phenotype correlation with p.Arg113His causes milder disease, especially if present homozygously (van der Lei et al. 2010). Severity of VWM does not correlate with eIF2B activity (Liu et al. 2011).

Megalencephalic leukoencephalopathy with subcortical cysts (MLC; MIM 604004) and mild clinical course was first described in 1995 (van der Knaap et al. 1995). The characteristic clinical finding in this white matter disease is macrocephaly developing from the age of 3–4 months. Head circumference rapidly evolves above the 97th percentile. Psychomotor development at that age is only slightly delayed, but problems become evident at the end of the first year of life. Children usually do learn to walk without support, but later than normal, between the age of 18 months and 3 years. Gait is ataxic, and patients also show intention tremor and dysmetria. Cognitive abilities are relatively spared. During the disease course, spasticity develops, and children become wheelchair-bound at the end of their first or in their second decade. Epilepsy is quite common, but usually easy to control. Often, seizures are triggered by mild head trauma. Mild falls can also lead to transient neurological symptoms such as aphasia, but recovery is complete, unlike in children with VWM.

MRI reveals diffuse white matter abnormalities with elevated signal in T2-weighted images. White matter appears swollen. Cerebellar white matter shows only mild changes. Basal ganglia are spared. In the early stages of disease, there is no atrophy, but this gradually develops over time. There are subcortical cysts, almost always in the anterior part of the temporal lobe, frequently also in the frontal and parietal subcortical white matter, best seen in FLAIR images (Fig. 27.5).

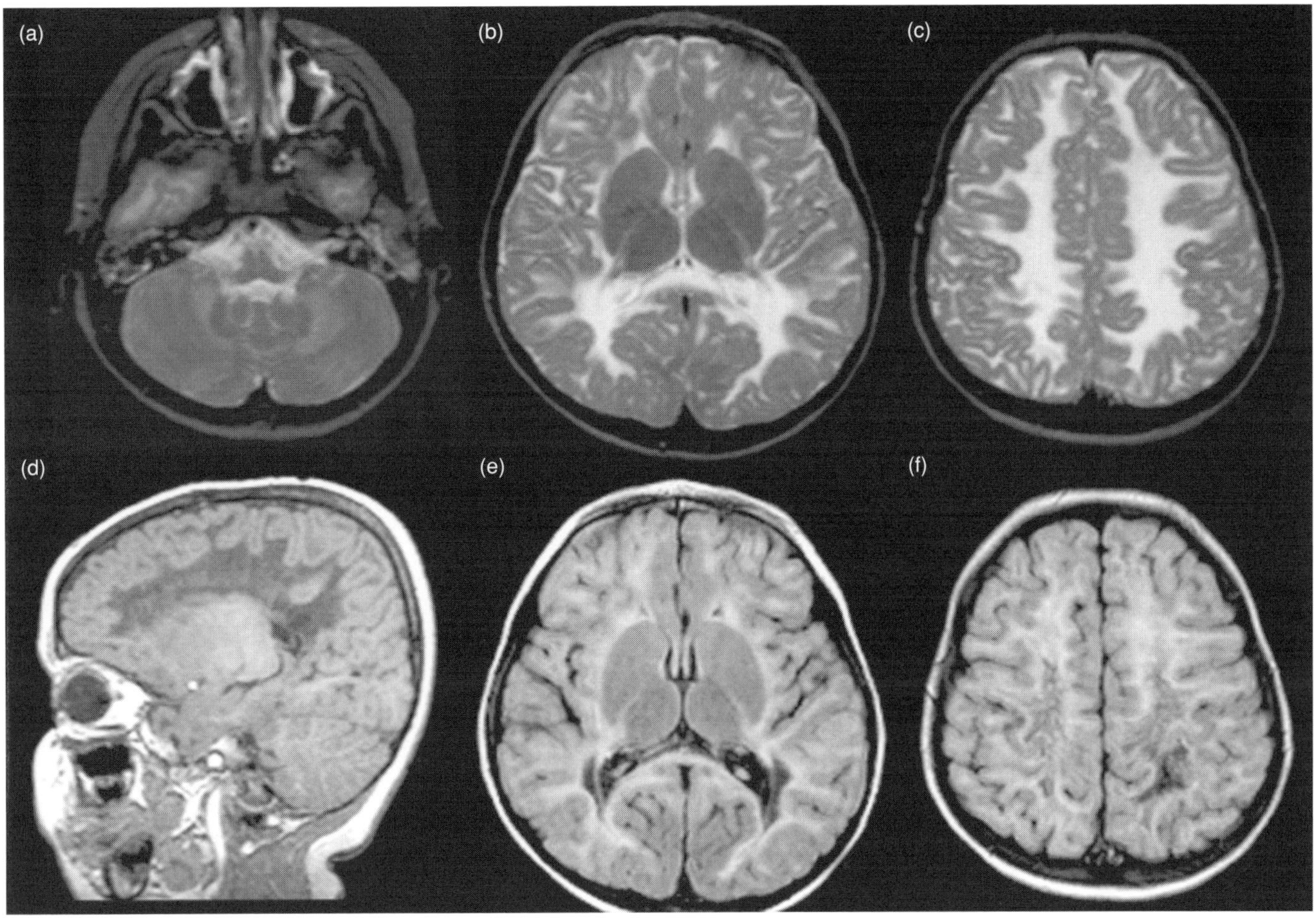

Fig. 27.4. MRI of a 3-year-old child with vanishing white matter (VWM) disease. **(a, b, c)** Axial T2-weighted images show diffuse hyperintense signal of the supratentorial white matter **(b, c)** and also faint signal abnormalities of the cerebellar white matter **(a)**. **(d)** The sagittal T1-weighted image demonstrates the radiating stripes within the white matter. **(e, f)** The cystic transformation of the white matter is best seen on the FLAIR images. (Images kindly provided by Professor Dr. van der Knaap, Amsterdam.)

Fig. 27.5. MRI of an 18 month-old child with megalencephalic leukoencephalopathy with subcortical cysts (MLC) due to compound heterozygous mutations in *MLC1*. **(a)** The white matter is diffusely hyperintense and appears swollen on the T2-weighted axial image. **(b)** The temporal cysts are best seen on this axial FLAIR image.

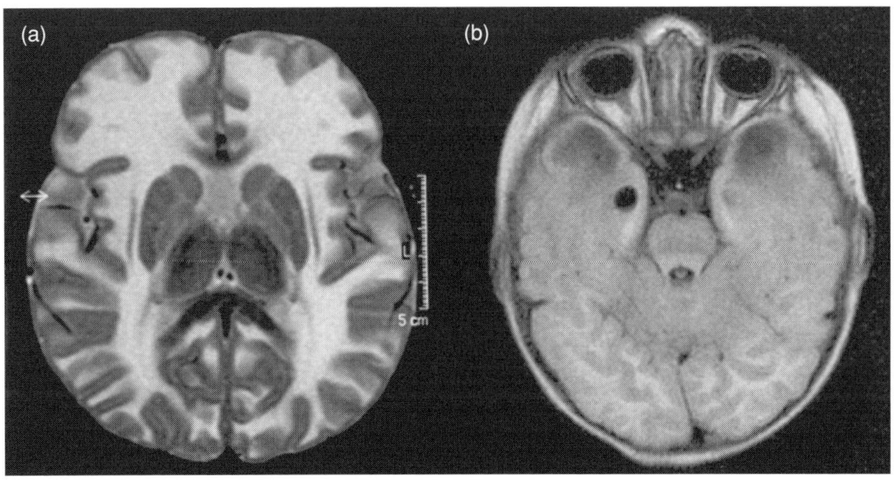

The MRI is diagnostic for MLC. There are no laboratory abnormalities. Two-thirds of the patients carry recessive mutations in *MLC1* coding for a transmembrane protein with hitherto unknown function, the rest carries mutations in the gene coding for GlialCAM (López-Hernández et al. 2011). With this gene, children carrying two mutations show the classical MLC phenotype, whereas children with one mutation show improvement of their MRI (van der Knaap et al. 2010).

Leukoencephalopathy with brainstem and spinal cord involvement and lactate elevation (LBSL; MIM 611105) is

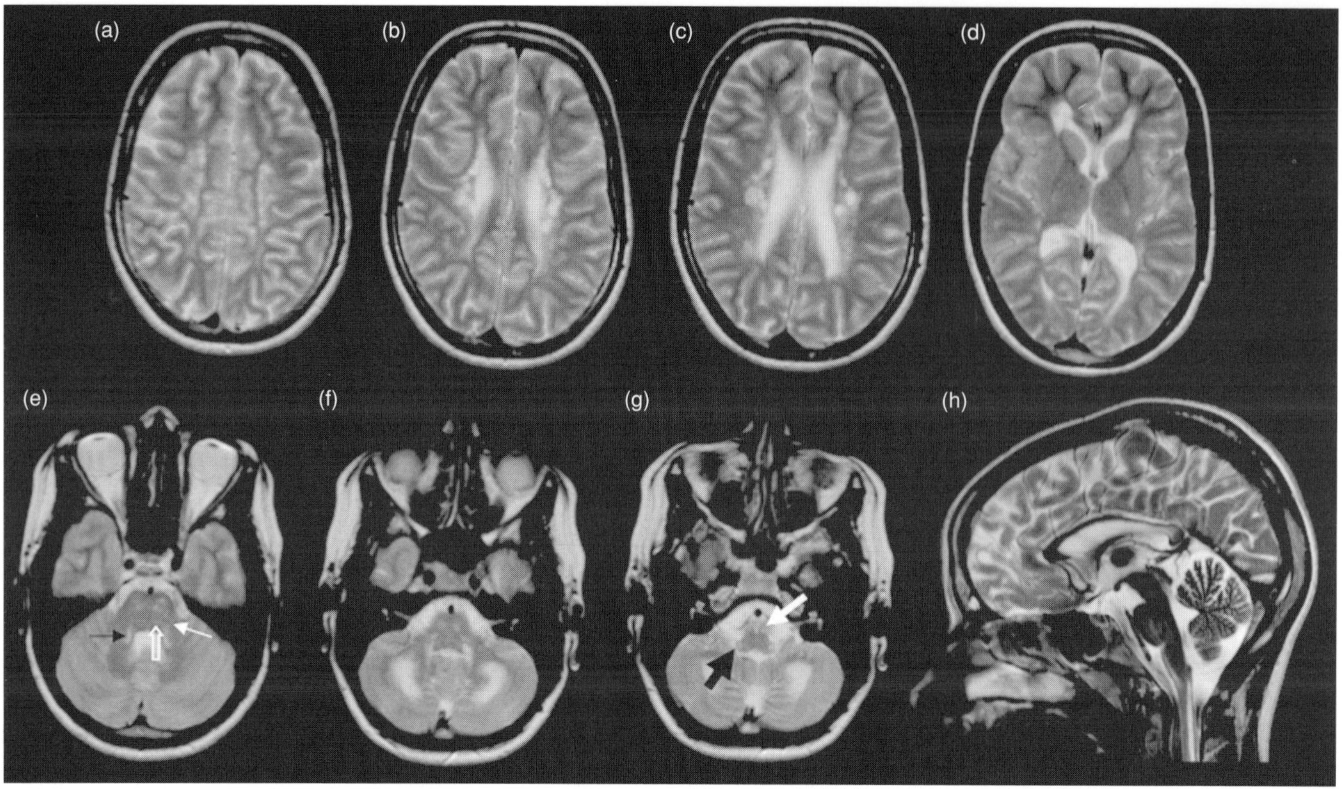

Fig. 27.6. T2-weighted images of a 16-year-old with leukoencephalopathy with brainstem and spinal cord involvement and lactate (LBSL). In the supratentorial white matter, there are patchy, partly confluent hyperintense patches in the centrum semiovale and in the frontal white matter adjacent to the ventricles **(a–d)**. There is symmetric hyperintensity in the posterior limb of the internal capsule **(d)**. Infratentorially, the cerebellar white matter is abnormal **(f, g)**. Within the brainstem, the internal intraparenchymal trajectories of the trigeminal nerves (white arrow), the middle cerebellar peduncles (black arrow), the inferior cerebellar peduncles (thick black arrow), the pyramidal tracts (thick white arrow) are involved **(e–g)**. Involvement of transverse pontine fibers (open arrow) is very faint, but present. The sagittal image demonstrates high signal of the posterior columns and the pyramidal tracts **(h)**.

another recently described autosomal recessive white matter disease (van der Knaap et al. 2003). Slowly progressive symptoms start in childhood or adolescence and include spasticity, mild cerebellar symptoms, and pain and paresthesias mainly of the legs. Romberg sign is positive, and vibration sense is absent or severely reduced. Many patients become wheelchair dependent during adult life. Cognition is normal to mildly impaired. LBSL is caused by compound heterozygous mutations in *DARS2* coding for the mitochondrial aspartyl-tRNA synthetase (Scheper et al. 2007).

MRI demonstrates typical abnormalities which allow making the diagnosis (Fig. 27.6): on T2-weighted images, the cerebral white matter shows sometimes inhomogeneous, sometimes confluent high signal with sparing of the U fibers. Dorsal columns and lateral corticospinal tracts of the myelum are also affected as well as the pyramids in the medulla oblongata. Supportive criteria are signal abnormalities in the splenium of the corpus callosum, the posterior limb of the internal capsule, the medial lemniscus in the brainstem, superior and inferior cerebellar peduncles, the intraparenchymal part of the trigeminal nerve, the mesencephalic trigeminal tracts, the anterior spinocerebellar tracts in the medulla, and in the cerebellar white matter. Proton MR spectroscopy usually shows elevated lactate, but this is not an obligate finding (van der Knaap et al. 2003).

Mitochondrial disorders

Mitochondrial disorders are a group of heterogeneous diseases with a multitude of possible symptoms and signs. They can manifest at any age with virtually any symptom. Cerebellar signs are common, and ataxia deteriorating with infections is one more frequent manifestation of a mitochondrial disorder in childhood. Recovery may be complete or incomplete, and over time, there is usually stepwise deterioration. Exclusive cerebellar symptoms are, however, rare in children with mitochondrial disorders. They usually have other neurological complaints such as epilepsy or extrapyramidal features.

Lactate elevation in body fluids is the most useful biochemical clue, although it may be absent or only present with exacerbation of the symptoms. Brain lactate can be quantified non-invasively with proton MR spectroscopy and does not correlate with CSF lactate in all patients. Alanine is often elevated in plasma, CSF or urine. Pyruvate levels are disproportionately elevated in pyruvate dehydrogenase deficiency (PDH). Citric acid intermediates may be found in urine. Sometimes it is possible to make a clinical diagnosis of one of the well-defined syndromes. Then, straightforward genetic testing is an option. Mostly, though, the overall picture is nonspecific, and muscle biopsy with assessment of activity of single enzymes including PDH and measurement of substrate

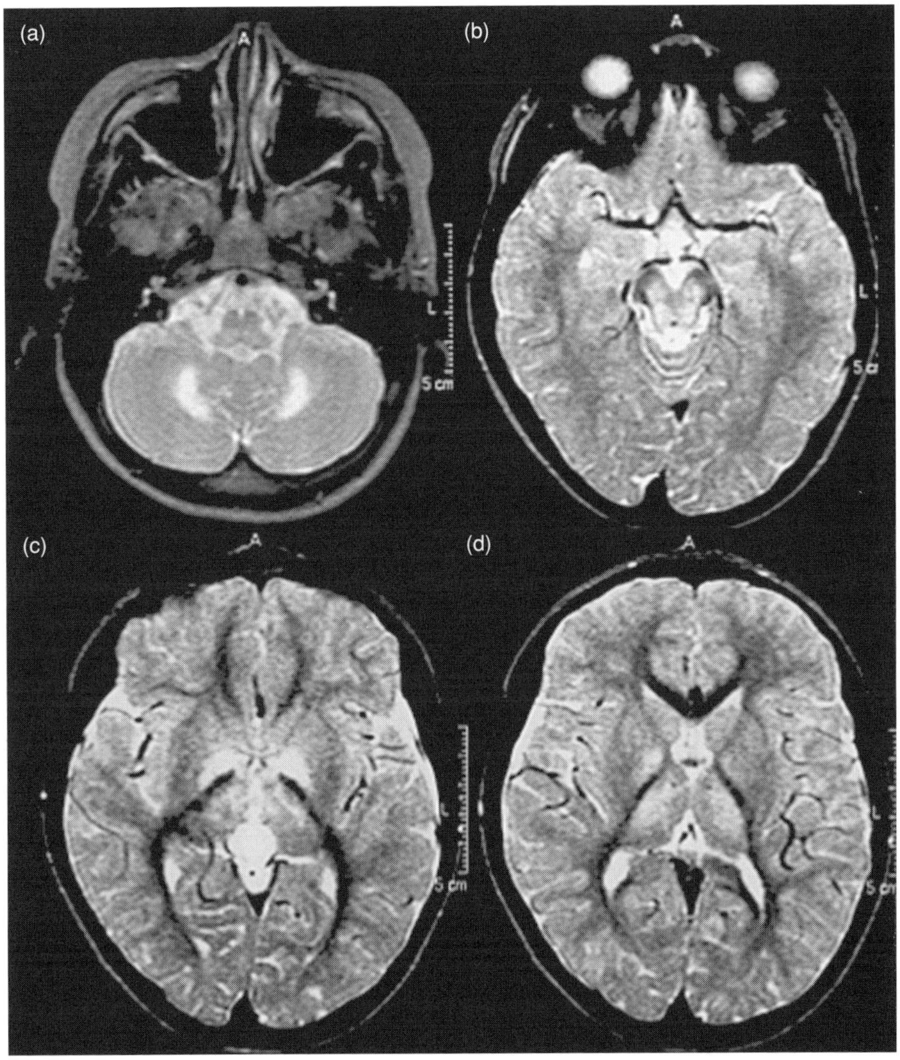

Fig. 27.7. MRI of a 5-year-old child with a large deletion of mitochondrial DNA, but no typical Kearns-Sayre syndrome. The axial T2-weighted images show several affected structures: **(a)** cerebellar white matter, **(b)** the mesencephalon besides the pyramidal tracts, **(c)** the globus pallidus and also part of the thalami and the head of the caudate nuclei. The supratentorial white matter is not affected.

oxidation rates in fresh tissue is the diagnostic procedure of choice. If a single enzyme deficiency is found, subsequent genetic investigation of the appropriate subunits and assembly factors will ensue. Other techniques include quantification of mitochondrial DNA (mtDNA) in muscle and especially liver. MRI shows a multitude of abnormalities including diffuse signal changes and cavitations of white matter, signal changes of the basal ganglia (often symmetric) and brainstem, diffuse cerebellar or global atrophy or stroke-like lesions with cortical edema, and T2 hyperintensity. Calcifications of basal ganglia and dentate nuclei are sometimes present (Fig. 27.7).

There are a few well-defined mitochondrial disorders with cerebellar signs as the prominent abnormality: MERRF (myoclonic epilepsy with ragged red fibers), NARP (neuropathy, ataxia, and retinitis pigmentosa), IOSCA (infantile-onset spinocerebellar ataxia), and the spectrum of POLG1-associated disorders, among them SANDOS (sensory ataxic neuropathy, dysarthria, and ophthalmoparesis), SCAE (spinocerebellar ataxia with epilepsy), and MIRAS (mitochondrial recessive ataxia syndrome) which are partly overlapping.

NARP (MIM 551500) is characterized by developmental delay, gait and appendicular ataxia, peripheral neuropathy, and retinitis pigmentosa. The disorder is usually slowly progressive. Patients harbor a missense mutation, T8993G/C, in *MTATP6* in the mtDNA coding for one of the subunits of the ATP synthase. For this mutation, severity correlates with the degree of heteroplasmy. If it is very high, patients develop Leigh syndrome, a much more severe disease. As is usual for mtDNA mutations, the disease is inherited via the maternal line. MRI shows variable abnormalities including supratentorial and cerebellar atrophy and signal abnormalities of the basal ganglia.

Kearns-Sayre syndrome (KSS; MIM 530000) is characterized by chronic-progressive external ophthalmoplegia, retinitis pigmentosa, and cardiac involvements (conduction block, cardiac hypertrophy). Many patients also show cerebellar ataxia. CSF protein levels are high. This disorder is due to large-scale deletions of the mtDNA; its occurrence is usually sporadic. MRI reveals T2 white matter hyperintensities of the U fibers and the deep white matter, of the globus pallidus, and the cerebellar white matter. Also mesencephalic and brainstem signal abnormalities may be seen. Cerebellar atrophy is possible. CT often shows calcifications, especially of the basal ganglia.

IOSCA (MIM 271745) is a very rare ataxia with early onset so far only reported in Finnish children (Koskinen et al. 1994).

Development in the first year of life is normal; in the second year of life, ataxia and hypotonia appear, and choreoathetosis develops. Tendon reflexes disappear over time, because of peripheral neuropathy. In the classic form, sensorineural deafness and external ophthalmoplegia develop by the age of 7 years. Later, optic atrophy becomes evident. Epilepsy with recurrent status epilepticus including epilepsia partialis continua develops is an important symptom that is difficult to manage. Pes cavus and scoliosis develop in many patients. Ambulation is usually lost in adolescence. MRI shows cerebellar atrophy; signal of cerebellar white matter may be elevated. During status epilepticus, cerebral cortex is often hyperintense on T2-weighted images and has a swollen aspect, reflecting cortical edema and resembling the abnormalities seen in mitochondrial encephalomyopathy, lactic acidosis, and stroke-like episodes (MELAS) or Alpers disease. Neuropathology has revealed severe atrophy of the posterior columns and spinocerebellar tracts of the spinal cord, similar to what can be found in Friedreich ataxia. All but one IOSCA patient are homozygous for the Y508C missense mutation in *C10orf2* which codes for the mitochondrial protein Twinkle (Nikali et al. 2005). Twinkle is a helicase important for maintenance of mtDNA. However, in children with IOSCA, no evidence for abnormal mitochondrial function was found until recently when complex I deficiency could be proven in brain tissue of an affected patient. Other missense mutations of *C10orf2* lead to dominant chronic progressive external ophthalmoplegia in adults.

MERRF (MIM 545000) is a rare mitochondrial disorder caused by missense mutations in the transfer RNA (tRNA) gene for lysine and also some other mitochondrial genes. A8344G in $tRNA^{Lys}$ accounts for 80–90% of all cases. Patients develop progressive myoclonic epilepsy, ataxia, and cognitive decline. Hearing loss is another frequent symptom.

Polymerase γ1 (**POLG1**; MIM 174763) is an enzyme important for replication and maintenance of the mtDNA. Mutations in this gene, in acting either a dominant or a recessive manner, have been shown to cause a multitude of disorders, some of them readily identifiable entities (Milone and Massie 2010). Dominant mutations are associated with chronic progressive external ophthalmoplegia, as with *C10orf2* mutations. Recessive mutations cause different clinical entities. The most important one in childhood is Alpers disease (MIM 203700), characterized by (recurrent) partial status epilepticus, epilepsia partialis continua, and liver involvement (Naviaux et al. 1999). Valproic acid may trigger acute, fatal liver failure; in other patients, liver failure is more insidious. Many children recover from their first status epilepticus, but suffer from moderate to severe ataxia and cognitive decline. Epilepsy may be controlled for months. Usually, status epilepticus relapses. Most children die months to years after the first manifestation. Isolated (sensory or cerebellar) ataxia, as found in adults, especially with a homozygous *W748S* mutation, is probably very rare in children as a manifestation of POLG1-related disorder if it exists at all – epilepsy and status epilepticus seem to be extremely frequent in children. Nevertheless, this mutation is said to be the most common cause of recessive progressive ataxia starting in adolescence or adulthood in Europe (Hakonen et al. 2005). Haplotype analysis has revealed that all chromosomes carrying *W748S* in combination with *E1143G* originate from a common ancient founder. MRI findings show global cerebral atrophy in later stages. In the acute phase, edema of cortex and ipsilateral thalamus are suggestive of Alpers disease, the localization of the cortical edema correlating with the EEG abnormalities. These consist of rhythmic high-amplitude delta with superimposed spikes and polyspikes (RHADS) in many, but not all, children (Wolf et al. 2009). Neuropathological studies show hepatic steatosis and cortical and thalamic degeneration with gliosis and subcortical neuronal loss.

Coenzyme Q10-related disorders

Coenzyme Q10 (CoQ10), also called ubiquinone, is a mobile lipophilic electron carrier critical for electron transfer in the mitochondrial respiratory chain. Whether or not (inherited) CoQ10 deficiency could lead to ataxia has been under discussion for many years (Quinzii et al. 2008). There were reports of patients with ataxia and low CoQ10 levels in muscle who showed variable clinical improvement after substitution of CoQ10. Some of these patients were later diagnosed with ataxia with oculomotor apraxia type I (Quinzii et al. 2005). Recently, CoQ10 has also been shown to be reduced in muscle of patients with a different mitochondrial disorder. Respiratory chain analysis shows decreased activity of complex II + III and complex I + III, reflecting the CoQ10 deficiency. These activities can be restored by adding CoQ10.

Recently, different defects of the complicated human CoQ10 biosynthesis were described (MIM 607426). None of these cause isolated cerebellar ataxia. The first molecular defect in the biosynthetic pathway to be described were recessive mutations in *COQ2* (MIM *609825), coding for parahydroxybenzoid-polyprenyltransferase in two siblings with encephalomyopathy and nephropathy starting in infancy (Mollet et al. 2007). Another sibling pair died shortly after birth from hepatopathy, renal failure, and anemia. A defect in *COQ9* led to a severe neonatal presentation with hypothermia, seizures, lactic acidosis, renal tubulopathy, and cardiac hypertrophy. Cerebral MRI revealed global atrophy (Duncan et al. 2009).

Several children with CoQ10 deficiency were described with epilepsy including epilepsia partialis continua, ataxia, and mental retardation. Lactate was mildly to moderately elevated. Mutations in *ADCK3* (*CABC1*) underlie this disorder (Lagier-Tourenne et al. 2008; Mollet et al. 2008). MRI shows cerebellar atrophy and, in the patients with epilepsy, edematous cortical areas, resembling the findings in IOSCA. ADCK3 is a presumed ancestral kinase involved in the biosynthesis of coenzyme Q10 although its exact role is still not known.

PDSS1, coding for trans-prenyltransferase, has been found to be mutated in a consanguineous family with early-onset sensorineural deafness, mental retardation, neuropathy, obesity, livedo reticularis, and mild aortic and mitral regurgitation (Mollet et al. 2007). Mutations in *PDSS2* coding for decaprenyl diphosphate synthase lead to Leigh syndrome and nephrotic syndrome (Lopez et al. 2006).

Supplementation of CoQ10 is unfortunately not invariably of benefit in children with defects of its biosynthesis. Some do improve substantially, others not. It is still a subject of debate as to the choice of tissue or body fluid in which coenzyme Q10 levels can be quantified most reliably. Many advocate measuring it in muscle tissue; others found a good correlation of muscle levels with the concentration in mononuclear cells. A simple and reliable test is not yet available.

Gray matter disorders

Niemann-Pick disease type C (NPC; MIM 257220 and 607625) is a neurodegenerative disorder presenting at all ages (Vanier 2010). The early-infantile form starts between ages 2 and 24 months, the late-infantile form between the ages of 2 and 6 years, the juvenile form between the ages of 6 and 15 years. Thereafter, the disease is labelled as adult form. Diagnosis may be difficult, as there is no reliably present biochemical marker nor typical imaging features. Half of the patients with NPC have neonatal cholestatic jaundice which is usually transient. Rapidly fatal neonatal liver disease is, however, possible. In the classic form of the disease, children develop normally in the early years, but are considered clumsy. Slow dementia may be difficult to ascertain, especially early in the disease. Ataxia develops, then also dysarthria, spasticity, dystonia, and swallowing difficulties. Epilepsy is common, especially in the later stages of disease. Psychosis is a late feature. The disease invariably progresses to a stage where all abilities and contact are lost. There are children and adolescents with pure cerebellar ataxia and, even years after onset, normal cognitive abilities. Patients with onset in the first 2 years of life show spastic ataxia and hepatosplenomegaly. Many do not learn to walk. Hepatosplenomegaly is absent in at least 10% of patients. Fetal hydrops or ascites are possible. Two symptoms are typical of NPC: gelastic cataplexy and vertical (mostly downward) supranuclear gaze palsy. In the first, children with NPC show sudden loss of tone when laughing. There may be only head nodding in some, others fall. This phenomenon is often mistaken for epilepsy. Vertical supranuclear gaze palsy is present in virtually all patients with the classic form of the disease, but may be absent in children with early disease onset or adults with late onset. Patients have difficulties walking up or down stairs and with reading. Oculocephalic reflex is normal.

MRI shows nonspecific findings (Fig. 27.8). Early in the disease course, it may be normal; slowly progressive supratentorial atrophy develops over time. In some, cerebellar atrophy is prominent from the beginning. Vague, ill-defined white matter abnormalities in the centrum semiovale reflect axonal compromise; these can be seen also in other gray matter disorders. Proton MR spectroscopy reveals a lipid peak in some, but not all patients; *N*-acetylaspartate (NAA) is decreased.

Histopathology shows foamy storage cells in the visceral organs. In bone marrow aspirates, sea-blue histiocytes and foamy cells are found. Also neuronal cells show storage material with distended cytoplasm, especially pyramidal neurons in the deeper cortical layers. They also store neurofibrillary tangles. In the cerebellum, there is loss of Purkinje and granule cells. The biochemical defect in NPC is a disruption in intracellular cholesterol trafficking. Cholesterol taken up by endocytosis accumulates in lysosomes and late endosomes. It cannot be esterified. Other glycolipids are also accumulating.

Of the patients with NPC 95% carry recessive mutations in *NPC1* (Carstea et al. 1997). This protein has its highest level of expression in the cerebellum and the pons. Its precise function has still not been fully elucidated, but it is involved in intracellular cholesterol transport. Most mutations in *NPC1* are private. One missense mutation, I1061T, is more frequent in patients from Western European descent and is also prevalent in Hispanic-Americans. Mutations in *NPC2* account for the remaining patients (Naureckiene et al. 2000). The NPC2 protein is a soluble, cholesterol-binding protein also involved in cholesterol trafficking.

NPC is suspected on clinical grounds. Plasma chitotriosidase activity is often moderately elevated, but much less than in patients with Gaucher disease. Filipine staining in cultured fibroblasts is abnormal, reflecting the intralysosomal accumulation of nonesterified cholesterol. Bone marrow aspirates show the typical storage cells, although the procedure is no longer widely performed. Mutation analysis first of *NPC1*, and if negative, of *NPC2*, will reveal the underlying mutations and allows prenatal diagnosis.

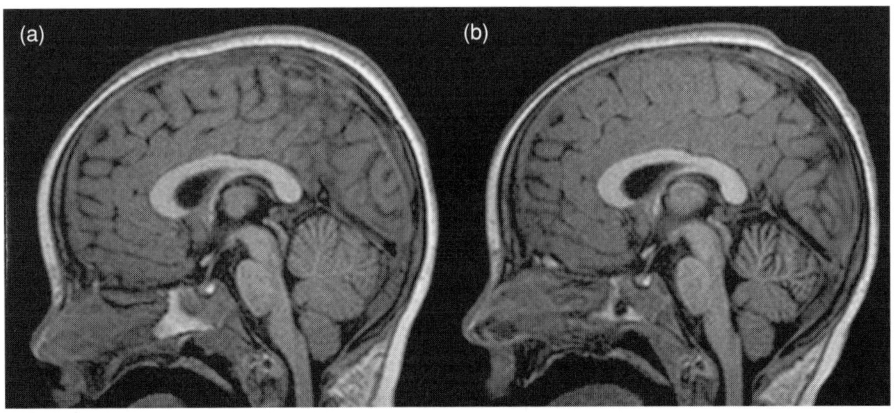

Fig. 27.8. Sagittal T1-weighted images of a child with Niemann Pick disease type C (NPC). **(a)** The first MRI is normal although the child had already severe ataxia and pyramidal signs. **(b)** 18 months later, at the age of 5 years, there is slight cerebellar atrophy.

Until recently, treatment has been purely symptomatic and supportive. Bone marrow transplantation had no effect on the neurological symptoms. As glycolipids are also stored in neurons, substrate-reducing therapy with Miglustat, similar to the approach in patients with Gaucher disease, has been tested and found to be beneficial – it stabilizes the disease course in 72% of patients. Its effect was first shown for adolescents and adults, then for children (Patterson et al. 2007). It is now recommended to start treatment in all patients as soon as they show neurological symptoms (Group et al. 2009). Side effects include, in particular, diarrhea and flatulence which can be managed by diet and medication. Patients with late disease onset profit the most from the treatment.

G_{M2} gangliosidosis (MIM 272800, 268800) is a heterogeneous disease due to deficiency of either hexosaminadase A (including Tay-Sachs disease), hexosaminidases A and B (including Sandhoff disease) or G_{M2} activator deficiency. The infantile form, Tay-Sachs and Sandhoff disease, starts after 3 to 5 months of age with mild hypotonia, then slowing of development and regression. Infants display a startle response to sudden acoustic stimuli with myoclonus. By the end of the first year of life, many of the children suffer from epilepsy. Macrocephaly develops from age 18 months. Ophthalmological examination reveals a cherry-red spot. MRI in these children shows hypomyelination secondary to early neuronal involvement and slightly increased T2 signal of the basal ganglia; thalami may be hypointense (Autti et al. 2007).

In the later-onset forms, ataxia and action myoclonus may be prominent symptoms, and the MRI shows cerebellar atrophy. Cognition is much less affected. These children may resemble patients with pure hereditary ataxia and lack a cherry-red spot, making the diagnosis less obvious. Others show mainly dementia and a combination of pyramidal, extrapyramidal, and cerebellar signs with general cerebral atrophy. Another late-onset variant mimicks spinal muscular atrophy type 3 with absence of upper motor neuron signs (Maegawa et al. 2006).

Ganglioside G_{M2} and other lipids accumulate in lysosomes. In Sandhoff disease, the lipids also accumulate in visceral organs, leading to hepatosplenomegaly. Mutations in *HEXA* lead to Tay-Sachs disease and later-onset variants of G_{M2} gangliosidosis. G269S in exon 7 causes late-onset disease (Cordeiro et al. 2000).

Late-infantile neuronal ceroid lipofuscinosis (CLN2; MIM 204500) is another lysosomal disorder usually starting between the ages of 2 and 4 years. Early development, especially language development, is often slightly delayed, but usually children come to attention with tonic-clonic seizures and ataxia. Action myoclonus may be prominent. Epilepsy is difficult to control, and myoclonic seizures develop. Ataxia rapidly progresses, and children also develop mild pyramidal signs and dementia. Pigmentary retinopathy is present, but clinically not evident until late in the disease course. EEG shows giant potentials triggered by slow photic stimulation. Some patients are much more mildly affected and show mainly ataxia and action myoclonus with only mild dementia. Other forms of neuronal ceroid lipofuscinosis may present similarly to CLN2, CLN5 (Finnish variant) and CLN6 being other variants with late-infantile onset, but different genetic basis (Mole et al. 2005); also CLN8 can present similarly to CLN2 (Reinhardt et al. 2010).

MRI in CLN2 shows, as in most gray matter disorders, nonspecific findings with mild supratentorial and also cerebellar atrophy. Periventricular white matter has an ill-defined slightly elevated signal on T2-weighted images.

CLN2 is caused by recessive mutations in *TPP1* (also called *CLN2*), coding for tripeptidylpeptidase 1, a serine protease involved in lysosomal protein degradation (Sleat et al. 1997). Some mutations are associated with a milder clinical course. TPP1 activity can be measured in white blood cells or dried blood spots. Ultrastructural examination of lymphocytes, skin or conjunctiva shows curvilinear inclusions.

Infantile neuroaxonal dystrophy (INAD; MIM 256600) shows a typical clinical course in most patients with normal development in the first 12–18 months and then gradual decline with prominent muscular hypotonia, development of cerebellar ataxia and nystagmus and later spasticity, dementia and swallowing difficulties. Tendon reflexes may be lost, and electromyography shows denervation. Epilepsy is not a common symptom of this disorder, unlike in most other neurodegenerative disorders of this age group. Ophthalmological examination often shows pigmentary retinopathy and optic atrophy (Aicardi and Castelein 1979; Nardocci et al. 1999).

MRI reveals cerebellar atrophy with high T2 signal of the cerebellar cortex, best seen in coronal FLAIR images, and often, especially later on in the disease, a hypointense signal of the pallidum on T2-weighted images (Fig. 27.9). This combination is typical of INAD, whereas high T2 signal intensity of the cerebellar cortex has been reported also with other disorders. EEG shows prominent beta activity, especially in early sleep stages, which is very helpful in the differential diagnosis.

Until recently, diagnosis of INAD could only be confirmed by demonstrating axonal swelling and spheroids in ultrastructural examination of biopsies of skin or conjunctiva. The underlying gene defect was found in 2006 when recessive mutations in *PLA2G6* were identified (Morgan et al. 2006). This gene codes for a phospholipase and also causes a subset of childhood forms of neurodegeneration with brain iron accumulation (NBIA). Cerebellar atrophy seems to be an important predictor for the presence of mutations in *PLA2G6*. The pathogenesis is not yet understood.

Other inborn errors of metabolism

L2-hydroxyglutaric aciduria (MIM 236792) is a rare organic aciduria characterized by urinary excretion of large amounts of 2-hydroxyglutaric acid. Affected patients usually show mental retardation becoming evident around 2 years of age and cerebellar signs – gait ataxia, intention tremor, dysmetria, saccadic speech, and a cerebellar eye movement disorder. Macrocephaly is present in half of the patients, and epilepsy is seen frequently (Steenweg et al. 2010). The disease may be

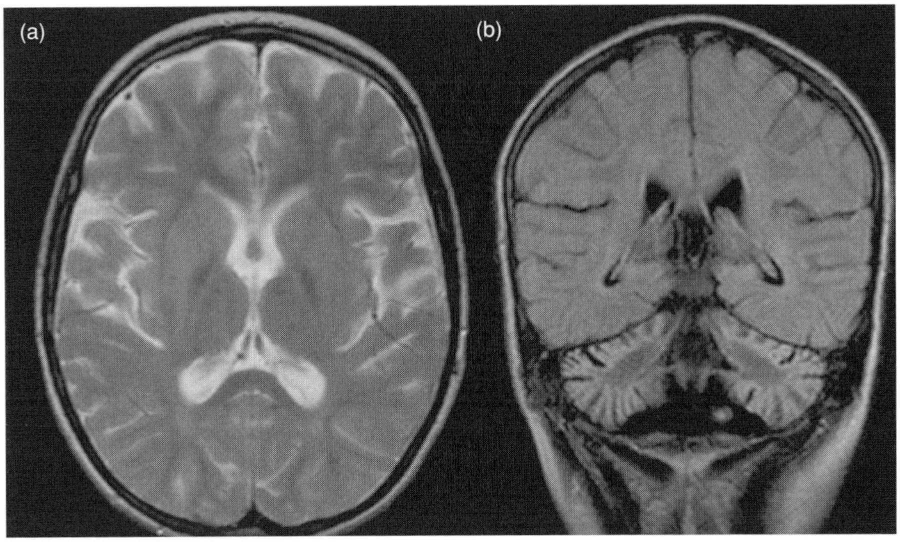

Fig. 27.9. (a) Axial T2-weighted and **(b)** coronal FLAIR MR images of a 6-year-old child with infantile neuroaxonal dystrophy (INAD). Note **(a)** the hypointense pallidum and **(b)** the hyperintense, atrophic cerebellar cortex.

stable for a long time, but is slowly progressive over time. Symptoms may be quite mild in single cases. Patients seem to be more prone to develop a brain tumor, and rapid deterioration of symptoms should prompt evaluation for a cerebral malignancy.

Diagnosis is suggested by typical MRI abnormalities – T2 hyperintensities predominantly of the subcortical white matter, the dentate nucleus, and the basal ganglia (Steenweg et al. 2009) – and the increased excretion of L2-hydroxyglutaric acid found by organic acid analysis. Recessive mutations in *L2HGDH* coding for L-2-hydroxyglutarate dehydrogenase which catalyzes the conversion of L-2-hydroxyglutaric acid to 2-ketoglutarate cause this disease (Rzem et al. 2004). This enzyme is located in mitochondria, and its exact function is still to be unravelled.

Refsum disease (MIM 266500) is a rare autosomal recessive disorder caused by peroxisome dysfunction. There are two different forms, caused by mutations in the genes coding for phytanoyl-CoA hydroxylase (adult Refsum disease 1) and for peroxin 7 (adult Refsum disease 2) (Jansen et al. 1997; van den Brink et al. 2003). Deficient function of other peroxisomal proteins causes the infantile form of Refsum disease with a completely different clinical and biochemical presentation.

Patients develop retinitis pigmentosa with night blindness (this is usually the earliest symptom) and concentric visual field constriction, miosis, peripheral sensorimotor demyelinating neuropathy, cerebellar ataxia, and often anosmia and sensorineural hearing loss. The neuropathy may be waxing and waning. Peripheral nerves may be thickened and palpable, and there is considerable distal amyotrophy. Cataracts may occur. Cardiac involvement with arrhythmias and cardiac failure is possible. Skin changes include dry skin and ichthyosis and are more pronounced in children. Symptoms start between the end of the first until the third decade and slowly deteriorate; onset in early childhood is possible. Laboratory investigations show elevated CSF protein and high plasma phytanic acid. This disease is important to recognize as it is treatable: phytanic acid is of exogenous origin, and a diet restricted in phytanic acid stops progression and can even improve symptoms. Major sources of phytanic acid are meat and dairy products from ruminants. Plasmapheresis to reduce the levels of plasma phytanic acid is also beneficial, especially at start of the dietary treatment or with very high phytanic acid levels, in order to obtain a quick response. If untreated, half of the patients die before the age of 30 years. There are no systematic data about neuroimaging. **Other peroxisomal disorders** may present with isolated ataxia or ataxia and peripheral neuropathy, even with normal cognitive development and no or mild MRI changes. This has been shown for example, for mutations in *PEX10* and *PEX2* (Régal et al. 2010; Sevin et al. 2011).

Congenital disorders of glycosylation (CDG) are a large and heterogeneous group of inborn errors of protein *N*-linked glycosylation (Jaeken et al. 2009). Diagnosis can be made with isoelectrofocusing of serum transferrine. Numerous different enzymes play a role in the complex process of protein glycosylation, and defects have been delineated for many of them. CDG type Ia (MIM 212065) is the first CDG syndrome which was described by Jaeken in Belgian twin sisters (Jaeken et al. 1984) and is also the most common subtype (Grunewald 2009). Clinical features of this subtype include cerebellar ataxia. Patients suffer from neurological symptoms including moderate to severe mental retardation, they show dysmorphic signs, the best known being inverted nipples and abnormal fat distribution, and most of the patients have evidence of multiorgan involvement. Hepatomegaly and mild proteinuria are common; hepatic or cardiac failure and nephrotic syndrome are exceptional. Clotting abnormalities are frequent, and patients may develop deep venous thrombosis. Severe infections may be a problem. The neurological picture including ataxia is overall stable, and, as a rule, children do not learn to walk. Stroke-like episodes have been reported. Retinitis pigmentosa and strabismus are also part of the clinical picture. Electrophysiological investigations show demyelinating polyneuropathy, and amyotrophy is common, especially in the legs. Imaging features are variable and nonspecific including pontocerebellar hypoplasia, cerebellar atrophy, and Dandy-Walker malformation.

The biochemical basis of CDG Ia is deficiency of phosphomannomutase (PMM) due to recessive mutations in the *PMM2* gene. Enzyme activity can be measured in leukocytes and fibroblasts. This enzyme catalyzes the conversion of mannose 6-phosphate to mannose 1-phosphate, the latter being necessary for the initial step of protein glycosylation (Matthijs et al. 1997).

REFERENCES

Aicardi J, Castelein P (1979) Infantile neuroaxonal dystrophy. Brain 102: 727–748.

Autti T, Joensuu R, Aberg L (2007) Decreased T2 signal in the thalami may be a sign of lysosomal storage disease. Neuroradiology 49: 571–578.

Carstea ED, Morris JA, Coleman KG, Loftus SK, Zhang D, Cummings C, et al. (1997) Niemann-Pick C1 disease gene: homology to mediators of cholesterol homeostasis. Science 277: 228–231.

Cordeiro P, Hechtman P, Kaplan F (2000) The GM2 gangliosidoses databases: allelic variation at the HEXA, HEXB, and GM2A gene loci. Genet Med 2: 319–327.

Duncan AJ, Bitner-Glindzicz M, Meunier B, Costello H, Hargreaves IP, Lopez LC, et al. (2009) A nonsense mutation in COQ9 causes autosomal-recessive neonatal-onset primary coenzyme Q10 deficiency: a potentially treatable form of mitochondrial disease. Am J Hum Genet 84: 558–566.

Eichler F, Grodd W, Grant E, Sessa M, Biffi A, Bley A, et al. (2009) Metachromatic leukodystrophy: a scoring system for brain MR imaging observations. Am J Neuroradiol 30: 1893–1897.

Ellis D, Malcolm S (1994) Proteolipid protein gene dosage effect in Pelizaeus-Merzbacher disease. Nat Genet 6: 333–334.

Garbern JY (2007) Pelizaeus-Merzbacher disease: Genetic and cellular pathogenesis. Cell Mol Life Sci 64: 50–65.

Garcia-Cazorla A, Wolf NI, Serrano M, Perez-Duenas B, Pineda M, Campistol J, et al. (2009) Inborn errors of metabolism and motor disturbances in children. J Inherit Metab Dis 32: 618–629.

Gieselmann V, Krageloh-Mann I (2010) Metachromatic leukodystrophy – an update. Neuropediatrics 41: 1–6.

Group N-CGW, Wraith JE, Baumgartner MR, Bembi B, Covanis A, Levade T, Mengel E, et al. (2009) Recommendations on the diagnosis and management of Niemann-Pick disease type C. Mol Genet Metab 98: 152–165.

Grunewald S (2009) The clinical spectrum of phosphomannomutase 2 deficiency (CDG-Ia). Biochim Biophys Acta 1792: 827–834.

Hakonen AH, Heiskanen S, Juvonen V, Lappalainen I, Luoma PT, Rantamaki M, et al. (2005) Mitochondrial DNA polymerase W748S mutation: a common cause of autosomal recessive ataxia with ancient European origin. Am J Hum Genet 77: 430–441.

Henneke M, Combes P, Diekmann S, Bertini E, Brockmann K, Burlina AP, et al. (2008) GJA12 mutations are a rare cause of Pelizaeus-Merzbacher-like disease. Neurology 70: 748–754.

Hudson LD, Puckett C, Berndt J, Chan J, Gencic S (1989) Mutation of the proteolipid protein gene PLP in a human X chromosome-linked myelin disorder. Proc Natl Acad Sci U S A 86: 8128–8131.

Jaeken J, Hennet T, Matthijs G, Freeze HH (2009) CDG nomenclature: time for a change! Biochim Biophys Acta 1792: 825–826.

Jaeken J, van Eijk HG, van der Heul C, Corbeel L, Eeckels R, Eggermont E (1984) Sialic acid-deficient serum and cerebrospinal fluid transferrin in a newly recognized genetic syndrome. Clin Chim Acta 144: 245–247.

Jansen GA, Ofman R, Ferdinandusse S, Ijlst L, Muijsers AO, Skjeldal OH, et al. (1997) Refsum disease is caused by mutations in the phytanoyl-CoA hydroxylase gene. Nat Genet 17: 190–193.

Koskinen T, Santavuori P, Sainio K, Lappi M, Kallio AK, Pihko H (1994) Infantile onset spinocerebellar ataxia with sensory neuropathy: a new inherited disease. J Neurol Sci 121: 50–56.

Lagier-Tourenne C, Tazir M, Lopez LC, Quinzii CM, Assoum M, Drouot N, et al. (2008) ADCK3, an ancestral kinase, is mutated in a form of recessive ataxia associated with coenzyme Q10 deficiency. Am J Hum Genet 82: 661–672.

Liu AR, van der Lei HD, Wang X, Wortham NC, Tang H, van Berkel CG, et al. (2011) Severity of Vanishing White Matter disease does not correlate with deficits in eIf2B activity or the integrity of eIF2B complexes. Hum Mutat, doi: 10.1002/humu.21535.

Lopez LC, Schuelke M, Quinzii CM, Kanki T, Rodenburg RJ, Naini A, et al. (2006) Leigh syndrome with nephropathy and CoQ10 deficiency due to decaprenyl diphosphate synthase subunit 2 (PDSS2) mutations. Am J Hum Genet 79: 1125–1129.

López-Hernández T, Ridder MC, Montolio M. Capdevila-Nortes X, Polder E, Sirisi S, et al. (2011) Mutant GlialCAM causes megalencephalic leukoencephalopathy with subcortical cysts, benign familial macrocephaly, and macrocephaly with retardation and autism. Am J Hum Genet 88: 422–432.

Maegawa GH, Stockley T, Tropak M, Banwell B, Blaser S, Kok F, et al. (2006) The natural history of juvenile or subacute GM2 gangliosidosis: 21 new cases and literature review of 134 previously reported. Pediatrics 118: e1550–1562.

Matthijs G, Schollen E, Pardon E, Veiga-Da-Cunha M, Jaeken J, Cassiman JJ, Van Schaftingen E (1997) Mutations in PMM2, a phosphomannomutase gene on chromosome 16p13, in carbohydrate-deficient glycoprotein type I syndrome (Jaeken syndrome). Nat Genet 16: 88–92.

Milone M, Massie R (2010) Polymerase gamma 1 mutations: clinical correlations. Neurologist 16: 84–91.

Mole SE, Williams RE, Goebel HH (2005) Correlations between genotype, ultrastructural morphology and clinical phenotype in the neuronal ceroid lipofuscinoses. Neurogenetics 6: 107–126.

Mollet J, Delahodde A, Serre V, Chretien D, Schlemmer D, Lombes A, et al. (2008) CABC1 gene mutations cause ubiquinone deficiency with cerebellar ataxia and seizures. Am J Hum Genet 82: 623–630.

Mollet J, Giurgea I, Schlemmer D, Dallner G, Chretien D, Delahodde A, et al. (2007) Prenyldiphosphate synthase, subunit 1 (PDSS1) and OH-benzoate polyprenyltransferase (COQ2) mutations in ubiquinone deficiency and oxidative phosphorylation disorders. J Clin Invest 117: 765–772.

Morgan NV, Westaway SK, Morton JE, Gregory A, Gissen P, Sonek S, et al. (2006) PLA2G6, encoding a phospholipase A2, is mutated in neurodegenerative disorders with high brain iron. Nat Genet 38: 752– 754.

Nardocci N, Zorzi G, Farina L, Binelli S, Scaioli W, Ciano C, et al. (1999) Infantile neuroaxonal dystrophy: clinical spectrum and diagnostic criteria. Neurology 52: 1472–1478.

Naureckiene S, Sleat DE, Lackland H, Fensom A, Vanier MT, Wattiaux R, et al. (2000) Identification of HE1 as the second gene of Niemann-Pick C disease. Science 290: 2298–2301.

Naviaux RK, Nyhan WL, Barshop BA, Poulton J, Markusic D, Karpinski NC, Haas RH (1999) Mitochondrial DNA polymerase gamma deficiency and mtDNA depletion in a child with Alpers' syndrome. Ann Neurol 45: 54–58.

Nikali K, Suomalainen A, Saharinen J, Kuokkanen M, Spelbrink JN, Lonnqvist T, Peltonen L (2005) Infantile onset spinocerebellar ataxia is caused by recessive mutations in mitochondrial proteins Twinkle and Twinky. Hum Mol Genet 14: 2981–2990.

Patterson MC, Vecchio D, Prady H, Abel L, Wraith JE (2007) Miglustat for treatment of Niemann-Pick C disease: a randomised controlled study. Lancet Neurol 6: 765–772.

Pronk JC, van Kollenburg B, Scheper GC, van der Knaap MS (2006) Vanishing white matter disease: a review with focus on its genetics. Ment Retard Dev Disabil Res Rev 12: 123–128.

Quinzii CM, Kattah AG, Naini A, Akman HO, Mootha VK, DiMauro S, Hirano M (2005) Coenzyme Q deficiency and cerebellar ataxia associated with an aprataxin mutation. Neurology 64: 539–541.

Quinzii CM, Lopez LC, Naini A, DiMauro S, Hirano M (2008) Human CoQ10 deficiencies. Biofactors 32: 113–118.

Régal L, Ebberink MS, Goemans N, Wanders RJ, De Meirleir L, Jaeken J, et al. (2010) Mutations in PEX10 are a cause of autosomal recessive ataxia. Ann Neurol 68: 259–263.

Reinhardt K, Grapp M, Schlachter K, Brück W, Gärtner J, Steinfeld R (2010) Novel CLN8 mutations confirm the clinical and ethnic diversity of late infantile neuronal ceroid lipofuscinosis. Clin Genet 77: 79–85.

Rzem R, Veiga-da-Cunha M, Noel G, Goffette S, Nassogne MC, Tabarki B, et al. (2004) A gene encoding a putative FAD-dependent L-2-hydroxyglutarate dehydrogenase is mutated in L-2-hydroxyglutaric aciduria. Proc Natl Acad Sci U S A 101: 16849–16854.

Scheper GC, van der Klok T, van Andel RJ, van Berkel CG, Sissler M, Smet J, et al. (2007) Mitochondrial aspartyl-tRNA synthetase deficiency causes leukoencephalopathy with brain stem and spinal cord involvement and lactate elevation. Nat Genet 39: 534–539.

Sedel F, Saudubray JM, Roze E, Agid Y, Vidailhet M (2008) Movement disorders and inborn errors of metabolism in adults: a diagnostic approach. J Inherit Metab Dis 31: 308–318.

Sevin C, Ferdinandusse S, Waterham HR, Wanders RJ, Aubourg P (2011) Autosomal recessive cerebellar ataxia caused by mutations in the PEX2 gene. Orphanet J Rare Dis 6: 8.

Sistermans EA, de Coo RF, De Wijs IJ, Van Oost BA (1998) Duplication of the proteolipid protein gene is the major cause of Pelizaeus-Merzbacher disease. Neurology 50: 1749–1754.

Sleat DE, Donnelly RJ, Lackland H, Liu CG, Sohar I, Pullarkat RK, Lobel P (1997) Association of mutations in a lysosomal protein with classical late-infantile neuronal ceroid lipofuscinosis. Science 277: 1802–1805.

Steenweg ME, Jakobs C, Errami A, van Dooren SJ, Adeva Bartolome MT, Aerssens P, et al. (2010) An overview of L-2-hydroxyglutarate dehydrogenase gene (L2HGDH) variants: a genotype-phenotype study. Hum Mutat 31: 380–390.

Steenweg ME, Salomons GS, Yapici Z, Uziel G, Scalais E, Zafeiriou DI, Ruiz-Falco ML, Mejaski-Bosnjak V, Augoustides-Savvopoulou P, Wajner M, Walter J, Verhoeven-Duif NM, Struys EA, Jakobs C and van der Knaap MS. (2009) L-2-Hydroxyglutaric aciduria: pattern of MR imaging abnormalities in 56 patients. Radiology 251: 856–865.

Timmons M, Tsokos M, Asab MA, Seminara SB, Zirzow GC, Kaneski CR, et al. (2006) Peripheral and central hypomyelination with hypogonadotropic hypogonadism and hypodontia. Neurology 67: 2066–2069.

Uhlenberg B, Schuelke M, Ruschendorf F, Ruf N, Kaindl AM, Henneke M, et al. (2004) Mutations in the gene encoding gap junction protein alpha 12 (connexin 46.6) cause Pelizaeus-Merzbacher-like disease. Am J Hum Genet 75: 251–260.

van den Brink DM, Brites P, Haasjes J, Wierzbicki AS, Mitchell J, Lambert-Hamill M, et al. (2003) Identification of PEX7 as the second gene involved in Refsum disease. Am J Hum Genet 72: 471–477.

van der Knaap MS, Barth PG, Stroink H, van Nieuwenhuizen O, Arts WF, Hoogenraad F, Valk J (1995) Leukoencephalopathy with swelling and a discrepantly mild clinical course in eight children. Ann Neurol 37: 324–334.

van der Knaap MS, Lai V, Kohler W, Salih MA, Fonseca MJ, Benke TA, et al. (2010) Megalencephalic leukoencephalopathy with cysts without MLC1 defect. Ann Neurol 67: 834–837.

van der Knaap MS, Pronk JC, Scheper GC (2006) Vanishing white matter disease. Lancet Neurol 5: 413–423.

van der Knaap MS, van der Voorn P, Barkhof F, Van Coster R, Krageloh-Mann I, Feigenbaum A, et al. (2003) A new leukoencephalopathy with brainstem and spinal cord involvement and high lactate. Ann Neurol 53: 252–258.

van der Lei HD, van Berkel CG, van Wieringen WN, Brenner C, Feigenbaum A, Mercimek-Mahmutoglu S, et al. (2010) Genotype-phenotype correlation in vanishing white matter disease. Neurology 75: 1555–1559.

Vanier MT (2010) Niemann-Pick disease type C. Orphanet J Rare Dis 5: 16.

Wolf NI, Harting I, Boltshauser E, Wiegand G, Koch MJ, Schmitt-Mechelke T, et al. (2005a) Leukoencephalopathy with ataxia, hypodontia, and hypomyelination. Neurology 64: 1461–1464.

Wolf NI, Sistermans EA, Cundall M, Hobson GM, Davis-Williams AP, Palmer R, et al. (2005b) Three or more copies of the proteolipid protein gene PLP1 cause severe Pelizaeus-Merzbacher disease. Brain 128: 743–751.

Wolf NI, Rahman S, Schmitt B, Taanman JW, Duncan AJ, Harting I, et al. (2009) Status epilepticus in children with Alpers' disease caused by POLG1 mutations: EEG and MRI features. Epilepsia 50: 1596–1607.

28
The Episodic Ataxias

Tracey D. Graves and Michael G. Hanna

The episodic ataxias are a group of autosomal dominant conditions where patients experience episodes of cerebellar ataxia. The most common are episodic ataxia type 1 (EA1) and type 2 (EA2). EA2 is more common and patients experience attacks lasting hours to days. In EA1 attacks are much shorter but patients may have multiple attacks in a day. Comparison is made between EA1 and EA2 in Table 28.1.

Episodic ataxia type 1

Classification

The ICD 10 classification is G11.9 Hereditary ataxia, unspecified.

Prevalence/incidence

Episodic ataxia type 1 is rarer than type 2, with an estimated prevalence of 1:1 000 000 (Joanna Jen, personal communication).

Epidemiology

It appears that the disease is distributed worldwide.

Definition of condition

Episodic ataxia type 1 is an autosomal dominant ion channel disorder (channelopathy) affecting the cerebellum and peripheral nerves. In keeping with other channelopathies, patients have intermittent symptoms, with little or no difficulties in between attacks and do not develop progressive deficits.

Aetiology including genetics

Linkage analysis in EA1 families implicated chromosome 12p13 (Litt et al. 1994) and the gene responsible was found to be *KCNA1* (Browne et al. 1994). This is a single-exon gene which encodes the delayed-rectifier potassium channel, $K_v1.1$, responsible for repolarizing nerves after depolarization. These channels are expressed at the node of Ranvier of myelinated axons, synaptic terminals and proximal dendrites and in the cerebellum are present at the axon terminal.

Mutations have been described throughout the gene and all affect highly conserved residues, usually resulting in amino acid substitutions. There are no obvious mutation hotspots or

TABLE 28.1
Comparison between episodic ataxia types 1 and 2

	Episodic ataxia type 1	Episodic ataxia type 2
Mode of inheritance	Autosomal dominant	Autosomal dominant
Age at onset	Early childhood	Before age 20
Features	Ataxia Dizziness often without vertigo Visual blurring No nystagmus	Ataxia, truncal instability which may persist between attacks, dysarthria, nystagmus May be associated with vertigo, nausea, vomiting & headache Weakness may occur during spells and can precede onset of episodic ataxia
Precipitating factors	Abrupt postural change, emotion, startle, vestibular stimulation, intercurrent infection	Physical or emotional stress, e.g., intercurrent infection
Duration	Brief, attacks last minutes	Attacks often last 30 minutes to hours
Frequency	Many per day	Variable, less frequent Not usually more than one in a day
Additional features	Neuromyotonia on EMG (continuous spontaneous muscle fibre activity). Myokymia seen clinically during and between episodes of ataxia Seizures may occur	Downbeating gaze-evoked nystagmus in all directions between episodes. Impaired vestibulo-ocular reflex, opticokinetic nystagmus and smooth pursuits. Some patients develop progressive cerebellar atrophy Dystonia rarely described Seizures may occur
Treatment	Phenytoin, carbamazepine	Acetazolamide
Gene	*KCNA1*	*CACNA1A*, allelic with FHM1 and SCA6

Adapted from Graves and Hanna (2005).

common mutations, therefore DNA-based diagnosis is by direct sequencing of the entire gene.

Pathophysiology

Cellular electrophysiology experiments, where mutant potassium channels are expressed in *Xenopus laevis* oocytes, showed that some mutations altered potassium channel function while others did not form functional channels. Some potassium channel mutations were also found to have a dominant negative effect on wild-type protein function. Hence, EA1 can be due to haploinsufficiency or dominant negative effects on channel function.

Clinical features

Episodes of ataxia are frequent and short-lasting and may be associated with a feeling of 'dizziness' which patients often find hard to precisely characterize. All patients tend to experience a profound sense of imbalance or dysequilibrium during an attack and want to sit or lie down. Sometimes the inter-attack myokymia may be exacerbated during an attack and patients may describe this as a 'tremor'. Attacks can be precipitated by sudden movement, emotion or intercurrent infection. Patients may have sensory warning symptoms prior to an attack (VanDyke et al. 1975; Brunt and van Weerden 1990). The age at onset of attacks is usually early childhood (2–15 years) and patients often experience multiple attacks in a day, with clustering of attacks. Patients have continuous peripheral nerve excitability, known as myokymia, between attacks. This is manifest as continuous fine muscular twitching movements which flit from place to place and involve the craniofacial and/or limb musculature. This is often prominent around the eyes and small hand muscles. Some patients experience periods (days or weeks) with prominent myokymia, followed by periods of remission, although the explanation for this is not clear. Contractures due to continuous muscle activity may occur (VanDyke et al. 1975; Hanson et al. 1977; Gancher and Nutt 1986). Severe contractures in newborn infants due to intense myokymic discharges which abate as the child gets older have been reported (Zuberi et al. 1999; Kinali et al. 2004).

There is an increased relative risk of seizures in patients with EA1 (Zuberi et al. 1999; Eunson et al. 2000). These include partial and generalized seizures, with varying response to anticonvulsant medications (VanDyke et al. 1975; Brunt and van Weerden 1990; Zuberi et al. 1999). In one pedigree the seizure phenotype (simple partial and generalized tonic-clonic seizures) was present in the absence of any ataxic episodes, although affected individuals displayed clinical and electrical myokymia (Eunson et al. 2000). This suggests that potassium channel dysfunction may lead to a phenotype indistinguishable from the idiopathic epilepsies.

The most reliable distinguishing feature between EA1 and EA2 is that the former displays myokymia. However, atypical families do occur; one from the US had long attack duration, additional seizures but no evidence of myokymia, interictal nystagmus or response to acetazolamide. A novel *KCNA1* mutation was identified (Lee et al. 2004).

Isolated neuromyotonia can also be due to *KCNA1* mutations, with hypertonia and hypertrophy of the affected musculature (Eunson et al. 2000). This can lead to delayed motor development with kyphosis and contractures, which may occur years before EA1 manifests (Kinali et al. 2004). A patient has been described with distal muscular atrophy and weakness (Klein et al. 2004). Therefore, the neuromuscular spectrum of the disease is broadening and there are likely to be further phenotypes associated with *KCNA1* mutations.

Diagnosis

Although the causative gene has been identified, diagnosis relies on a thorough clinical history, including witness accounts (+/– video footage) of attacks. A dominant family history may be evident, although *de novo* mutations may occur. It is also apparent that parents who believe themselves to be asymptomatic may, on direct questioning, give a history of ataxic spells during early life and display myokymia. A description of the attacks should reveal symptoms of frequent, short-lasting episodes of ataxia and dizziness and persistent myokymia (see Table 28.1). Myokymia can be visualized in the outstretched arms as fine, low-amplitude side-to-side movements of the fingers. Asking the patient to rest the elbows on a flat surface with the hands relaxed and the wrist in slight flexion will enhance visualization of the small non-rhythmic, jerky finger movements. Myokymia can also be seen around the eyes.

Differential diagnosis

Although there is a differential diagnosis for EA per se, the brief attacks and co-occurrence of myokymia mean that EA1 is a distinct clinical entity. However, one of the biggest problems is delayed or missed diagnosis as patients, in particular, children, find it extremely difficult to describe their symptoms. Given that attacks are so brief and that physical signs may be absent, or hidden unless specifically elicited, the most common misdiagnoses would be epilepsy or functional disorders.

Treatment and management

Sodium channel blockers such as phenytoin can be used to treat myokymia (VanDyke et al. 1975; Hanson et al. 1977; Gancher and Nutt 1986) but carbamazepine treats both the ataxia and the myokymia and is therefore superior (Zuberi et al. 1999). Acetazolamide has been used (Lubbers et al. 1995), but is less effective in EA1 than in EA2 (Zuberi et al. 1999). One pedigree with a severe truncation mutation (*R417X*) showed treatment resistance with an acute deterioration in symptoms on lamotrigine (Eunson et al. 2000).

Investigations including imaging

Neuroimaging is normal and has no role in the diagnosis. Electromyogram (EMG) shows peripherally induced myokymia, even in muscles not clinically affected, and rhythmically and semi-rhythmically occurring single action potentials (Brunt and van Weerden 1990). EMG is unpleasant and not usually recommended in children. The definitive diagnostic test remains genetic testing for mutations in the potassium channel gene, *KCNA1*.

SHORT- AND LONG-TERM OUTCOMES

Both the ataxia and myokymia are well treated with carbamazepine, so if this can be tolerated, patients can lead a near normal life. The main issue remains delayed diagnosis, with many patients diagnosed with epilepsy or psychiatric disorders, before the correct diagnosis is made. In some families, the attacks are too mild to seek medical attention and are put down to their 'familial trait'. Although symptoms can be very disabling in childhood, attack frequency will often reduce with age and may cease completely in adulthood in some pedigrees. Lifespan is not shortened.

ECONOMIC ASPECTS

The phenotype is very variable, tending to improve with age, such that many patients continue a normal school and working life. However, some patients find it difficult to gain or maintain employment.

COMORBIDITIES

Those with classic EA1, when well controlled, can lead a normal life. Patients may suffer problems due to associated problems such as epilepsy or contractures (see above).

SERVICE IMPLICATIONS

Given its rarity, the diagnosis of EA1 relies on a high index of clinical suspicion and is therefore unlikely to impact greatly on paediatric services. The provision of a country-wide referral system to a subspecialized clinic may provide better use of resources and give expert care to patients.

IMPLICATIONS FOR FUTURE RESEARCH

As in all rare diseases, the identification of patients and their genetic abnormalities may provide insights into potassium channel function and is likely to widen the phenotypic spectrum of EA1.

Episodic ataxia type 2

Families with prolonged episodes of cerebellar ataxia have long been recognized. Attacks are precipitated by exercise and emotional or physical stress (Gancher and Nutt 1986; Koller and Bahamon-Dussan 1987; von Brederlow et al. 1995) and prevented by acetazolamide (Griggs et al. 1978; Zasorin et al. 1983). Patients have selective cerebellar vermis atrophy on MRI (Vighetto et al. 1988). EEG abnormalities are also seen (Van Bogaert and Szliwowski 1996), including nonspecific intermittent rhythmic delta activity and bursts of spike and wave activity, which could lead to a misdiagnosis of epilepsy (Neufeld et al. 1996).

CLASSIFICATION

The ICD 10 classification is G11.9 Hereditary ataxia, unspecified.

PREVALENCE/INCIDENCE

The estimated prevalence is ten times greater than that of EA1 at 1:100 000 (Joanna Jen, personal communication).

EPIDEMIOLOGY

It appears that the disease is distributed worldwide.

DEFINITION OF CONDITION

EA2 is an autosomal dominant channelopathy affecting the cerebellum. As distinct from EA1, patients may develop progressive cerebellar ataxia in later life, leading to reduced mobility and dysarthria.

AETIOLOGY INCLUDING GENETICS

Linkage to 19p13 (Vahedi et al. 1995; von Brederlow et al. 1995) resulted in identification of the causative gene, *CACNA1A* (Ophoff et al. 1996). This is a large gene which encodes the P/Q-type calcium channel α-subunit; this is functionally the most important and includes the ion channel pore and voltage sensor. The α-subunit co-assembles with $\alpha_2\delta$ and β-subunits to form functional calcium channels. These are expressed throughout the brain in a presynaptic distribution, with particularly high expression levels in the cerebellum (Stea et al. 1994; Tanaka et al. 1995) and the peripheral nerve terminal (Uchitel et al. 1992) and play an important role in controlling the release of both inhibitory (Stephens et al. 2001) and excitatory (Reid et al. 1998) neurotransmitters. Since identification of the gene, many mutations have been identified. Most are single base pair substitutions which are private to individual pedigrees and there are no common recurrent mutations. Mutations are distributed throughout the gene and there is no correlation between either the site or type of mutation and the clinical phenotype. The combination of the size of *CACNA1A* and the lack of mutation hotspots makes genetic testing difficult. DNA-based diagnosis was until recently only available on a research basis but is now becoming more widely available. Recently, multi-exonic deletions and duplications have been identified (Riant et al. 2008; Labrum et al. 2009), meaning that a cheaper and quicker screening test (MPLA) could be employed as a first-pass technique in mutation identification, which hopefully will result in more patients receiving a genetic diagnosis.

PATHOPHYSIOLOGY

Mutations which have been characterized electrophysiologically using *in vitro* assays have shown reduced current density (Jen et al. 2001; Wappl et al. 2002) or calcium conductance (Wappl et al. 2002), although some mutations lead to reduced protein expression (Spacey et al. 2004) or impaired membrane trafficking (Imbrici et al. 2004). This suggests that haploinsufficiency is an important mechanism in disease pathogenesis.

Clinical features

Patients usually present in early childhood to adolescence, although the age at onset is variable, even between family members. Very rarely, a late-onset form may occur (Imbrici et al. 2005). Episodes of ataxia often manifest once walking is attempted, i.e. between the ages of 1 and 2 years, where it is observed that an affected child has intermittent problems with balance. Parents may also notice triggers or precipitating factors, such as tiredness, stress or emotion. Some parents described that the child becomes generally 'floppy' or hypotonic during an attack. Attacks typically consist of ataxia, vertigo and dysarthria lasting between 10 minutes and many hours. There may be associated dizziness, headache, diplopia, tinnitus or dystonia. Attack frequency is very variable, for example we have observed patients with weekly attacks and patients with only a few attacks over many years. The frequency and severity of attacks can be variable between family members and attacks may become less frequent with age. Although there are usually no symptoms between attacks, patients often display interictal nystagmus, classically in the downbeat direction, although this is often absent in childhood. Other clinical signs include hypometric saccades (Engel et al. 2004), impaired vestibulo-ocular reflex (VOR) (Wiest et al. 2001) and loss of VOR suppression (Baloh et al. 1997). The natural history is variable between pedigrees. An international study into the natural history of the disease is under way (Joanna Jen, personal communication). Patients may develop a progressive cerebellar syndrome (Denier et al. 1999) in addition to paroxysmal ataxia. Approximately 50% of patients complain of headaches indistinguishable from migraine (Baloh et al. 1997). It is probable that a proportion of patients previously termed as suffering with basilar migraine have EA2.

Mutations in *CACNA1A* also lead to familial hemiplegic migraine (FHM1), a severe autosomal dominant subtype of migraine. Aura symptoms include hemiplegia, which may be prolonged, and some mutations are associated with cerebral oedema following minor head injury (Kors et al. 2001), coma (Ducros et al. 2001; Beauvais et al. 2004) and death (Kors et al. 2001). A proportion of patients also develop a progressive cerebellar syndrome (Terwindt et al. 1998; Ducros et al. 1999, 2001), analogous to that seen in EA2 pedigrees. A CAG trinucleotide repeat expansion in exon 47 of *CACNA1A* leads to spinocerebellar ataxia type 6 (SCA6) (Zhuchenko et al. 1997). The same abnormally expanded CAG repeats can also be occasionally associated with an EA2 phenotype (Jodice et al. 1997). Since identification of the gene, the phenotypic spectrum of disease associated with *CACNA1A* mutations has broadened and the boundaries between these conditions have blurred.

Patients may complain of subjective feelings of weakness prior to an attack, but clinical weakness is rare. However, some pedigrees do display genuine weakness as a manifestation of an attack, as hemiplegia (Jen et al. 1999) or diffuse weakness (Jen et al. 2004), accompanied by jitter and block on EMG, indicating impaired neuromuscular transmission (Maselli et al. 2003). Indeed, one patient was initially diagnosed with myasthenia gravis (Jen et al. 2001). Attacks of EA2 are often precipitated by stress; however, one pedigree has been reported in which fever-induced attacks were common (Subramony et al. 2003). Some mutations are associated with segmental dystonia, for example writer's cramp or blepharospasm (Guida et al. 2001; Spacey et al. 2004).

Although the association of EA and epilepsy is more apparent in EA1, there is increasing evidence that epilepsy is also more prevalent in EA2. A patient with a complicated phenotype of EA2, mental retardation, generalized and absence seizures and a primary generalized spike wave EEG had a C-terminal nonsense mutation in *CACNA1A* (Jouvenceau et al. 2001). A further large family with an EA2 and epilepsy phenotype has strengthened the association (Imbrici et al. 2004) and other groups have also described patients with EA2 and seizures (Jen et al. 2004; Kaunisto et al. 2004). We recently reported an excess of *CANCA1A* polymorphisms in patients with EA2 and epilepsy leading to a reduction in calcium channel function in vivo (Rajakulendran et al. 2010).

Learning difficulties have been reported in 11% of mutations; however, this is likely to be an underestimate, as it is only mentioned if severe. In a recent series, we found that 30% of patients had learning difficulties, although not all had mutations in *CACNA1A* (Rajakulendran et al. 2010). We suspect that if specific neurocognitive testing were undertaken in patients with EA2, the actual proportion would be much greater.

Diagnosis

Although the causative gene has been identified, diagnosis relies on a thorough clinical history, including witness accounts (+/– video recording) of attacks. A thorough description of attacks should reveal symptoms of ataxia, dysarthria, vertigo and nausea. Supportive features for the diagnosis include appropriate length of attacks, age at onset, triggers, response to acetazolamide and interictal nystagmus. Recently, diagnostic criteria have been suggested (Jen et al. 2004). There should be no clinical or electrophysiological evidence of myokymia. Although autosomal dominant inheritance is usual, new mutations do occur (Yue et al. 1998), hence lack of a family history does not exclude the diagnosis. It is also apparent that parents who feel that they are asymptomatic may, on direct questioning, give a history of ataxic spells and display interictal nystagmus.

Differential diagnosis

The differential diagnosis for EA2 is between the other episodic neurological disorders, including epilepsy, migraine and the paroxysmal dyskinesias. More rarely, inherited metabolic disorders, including those of mitochondrial oxidative metabolism (e.g. pyruvate carboxylase deficiency and pyruvate dehydrogenase deficiency), the urea cycle (e.g. ornithine transcarbamylase deficiency), or aminoacidurias (e.g. Hartnup disease) can lead to prolonged attacks of ataxia.

Treatment and management

Acetazolamide is the mainstay of therapy and may completely ameliorate attacks in selected patients (Griggs et al. 1978). Treatment requires regular monitoring of renal function and yearly imaging of the renal tract to identify calculi, although these are generally not clinically significant. Side effects such as nausea and paraesthesiae can be minimized by the gradual introduction of acetazolamide in minute doses, increasing in small increments over a protracted time period. Some patients develop significant mood disturbance (usually depression) on commencing acetazolamide necessitating its withdrawal. Patients unresponsive to acetazolamide may respond to 4-aminopyridine (Strupp et al. 2004). Anecdotal evidence suggests that dichlorphenamide is also effective. Whether treatment of attacks has any effect on the natural history of the disease is currently unknown. A large-scale international clinical trial comparing treatments is planned (Joanna Jen, personal communication).

Investigations including imaging

Depending upon the age at which the patient is scanned, brain MRI will often show cerebellar atrophy (Vighetto et al. 1988), consistent with the interictal nystamus and progressive cerebellar ataxia which may develop in this condition.

Short- and long-term outcomes

If patients are able to tolerate acetazolamide, then both the attack frequency and severity can be drastically reduced, although most patients will still have some attacks. Approximately 30% will develop progressive cerebellar ataxia, which can be very disabling.

Economic aspects

Although the attack frequency in EA2 is less than in EA1, the attacks are much more prolonged and debilitating, requiring days off of school or work, which may be incompatible with continued employment.

Comorbidities

Coexisting migraine may also lead to disability. Several mutations have been associated with learning difficulties (Denier et al. 1999; Jouvenceau et al. 2001; van den Maagdenberg et al. 2002; Jen et al. 2004; Veneziano et al. 2009) (see above). Those developing progressive cerebellar ataxia in middle age can have problems with speech and mobility.

Service implications

As genetic testing becomes easier and more widely available, increasing numbers of patients will be identified and the phenotypic spectrum is likely to grow further. The main factor in achieving a diagnosis though, remains a high index of clinical suspicion, in order that the genetic test is sent in the first place. Once a family mutation is known, testing of other affected family members becomes easier.

Implications for future research

So far, the effects of disease-causing mutations on calcium channel function have been tested in isolated cell models. Their effect on neurotransmitter release is likely to be complicated and dependent upon networks of different cell types. Therefore, mutations need to be studied in cultured mammalian cerebellar and other neuronal cell cultures.

Other episodic ataxias

There are patients who have symptoms which do not fit neatly into either of the categories of EA1 or EA2. In addition, there are isolated pedigrees with clinically distinct syndromes, which are summarised in Table 28.2.

Episodic ataxia type 3

In one Canadian pedigree, patients had vertigo and tinnitus, not usually seen in EA1 and lacked the interictal nystagmus characteristic of EA2. The age at onset was considered too late for either EA1 or EA2; EA3 therefore is not a disease to consider in children. The duration of attacks was intermediate between EA1 and EA2 and patients responded to acetazolamide (Steckley et al. 2001). A genome-wide screen showed linkage to chromosome 1q42, but no mutations were identified (Cader et al. 2005).

Episodic ataxia type 4

Initially described in two autosomal dominant North Carolina families (Farmer and Mustian 1963), the age at onset ranged from the third to the sixth decade, so EA4 is not a differential diagnosis of EA in children. Symptoms included episodic attacks of horizontal diplopia, oscillopsia, ataxia, nausea, vertigo and tinnitus, gradually becoming constant. Attacks were precipitated by sudden movement of the head, fatigue or by observing movement in the peripheral vision, and alleviated by lying down with eyes closed; acetazolamide was ineffective. Eye movement abnormalities included gaze-evoked nystagmus, abnormal smooth pursuits, reduced optokinetic nystagmus, failure of VOR suppression and strabismus. Linkage was excluded to the known autosomal dominant cerebellar ataxias (Damji et al. 1996).

Episodic ataxia type 5

The auxiliary calcium channel β4-subunit encoded by *CACNB4* has a crucial role in membrane trafficking and function of $Ca_v2.1$ in neurons. A *CACNB4* mutation was identified in five affected but also two unaffected members of a French-Canadian family with an EA2 phenotype, but no mutations in *CACNA1A*. The age at onset was not specified. The mutation had no effect on P/Q-type calcium channel function *in vitro* (Escayg et al. 2000). Further mutations have not been identified (in total 106 patients screened), suggesting that these may be polymorphisms or a very rare cause of an EA2-like phenotype (Graves and Hanna 2008).

Episodic ataxia type 6

A new disease-associated gene has been identified in a patient with episodic ataxia, hemiplegic migraine and seizures.

TABLE 28.2
Summary of the different episodic ataxias

	EA1	EA2	EA3	EA4	EA5	EA6	EA7	EA8	Other EAs
OMIM	160120	108500	606554	606552	601949	600111	611907	unassigned	unassigned
Attack duration	sec–min	hours	1 min–6h	brief	hours	hours–days	hours–days	minutes	hours–days
Age at onset (y)	<20	<20	1–42	23–60	<20	5	<20	40–64	after 30
Myokymia	usual	no	usual	no	no	no	no	no	no
Nystagmus	no	usual	occasional	usual	usual	no	no	yes	usual
Epilepsy	occasional	infrequent	occasional	occasional	usual	yes	no	no	no
Tinnitus	infrequent	no	usual	occasional	no	no	no	no	no
Vertigo	no	yes	yes	yes	yes	no	yes	yes	yes
Acetazolamide	occasional	usual	usual	no	transient	no	no	no	occasional
Inheritance	AD	AD	AD	AD	AD	sporadic	AD	AD/AR	multiple
Chromosomal locus	12q13	19p13	1q42	unknown	2q22–q23	5p13	19q13	13p12–13	unknown
Gene	*KCNA1*	*CACNA1A*	unknown	unknown	*CACNB4*	*SLC1A3*	unknown	unknown	unknown
Protein	$K_v1.1$	$Ca_v2.1$	unknown	unknown	$Ca_v2.1$	EAAT1	unknown	unknown	unknown
Reference	Browne et al. 1994	Ophoff et al. 1996	Cader et al. 2005	Damji et al. 1996	Escayg et al. 2000	Jen et al. 2005	Kerber et al. 2007	Cha et al. 2007	

AD, autosomal dominant; AR, autosomal recessive. Modified from Jen et al. (2007).

Throughout his life, the proband had episodes of ataxia lasting days, provoked by febrile illness. He later developed hemiplegic migraine and coma. MRI during an episode of coma showed mild cerebellar atrophy and cortical hyperintensity, contralateral to the hemiparesis. EEG showed a left frontotemporal epileptiform focus; he later developed complex partial seizures. He had truncal ataxia, generalized hyperreflexia but with flexor plantar responses. There was no nystagmus but eye movements were abnormal with reduced smooth pursuits, optokinetic nystagmus and failure of fixation-suppression of the VOR. A novel *de novo* mutation in *SLC1A3*, which encodes the excitatory amino acid transporter type 1 (EAAT1), was identified (Jen et al. 2005). Excitatory amino acid transporters are the sole means of removing glutamate from the extracellular fluid and are therefore critical to the control of neurotransmission. Functional analysis using a glutamate uptake assay showed reduced uptake via mutant transporters and a dominant negative effect on wild-type cell surface expression. The mutation therefore causes disease by both reduced protein expression and function, leading to reduced glutamate reuptake (Jen et al. 2005). Recently, another affected pedigree has been identified. Patients had onset before age 14 with a syndrome indistinguishable from EA2 (de Vries et al. 2009). Again, glutamate reuptake was moderately reduced.

Episodic ataxia type 7

Six affected members of a US pedigree experienced episodes of ataxia, dysarthria and weakness, lasting hours to days, which were triggered by exercise or excitement. The phenotype was similar to that of EA2, with age at onset before age 20. However, there was no interictal nystagmus or ataxia. Two patients had vertigo as part of their attacks. Linkage was demonstrated to chromosome 19q13, although no pathogenic mutations were identified (Kerber et al. 2007).

Episodic ataxia type 8

Another late-onset syndrome of vertical oscillopsia and slowly progressive gait ataxia has also been described. This is therefore not relevant to paediatric practice, but is included for completeness. Attacks were intermediate in length between EA1 and EA2, lasting between 5 and 60 minutes. In common with EA2, attacks were triggered by exertion, alcohol and caffeine; however, treatment with acetazolamide was ineffective and no pathogenic mutations were found in *CACNA1A*. Patients all had downbeat nystagmus and most had abnormal smooth pursuit eye movements. All probands had normal brain MRI (Cha et al. 2007).

Conclusions

The episodic ataxias are rare conditions, but are more common than many other neurological conditions. Wider access to genetic testing will provide a more accurate assessment of prevalence and allow many more patients to be identified. Providing the correct diagnosis can remove uncertainty and stigma, obviate the need for unnecessary investigations and by providing appropriate treatment, lead to amelioration of symptoms. They are therefore a very rewarding group of conditions to diagnose and treat.

Vignettes

Case 1

From 6 months to 5 years the patient had epileptic seizures with impairment of awareness and apnoea. At age 5 he developed episodes, beginning with a tingling sensation rising up the legs, progressing to ataxia and dizziness with dysarthria and retained awareness. The attacks last between 30 seconds and 2 minutes. They occurred up to three times per day and were triggered by sudden movement, anxiety and exercise. Secondary generalized seizures occurred once a month and were not controlled by carbamazepine or lamotrigine but responded to acetazolamide, which also reduced the frequency of episodic ataxia attacks. His father had similar attacks of ataxia until age 15 and his paternal uncle continues to have attacks. His paternal grandmother also has epilepsy and she and her sister continue to have episodic ataxia.

Diagnosis: EA1 F414S *KCNA1* mutation (Graves et al. 2010).

Case 2

This patient had onset of attacks at age 2 years. The attacks was precipitated by exercise and stress and consisted of him being noted to be pale and unsteady, associated with vertigo, nausea and vomiting, which was worse on movement and occasionally associated with headache. He would then sleep for at least an hour. Attacks occurred every 3–5 weeks as a toddler increasing to fortnightly in his teenage years. Treatment with acetazolamide reduced the attacks to three to four per year. There was no therapeutic benefit from sodium valproate or carbamazepine. Interictal examination revealed gaze-evoked nystagmus, which was upbeat on upgaze, and broken smooth pursuit eye movements. These abnormalities had been present since the age of 4. There was no interictal gait or limb ataxia. An electronystagmogram showed saccadic dysmetria, bilateral gaze-evoked nystagmus and hypomobile opticokinetic nystagmus. An MRI was normal and an EEG showed generalized spike wave discharge. His parents both have migraine but not EA2.

Diagnosis: EA2 L621R *CACNA1A* mutation (Rajakulendran et al. 2010).

Case 3

Episodes of 'clumsiness' began at the age of 10. There was sudden onset of dizziness and the inability to sit or stand, with associated nausea. Examination showed reduced balance on heel toe walking and mild dysdiadochokinesis. At the age of 11, she experienced typical absence seizures with ictal EEG recordings consistently showing 3Hz generalized spike and wave discharges. A few months later, she experienced attacks of vertigo, nausea and vomiting. Initially they occurred weekly and would last up to 4 hours. Sleep would help in resolution of attack. Examination during one such episode revealed ataxia, problems with sitting balance (she was unable to sit without falling) and gaze-evoked nystagmus. Initial treatment with acetazolamide resulted in a marked improvement, although attacks were not completely abolished. Over the years, the attack frequency varied from twice monthly to periods of 6 months when she was attack free. The duration of the attacks diminished with age. MRI at 18 years old demonstrated slight atrophy of the cerebellum, in particular the vermis. There was no family history.

Diagnosis: EA2 and absence epilepsy with heterozygous deletion of *CACNA1A* exons 39–47 (Labrum et al. 2009).

Case 4

Since the age of 5, this patient had intermittent severe generalized throbbing headache with photophobia and phonophobia. These would be preceded by a prolonged aura (up to 6 hours) of vertigo, nausea and vomiting, ataxia, dysarthria and feeling very tired. There were no associated visual or sensory symptoms. She was always poor at sport. At the age of 4 she developed stereotyped attacks consisting of feeling extremely dizzy and lightheaded, as if she was on a boat, her legs felt like jelly, making it difficult to walk, sometimes leading to falls. She would vomit multiple times (even if lying still or with empty stomach), her speech sounded as if drunk and her limbs were uncoordinated. Attacks were precipitated by emotional stress, physical exertion, caffeine, menstruation, and could be paroxysmal. The frequency was variable, at its worst five per week and a best of 6 months attack free on treatment. Interictal symptoms included mild clumsiness and poor balance. On examination, she had mild dysarthria, finger-nose ataxia, dysdiadochokinesis and heel-shin ataxia. Eye movements were abnormal with square wave jerks, horizontal nystagmus on lateral gaze, downbeat nystagmus on down gaze and jerky pursuits. MRI at age 30 showed mild cerebellar hemisphere atrophy. Acetazolamide was only slightly effective, but dichlorphenamide led to 6 months of freedom from attack. Topiramate was an effective migraine prophylaxis. Her sons had delayed motor milestones and behavioural problems with similar but less severe attacks. Her father was diagnosed with cerebellar ataxia in his 20s and was wheelchair bound at the end of his life; he died aged 66.

Diagnosis: EA unknown type. No mutations identified in genes for EA1, EA2, EA5 or EA6.

Acknowledgements

The authors' research work is undertaken at University College London Hospitals/University College London, which received a proportion of funding from the Department of Health's National Institute for Health Research Biomedical Research Centres funding scheme. M.G. Hanna receives research funding from the Medical Research Council, MRC Centre grant (G0601943), from the Muscular Dystrophy Campaign Centre Grant and from the Consortium for Clinical Investigation of

Neurological Channelopathies (CINCH) NIH grant no. 1 U45 RR198442–01. M.G. Hanna provides the UK national patient referral centre for neurological channelopathies funded by the UK Department of Health National Commissioning Group. The authors wish to thank all clinical colleagues who have referred patients to this centre.

REFERENCES

Baloh RW, Yue Q, Furman JM, Nelson SF (1997) Familial episodic ataxia: clinical heterogeneity in four families linked to chromosome 19p. Ann Neurol 41(1): 8–16.

Beauvais K, Cave-Riant F, De Barace C, Tardieu M, Tournier-Lasserve E, Furby A (2004) New CACNA1A gene mutation in a case of familial hemiplegic migraine with status epilepticus. Eur Neurol 52(1): 58–61.

Browne DL, Gancher ST, Nutt JG, Brunt ER, Smith EA, Kramer P, Litt M (1994) Episodic ataxia/myokymia syndrome is associated with point mutations in the human potassium channel gene, KCNA1. Nat Genet 8(2): 136–140.

Brunt ER, van Weerden TW (1990) Familial paroxysmal kinesigenic ataxia and continuous myokymia. Brain 113 (Pt 5): 1361–1382.

Cader MZ, Steckley JL, Dyment DA, McLachlan RS, Ebers GC (2005) A genome-wide screen and linkage mapping for a large pedigree with episodic ataxia. Neurology 65(1): 156–158.

Cha YH, Lee H, Jen JC, Kattah JC, Nelson SF, Baloh RW (2007) Episodic vertical oscillopsia with progressive gait ataxia: clinical description of a new episodic syndrome and evidence of linkage to chromosome 13q. J Neurol Neurosurg Psychiatr 78(11): 1273–1275.

Damji KF, Allingham RR, Pollock SC, Small K, Lewis KE, Stajich JM, et al. (1996) Periodic vestibulocerebellar ataxia, an autosomal dominant ataxia with defective smooth pursuit, is genetically distinct from other autosomal dominant ataxias. Arch Neurol 53(4): 338–344.

de Vries B, Mamsa H, Stam AH, Wan J, Bakker SL, Vanmolkot KR, Haan J, et al. (2009) Episodic ataxia associated with EAAT1 mutation C186S affecting glutamate reuptake. Arch Neurol 66(1): 97–101.

Denier C, Ducros A, Vahedi K, Joutel A, Thierry P, Ritz A, et al. (1999) High prevalence of CACNA1A truncations and broader clinical spectrum in episodic ataxia type 2. Neurology 52(9): 1816–1821.

Ducros A, Denier C, Joutel A, Vahedi K, Michel A, Darcel F, et al. (1999) Recurrence of the T666M calcium channel CACNA1A gene mutation in familial hemiplegic migraine with progressive cerebellar ataxia. Am J Hum Genet 64(1): 89–98.

Ducros A, Denier C, Joutel A, Cecillon M, Lescoat C, Vahedi K, et al. (2001) The clinical spectrum of familial hemiplegic migraine associated with mutations in a neuronal calcium channel. N Engl J Med 345(1): 17–24.

Engel KC, Anderson JH, Gomez CM, Soechting JF (2004) Deficits in ocular and manual tracking due to episodic ataxia type 2. Mov Disord 19(7): 778–787.

Escayg A, De Waard M, Lee DD, Bichet D, Wolf P, Mayer T, et al. (2000) Coding and noncoding variation of the human calcium-channel beta4-subunit gene CACNB4 in patients with idiopathic generalized epilepsy and episodic ataxia. Am J Hum Genet 66(5): 1531–1539.

Eunson LH, Rea R, Zuberi SM, Youroukos S, Panayiotopoulos CP, Liguori R, et al. (2000) Clinical, genetic, and expression studies of mutations in the potassium channel gene KCNA1 reveal new phenotypic variability. Ann Neurol 48(4): 647–656.

Farmer TW, Mustian VM (1963) Vestibulocerebellar ataxia. A newly defined hereditary syndrome with periodic manifestations. Arch Neurol 8: 471–480.

Gancher ST, Nutt JG (1986) Autosomal dominant episodic ataxia: a heterogeneous syndrome. Mov Disord 1(4): 239–253.

Graves TD, Hanna MG (2005) Neurological channelopathies. Postgrad Med J 81(951): 20–32.

Graves TD, Hanna MG (2008) Episodic ataxia: SLC1A3 and CACNB4 do not explain the apparent genetic heterogeneity. J Neurol 255(7): 1097–1099.

Graves TD, Rajakulendran S, Zuberi SM, Morris HR, Schorge S, Hanna MG, Kullmann DM (2010) Nongenetic factors influence severity of episodic ataxia type 1 in monozygotic twins. Neurology 75(4): 367–372.

Griggs RC, Moxley RT, 3rd, Lafrance RA, McQuillen J (1978) Hereditary paroxysmal ataxia: response to acetazolamide. Neurology 28(12): 1259–1264.

Guida S, Trettel F, Pagnutti S, Mantuano E, Tottene A, Veneziano L, et al. (2001. Complete loss of P/Q calcium channel activity caused by a CACNA1A missense mutation carried by patients with episodic ataxia type 2. Am J Hum Genet 68(3): 759–764.

Hanson PA, Martinez LB, Cassidy R (1977) Contractures, continuous muscle discharges, and titubation. Ann Neurol 1(2): 120–124.

Imbrici P, Eunson LH, Graves TD, Bhatia KP, Wadia NH, Kullmann DM, Hanna MG (2005) Late-onset episodic ataxia type 2 due to an in-frame insertion in CACNA1A. Neurology 65(6): 944–946.

Imbrici P, Jaffe SL, Eunson LH, Davies NP, Herd C, Robertson R, et al. (2004) Dysfunction of the brain calcium channel CaV2.1 in absence epilepsy and episodic ataxia. Brain 127(Pt 12): 2682–2692.

Jen J, Yue Q, Nelson SF, Yu H, Litt M, Nutt J, Baloh RW (1999) A novel nonsense mutation in CACNA1A causes episodic ataxia and hemiplegia. Neurology 53(1): 34–37.

Jen J, Wan J, Graves M, Yu H, Mock AF, Coulin CJ, et al. (2001) Loss-of-function EA2 mutations are associated with impaired neuromuscular transmission. Neurology 57(10): 1843–1848.

Jen J, Kim GW, Baloh RW (2004) Clinical spectrum of episodic ataxia type 2. Neurology 62(1): 17–22.

Jen JC, Wan J, Palos TP, Howard BD, Baloh RW (2005) Mutation in the glutamate transporter EAAT1 causes episodic ataxia, hemiplegia, and seizures. Neurology 65(4): 529–534.

Jen JC, Graves TD, Hess EJ, Hanna MG, Griggs RC, Baloh RW (2007) Primary episodic ataxias: diagnosis, pathogenesis and treatment. Brain 130(Pt 10): 2484–2493.

Jodice C, Mantuano E, Veneziano L, Trettel F, Sabbadini G, Calandriello L, et al. (1997) Episodic ataxia type 2 (EA2) and spinocerebellar ataxia type 6 (SCA6) due to CAG repeat expansion in the CACNA1A gene on chromosome 19p. Hum Mol Genet 6(11): 1973–1978.

Jouvenceau A, Eunson LH, Spauschus A, Ramesh V, Zuberi SM, Kullmann DM, Hanna MG (2001) Human epilepsy associated with dysfunction of the brain P/Q-type calcium channel. Lancet 358(9284): 801–807.

Kaunisto MA, Harno H, Kallela M, Somer H, Sallinen R, Hamalainen E, et al. (2004) Novel splice site CACNA1A mutation causing episodic ataxia type 2. Neurogenetics 5(1): 69–73.

Kerber KA, Jen JC, Lee H, Nelson SF, Baloh RW (2007) A new episodic ataxia syndrome with linkage to chromosome 19q13. Arch Neurol 64(5): 749–752.

Kinali M, Jungbluth H, Eunson LH, Sewry CA, Manzur AY, Mercuri E, et al. (2004) Expanding the phenotype of potassium channelopathy: severe neuromyotonia and skeletal deformities without prominent Episodic Ataxia. Neuromuscul Disord 14(10): 689–693.

Klein A, Boltshauser E, Jen J, Baloh RW (2004). Episodic ataxia type 1 with distal weakness: a novel manifestation of a potassium channelopathy. Neuropediatrics 35(2): 147–149.

Koller W, Bahamon-Dussan J (1987) Hereditary paroxysmal cerebellopathy: responsiveness to acetazolamide. Clin Neuropharmacol 10(1): 65–68.

Kors EE, Terwindt GM, Vermeulen FL, Fitzsimons RB, Jardine PE, Heywood P, et al. (2001) Delayed cerebral edema and fatal coma after minor head trauma: role of the CACNA1A calcium channel subunit gene and relationship with familial hemiplegic migraine. Ann Neurol 49(6): 753–760.

Labrum RW, Rajakulendran S, Graves TD, Eunson LH, Bevan R, Sweeney MG, et al. (2009) Large scale calcium channel gene rearrangements in episodic ataxia and hemiplegic migraine: implications for diagnostic testing. J Med Genet 46(11): 786–791.

Lee H, Wang H, Jen JC, Sabatti C, Baloh RW, Nelson SF (2004) A novel mutation in KCNA1 causes episodic ataxia without myokymia. Hum Mutat 24(6): 536.

Litt M, Kramer P, Browne D, Gancher S, Brunt ER, Root D, et al. (1994) A gene for episodic ataxia/myokymia maps to chromosome 12p13. Am J Hum Genet 55(4): 702–709.

Lubbers WJ, Brunt ER, Scheffer H, Litt M, Stulp R, Browne DL, van Weerden TW (1995) Hereditary myokymia and paroxysmal ataxia linked to chromosome 12 is responsive to acetazolamide. J Neurol Neurosurg Psychiatr 59(4): 400–405.

Maselli RA, Wan J, Dunne V, Graves M, Baloh RW, Wollmann RL, Jen J (2003) Presynaptic failure of neuromuscular transmission and synaptic remodeling in EA2. Neurology 61(12): 1743–1748.

Neufeld MY, Nisipeanu P, Chistik V, Korczyn AD (1996) The electroencephalogram in acetazolamide-responsive periodic ataxia. Mov Disord 11(3): 283–288.

Ophoff RA, Terwindt GM, Vergouwe MN, van Eijk R, Oefner PJ, Hoffman SM, et al. (1996) Familial hemiplegic migraine and episodic ataxia type-2 are caused by mutations in the Ca2+ channel gene CACNL1A4. Cell 87(3): 543–552.

Rajakulendran S, Graves TD, Labrum RW, Kotzadimitriou D, Eunson L, Davis MB, et al. (2010) Genetic and functional characterisation of the P/Q calcium channel in episodic ataxia with epilepsy. J Physiol 588(Pt 11): 1905–1913.

Reid CA, Bekkers JM, Clements JD (1998) N- and P/Q-type Ca2+ channels mediate transmitter release with a similar cooperativity at rat hippocampal autapses. J Neurosci 18(8): 2849–2855.

Riant F, Mourtada R, Saugier-Veber P, Tournier-Lasserve E (2008) Large CACNA1A deletion in a family with episodic ataxia type 2. Arch Neurol 65(6): 817–820.

Spacey SD, Hildebrand ME, Materek LA, Bird TD, Snutch TP (2004) Functional implications of a novel EA2 mutation in the P/Q-type calcium channel. Ann Neurol 56(2): 213–220.

Stea A, Tomlinson WJ, Soong TW, Bourinet E, Dubel SJ, Vincent SR, Snutch TP (1994) Localization and functional properties of a rat brain alpha 1A calcium channel reflect similarities to neuronal Q- and P-type channels. Proc Natl Acad Sci U S A 91(22): 10576–10580.

Steckley JL, Ebers GC, Cader MZ, McLachlan RS (2001) An autosomal dominant disorder with episodic ataxia, vertigo, and tinnitus. Neurology 57(8): 1499–1502.

Stephens GJ, Morris NP, Fyffe RE, Robertson B (2001) The Cav2.1/alpha1A (P/Q-type) voltage-dependent calcium channel mediates inhibitory neurotransmission onto mouse cerebellar Purkinje cells. Eur J Neurosci 13(10): 1902–1912.

Strupp M, Kalla R, Dichgans M, Freilinger T, Glasauer S, Brandt T (2004) Treatment of episodic ataxia type 2 with the potassium channel blocker 4-aminopyridine. Neurology 62(9): 1623–1625.

Subramony SH, Schott K, Raike RS, Callahan J, Langford LR, Christova PS, et al. (2003). Novel CACNA1A mutation causes febrile episodic ataxia with interictal cerebellar deficits. Ann Neurol 54(6): 725–731.

Tanaka O, Sakagami H, Kondo H (1995) Localization of mRNAs of voltage-dependent Ca(2+)-channels: four subtypes of alpha 1- and beta-subunits in developing and mature rat brain. Brain Res Mol Brain Res 30(1): 1–16.

Terwindt GM, Ophoff RA, Haan J, Vergouwe MN, van Eijk R, Frants RR, Ferrari MD (1998) Variable clinical expression of mutations in the P/Q-type calcium channel gene in familial hemiplegic migraine. Dutch Migraine Genetics Research Group. Neurology 50(4): 1105–1110.

Uchitel OD, Protti DA, Sanchez V, Cherksey BD, Sugimori M, Llinas R (1992) P-type voltage-dependent calcium channel mediates presynaptic calcium influx and transmitter release in mammalian synapses. Proc Natl Acad Sci U S A 89(8): 3330–3333.

Vahedi K, Joutel A, Van Bogaert P, Ducros A, Maciazeck J, Bach JF, Bousser MG, Tournier-Lasserve E (1995) A gene for hereditary paroxysmal cerebellar ataxia maps to chromosome 19p. Ann Neurol 37(3): 289–293.

Van Bogaert P, Szliwowski HB (1996) EEG findings in acetazolamide-responsive hereditary paroxysmal ataxia. Neurophysiol Clin 26(5): 335–340.

van den Maagdenberg AM, Kors EE, Brunt ER, van Paesschen W, Pascual J, Ravine D, et al. (2002) Episodic ataxia type 2. Three novel truncating mutations and one novel missense mutation in the CACNA1A gene. J Neurol 249(11): 1515–1519.

VanDyke DH, Griggs RC, Murphy MJ, Goldstein MN (1975) Hereditary myokymia and periodic ataxia. J Neurol Sci 25(1): 109–118.

Veneziano L, Guida S, Mantuano E, Bernard P, Tarantino P, Boccone L, et al. (2009) Newly characterised 5′ and 3′ regions of CACNA1A gene harbour mutations associated with Familial Hemiplegic Migraine and Episodic Ataxia. J Neurol Sci 276(1–2): 31–37.

Vighetto A, Froment JC, Trillet M, Aimard G (1988) Magnetic resonance imaging in familial paroxysmal ataxia. Arch Neurol 45(5): 547–549.

von Brederlow B, Hahn AF, Koopman WJ, Ebers GC, Bulman DE (1995) Mapping the gene for acetazolamide responsive hereditary paryoxysmal cerebellar ataxia to chromosome 19p. Hum Mol Genet 4(2): 279–284.

Wappl E, Koschak A, Poteser M, Sinnegger MJ, Walter D, Eberhart A, et al. (2002) Functional consequences of P/Q-type Ca2+ channel Cav2.1 missense mutations associated with episodic ataxia type 2 and progressive ataxia. J Biol Chem 277(9): 6960–6966.

Wiest G, Tian JR, Baloh RW, Crane BT, Demer JL (2001) Otolith function in cerebellar ataxia due to mutations in the calcium channel gene CACNA1A. Brain 124(Pt 12): 2407–2416.

Yue Q, Jen JC, Thwe MM, Nelson SF, Baloh RW (1998) De novo mutation in CACNA1A caused acetazolamide-responsive episodic ataxia. Am J Med Genet 77(4): 298–301.

Zasorin NL, Baloh RW, Myers LB (1983) Acetazolamide-responsive episodic ataxia syndrome. Neurology 33(9): 1212–1214.

Zhuchenko O, Bailey J, Bonnen P, Ashizawa T, Stockton DW, Amos C, et al. (1997) Autosomal dominant cerebellar ataxia (SCA6) associated with small polyglutamine expansions in the alpha 1A-voltage-dependent calcium channel. Nat Genet 15(1): 62–69.

Zuberi SM, Eunson LH, Spauschus A, De Silva R, Tolmie J, Wood NW, et al. (1999) A novel mutation in the human voltage-gated potassium channel gene (Kv1.1) associates with episodic ataxia type 1 and sometimes with partial epilepsy. Brain 122 (Pt 5): 817–825.

29
Neurocutaneous Syndromes with Cerebellar Involvement

Thierry A.G.M. Huisman

Introduction
The neurocutaneous syndromes or phakomatoses encompass a heterogeneous group of congenital disorders that are characterized by various combinations of hamartous malformations and tumors of the skin, central and peripheral nervous system, and visceral organs. Currently more than 40 disorders have been identified (Herron et al. 2000; Lin and Barker 2006). Despite the fact that these disorders are very distinct from each other, they have in common that the observed lesions are all ectodermal in origin and result from a defective tumor suppressor gene (Korf 2004).

The more common neurocutaneous disorders are neurofibromatosis type 1 (von Recklinghausen disease), neurofibromatosis type 2 (MISME syndrome), tuberous sclerosis complex (Bourneville-Pringle disease), encephalo-trigeminal angiomatosis (Sturge-Weber-Dimitri syndrome), and retinocerebellar angiomatosis (von Hippel-Lindau syndrome). A number of less frequent neurocutaneous disorders have been identified, too many to discuss in detail.

Neuroimaging plays a central role in the evaluation and classification of the various neurocutaneous disorders. Cross-sectional imaging including computed tomography (CT) and magnetic resonance imaging (MRI) allows identification of degree and quality of pathology, helps to monitor disease progression, and guides therapeutic (neurosurgical) interventions. Most reports have focused on the cerebral findings; significantly less is known about posterior fossa involvement. This is partially due to the fact that not all phakomatoses appear to affect the supra- and infratentorial brain simultaneously, infratentorial lesions may go undetected because clinical findings are less 'disabling' or less 'prominent' on clinical examination, and finally the posterior fossa is more difficult to image because of its smaller size and higher susceptibility to artifacts both on CT and MRI. The impact of the cerebellum on neurocognitive development and overall function should, however, not be underestimated. Next to obvious focal lesions, such as hamartomas or neoplasms, a diffuse impaired or altered cerebellar gray and white matter development should be ruled out (Arulrajah et al. 2009, 2010; Ertan et al. 2010).

In the current chapter, the cerebellar manifestations of the common neurocutaneous disorders will be discussed as well as two rare phakomatoses that are known to affect the cerebellum (PHACE syndrome) and ataxia-telangiectasia (Louis-Bar syndrome). This chapter is primarily summarizing the key clinical features and matching diagnostic neuroimaging findings. It would go beyond the scope of this chapter to discuss the numerous neuropsychological evaluation and treatment options available, because they are subject to continuous changes and improvements.

Neurofibromatosis type 1
Neurofibromatosis type I (NF1) also known as von Recklinghausen disease or peripheral neurofibromatosis, is the most common neurocutaneous disorder with an incidence of 1 in 3000–4000. NF1 is an autosomal dominant genetic disease with a high penetrance rate (up to 100%) and high phenotypic variability. As many as 50% of cases are de novo mutations. NF1 results from a deficient tumor suppressor, neurofibromin, which is encoded on chromosome 17q11.2.

The findings in NF1 can be divided into three categories: cutaneous lesions, central nervous system (CNS) tumors, and mesodermal dysplasia.

The cutaneous features include hyperpigmented café-au-lait macules, skin-fold freckles, and neurofibromas. The café-au-lait macules are usually noticed in the first months of life. Six or more spots larger than 5mm before puberty and skin-fold freckles appearing between 3–5 years indicate NF1. Neurofibromas are benign tumors of the nerve sheath consisting of a mixture of proliferated Schwann cells, fibroblasts, and pericytes (Yohay 2006). Neurofibromas may occur anywhere in the body anywhere along the nerve from the dorsal root ganglion to the terminal nerve branches. They may be solitary and nodular or diffuse, affecting multiple nerves simultaneously (plexiform neurofibromas) (Korf 2004). Focal neurofibromas are usually not present in young children but appear later in life, while plexiform neurofibromas are usually congenital (Korf 2004). Large plexiform neurofibromas may displace and encase vascular structures or the tracheo-bronchial tree or extend through foramina into the spinal canal (Fig. 29.1a).

Central nervous system lesions are seen in 15–20% of patients. In addition, there is a four-fold increased risk of developing CNS neoplasm (Herron et al. 2000). Typical intracranial lesions include optic pathway gliomas (Figs 29.1b,c) (most frequently low-grade pilocytic astrocytomas), brainstem and tectal gliomas, rarely cranial nerve tumors, and characteristic focal areas of myelin vacuolization or neurofibromatosis spots. These latter lesions are also known as unidentified bright objects (UBOs) because they are bright on T2-weighted MR

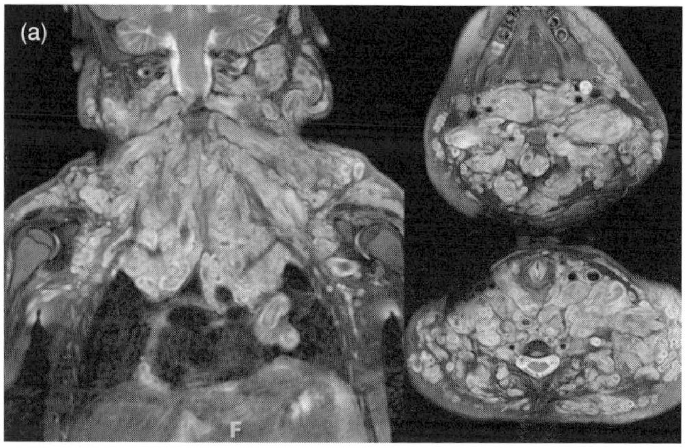

Fig. 29.1(a). Coronal and axial T2-weighted fat-saturated MRI of a child with neurofibromatosis type 1. Innumerous T2-hyperintense neurofibromas are seen in the neck, paraspinal tissues and upper chest. The lesions encase the neck vessels and airways. There is additional, intraspinal extension through the widened neuroforamina with compression of the spinal cord.

imaging, and non-enhancing (Figs 29.1b,d). These lesions are found in 43–93% of pediatric NF patients, are usually multiple and found in the basal ganglia, internal capsule, brainstem, cerebellum, and dentate nuclei (Fig. 29.1b). These lesions appear by 3 years of age, and increase in number and size until 10–12 years before they again regress (Rodriguez and Young Poussaint 2004). They are typically asymptomatic; no malignant degeneration occurs.

Mesodermal dysplasia is linked to various skeletal pathologies including fractures and pseudoarthrosis of long bones (especially the tibia), sphenoid and vertebral dysplasia, short stature and scoliosis (Korf 2004; Yohay 2006).The defective connective tissue also leads to dural ectasia, arachnoid cysts, and meningoceles (Lin and Barker 2006).

Moreover, there is an increased risk for cardiovascular abnormalities (Fig. 29.1e) including vasculopathy, intracranial aneurysms, moyamoya syndrome, hypertension, and congenital heart defects. Macrocephaly is noted in up to 50% of all children, most frequently due to a large brain size (Rodriguez and

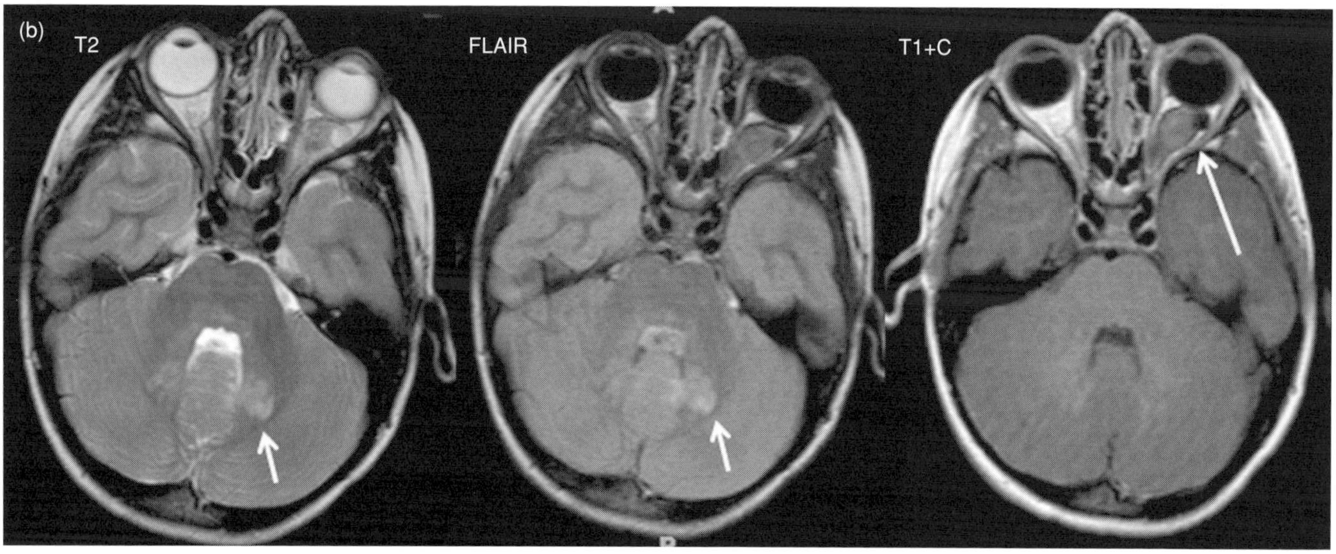

Fig. 29.1(b). Axial T2, fluid attenuated inversion recovery (FLAIR) and contrast-enhanced axial T1-weighted MRI in a child with confirmed neurofibromatosis type 1. The unidentified bright objects within the dentate nuclei are T2 and FLAIR hyperintense and do not show any degree of contrast enhancement (arrows). In addition, a mildly enhancing optic nerve glioma is noted (large arrow).

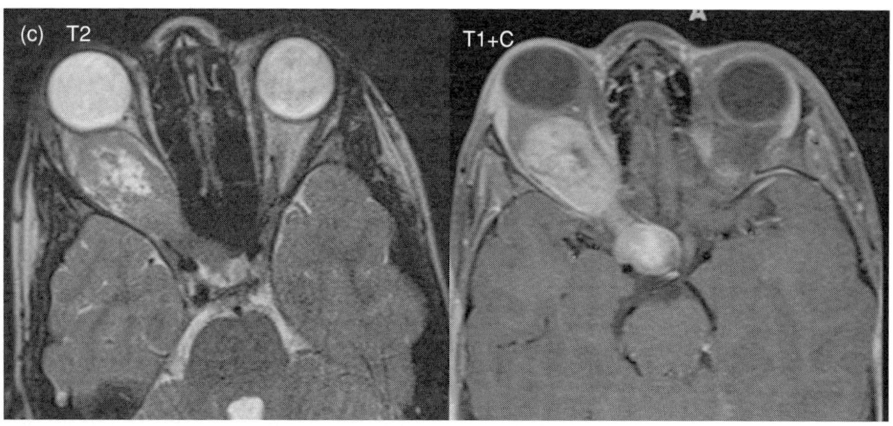

Fig. 29.1(c). Axial T2 and contrast-enhanced T1-weighted MRI of the orbits. A partially degenerated, necrotic, inhomogeneously enhancing right optic glioma is seen extending through the widened optic canal towards the optic chiasm in a child with confirmed neurofibromatosis type 1.

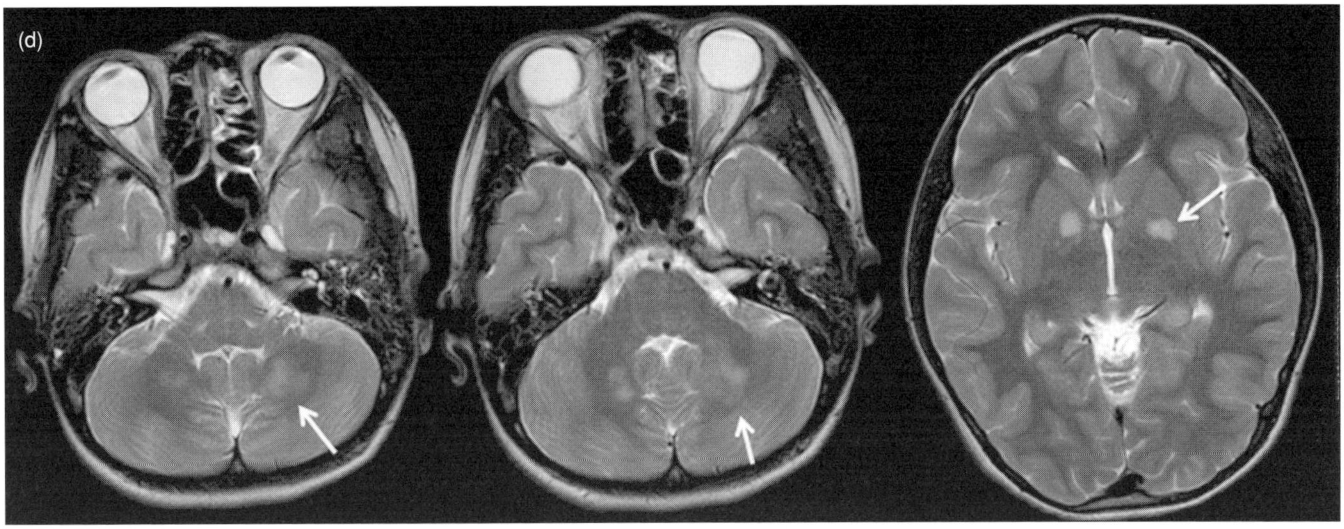

Fig. 29.1(d). Axial T2-weighted MRI in a young child with confirmed neurofibromatosis type 1. Multiple T2-hyperintense focal lesions (unidentified bright objects) are seen in the cerebellar hemispheres and peduncles, dentate nuclei and basal ganglia (arrows). No mass effect is noted.

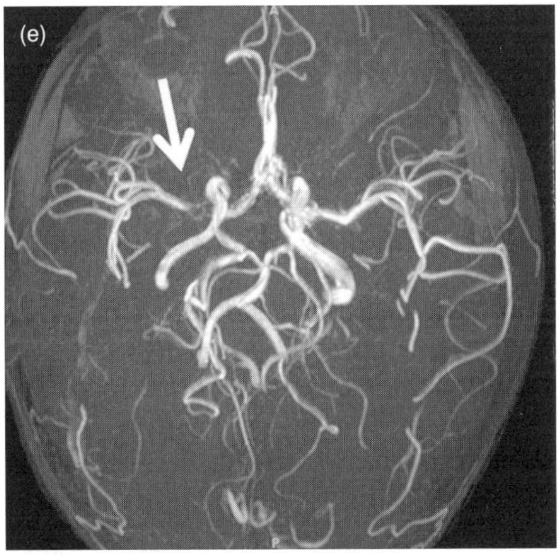

Fig. 29.1(e). Axial MR angiography image of the circulus arteriosus Willisi in a child with neurofibromatosis type 1. High-grade stenosis of the right proximal middle cerebral artery (arrow) is seen as well as moyamoya-like collaterals along the affected stenotic vessels.

Young Poussaint 2004; Yohay 2006). Approximately 50% of children with NF1 present with mental retardation (UK: learning disability) (Korf 2004). Neuroendocrine symptoms and visual disturbances typically result from local compression by an enlarging glioma.

Malignant degeneration of NF1 lesions are reported to occur in up to 10% of patients. Most frequently, malignant degeneration of a plexiform neurofibroma occurs, resulting in aggressive malignant peripheral nerve sheath tumors. Malignant degeneration should be suspected if the neurofibromas rapidly enlarge or become painful. NF1 patients are also reported to be at increased risk for leukemia and rhabdomyosarcoma (Korf 2004).

Cerebellar gliomas are rarely seen in NF1 but unfortunately appear to have a higher propensity for malignant degeneration (Ilgren et al. 1985; Carella and Medicamento 1997; Vinchon et al. 2000). The true incidence of cerebellar gliomas is unknown. Pascual-Castroviejo reviewed a series of 600 NF1 patients covering a survey period of 39 years and found five patients with posterior fossa tumors (0.83%) (Pascual-Castroviejo 2010) (Fig. 29.1f).

Neuroimaging typically relies on the high soft tissue contrast of MRI to identify, localize, and characterize the previously described NF1 lesions. Optic pathway gliomas have variable degrees of contrast enhancement; the anterior pathway gliomas may show avid enhancement while the more posterior lesions usually do not enhance but appear T2-hyperintense. The neurofibromas are typically T1-hypointense, T2-hyperintense, with variable degrees of contrast enhancement. MR angiography sequences should be considered to exclude intracranial vascular lesions. ^{1}H MR spectroscopy can be helpful to differentiate focal gliomas from UBOs. Near normal spectra are found in UBOs, with a slightly decreased *N*-acetylasparate/choline and *N*-acetylasparate/creatine ratio. In particular no increased choline is found in the UBOs, in contrast to elevated choline levels in gliomas (Lin and Barker 2006). Diffusion tensor imaging (DTI) has shown that the apparent diffusion coefficient (ADC) is significantly increased and fractional anisotropy decreased in UBOs, which would support the thesis that UBOs result from myelin vacuolization and/or axonal disruption (Huisman, personal research data). Tractography studies showed that UBOs do not lead to significant changes in white matter trajectories such as tract displacement or destruction (Huisman, personal research data). More interestingly, several studies showed that the ADC values are also increased in the normal-appearing white matter of children with NF1 (Alkan et al. 2005; Eastwood et al. 2001; Goh et al. 2004). The significance of this finding is still unclear but could possibly give insight into the increased incidence of developmental delay in NF1 patients. CT may be helpful for identification of bony lesions as well as possible calcifications.

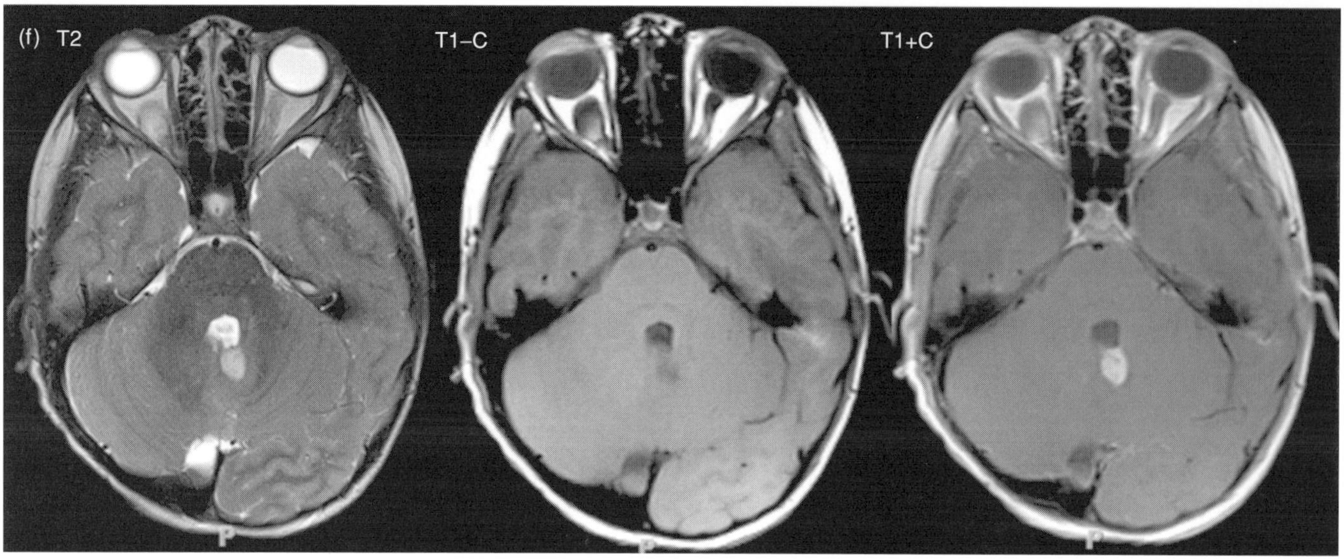

Fig. 29.1(f). Axial T2-, pre- and postcontrast T1-weighted MRI of the posterior fossa in a child with neurofibromatosis type 1. A T2-hyperintense, T1-hypointense, strongly enhancing, well-circumscribed focal lesion is seen dorsal to the fourth ventricle within the vermis. Histological study confirmed a pilocytic astrocytoma. In addition, a right optic nerve glioma is noted.

Neurofibromatosis type 2

Neurofibromatosis type 2 (NF2) also known as central neurofibromatosis, vestibular schwannoma neurofibromatosis or multiple inherited schwannomas, meningiomas, and ependymomas (MISME) syndrome is very different from NF1 and has only few overlapping features. NF2 patients have only minimal skin lesions and the prevalence of NF2 is much lower compared with NF1 (1:40 000). NF2 is an autosomal dominant disorder with complete penetrance. The defective tumor suppressor protein, merlin or schwannomin, is encoded on chromosome 22q12.2. In 50% of cases disease results from a spontaneous mutation (Korf 2004; Rodriguez and Young Poussaint 2004; Lin and Barker 2006).

As the acronym MISME suggests, NF2 is characterized by multiple schwannomas, typically affecting the vestibular nerves bilaterally (Fig. 29.2). Less frequently other cranial nerves may be involved, especially the trigeminal nerve. Schwannomas may also occur along the spinal nerves, frequently extending through the neural foramina into the spinal canal with resultant spinal cord compression. In contrast to the neurofibromas, these schwannomas have no malignant potential. In addition, schwannomas displace rather than infiltrate nerve roots because they originate from the Schwann cells that encircle the nerves. Consequently surgical resection is frequently possible (Lin and Barker 2006). Next to the schwannomas, meningiomas can be seen throughout the entire CNS including intraventricular locations. Finally, there is an increased prevalence of ependymomas, frequently affecting the spinal cord.

Cutaneous manifestations are much less common in NF2 than in NF1; however, plaque-like cutaneous schwannomas may occur. Café-au-lait spots are rarely present (Yohay 2006). Juvenile subcapsular lenticular opacities, cataracts, corneal

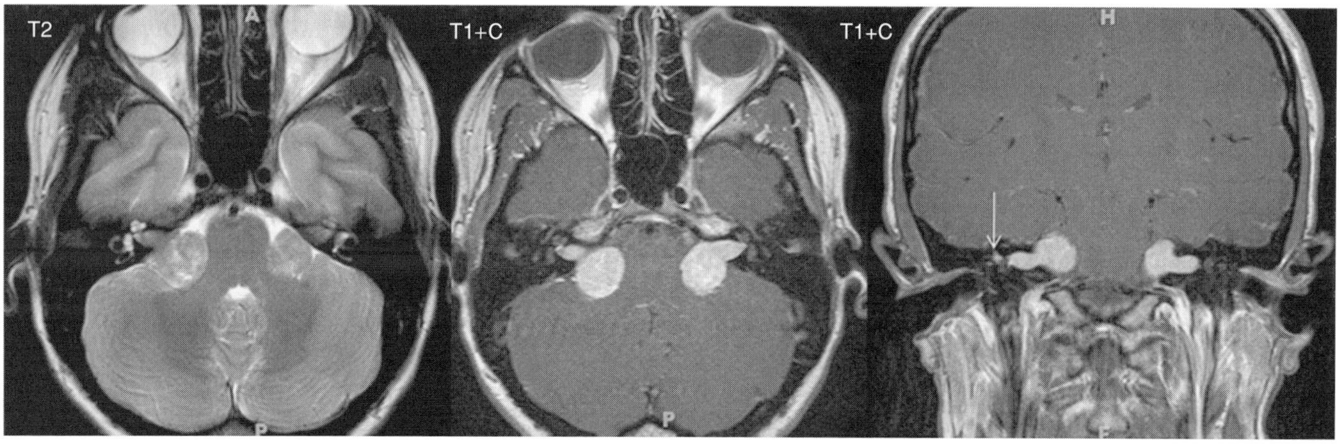

Fig. 29.2. Axial T2-, contrast-enhanced axial and coronal T1-weighted MRI of the posterior fossa in a child with neurofibromatosis type 2. Bilateral T2-heterogeneous, strongly enhancing vestibular schwannomas are identified extending from the widened internal auditory canal into the cerebello-pontine angles. The middle cerebellar peduncles are compressed. Tumor extension is seen into the right vestibulum of the inner ear (arrow).

scarring, and retinal hamartomas may be seen. In contrast to NF1, NF2 is not linked with UBOs, skeletal dysplasia, developmental delay, or microcephaly. There is no increased risk for systemic malignancies.

Patients typically present with hearing loss during early adulthood due to the vestibular schwannomas, or with symptoms of cord compression.

Cerebellar symptoms usually result from direct compression of cerebellar structures by large vestibular schwannomas located within the cerebello-pontine angle (Pothula et al. 2001). No focal intraaxial cerebellar tumors have been linked to NF2.

MRI plays an essential role in the identification of the schwannomas, meningiomas, and ependymomas. In addition, follow-up MR examinations should be considered to study spontaneous evolution. Vestibular schwannomas may be stable for many years (dormant), or may undergo cystic degeneration or phases of rapid growth. Schwannomas are typically T2-hyperintense with strong contrast enhancement. Meningiomas are usually T1- and T2-isointense to gray matter with strong contrast enhancement. Ependymomas are typically T2-hyperintense, T1-isointense with strong contrast enhancement.

Tuberous sclerosis complex

Tuberous sclerosis complex (TSC), also known as Bourneville-Pringle disease, is an autosomal dominant disorder with a prevalence of 1:6000–10 000 patients. At least two genetic defects have been identified, one localized on chromosome 9q34, encoding for *TSC1* or hamartin, and a second on chromosome 16p13.3 encoding for *TSC2* or tuberin (Lin et al. 2003; Smirniotopoulos 2004). Clinically patients present with a triad of seizures, mental retardation (UK: learning disability) and facial angiofibromas. The majority of patients (>75%) have learning difficulties, cognitive impairment, and behavioral problems (Lin and Barker 2006).

TSC is a classic neurocutaneous disorder with simultaneous involvement of the skin and multiple organs (heart, kidneys, lungs, eyes) and the CNS. The skin lesions include hypomelanotic macules, subcutaneous shagreen patches, ungual or periungual fibromas, and facial angiofibromas. Angiomyolipomas and cysts are seen in the kidneys, rhabdomyomas in the heart, and lymphangiomyomatosis in the lungs. In addition, retinal nodular hamartomas and achromic patches occur (Lin et al. 2003; Smirniotopoulos 2004).

The CNS lesions include cortical tubers, subependymal nodules, radial glial bands or cerebral white matter migration lines, and giant cell astrocytomas. The cortical tubers and subependymal nodules are seen in nearly all patients and may calcify with age. The radial glial bands are also seen in nearly all TSC patients (Fig. 29.3a). They represent islets or bands of arrested disordered neurons intermixed with glial cells. Giant cell astrocytomas are seen in about 15% of patients and may be complicated by supratentorial hydrocephalus due to their typical close proximity to the foramen of Monro.

All TSC lesions are easily diagnosed on MRI. The cortical tubers change their relative signal intensities with progressing white matter myelination and typically enlarge the affected gyrus. The hyperintense signal on T2-weighted and fluid-attenuated inversion recovery (FLAIR) MR images give the appearance of 'empty gyri'. Calcifications may appear on follow-up. The subependymal nodules are typically located along the lateral ventricles and may show calcifications which are best seen on CT. The white matter migration lines are best seen on FLAIR images as hyperintense, ill-defined bands that extend from the ventricles towards the overlying cortex. The giant cell astrocytomas are T2-hyperintense, highly vascularized tumors with avid contrast enhancement and prominent tumor vessels (Lin et al. 2003; Smirniotopoulos 2004).

Functional MRI studies of the cortical tubers showed decreased *N*-acetylasparate/creatine and increased myoinositol/creatine ratio, increased ADC values, and a focal hypoperfusion (Lin and Barker 2006). In addition, the ADC values of the normal-appearing white matter proved to be increased in TSC patients. These findings suggest that myelination is delayed or impaired in TSC patients, which could explain global neurocognitive deficits (Arulrajah et al. 2009).

Cerebellar involvement is seen in up to 33% of TSC patients. Cortical tubers and focal atrophy have been described (Ertan et al. 2010). The cerebellar cortical tubers differ from the supratentorial tubers in their imaging features. They are triangular in shape with a broad base towards the cerebellar cortex (Fig. 29.3b). In contrast to the supratentorial tubers, most cerebellar tubers show a mild to moderate 'zebra-like' contrast enhancement (Ertan et al. 2010) (see Fig. 29.3c). Several studies have shown that cerebellar lesions, in particular the number of cerebellar tubers, are correlated with increased autistic behavior. Children with right cerebellar lesions proved to have higher social isolation and communicative and developmental disturbance compared with children with left-sided cerebellar lesions (Weber et al. 2000; Eluvathingal et al. 2006).

Sturge-Weber-Dimitri syndrome

Sturge-Weber-Dimitri syndrome (SWDS) also known as encephalo-trigeminal angiomatosis, is a congenital neurocutaneous disorder of unknown inheritance with an estimated prevalence of 1:50 000 (Thomas-Sohl et al. 2004). SWDS is characterized by angiomas involving the facial skin, ocular choroid, and leptomeninges (pia mater). Persistence of the embryonic precirculatory venous plexus, defective development of normal cortical veins, and redirection of the venous blood flow into the developing leptomeninges result in a chronic cortical venous hypertension with progressive venous ischemic injury, and subsequent progressive atrophy of the cortex and subcortical white matter (Smirniotopoulos 2004; Lin and Barker 2006). Clinically, patients present with seizures, developmental delay, cognitive impairment, visual field defects, headache, and stroke-like symptoms (Thomas-Sohl et al. 2004). One of the characteristic features is the facial, cutaneous vascular malformation (port-wine stain) located in the ophthalmic and maxillary subdivision of the trigeminal nerve ipsilateral to the side of leptomeningeal angiomatosis. In

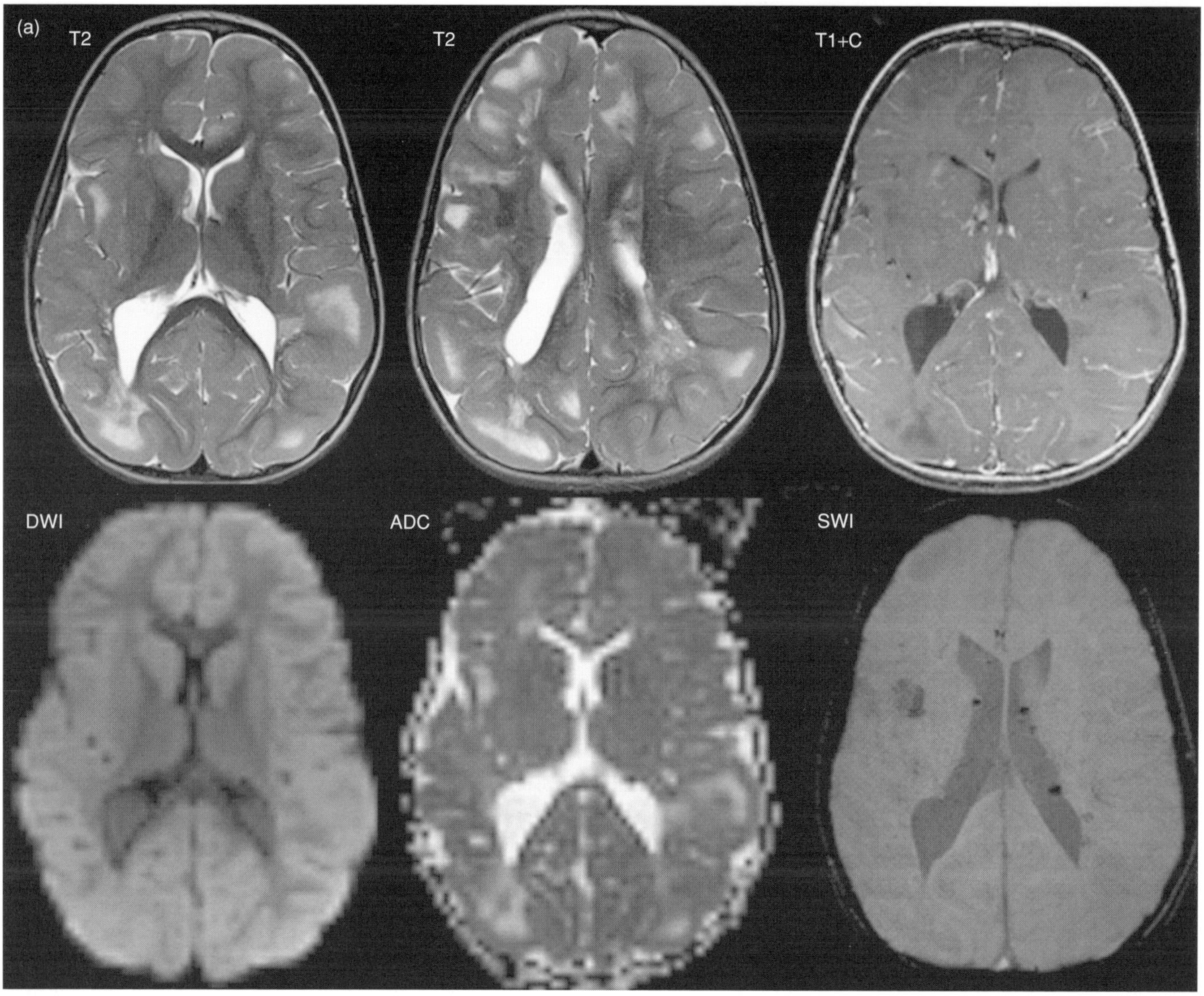

Fig. 29.3(a). Axial T2, contrast-enhanced T1-, diffusion-(DWI/ADC) and susceptibility-weighted (SWI) MRI in a child with confirmed diagnosis of tuberous sclerosis complex. Multiple slightly expansive T2-hyperintense cortical/subcortical tubers (empty gyri) are seen within both cerebral hemispheres as well as several calcified, SWI-hypointense subependymal nodules. A radial glial band is seen along the left trigonum of the lateral ventricle, extending towards an overlying subcortical tuber.

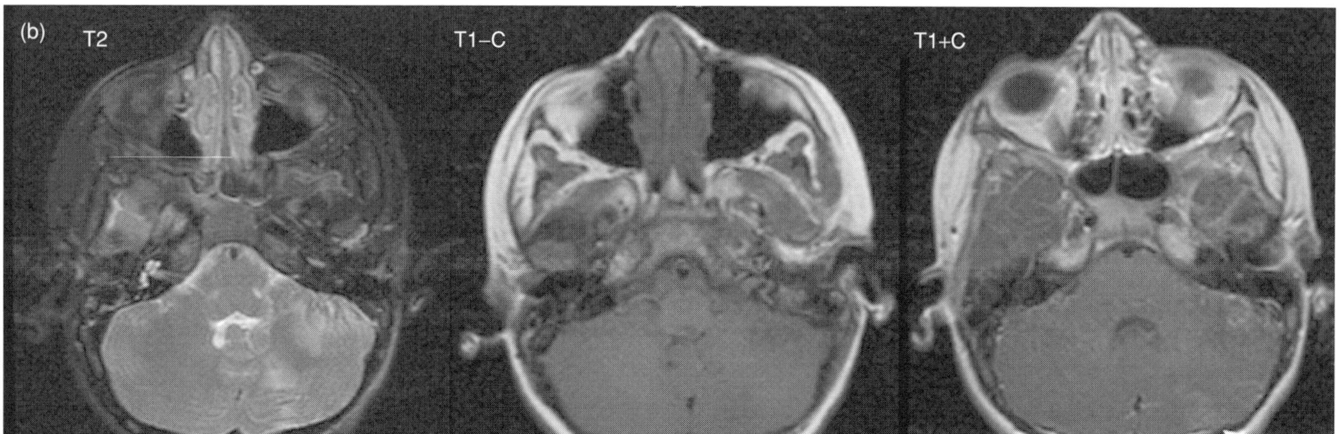

Fig. 29.3(b). Axial T2-, pre- and postcontrast T1-weighted MRI in a child with confirmed tuberous sclerosis complex. Cerebellar subcortical, contrast enhancing, wedge-shaped tubers are seen in the left cerebellar hemisphere (arrow).

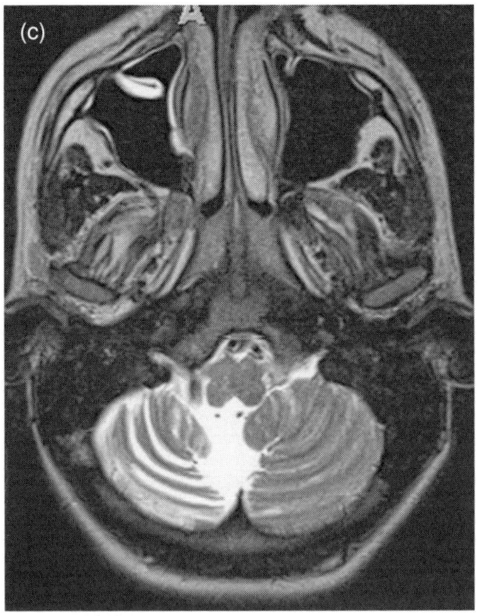

Fig. 29.3(c). Axial T2-weighted MRI of the cerebellum in a child with confirmed tuberous sclerosis complex. Moderate degree of right cerebellar atrophy is seen with widening of the cerebellar fissures. The left cerebellar hemisphere is unremarkable.

addition, congenital glaucoma, choroidal angiomas, scleral or episcleral telangiectasia, and an enlarged eye globe (buphthalmus) may be noted. The intracranial manifestations include the previously mentioned leptomeningeal angiomatosis with underlying cortical/subcortical atrophy which typically affects the occipital lobe but may extend anteriorly or even affect both hemispheres simultaneously (15%). The choroid plexus within the lateral ventricle is usually enlarged (Fig. 29.4a) and the ipsilateral intramedullary veins are enlarged as result of shunting of venous blood towards the deep venous system. The diploic space of the overlying skull may be widened (Smirniotopoulos 2004; Thomas-Sohl et al. 2004; Lin and Barker 2006) (see Fig. 29.4b).

Simultaneous supra- and infratentorial involvement including cerebellar leptomeningeal angiomatosis, atrophy and developmental venous anomalies are seen in up to 40% of patients (Arulrajah et al. 2009; Smith-Pearl et al. 2009) (see Fig. 29.4c).

On neuroimaging, the leptomeningeal angiomatosis is best seen on contrast-enhanced FLAIR MR sequences, with prominent sulcal enhancement overlying an atrophic thinned or interrupted cortex. Intracortical calcifications are well seen on susceptibility-weighted imaging (hypointense) and appear hyperdense on CT (tram tracks; see Fig. 29.4d). The adjacent subcortical white matter may be T2-hypointense which is believed to result either from an abnormal myelination or increased amount of deoxygenated venous blood within the venous capillaries. Dilated intramedullary veins are easily depicted on susceptibility weighted imaging (SWI) (Smirniotopoulos 2004; Thomas-Sohl et al. 2004; Lin and Barker 2006). Early studies in neonates may appear negative or show only minimal findings. Follow-up studies are helpful to show disease progression. One-sided periventricular white matter hyperechogenicity on ultrasonography can be an early sign of SWDS in neonates with a cutaneous nevus (Stranzinger and Huisman 2007).

Functional MR sequences including ^{1}H magnetic resonance spectroscopy (MRS) and difusion-weighted images (DWI)/DTI show the extent of white matter injury. In regions of cerebral atrophy, *N*-acetylasparate is decreased suggesting neuronal loss, while choline is elevated indicating abnormal myelination (Moore et al. 1998; Lin et al. 2003). These findings are supported by DWI/ADC studies showing increased ADC values in normal-appearing white matter distant from the area of leptomeningeal angiomatosis. In addition, increased ADC values are seen in the pons and cerebellar white matter. These findings may explain the observed neurocognitive deficits (Smith-Pearl et al. 2009; Arulrajah et al. 2010).

Von Hippel-Lindau syndrome

Von Hippel-Lindau (VHL) syndrome, also known as retinocerebellar angiomatosis or hemangioblastomatosis, is a congenital autosomal dominant phakomatosis with variable penetrance (Lin and Barker 2006; Jensen et al. 2009). VHL syndrome results from a deletion or mutation of a tumor suppressor gene localized on chromosome 3p25–26. Most patients inherit VHL syndrome; however, 20% result from a spontaneous mutation. The incidence is 1:36 000–60 000 (Korf 2004; Smirniotopoulos 2004; Lin and Barker 2006; Jensen et al. 2009).

VHL syndrome is not a classic neurocutaneous disorder because of the lack of cutaneous stigmata. Retinal hemangioblastomas are however noted in 25–60% of patients. Hemorrhages may cause retinal detachment or present as a blind spot (Smirniotopoulos 2004). The typical CNS lesions are predominantly infratentorial with benign hemangioblastomas in the cerebellum (65%), brainstem (20%), or spinal cord (15%) (Herron et al. 2000; Lin and Barker 2006). Most cerebellar hemangioblastomas appear pial based and are consequently in peripheral location (Fig. 29.5a). Cerebellar hemangioblastomas may be solitary or multiple (Lin and Barker 2006). Multiple hemangioblastomas are almost always associated with VHL syndrome. In particular, multilevel, nerve root hemangioblastomas should not be mistaken for drop metastases (Smirniotopoulos 2004). Low-grade adenocarcinomas may arise within the endolymphatic sac (10% of patients), are highly vascular and locally aggressive with erosion and destruction of the adjacent petrous bone (Smirniotopoulos 2004; Lin and Barker 2006). Neurological symptoms usually result from local compression of adjacent functional centers. Bulbar symptoms or obstructive hydrocephalus have been reported in lower brainstem hemangioblastomas (Pavesi et al. 2010). The risk of intracerebral hemorrhage is low (Jensen et al. 2009). An important indicator for the probability of hemorrhage is tumor size. Spontaneous or postoperative hemorrhage have been reported to occur exclusively in large tumors. Hemangioblastomas smaller than 1.5cm harbor virtually no risk of spontaneous hemorrhage (Gläsker and van Velthoven 2005).

Patients with VHL syndrome may have additional benign or malignant lesions outside the CNS. Multiple organs can be

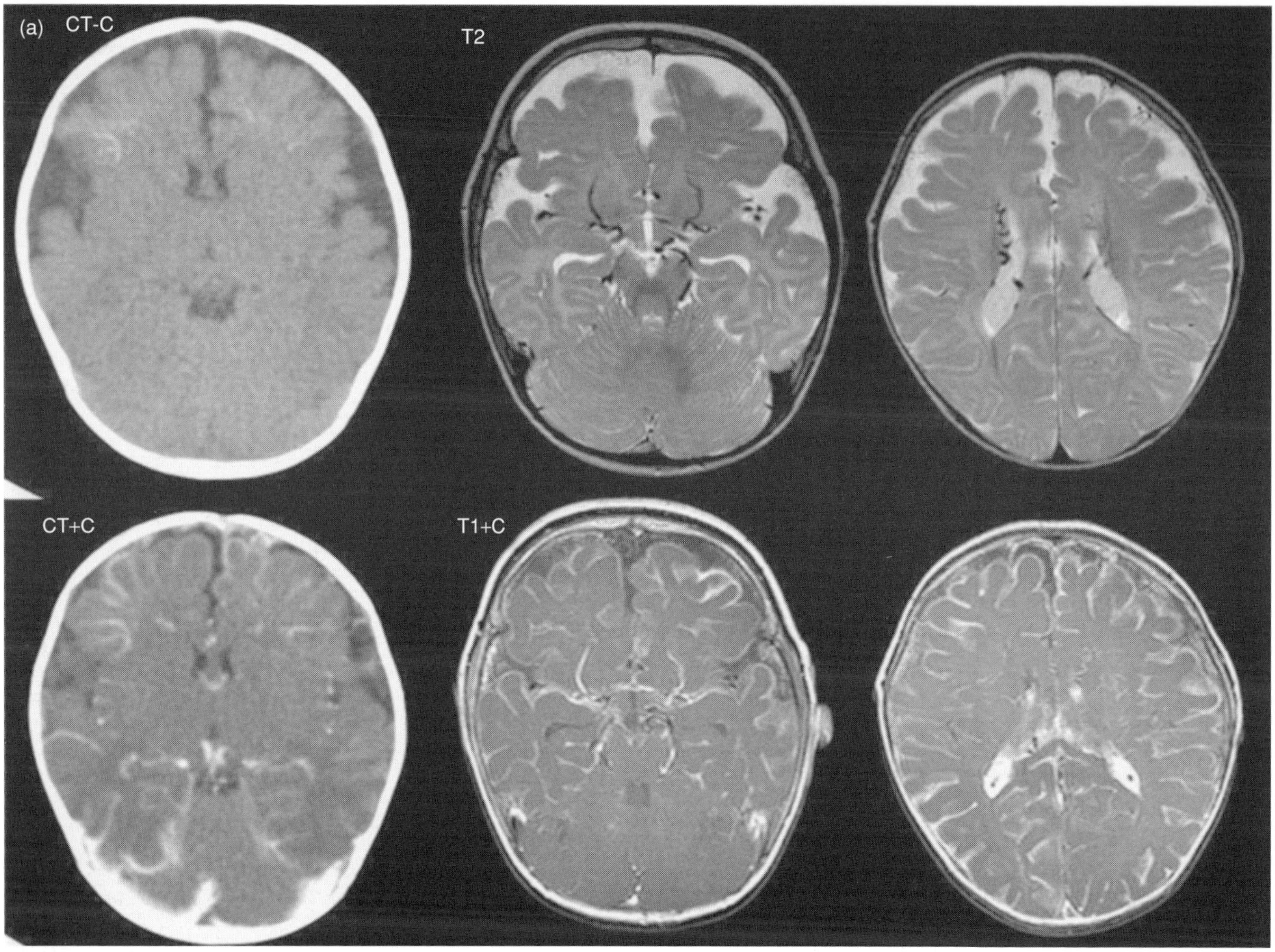

Fig. 29.4(a). Axial pre- and postcontrast CT, and axial T2-, and contrast-enhanced T1-weighted MRI in a 4-month-old boy with confirmed Sturge-Weber syndrome. CT shows subcortical frontal lobe calcifications; MRI shows prominent subependymal veins and a moderately increased leptomeningeal enhancement consistent with a bilateral leptomeningeal angiomatosis. The choroid plexus is typically enlarged in the lateral ventricles.

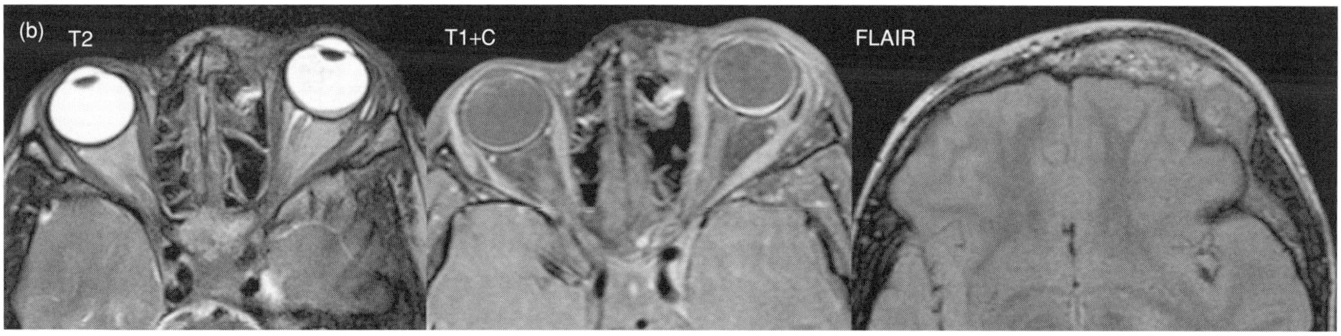

Fig. 29.4(b). Axial T2, contrast-enhanced T1 and FLAIR images in a child with Sturge-Weber syndrome. Mild thickening and increased contrast enhancement of the retinal choroid in the left eye globe are seen, as well as widening of the diploe in the adjacent left frontal bone.

involved. Cysts or clear-cell carcinomas are seen in the kidneys, cysts, islet cell tumors or microcystic serous adenomas in the pancreas, pheochromocytomas in the adrenal glands, and papillary cystadenomas in the testicles (male patients) or broad ligament of the uterus (female patients).

VHL patients should receive life-long screening including brain, spine, and abdominal studies. Renal cell carcinoma develops in 45–50% of all VHL patients and is the leading cause of death (Herron et al. 2000; Smirniotopoulos 2004; Jensen et al. 2009).

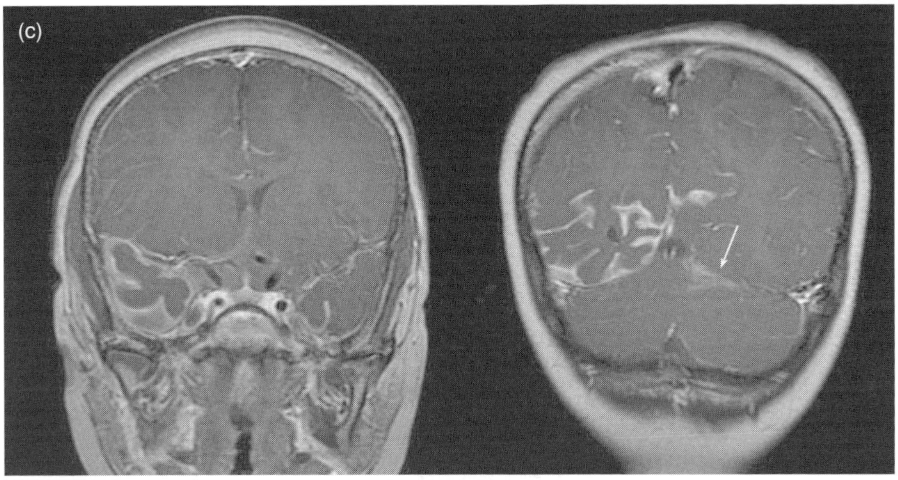

Fig. 29.4(c). Coronal contrast-enhanced T1-weighted MRI in a child with confirmed Sturge-Weber syndrome. Simultaneous supra- and infratentorial contrast enhancing leptomeningeal angiomatosis is seen affecting right temporal and occipital lobes as well as left cerebellar hemisphere (arrow).

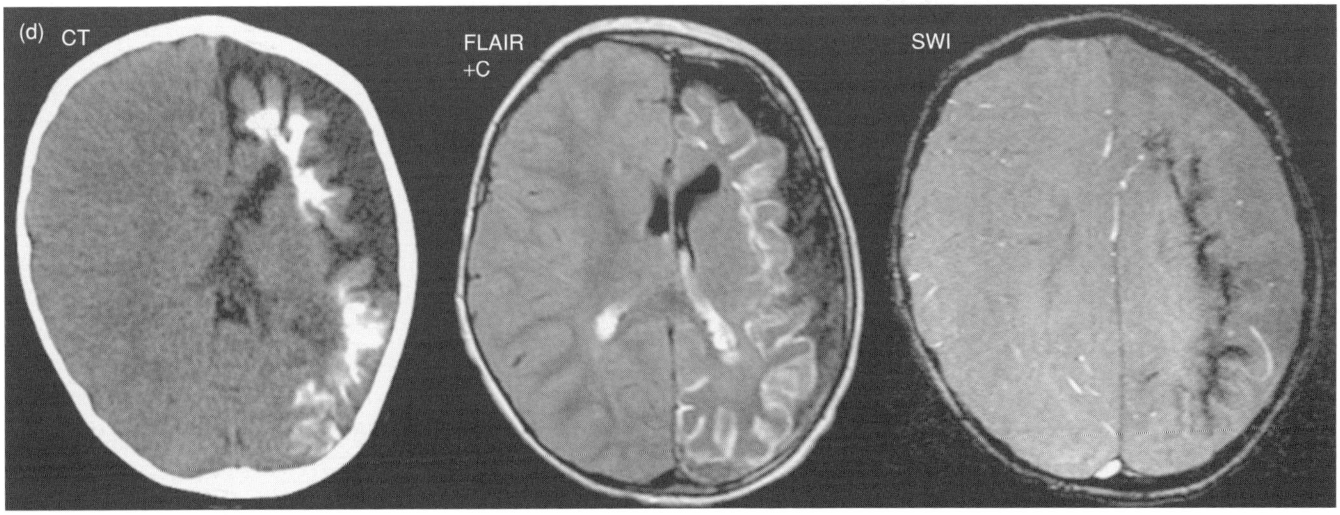

Fig. 29.4(d). Axial non-contrast-enhanced CT, contrast-enhanced fluid attenuated inversion recovery (FLAIR) and susceptibility weighted imaging (SWI) of a young child with confirmed Sturge-Weber syndrome. Dense cortical and subcortical calcifications (SWI-hypointense) are seen along the atrophic left cerebral hemisphere. A left cortical, tram-like enhancement is seen on contrast-enhanced FLAIR as well as mildly enlarged choroid plexus.

On neuroimaging, hemangioblastomas typically present with a peripherally located, sharply demarcated, strongly enhancing solid tumor nodule surrounded by a non-enhancing fluid-filled pseudocyst. The pseudocyst is not lined by a classic cyst wall; the fluid is trapped by the adjacent, compressed brain tissue. Cerebellar hemangioblastomas may change their appearance over time. Slater showed that early cerebellar hemangioblastomas present as a solid nodule and only develop an enlarging cyst on follow-up (Slater et al. 2003). MRI may show mildly dilated feeding arteries (Fig. 29.5b) due to the high tumor vascularity (Smirniotopoulos 2004). Perifocal vasogenic or venous edema may surround the lesion. Conventional catheter angiography can be helpful to identify additional lesions, especially if they are small. Dilated feeding arteries and especially the capillary tumor blush facilitates angiographic detection.

PHACE syndrome

PHACE is a rare neurocutaneous disorder characterized by posterior fossa malformations, facial hemangiomas, arterial anomalies, coarctation of the aorta/cardiac defects, and eye abnormalities (Frieden et al. 1996). The acronym PHACE may be expanded to PHACES if additional ventral developmental defects are noted such as clefts of the sternum or supraumbilical raphe (Metry et al. 2001). Nearly 90% of patients are female (Edelstein et al. 2004; Heyer et al. 2006). Migraine, seizures, developmental delay, mental retardation, and hemiparesis are seen in 90% of PHACE patients with intracerebral anomalies (Edelstein et al. 2004). The pathogenesis of PHACE syndrome is unknown (Edelstein et al. 2004; Heyer et al. 2006).

The facial hemangiomas are present at birth and may be either focal or plaque-like segmental. Four different patterns of extension have been identified: the frontotemporal region; the maxillary region respecting the nasomedial sulcus; the mandible, chin, and lower lip; and the medial frontal scalp, nasal bridge, and philtrum. If the mandibular region is affected, an increased risk for subglottic hemangiomas has been reported (7% of patients) (Poetke et al. 2002). The facial hemangioma seen in PHACE syndrome should not be mistaken for the port

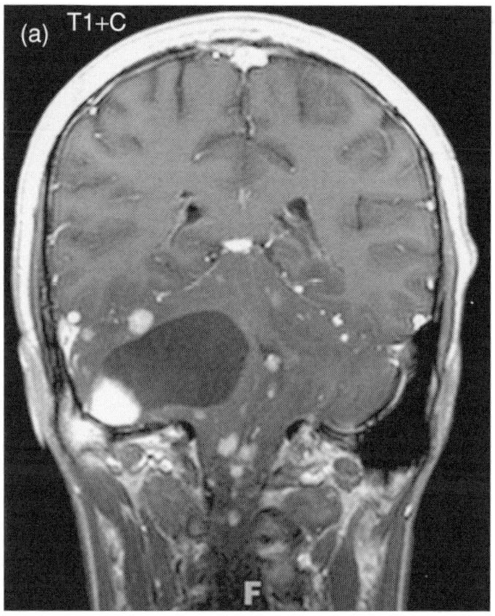

Fig. 29.5(a). Coronal contrast-enhanced T1-weighted MRI of an adolescent with confirmed von Hippel-Lindau syndrome. Multiple contrast-enhancing solid nodules are seen within both hemispheres in typical predominantly peripheral location. One right cerebellar lesion has a large cystic component. Typically the pseudocyst wall does not enhance. Additional lesions are seen along the spinal cord.

wine stain seen in SWDS. The facial hemangiomas seen in PHACE syndrome are characterized by a phase of rapid neonatal growth (proliferative phase) followed by a phase of slow regression. In contrast, the capillary malformations as seen in SWDS typically grow commensurately with the child and never regress spontaneously.

A spectrum of posterior fossa anomalies may be seen. Most frequently Dandy-Walker malformations are encountered (30–81% of patients) followed by hypoplasia or agenesis of the cerebellum and vermis (Edelstein et al. 2004). In addition, partial or complete hypoplasia/agenesis of the corpus callosum, abnormalities of the septum pellucidum, arachnoidal cysts, and rarely focal dysplasia of the cerebral cortex have been described (Edelstein et al. 2004).

Arterial anomalies are seen in at least one-third of patients (Edelstein et al. 2004; Heyer et al. 2006). Cerebrovascular pathology is categorized into congenital vascular anomalies and progressive vascular disorders. The spectrum of congenital anomalies is wide and includes aberrant origins or course of cerebral vessels, agenesis or hypoplasia of the carotid and vertebral arteries, saccular aneurysms, arterial dysplasias, persisting fetal anastomoses, and intracranial arteriovenous malformations. Stenosis or occlusion of major intracranial arteries results from a progressive vasculopathy. Ischemic stroke with focal neurological deficit may result. The vascular lesions are most frequently noted ipsilateral to the facial hemangioma (Fig. 29.6); however, bilateral involvement has also been described.

Cardiac or aortic anomalies are seen in 30% of patients. Aortic coarctation is most frequently seen. The spectrum of cardiac anomalies includes persistent ductus arteriosus, ventricular and atrial septal effect's and pulmonary stenosis (Heyer et al. 2006).

Eye abnormalities include micropthalmos, coloboma, iris hypoplasia, posterior segment abnormalities, retinal vascular abnormalities, persistent fetal retinal vessels, and optic nerve hypoplasia.

If a large facial hemangioma is identified in a neonate and PHACE syndrome is suspected, neuroimaging is indicated to exclude or confirm intracranial pathology. In addition, serial neuroimaging should be considered to rule out or to follow progressive occlusive vasculopathy. Early recognition of critical stenosis or occlusion of intracranial arteries may guide surgical revascularization in order to prevent irreversible ischemic injury (Heyer et al. 2006). Neuroimaging is fairly straightforward and takes advantage of both anatomical and functional MR sequences.

Louis-Bar syndrome or ataxia-telangiectasia

Ataxia-telangiectasia (AT) is a rare autosomal recessive neurocutaneous disorder characterized by progressive cerebellar degeneration, cerebellar ataxia, oculocutaneous telangiectasias, increased sensitivity to ionizing radiation, progressive immunodeficiency, and an increased risk for lymphoreticular malignancies (lymphoma and leukemia) (Herron et al. 2000; Edelstein et al. 2004; Jensen et al. 2009). The incidence is estimated at 1:40 000–100 000.

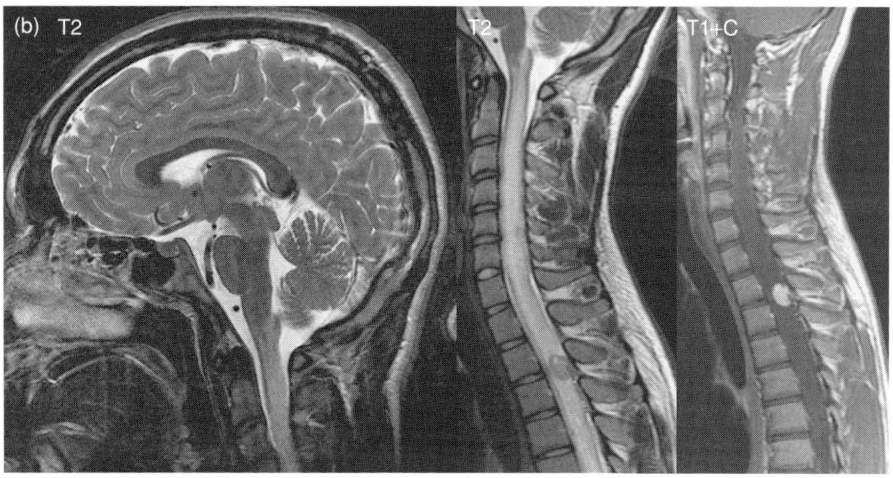

Fig. 29.5(b). Sagittal T2-weighted MRI of the brain and T2- and contrast-enhanced T1-weighted MRI of the spine in a young adult with von Hippel-Lindau syndrome shows two contrast-enhancing, highly vascularized hemangioblastomas along the spinal cord. Extensive vasogenic or venous edema is noted in the cervical spinal cord, extending into the lower brainstem. In addition, mildly enlarged feeding vessels are seen dorsally to the solid tumor nodule.

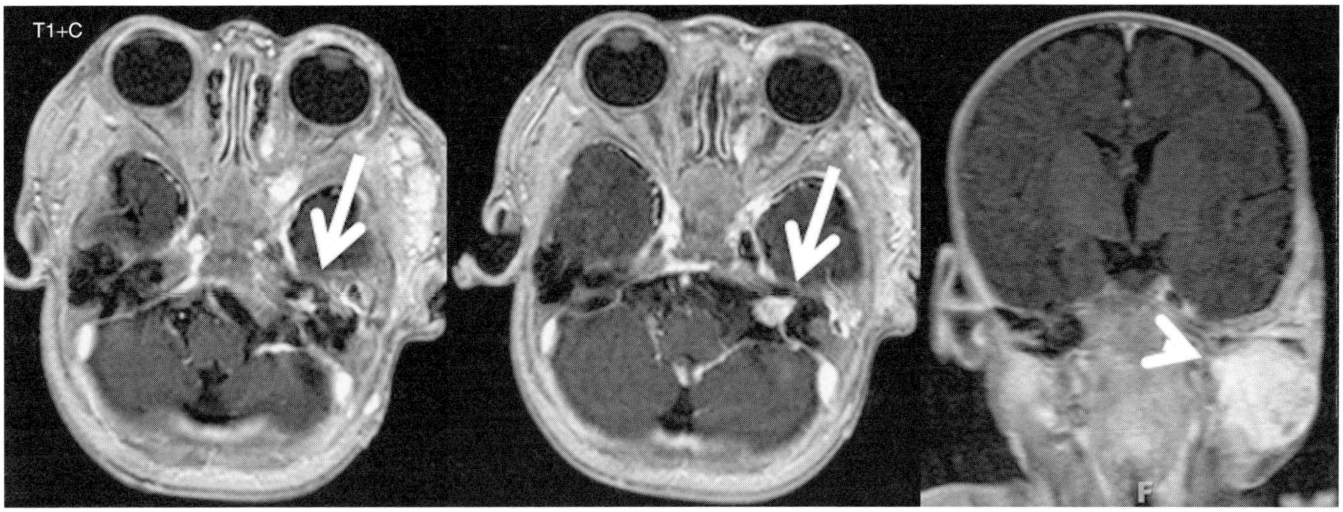

Fig. 29.6. Axial and coronal contrast-enhanced T1-weighted MRI of a young child with PHACE association. A large left-sided strongly enhancing facial hemangioma (arrowhead) is seen in combination with an equally strong enhancing hemangioma in the ipsilateral inner auditory canal extending into the cochlea (arrows).

The diagnostic criteria include an ataxic gait in the first 3 years of life; oculomotor signs and dysarthria by early school years; progressive limb ataxia, swallowing disorder, and peripheral neuropathy. In addition, at least one finding out of the following should be present: ocular telangiectasia; elevated serum alpha-fetoprotein after 1 year of age; spontaneous or radiation-induced chromosomal breakage (Jensen et al. 2009). Mucocutaneous telangiectasias are first noted on the bulbar conjunctiva, later followed by lesions in the face, neck, and palate (Edelstein et al. 2004).

Patients have a significantly reduced life expectancy because of the increased risk for malignancies, pneumonia, and intracranial hemorrhage related to the intracranial vascular abnormalities (Jensen et al. 2009).

Histologically, the cerebellum shows atrophy of all cortical layers and severe Purkinje cell loss in the vermis and cerebellar hemispheres. The neuronal degeneration most likely results from a mutation of the designated ataxia-telangiectasia mutated or *ATM* gene. ATM expression is especially high in areas of Purkinje cell precursors. Consequently, an *ATM* mutation will result in a faulty cerebellar neurogenesis (Edelstein et al. 2004). In addition, ATM is activated in response to double-strand DNA breaks. *ATM* mutations are also believed to result in defective repair of these DNA breaks, which may explain the increased radiosensitivity of AT patients (Edelstein et al. 2004). The high sensitivity to ionizing radiation increases the risk for malignancies 100 to 1200 times. Consequently, 10–15% of all AT patients suffer from lymphoreticular malignancies by early adulthood (Edelstein et al. 2004). In addition, there is an increased risk for malignant intracranial tumors such as medulloblastomas and gliomas.

A small or absent thymus is related to a higher incidence of sinus and pulmonary infections, with secondary complications such as bronchiectasis and pulmonary arteriovenous fistulae (Edelstein et al. 2004).

Telangiectatic vessels are seen in the leptomeninges as well as an abnormal cortical vasculature (Edelstein et al. 2004).

Neuroimaging reveals cerebellar cortical atrophy, especially affecting the superior vermis, as well as atrophy of the dentate and olivary nuclei and degeneration of the posterior columns. The atrophy is typically progressive over time with increasing widening of the cerebellar fissures. Intraparenchymal hemorrhages may result from ruptured parenchymal telangiectasias. Chronic inflammatory sinus disease may be seen as well as a small or absent thymus in the upper mediastinum. Radiographic studies including CT should be avoided to minimize the risk for radiation-induced malignancies.

REFERENCES

Alkan A, Sigirci A, Kutlu R, Ozcan H, Erdem G, Aslan M, et al. (2005) Neurofibromatosis type 1: Diffusion weighted imaging findings of brain. Eur J Radiol 56: 229–234.

Arulrajah S, Ertan G, Jordan L, Tekes A, Khaykin E, Izbudak I, Huisman TA (2009) Magnetic resonance imaging and diffusion-weighted imaging of normal appearing white matter in children and young adults with tuberous sclerosis complex. Neuroradiology 51: 781–786.

Arulrajah S, Ertan G, Comi A, Tekes A, Lin DL, Huisman TA (2010) MRI with diffusion-weighted imaging in children with simultaneous supra- and infratentorial manifestations of Sturge-Weber syndrome. J Neuroradiol 37: 51–59.

Carella A, Medicamento N (1997) malignant evolution of presumed benign lesions in the brain in neurofibromatosis: case report. Neuroradiology 39: 639–641.

Eastwood JD, Fiorella DJ, MacFall JF, Delong DM, Provenzale JM, Greenwood RS (2001) Increased brain apparent diffusion coefficient in children with neurofibromatosis type 1. Radiology 219: 354–358.

Edelstein S, Naidich TP, Newton TH (2004) The rare phakomatoses. Neurimag Clin N Am 14: 185–217.

Eluvathingal TJ, Behen ME, Chugani HT, Janisse J, Bernardi B, Chakraborty P, et al. (2006) Cerebellar lesions in tuberous sclerosis complex: Neurobehavioral and neuroimaging correlates. J Child Neurol 21: 846–851.

Ertan G, Arulrajah S, Tekes A, Jordan L, Huisman TA (2010) Cerebellar abnormality in children and young adults with tuberous sclerosis complex: MR and diffusion weighted imaging findings. J Neuroradiol 37: 231–238.

Frieden IJ, Reese V, Cohen D (1996) PHACE syndrome: the association of posterior fossa brain malformations, hemangiomas, arterial anomalies, coarctation of the aorta and cardiac defects, and eye abnormalities. Arch Dermatol 132: 307–311.

Gläsker S, van Velthoven V (2005) Risk of hemorrhage in hemangioblastomas of the central nervous system. Neurosurgery 57(1): 71–76.

Goh WH, Khong P-L, Leung CS, Wong VC (2004) T2-weighted hyperintensities (unidentified bright objects) in children with neurofibromatosis 1: Their impact on cognitive function. J Child Neurol 19: 853–858.

Herron J, Darrah R, Quaghebeur G (2000) Intra-cranial manifestations of the neurocutaneous syndromes. Clin Radiol 55: 82–98.

Heyer GL, Millar WS, Ghatan S, Garzon MC (2006) The neurologic aspects of PHACE: Case report and review of the literature. Pediatr Neurol 35: 419–424.

Ilgren EB, Kinnier-Wilson LM, Stiller CA (1985) Gliomas in neurofibromatosis: a series of 89 cases with evidence for increased malignancy in associated cerebellar astrocytomas. Pathol Annu 79: 582–588.

Jensen L, Heath KJ, Byard RW (2009) Sudden death and the forensic evaluation of neurocutaneous syndromes. J Forensic Leg Med 16: 369–374.

Korf BR (2004) The phakomatoses. Neuroimag Clin N Am 14: 139–148.

Lin DDM, Barker PB (2006) Neuroimaging of phakomatoses. Semin Pediatr Neurol 13: 48–62.

Lin DD, Barker PB, Kraut MA, Comi A (2003) Early characteristics of Sturge-Weber syndrome shown by perfusion MR imaging and proton MR spectroscopic imaging. AJNR Am J Neuroradiol 24: 1912–1915.

Metry DW, Dowd CF, Barkovich AJ, Frieden IJ (2001) The many faces of PHACE syndrome. J Pediatr 139: 117–123.

Moore GJ, Slovis TL, Chugani HT (1998) Proton magnetic resonance spectroscopy in children with Sturge-Weber syndrome. J Child Neurol 13: 332–335.

Pascual-Castroviejo I, Pascual-Pascual SI, Viano J, Carceller F, Gutierrez-Molina M, Morales C, Frutos-Martinez R (2010) Posterior fossa tumors in children with neurofibromatosis type 1 (NF1) Childs Nerv Syst 26: 1599–1603.

Pavesi G, Berlucchi S, Munari M, Manara R, Scienza R, Opocher G (2010) Clinical and surgical features of lower brain stem hemangioblastomas in von Hippel-Lindau disease. Acta Neurochir 152: 287–292.

Poetke M, Frommeld T, Berlien HP (2002) PHACE syndrome: new views on diagnostic criteria. Eur J Pediatr Surg 12: 366–374.

Pothula VB, Lesser T, Mallucci C, May P, Foy P (2001) Vestibular schwannomas in children. Otol Neurotol 22: 903–907.

Rodriguez D, Young Poussaint T (2004) Neuroimaging findings in neurofibromatosis type 1 and 2. Neuroimag Clin N Am 14: 149–170.

Smirniotopoulos JG (2004) Neuroimaging of phakomatoses: Sturge-Weber syndrome, tuberous sclerosis, von Hippel-Lindau syndrome. Neuroimag Clin N Am 14: 171–183.

Smith-Pearl M, Abdalla WM, Lin DD, Comi AM, Boltshauser E, Gailloud P, Huisman TA (2009) Sturge-Weber syndrome with cerebellar involvement. J Neuroradiol 36: 57–60.

Slater A, Moore NR, Huson SM (2003) The natural history of cerebellar hemangioblastomas in von Hippel-Lindau disease. AJNR Am J Neuroradiol 24: 1570–1574.

Stranzinger E, Huisman TA (2007) Sturge-Weber. Early manifestation and visualization of disease course. Radiologe 47: 1126–1130.

Thomas-Sohl KA, Vaslow DF, Maria BL (2004) Sturge-Weber syndrome: a review. Pediatr Neurol 30: 303–310.

Vinchon M, Soto-Ares G, Ruchoux M-M, Dhellemmas P (2000) Cerebellar gliomas in children with NF1: pathology and surgery Childs Nerv Syst 16: 417–420.

Weber AM, Egelhoff JC, McKellop JM, Franz DN (2000) Autism and the cerebellum: evidence from tuberous sclerosis. J Autism Dev Disord 30: 511–517.

Yohay K (2006) Neurofibromatosis types 1 and 2. Neurologist 12: 86–93.

Part 6
Cerebellar Disruptions

30
Prenatal Cerebellar Disruptions

Andrea Poretti and Eugen Boltshauser

Disruptions are defined as morphological defects of an organ, part of an organ, or a larger region of the body resulting from an extrinsic breakdown of, or an interference with, an originally normal developmental process (Reardon and Donnai 2007). *Malformations* are defined as morphological defects of an organ, part of an organ, or a larger region of the body resulting from an intrinsically abnormal developmental process. It may well be that genetic factors contribute to the susceptibility to disruptions such as autosomal dominant porencephaly in *COL4A1* mutation (de Vries et al. 2009).

Typical disruptive mechanisms include a number of infectious agents (classically toxoplasmosis, rubella virus, cytomegalovirus, herpes virus, and human immunodeficiency virus), haemorrhages (in part favoured by cerebrovascular anomalies, congenital tumours or infections, and maternal septic shock), ischemias, mechanical effects (amnion rupture sequence, mechanical effects due to invasive procedures for prenatal diagnosis), drugs with teratogenic effects, e.g., alcohol, cocaine, isoretinoin, phenytoin, valproic acid, warfarin), and maternal conditions (such as maternal diabetes mellitus type 1 or maternal phenylketonuria) (Lammens et al. 2006). Typical examples of disruptions are twin disruption sequence (Zankl et al. 2004), amnion rupture sequence (Van Allen et al. 1987), and hydranencephaly (Van Allen 1992).

Disruptive mechanisms can affect the cerebrum and/or the cerebellum. However, cerebrum and cerebellum have variable vulnerability to the different disruptive factors in the prenatal period. On the basis of the disorders described, it appears that in the prenatal period the cerebellum is particularly vulnerable to infections and haemorrhages (Boltshauser 2001). Prenatal cerebellar ischemic stroke is, however, rare (Ansari et al. 2011). Perinatally, the cerebellum is vulnerable in extremely preterm babies, whereas metabolic and toxic insults particularly affect the cerebellum in the postnatal period. However, the cerebellum is mostly resistant to pre-, peri-, and postnatal hypoxic-ischemic events (Steinlin et al. 1998; Boltshauser 2001; Poretti et al. 2008a) and reports of cerebellar involvement in perinatal hypoxia in neonates at term are few (Table 30.1) (Sargent et al. 2004; Connolly et al. 2007; Limperopoulos et al. 2009). Central to the cerebellum's susceptibility to disruptions is its protracted developmental process, which extends from 4 weeks of gestation until at least 2 years postnatal (ten Donkelaar et al. 2003).

The prenatal cerebellar disruptions which are discussed in this chapter are global cerebellar hypoplasia, cerebellar cleft, unilateral cerebellar hypoplasia, and vanishing cerebellum in myelomeningocele. Cerebellar agenesis has been discussed separately (see Chapter 7). Indeed, some disorders such as global cerebellar hypoplasia, cerebellar agenesis, and cerebellar cortical dysplasia may be due to a 'malformation' as well as to a 'disruption'.

TABLE 30.1
Cerebellar vulnerability

Conditions	Cerebellar vulnerability
Hypoxic-ischemic events including perinatal asphyxia at term	(+)
Postnatal infections	+
Prematurity (<30 weeks gestational age)	+
Prenatal infections (in particular cytomegalovirus)	++
Prenatal hemorrhages	+++
Toxicity/selected drugs	+++
Metabolic disorders	++++

From Poretti A et al. Eur J Paediatr Neurol 2009; 13: 397–407.

Global cerebellar hypoplasia

The term 'global cerebellar hypoplasia' describes a cerebellum with reduced volume, while cerebellar shape is (near) normal, the cerebellar structures do not fill a normally configurated posterior fossa, or a small cerebellum is found within a small posterior fossa (Boltshauser 2004). In this section we will discuss only global cerebellar hypoplasia due to prenatal cerebellar disruptions. For a comprehensive review of cerebellar hypoplasia see Chapter 8.

Global cerebellar hypoplasia is a heterogeneous condition and can be due to a variety of causes, both malformations and disruptions (Sarnat and Alcala 1980). Typical causes of *malformations* include chromosomal aberrations, several metabolic disorders, isolated genetic cerebellar hypoplasias, complex genetic malformations or migration disorders such as lissencephaly, some types of congenital muscular dystrophies, and pontocerebellar hypoplasias. However, prenatal infections, particularly cytomegalovirus (CMV), are typical causes of *disruptions* (Barkovich and Lindan 1994; de Vries et al. 2004), while exposure to teratogenic drugs such as anticonvulsant drugs (Squier et al. 1990) or cocaine (Bellini et al. 2000) can probably cause both *malformations* and *disruptions* depending on the drug and the time of the insult.

Prenatal cytomegalovirus infection

In general, several potential pathogenetic mechanisms by which CMV may injure the central nervous system have been suggested (Cheeran et al. 2009). Because CMV can infect endothelial cells of CNS capillaries and other vessels, it has been postulated that a viral angiitis may be responsible for perfusion failure of the developing brain, causing cerebral tissue ischemia and infarction, particularly in the periventricular region (Marques Dias et al. 1984). Such lesions during fetal development may interfere with radial glial cells or their fibres, leading to migration disorders. However, recent studies reported that CMV acts as a teratogen, disrupting normal cellular differentiation, and induces apoptosis (Cheeran et al. 2009). A wide variety of cells in the central nervous system including astrocytes, oligodendrocytes, neurons, and endothelial cells can be infected by CMV (Odeberg et al. 2006; Luo et al. 2008; Cheeran et al. 2009). Typically, CMV infects the cells in the ventricular and periventricular zones, where the neural stem cells are located (Cheeran et al. 2009). Therefore, CMV can disrupt their health and function causing neuronal migration abnormalities and inducing loss of these cells due to inhibition of the cell cycle or increased cell death by apoptosis (Odeberg et al. 2006). CMV can inhibit the differentiation of neural precursor cells into neurons and may disrupt the maturation of oligodendrocytes (Cheeran et al. 2009). Additionally, alterations in the micro-environment of the developing brain due to cytokines generated by resident glial cells and infiltrating immune cells may induce apoptosis of cells in the fetal brain (Cheeran et al. 2009).

Approximately 1% of all newborn infants are congenitally infected with CMV (Jones 2003). However, only 10% of these will have typical symptoms at birth such as hepatomegaly, splenomegaly, and petechiae. CNS manifestations are common and include lethargy, poor feeding, seizures, hyper- or hypotonia, microcephaly, chorioretinitis, and sensorineural deafness. About 10–15% of the asymptomatic and almost all symptomatic newborn infants develop neurological impairments, sensorineural hearing loss, and decreased vision. The severity of the neurological symptoms is highly variable and usually correlates with the timing of the infection during the pregnancy. At the severe end of the spectrum are profound mental retardation, spasticity, and seizures; at the mild end behavioral and motor coordination problems. The neurological symptoms seem to be related particularly to the cerebral and less to the cerebellar abnormalities.

Distinct neuroimaging findings in congenital CMV infection include multifocal lesions, predominantly involving the deep parietal white matter with relative sparing of both the arcuate fibres and the white matter adjacent to the ventricles (Fig. 30.1) (Barkovich and Lindan 1994; de Vries et al. 2004; van der Knaap et al. 2004; Mejaski-Bosnjak 2008; van der Voom et al. 2009; Fink et al. 2010). In the affected white matter apparent diffusion coefficient (ADC) values were increased, fractional anisotropy (FA) and magnetization transfer ratio (MTR) values were reduced, concentrations of total *N*-acetylaspartate and choline-containing compounds were reduced, and myoinositol concentrations were slightly increased (van der Voom et al. 2009). These changes reflect loss of tissue in the injured white matter with damage to myelin and axonal membranes in the white matter with losses of oligodendrocytes, myelin sheaths and axons. This suggests that the pathology of white matter lesions in congenital CMV infections is characterized by axonal loss, lack of myelin deposition due to damage, loss of oligodendrocytes within the developing white matter, and astrogliosis (van der Voom et al. 2009). Additional typical neuroimaging findings are focal enlargement of the anterior temporal horn and subcortical cysts. Early infections affect neuronal growth and migration including gyral abnormalities such as lissencephaly, pachygyria, and polymicrogyria in most patients (Fig. 30.1) (Barkovich and Lindan 1994; de Vries et al. 2004; van der Knaap et al. 2004). On the basis of the gyral abnormalities it is possible to determine the timing of the infection. If lissencephaly is present, the infection is more likely to have occurred before 16–18 weeks, whereas in the case of polymicrogyria the infection probably occurred between 18 and 24 weeks of gestation (de Vries et al. 2004). Additional inconsistent neuroimaging findings of early infections are cerebellar hypoplasia and calcification (Fig. 30.1) (Barkovich and Lindan 1994; de Vries et al. 2004; van der Knaap et al. 2004). The severity of the cerebellar abnormalities also usually correlates with the timing of the infection during the pregnancy and the appearance of the cerebral hemispheres. In patients with complete lissencephaly and thin cerebral cortex, the cerebellum is small and shrunken, with thin cortex and shallow sulci, the hemispheres are extremely small, and the vermis is not seen at all; cerebellar calficication can be present (Patel and Barkovich 2002). In patients with diffuse polymicrogyria, the cerebellum is nearly normal in size, with much milder dysplasia of the folial pattern (Patel and Barkovich 2002). In seven patients with less prominent clinical signs (microcephaly, hearing deficits, and minor neurological impairment), very likely due to a CMV infection in the third trimester, Steinlin et al. did not detect cerebellar involvement (Steinlin et al. 1996). Indeed, late-onset infections do not affect neuronal migration and organization, but mainly lead to cerebral white matter lesions (Barkovich and Lindan 1994; de Vries et al. 2004; van der Knaap et al. 2004; van der Voom et al. 2009).

Because postnatal CMV infection is very common it is important that the diagnostic test is performed in the first 3 weeks after birth. A positive test thereafter can indicate either a pre-, peri-, or postnatal infection. If the patient presents beyond the neonatal period, the diagnosis may be confirmed by presence of CMV-DNA in dried blood during newborn bloodspot screening.

In a neonate with congenital infection, the differential diagnosis includes any of the TORCH (toxoplasmosis, rubella, CMV, herpes simplex) agents. In particular, congenital toxoplasmosis can mimic congenital CMV infection. In this case, the MRI pattern of CMV infection can be helpful. However, this MRI pattern can also be caused by loss-of-function mutations in the gene encoding the RNASET2 glycoprotein (Henneke et al. 2009).

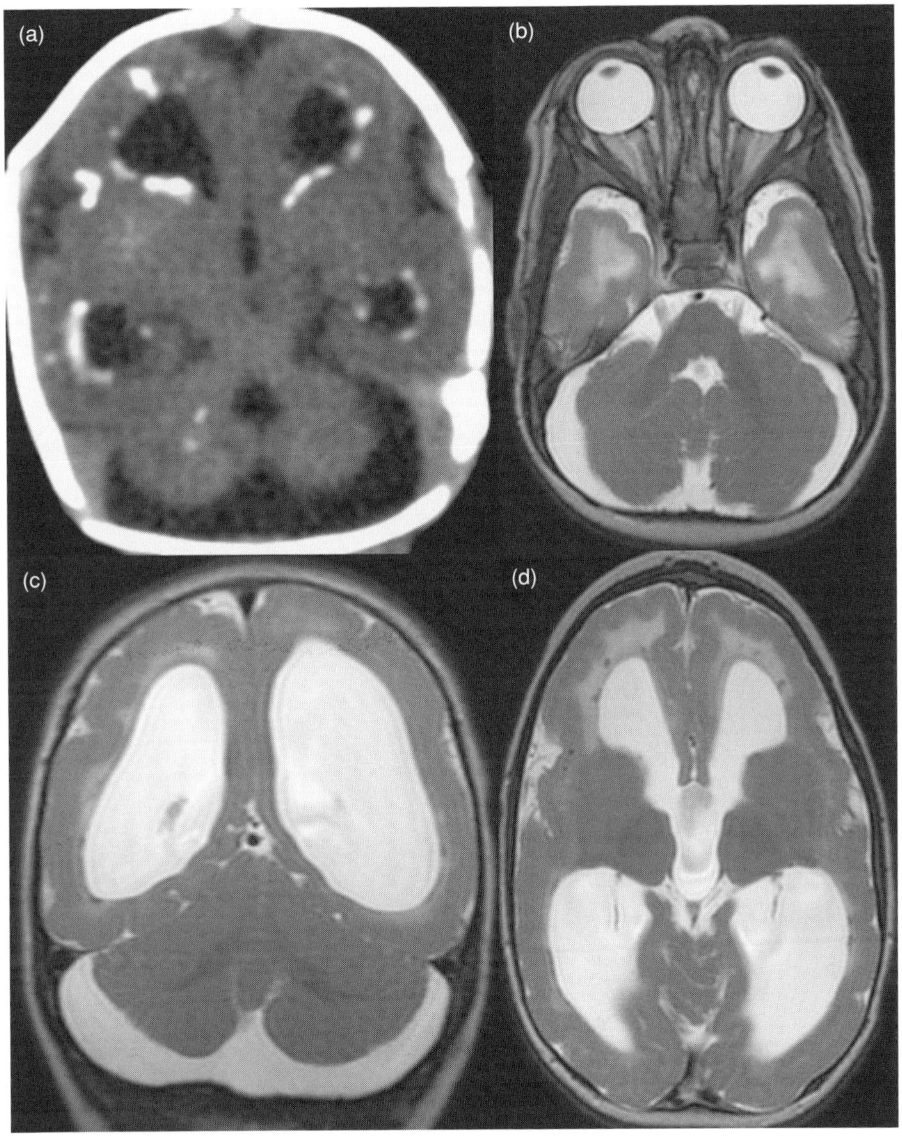

Fig. 30.1. Congenital cytomegalovirus infection. **(a)** axial CT on day 2 showing ventriculomegaly, cerebellar hypoplasia, and periventricular hyperdensities representing calcification; **(b)** axial T2-weighted MRI at the age of 14 months revealing cerebellar hypoplasia as well as hyperintensity of the white matter and polymicrogyria of both temporal lobes; **(c)** coronal T2-weighted MRI demonstrating global cerebellar hypoplasia, enlarged lateral ventricles, hyperintensity of the white matter, and cortical gyral anomalies such as pachygyria and polymicrogyria; **(d)** axial T2-weighted image demonstrating enlarged lateral and third ventricles, hyperintensity of the white matter, cortical gyral anomalies such as pachygyria and polymicrogyria, and periventricular hypointensities suggestive of calcification. (Reprinted with permission from Poretti A et al. Eur J Paediatr Neurol 2009; 13: 397–407.)

Cerebellar cleft

Cerebellar clefts are characterized by a cleft affecting principally the cortical gray matter of one cerebellar hemisphere and extending from the surface into the parenchyma (Fig. 30.2) (Poretti et al. 2008b, 2009b). Malorientation of the cerebellar foliation, irregular gray/white matter junction, and a lack of the normal architecture of the white matter confined only to the region adjacent to the cleft are additional typical neuroimaging findings. Cerebellar clefts are probably not rare, but under-recognized: only 18 patients had been previously reported (Poretti et al. 2008b, 2009b; Boddaert et al. 2010).

We suggest that cerebellar clefts may be the result of a prenatally acquired local event, mostly a haemorrhage. Our hypothesis is supported by the following observations: in two cases a fetal cerebellar haemorrhage could be detected in the 24th week of gestation (Fig. 30.3); history of prenatal injury in one child reported by Boddaert et al. (2010); the unilaterality of both cerebellar clefts and dysplasia (in contrast to the global cerebellar cortical dysplasia with probably a genetic origin; Demaerel et al. 1998; Demaerel 2002); the associated supratentorial abnormalities (schizencephaly (Fig. 30.4) and sparse bilateral, asymmetric, paratrigonal subependymal heterotopia) may be caused by vascular disruptions such as focal haemorrhage or ischemia (Barkovich and Kjos 1992; Takano et al. 1999; Dale and Coleman 2002; Battaglia et al. 2003a, 2003b; Curry et al. 2005); the lack of dysmorphic features, congenital malformations in other organ systems or recurrence in other family members. Other causes such as a transient hypotension in early fetal life or an ischemic event seem to be unlikely: none of the clefts was localized in a cerebellar watershed zone.

Increasing experience with prenatal ultrasound (Ranzini et al. 1998; Robins et al. 1998; Sharony et al. 1999; Hiller et al. 2003; Yuksel and Batukan 2003; Ortiz et al. 2004; Lerner et al. 2006) and greater availability of fetal MRI (Gorincour et al. 2006; Malinger et al. 2006, 2009; Nomura et al. 2009) has demonstrated the prenatal occurrence of cerebellar haemorrhages. Possible causes include cerebrovascular anomaly (Sharony et al. 1999; Lerner et al. 2006), tumour, congenital

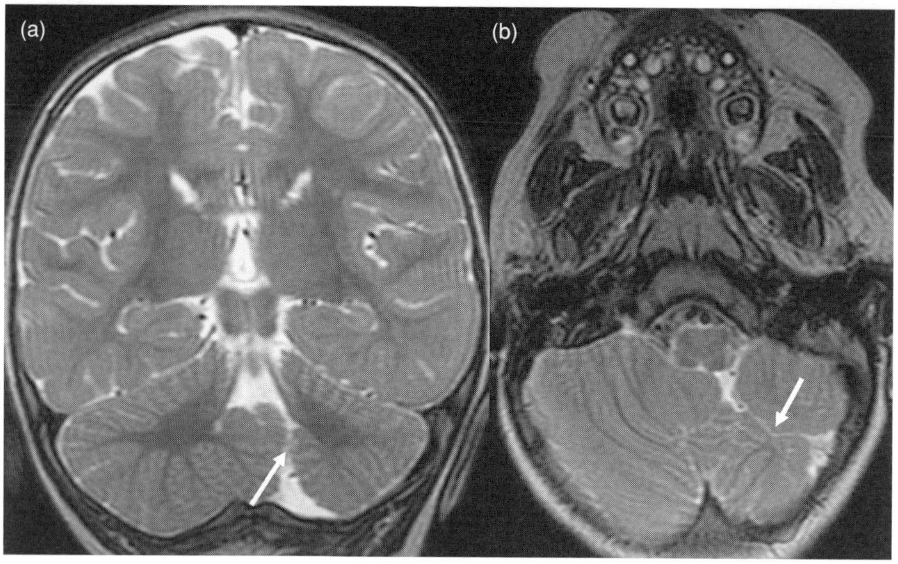

Fig. 30.2. Unilateral cerebellar cleft in a child aged 1 year 6 months. **(a)** Coronal T2-weighted MRI revealing a left paravermian cleft extending to lateral recessus of the fourth ventricle; **(b)** axial T2-weighted MRI showing a left sided cleft, malorientation of the adjacent cerebellar folia, and abnormal arborization of the white matter. (Reprinted with permission from Poretti A et al. Neuropediatrics 2008; 39: 106–112.)

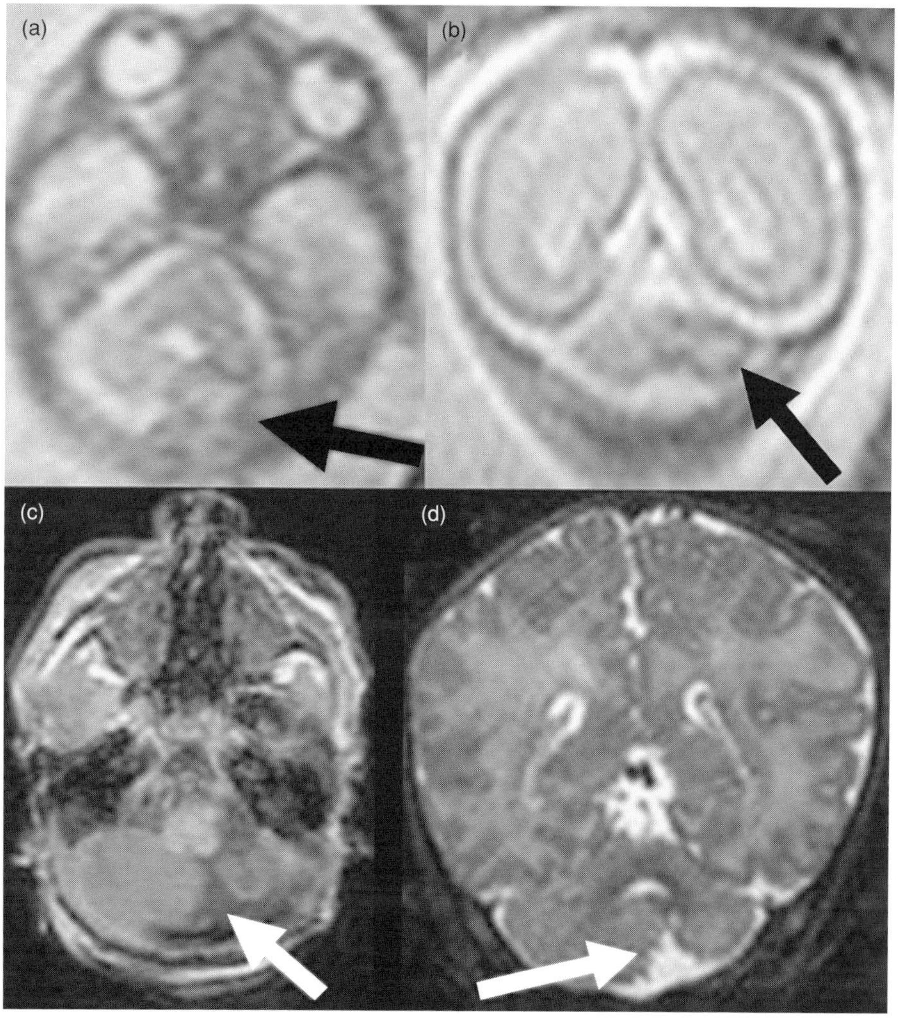

Fig. 30.3. (a, b) Axial and coronal T2-weighted fetal MRI at 24 weeks of gestation showing hypointensity and irregular contour of the left cerebellar hemisphere suggestive of hemorrhage. **(c, d)** axial T1-weighted MRI and coronal T2-weighted MRI of the same patient 1 month after birth demonstrating a paravermian cleft reaching to the fourth ventricle and clear volume reduction of the left cerebellar hemisphere. (Reprinted with permission from Poretti A et al. Neuropediatrics 2008; 39: 106–112.)

infection including cytomegalovirus (Ortiz et al. 2004) and B-19 parvovirus (Glenn et al. 2007), or maternal septic shock (Nomura et al. 2009). In most cases the aetiology remains unidentified (Robins et al. 1998; Hiller et al. 2003; Yuksel and Batukan 2003; Gorincour et al. 2006; Malinger et al. 2006). Cerebellar haemorrhages were detected between 18 and 24 weeks of gestation. In the two cases with cerebellar clefts they were found at 24 weeks of gestation. Merrill et al. reported

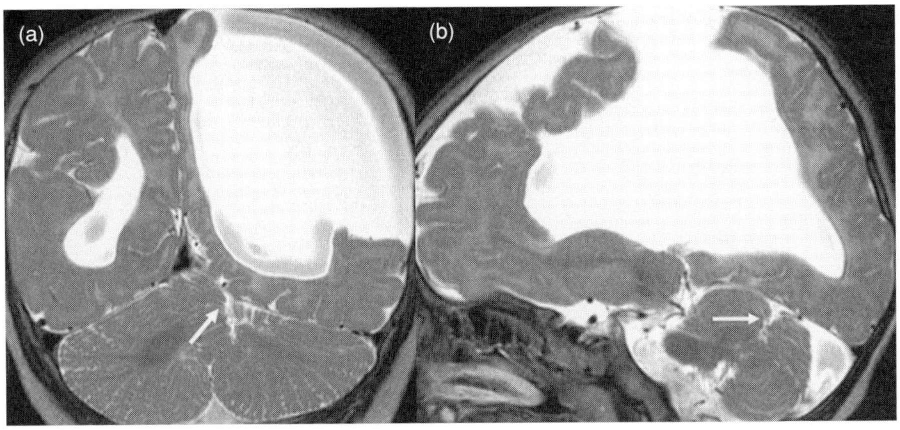

Fig. 30.4. Child at the age of 8 months. **(a)** coronal T2-weighted MRI showing a cleft in the left cerebellar hemisphere and bilateral open lip schizencephaly; **(b)** parasagittal T2-weighted MRI demonstrating a cleft in the superior left cerebellar hemisphere and malorientation of the cerebellar folia. (Reprinted with permission from Poretti A et al. Neuropediatrics 2008; 39: 106–112.)

that cerebellar haemorrhages may occur within germinal matrices located in the subpial external granule cell layer, which is thickest at 24 weeks' gestation and begins to involute at 30 weeks' gestation (Merrill et al. 1998). It seems plausible that the period between the 20th and 24th weeks of gestation is the most vulnerable for cerebellar haemorrhages.

Cerebellar haemorrhages are also a known complication of very low birthweight preterm infants, with up to 19% of infants born under 750g developing ultrasonographic evidence of a cerebellar haemorrhage (Johnsen et al. 2005; Limperopoulos et al. 2005; Dyet et al. 2006; Sehgal et al. 2009; Steggerda et al. 2009). Concomitant supratentorial lesions are common, but in about 25% of cases haemorrhage is confined to the cerebellum (Limperopoulos et al. 2005). Risk factors include multiple gestations, twin to twin transfusion, emergency cesarean delivery, fetal heart rate abnormalities, need for cardiotropins, neonatal sepsis, and patent ductus arteriosus (Limperopoulos et al. 2005; Sehgal et al. 2009). Two of our patients were born preterm at 24 and 30 weeks' gestation, respectively, after a twin pregnancy with twin to twin transfusion in one case (Poretti et al. 2009b). One infant developed bilateral intraparenchymal cerebellar haemorrhages seen on MRI 3 weeks after birth at 32 weeks post-menstrual age. At the age of 14 months, the MRI showed bilateral cerebellar clefts. In the other, an intraparenchymal cerebellar haemorrhage in the left hemisphere was detected on MRI at the age of 4 months (corrected age 40 weeks of gestation) (Poretti et al. 2009b). At the age of 1 year 10 months, the MRI showed a cerebellar cleft (Poretti et al. 2009b). Therefore, cerebellar clefts can represent residual changes also after neonatal cerebellar haemorrhage in preterm infants.

The clinical presentation was highly variable. Typical cerebellar signs included truncal ataxia in five cases (mild to minimal), dysarthria and minimal limb ataxia in four, and ocular motor apraxia and general muscular hypotonia in three. Truncal muscular hypotonia, spasticity, and epileptic seizures were found only in the two patients with associated schizencephaly. Eight patients had mental retardation (particularly severe in one patient with extensive supratentorial abnormalities). Other nonspecific findings included speech impairment (6), various behavioral changes (5), and other ocular movement disorders (2). Altogether, neurological outcome in children with cerebellar clefts depends mainly on supratentorial lesions.

The clefts were located in the left cerebellar hemisphere in 10 cases, in the right in four, and bilaterally in one (Figs 30.2, 30.3, 30.4). Precise localization was difficult because they traverse different lobules. In all patients the vermis was not involved. Malorientation of the cerebellar foliation, an irregular gray/white matter junction, and a lack of the normal architecture of the white matter confined only to the region adjacent to the cleft were consistently present. In all patients the affected hemispheres were reduced in volume (severe in one, moderate in five, mild in seven, and minimal in two), resulting in asymmetric sizes of the cerebellar hemispheres. Extension of the cleft into the fourth ventricle was seen in six patients.

Supratentorial abnormalities were found in five cases: schizencephaly (Fig. 30.4) and sparse bilateral, asymmetric, paratrigonal subependymal heterotopia in two cases mild ventriculomegaly and an atretic occipital encephalocele in one.

Unilateral cerebellar hypoplasia

Unilateral cerebellar hypoplasia (UCH) is a rare finding representing a spectrum ranging from 'complete' aplasia (unilateral absence of one cerebellar hemisphere) through subtotal asymmetric hypoplasia to mild asymmetry in the size of the cerebellar hemispheres (Poretti et al. 2009a, 2010) (Figs 30.5, 30.6). In our experience, minor asymmetry of the cerebellar hemispheres is occasionally seen as an incidental finding without clinical significance. However, a severe UCH is expected to be of clinical relevance.

UCH was first described by Strong in the postmortem examination of a 3-year-old girl with mental retardation (Strong 1915). Since then additional pathological reports have been published (Mackiewicz 1935; Tennstedt 1965; Simon and Kafritsas 1992). The advent of CT and MRI has facilitated the recognition of this lesion in vivo and 31 non-neuropathological cases have since been published (Mendelsohn et al. 1983; Harbord et al. 1989; Altman et al. 1992; Meyer et al. 1994; Boltshauser et al. 1996; Robins et al. 1998; Mancini et al. 2001; Erdogan et al. 2002; McCollom and Rashidian 2003; Sztriha and Johansen 2005; Gallini et al. 2006; Gross-Tsur

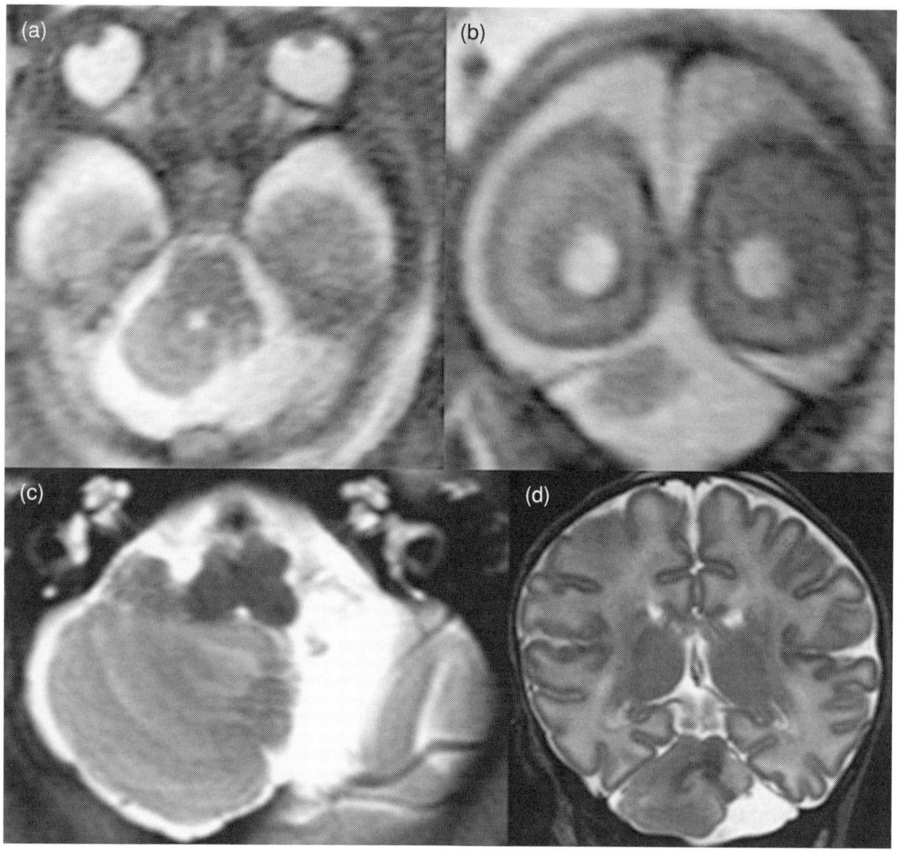

Fig. 30.5. Fetal MRI at 21 weeks of gestation. **(a, b)** Axial T2-weighted and coronal T2-weighted MRI showing severe hypoplasia of the left cerebellar hemisphere. Postnatal follow-up MRI at 1 month. **(c)** Axial T2-weighted MRI showing almost complete absence of the left cerebellar hemisphere, normal structure of the vermis, and an asymmetric brainstem (volume reduced contralateral to the hypoplastic cerebellar hemisphere) and asymmetric posterior fossa (volume reduced ipsilateral to the hypoplastic cerebellar hemisphere); **(d)** coronal T2-weighted MRI demonstrating severe hypoplasia of the left cerebellar hemisphere. (Reprinted with permission from Poretti A et al. Dev Med Child Neurol 2010; 52: 718–724.)

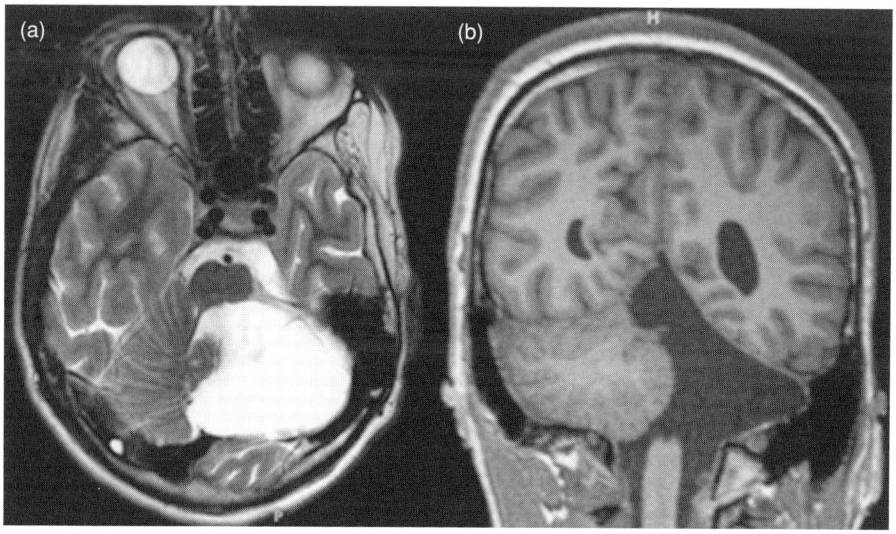

Fig. 30.6. Patient with severe unilateral cerebellar hypoplasia at 6 years 10 months. **(a)** Axial T2-weighted MRI showing almost complete absence of the left cerebellar hemisphere and the normal structure of the right cerebellar hemisphere; **(b)** coronal T1-weighted MRI presenting almost complete absence of the left cerebellar hemisphere and the normal structure on the right. Additionally, there is a mild asymmetry in the size of the lateral ventricles. (Reprinted with permission from Poretti A et al. Dev Med Child Neurol 2010; 52: 718–724.)

et al. 2006; Malinger et al. 2006, 2009, Poretti et al. 2010; Benbir et al. 2011).

UCH has been previously described occurring prenatally from 21 weeks of gestation in seven cases (Robins et al. 1998; McCollom and Rashidian 2003; Gallini et al. 2006; Malinger et al. 2006, 2009; Poretti et al. 2010). In two cases, normal brain anatomy was reported from the first ultrasound and UCH was diagnosed later (Robins et al. 1998; McCollom and Rashidian 2003). These findings argue strongly for a prenatally acquired lesion (disruption) rather than a malformation.

The pathogenesis of the disruptive event resulting in UCH is debatable; however a haemorrhagic event is likely. Prenatal cerebellar haemorrhages had been reported and in these cases they were mostly detected between 18 and 24 weeks of gestation (Ranzini et al. 1998; Robins et al. 1998; Sharony et al. 1999; Hiller et al. 2003; Yuksel and Batukan 2003; Ortiz et al. 2004; Lerner et al. 2006; Gorincour et al. 2006; Malinger et al. 2006, 2009; Nomura et al. 2009). Follow-up examinations after fetal cerebellar haemorrhage have shown a gradual reduction in the size of the affected hemisphere (Ranzini et al. 1998;

Malinger et al. 2006, 2009). Haemosiderin deposition was not seen on follow-up imaging in any of the cases. Indeed, in preterm infants with cerebellar haemorrhage haemosiderin is no longer detectable 6 weeks after its occurrence. This is probably due to the high permeability of the blood–brain barrier to haemosiderin-loaded macrophages.

The clinical presentation of UCH is variable. Of the 26 cases described, a follow-up was reported in 22 cases (mean age 6.1 years, range 6 months to 38 years) (Harbord et al. 1989; Boltshauser et al. 1996; Robins et al. 1998; Mancini et al. 2001; Erdogan et al. 2002; McCollom and Rashidian 2003; Sztriha and Johansen 2005; Gallini et al. 2006; Gross-Tsur et al. 2006; Poretti et al. 2010; Benbir et al. 2011). Typical cerebellar signs were present in eight patients: truncal ataxia in seven, muscular hypotonia in five, and limb ataxia in four. Squint was found in six cases, head nodding in two. These neurological symptoms vary in severity, but are mostly mild.

Cognitive outcome was reported in 14 of 18 cases (Boltshauser et al. 1996; Mancini et al. 2001; Erdogan et al. 2002; Sztriha and Johansen 2005; Gross-Tsur et al. 2006; Poretti et al. 2010). Normal cognitive development has been reported in seven cases (IQ results were documented only in three cases): the full-scale IQ ranges were 88 to 108 (Poretti et al. 2010). Therefore severe UCH is compatible with a favorable cognitive outcome. In the other cases, mental retardation (UK: learning disability) of differing severity was reported with IQ scores (if measured or documented) ranging between 60 and 74 (Boltshauser et al. 1996; Gross-Tsur et al. 2006; Poretti et al. 2010). Cognitive functions were often, but not consistently, impaired when the cerebellar vermis was involved. Conversely, patients with lesions confined to the cerebellar hemispheres had a favorable outcome with normal cognitive functions (Poretti et al. 2010).

A detailed neuropsychological assessment was performed in five cases (Gross-Tsur et al. 2006; Poretti et al. 2010). Four children had difficulties in spatial cognition, one each in memory and executive functions, graphomotor and arithmetic skills, and social perception and comprehension, respectively. Language and speech disorders were prevalent, and described in six patients: dysarthria and expressive language disorder (2) and dysprosody and no expressive language (1). Behavioral disorders were noted in four: attention-deficit hyperactivity disorder, depressive mood, anxiety, and catatonia with obsessive-compulsive disorder. This pattern of deficits overlaps with the symptom profile of the cerebellar cognitive affective syndrome (Schmahmann and Sherman 1998). However, in patients with severe UCH it seems to be less specific than in patients with postnatally acquired cerebellar lesions.

The characteristic MRI finding is an asymmetry of the cerebellar hemispheres ranging from aplasia to mild hypoplasia of a cerebellar hemisphere (Figs 30.5, 30.6). The vermis was involved in 12 of 20 patients with information about vermis involvement. This is in contrast to cerebellar clefts, another form of prenatal cerebellar disruption, affecting only the cerebellar hemispheres. The volume of the posterior fossa was variable and could be clearly enlarged, normal, or reduced ipsilateral to the hypoplastic hemisphere (Fig. 30.5). In almost all the patients a brainstem asymmetry was easily recognizable. This asymmetry included hypoplasia of the ipsilateral middle and superior cerebellar peduncles and superior colliculus, a highly asymmetric pons with absent contralateral olivary body, and contralateral reduction of the red nucleus and the substantia nigra (Figs 30.5, 30.6), as comprehensively reported by Strong, and these are considered to be secondary changes (Strong 1915).

Vanishing cerebellum in myelomeningocele

In myelomeningocele, prenatal hindbrain herniation through the foramen magnum is a secondary result of prolonged prenatal CSF leak. This herniation may result in parenchymal damage due to ischemia, presumably induced by mechanical distortion. When tissue loss is severe, grossly reduced or virtually no cerebellum may be present, as seen in a minority of patients

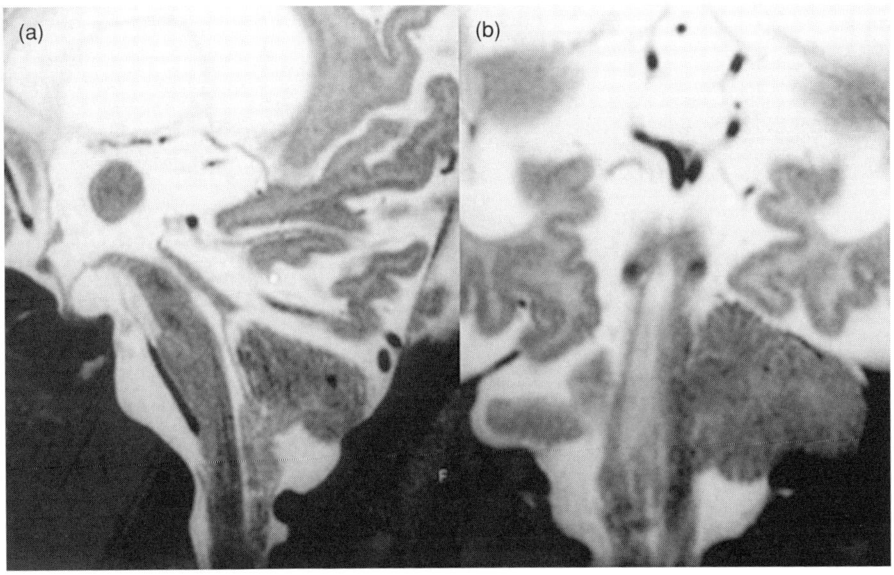

Fig. 30.7. Vanishing cerebellum in a 5-month-old infant with myelomeningocele. **(a)** Sagittal T2-weighted MRI demonstrating a very small posterior fossa and a lack of pontine prominence; **(b)** coronal T2-weighted MRI showing marked destruction of the right cerebellar hemisphere. (Reprinted with permission from Boltshauser E et al. Eur J Paediatr Neurol 2002; 6: 109–113.)

(Fig. 30.7). This infrequent observation was called 'vanishing cerebellum in Chiari II malformation' by Sener (Sener 1995). However, this designation does not reflect the remarkable asymmetry of tissue damage for which we have no obvious explanation. The damage basically involves one hemisphere, sparing the vermis. Boltshauser et al. reported three patients with this phenomenon (Boltshauser et al. 2002). In one patient, vanishing cerebellum was already detectable at 25 weeks of gestation by prenatal ultrasonography and the tissue damage was remarkably asymmetric in all patients. An appropriately tested child showed severe cognitive impairments. However, the other two patients could not be adequately assessed (one patient died early and another was still too young for final assessment). Therefore no conclusion on the cognitive consequence of vanishing cerebellum can be drawn from the available literature. However, we hypothesize that vanishing cerebellum impairs cognitive development (Boltshauser et al. 2002).

REFERENCES

Altman NR, Naidich TP, Braffman BH (1992) Posterior fossa malformations. AJNR Am J Neuroradiol 13: 691–724.

Ansari SA, Hunter JV, Nassif LM, Clark GD, Ramocki MB (2011) Bilateral in utero cerebellar infarction. J Child Neurol 26: 895–899.

Barkovich AJ, Kjos BO (1992) Gray matter heterotopias: MR characteristics and correlation with developmental and neurologic manifestations. Radiology 182: 493–499.

Barkovich AJ, Lindan CE (1994) Congenital cytomegalovirus infection of the brain: imaging analysis and embryologic considerations. AJNR Am J Neuroradiol 15: 703–715.

Battaglia G, Pagliardini S, Saglietti L, Cattabeni F, Di Luca M, Bassanini S, Setola V (2003a) Neurogenesis in cerebral heterotopia induced in rats by prenatal methylazoxymethanol treatment. Cereb Cortex 13: 736–748.

Battaglia G, Bassanini S, Granata T, Setola V, Giavazzi A, Pagliardini S (2003b) The genesis of epileptogenic cerebral heterotopia: clues from experimental models. Epileptic Disord 5 Suppl 2: S51–58.

Bellini C, Massocco D, Serra G (2000) Prenatal cocaine exposure and the expanding spectrum of brain malformations. Arch Intern Med 160: 2393.

Benbir G, Kara S, Yalcinkaya BC, Karhkaya G, Tuysuz B, Kocer N, Yalcinkaya C (2011) Unilateral cerebellar hypoplasia with diferent clinical features. Cerebellum 10: 49–60.

Boddaert N, Desguerre I, Bahi-Buisson N, Romano S, Valayannopoulos V, Saillour Y, et al. (2010) Posterior fossa imaging in 158 children with ataxia. J Neuroradiol 37: 220–230.

Boltshauser E, Steinlin M, Martin E, Deonna T (1996) Unilateral cerebellar aplasia. Neuropediatrics 27: 50–53.

Boltshauser E (2001) Cerebellar imaging – an important signpost in paediatric neurology. Childs Nerv Syst 17: 211–216.

Boltshauser E, Schneider J, Kollias S, Waibel P, Weissert M (2002) Vanishing cerebellum in myelomeningocoele. Eur J Paediatr Neurol 6: 109–113.

Boltshauser E (2004) Cerebellum-small brain but large confusion: a review of selected cerebellar malformations and disruptions. Am J Med Genet A 126A: 376–385.

Cheeran MC, Lokensgard JR, Schleiss MR (2009) Neuropathogenesis of congenital cytomegalovirus infection: disease mechanisms and prospects for intervention. Clin Microbiol Rev 22: 99–126.

Connolly DJ, Widjaja E, Griffiths PD (2007) Involvement of the anterior lobe of the cerebellar vermis in perinatal profound hypoxia. AJNR Am J Neuroradiol 28: 16–19.

Curry CJ, Lammer EJ, Nelson V, Shaw GM (2005) Schizencephaly: heterogeneous etiologies in a population of 4 million California births. Am J Med Genet A 137A: 181–189.

Dale ST, Coleman LT (2002) Neonatal alloimmune thrombocytopenia: antenatal and postnatal imaging findings in the pediatric brain. AJNR Am J Neuroradiol 23: 1457–1465.

de Vries LS, Gunardi H, Barth PG, Bok LA, Verboon-Maciolek MA, Groenendaal F (2004) The spectrum of cranial ultrasound and magnetic resonance imaging abnormalities in congenital cytomegalovirus infection. Neuropediatrics 35: 113–119.

de Vries LS, Koopman C, Groenendaal F, Van Schooneveld M, Verheijen FW, Verbeek E, et al. (2009) COL4A1 mutation in two preterm siblings with antenatal onset of parenchymal hemorrhage. Ann Neurol 65: 12–18.

Demaerel P (2002) Abnormalities of cerebellar foliation and fissuration: classification, neurogenetics and clinicoradiological correlations. Neuroradiology 44: 639–646.

Demaerel P, Lagae L, Casaer P, Baert AL (1998) MR of cerebellar cortical dysplasia. AJNR Am J Neuroradiol 19: 984–986.

Dyet LE, Kennea N, Counsell SJ, Maalouf EF, Ajayi-Obe M, Duggan PJ, et al. (2006) Natural history of brain lesions in extremely preterm infants studied with serial magnetic resonance imaging from birth and neurodevelopmental assessment. Pediatrics 118: 536–548.

Erdogan N, Kocakoc E, Bekar D, Ozturk (2002) Unilateral absence of cerebellar hemisphere: a case report. Neuroradiology 44: 49–51.

Fink KR, Thapa MM, Ishak GE, Pruthi S (2010) Neuroimaging of pediatric central nervous system cytomegalovirus infection. Radiographics 30: 1779–1796.

Gallini F, Luciano R, Pane M, De Carolis MP, Romagnoli C, Mercuri E (2006) Crossed cerebellar atrophy of prenatal onset. Childs Nerv Syst 22: 734–736.

Glenn OA, Bianco K, Barkovich AJ, Callen PW, Parer JT (2007) Fetal cerebellar hemorrhage in parvovirus-associated non-immune hydrops fetalis. J Matern Fetal Neonatal Med 20: 769–772.

Gorincour G, Rypens F, Lapierre C, Costa T, Audibert F, Robitaille Y (2006) Fetal magnetic resonance imaging in the prenatal diagnosis of cerebellar hemorrhage. Ultrasound Obstet Gynecol 27: 78–80.

Gross-Tsur V, Ben-Bashat D, Shalev RS, Levav M, Sira LB (2006) Evidence of a developmental cerebello-cerebral disorder. Neuropsychologia 44: 2569–2572.

Harbord MG, Finn JP, Hall-Craggs MA, Brett EM, Baraitser M (1989) Moebius' syndrome with unilateral cerebellar hypoplasia. J Med Genet 26: 579–582.

Henneke M, Diekmann S, Ohlenbusch A, Kaiser J, Engelbrecht V, Kohlschutter A, et al. (2009) RNASET2-deficient cystic leukoencephalopathy resembles congenital cytomegalovirus brain infection. Nat Genet 41: 773–775.

Hiller LT, McGahan JP, Bijan B, Melendres G, Towner D (2003) Sonographic detection of in utero isolated cerebellar hemorrhage. J Ultrasound Med 22: 649–652.

Johnsen SD, Bodensteiner JB, Lotze TE (2005) Frequency and nature of cerebellar injury in the extremely premature survivor with cerebral palsy. J Child Neurol 20: 60–64.

Jones CA (2003) Congenital cytomegalovirus infection. Curr Probl Pediatr Adolesc Health Care 33: 70–93.

Lammens M, ten Donkelaar HJ, van Gut JM, van Noort G, Willemsen M, Hamel B (2006) Causes of congenital malformations. In: ten Donkelaar HJ, Lammens M, Hori A, editors. Clinical neuroembryology: development and developmental disorders of the human central nervous system. Berlin: Springer. p 106–109.

Lerner A, Gilboa Y, Gerad L, Malinger G, Kidron D, Achiron R (2006) Sonographic detection of fetal cerebellar cavernous hemangioma with in-utero hemorrhage leading to cerebellar hemihypoplasia. Ultrasound Obstet Gynecol 28: 968–971.

Limperopoulos C, Benson CB, Bassan H, Disalvo DN, Kinnamon DD, Moore M, et al. (2005) Cerebellar hemorrhage in the preterm infant: ultrasonographic findings and risk factors. Pediatrics 116: 717–724.

Limperopoulos C, Robertson RL, Sullivan NR, Bassan H, du Plessis AJ (2009) Cerebellar injury in term infants: clinical characteristic, magnetic resonance imaging findings, and outcome. Pediatr Neurol 41: 1–8.

Luo MH, Schwartz PH, Fortunado EA (2008) Neonatal enural progenitor cells and their neuronal and glial cell derivates are fully permissive for human cytomegalovirus infection. J Virol 20: 9994–10007.

Mackiewicz S (1935) Über einen Fall von halbseitiger Aplasie des Kleinhirns. Schweiz Arch Neurochir Neurol Psychiatr 36: 81–111.

Malinger G, Zahalka N, Kidron D, Ben-Sira L, Lev D, Lerman-Sagie T (2006) Fatal outcome following foetal cerebellar haemorrhage associated with placental thrombosis. Eur J Paediatr Neurol 10: 93–96.

Malinger G, Lev D, Lerman-Sagie T (2009) The fetal cerebellum. Pitfalls in diagnosis and management. Prenat Diagn 29: 372–380.

Mancini J, Lethel V, Hugonenq C, Chabrol B (2001) Brain injuries in early foetal life: consequences for brain development. Dev Med Child Neurol 43: 52–55.

Marques Dias MJ, Harmant-van Rijckevorsel G, Landrieu P, Lyon G (1984) Prenatal cytomegalovirus disease and cerebral microgyria: evidence for perfusion failure, not disturbance of histogenesis, as the major cause of fetal cytomegalovirus encephalopathy. Neuropediatrics 15: 18–24.

McCollom D, Rashidian J (2003) Prenatal diagnosis of unilateral cerebellar hypoplasia. Journal of Diagnostic Medical Sonography 19: 120–123.

Mendelsohn DB, Hertzanu Y, Glass RB, Spiro F (1983) Unilateral cerebellar hypoplasia. J Comput Assist Tomogr 7: 1077–1078.

Merrill JD, Piecuch RE, Fell SC, Barkovich AJ, Goldstein RB (1998) A new pattern of cerebellar hemorrhages in preterm infants. Pediatrics 102: E62.

Mejaski-Bosnjak V (2008) Congenital CMV infection: a common cause of childhood disability. Dev Med Child Neurol 50: 403.

Meyer BU, Roricht S, Machetanz J (1994) Reduction of corticospinal excitability by magnetic stimulation over the cerebellum in patients with large defects of one cerebellar hemisphere. Electroencephalogr Clin Neurophysiol 93: 372–379.

Nomura ML, Barini R, de Andrade KC, Faro C, Marins M (2009) Prenatal diagnosis of isolated fetal cerebellar hemorrhage associated with maternal septic shock. Prenat Diagn 29: 169–171.

Odeberg J, Wolmer N, Falci S, Westgren M, Seiger A, Söderberg-Nauclér C (2006) Human cytomegalovirus inhibits neuronal differentiation and induces apoptosis in human neural precursor cells. J Virol 80: 8929–8939.

Ortiz JU, Ostermayer E, Fischer T, Kuschel B, Rudelius M, Schneider KT (2004) Severe fetal cytomegalovirus infection associated with cerebellar hemorrhage. Ultrasound Obstet Gynecol 23: 402–406.

Patel S, Barkovich AJ (2002) Analysis and classification of cerebellar malformations. AJNR Am J Neuroradiol 23: 1074–1087

Poretti A, Wolf NI, Boltshauser E (2008a) Differential diagnosis of cerebellar atrophy in childhood. Eur J Paediatr Neurol 12: 155–167.

Poretti A, Leventer RJ, Cowan FM, Rutherford MA, Steinlin M, Klein A, et al. (2008b) Cerebellar cleft: a form of prenatal cerebellar disruption. Neuropediatrics 39: 106–112.

Poretti A, Prayer D, Boltshauser E (2009a) Morphological spectrum of prenatal cerebellar disruptions. Eur J Paediatr Neurol 13: 397–407.

Poretti A, Huisman TA, Cowan FM, Del Giudice E, Jeannet PY, Prayer D, et al. (2009b) Cerebellar cleft: confirmation of the neuroimaging pattern. Neuropediatrics 40: 228–233.

Poretti A, Limperopoulos C, Roulet-Perez E, Wolf NI, Rauscher C, Prayer D, et al. (2010) Outcome of severe unilateral cerebellar hypoplasia. Dev Med Child Neurol 52: 718–724.

Ranzini AC, Shen-Schwarz S, Guzman ER, Fisher AJ, White M, Vintzileos AM (1998) Prenatal sonographic appearance of hemorrhagic cerebellar infarction. J Ultrasound Med 17: 725–727.

Reardon W, Donnai D (2007) Dysmorphology demystified. Arch Dis Child Fetal Neonatal Ed 92: F225–229.

Robins JB, Mason GC, Watters J, Martinez D (1998) Case report: cerebellar hemi-hypoplasia. Prenat Diagn 18: 173–177.

Sarnat HB, Alcala H (1980) Human cerebellar hypoplasia: a syndrome of diverse causes. Arch Neurol 37: 300–305.

Sargent MA, Poskitt KJ, Roland EH, Hill A, Hendson G (2004) Cerebellar vermian atrophy after neonatal hypoxic-ischemic encephalopathy. AJNR Am J Neuroradiol 25: 1008–1015.

Schmahmann JD, Sherman JC (1998) The cerebellar cognitive affective syndrome. Brain 121: 561–579.

Sehgal A, El-Naggar W, Glanc P, Asztalos E (2009) Risk factors and ultrasonographic profile of posterior fossa haemorrhages in preterm infants. J Paediatr Child Health 45: 215–218.

Sener RN (1995) Cerebellar agenesis versus vanishing cerebellum in Chiari II malformation. Comput Med Imaging Graph 19: 491–494.

Sharony R, Kidron D, Aviram R, Beyth Y, Tepper R (1999) Prenatal diagnosis of fetal cerebellar lesions: a case report and review of the literature. Prenat Diagn 19: 1077–1080.

Simon M, Kafritsas D (1992) Unilateral cerebellar hypoplasia. Clin Neuropathol 11: 71–73.

Squier W, Hope PL, Lindenbaum RH (1990) Neocerebellar hypoplasia in a neonate following intra-uterine exposure to anticonvulsants. Dev Med Child Neurol 32: 737–742.

Steggerda SJ, Leijser LM, Wiggers-de Bruine FT, van der Grond J, Walther FJ, van Wezel-Meijler G (2009) Cerebellar injury in preterm infants: incidence and findings on US and MR images. Radiology 252: 190–199.

Steinlin MI, Nadal D, Eich GF, Martin E, Boltshauser EJ (1996) Late intrauterine cytomegalovirus infection: clinical and neuroimaging findings. Pediatr Neurol 15: 249–253.

Steinlin M, Blaser S, Boltshauser E (1998) Cerebellar involvement in metabolic disorders: a pattern-recognition approach. Neuroradiology 40: 347–354.

Strong OS (1915) A case of unilateral cerebellar agenesis. J Comp Neurol 25: 361–391.

Sztriha L, Johansen JG (2005) Spectrum of malformations of the hindbrain (cerebellum, pons, and medulla) in a cohort of children with high rate of parental consanguinity. Am J Med Genet A 135A: 134–141.

Takano T, Takikita S, Shimada M (1999) Experimental schizencephaly induced by Kilham strain of mumps virus: pathogenesis of cleft formation. Neuroreport 10: 3149–3154.

ten Donkelaar HJ, Lammens M, Wesseling P, Thijssen HO, Renier WO (2003) Development and developmental disorders of the human cerebellum. J Neurol 250: 1025–1036.

Tennstedt A (1965) Kleinhirnaplasie beim Erwachsenen. Zentralbl Allg Pathol 107: 301–304.

Van Allen MI (1992) Structural anomalies resulting from vascular disruption. Pediatr Clin North Am 39: 255–277.

Van Allen MI, Curry C, Gallagher L (1987) Limb body wall complex: I. Pathogenesis. Am J Med Genet 28: 529–548.

van der Knaap MS, Vermeulen G, Barkhof F, Hart AA, Loeber JG, Weel JF (2004) Pattern of white matter abnormalities at MR imaging: use of polymerase chain reaction testing of Guthrie cards to link pattern with congenital cytomegalovirus infection. Radiology 230: 529–536.

van der Voom JP, Pouweis R, Vermeulen RJ, Barkhof F, van der Knaap MS (2009) Quantitative MR imaging and spectroscopy in congenital cytomegalovirus infection and periventricular leukomalacia suggests a comparable neuropathological substrate of the cerebral white matter lesions. Neuropediatrics 40: 168–173.

Yuksel A, Batukan C (2003) Fetal cerebellar hemorrhage in a severely growth-restricted fetus: natural history and differential diagnosis from Dandy-Walker malformation. Ultrasound Obstet Gynecol 22: 178–181.

Zankl A, Brooks D, Boltshauser E, Largo R, Schinzel A (2004) Natural history of twin disruption sequence. Am J Med Genet A 127A: 133–138.

31
Cerebellar Injury in the Preterm Infant

Catherine Limperopoulos

Preterm birth is associated with a high risk for brain injury and extensive long-term neurodevelopmental disability. Because improved survival and the increased sensitivity and availability of advanced neuroimaging techniques in the critically ill neonate have forced a re-evaluation of preterm-related brain injury, our understanding of such injury and its long-term sequelae has changed dramatically. Until recently, both clinical and basic research studies on the preterm brain focused almost exclusively on cerebral injury, and in particular injury to the developing white matter. In contrast to this predominant focus on cerebral injury, recent studies in preterm infants have described a previously under-recognized high incidence of cerebellar injury that is associated with pervasive developmental disabilities. This chapter will begin by providing a brief overview of cerebellar development, followed by a discussion of the developmental vulnerability of the premature cerebellum. The incidence, risk factors, and impact of preterm birth on cerebellar and cerebral development are then examined. Finally, the functional consequences of cerebellar injury in ex-preterm survivors, and the role of early-life cerebellar injury in cognitive-affect disturbances, are explored.

Normal development of the cerebellum

Although a comprehensive overview of cerebellar development is beyond the scope of this chapter, a brief overview of normal development of the cerebellum is warranted to provide a conceptual framework within which to discuss cerebellar injury in the preterm infant. Embryologically, the cerebellum is one of the first brain structures to arise at around 4 weeks' gestation, and it is one of the last structures to reach its mature configuration (Ten Donkelaar and Lammens 2009). In the earliest part of this process, critical neural infrastructure is laid down, upon which subsequent and ongoing fine-tuning of neuronal networks occurs.

A number of critical, sequential developmental events occur in the immature brain in a precisely programmed fashion (Kostovic et al. 2002; Price et al. 2006; Rakic 2006; Rakic et al. 2007; Bystron et al. 2008). In the mid-first trimester, cerebellar precursor cells arise in the ventricular zone around the fourth ventricle (primary neuroepithelium) (Miale and Sidman 1961; Baader et al. 1996) from where they migrate to their mature location. Early migration of Purkinje cells occurs along guiding radial glia (Hatten 1990) into the primordial cerebellum. Precursor cells also migrate from the ventricular zone to the lateral rhombic lips where mitotic activity continues. Two distinct migrations follow thereafter. First, neurons of the future brainstem nuclei migrate in a ventral direction to their pontine and medullary destinations. Second, at the end of the first trimester migration of future granular cells takes place tangentially from the rhombic lips over the surface of the cerebellum to form the external granular layer, where a secondary neuroepithelium is established and neuronal proliferation continues through the third trimester (Miale and Sidman 1961; Rivas and Hatten 1995; Wingate 2001). The external granular layer is at its thickest around 24 weeks and, from 30 weeks' gestation, it begins to involute along two pathways (Rakic and Sidman 1970; Kollias et al. 1993). The first pathway is via centripetal migration through the molecular and Purkinje cell layers to form the internal granular layer (Hatten 1990). The second path is through an activation of apoptosis, which removes remaining external granular neurons (Nat et al. 2001). Involution of the external granular layer is completed by 12 months postnatally, and the cerebellar cortex reaches its final three-layer organization at around 12 months as well. Migration, proliferation, and arborization of the cerebellar neurons are complete by 20 months of life.

Vulnerability of the developing cerebellum

Cerebellar maturation and adaptation follows a highly orchestrated series of programmed developmental processes of migration, proliferation, and arborization (described above), which may place the immature cerebellum at risk for injury. Nowhere is cerebellar development more dynamic and complex than in fetal life and the early postnatal years. This protracted developmental course exposes the cerebellum to a host of potential insults capable of derailing its developmental program (Hamre and West 1993; Bautista et al. 1995; Fukuda et al. 1996; Ulupinar and Yucel 2005; Ulupinar et al. 2006). The high-energy demands of the developing cerebellum are normally supported by an intact posterior fossa circulation. The abundant activity in the primary and secondary germinal matrices in the cerebellum is maintained by a responsive, transient and fragile vascular system, similar to that found around the lateral ventricles (Pape and Wigglesworth 1979). In vivo normal MRI studies have demonstrated that cerebellar growth is particularly exuberant over the third trimester (Limperopoulos et al. 2005b), unparalleled in comparison to other cerebral structures. The cerebellum demonstrates an exponential growth in foliation and the surface area of the cerebellar cortex increases more that 30-fold from 24 weeks of gestation to term (Rakic and Sidman 1970; Lemire et al. 1985). For many extremely preterm infants (<25 weeks' gestational age) these critical phases of cerebellar development will occur in the hazards of an extrauterine environment, namely the neonatal intensive care unit. It is possible that very early exposure to extrauterine life can disturb the highly regulated processes that govern normal cerebellar development, and, of particular significance, accelerated late gestation growth appears to be impeded by premature extrauterine life (described later). The mechanisms underlying this cerebellar growth restriction remain unknown and await further study.

Cerebellar injury in the preterm infant: Incidence and risk factors

Early neuropathologic studies reported an incidence of cerebellar injury as high as 25% in preterm infants <1500 grams, usually associated with complicated births, a striking clinical presentation, and high mortality (Grunnet and Shields 1976; Martin et al. 1976; Pape et al. 1976; Perlman et al. 1983; Bejar et al. 1985). Although subsequent clinical studies reported a lower incidence of cerebellar injury in surviving preterm infants, more recent reports suggest that cerebellar injury occurs in up to 19% of preterm infants <32 weeks' gestational age (Steggerda et al. 2009), with a predilection in extremely preterm infants (<750 grams) (Limperopoulos et al. 2005a). Given the relative insensitivity of the traditional anterior fontanel cranial ultrasound approach to the posterior fossa, it was not until the advent of the mastoid foramen views (present at the junction of the temporal, parietal, and occipital bones) (Merrill et al. 1998; Di Salvo 2001; Limperopoulos et al. 2005a; Steggerda et al. 2009) that a striking high incidence of cerebellar lesions was reported in preterm infants. Despite the increased sensitivity of mastoid views for cerebellar hemorrhage, a recent study showed that mastoid foramen views detected only 50% of the cerebellar lesions detected by MRI in preterm infants (Steggerda et al. 2009). Further, punctate hemorrhagic lesions may remain undetected even when the mastoid approach is used. Therefore, the use of MRI is strongly advocated as a primary diagnostic tool for confirming the presence and topography of cerebellar injury (Steggerda et al. 2009).

Cerebellar lesions in the preterm infant are usually clinically silent in onset (Merrill et al. 1998; Steggerda et al. 2009), although a recent report described unexplained motor agitation in the days preceding the diagnosis of cerebellar injury (Ecury-Goossen et al. 2010). On average, cerebellar injury is detected at a median age of 2.5–5 days (range: 1–12 days) (Limperopoulos et al. 2005a; Sehgal et al. 2009). Cerebellar injury most commonly occurs with a prominent hemorrhagic component, and can present with or without associated supratentorial injury. Cerebellar hemorrhagic injury frequently occurs with intraventricular hemorrhage (77%). However, concomitant posthemorrhagic hydrocephalus and supratentorial parenchymal injury (e.g., periventricular hemorrhagic infarction and periventricular white matter injury) may also occur in a subset of preterm infants with cerebellar injury (Bodensteiner and Johnsen 2005; Johnsen et al. 2005; Limperopoulos et al. 2005a, 2007; Messerschmidt et al. 2005, 2008; Sehgal et al. 2009).

Cerebellar infarction has also been described as an important complication of extreme preterm birth with no apparent evidence for prior hemorrhage (Mercuri et al. 1997; Bodensteiner and Johnsen 2005). The topography of injury, primarily inferior bilateral (60%), suggests a vascular distribution primarily involving the inferior cerebellar arteries (Mercuri et al. 1997; Bodensteiner and Johnsen 2005). Cerebellar infarction has been invariably associated with supratentorial white matter injury, suggesting that the etiology of cerebellar and cerebral injury is likely to be similar.

Cerebellar injury is often accompanied by subsequent cerebellar atrophy in 37% of affected infants which is detectable about 2 months following the initial injury (Limperopoulos et al. 2005a; Steggerda et al. 2009). Available data (Bodensteiner and Johnsen 2005; Johnsen et al. 2005; Limperopoulos et al. 2005a; Messerschmidt et al. 2005, 2008; Bednarek et al. 2008; Sehgal et al. 2009; Steggerda et al. 2009) suggest a wide range of severity of cerebellar injuries in preterm infants, ranging from mild punctate lesions and focal unilateral lesions, to more extensive bihemispheric and vermian lesions, to near-total destruction of the cerebellum (Fig. 31.1). In some reports, severe cerebellar lesions have been described in association with hypoplasia/atrophy of the brainstem (Johnsen et al. 2002; Bodensteiner and Johnsen 2006).

A number of perinatal risk factors have been associated with cerebellar injury. Extreme preterm birth has been repeatedly identified as an important risk factor in both clinical and postmortem studies (Grunnet and Shields 1976; Limperopoulos et al. 2005a; Messerschmidt et al. 2008; Sehgal et al. 2009). Grunnet et al. (Grunnet and Shields 1976) demonstrated that 75% of cases with cerebellar hemorrhage were less than 28 weeks' gestation. Other risk factors include a combination of factors: maternal/antenatal (e.g., assisted conception), intrapartum (e.g., fetal heart rate abnormalities; emergent cesarean section) and early postnatal (e.g., pressor-inotrope support, prolonged ventilation) (Limperopoulos et al. 2005a; Messerschmidt et al. 2008; Sehgal et al. 2009). These data are summarized in Table 31.1. Taken together, determinants of cerebellar injury are multifactorial and collectively point to a greater degree of fetal/early-neonatal illness that precedes the development of cerebellar injury. Large prospective studies are needed to delineate the antecedents of cerebellar injury.

Pathogenesis of cerebellar injury in the preterm infant

The precise mechanisms underlying direct cerebellar injury in the preterm infant remain poorly understood; however, several hypotheses have been put forth. The etiology is likely to be multifactorial. Germinal matrix hemorrhage has been implicated in a number of ways, including direct hemorrhage into the primary and secondary cerebellar germinal matrices (described above), a mechanism supported by its common co-occurrence with germinal matrix-intraventricular hemorrhage (GM-IVH) (Pape et al. 1976); blood from large supratentorial GM-IVH lesions 'dissecting' from the fourth ventricle into the vermis or from the posterior fossa subarachnoid space into the cerebellar

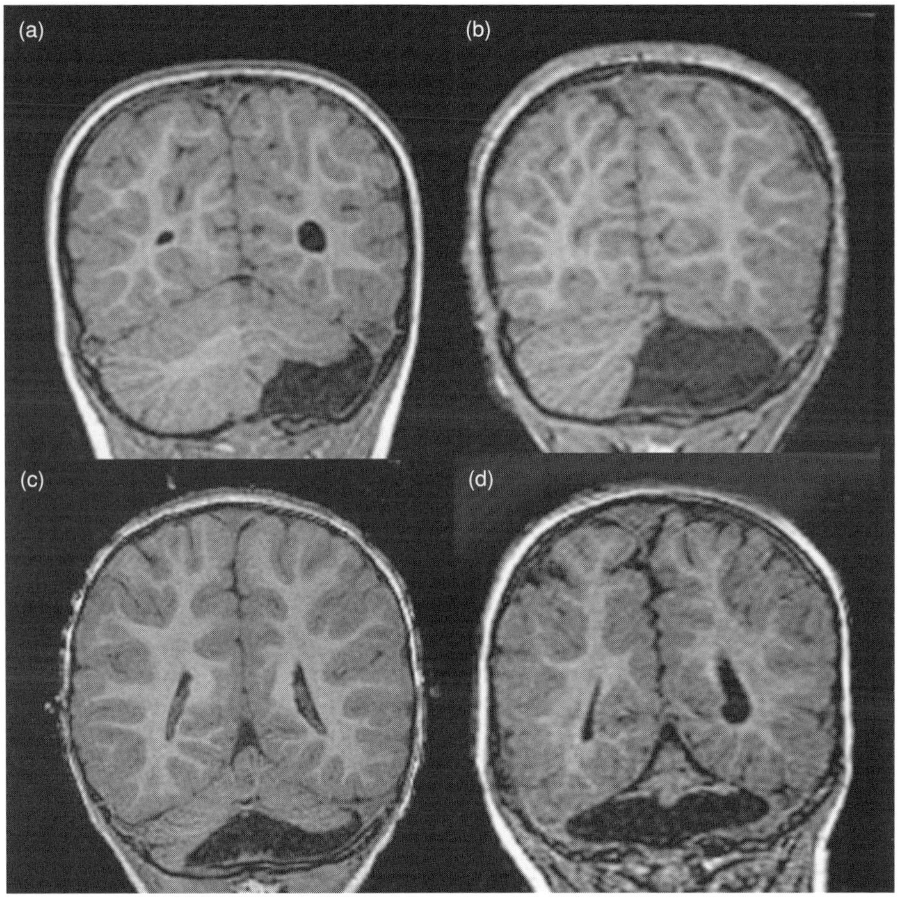

Fig. 31.1. Spectrum of direct cerebellar injury in preterm infants. **(a)** Mild-moderate unilateral cerebellar injury; **(b)** severe unilateral cerebellar injury. **(c)** infero-medial cerebellar injury; **(d)** severe bilateral cerebellar and vermis injury. (Reproduced with permission from *Pediatrics* (2007), 120(3): 584–593.)

TABLE 31.1
Perinatal risk factors associated with cerebellar injury in the preterm infant

Antenatal	Intrapartum	Postnatal
Assisted conception (Limperopoulos et al. 2005a)	Abnormal fetal heart rate (Limperopoulos et al. 2005a; Sehgal et al. 2009)	High-frequency ventilation (Limperopoulos et al. 2005a)
Multiple gestation (Sehgal et al. 2009)	Emergent cesarean section (Limperopoulos et al. 2005a; Messerschmidt et al. 2008)	Early intubation (Limperopoulos et al. 2005a)
Antenatal steroids (Messerschmidt et al. 2008; Sehgal et al. 2009)	Apgar score at 1 minute (Limperopoulos et al. 2005a; Messerschmidt et al. 2008)	Pressor-inotrope support (Limperopoulos et al. 2005a; Messerschmidt et al. 2008; Sehgal et al. 2009)
	Apgar score at 5 minutes (Limperopoulos et al. 2005a)	Volume expanders (Limperopoulos et al. 2005a)
		Patent ductus arteriosus (Limperopoulos et al. 2005a)
		Pulmonary hemorrhage (Limperopoulos et al. 2005a)
		Highest mean arterial pressure (Sehgal et al. 2009)
		*Lowest pH (Limperopoulos et al. 2005a)
		Lowest plasma bicarbonate (Limperopoulos et al. 2005a)
		*Lowest white blood cell count (Limperopoulos et al. 2005a)
		*Lowest hematocrit (Limperopoulos et al. 2005a)
		*Lowest platelet count (Limperopoulos et al. 2005a; Sehgal et al. 2009)
		Culture proven sepsis (Sehgal et al. 2009)

* first 5 days of life.

hemispheres (Grunnet and Shields 1976); and blood products adjoining the two cerebellar germinal matrices causing direct injury to the rapidly proliferating cells (Messerschmidt et al. 2005). Cerebellar hypoxia-ischemia/reperfusion insults have also been proposed as mechanisms (Pape et al. 1976; Mercuri et al. 1997). Both arterial (Mercuri et al. 1997) and venous vaso-occlusion with secondary hemorrhagic transformation have been suggested. Cerebellar hemorrhagic injury has been described in the presence of increased cerebral venous pressure, such as extracorporeal membrane oxygenation (Bulas et al. 1991; Evans et al. 1994) and with the use of earlier face mask ventilation (Pape et al. 1976). Global hypoperfusion of the cerebellum may also play a role in the genesis of cerebellar injury. Neuropathologic studies have reported a high incidence of cerebellar necrotic lesions in preterm infants (Skullerud and Westre 1986; Armstrong et al. 1987). Cystic leukomalacia has been reported in the superficial white matter of the cerebellar folia in extremely preterm infants with severe systemic hypotension (Tsuru et al. 1995). Injury to the immature cerebellar folia is believed to arise from border-zone ischemia between the posterior inferior and superior cerebellar artery territories. Finally, the potential role of acquired early cerebellar injury after birth in the pathogenesis of subsequent developmental failure (i.e., cerebellar hypolasia) has also been proposed and referred to as disturbed cerebellar development (Boltshauser 2004; Messerschmidt et al. 2005, 2008).

Impaired cerebellar development after preterm birth

Impaired cerebellar development in preterm infants may be grouped into two broad categories, that occurring in infants with or without evidence of direct cerebellar injury in the neonatal period. Combinations of direct and indirect cerebellar injury may also occur. These two forms of cerebellar injury are summarized below.

Direct injury to the cerebellum (described earlier) is often hemorrhagic and usually affects subsequent cerebellar growth, often to a striking degree (Evans et al. 1994; Bodensteiner and Johnsen 2005; Johnsen et al. 2005; Messerschmidt et al. 2008), through a combination of initial tissue loss (cerebellar atrophy) and subsequent cerebellar growth failure (cerebellar disruption). The initial injury to the cerebellum is often not fully appreciated by cranial ultrasonography, which detects the hemorrhagic component but not the surrounding ischemic injury (Fig. 31.2) (Volpe et al. 1983; Gould et al. 1987; Perlman and Volpe 1987). Hemosiderin deposits on the surface of the cerebellum may damage underlying structures and may further impair cerebellar growth and development. Subsequent cerebellar atrophy and disruption has been reported in older infants with superficial cerebellar siderosis (Hughes and Oppenheimer 1969; Bourgouin et al. 1992; Castro Conde et al. 2005; Messerschmidt et al. 2008; Steggerda et al. 2009). The neurotoxic effects of extravascular blood may be particularly pronounced in the developing external granular germinal layer during the critical third trimester period characterized by rapid neuronal proliferation and migration.

Indirect injury to the cerebellum (underdevelopment) is the second category of cerebellar growth impairment and is increasingly recognized in basic (Rees et al. 1997, 2009; Ulupinar and Yucel 2005; Ulupinar et al. 2006) and clinical studies (Limperopoulos et al. 2005b, 2005c; Shah et al. 2006). The successful application of advanced MRI techniques in preterm infants has provided important insights into our understanding of indirect cerebellar injury. A particularly rapid growth period (177%) for the immature cerebellum during the third trimester of gestation has been described, a growth rate that far exceeds that of the cerebral hemispheres (107%) (Limperopoulos et al. 2005b). However, when compared with term infants, significant growth impairment is evident in preterm infants as early as term equivalent age, even in the absence of direct cerebellar injury. Using diffusion tensor imaging, significant alterations in water diffusion have been reported in the cerebellar gray and white matter of preterm infants with supratentorial intraventricular hemorrhage (Tam et al. 2009). Cerebellar volume has been shown to decrease by 3.11% during late adolescence in individuals born very preterm (<33 weeks' gestation) (Parker et al. 2008), compared with term-born controls in whom cerebellar volume remained stable over the same period. Interestingly, this significant difference in developmental growth patterns between the two groups was confined to the cerebellum. Potential mechanisms of indirect injury to the cerebellum include injury below the resolution of current clinical MRI, or deficient maternal-placental growth factors. Autopsy

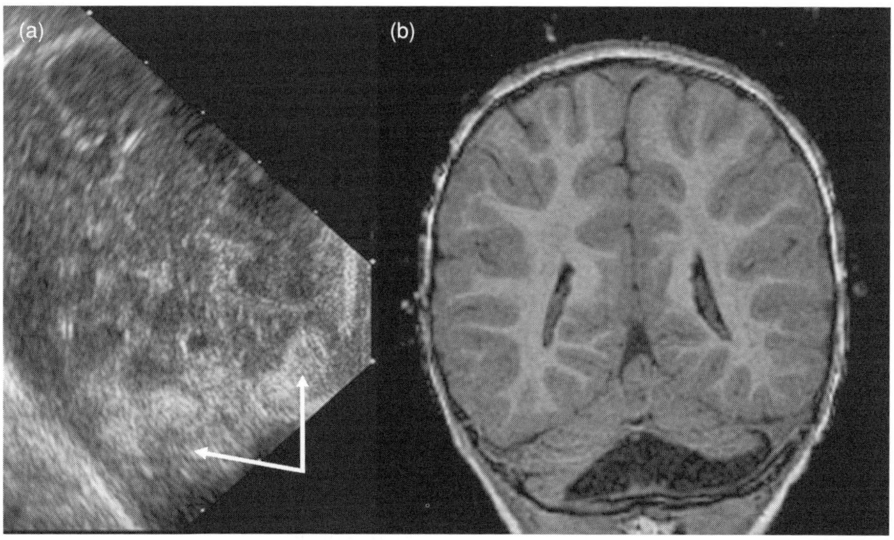

Fig. 31.2. Evolution of bilateral cerebellar and vermis hemorrhagic injury in a 26-week preterm infant. **(a)** Acute bilateral cerebellar hemispheric and vermis echodensities on ultrasonography (mastoid view) depicts the initial hemorrhagic component (arrows) of the injury. **(b)** Follow-up MRI study at 20 months shows significant bilateral cerebellar hemisphere and vermis atrophy. (Reproduced with permission from *Pediatrics* (2005), 116(3): 717–24.)

studies show evidence of microscopic injury to the dentate nucleus and cerebellar cortex in preterm infants, with neuronal loss in 25–30% and gliosis in up to 45% (Pierson et al. 2007). Potential mediators of injury include repeated hypo-/hyperoxygenation, apnea and bradycardia, patent ductus arteriosus, ventilatory support, pharmacologic agents, infection-inflammation, and other factors related to a compromised cerebral circulation (Weir et al. 1999; Limperopoulos et al. 2005a; Ulupinar and Yucel 2005; Thomson et al. 2006; Ulupinar et al. 2006; Rees et al. 2009).

In summary, these data support the notion that both direct and indirect mechanisms of cerebellar injury seem to arrest cerebellar growth and development in the preterm infant. The determinants and consequences of this preterm-related cerebellar growth impairment remain poorly understood and warrant further study.

Impact of direct cerebellar injury on cerebral development

In the late second trimester, when most cerebellar injuries occur in preterm born infants, major developmental events are yet to occur in the developing cerebrum. Although neuronal migration is in large part completed by 24 weeks' gestation, cerebral cortical organization, particularly synaptogenesis, dendritic outgrowth and arborization, and axonal sprouting are yet to occur during the third trimester and beyond (Huttenlocher 1979; Huttenlocher and Dabholkar 1997). These events in cerebral cortical development are critically dependent upon appropriate neuronal activation from structures such as the cerebellum. In addition to the surge of developmental events that occur in the third trimester, the cerebellum has multiple integrated feed-forward and feed-back connections with remote, usually contralateral regions of the cerebral hemisphere (Ramnani 2006). Withdrawal of this support is likely to disrupt the development of these critical connections. Transneuronal viral vectors in nonhuman primates have described projection pathways from the dentate pass through the contralateral thalamus to the frontal cortex (prefrontal, premotor, and primary motor) and to the posterior parietal cortex (Middleton and Strick 2001; Kelly and Strick 2003). In addition, pathways from the vermis and fastigial nuclei (the limbic cerebellum) have been delineated via the hypothalamus to the cerebral limbic centers (Stoodley and Schmahmann 2009a). Interruption of any of these cerebellar projection pathways following cerebellar injury is likely to result in decreased cerebral activation.

The potential role for disturbed cerebellar development following early-life cerebellar injury has recently been explored using advanced MRI techniques. Limperopoulos and colleagues (Limperopoulos et al. 2005b) demonstrated that cerebellar injury in the preterm infant is associated with impaired growth of the uninjured contralateral cerebral hemisphere, as early as term equivalent. The same investigators have also examined the regional specificity of such crossed cerebellocerebral diaschisis on remote growth effects in the cerebrum after prematurity-related cerebellar injury. Unilateral cerebellar injury was associated with significantly decreased volume in specific target regions for cerebellar projection pathways, including the dorsolateral prefrontal, premotor, sensorimotor, and midtemporal gray and white matter regions (Limperopoulos et al. 2010). Factors associated with this impaired cerebral growth included lower gestational age, severity of the initial cerebellar injury, and age at the time of the MRI study. These data suggest that regional cerebral growth impairment is due to interruption of cerebellocerebral pathways with loss of neuronal activation critical for development in these cerebral regions. Ongoing research is needed to better elucidate the functional significance of theses regional cerebral impairments in ex-preterm children with cerebellar injury.

The cerebellum and higher order functions

Over the past decades, our understanding of the role of the cerebellum in motor control and coordination has been repeatedly challenged by increasing recognition that the cerebellum has an important role in higher order functions. An extensive overview of the cerebellum and its critical role in higher order functions is described elsewhere in this book. Briefly, Schmahmann and Sherman (1997) provided the first comprehensive description of a distinct 'cerebellar cognitive-affective syndrome', a syndrome characterized by 'higher-order' dysfunction following cerebellar injury in adults, including executive, visual-spatial, and linguistic dysfunction, as well as impaired attention. The cerebellum's contribution to higher cognitive function, affect and behavior has since been corroborated by others and is now increasingly endorsed (Schmahmann and Sherman 1998; Levisohn et al. 2000; Rapoport et al. 2000; Riva and Giorgi 2000; Beldarrain 2002; Molinari et al. 2002; Steinlin et al. 2003; Ito 2006; Schmahmann et al. 2007; Stoodley and Schmahmann, 2009b). Similar findings have also been described in older children with acquired and developmental cerebellar lesions (Merrill et al. 1998; Riva and Giorgi 2000; Bolduc and Limperopoulos 2009) as well as attention-deficit hyperactivity syndrome, autism spectrum disorders, and schizophrenia (Courchesne et al. 1994; Bishop 2002; Seidman et al. 2005). Noteworthy is the fact that these socio-affective changes are most prominent when the vermis and paravermian regions of the cerebellum are injured. Conversely, the lateral hemispheres of the cerebellum are believed to be involved in higher cognitive function and motor function. Relevant to preterm children is a developmental form of the cerebellar cognitive affective disorder described below.

Functional consequences of cerebellar injury in preterm survivors

Until recently, the neurodevelopmental outcome of preterm survivors following direct cerebellar injury remained poorly defined. Available data were limited by small sample sizes, combined preterm and term infants, a broad age range at testing, and a lack of a standardized approach to outcome ascertainment (Williamson et al. 1985; Chadduck et al. 1995; Mercuri et al. 1997; Johnsen et al. 2002, 2005; Miall et al.

2003; Bodensteiner and Johnsen 2005; Bednarek et al. 2008). Moreover, earlier outcome studies primarily described an extensive form of cerebellar injury that occurred in combination with supratentorial parenchymal injury. A high prevalence of profound neurologic impairment, including microcephaly, spastic quadriplegia and diplegia, hypotonia, dystonia, ataxia, and seizures, was reported among survivors (Johnsen et al. 2002, 2005; Bodensteiner and Johnsen, 2005).

More recently, outcome studies have begun to incorporate a multidimensional approach for evaluating the impact of early-life cerebellar injury in survivors of preterm birth using more rigorous study designs. Converging lines of evidence point to a significantly increased risk for developmental disabilities among preterm born children with cerebellar injury when compared with their age-matched preterm-born peers with normal imaging studies. Limperopoulos and colleagues (Limperopoulos et al. 2007) compared neurodevelopmental outcome in 35 preterm infants with isolated cerebellar hemorrhagic injury with 35 age-matched controls. Children underwent formal neurologic examinations and a battery of standardized outcome evaluations at a mean age of 32 months. Neurologic abnormalities were present in 66% of cases with isolated cerebellar hemorrhagic injury compared with 5% of the infants in the control group. Abnormalities included hypotonia in all children with cerebellar injury, regional/focal hypertonia in 11%, and motor asymmetries in 6%. In addition, 37% had an abnormal gait, 23% had extraocular abnormalities, and 17% had visual field defects and microcephaly. Children with isolated cerebellar injury had significantly lower mean scores on all tested measures compared with controls. Severe motor disabilities were reported in 48%, the presence of expressive and receptive language deficits ranged from 37% to 42%, and cognitive impairments were present in 40%. A surprisingly high prevalence of early signs of autistic features was noted in 42%, and over one-third demonstrated internalizing behavioral problems (e.g., withdrawn, somatic complaints, anxious and depressed). Of particular note is the fact that these social-behavioral problems were almost exclusively associated with injury to the vermis. Interestingly, preterm infants with cerebellar hemorrhagic injury and supratentorial parenchymal injury were not at overall greater risk for neurodevelopmental disabilities, although neuromotor impairment was more severe. These data strongly support an under-recognized role for cerebellar injury in the high prevalence of pervasive neurodevelopmental disabilities as well as social, affective, and behavioral dysfunction in survivors of preterm-born.

A second case-control study by Messerschmidt et al. (Messerschmidt et al. 2008) on 31 preterm infants with cerebellar injury and 31 age- and sex-matched controls with normal cerebellar development (24–36 month age range) showed that children with cerebellar injury had significantly poorer neuromotor and cognitive development compared with controls. In addition, the distribution of cerebral palsy was different between the groups. Mixed cerebral palsy (spastic-ataxic, spastic-dyskinetic) was diagnosed in 48%. Additionally, the frequencies of microcephaly and epilepsy were found to be significantly higher in children with cerebellar injury. Noteworthy is the fact that the cohort described by Messerschmidt had associated supratentorial injury, which was comparable in both groups.

The functional impact of indirect injury to the cerebellum in survivors of preterm birth has only recently been explored. In ex-preterm-born adolescents without evidence of direct cerebellar injury, MRI measures of cerebellar volume have been shown to be inversely related to adverse cognitive and neuropsychiatric outcome (Allin et al. 2001; Parker et al. 2008), particularly when this volume decrease involved the lateral hemispheres (Allin et al. 2001, 2005). Reductions in cerebellar volume in very preterm-born adolescents also correlated with reduced self-reporting of mental wellbeing (e.g., concentration, feeling worthless, feeling confident, overcoming difficulties) (Parker et al. 2008). These data corroborate previous reports in adults that implicate the cerebellum in cognition and in the regulation of emotions, affect, and behavior in adults.

In summary, accumulating evidence suggests an increased risk among extremely preterm infants with cerebellar injury for significant and far-reaching developmental consequences by preschool age. Long-term follow-up studies are urgently needed to better elucidate the extent to which theses deficits are transient or persistent in nature, and to define the true prevalence of autism spectrum disorders in this vulnerable population. Additionally, the structure-function relationship between cerebellar topography and domain-specific developmental disabilities warrants further study.

Summary and conclusions

To date, it has been established that cerebellar injury occurs in the smallest, sickest preterm infants. Cerebellar underdevelopment occurs on a continuum of severity ranging from mild to severe, near complete destructive injury. The developmental consequences of direct cerebellar injury far exceed the motor domain and include pervasive neurodevelopmental sequelae in the areas of cognitive, behavioral, and affective function. Studies are needed to expand our understanding of the acute antecedents and sequelae of prematurity-related cerebellar injury. Likewise, longitudinal studies are needed to further delineate the true nature and severity of these developmental cognitive affective deficits following cerebellar injury. The precise structure-function relationships between these observations are not yet known. The relative contribution of direct cerebellar injury versus the role of secondary trophic withdrawal in supratentorial regions to the high prevalence of pervasive neurodevelopmental impairments experienced by survivors awaits further study. A better understanding of the causes and functional consequences of cerebellar injury in the surviving preterm infant will provide clinicians with accurate information to allow for informed prognostic counseling of future families, and facilitate the development of more effective and individually tailored early intervention programs. Finally, given the well-documented protracted development course of the cerebellum and its highly plastic properties, together with the recent successful application of advanced magnetic resonance imaging techniques, the effectiveness of targeted early intervention strategies can be studied.

REFERENCES

Allin M, Matsumoto H, Santhouse AM, Nosarti C, AlAsady MH, Stewart AL, et al. (2001) Cognitive and motor function and the size of the cerebellum in adolescents born very pre-term. Brain 124(Pt 1): 60–66.

Allin MP, Salaria S, Nosarti C, Wyatt J, Rifkin L, Murray RM (2005) Vermis and lateral lobes of the cerebellum in adolescents born very preterm. Neuroreport 16(16): 1821–1824.

Armstrong DL, Sauls CD, Goddard-Finegold J (1987) Neuropathologic findings in short-term survivors of intraventricular hemorrhage. Am J Dis Child 141: 617–621.

Baader SL, Schilling ML, Rosengarten B, Pretsch W, Teutsch HF, Oberdick J, Schilling K (1996) Purkinje cell lineage and the topographic organization of the cerebellar cortex: a view from X inactivation mosaics. Dev Biol 174(2): 393–406.

Bautista JR, Rubin SA, Moran TH, Schwartz GJ, Carbone KM (1995) Developmental injury to the cerebellum following perinatal Borna disease virus infection. Brain Res Dev Brain Res 90(1–2): 45–53.

Bednarek N, Akhavi A, Pietrement C, Mesmin F, Loron G, Morville P (2008) Outcome of cerebellar injury in very low birth-weight infants: 6 case reports. J Child Neurol 23(8): 906–911.

Bejar R, Coen RW, Ekpoudia I, James HE, Gluck L (1985) Real time ultrasound diagnosis of hemorrhagic pathological conditions in the posterior fossa of preterm infants. Neurosurgery 16(3): 281–289.

Beldarrain MG (2002) The cerebellum may be directly involved in cognitive functions. Neurology 59(5): 791; author reply.

Bishop DV (2002) Cerebellar abnormalities in developmental dyslexia: cause, correlate or consequence? Cortex 38(4): 491–498.

Bodensteiner JB, Johnsen SD (2005) Cerebellar injury in the extremely premature infant: newly recognized but relatively common outcome. J Child Neurol 20(2): 139–142.

Bodensteiner JB, Johnsen SD (2006) Magnetic resonance imaging (MRI) findings in children surviving extremely premature delivery and extremely low birthweight with cerebral palsy. J Child Neurol 21(9): 743–747.

Bolduc ME, Limperopoulos C (2009) Neurodevelopmental outcomes in children with cerebellar malformations: a systematic review. Dev Med Child Neurol 51(4): 256–267.

Boltshauser E (2004) Cerebellum-small brain but large confusion: a review of selected cerebellar malformations and disruptions. Am J Med Genet A 126(4): 376–385.

Bourgouin PM, Tampieri D, Melancon D, del Carpio R, Ethier R (1992) Superficial siderosis of the brain following unexplained subarachnoid hemorrhage: MRI diagnosis and clinical significance. Neuroradiology 34(5): 407–410.

Bulas DI, Taylor GA, Fitz CR, Revenis ME, Glass P, Ingram JD (1991) Posterior fossa intracranial hemorrhage in infants treated with extracorporeal membrane oxygenation: sonographic findings. AJR Am J Roentgenol 156(3): 571–575.

Bystron I, Blakemore C, Rakic P (2008) Development of the human cerebral cortex: Boulder Committee revisited. Nat Rev Neurosci 9(2): 110–122.

Castro Conde JR, Martinez ED, Rodriguez RC, Rodriguez De Hoyos AL (2005) CNS siderosis and Dandy-Walker variant after neonatal alloimmune thrombocytopenia. Pediatr Neurol 32(5): 346–349.

Chadduck WM, Duong DH, Kast JM, Donahue DJ (1995) Pediatric cerebellar hemorrhages. Childs Nerv Syst 11(10): 579–583.

Courchesne E, Townsend J, Saitoh O (1994) The brain in infantile autism: posterior fossa structures are abnormal. Neurology 44(2): 214–223.

Di Salvo DN (2001) A new view of the neonatal brain: clinical utility of supplemental neurologic US imaging windows. Radiographics 21(4): 943–955.

Ecury-Goossen GM, Dudink J, Lequin M, Feijen-Roon M, Horsch S, Govaert P (2010) The clinical presentation of preterm cerebellar haemorrhage. Eur J Pediatr 169(10): 1249–1253.

Evans MJ, McKeever PA, Pearson GA, Field D, Firmin RK (1994) Pathological complications of non-survivors of newborn extracorporeal membrane oxygenation. Arch Dis Child 71(2): F88–92.

Fukuda K, Aihara N, Sagar SM, Sharp FR, Pitts LH, Honkaniemi J, Noble LJ (1996) Purkinje cell vulnerability to mild traumatic brain injury. J Neurotrauma 13(5): 255–266.

Gould SJ, Howard S, Hope PL, Reynolds EO (1987) Periventricular intraparenchymal cerebral haemorrhage in preterm infants: the role of venous infarction. J Pathol 151: 197–202.

Grunnet ML, Shields WD (1976) Cerebellar hemorrhage in the premature infant. J Pediatr 88(4 Pt 1): 605–608.

Hamre KM, West JR (1993) The effects of the timing of ethanol exposure during the brain growth spurt on the number of cerebellar Purkinje and granule cell nuclear profiles. Alcohol Clin Exp Res 17(3): 610–622.

Hatten ME (1990) Riding the glial monorail: a common mechanism for glial-guided neuronal migration in different regions of the developing mammalian brain. Trends Neurosci 13(5): 179–184.

Hughes JT, Oppenheimer DR (1969) Superficial siderosis of the central nervous system. A report on nine cases with autopsy. Acta Neuropathol 13(1): 56–74.

Huttenlocher PR (1979) Synaptic density in human frontal cortex – developmental changes and effects of aging. Brain Res 163(2): 195–205.

Huttenlocher PR, Dabholkar AS (1997) Regional differences in synaptogenesis in human cerebral cortex. J Comp Neurol 387(2): 167–178.

Ito M (2006) Cerebellar circuitry as a neuronal machine. Prog Neurobiol 78(3–5): 272–303.

Johnsen SD, Tarby TJ, Lewis KS, Bird R, Prenger E (2002) Cerebellar infarction: an unrecognized complication of very low birthweight. J Child Neurol 17(5): 320–324.

Johnsen SD, Bodensteiner JB, Lotze TE (2005) Frequency and nature of cerebellar injury in the extremely premature survivor with cerebral palsy. J Child Neurol 20(1): 60–64.

Kelly RM, Strick PL (2003) Cerebellar loops with motor cortex and prefrontal cortex of a nonhuman primate. J Neurosci 23(23): 8432–8444.

Kollias SS, Ball WS, Jr, Prenger EC (1993) Cystic malformations of the posterior fossa: differential diagnosis clarified through embryologic analysis. Radiographics 13(6): 1211–1231.

Kostovic I, Judas M, Rados M, Hrabac P (2002) Laminar organization of the human fetal cerebrum revealed by histochemical markers and magnetic resonance imaging. Cereb Cortex 12(5): 536–544.

Lemire R, Loeser J, Leech R, Alvord E (1985) Normal and abnormal development of the human nervous system. Hagerstown, MD: Harper & Row.

Levisohn L, Cronin-Golomb A, Schmahmann JD (2000) Neuropsychological consequences of cerebellar tumour resection in children: cerebellar cognitive affective syndrome in a paediatric population. Brain 123(Pt 5): 1041–1050.

Limperopoulos C, Benson CB, Bassan H, Disalvo DN, Kinnamon DD, Moore M, et al. (2005a) Cerebellar hemorrhage in the preterm infant: ultrasonographic findings and risk factors. Pediatrics 116(3): 717–724.

Limperopoulos C, Soul JS, Gauvreau K, Huppi PS, Warfield SK, Bassan H, et al. (2005b) Late gestation cerebellar growth is rapid and impeded by premature birth. Pediatrics 115(3): 688–695.

Limperopoulos C, Soul JS, Haidar H, Huppi PS, Bassan H, Warfield SK, et al. (2005c) Impaired trophic interactions between the cerebellum and the cerebrum among preterm infants. Pediatrics 116(4): 844–850.

Limperopoulos C, Bassan H, Gauvreau K, Robertson RL, Jr., Sullivan NR, Benson CB, et al. (2007) Does cerebellar injury in premature infants contribute to the high prevalence of long-term cognitive, learning, and behavioral disability in survivors? Pediatrics 120(3): 584–593.

Limperopoulos C, Chilingaryan G, Guizard N, Robertson RL, du Plessis AJ (2010) Cerebellar injury in the premature infant is associated with impaired growth of specific cerebral regions. Pediatr Res 68: 145–150.

Martin R, Roessmann U, Fanaroff A (1976) Massive intracerebellar hemorrhage in low-birth-weight infants. J Pediatr 89(2): 290–293.

Mercuri E, He J, Curati WL, Dubowitz LM, Cowan FM, Bydder GM (1997) Cerebellar infarction and atrophy in infants and children with a history of premature birth. Pediatr Radiol 27(2): 139–143.

Merrill JD, Piecuch RE, Fell SC, Barkovich AJ, Goldstein RB (1998) A new pattern of cerebellar hemorrhages in preterm infants. Pediatrics 102(6): E62.

Messerschmidt A, Brugger PC, Boltshauser E, Zoder G, Sterniste W, Birnbacher R, Prayer D (2005) Disruption of cerebellar development: potential complication of extreme prematurity. AJNR Am J Neuroradiol 26(7): 1659–1667.

Messerschmidt A, Fuiko R, Prayer D, Brugger PC, Boltshauser E, Zoder G, et al. (2008) Disrupted cerebellar development in preterm infants is associated with impaired neurodevelopmental outcome. Eur J Pediatr 167(10): 1141–1147.

Miale IL, Sidman RL (1961) An autoradiographic analysis of histogenesis in the mouse cerebellum. Exp Neurol 4: 277–296.

Miall LS, Cornette LG, Tanner SF, Arthur RJ, Levene MI (2003) Posterior fossa abnormalities seen on magnetic resonance brain imaging in a cohort of newborn infants. J Perinatol 23(5): 396–403.

Middleton FA, Strick PL (2001) Cerebellar projections to the prefrontal cortex of the primate. J Neurosci 21(2): 700–712.

Molinari M, Filippini V, Leggio MG (2002) Neuronal plasticity of interrelated cerebellar and cortical networks. Neuroscience 111(4): 863–870.

Nat R, Voiculescu B, Stanciu C, Vidulescu C, Cergan R, Badiu C, Popescu LM (2001) Apoptosis in human embryo development: 2. Cerebellum. J Cell Mol Med 5(2): 179–187.

Pape KE, Wigglesworth JS (1979) Birth trauma. In: Haemorrhage, Ischemia, and the Perinatal Brain. Philadelphia: J.B. Lippincott Co.; 61–84.

Pape KE, Armstrong DL, Fitzhardinge PM (1976) Central nervous system patholgoy associated with mask ventilation in the very low birthweight infant: a new etiology for intracerebellar hemorrhages. Pediatrics 58(4): 473–483.

Parker J, Mitchell A, Kalpakidou A, Walshe M, Jung HY, Nosarti C, et al. (2008) Cerebellar growth and behavioural & neuropsychological outcome in preterm adolescents. Brain 131(Pt 5): 1344–1351.

Perlman JM, Volpe JJ (1987) Are venous circulatory abnormalities important in the pathogenesis of hemorrhagic and/or ischemic cerebral injury? Pediatrics 80(5): 705–711.

Perlman JM, Nelson JS, McAlister WH, Volpe JJ (1983) Intracerebellar hemorrhage in a premature newborn: diagnosis by real-time ultrasound and correlation with autopsy findings. Pediatrics 71(2): 159–162.

Pierson CR, Folkerth RD, Billiards SS, Trachtenberg FL, Drinkwater ME, Volpe JJ, Kinney HC (2007) Gray matter injury associated with periventricular leukomalacia in the premature infant. Acta Neuropathol 114(6): 619–631.

Price DJ, Kennedy H, Dehay C, Zhou L, Mercier M, Jossin Y, et al. (2006) The development of cortical connections. Eur J Neurosci 23(4): 910–920.

Rakic P (2006) A century of progress in corticoneurogenesis: from silver impregnation to genetic engineering. Cereb Cortex 16 Suppl 1: i3–17.

Rakic P, Sidman RL (1970) Histogenesis of cortical layers in human cerebellum, particularly the lamina dissecans. J Comp Neurol 139(4): 473–500.

Rakic P, Hashimoto-Torii K, Sarkisian MR (2007) Genetic determinants of neuronal migration in the cerebral cortex. Novartis Found Symp 288: 45–53; discussion 53–58, 96–98.

Ramnani N (2006) The primate cortico-cerebellar system: anatomy and function. Nat Rev Neurosci 7(7): 511–522.

Rapoport M, van Reekum R, Mayberg H (2000) The role of the cerebellum in cognition and behavior: a selective review. J Neuropsychiatry Clin Neurosci 12(2): 193–198.

Rees S, Stringer M, Just Y, Hooper SB, Harding R (1997) The vulnerability of the fetal sheep brain to hypoxemia at mid-gestation. Brain Res Dev Brain Res 103(2): 103–118.

Rees SM, Loeliger MM, Munro KM, Shields A, Dalitz PA, Dieni S, et al. (2009) Cerebellar development in a baboon model of preterm delivery: impact of specific ventilatory regimes. J Neuropathol Exp Neurol 68(6): 605–615.

Riva D, Giorgi C (2000) The cerebellum contributes to higher functions during development: evidence from a series of children surgically treated for posterior fossa tumours. Brain 123(Pt 5): 1051–1061.

Rivas RJ, Hatten ME (1995) Motility and cytoskeletal organization of migrating cerebellar granule neurons. J Neurosci 15(2): 981–989.

Schmahmann JD, Sherman JC (1997) Cerebellar cognitive affective syndrome. Int Rev Neurobiol 41: 433–440.

Schmahmann JD, Sherman JC (1998) The cerebellar cognitive affective syndrome. Brain 121(Pt 4): 561–579.

Schmahmann JD, Weilburg JB, Sherman JC (2007) The neuropsychiatry of the cerebellum – insights from the clinic. Cerebellum 6(3): 254–267.

Sehgal A, El-Naggar W, Glanc P, Asztalos E (2009) Risk factors and ultrasonographic profile of posterior fossa haemorrhages in preterm infants. J Paediatr Child Health 45(4): 215–218.

Seidman LJ, Valera EM, Makris N (2005) Structural brain imaging of attention-deficit/hyperactivity disorder. Biol Psychiatry 57(11): 1263–1272.

Shah DK, Anderson PJ, Carlin JB, Pavlovic M, Howard K, Thompson DK, et al. (2006) Reduction in cerebellar volumes in preterm infants: relationship to white matter injury and neurodevelopment at two years of age. Pediatr Res 60(1): 97–102.

Skullerud K, Westre B (1986) Frequency and prognostic significance of germinal matrix hemorrhage, periventricular leukomalacia, and pontosubicular necrosis in preterm neonates. Acta Neuropathol (Berl) 70(3): 257–261.

Steggerda SJ, Leijser LM, Wiggers-de Bruine FT, van der Grond J, Walther FJ, van Wezel-Meijler G (2009) Cerebellar injury in preterm infants: incidence and findings on US and MR images. Radiology 252(1): 190–199.

Steinlin M, Imfeld S, Zulauf P, Boltshauser E, Lovblad KO, Ridolfi Luthy A, et al. (2003) Neuropsychological long-term sequelae after posterior fossa tumour resection during childhood. Brain 126(Pt 9): 1998–2008.

Stoodley CJ, Schmahmann JD (2009a) Functional topography in the human cerebellum: a meta-analysis of neuroimaging studies. Neuroimage 44(2): 489–501.

Stoodley CJ, Schmahmann JD (2009b) The cerebellum and language: evidence from patients with cerebellar degeneration. Brain Lang 110(3): 149–153.

Tam EW, Ferriero DM, Xu D, Berman JI, Vigneron DB, Barkovich AJ, Miller SP (2009) Cerebellar development in the preterm neonate: effect of supratentorial brain injury. Pediatr Res 66(1): 102–106.

Ten Donkelaar HJ, Lammens M (2009) Development of the human cerebellum and its disorders. Clin Perinatol 36(3): 513–530.

Thomson MA, Yoder BA, Winter VT, Giavedoni L, Chang LY, Coalson JJ (2006) Delayed extubation to nasal continuous positive airway pressure in the immature baboon model of bronchopulmonary dysplasia: lung clinical and pathological findings. Pediatrics 118(5): 2038–2050.

Tsuru A, Mizuguchi M, Takashima S (1995) Cystic leukomalacia in the cerebellar folia of premature infants. Acta Neuropathol 90: 400–402.

Ulupinar E, Yucel F (2005) Prenatal stress reduces interneuronal connectivity in the rat cerebellar granular layer. Neurotoxicol Teratol 27(3): 475–484.

Ulupinar E, Yucel F, Ortug G (2006) The effects of prenatal stress on the Purkinje cell neurogenesis. Neurotoxicol Teratol 28(1): 86–94.

Volpe JJ, Herscovitch P, Perlman JM, Raichle ME (1983) Positron emission tomography in the newborn: extensive impairment of regional cerebral blood flow with intraventricular hemorrhage and hemorrhagic intracerebral involvement. Pediatrics 72(5): 589–601.

Weir FJ, Ohlsson A, Myhr TL, Fong K, Ryan ML (1999) A patent ductus arteriosus is associated with reduced middle cerebral artery blood flow velocity. Eur J Pediatr 158(6): 484–487.

Williamson WD, Percy AK, Fishman MA, Cheek WR, Desmond MM, LaFevers N, Thurber SD (1985) Cerebellar hemorrhage in the term neonate: developmental and neurologic outcome. Pediat Neurol 1(6): 356–360.

Wingate RJ (2001) The rhombic lip and early cerebellar development. Curr Opin Neurobiol 11(1): 82–88.

Part 7
Vascular Disorders, Tumours, and Paraneoplastic Cerebellar Syndromes

32 Vascular Disorders of the Posterior Fossa

Maja Steinlin

Vascular pathology of the cerebellum is a component of stroke problems in childhood and is comparable with supratentorial cerebrovascular problems. However, there are some specific localization and age-related characteristics for childhood stroke in the infratentorial region. Isolated cerebellar haemorrhagic strokes occur more frequently than ischaemic strokes. The ratio of infratentorial to supratentorial aneurysms is higher in childhood than in adulthood. Vascular malformations such as arteriovenous malformations (AVMs), arteriovenous fistula (AVFs), and developmental venous anomalies (DVA) occur as frequently in children as in adults. In comparison with young adults, ischaemic infratentorial events occur less frequently in children.

Ischaemic stroke

Infratentorial ischaemic stroke in childhood accounts for 5–15% of childhood strokes (Delsing et al. 2001; Matta et al. 2006). This is significantly lower than in young adults (32%) (Bigi et al. 2011). Generally, infratentorial ischaemic stroke shares the same pathological characteristics as supratentorial stroke (Fox and Fullerton 2010), but there are some specific differences in terms of aetiology and presentation.

Aetiology

Basilar artery thrombosis and dissection of basilar or vertebral arteries account for the majority of infratentorial ichaemic stroke in childhood (Ganesan et al. 2002 and author's unpublished results). For both aetiologies, coexisting risk factors of infection and coagulopathies are most important. Further underlying conditions of systemic autoimmune disease, vascular malformations, and hypotension are also significant. Children with sickle cell anaemia and stroke demonstrate an anterior-posterior gradient in localization of ischaemic lesions (Pegelow et al. 2002). Few lesions occur in the occipital lobe (1.7%), slightly more in the cerebellum (5.5%), compared to 81% of affected children having lesions in the frontal lobe. The two most frequent aetiologies for supratentorial stroke, i.e., transient focal arteriopathy and cardiac conditions, are usually not implicated in infratentorial stroke of childhood. However, as paediatric stroke is often due to multiple risk factors, and as aetiologies causing supratentorial stroke can never be excluded for infratentorial lesions, evaluation of children with infratentorial stroke should be as thorough as for supratentorial stroke (Amlie-Lefond et al. 2008).

Moyamoya disease is rarely encountered in the posterior circulation; however, there are important aspects of posterior circulation in moyamoya disease that should be discussed.

The main feature of moyamoya disease is bilateral steno-occlusive changes at and around the internal carotid artery (ICA) bifurcation along with a distribution of abnormal netlike vessels in the basal regions. Changes similar to those around the ICA can also be found in the posterior circulation. Mugikura et al. demonstrated in childhood moyamoya disease that, with increasing degree of stenotic processes of the ICA, the posterior cerebral artery (PCA) also becomes involved (Mugikura et al. 1999). In SPECT and MR analyses of the posterior circulation in moyamoya disease, the presence of stenotic processes in the PCAs is seen to lead to a lack of posterior-anterior leptomeningeal collaterals, which usually have a preventive effect for ischaemic lesions. In cases with posterior circulation involvement, ischaemic lesions are observed not only in posterior watershed areas and PCA territory, but also in parietal, temporal and frontal lobes (Yamada et al. 1996).

Presentation

In our group of 25 children with posterior circulation stroke, taken from the Swiss Neuropaediatric Stroke Registry (SNPSR), paediatric National Institutes of Health score at presentation was comparable with those presenting with supratentorial stroke, i.e., 7 (range 1–25) and 6 (range 1–27), respectively. Children with basilar thrombosis manifest with obtundation, vomiting and neurological signs of spastic quadriplegia or ataxia (Luchini et al. 1992). Because of these unspecific symptoms, diagnosis is often delayed. Infratentorial strokes due to dissection present less severely, usually with focal symptoms such as ataxia, hemisyndromes or cranial nerve deficits (Ganesan et al. 2002).

Diagnosis

Magnetic resonance imaging (MRI) with diffusion-weighted sequences (Fig. 32.1) is mandatory in the diagnosis of infratentorial stroke. It is well recognized that infratentorial ischaemic lesions are frequently missed using computed tomography (CT) (Bürki et al. 2010). Careful angiographic imaging should be performed to investigate underlying causes, especially dissection or basilar thrombosis, which are the most frequent. The most sensitive imaging for dissection are fat-suppressed sequences of cervical and craniocervical regions. Contrast-enhanced vascular imaging from the aortic arch to brain are also helpful.

Infratentorial ischaemic strokes in childhood are less commonly confined to one site; of the 25 children from the SNPSR

(a) (b) (c) (d)

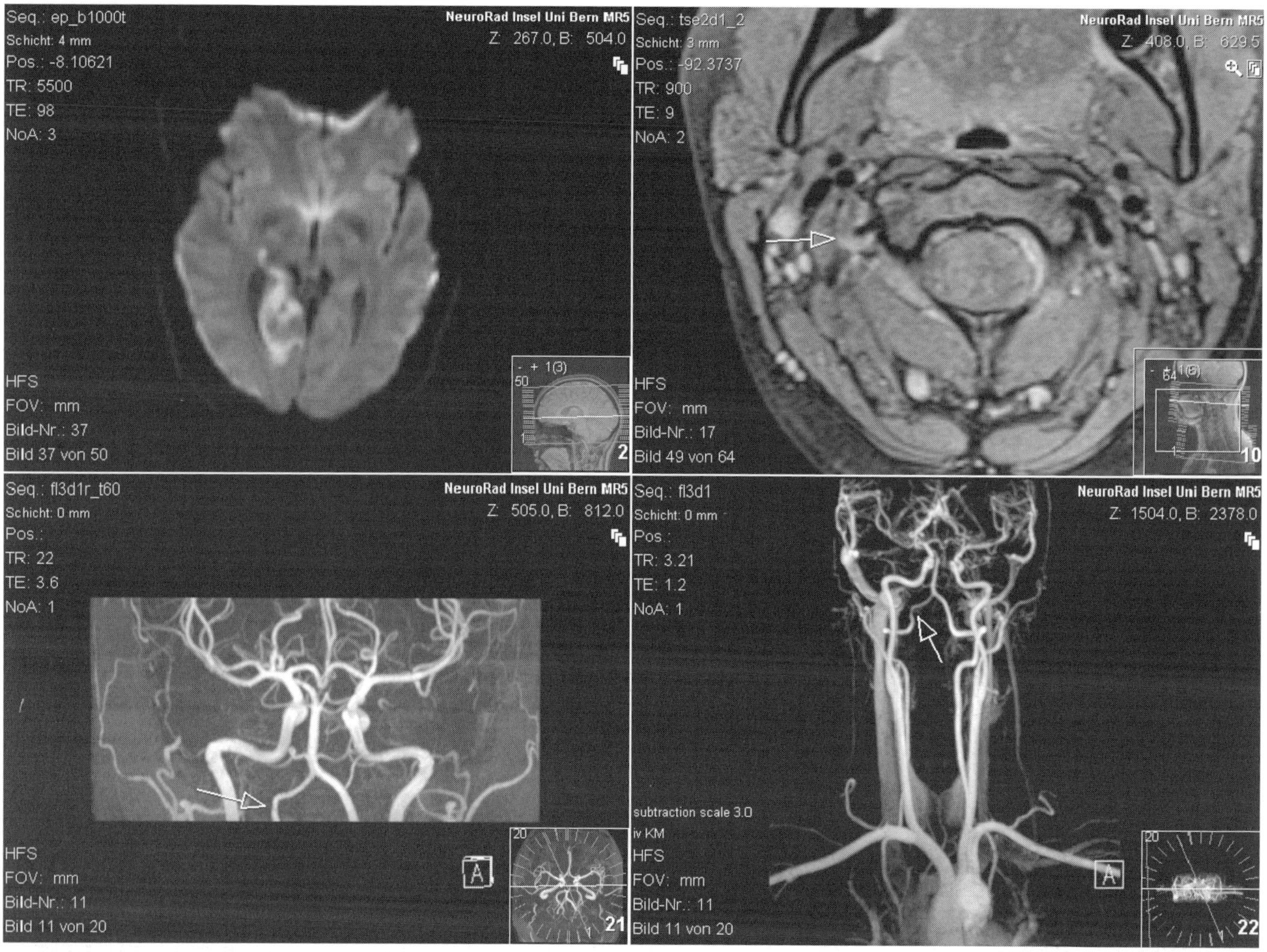

Fig. 32.1. Unilateral dissection of the right vertebral artery with subsequent infarction of the right posterior cerebral artery: **(a)** DWI (bright signal) indicates acute infarction. **(b)** T1-weighted fat-saturated axial images of the neck shows haematoma inside the wall of the enlarged right vertebral artery (arrow). **(c)** Time-of-flight angiography and **(d)** magnetic resonance luminography of the neck vessels shows a stenosis of the right vertebral artery at the dural entrance.

only 6 had isolated cerebellar lesions. Additional areas of involvement were most frequently the pons and mesencephalon.

Treatment

Indications for treatment are similar to that of supratentorial strokes: basic supportive therapies are mandatory, especially careful control of body temperature, blood pressure and glucose. Infratentorial ischaemic lesions are known to be at a high risk for developing malignant oedema, thus careful observation of these children, and if necessary decompressive surgery are important. However, in our own group of 25 children, oedema developed in only one case of bilateral cerebellar ischaemia. Platelet antiaggregation is the treatment of choice. There are some special indications for heparinization, i.e., in extracranial arterial dissection and cardiac embolic strokes. The indications for thrombolysis in childhood are not known. As clinical presentations for basilar thrombosis are frequently severe, and the therapeutic window for thrombolysis may be up to 24 hours, many children with basilar thrombosis receive this treatment. However, in our group of seven children with basilar thrombosis, outcome did not appear dependent on the type of treatment given, whether thrombolysis, heparinization or platelet antiaggregation. Because of risk of further embolic ischaemic events, in cases of extracranial arterial dissection heparinization is recommended. For all other children antiplatelet aggregation seems to be the treatment of choice (Royal College of Physicians 2004; Roach et al. 2008).

Outcome

Outcome in our group of children with infratentorial ischaemia showed a modified Rankin score (0–6) of 1.25, which is slightly better than for supratentorial stroke of 2.0. Despite the severe symptoms during the acute phase in children with basilar thrombosis, the outcome in these children is not as detrimental as might be expected. In our group of seven patients all had mild to moderate residual neurological problems such as ataxia or tetraspasticity; all attended normal school, with special help for two. Children with underlying dissections or other aetiologies have less prominent symptoms at presentation and their outcome is slightly better. Although the majority of these children have normal to low normal IQ, about half of them have cognitive deficits (processing speed, attention/concentration), which interfere significantly with their daily life. In the group of children reported by Ganesan et al., 12/22 were normal but only one was considered to be significantly cognitively impaired (Ganesan et al. 2002). Long-term follow-up and support, especially for cognitive problems, is important for these children.

Haemorrhagic stroke

Cerebellar haemorrhagic stroke in childhood is in most cases due to arteriovenous malformations, with fewer due to cavernomas and rupture of aneurysms of the posterior circulation.

Arteriovenous malformations

Arteriovenous malformations (AVMs) are a compact collection of abnormal thin-walled vessels connecting arteries to veins without an intervening capillary network. They are the expression of a malformation during the late somite stage of the fourth week of embryonic life. AVMs have an early postnatal growth potential. Increase in size with age results in progressive dilation of the feeding arteries and draining veins.

There is increasing evidence that the *incidence* of AVMs in children is about 1:100 000 and about 10–20% become symptomatic during childhood (Kondziolka et al. 1992). Boys and girls are about equally affected (Stapf et al. 2003). Cerebellar AVMs account for about 15% of all AVMs in children, as in a series of 132 reported by Humphreys, 13% had cerebellar and 10% pontine AVMs (Humphreys 1986). The most frequent *localization* is in the cerebellar hemisphere, but AVMs in the vermis and fourth ventricle are also reported. Some cerebellar AVMs spread to the brainstem. Considering the higher volume of the cerebrum, infratentorial AVMs have about the same frequency as supratentorial AVMs.

Presentation: Most cerebellar AVMs present with acute bleeding (Khaw et al. 2004; Stapf et al. 2003) (Fig. 32.2).

(a) (b) (c) (d)

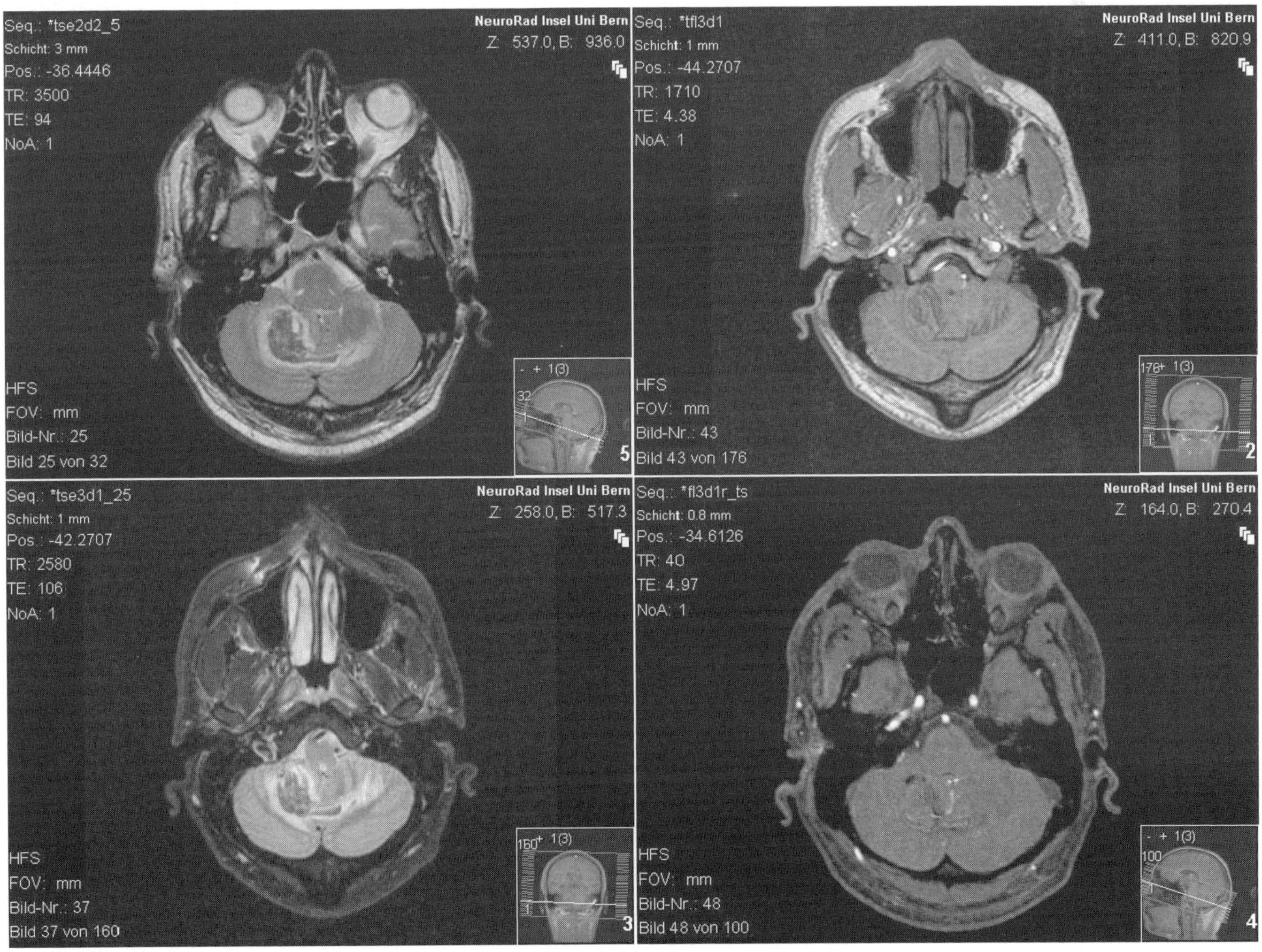

Fig. 32.2. Right cerebellar arteriovenous malformation (AVM): hyperacute haemorrhage of the right cerebellar hemisphere T2-weighted dark **(a, c)**, T1-weighted **(b)** isointense signal indicates deoxyhaemoglobin. Because of compression of the AVM by the haematoma, time-of-flight magnetic resonance angiography detects only subtle flow signals of the AVM **(d)**.

Children have a higher frequency of bleeding but a lower frequency of seizures compared with adults under 50, a relationship which is reversed in adults older than 50 years (Stapf et al. 2003). Rare cases are reported in which presentation is more insidious, with symptoms such as headache, ataxia and even mutism in a case of AVM within the vermis (Al-Anazi et al. 2001; Sugita et al. 2003).

Whether in children the risk of hemorrhage is higher in cerebellar AVMs than in supratentorial AVMs is still not known (Khaw et al. 2004; Arnaout et al. 2009). Khaw et al. showed the yearly risk of haemorrhage to be 11.6%. Additional concomitant abnormalities may contribute to this high risk. Although Stapf et al. showed that children with AVMs have a significantly lower incidence of coexisting aneurysms (Stapf et al. 2003), in the series of Griffiths et al. in 10 of 14 cases with cerebellar AVMs which presented with acute hemorrhage, findings including intranidal aneurysm, venous aneurysm or outflow obstructions could be detected by angiography (Griffiths et al. 1998). One might speculate that an increase of additional vascular malformations in childhood cerebellar AVMs might increase the risk of hemorrhage.

Diagnosis: The criterion standard for diagnostic work-up of cerebellar AVMs is still conventional angiography (Fig. 32.3). AVMs are usually supplied by ipsilateral cerebellar arteries to the nidus, most frequently the superior cerebellar artery is reported, but also supply from anterior inferior or posterior cerebellar arteries, in rare cases even from the external carotid artery. Venous drainage is usually but not exclusively in a posterior direction. Accompanying aneurysms can be detected within the nidus or outflow vessels, but almost never in the feeding arteries (Grifffiths et al. 1998). Because of the high risk of bleeding in cerebellar AVMs, treatment must be evaluated carefully. In children, an interventional or surgical approach is preferable to radiotherapy. Ideally there should be an interdisciplinary discussion about the best treatment option for individual cases. In about 1.5%, spontaneous

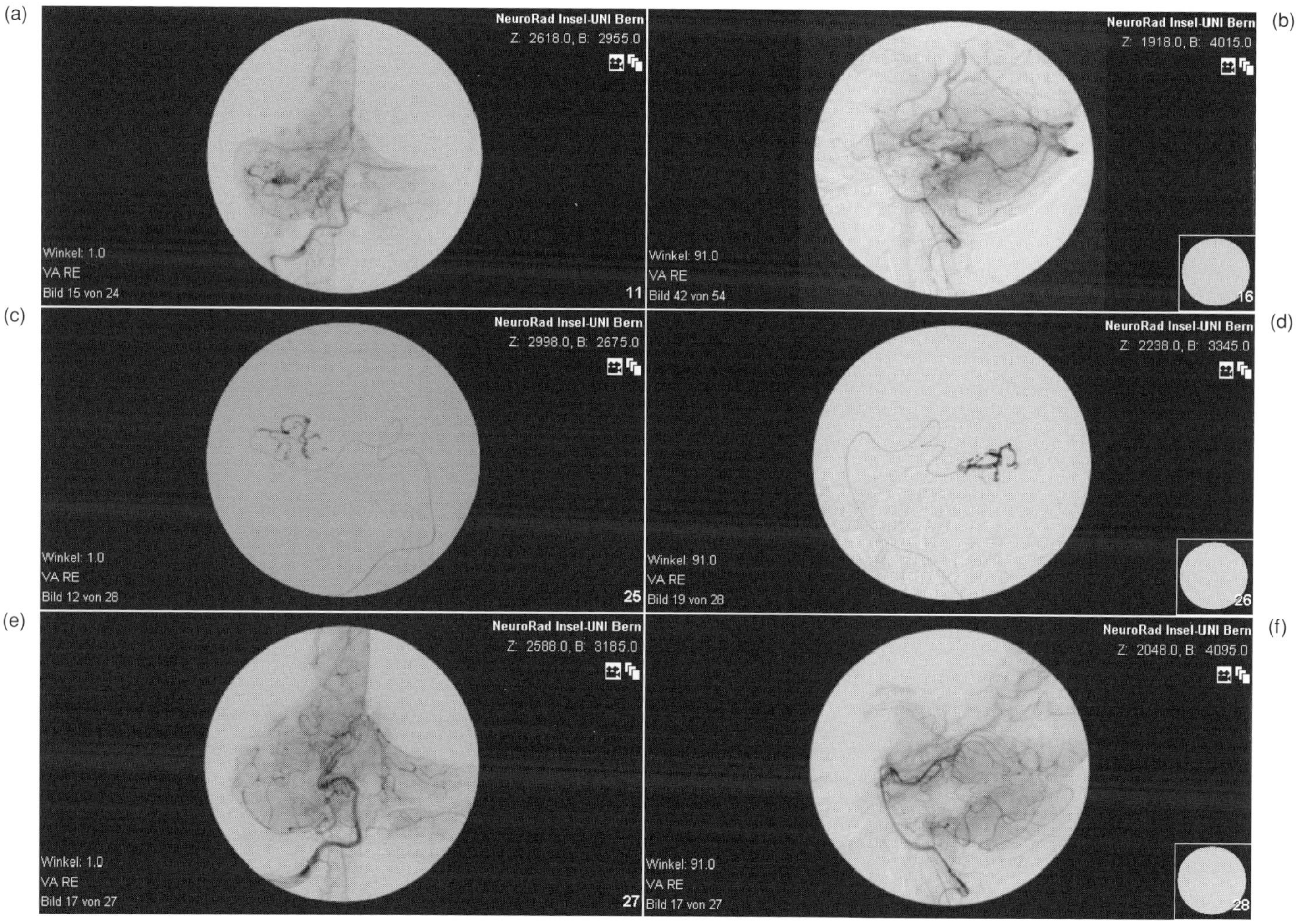

Fig. 32.3. Digital subtraction angiography (DSA) of a right cerebellar arteriovenous malformation (AVM) in **(a)** Towne and **(b)** lateral projection, supplied by feeders from the right posterior inferior cerebellar artery (PICA) and superior cerebellar artery (SCA). **(c, d)** DSA of glue injection into the nidus of the AVM with the tip of the microcatheter in the main feeder of the right SCA. **(e, f)** DSA following two glue embolizations via SCA and PCA reveals devascularization of the AVM.

occlusion of cerebellar AVMs can be observed (Panciani et al. 2008).

Mortality: Mortality is high due to the space-occupying consequences of acute bleeding in cerebellar AVMs. In a series of 17 children with acute haemorrhage due to cerebellar AVMs, 6 children died within a week of presentation; the size of the acute haematoma was a reasonable predictor of outcome (Griffiths et al. 1998). Acute decompression and/or evacuation of a haematoma is indicated and may decrease mortality and morbidity.

Outcome: The outcome for children who survive after acute infratentorial hemorrhage seems to be more optimistic than in adults. In our own series of eight surviving children after acute cerebellar haemorrhage (Wingeier et al. 2010), all of them showed mild motor (ataxic) difficulties and six had restricted oculomotor movements. However, these neurological symptoms caused only minimal interference to their daily life. Neuropsychological testing revealed reduced reaction times in all cases, semantic and phonemic word fluency problems in many, and in one a disexecutive syndrome was apparent. Children with vermal lesions showed cerebellar cognitive affective syndrome. In summary, the mortality for haemorrhagic cerebellar stroke due to AVMs of more than 30% is high; however, survivors have low levels of morbidity.

Arteriovenous fistulas

Arteriovenous fistulas (AVF) are characterized by the presence of one to three dilated feeding arteries opening to a dilated vein, often associated with a large venous pouch. Intradural AVFs are always on the surface of the supra-or infratentorial cortex. Cerebral AVFs account for 4.7% of all intracranial AVMs. In a series of 52 children with AVFs, only 11 were infratentorial and three had supra- and infratentorial localizations (Weon et al. 2005). Yoshida et al. reported 14 children with infratentorial AVFs, there was a male to female predominace of 1.8:1, and an even higher male predominance of 7:1 after excluding the six children with hereditary haemorrhagic teleangiectasias (Yoshida et al. 2004). Posterior fossa AVFs with tentorial and petrosial draining have not been reported in children.

Presentation: The manifestation of infratentorial AVFs has been reported as follows: only one occurred during the neonatal period, 50% occurred in infancy, and 43% in childhood. Symptoms and signs were typically macrocrania in infants and headache, neurological deficits without or with haemorrhage in children. Probably because of the thickness of the venous varix, haemorhage is uncommon. Hemorrhage may be intracerebral, subarachnoid or intraventricular. In about one-third of children there was cardiac overload at presentation, but only two children presented with additional neurological symptoms (Yoshida et al. 2004).

Diagnosis: Diagnosis is usually made by conventional angiography. Supply to the symptomatic fistula from the basilar artery is seen in the majority, but also occurs from the posterior inferior and anterior cerebellar arteries. Most children have one or two feeding arteries, but three and more are possible.

Treatment: The treatment of choice in the majority of children is by endovascular occlusion of the feeding arteries. In most children more than one intervention session is needed to achieve complete occlusion.

Outcome: The outcome of these children is rather good; in the series of Yoshida, 71% were neurologically normal. Those with moderate to severe outcomes were those with significant symptoms at presentation. In the two mortalities, occlusion of fistula was incomplete (Yoshida et al. 2004).

Rendu-Osler disease or hereditary haemorrhagic telangiectasia

Hereditary haemorrhagic telangiectasias (*HHT1* MIM #187300; *HHT2* MIM #600376; *HHT3* MIM %601101) are mucocutaneous and visceral telangiectasias, which lead to recurrent epistaxis and mucocutaneous and gastrointestinal hemorrhage in adults. These classic symptoms are unusual before puberty. However, multiple small AVMs or AVFs are highly suggestive of HHT (Matsubara et al. 2000).

HHT is an autosomal dominant angiodysplasia with high penetrance and variable expressivity. To date, two responsible genes on chromosome 9 and 12, and one gene locus on chromosome 5, are known. Because of the accompanying expression of the capillary remodelling disorder of HHT, many patients also have arteriovenous malformations or fistulas in the pulmonary, hepatic or cerebral circulation (Figs 32.4 and 32.5) (Plauchu and Dupuis-Girod 2009; Faughnan et al. 2011). Willinsky reported that 28% of patients with multiple central nervous system AVMs did have HHT (Willinsky et al. 1990). Identification of multiple AVMs or AVFs in a child should alert suspicion of underlying HHT. Further cerebral complications of HHT include brain abscesses or embolic stroke. All three complications can affect the cerebellum.

Cavernous malformations

Cavernous malformations (*CCM1* MIM #116860; *CCM2* MIM #603284; *CCM3* MIM #603265) are well-circumscribed tumours of dilated and hypertrophied capillary beds, without arteriovenous shunting. They are thought to be congenital anomalies arising in the 3rd to 8th gestational week. However, they may expand like tumours by reactive angiogenesis, influenced by angiogenetic proteins expressed by the cavernoma. As many as 8–44% of cavernomas are accompanied by other vascular malformations such as capillary telangiectasias and AVMs. The incidence of cavernomas is suggested to be lower than 1% of the population. A female preponderance of 2:1–1.5 in childhood is noted in several reports (Lena et al. 2007). Radiotherapy of the brain in children increases the risk for development of cavernomas (Burn et al. 2007).

There are familial autosomal dominant traits for cavernomas and to date three different genes (*CCM1*, *CCM2*, and *CCM3*) have been identified (Felbor et al. 2006). All genetic forms have a higher rate of multiple lesions (60% versus 10% in the sporadic forms) (Houtteville 1997), thus the likelihood of a cavernoma in the posterior fossa is increased. Familial forms are characterized by a more aggressive course

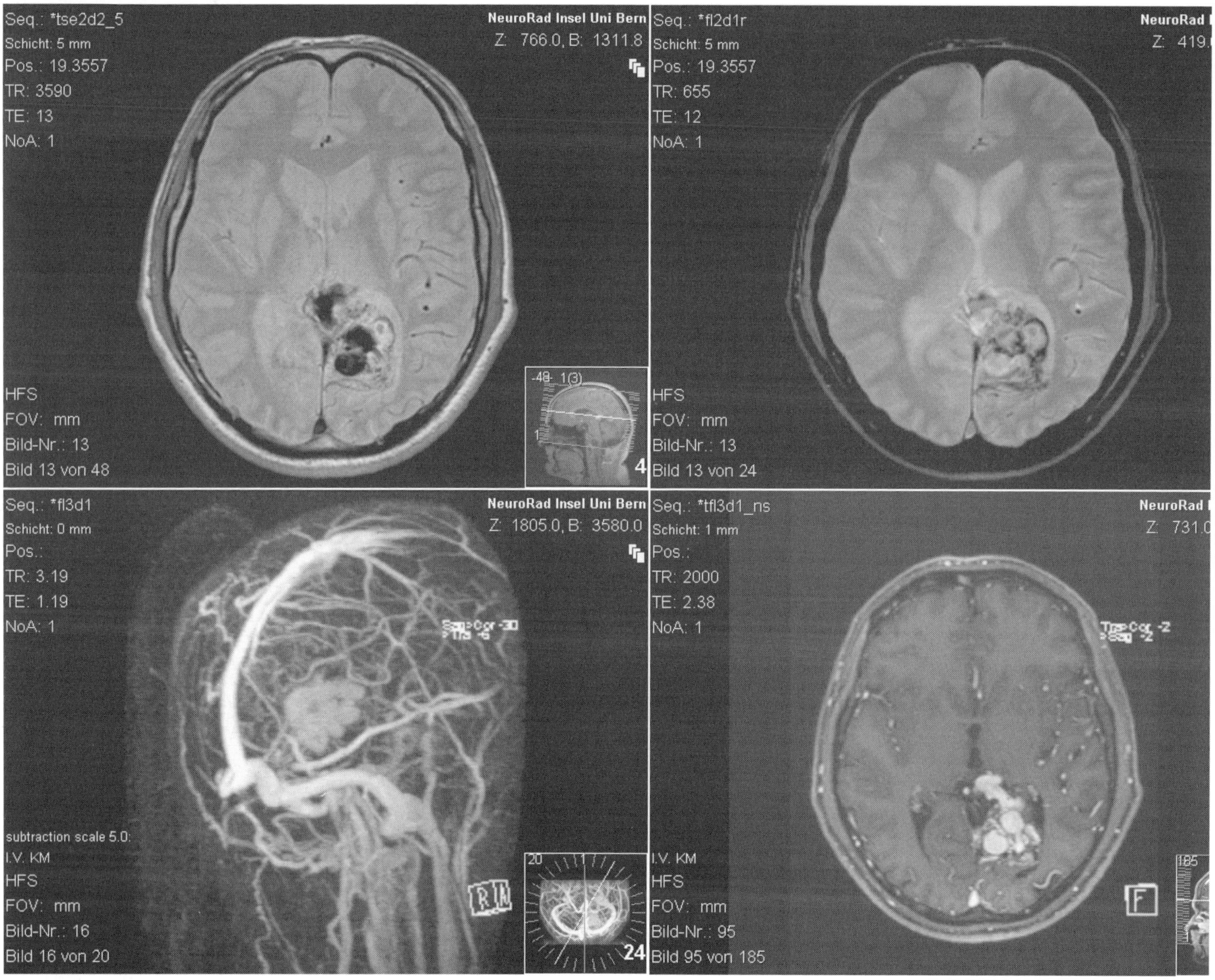

Fig. 32.4. Rendu-Osler disease with a left occipital arteriovenous malformation draining via enlarged periatrial veins mainly into the internal cerebral venous system.

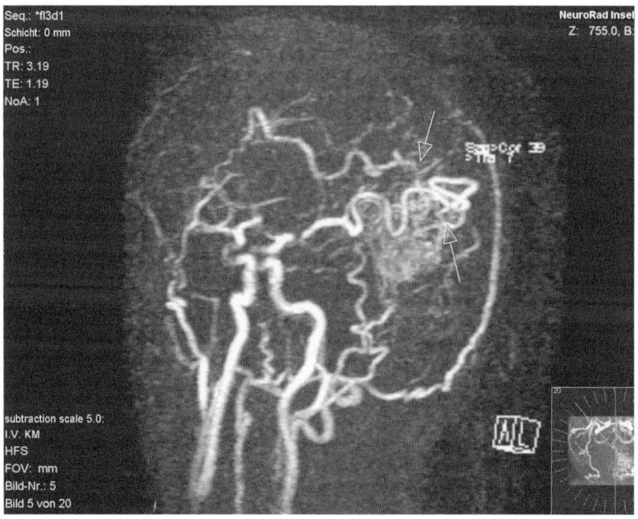

Fig. 32.5. Time-resolved contrast-enhanced MRA (TWIST-MRA) with high temporal resolution confirms branches of the middle cerebral and pericallosal arteries as main feeders of the arteriovenous malformation, with an additional blood supply from dural branches of the posterior meningeal artery.

(haemorrhage and neurological deficit) and, in particular, cavernomas related to *CCM3* have a high risk of bleeding. Familial forms have presented at younger ages, but the majority only present in adulthood (Houtteville 1997).

About 20% of all cavernomas in children are located in the posterior fossa, most of them in the pons or medulla (Lena et al. 2007).

Presentation

The presentation of cerebellar cavernomas include symptoms related to acute focal hemorrhage. In contrast to the acute bleed by AVMs or aneurysms, the mass of the haematoma is usually not as significant, thus the symptoms not as prominent. Most children present with headache and acute cerebellar symptoms such as ataxia, nystagmus or vertigo. Cerebellar cavernomas may also present as a space-occupying lesion, due to growth, without acute bleeding. In comparison to supratentorial cavernomas, infratentorial cavernomas have a two-fold increased rate of haemorrhage per patient and per year (Cantu et al. 2005). Thus, surgical excision of cerebellar cavernomas is the rule.

Brainstem cavernomas comprise a subset of posterior fossa cavernomas, occurring more frequent than cerebellar cavernomas (Lena et al. 2007). Presenting symptoms are more severe and are usually focal neurological deficits, corresponding to the location of the cavernoma (Scott et al. 1992; Di Rocco et al. 1997; Lena et al. 2002). Similar to cerebellar cavernomas, brainstem cavernomas have a higher hemorrhage risk than in other locations (Hauck et al. 2009). There is a significant higher morbidity after rebleeding compared to first time haemorrhage (Di Rocco et al. 1997).

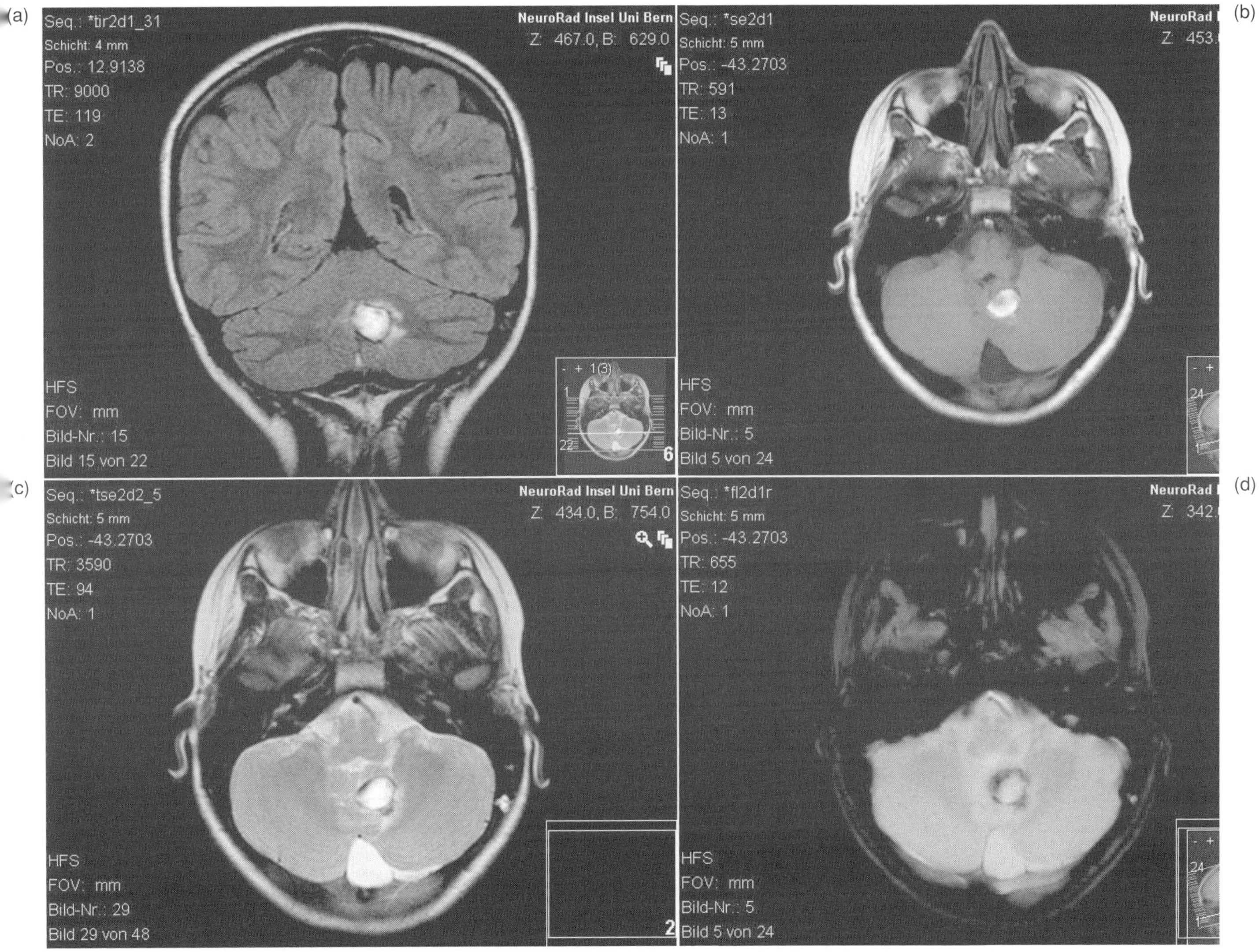

Fig. 32.6. Subacute haemorrhage from a cerebellar cavernoma: inhomogeneous T1-weighted **(a, b, d)** and T2-weighted **(c)** hypersignal indicates the degradation of (met-)haemoglobin. The hypointense rim on T2-weighted **(c)** and gradient-echo sequences **(d)** indicates haemosiderin deposition.

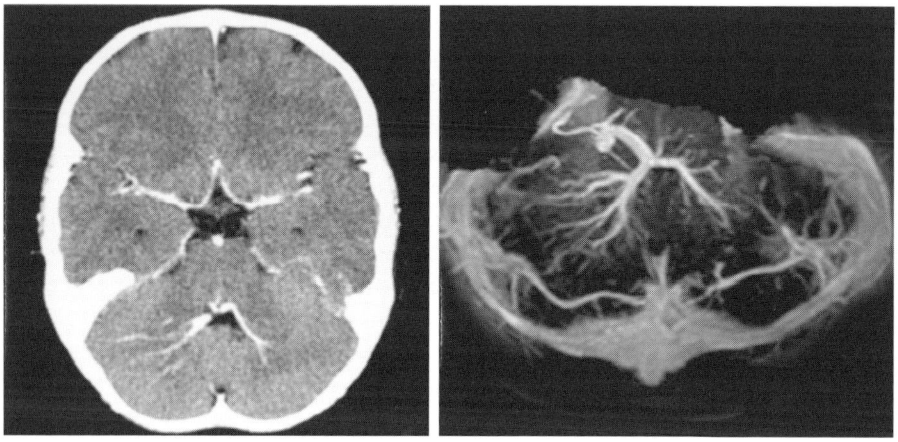

Fig. 32.7. Developmental venous anomaly (DVA) in the right cerebellar hemisphere. Angio-CT (left) and magnetic resonance venography (right) show the characteristic caput medusae (dendritic transcortical veins draining into the right sigmoid sinus).

Diagnosis

The criterion standard for diagnosis of cavernoma is MRI (Fig. 32.6). As these are low-flow vascular malformations without arteriovenous shunting they are not detectable by conventional angiography.

Treatment

Considering the high risk of hemorrhage in infratentorial cavernomas, the current consensus is that these cavernomas should be totally resected after becoming symptomatic. Because of advances in modern surgical approaches, surgery even in an unfavourable location such as the brainstem is related to a small risk of residual deficit (Bruneau et al. 2006). Cavernomas have no arteriovenous connections and hence are unsuitable for interventional embolization.

Outcome

The outcome for children after symptomatic presentation and appropriate treatment is favourable. The majority of children are asymptomatic; and even in cases with brainstem cavernomas, improvement of symptoms is usual. In the series reported by Lena et al. only one of nine children showed worsening after the operation, with one child dying after rehemorrhaging. All others were asymptomatic or improved after surgery (Lena et al. 2002).

Developmental venous anomalies

Developmental venous anomalies (DVAs) rarely become symptomatic and present by haemorrhagic stroke.

DVAs are enlarged veins, which are thought to originate from a developmental arrest of fetal veins (Topper et al. 1999) or from a transient venous hypertension during the late embryonic stage (Nomura et al. 2006). Infratentorial venous anomalies occur always in the cerebellum, and are encountered only as tectum derivatives such as metencephalum, mesencephalum and telencephalum (Berenstein and Lasjaunias 1992).

Cerebellar DVAs are less frequent than supratentorial DVAs. They usually drain into the vein of Galen, the sinus petrosus, the torcula or lateral sinus (Fig. 32.7).

Presentation

About 1–16% of DVAs may bleed; infratentorial and deep DVA seem to have a higher incidence of haemorrhage (Uchino et al. 1996). However, haemorrhage of DVAs is rarely life threatening, even when combined with cavernomas. In 8–33% of cases, DVAs are associated with a cavernoma (Fleetwood and Steinberg 2002), and in some cases these cavernomas are shown to be acquired and not congenital (Campeau and Lane 2005). Further, the new development of cerebellar AVMs draining into DVAs has been reported (Nussbaum et al. 1998). These findings suggest that venous outflow disturbance and venous hypertension are important in the pathogenesis of cavernomas and arteriovenous malformations.

As they consist of a compensatory drainage system they should not be ligated, embolized or resected (Mori et al. 1994).

Aneurysms

Aneurysms are acquired fusiform or saccular abnormalities of vessels, with a lack of the intima and thinning of the vascular wall. The incidence of childhood aneurysms is low, they account for about 1–2% of all aneurysms. However, they can occur at any age from the neonatal period onwards.

In childhood, aneurysms are predominantly peripheral and distal to the circle of Willis. About three-quarters are giant aneurysms, a greater proportion than for those arising in adulthood. The frequency of posterior circulation aneurysms is 20–30%, higher than in adults (Huang et al. 2005; Lasjaunias et al. 2005). In a large series of 59 children reported by Lasjaunias, 20 children had 23 posterior circulation aneurysms; their characteristics were similar to the anterior circulation aneurysms with a female preponderance (5:1) below the age of 2 years, switching to a male preponderance of 3:2 during childhood.

In the same series 18 of 23 aneurysms were considered to be *fusiform dissecting aneurysms* (large, fusiform and partially thrombosed), involving the PCA, PICA, and basilar and vertebral arteries. They represent acute, subacute or chronic recurrent dissection of the arterial wall due to non-infectious aetiology. There was an equal distribution of anterior and posterior dissecting aneurysms.

Besides large fusiform dissecting aneurysms, *saccular or congenital aneurysms* are the most frequent type in childhood, and are thin-walled endothelial-lined fibrous sacs often located at arterial bifurcations (Allison et al. 1998). In the series of Lasjaunias, three were located on the basilar tip and one in the posterior communicating artery. In the series of Allison, 8 of 18 congenital aneurysms were located in the posterior circulation (overall frequency in posterior circulation aneurysm, 44%), in the PICA, PCA, or posterior cerebellar superior and basilar arteries. Many disorders are associated with congenital aneurysm in childhood, including Ehlers-Danlos syndrome, Marfan syndrome, polycystic kidney disease, and neurofibromatosis. Familial aneurysms seldom present during childhood.

Infectious and traumatic aneurysms are not limited to bifurcations and are more frequent in children than in adults, though rare. There was only one each of traumatic and infectious causes in the series reported by Lasjaunias et al. (2005). In the series reported by Allison et al., there were four infectious aneurysms (due to *Pseudomas*, HIV and *Aspergillus*) of the posterior circulation, three located in the basilar artery and one in the vertebral artery. Traumatic aneurysms are considered pseudoaneurysms because of lack of endothelial lining (Allison et al. 1998), they tend to be supratentorial (none were in the posterior circulation in the series of Allison, and one in the series of Lasjaunias). They are not related to bifurcation sites and typically do not have a neck.

Presentation

The presentation of children with posterior circulation aneurysms is with infratentorial subarachnoid haemorrhage (SAH) in the majority, frequently combined with severe headache, meningeal signs, vomiting and obtundation which might progress to coma. Blood can be detected in the fourth ventricle (85%) and subarachnoid space (65%). In children younger than 5 years of age, the typical history of acute headache is rarely reported. As children tend more frequently to have giant aneurysms, presentation by focal signs occurs in about 20%. For aneurysms of the posterior fossa with the arteries in close proximity to the cranial nerves, focal symptoms as third or fourth nerve palsy, facial palsy, and hearing deficits may occur. Cerebellar symptoms such as vertigo, vomiting, and gait instability may also be evident.

Treatment

Initial treatment during the acute phase of subarachnoid haemorrhage should be directed at controlling symptoms and complications. Because of possible compression in the posterior fossa the risk for acute hydrocephalus and/or upward herniation are high. Surgical decompression and/or evacuation of haematoma are important for many children. Vasospasm causing delayed cerebral ischaemia is not a typical problem associated with SAH in the paediatric age group. In a series reported by Aryan, only 16% were affected, all of them older than 9 years (Aryan et al. 2005). The greater tolerance in younger children is thought to be related to relatively better collateral circulation (Huang et al. 2005).

Diagnosis

The criterion standard for further diagnostic work-up is conventional angiography (Fig. 32.8). As with AVMs, an interdisciplinary team should discuss treatment options as to whether interventional, neurosurgical or a combination of both are best for the individual child.

Outcome

Mortality for aneurysms in childhood overall is 10% lower than in adults, which appears to be related to the lower risk of vasospasm (Lasjaunias et al. 1997). Outcome for surviving children after infratentorial aneurysm has not been well studied.

Neonates

Neonates are a special group presenting with symptomatic aneurysms: van Raay et al. (2009) report a literature review of 17 neonates (10 girls and 7 boys) with 19 aneurysms, 28% of which were in the posterior circulation (PCA, PICA, basilar artery, superior cerebellar artery), four were saccular and one fusiform. Of these five, two had a history of mildly traumatic birth. *Presentation* was by subarachnoid hemorrhage in all cases, symptoms were extremely variable and unspecific with irritability ranging to coma, vomiting, apnoea, fever, bulging fontanelle, and increasing head size. Three of the five children died, the other two having favourable outcome. The *aetiology* of aneurysms presenting in the neonatal period remains controversial: some are of congenital origin with possible pathology of internal elastic lamina or muscular media; for some a traumatic component might be of importance.

Acknowledgement

Professor Gerhard Schroth, Department of Neuroimaging, University Hospital Bern, Switzerland is acknowledged for the illustrations that appear in this chapter. Thanks also to Avril Castagna Sloane, MD, for help in the preporation of this manuscript.

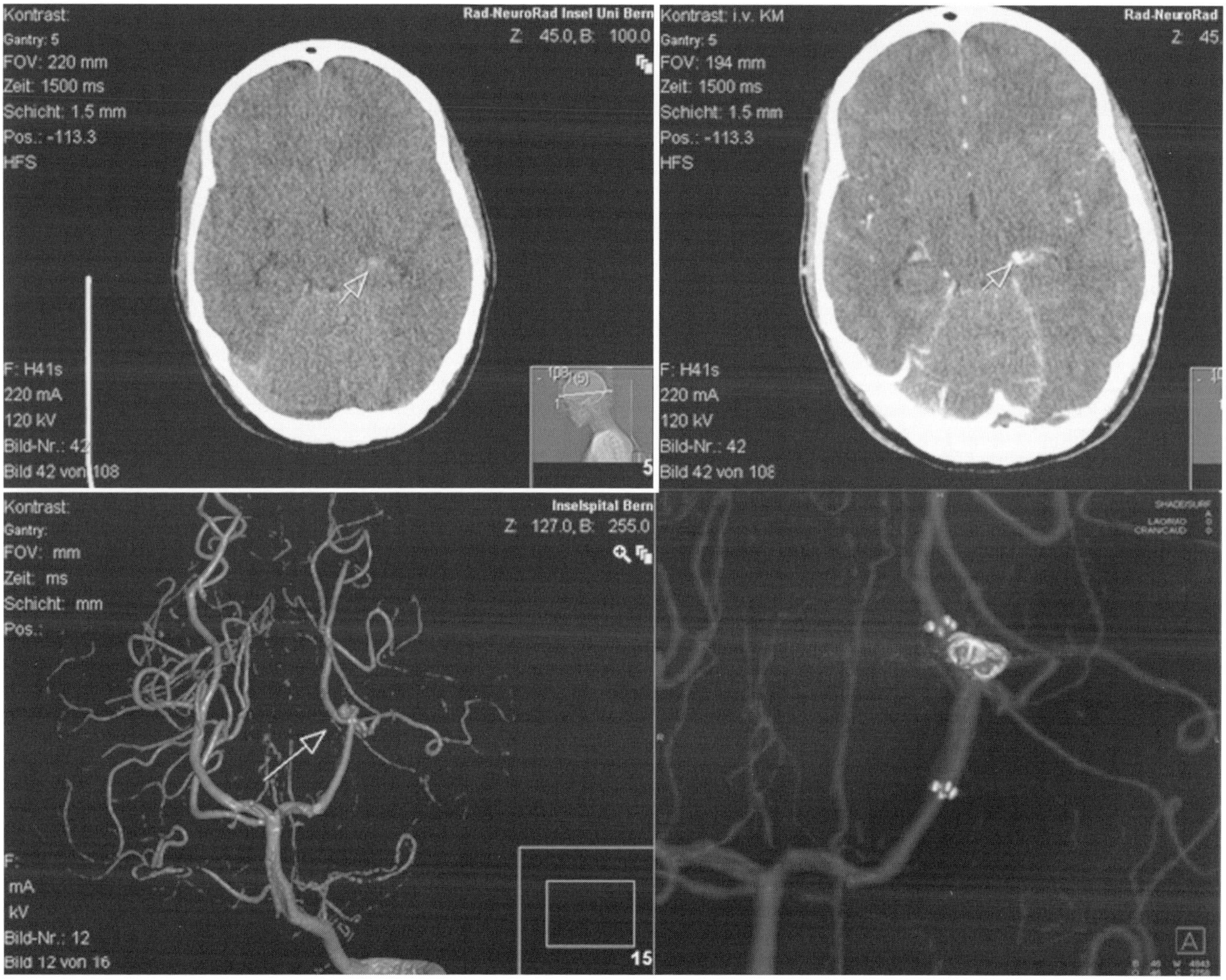

Fig. 32.8. Non-contrast-CT (upper left image) indicates subtle subarachnoid haemorrhage (SAH) in the perimesencephal cistern (Fisher I). Angio-CT (upper right image) indicates an aneurysm in the ambient cistern as source of the SAH. Three-dimensional rotation angiography (lower row) confirms a bilobulated aneurysm of the left posterior cerebral artery arising with a broad neck from the branching into the calcarine and occipitotemporal arteries. Three-dimensional digital abstraction angiography after endovascular treatment shows the electrolytically detachable coils in the aneurysm and normal flow through the adjacent posterior cerebral artery protected by a neuroform stent, which bridges the wide neck of the aneurysm and keeps the coils inside the aneurysm. (See color plate 27).

REFERENCES

Al-Anazi A, Hassounah M, Sheikh B, Barayan S (2001) Cerebellar mutism caused by arteriovenous malformation of the vermis. Br J Neurosurg 15: 47–50.

Allison J, Davis PC, Sato Y, James CA, Haque SS, Angtuaco EJC, Glasier CM (1998) Intracranial aneurysms in infants and children. Pediatr Radiol 28: 223–229.

Amlie-Lefond C, Sébire G, Fullerton HJ (2008) Recent developments in childhood arerial ischaemic strokes. Lancet Neurol 7: 425–435.

Arnaout O, Gross B, Eddleman C, Bendok B, Getch C, Hunt H (2009) Posterior fossa arteriovenous malformations. Neurosurg Focus 26: E 12.

Aryan HE, Gianmotta SL, Fukushima T, Park MS, Osgur BM, Levy ML (2005) Aneruysms in children: Review of 15 years' experience. J Clin Neurosci 13: 188–192.

Berenstein A, Lasjaunias P (1992) Endovascular treatment of cerebral intracranial lesions. In: Surgical Neuroangiography Vol 4. Berlin, Heidelberg, New York: Springer.

Bigi S, Fischer U, Wehrli E, Mattle HP, Boltshauser E, Bürki S, et al. (2011) Acute ischaemic stroke in children versus young adults. Ann Neurol 70: 245–254.

Bruneau M, Bijlenga P, Reverdin A, Rilliet L, Villemure JG, Porchet F, deTribolet N (2006) Early surgery for brainstem cavernomas. Acta Neurochir 148: 405–414.

Bürki S, Roellin K, Remonda L, Gubser Mercati D, Jeannet PY, Keller E et al. (2010) Neuroimaging in childhood arterial ischaemic stroke: evaluation of imaging modalities and aetiologies. Dev Med Child Neurol 52: 1033–1037.

Burn S, Gunny R, Phipps K, Gaze M, Hayward R (2007) Incidence of cavernoma developmental in children after radiotherapy for brain tumors. J Neurosurg 106: 379–383.

Campeau NG, Lane JI (2005) De novo Development of lesion with the appearance of cavernous malformation adjacent to an exsting developmental venous anomaly. Am J Neuroradiol 26: 156–169.

Cantu C, Murillo-Bonilla L, Arauz A, Higuera J, Padilla J, Barinagarrementeria F (2005) Predictive factors for intracerebral haemorrhage in patients with cavernous angiomas. Neurol Res 27, 314–318.

Delsing BJ, Catsman-Berrevoets CE, Appel IM (2001) Early prognostic indicators of outcome in ischemic childhood stroke. Pediatr Neurol 24: 283–289.

Di Rocco C, Iannelli A, Tamburrini G (1997) Surgical management of paediatric cerebral cavernomas. J Neurosug Sci 41: 343–347.

Faughnan ME, Palda VA, Garcia-Tsao G, Geisthoff UW, McDonald J, Proctor DD, et al. (2011) International Guidelines for the diagnosis and management of hereditary hemorrhagic telangiectasia. J Med Genet 48: 73–87.

Felbor U, Sure U, Grimm T, Bertalanffy H (2006) Genetics of cerebral cavernous angioma. Zentralbibl Neurochir 67: 110–116.

Fleetwood IG, Steinberg GK (2002) Arteriovenous malformations. Lancet 359: 863–873.

Fox CH, Fullerton HJ (2010) Recent advances in childhood ischemic stroke. Curr Atheroscler Repn 12: 217–224.

Ganesan V, Chong WK, Cox TC, Chawda J, Prengler M, Kirkham FJ (2002) Posterior circulation stroke in childhood: Risk factors and recurrence. Neurology 59: 1552–1556.

Griffiths PD, Blaser S, Armstrong D, Chuang S, Humphreys RP, Harwood-Nash D (1998) Cerebellar arteriovenous malformations in children. Neuroradiology 40: 324–331.

Hauck EF, Barnett SL, White JA, Samson D (2009) Symptomatic brainstem cavernomas. Neurosurg 64: 61–71.

Houtteville JP (1997) Brain cavernoma: a dynamic lesion. Surg Neurol 48: 610–614.

Huang J, McGirt MJ, Gailloud P, Tamargo RJ (2005) Intracranial aneurysms in the pediatric population: case series and literature review. Surg Neurol 63: 424–433.

Humphreys RP (1986) Hemorrhagic stroke in childhood. J Pediatr Neurosci 2: 1–10.

Khaw AV, Mohr JP, Sciacca RR, Schumacher HC, Hartmann A, Pile-Spellman J, et al. (2004) Association of infratentorial brain arteriovenos malformations with hemorrhage at initial presentation. Stroke 35: 660–663.

Kondziolka D, Humphreys RP, Hoffman HJ, Hendrik EB, Drake JM (1992) Arteriovenous malformations of he brain in children: a forty year experience. Can J Neurol Sci 19: 40–45.

Lasjaunias PL, Campi A, Rodesch G, Alvarez H, Kanaan I, Taylor W (1997) Aneurysmal disease in children: review of 20 cases with intracranial arterial localisations. Interv Neuroradiol 3: 215–229.

Lasjaunias P, Wuppalapati S, Alvarez H, Rodesch G, Ozanne A (2005) Intracranial aneurysms in children aged under 15 years: review of 59 consecutive childen with 75 aneurysms. Childs Nerv Syst. 21: 437–450.

Lena G, Paz-Paredes A, Choux M (2002) Brain stem cavernomas in children. Nine case reports and literature review. Neurochirurgie 28: 319–325.

Lena G, Ternier J, Paz-Paredes A, Scavarda D (2007) Central nervous system cavernomas in children. Neurochirurgie 53: 223–237.

Luchini P, Guida F, di Paola F, Bocca A, Longati P (1992) Vertebrobasilar infarcts in infancy: a case report and review of the literature. Childs Nerv System 8: 426–429.

Matsubara S, Manza JL, ter Brugge K, Willinsky RA, Montanera W, Faughnan ME (2000) Angiographic and clnical characteristics of patients with cerebral artriovenous malformations associated with hereditary haemorrhagic teleangiectasia. AJNR Am J Neuroradiol 21: 1016–1020.

Matta AP, Galvao KR, Oliveira BS (2006) Cerebrovascular disorders in childhood etiology, clinical presentation and neuroimaging findings in a case series study. Arq Neuropsiquiatr 64: 181–185.

Mori K, Seike M, Kurisaka M, Kamimura Y, Morimoto M (1994) Venous malformation in the posterior fossa: guidelines for treatment. Acra Neurochir (Wien) 126: 107–112.

Mugikura S, Takahashi S, Higano S, Shirane R, Kurihara N, Furuta S, et al. (1999) The relationship between cerebral infarction an angiographic characteristics in childhood moyamoya disease. AJNR Am J Neuroradiol 20: 336–343.

Nomura S, Kato S, Ishihara H, Yoneda H, Ideguchi M, Suzuki M (2006) Association of intra- and extradural developmental venous anomalies, so-called venous angioma and sinus pericranii. Childs Nerv Syst 22: 428–431.

Nussbaum ES, Heros RC, Madison MT, Awasthi D, Truwit CL (1998) The pathogenesis of arteriovenous malformations: insights provided by a case of multiple arteriovenous malformations developing in relation to a developmental venous anomaly. Neurosurg 43: 347–351, discussion 351–352.

Panciani PP, Fontanella M, Carlino C, Bergui M, Ducati A (2008) Progressive spontaneous occlusion of a cerebellar AVM: Pathogenetic hypothesis and review of literature. Clin Neurol Neurosurg 110: 502–510.

Pegelow CH, Macklin EA, Moser FG, Wang WC, Bello JA, Miller ST, et al. (2002) Longitudinal changes in brain magnetic resonance imaging findings in children with sickle cell disease. Blood 99: 3014–3018.

Plauchu H, Dupuis-Girod S (2009) Hereditary hemorrhagic teleangiectasia. Rev Prat 20: 899–903.

Roach ES, Golomb MR, Adams R, Biller J, Daniels S, Ferreiro D, et al. (2008) American heart association Stroke Council, Council on cardiovascular disease in the young: Management of stroke in infants and children: a scientific statement from a Special Writing Group of the American Heart Association Stroke Council and the Council on Cardiovascular Disease in the Young. Stroke 39: 2644–2691.

Royal College of Physicians (2004) Stroke in childhood. Clinical guidelines for diagnosis, management and rehabilitation. (Paediatric Stroke Working Group, Chairman: V. Ganesan.) Royal College of Physicians of London. www.childstroke.org.uk.

Scott RM, Barnes P, Kupsky W, Adelman LS (1992) Cavernous angiomas of the central nervous system in children. J Neurosurg 76: 38–46.

Stapf C, Khaw AV, Sciacca RR, Hofmeister C, Schumacher HC, Pile-Spellman J, et al. (2003) Effect of age on clinical and morphological characteristics in patients with brain arteriovenous malformation. Stroke 34: 2664–2670.

Sugita K, Suga S, Tanaka Y (2003) A juvenile case of cerebellar arteriovenous malformation (AVM) with gradual onset of headache and ataxia. Bull Tokyo Dent Coll 44: 17–19.

Topper R, Jurgens E, Ruel J, Thron A (1999) Clinical significance of intracranial developmental venous anomalies. J Neurol Neurosurg Psychiatry 67: 234–238.

Uchino A, Hasuo K, Matsumoto S, Fujii K, Fukui M, Horino K, et al. (1996) Cerebral venous angiomas associated with hemorrhagic lesions. Their MRI manifestations. Clin Imaging 20: 157–163.

Van Raay Y, Darteyre S, DiRocco F, Goodden J, Papouin M, Brunelle F, et al. (2009) Neonatal ruptured intracranial aneurysms: case report and literature review. Childs Nerv Syst 8: 1025–1033.

Weon YC, Yoshida M, Sachet M, Mahadevan H, Alvarez G, Rodesch G, Lasjaunias P (2005) Supratentorial cerebral arteriovenous fistulas (AVFs) in children: review of 41 cases with 63 non choroidal single hole AVFs. Acta Neurochir 147: 17–31.

Willinsky RA, Lasjaunias P, Terbrugge K, Burrow P (1990) Multiple cerebral arteriovenous malformations (AVMs). Review of our experience from 203 patients with cerebral vascular lesions. Neuroradiology 32: 207–210.

Wingeier K, Bigi S, El-Koussy M, Heinks-Maidonado T, Boltshauser E, Steinlin M (2011) Long-term sequelae after aquired pediatric hemorrhagic cerebellar lesions. Childs Nerv Syst 27(6): 923–31.

Yamada I, Nurata Y, Umehara I, Suzuki S, Matsushima Y (1996) SPECT and MR evaluations of the posterior circulation in moyamoya disease. J Nucl Med 7: 1613–1617.

Yoshida Y, Weon YC, Sachet M, Mahadevan J, Alvarez H, Rodesch G, Lasjaunias P (2004) Posterior cranial fossa single-hole arteriovenous fistulae in children: 14 consecutive cases. Neuroradiol 46: 474–481.

33
Posterior Fossa Tumours

Michael A. Grotzer

Brain tumours are the most common solid tumours in children (Gurney and Kadan-Lottick 2001). The leading cause of cancer-related morbidity and mortality in children, they differ from primary central nervous system (CNS) tumours occurring in adults in histology, localization, management, and prognosis (Merchant et al. 2010). Because the developing brain is highly vulnerable to treatment-induced cognitive and endocrine sequelae, particularly from radiotherapy, contemporary strategies for the management of childhood brain tumours incorporate both age-specific and histology-specific approaches. Ongoing studies focus not only on the duration, but also on the quality of survival (Packer 2008).

Epidemiology

The incidence rate of childhood primary nonmalignant and malignant CNS tumours (ages 0–19 years) is 4.71 cases per 100 000 person-years. The rate is slightly higher in males (4.75 per 100 000 person-years) than females (4.66 per 100 000 person-years) (CBTRUS 2010). The reported incidence of primary malignant brain tumours among children in the United States increased by 35% during the period from 1973 through 1994 (Ries et al. 1998). It has been suggested that this increase may be due, to some extent, to improved detection and reporting coincident with the availability of high-resolution neuro-imaging beginning in the 1980s (Smith et al. 1998). But these observations also raised serious concerns that environmental factors may play a substantial causative or contributory role. Despite these concerns, multiple epidemiological studies, including those investigating maternal nutritional intake, parental occupational exposure, and children's diet and exposure to electromagnetic fields, do not establish direct links between such factors and the development of childhood brain tumours (Feychting et al. 2000; Lubin et al. 2000; Connelly and Malkin 2007).

Etiology

The percentage of childhood CNS tumours due to hereditary factors has been estimated at 2% (Narod et al. 1991). However, certain brain tumours have a clearly higher probability to be caused by hereditary factors. The most frequent association is with the neurocutaneous disorders (Ruggieri et al. 2008). In neurofibromatosis type 1 (NF1), astrocytomas are the most common CNS tumours. They may arise in all parts of the brain, but the most common sites are the optic nerves and chiasm, and to a lesser extent the posterior fossa (Friedman et al. 1999). NF2 predisposes to bilateral vestibular schwannomas (acoustic neuromas) and to a lesser extent to trigeminal schwannomas, ependymomas, and meningiomas (Friedman et al. 1999). The brain lesions in the tuberous sclerosis complex include cortical dysplasia (cortical tubers), subependymal nodules, and subependymal giant cell astrocytomas (Roach et al. 1998). In patients with Von Hippel-Lindau disease, CNS hemangioblastomas (cerebellar, brainstem, spinal) have been observed (Friedrich 1999; Hussein 2007). These tumours are histologically benign and do not tend to metastasize.

Endogenous immunosuppression as in the Wiskott-Aldrich syndrome, ataxia-telangiectasia, and exogenous immunosuppression as in organ-transplant recipients and HIV infection have been associated with an increased risk of CNS malignancies (Granovsky et al. 1998; Varan et al. 2004). Virtually all of these CNS tumours were B-cell lymphomas.

The best confirmed exogenous risk factor for childhood brain tumours is ionizing radiation. Prenatal diagnostic X-ray exposure has been related to CNS tumours in childhood (Shu et al. 1994). Several other reports have described the occurrence of gliomas, meningiomas, and other brain tumours in children who received radiation therapy to the head for tinea capitis and for prior malignancies (Shore et al. 1976; Liwnicz et al. 1985; Shapiro et al. 1989; Relling et al. 1999). The estimated cumulative risk of a second malignant brain tumour after childhood leukemia is 0.3% by 5 years, 0.5–0.8% by 10 years, and 3% by 30 years after treatment (Jenkinson and Hawkins 1999; Hijiya et al. 2007).

Pathophysiology and pathogenesis

The factors responsible for the initiation and progression of childhood nervous system tumours are still poorly understood. While a model of tumour progression has been proposed for malignant gliomas in adults, it is unlikely that this model is applicable to gliomas in infants. Malignant transformation for low-grade astrocytoma to malignant glioma is distinctively uncommon in children but not in adults. The high incidence of tumours in the first years of life suggests that tumour suppressor genes, which are involved in normal development, play a major role in tumorigenesis.

Clinical features

Clinical presentation depends on the age of the child and tumour location more than on histology. Congenital CNS tumours may cause obstetric complications including prolonged labor, failure to progress, fetal distress, or dystocia. Macrocephaly is the most common finding at presentation (Raisanen and

Davis 1993; Fort and Rushing 1997). Brain tumours in infants are notorious for their protean clinical manifestations, which may include irritability, listlessness, vomiting, failure to thrive, and progressive macrocephaly (Pollack 1994; Dobrovoljac et al. 2002). Hydrocephalus is compensated by open fontanels and split sutures and less likely to produce classic signs of increased intracranial pressure. Older children whose sutures have closed are more likely than infants to have localizing neurological findings. However, the majority of these children present with symptoms of increased intracranial pressure (ICP) including recurrent headache, nausea, or vomiting without focal deficits. Symptoms of increased ICP are particularly common with tumours of the posterior fossa, pineal region, and suprasellar region, which often obstruct the cerebral ventricles, producing hydrocephalus (Pollack 1994).

In contrast to the general signs and symptoms reviewed above, several paediatric brain tumours do have relatively characteristic clinical features. Diffuse pontomedullary brainstem tumours typically show a triad of mid-cranial nerve palsies (typically VI and VII), ataxia, and long tract signs.

Classification

The 2007 revision of the World Health Organization (WHO) *Classification of Tumors of the Nervous System* represents an international effort to achieve a general consensus on tumour nosology based on standard light microscopy and tumour location (Louis et al. 2007). The diagnostic categories of childhood brain tumours for which there is a high level of inter-observer diagnostic consistency include medulloblastoma, ependymoma, germinoma, teratoma, craniopharyngioma, and pilocytic astrocytoma. In contrast, diagnosis in astrocytoma, oligodendroglioma, and mixed glioma may be more difficult and less reliable in smaller institutions (Childhood Brain Tumor Consortium 1988; Bruner et al. 1998). Accordingly, recent clinical trials mandate centralized histological review. Whereas in adults the vast majority of brain tumours arise in the cerebral hemispheres, approximately 50% of brain tumours in children older than 1 year develop infratentorially.

Diagnostic criteria/process

Computed tomography (CT) or magnetic resonance imaging (MRI), performed with and without intravenous contrast, may be employed to diagnose the presence of brain tumours. Neuroimaging techniques are sufficient to diagnose typical cases of diffuse intrinsic brainstem gliomas (Albright et al. 1993). However, for all other posterior fossa tumours, neuroimaging techniques do not eliminate the need to obtain a histological diagnosis. MRI is preferred under most circumstances, providing superior resolution and multiplanar imaging capabilities, and avoiding the 'spray' artifact from the clivus or the petrous ridge that may obscure a CT image of the posterior fossa, where 50% of paediatric tumours arise (Vezina 1997).

Postoperative MRI provides an objective assessment of residual tumour volume, which for medulloblastoma, ependymoma, and other types of childhood brain tumours is of major prognostic significance. Postoperative neuroimaging should be performed within 24–72 hours of surgery to minimize interpretative difficulties caused by surgically induced postoperative reactive enhancement, generally assumed to commence after 48 hours (Albert et al. 1994; Jaspan and Griffiths 2004).

Staging procedures vary depending on tumour histology and location. Cerebellar low-grade gliomas do not disseminate through the subarachnoid space, so that imaging of spine and examination of CSF cytology should be limited to patients with symptoms and signs indicating spinal disease. In all other patients, every attempt should be made to undertake preoperative whole-neuroaxial imaging because, postoperatively, blood tracking down into the spinal sac will provide potential pitfalls in the assessment of the presence of CSF tumour spread. If preoperative imaging cannot be undertaken, the spine should be examined at least 14 days after surgery (Jaspan and Griffiths 2004).

Controversy exists regarding the frequency, extent (head ± spine) and ultimate value of surveillance imaging for specific tumour types. The recommendations of the Neurology and Tumor Imaging Committees of the Children's Cancer Group represent an effort to standardize the surveillance evaluation of children with CNS tumours (Kramer et al. 1994). Standard surveillance schedules may facilitate the comparison of multi-institutional cooperative study data, directing treatment, and understanding tumour behaviour. For tumours with the potential to grow rapidly (e.g., medulloblastoma, glioblastoma multiforme) more frequent neuroimaging surveillance may be warranted, especially if a specific study question will be answered or early presymptomatic detection of recurrence or progression will have a favourable impact on quality or duration of survival (Steinbok et al. 1996).

Differential diagnosis

The differential diagnosis of paediatric brain tumours is that of intracranial mass lesions, including vascular malformations, infectious processes or focal demyelinating diseases. Arterial aneurysm and cerebral arteriovenous malformation are the most common causes of spontaneous subarachnoid or intraventricular hemorrhage in childhood. However, acute intracranial hemorrhage can also be a manifestation of new-onset or recurrent medulloblastoma, atypical teratoid/rhabdoid tumour, or malignant glioma. MRI is often capable of evaluating time of onset as well as the involved vasculature. In addition, arteriography may help to rule out a vascular malformation and aid in operative planning by demonstrating the blood supply of the tumour and its proximity to major vascular structures.

Treatment

Current approaches to treatment for brain tumours of childhood are determined by histological tumour type, underlying genetic defects, clinical staging, tumour localization, and age. Some of these therapeutic strategies are discussed in greater detail below.

Medulloblastoma

Medulloblastoma constitute 20–25% of paediatric CNS tumours and are the most common malignant brain tumour in childhood (Packer and Vezina 2008; Dhall 2009). The incidence is highest at age 1–4 years, slightly lower among infants and at age 5–9 years, but falls to around half its peak by age 10–14 years. The male/female ratio is 1.6–1.7 to one (Stiller and Bleyer 2004). The classical medulloblastoma usually arises from the cerebellar vermis (Fig. 33.1). The desmoplastic type arises more often from the cerebellar hemispheres and occurs more frequently in adolescents and adults.

The clinical presentation of medulloblastoma is dominated by signs and symptoms of obstructive hydrocephalus and increased intracranial pressure: headache, nausea and vomiting; drowsiness and other behaviour changes; and ataxia. However, these characteristics are often indistinguishable from other posterior fossa tumours, including ependymoma and cerebellar astrocytoma.

Preoperative management issues are dominated by, but not limited to, the assessment and treatment of increased intracranial pressure. Patients with papilledema and significant visual impairment require emergency placement of an external ventricular drain followed immediately by tumour resection. Prolonged delay between ventricular drainage and tumour resection significantly increases the risk of transtentorial upward herniation. For patients with less severe signs and symptoms of increased intracranial pressure, corticosteroids may be used to relieve symptoms, reduce tumour swelling, and permit further surgical planning.

There are three surgical objectives in medulloblastoma treatment. First, sufficient tissue must be obtained to permit accurate histopathological diagnosis. Second, tumour removal should be complete or near complete since complete tumour removal favourably influences prognosis (Zeltzer et al. 1999). Third, every effort should be made to re-establish normal CSF flow. The majority of children with medulloblastoma will not need a permanent ventriculoperitoneal shunt. The incidence of tumour dissemination to the abdomen by ventriculoperitoneal shunt is extremely uncommon and the importance of this unusual complication has been exaggerated (Berger et al. 1991).

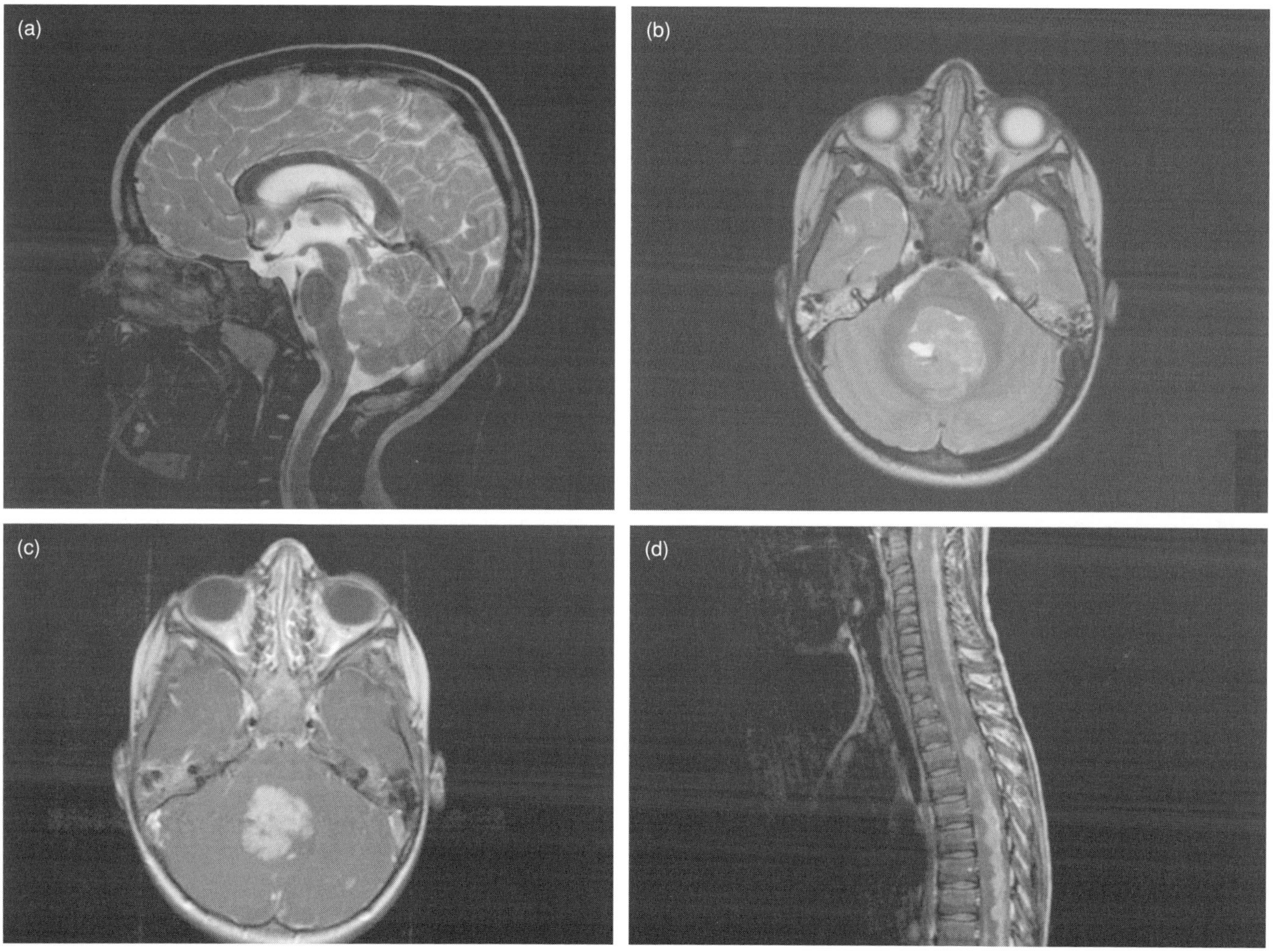

Fig. 33.1. Medulloblastoma in a 3-year-old child. T2-weighted MR images in **(a)** the sagittal plane and **(b)** the axial plane show the fourth ventricle mass arising from the cerebellar vermis. **(c)** Axial T1-weighted image following contrast injection shows enhancement of the main lesion and nodular cerebellar and pial metastases. **(d)** Sagittal T1-weighted image following contrast injection shows enhancement of nodular spinal metastases. (Courtesy of Ianina Scheer, Neuroradiology Department, University Children's Hospital of Zurich, Switzerland.)

Two postoperative complication syndromes deserve attention. (1) The syndrome of aseptic meningitis may occur in up to 5% of patients undergoing posterior fossa surgery and is not limited to those with medulloblastoma (Dubey et al. 2009). Symptoms of fever and meningism, ranging from mild to severe in intensity, develop 5–10 days after surgery. Although this complication may occur more frequently in patients with large postoperative pseudomeningoceles under tension, there are no clinical features that reliably distinguish this syndrome of presumed chemical meningitis from bacterial meningitis. Therefore, analysis and culture of cerebrospinal fluid (CSF) is essential. If no infectious cause is identified, this complication is effectively treated with corticosteroids. (2) The syndrome of cerebellar mutism after resection of posterior fossa tumours was first noted in the early 1980s (Hirsch et al. 1979; Wisoff and Epstein 1984). Several studies thereafter indicate that this syndrome is not rare, and occurs in up to 25% of children with large midline cerebellar tumours, usually after approaches that involve the vermis (Pollack 1997; Robertson et al. 2006). Complete or near-complete loss of speech is usually accompanied by severe lower cranial nerve, cerebellar, visual (Liu et al. 1998), and motor abnormalities (Kedar 1997; Liu et al. 1998). This disorder is apparent within the first 1–4 days after surgery. Most patients with this syndrome recover functional speech during a period of several weeks to months, although residual speech, lower cranial nerve, and motor coordination dysfunctions are common.

Clinical prognostic factors for medulloblastoma include metastatic stage as the most important, followed by residual tumour bulk, and patient's age at diagnosis (Garton et al. 1990; Cohen et al. 1995; Albright et al. 1996; Zeltzer et al. 1999). Accordingly, three tumour staging studies are important for medulloblastoma: (1) neuraxis staging evaluation by spinal MRI (preoperatively or 14 days after surgery) to identify metastatic tumour aggregates; (2) CSF cytological examination (intraoperatively or 14 days after surgery) to identify leptomeningeal tumour spread; and (3) postoperative neuroimaging to assess residual tumour. Based on results of these studies, medulloblastoma patients can be broadly separated into two groups: standard-risk patients (no evidence of metastatic disease, $\leq 1.5cm^3$ residual tumour, older than 3 years at diagnosis); and high-risk patients (evidence of leptomeningeal tumour spread, $>1.5cm^3$ residual tumour, younger than 3 years at diagnosis).

Clinical prognostic factors alone are not sufficient to identify reliably a low-risk group and a very high-risk group of patients which may need significantly different therapy regimens than standard- and high-risk medulloblastoma. Accordingly, biological studies of large, representative and relatively homogeneously treated medulloblastoma patients are of great interest (Crawford et al. 2007; Pizer and Clifford 2009). Independent research groups have shown that a high mRNA expression level of the tropomyosin receptor kinase C (TrkC) is a powerful predictor of favourable clinical outcome in medulloblastoma patients (Kim et al. 1999; Grotzer et al. 2000; Rutkowski et al. 2007). Amplification of the *c-myc* gene and high level of the c-Myc gene product have both been used as biological indicators of poor prognosis (Herms et al. 2000; Grotzer et al. 2001; Rutkowski et al. 2007). Other biological prognostic markers include the large cell/anaplastic (LC/A) phenotype, indicative of a very aggressive clinical behaviour and outcome (Eberhart et al. 2004; Stearns et al. 2006), and the beta-catenin status (Fattet et al. 2009).

Five general trends for treating medulloblastoma patients have emerged. (1) High-risk patients are treated with radiation including 36Gy craniospinal radiation and chemotherapy. (2) Standard-risk patients may be treated with less intensive approaches including reduced craniospinal radiation, in order to reduce significant treatment-associated toxicities. (3) Infants and children less than 3 or 4 years of age may be treated with intensive chemotherapy alone to postpone or avoid the neurotoxic effects of radiation on the developing brain. Newer protocols combine systemic and intrathecal chemotherapy with confocal radiation to the tumour bed (Rutkowski et al. 2010). (4) For recurrent tumours, the introduction of high-dose chemotherapy followed by peripheral blood stem cell (PBSC) rescue resulted in slightly increased survival rates, especially for patients with minimal residual disease before high-dose chemotherapy. However, the prognosis for recurrent medulloblastoma remains very poor (Gajjar and Pizer 2010). (5) A better understanding of the biological characteristics of medulloblastoma including the cells of origin and the aberrant cellular signaling pathways involved will be the promise of dramatically changing tumour stratification and treatment in the near future (Crawford et al. 2007; Packer and Vezina 2008; Pizer and Clifford 2009).

Radiation therapy is the mainstay of medulloblastoma treatment. Cumulative local tumour doses should be approximately 56Gy. Doses less than 50Gy have been shown to be less effective (Silverman and Simpson 1982). Radiation should also be delivered to the entire craniospinal axis, regardless of the tumour metastatic stage (Jenkin 1996). Treatment with craniospinal (36Gy) and local boost radiotherapy (total dose 54Gy) without adjuvant chemotherapy results in long-term disease control in approximately 60% of children with medulloblastoma (Evans et al. 1990). However, after whole-brain radiotherapy, many children will have significant long-term neuro-cognitive sequelae, including demonstrable drops in overall intelligence. This decline in intelligence is influenced by age at irradiation and dose (Silber et al. 1992; Mulhern et al. 2004, 2005).

Chemotherapy has an important role in the treatment of high-risk medulloblastoma. This has been proven by several prospective studies (Evans et al. 1990; Packer et al. 1994a; Bailey et al. 1995). Medulloblastomas are responsive to a variety of chemotherapeutic agents, including cisplatin, cyclophosphamide, vincristine, CCNU, and busulfan (Friedman et al. 1991). Incorporation of cisplatin, CCNU and vincristine into a post-radiation chemotherapy regimen for high-risk patients resulted in 5-year survival rates in excess of 80% (Packer 1990). Of note, this survival rate was significantly higher than survival rates for standard-risk patients treated with radiation therapy alone (i.e., historical controls). This and other single-institution studies have provided strong indirect support for the use of effective adjuvant chemotherapy for all medulloblastoma patients.

Low-grade glioma

Low-grade glioma/astrocytomas can occur anywhere within the CNS. The predominant histology of cerebellar astrocytomas is pilocytic, whereas dorsally exophytic low-grade gliomas are fibrillary by and large. Cerebellar pilocytic astrocytomas are usually large at presentation and may appear as cystic with a mural nodule of tumour (50%), solid with cystic/necrotic foci (40%) or purely solid (Jaspan and Griffiths 2004) (Fig. 33.2). Cerebellar pilocytic astrocytoma has perhaps the best prognosis of any brain tumour, with 10-year survival rates approaching 100% (Sutton et al. 1996). The prognosis of pilocytic astrocytomas is determined by the extent of resection. If the post-operative MRI shows resectable tumour, re-exploration may be indicated to achieve complete resection.

With improved survival rates in paediatric brain tumours, awareness of significant tumour-related and/or therapy-related long-term neurological, cognitive, emotional, or behavioural complications has increased (Mulhern et al. 2004).

Ependymoma

Ependymoma constitute approximately 10% of posterior fossa tumours in childhood. These tumours are derived from ependymal cells lining the ventricles or from the ependymal cell rests, which may sometimes occur quite distant from the ventricles. The floor of the fourth ventricle is the most common site, and the tumour typically fills the entire fourth ventricle (Fig. 33.3). Some tumours have a tendency to extend out through the foramina of Magendie or Luschka in a toothpaste-like fashion (Jaspan and Griffiths 2004).

Ependymoma behave primarily as localized, slow-growing, relatively noninvasive neoplasms (Packer 2005; Kilday et al. 2009; Zacharoulis and Moreno 2009). Five-year relapse-free survivals range from 30% to 70% (Packer 2005). Two primary factors correlate best with progression-free survival: the amount

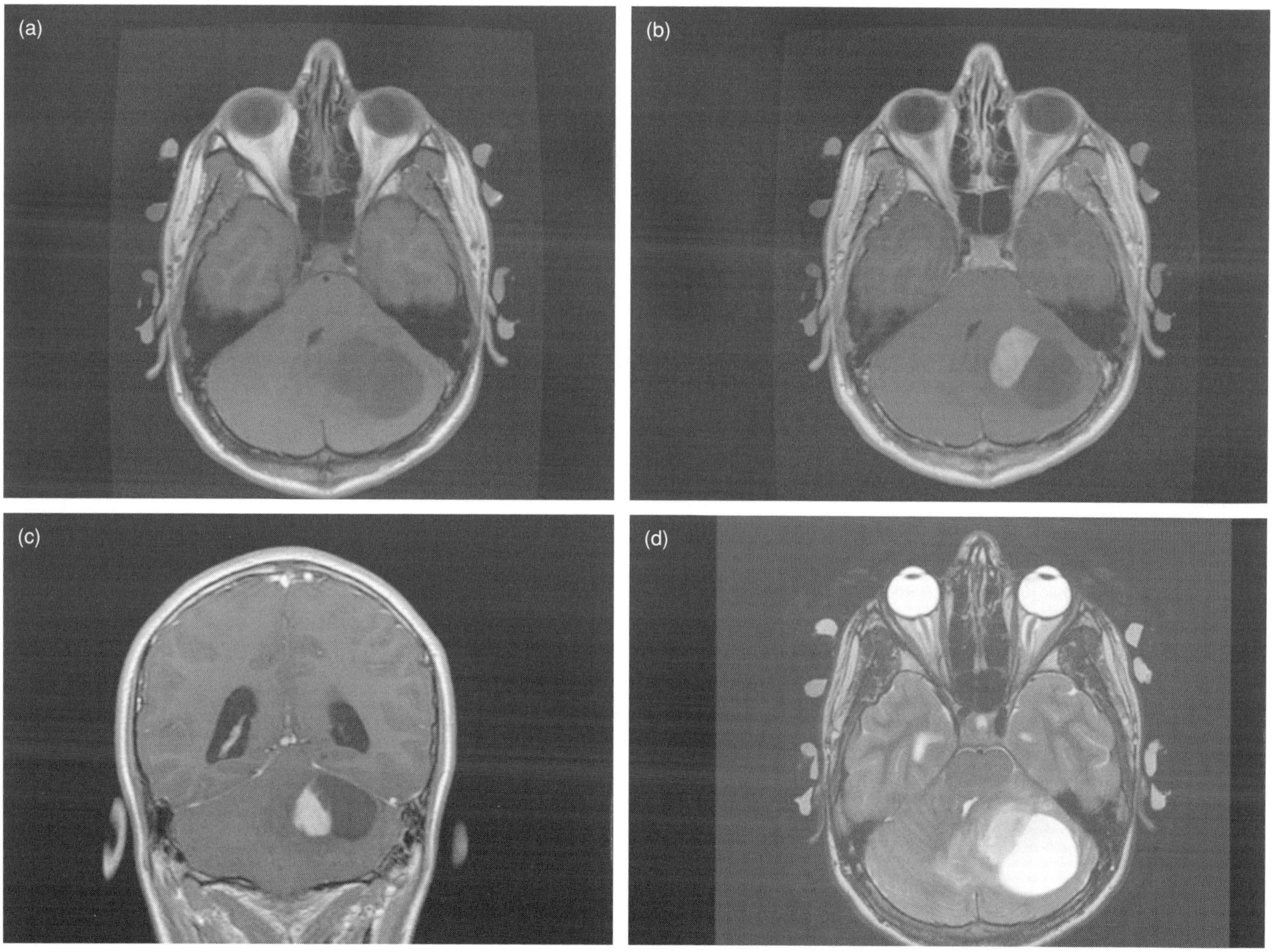

Fig. 33.2. Pilocytic cerebellar astrocytoma in a 7-year-old child. **(a)** Axial T1-weighted image before and **(b)** following contrast injection show a cerebellar hemispheric T1-hypointense cystic tumor with a mural nodule. **(c)** Coronal T1-weighted MR image following contrast injection. **(d)** Axial T2-weighted MR image. (Courtesy of Ianina Scheer, Neuroradiology Department, University Children's Hospital of Zurich, Switzerland.)

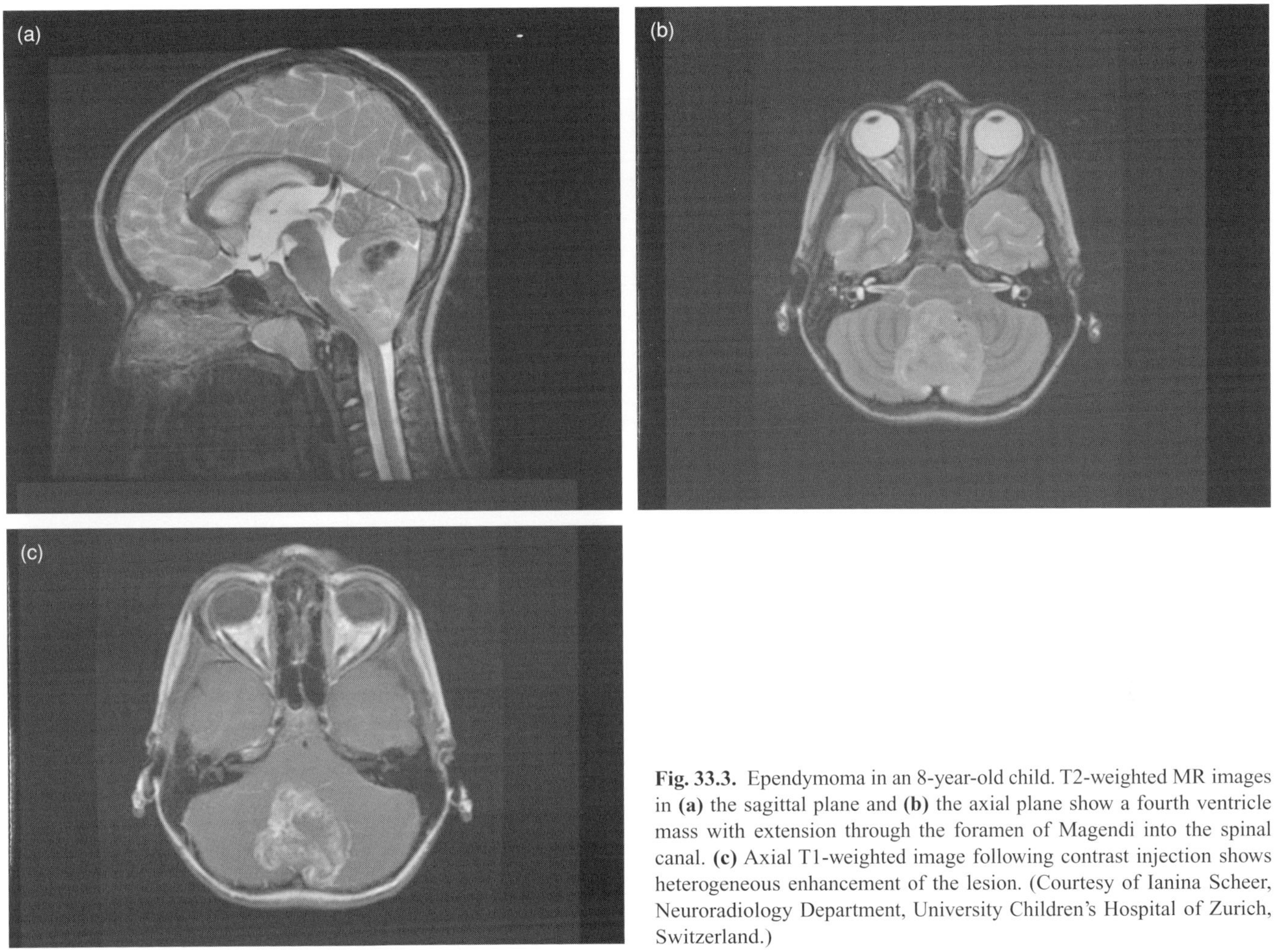

Fig. 33.3. Ependymoma in an 8-year-old child. T2-weighted MR images in **(a)** the sagittal plane and **(b)** the axial plane show a fourth ventricle mass with extension through the foramen of Magendi into the spinal canal. **(c)** Axial T1-weighted image following contrast injection shows heterogeneous enhancement of the lesion. (Courtesy of Ianina Scheer, Neuroradiology Department, University Children's Hospital of Zurich, Switzerland.)

of residual disease after initial surgery, and histological features of aggressivity. The challenge in ependymoma is local control, since metastatic relapses occur rarely. However, surgery is often difficult, and complete removal is achieved in less than 50% of the patients. Ependymomas are often located close to brainstem structures, which increases the risk of high morbidity when complete resection is attempted.

The frequency of gross total resections can be increased by sophisticated technologies including ultrasonic cavitrons, argon lasers, by experience of the neurosurgeon with children, and by the intent and preoperative plan to perform a radical surgical resection (Allen et al. 1998). The availability of intraoperative neuroimaging may provide immediate confirmation of the degree of resection and allow the surgeon to reoperate, immediately, if necessary (Wirtz et al. 2000).

Involved-field radiotherapy represents standard therapy for children older than 18 months who have intracranial ependymomas. In patients without disseminated disease at diagnosis, the pattern of relapse is local in the vast majority of cases. Therefore, prophylactic craniospinal irradiation is not recommended. Currently evaluated strategies to enhance local tumour control in patients with residual or progressive disease include radiosurgery (Grabb et al. 1996) and proton beam radiotherapy (MacDonald and Yock 2010). Proton radiation therapy is a form of radiation with physical properties that can provide an advantage in normal tissue sparing compared to the more commonly used photon therapy. At present, proton radiation is limited to selected centres. However, knowledge of its advantages, especially in very young children, has spread rapidly and its availability is becoming more widespread (MacDonald and Yock 2010).

Ependymoma are considered as relatively chemotherapy-resistant tumours. However, a pilot study including 19 children with newly diagnosed ependymoma reported a 74% 5-year progression-free survival after radiotherapy and chemotherapy (Needle et al. 1997). This is higher than published results for radiotherapy alone. Based on this provocative finding, current clinical trials use chemotherapy for patients whose postoperative imaging studies are positive for residual tumour, or even for all patients. For patients with recurrent ependymoma, options for further therapy other than reresection are few; usually, maximal irradiation has already been administered, and chemotherapy including high-dose chemotherapy is of modest benefit to only a minority of patients (Mason et al. 1998; Shih et al. 2008).

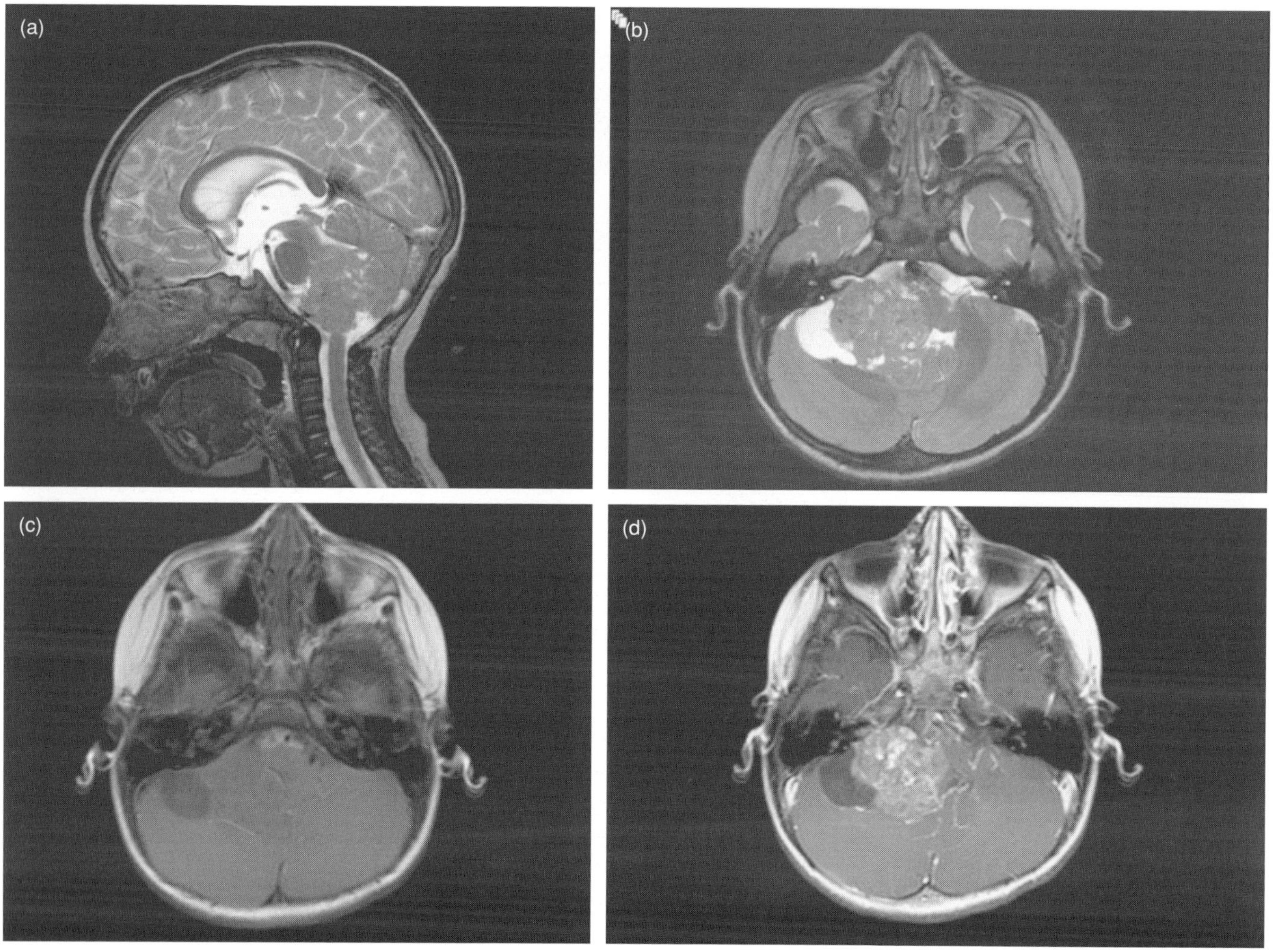

Fig. 33.4. Atypical teratoid/rhabdoid tumor in a 2-year-old child. T2-weighted MR images in **(a)** the sagittal plane and **(b)** the axial plane show the heterogeneous mass in the cerebello-pontine angle with cysts. **(c)** Axial T1-weighted image before and **(d)** following contrast injection show heterogeneous enhancement of the lesion (Courtesy of Ianina Scheer, Neuroradiology Department, University Children's Hospital of Zurich, Switzerland.)

Atypical teratoid/rhabdoid tumour

Central nervous system atypical teratoid/rhabdoid tumour (AT/RT) is a highly malignant embryonal tumour in young children. Infratentorial tumours can be located in the cerebellar hemispheres, cerebellopontine angle, and brainstem (Fig. 33.4). Seeding of AT/RT via the CSF may be found in more than 20% of the patients at presentation. CNS AT/RT is characterized by the presence of rhabdoid cells, with or without fields resembling classic primitive neuroectodermal tumour, epithelial tissue, and neoplastic mesenchyme (Rorke et al. 1996). The unique clinical, biological and histological features of this tumour have been defined over the past decade (Biegel et al. 2002; Judkins et al. 2004). It is similar to the renal malignant rhabdoid tumour of infancy in its aggressiveness, in some histological features, and in the loss of function of *hSNF5/INI1*, a recently described candidate tumour suppressor gene on chromosome 22 (Versteege et al. 1998; Reddy 2005). Experience to date indicates that infants and children with CNS AT/RT respond very poorly to chemotherapy and radiotherapy (Burger et al. 1998; Bambakidis et al. 2002; Hilden et al. 2004; Tekautz et al. 2005). In one of the largest reported series of patients with primary CNS AT/RT, only 6 of 36 children who received chemotherapy showed objective responses (>50% reduction in tumour mass) to chemotherapy and only 2 of 10 patients showed objective responses to radiotherapy (Rorke et al. 1996). More recently, aggressive therapy including intensive multi-agent chemotherapy, high-dose chemotherapy with stem cell rescue and intrathecal chemotherapy combined with early involved-field irradiation has prolonged the natural history in a subset of children (Hilden et al. 2004). However, the prognosis for children presenting with CNS AT/RT before the age of 3 years is still dismal (Hilden et al. 2004; Tekautz et al. 2005).

Dysplastic gangliocytoma of the cerebellum (Lhermitte-Duclos disease)

Dysplastic gangliocytoma of the cerebellum is a rare, slowly growing cerebellar mass (Lhermitte and Duclos 1920; Capone Mori et al. 2003; Eberhart et al. 2007). Histologically, the

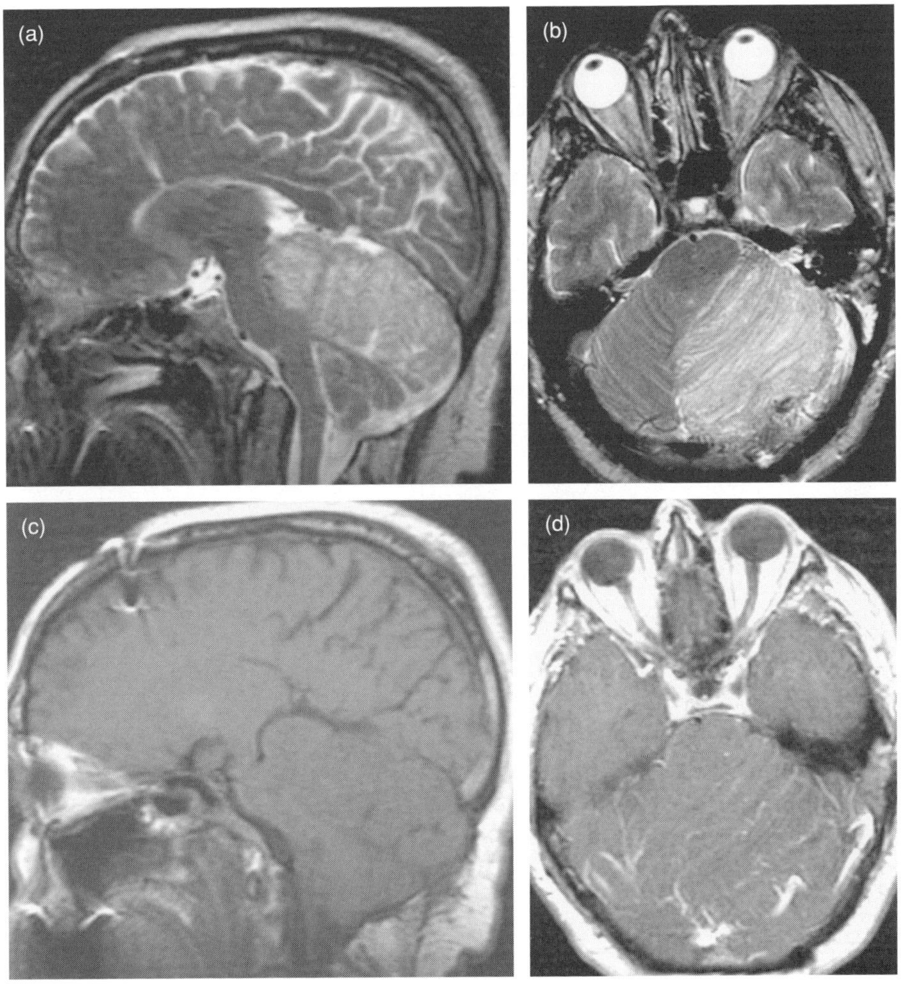

Fig. 33.5. Dysplastic gangliocytoma of the cerebellum (Lhermitte-Duclos disease) in an adult, representative of the typical pattern seen in this disorder at all ages. T2-weighted MR-images in **(a)** the sagittal plane and **(b)** the axial plane show the mass effect of the lesion, and the characteristic striated pattern of hyperintensity – 'tiger stripes'. **(c)** T1-weighted image in the sagittal plane shows the expanded superior aspect of the cerebellum and the abnormally thickened folia. **(d)** T1-weighted image following contrast injection shows lack of enhancement. (Courtesy of Jeremy D. Schmahmann, and Neuroradiology Department, Massachusetts General Hospital.)

lesion of Lhermitte-Duclos disease (LDD) is composed of dysplastic ganglion cells that are mostly confined to the internal granule cell layer (Abel et al. 2005). MR imaging is often sufficient for diagnosis (Fig. 33.5). Characteristic features consist of a typically striated pattern of hyperintensity on T2-weighted images with no gadolinium contrast enhancement (Thomas et al. 2007). The pathogenesis of dysplastic gangliocytoma of the cerebellum remains controversial, and the debate as to whether it represents a neoplastic or hamartomatous lesion is still ongoing. It has recently been reported that dysplastic gangliocytoma of the cerebellum is associated with the autosomal-dominant, familial, multiple hamartoma-neoplasia syndrome (or Cowden syndrome), and both conditions are associated with germline mutations in the *PTEN* gene, a tumour suppressor gene on chromosome 10q23 (Nelen et al. 1996; Koch et al. 1999; Zhou et al. 2003; Derrey et al. 2004; Perez-Nunez et al. 2004). Patients with dysplastic gangliocytoma of the cerebellum require long-term observation even when the initial tumour resection appeared near-total (Hashimoto et al. 1997).

Brainstem glioma

Brainstem gliomas account for 25–30% of all infratentorial paediatric brain tumours. They occur particularly in the first decade of life, with a mean age of 7 years. There are two major classes of brainstem gliomas: (1) diffuse intrinsic brainstem gliomas, typically centred in the pons and upper medulla, which carry a uniformly poor prognosis; and (2) focal brainstem gliomas, typically located in the upper midbrain or lower medulla, which often carry an excellent prognosis (Barkovich et al. 1990; Donaldson et al. 2006).

Diffuse intrinsic brainstem gliomas constitute approximately 70% of all brainstem neoplasms. The MRI characteristics of these tumours include diffuse infiltrative enlargement of the pons and/or rostral medulla with no or only minimal contrast enhancement (Vezina 1997; Jaspan and Griffiths 2004) (Fig. 33.6). T1 MRI sequences usually show mass effect and reduced signal compared with normal brain. T2 MRI sequences often reveal high-signal regions of tumour infiltration with rostral extension into the midbrain and brachium pontis and lateral extension into the cerebellar peduncles. Brainstem enlargement may be unilateral and is often asymmetric at initial diagnosis. The fourth ventricle is usually distorted; however, obstructive hydrocephalus is distinctly uncommon at initial presentation. The clinical presentation of diffuse pontomedullary brainstem gliomas typically includes one or more of the following abnormalities: (1) cranial nerve palsies – typically VI and VII; (2) ataxia; and (3) long tract signs, including

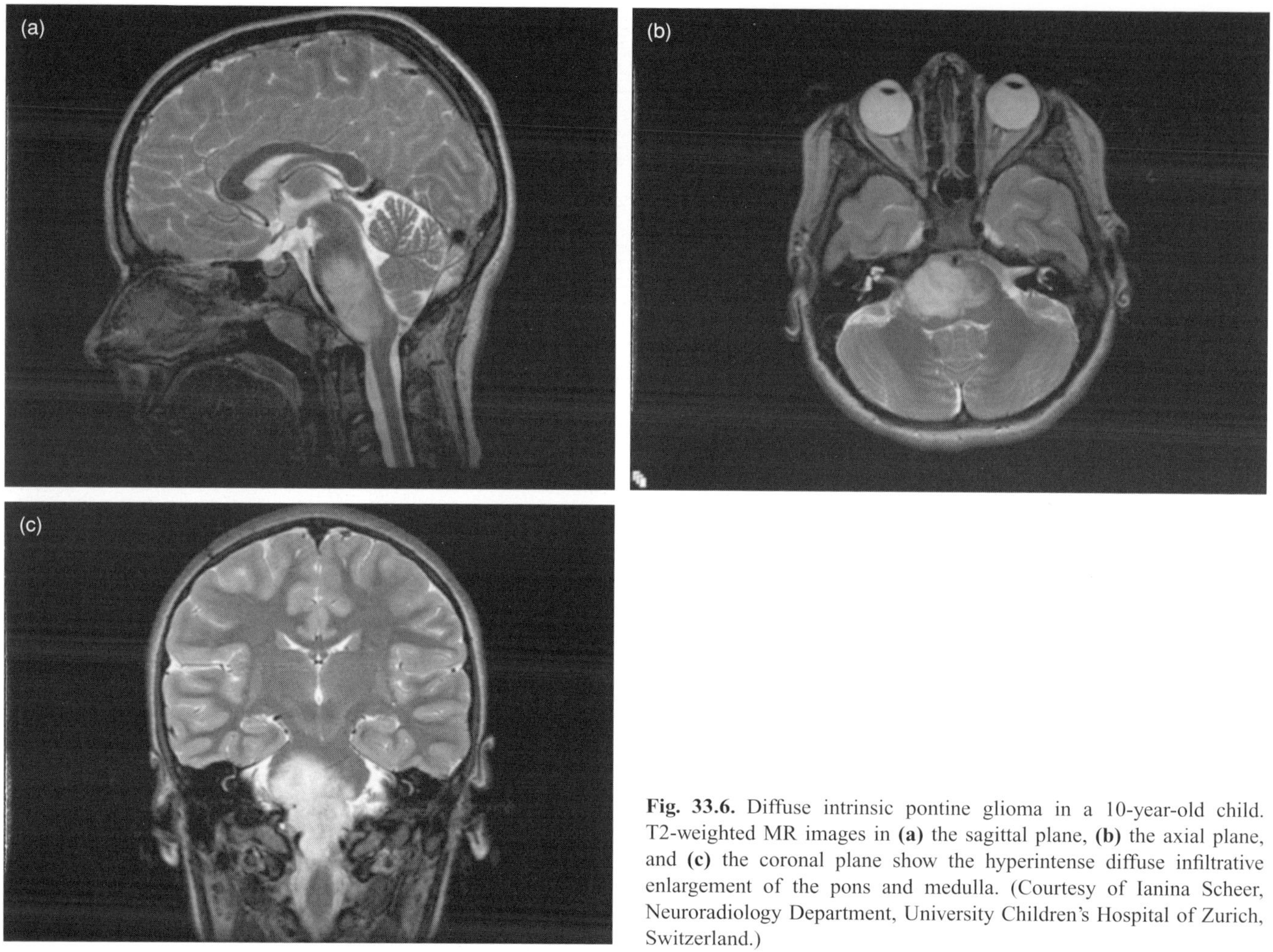

Fig. 33.6. Diffuse intrinsic pontine glioma in a 10-year-old child. T2-weighted MR images in **(a)** the sagittal plane, **(b)** the axial plane, and **(c)** the coronal plane show the hyperintense diffuse infiltrative enlargement of the pons and medulla. (Courtesy of Ianina Scheer, Neuroradiology Department, University Children's Hospital of Zurich, Switzerland.)

hyperreflexia and extensor plantar responses. The prediagnostic symptomatic interval is usually less than 3 months.

In many centres, current management for these tumours avoids routine diagnostic biopsy when the clinical and neuroimaging features typical of diffuse pontomedullary brainstem gliomas are identified. Diagnostic biopsy is clearly indicated for brainstem mass lesions with an unusual MRI appearance or an atypical clinical course. Examples of these circumstances include the young child with a several-year history of slowly progressive clumsiness and facial asymmetry who may have a ganglioglioma of the brainstem, or the adolescent with acute onset of facial weakness, ataxia, fever, and CSF pleiocytosis who may have focal brainstem encephalitis.

In general, there is no defined role for the routine resection of diffuse intrinsic brainstem gliomas. Early in the clinical course, tumour cells infiltrate widely throughout brainstem structures but still permit neurological function to remain at normal or near-normal levels. Consequently, removal of tumour is likely to result in severe neurological deficits. However, some diffuse pontomedullary brainstem gliomas may have a cystic projection dorsally or laterally. These surface projections may provide a limited opportunity for tumour resection; however, it is uncommon that more than 50% of the tumour can be removed and it is unlikely that limited debulking affects progression-free or total survival.

Diffuse brainstem gliomas are among the least responsive and most resistant childhood solid tumours (Hargrave et al. 2006). Conventional treatment consists of 55Gy involved-field radiation therapy administered in single daily fractions of approximately 1.8–2Gy. This approach results in median survival of 9–13 months from diagnosis (Jennings et al. 1996). Despite encouraging single-institution reports suggesting prolonged progression-free survival for children treated with hyperfractionated radiation therapy in which total radiation doses reached 78Gy, larger cooperative trials failed to demonstrate a significant advantage for hyperfractionated radiation (Packer et al. 1994b; Kaplan et al. 1996; Mandell et al. 1999).

Results from chemotherapy trials have been similarly disappointing (Hargrave et al. 2006). Pre-radiation single-agent or combination chemotherapy infrequently produces objective (i.e., radiographic) response rates that exceed 25% (Jennings et al. 1996). Furthermore, it is at best uncertain and at worst unlikely that even these limited response rates will translate into significantly longer survival. Even when the most aggressive chemotherapy approaches are used, such as high-dose chemotherapy followed by PBSC reinfusion, results are usually

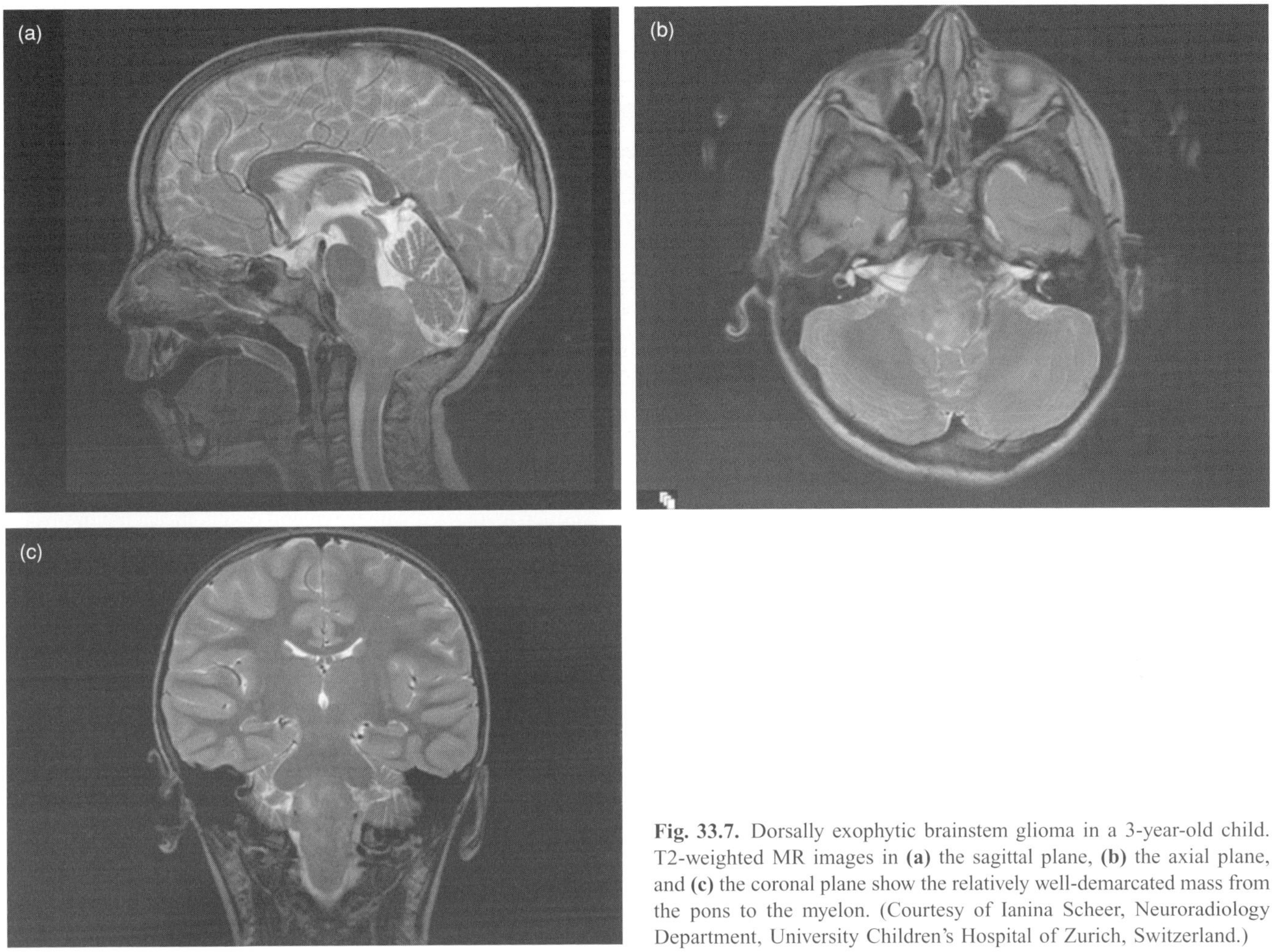

Fig. 33.7. Dorsally exophytic brainstem glioma in a 3-year-old child. T2-weighted MR images in **(a)** the sagittal plane, **(b)** the axial plane, and **(c)** the coronal plane show the relatively well-demarcated mass from the pons to the myelon. (Courtesy of Ianina Scheer, Neuroradiology Department, University Children's Hospital of Zurich, Switzerland.)

limited to relatively brief duration responses and few instances of significant tumour reduction lasting 12 months or longer (Bouffet et al. 2000). Based on these findings, it is difficult to support the use of chemotherapy in brainstem gliomas outside the setting of formal cooperative group studies. However, the extremely poor prognosis for these patients justifies the search for more effective antineoplastic agents.

Dorsally exophytic tumours arise from the floor of the fourth ventricle, often completely fill the ventricle, and the patient may have neurological signs for many years before developing symptoms of obstructive hydrocephalus (Fig. 33.7). MRI demonstrates a well-demarcated lesion, hypointense on T1-weighted images and hyperintense on T2-weighted images with gadolinium enhancement. Usually these are low-grade astrocytomas, and if near-total surgical tumour removal is achieved no treatment other than close observation is necessary. Use of local radiation therapy or chemotherapy should be limited to rare cases of higher-grade gliomas and cases of significant tumour growth after surgery (Pollack et al. 1993).

Cervicomedullary tumours occupy the inferior two-thirds of the medulla and the upper part of the cord and are usually low-grade gliomas. They tend to extend from the epicentre in conformance with the anatomical barriers (Robertson et al. 1994). Intratumoral cysts are infrequent. The clinical course typically runs for several years. Surgical resection of these tumours is indicated upon clinical or radiographic evidence of tumour growth. Although near-total resection is possible, the poorly defined interface between tumour and normal brainstem precludes complete surgical removal of these tumours. Long-term follow-up indicates that many patients will not have evidence of growth for more than 5 years. When growth occurs, the rate of growth is often extremely slow, and malignant transformation has not been observed. Therefore, a conservative management approach is justified.

Cystic nodular brainstem tumours may be found in any region of the brainstem but are most often found in the midbrain. These tumours have a radiographic appearance that is identical to their cerebellar counterparts and their histology is invariably juvenile pilocytic astrocytoma. Resection of the mural nodule is usually curative.

Tectal glioma differ from other brainstem tumours in nature, presentation, and clinical course (Daglioglu et al. 2003; Stark et al. 2005; Ternier et al. 2006). Tectal gliomas usually become symptomatic as late-onset hydrocephalus, whereas focal neurological deficits are rare. Magnetic resonance imaging typically reveals a dorsally exophytic mass extending from the quadrigeminal plate with symmetric periaqueductal T2-hyperintensity and T1-isointensity. Differential diagnosis includes germ cell tumours and pineal cysts. After hydrocephalus has been managed (e.g., with endoscopic third ventriculostomy), these children require prolonged, close clinical and radiological surveillance. Although their growth pattern is slow and their histological features are low-grade, a proportion of these tumours (especially the ones with a volume greater than $10cm^3$ at presentation) will continue to grow and will eventually require treatment (Ternier et al. 2006).

Treatment-related adverse events

In children treated for brain tumours, chronic neurocognitive effects are especially challenging (Mulhern et al. 2004; Duffner 2010). Many of the sequelae of treating childhood brain tumours manifest several years after diagnosis, which mandates long-term follow-up of these patients. Sequential assessments of neurocognitive function demonstrated progressive deterioration during 6 years after whole-brain radiotherapy (Jankovic et al. 1994).

1. Deterioration in intelligence has been demonstrated after 18Gy whole-brain radiotherapy in children with acute lymphatic leukemia (Jankovic et al. 1994). Accordingly, there is no doubt that whole-brain radiation doses of 24–36Gy as commonly used in children with medulloblastoma and other brain tumours have significant negative effects on future cognitive development. This was demonstrated by Mulhern et al. in a meta-analysis of 22 studies with a total of 544 patients (Mulhern et al. 1992). They also showed that the most critical factors influencing intellectual outcome are dose of irradiation and young age at time of irradiation. Accordingly, current therapeutic strategies try to omit or delay whole-brain irradiation in children younger than 3 years and try to reduce radiation doses. Additional risk factors for cognitive decline include perioperative complications, possibly hydrocephalus, and chemotherapy (especially methotrexate) (Duffner 2010). Accurate assessment of the effect of changes in cranial radiation on neurocognitive development in young children is complicated by important methodological and study design problems. A common concern is that measurement of IQ, per se, is neither a sensitive nor a specific way to assess the cognitive impairments of these patients (Jenney 1998). Accordingly, efforts have been made to establish and validate reliable and easy-to-use instruments for assessing IQ, and also other neuropsychological aspects (Bradlyn et al. 1996; Mulhern et al. 2004).
2. Leukoencephalopathy is a late treatment complication most often associated with parenteral or intrathecal methotrexate (MTX) and radiation therapy (Duffner 2004; Reddick et al. 2005) (Fig. 33.8). Young age is also an important risk factor; however, leukoencephalopathy affects patients of all ages. Additional neurotoxic mechanisms include internal hydrocephalus and damaged cerebellar structures affecting neuronal circuits (Rueckriegel et al. 2010). The clinical expression of leukoencephalopathy ranges from mild evidence of white matter injury on neuroimaging studies to severe necrotizing leukoencephalopathy with profound neurological impairment and, in some cases, death. Mild or subclinical cases are more common than severe necrotizing leukoencephalopathy.
3. Radiation necrosis is often a serious treatment complication (Fouladi et al. 2004; Lawrence et al. 2010). First, it may cause significant and persistent neurological injury. Second, it may produce progressive cerebral edema and

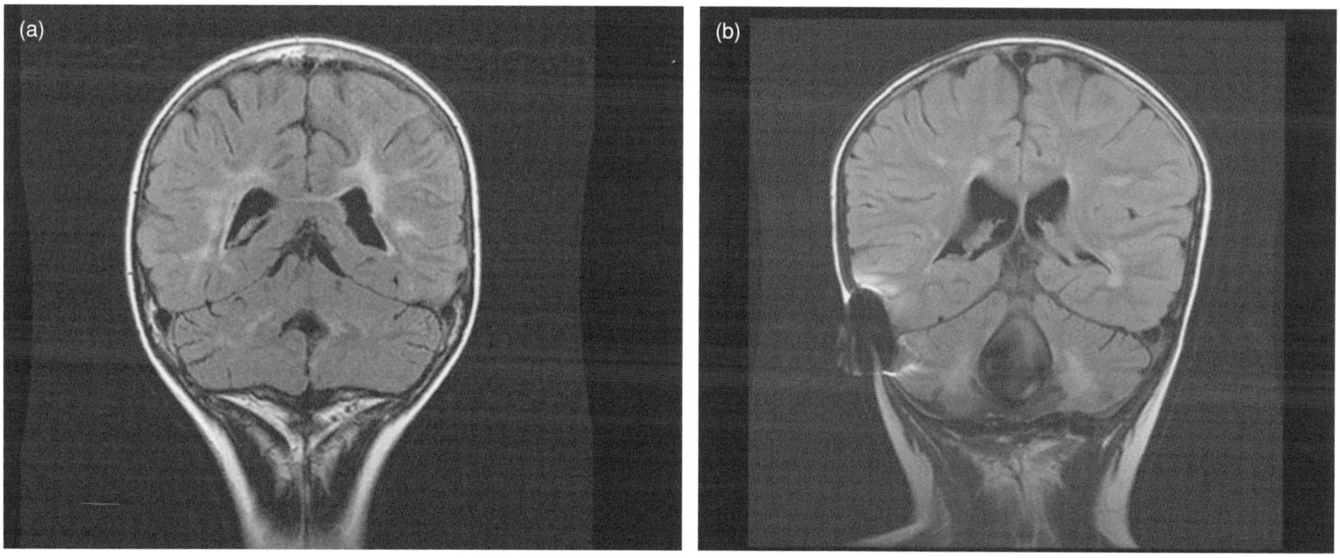

Fig. 33.8. Leukoencephalopathy in **(a)** a 10-year-old child and **(b)** a 14-year-old treated with craniospinal irradiation and multi-agent chemotherapy because of a medulloblastoma. FLAIR MR images in the coronal plane showing white matter changes. (Courtesy of Ianina Scheer, Neuroradiology Department, University Children's Hospital of Zurich, Switzerland.)

mass effect requiring prolonged corticosteroid use or surgery. Third, it may be confused with tumour growth, resulting in the inappropriate use of anti-tumour therapies. The onset of radiation necrosis clinical signs and symptoms is usually identified from 2–3 years after radiation, though confirmed cases have been detected as early as 9 months and as late as 16 years after radiation. The signs and symptoms are strongly related to the site of radiation necrosis. Radiation necrosis is often difficult to distinguish from recurrent tumour by CT or MRI. However, modern advancements with magnetic resonance spectroscopy, diffusion-weighted imaging, and positron emission tomography (PET) are providing the ability to distinguish viable tumour from necrotic tissue (Yang and Aghi 2009).

4. Endocrinopathies are very common in children who have received radiation therapy for brain tumours (Oberfield et al. 1997; Walter et al. 1999; Darzy and Shalet 2009; Diller et al. 2009). They include growth hormone deficiency and thyroid and gonadal dysfunction. Growth hormone deficiency is seen in the majority of children who have received whole-brain irradiation (Darzy and Shalet 2009; Diller et al. 2009). Growth may be further impaired by spinal irradiation, which directly affects the vertebral body growth centre (Sklar 1997; Darzy and Shalet 2009). Thyroid dysfunction is also common (Schmiegelow et al. 2003; Schmiegelow 2006).
5. Second malignancies including malignant glioma and meningiomas may develop as a consequence of radiation therapy for brain tumours (Helseth et al. 1999; Armstrong et al. 2009). Recent reports raise concerns that the addition of adjuvant chemotherapy may increase the risk for second malignancies in long-term survivors of childhood brain tumours (Duffner et al. 1998; Little et al. 1998). This may be especially true after prolonged use of alkylating agents and etoposide with or without irradiation.
6. An increasing number of clinical studies have demonstrated cognitive deficits in children with posterior fossa tumours. These long-term problems have been described by Schmahmann et al. as 'cerebellar cognitive affective syndrome', confirming the importance of the cerebellum for nonmotor functions (Schmahmann and Sherman 1998). The cerebellar cognitive affective syndrome is characterized by problems of executive functions, impaired spatial cognition, linguistic difficulties, and personality changes. In two subsequent paediatric series of patients who underwent resection of a cerebellar tumour without adjuvant therapy, impairments in planning and sequencing, visual-spatial functions, expressive language, verbal memory, and modulation of affect were described (Levisohn et al. 2000; Riva and Giorgi 2000). Steinlin et al. reported significant problems for attention, memory, processing speed, visuoconstructive abilities and verbal fluency (Steinlin et al. 2003). Additional studies found impairments in interpersonal relationships, school functions, and behaviour (Aarsen et al. 2004, 2006; Zuzak et al. 2008). The behavioural changes that were described included anxiety and depression, but also psychoticism, hostility, and delinquent and aggressive behaviour. These different neurobehavioural profiles could be grouped into two domains, reflecting either exaggeration or diminution of responses to the internal or external environment. Schmahmann et al. described these opposite behaviours in adults and children with both congenital and acquired cerebellar disorders as 'dysmetria of thought' (Schmahmann et al. 2007).

REFERENCES

Aarsen FK, Van Dongen HR, Paquier PF, Van Mourik M, Catsman-Berrevoets CE (2004) Long-term sequelae in children after cerebellar astrocytoma surgery. Neurology 62: 1311–1316.

Aarsen FK, Paquier PF, Reddingius RE, Streng IC, Arts WF, Evera-Preesman M, Catsman-Berrevoets CE (2006) Functional outcome after low-grade astrocytoma treatment in childhood. Cancer 106: 396–402.

Abel TW, Baker SJ, Fraser MM, Tihan T, Nelson JS, Yachnis AT, et al. (2005) Lhermitte-Duclos disease: a report of 31 cases with immunohistochemical analysis of the PTEN/AKT/mTOR pathway. J Neuropathol Exp Neurol 64: 341–349.

Albert FK, Forsting M, Sartor K, Adams HP, Kunze S (1994) Early postoperative magnetic resonance imaging after resection of malignant glioma: objective evaluation of residual tumor and its influence on regrowth and prognosis. Neurosurgery 34: 45–60.

Albright AL, Packer RJ, Zimmerman RA, Rorke LB, Boyett J, Hammond GD (1993) Magnetic resonance scans should replace biopsies for the diagnosis of diffuse brain stem gliomas: a report from the Children's Cancer Group. Neurosurgery 33: 1026–1029.

Albright AL, Wisoff JH, Zeltzer PM, Boyett JM, Rorke LB, Stanley P (1996) Effects of medulloblastoma resections on outcome in children: a report from the Children's Cancer Group. Neurosurgery 38: 265–271.

Allen J, Siffert J, Hukin J (1998) Clinical manifestations of childhood ependymoma: a multitude of syndromes. Pediatr Neurosurg 28: 49–55.

Armstrong GT, Liu Q, Yasui Y, Huang S, Ness KK, Leisenring W, et al. (2009) Long-term outcomes among adult survivors of childhood central nervous system malignancies in the Childhood Cancer Survivor Study. J Natl Cancer Inst 101: 946–958.

Bailey CC, Gnekow A, Wellek S, Jones M, Round C, Brown J, et al. (1995) Prospective randomised trial of chemotherapy given before radiotherapy in childhood medulloblastoma. International Society of Paediatric Oncology (SIOP) and the (German) Society of Paediatric Oncology (GPO): SIOP II. Med Pediatr Oncol 25: 166–178.

Bambakidis NC, Robinson S, Cohen M, Cohen AR (2002) Atypical teratoid/rhabdoid tumors of the central nervous system: clinical, radiographic and pathologic features. Pediatr Neurosurg 37: 64–70.

Barkovich AJ, Krischer J, Kun LE, Packer R, Zimmerman RA, Freeman CR, et al. (1990) Brain stem gliomas: a classification system based on magnetic resonance imaging. Pediatr Neurosurg 16: 73–83.

Berger MS, Baumeister B, Geyer JR, Milstein J, Kanev PM, LeRoux PD (1991) The risks of metastases from shunting in children with primary central nervous system tumors. J Neurosurg 74: 872–877.

Biegel JA, Tan L, Zhang F, Wainwright L, Russo P, Rorke LB (2002) Alterations of the hSNF5/INI1 gene in central nervous system atypical teratoid/rhabdoid tumors and renal and extrarenal rhabdoid tumors. Clin Cancer Res 8: 3461–3467.

Bouffet E, Raquin M, Doz F, Gentet JC, Rodary C, Demeocq F, et al. (2000) Radiotherapy followed by high dose busulfan and thiotepa: a prospective assessment of high dose chemotherapy in children with diffuse pontine gliomas. Cancer 88: 685–692.

Bradlyn AS, Ritchey AK, Harris CV, Moore IM, O'Brien RT, Parsons SK, et al. (1996) Quality of life research in pediatric oncology. Research methods and barriers. Cancer 78: 1333–9.

Bruner JM, Inouye L, Fuller GN, Langford LA (1998) Diagnostic discrepancies and their clinical impact in a neuropathology referral practice. Cancer 79: 796–803.

Burger PC, Yu IT, Tihan T, Friedman HS, Strother DR, Kepner JL, et al. (1998) Atypical teratoid/rhabdoid tumor of the central nervous system: a highly malignant tumor of infancy and childhood frequently mistaken for medulloblastoma: a Pediatric Oncology Group study. Am J Surg Pathol 22: 1083–1092.

Capone Mori A, Hoeltzenbein M, Poetsch M, Schneider JF, Brandner S, Boltshauser E (2003) Lhermitte-Duclos disease in 3 children: a clinical long-term observation. Neuropediatrics 34: 30–35.

CBTRUS (2010) Central Brain Tumor Registry of the United States statistical report: primary brain and central nervous system tumors diagnosed in the United States, 2004–2006 (http://www.cbtrus.org).

Childhood Brain Tumor Consortium (1988) A study of childhood brain tumors based on surgical biopsies from ten North American institutions: sample description. J Neurooncol 6: 9–23.

Cohen BH, Zeltzer PM, Boyett JM, Allen JC, Finlay JL, McGuire-Cullen P, et al. (1995) Prognostic factors and treatment results for supratentorial primitive neuroectodermal tumors in children using radiation and chemotherapy: a Childrens Cancer Group randomized trial. J Clin Oncol 13: 1687–1696.

Connelly JM, Malkin MG (2007) Environmental risk factors for brain tumors. Curr Neurol Neurosci Rep 7: 208–214.

Crawford JR, MacDonald TJ, Packer RJ (2007) Medulloblastoma in childhood: new biological advances. Lancet Neurol 6: 1073–1085.

Daglioglu E, Cataltepe O, Akalan N (2003) Tectal gliomas in children: the implications for natural history and management strategy. Pediatr Neurosurg 38: 223–231.

Darzy KH, Shalet SM (2009) Hypopituitarism following radiotherapy revisited. Endocr Dev 15: 1–24.

Derrey S, Proust F, Debono B, Langlois O, Layet A, Layet V, et al. (2004) Association between Cowden syndrome and Lhermitte-Duclos disease: report of two cases and review of the literature. Surg Neurol 61: 447–454.

Dhall G (2009) Medulloblastoma. J Child Neurol 24: 1418–1430.

Diller L, Chow EJ, Gurney JG, Hudson MM, Kadin-Lottick NS, Kawashima TI, et al. (2009) Chronic disease in the Childhood Cancer Survivor Study cohort: a review of published findings. J Clin Oncol 27: 2339–2355.

Dobrovoljac M, Hengartner H, Boltshauser E, Grotzer MA (2002) Delay in the diagnosis of paediatric brain tumours. Eur J Pediatr 161: 663–667.

Donaldson SS, Laningham F, Fisher PG (2006) Advances toward an understanding of brainstem gliomas. J Clin Oncol 24: 1266–1272.

Dubey A, Sung WS, Shaya M, Patwardhan R, Willis B, Smith D, Nanda A (2009) Complications of posterior cranial fossa surgery – an institutional experience of 500 patients. Surg Neurol 72: 369–375.

Duffner PK (2004) Long-term effects of radiation therapy on cognitive and endocrine function in children with leukemia and brain tumors. Neurologist 10: 293–310.

Duffner PK (2010) Risk factors for cognitive decline in children treated for brain tumors. Eur J Pediatr Neurol 14: 106–115.

Duffner PK, Krischer JP, Horowitz ME, Cohen ME, Burger PC, Friedman HS, Kun LE (1998) Second malignancies in young children with primary brain tumors following treatment with prolonged postoperative chemotherapy and delayed irradiation: A Pediatric Oncology Group Study. Ann Neurol 44: 313–316.

Eberhart CG, Kratz J, Wang Y, Summers K, Stearns D, Cohen K, et al. (2004) Histopathological and molecular prognostic markers in medulloblastoma: c-myc, N-myc, TrkC, and anaplasia. J Neuropathol Exp Neurol 63: 441–449.

Eberhart CG, Wiestler OD, Eng C (2007) Cowden disease and dysplastic gangliocytoma of the cerebellum/Lhermitte-Duclos disease. In: Louis DN, Ohgaki H., Wiestler OD, Cavenee WK, editors. WHO Classification of Tumours of the Central Nervous System: WHO; 226–228.

Evans AE, Jenkin DT, Sposto R, Ortega J, Wilson CB, Wara W, et al. (1990) The treatment of medulloblastoma: results of a prospective randomized trial of radiation therapy with and without CCNU, vincristine and prednisone. J Neurosurg 72: 572–582.

Fattet S, Haberler C, Legoix P, Varlet P, Lellouch-Tubiana A, Lair S, et al. (2009) Beta-catenin status in paediatric medulloblastomas: correlation of immunohistochemical expression with mutational status, genetic profiles, and clinical characteristics. J Pathol 218: 86–94.

Feychting M, Floderus B, Ahlbom A (2000) Parental occupational exposure to magnetic fields and childhood cancer (Sweden). Cancer Causes Control 11: 151–156.

Fort DW, Rushing EJ (1997) Congenital central nervous system tumors. J Child Neurol 12: 157–164.

Fouladi M, Chintagumpala M, Laningham FH, Ashley D, Kellie SJ, Langston JW, et al. (2004) White matter lesions detected by magnetic resonance imaging after radiotherapy and high-dose chemotherapy in children with medulloblastoma or primitive neuroectodermal tumor. J Clin Oncol 22: 4551–4560.

Friedman HS, Oakes WJ, Bigner SH, Wikstrand CJ, Bigner DD (1991) Medulloblastoma: tumor biological and clinical perspectives. J Neurooncol 11: 1–15.

Friedman JM, Gutmann DH, MacCollin M, Riccardi VM (1999) Neurofibromatosis. Phenotype, Natural History, and Pathogenesis, 3rd edition. Baltimore and London: Johns Hopkins University Press.

Friedrich CA (1999) Von Hippel-Lindau syndrome. A pleomorphic condition. Cancer 86: 2478–2482.

Gajjar A, Pizer B (2010) Role of high-dose chemotherapy for recurrent medulloblastoma and other CNS primitive neuroectodermal tumors. Pediatr Blood Cancer 54: 649–651.

Garton GR, Schomberg PJ, Scheithauer BW, Shaw EG, Ilstrup DM, Blackwell CR, et al. (1990) Medulloblastoma – prognostic factors and outcome of treatment: review of the Mayo Clinic experience. Mayo Clin Proc 65: 1077–1086.

Grabb PA, Lunsford LD, Albright AL, Kondziolka D, Flickinger JC (1996) Stereotactic radiosurgery for glial neoplasms of childhood. Neurosurgery 38: 696–701.

Granovsky MO, Mueller BU, Nicholson HS, Rosenberg PS, Rabkin CS (1998) Cancer in human immunodeficiency virus-infected children: a case series from the Children's Cyncer Group and th National Cancer Institue. J Clin Oncol 16: 1729–1735.

Grotzer MA, Hogarty MD, Janss AJ, Liu X, Zhao H, Eggert A, et al. (2001) MYC messenger RNA expression predicts survival outcome in childhood primitive neuroectodermal tumor/medulloblastoma. Clin Cancer Res 7: 2425–2433.

Grotzer MA, Janss AJ, Fung K, Biegel JA, Sutton LN, Rorke LB, et al. (2000) TrkC expression predicts good clinical outcome in primitive neuroectodermal brain tumors. J Clin Oncol 18: 1027–1035.

Gurney JG, Kadan-Lottick N (2001) Brain and other central nervous system tumors: rates, trends, and epidemiology. Curr Opin Oncol 13: 160–166.

Hargrave D, Bartels U, Bouffet E (2006) Diffuse brainstem glioma in children: critical review of clinical trials. Lancet Oncol 7: 241–248.

Hashimoto H, Iida J, Masui K, Nishi N, Sakaki T (1997) Recurrent Lhermitte-Duclos disease – case report. Neurol Med Chir (Tokyo) 37: 692–696.

Helseth E, Due-Tonnessen B, Wesenberg F, Lote K, Lundar T (1999) Posterior fossa medulloblastoma in children and young adults (0–19 years): survival and performance. Childs Nerv Syst 15: 451–455.

Herms J, Neidt I, Luscher B, Sommer A, Schurmann P, Schroder T, et al. (2000) C-MYC expression in medulloblastoma and its prognostic value. Int J Cancer 89: 395–402.

Hijiya N, Hudson MM, Lensing S, Zacher M, Onciu M, Behm FG, et al. (2007) Cumulative incidence of secondary neoplasms as a first event after childhood acute lymphoblastic leukemia. JAMA 297: 1207–1215.

Hilden JM, Meerbaum S, Burger P, Finlay J, Janss A, Scheithauer BW, et al. (2004) Central nervous system atypical teratoid/rhabdoid tumor: results of therapy in children enrolled in a registry. J Clin Oncol 22: 2877–2884.

Hirsch JF, Renier D, Czernichow P, Benveniste L, Pierre-Kahn A (1979) Medulloblastoma in childhood. Survival and functional results. Acta Neurochir (Wien) 48: 1–15.

Hussein MR (2007) Central nervous system capillary haemangioblastoma: the pathologist's viewpoint. Int J Exp Pathol 88: 311–324.

Jankovic M, Brouwers P, Valsecchi MG, Van Veldhuizen A, Huisman J, Kamphuis R, et al. (1994) Association of 1800 cGy cranial irradiation with intellectual function in children with acute lymphoblastic leukaemia. ISPACC. International Study Group on Psychosocial Aspects of Childhood Cancer. Lancet 344: 224–227.

Jaspan T, Griffiths PD (2004) Diagnostic imaging. In: Brain and Spinal Tumors of Childhood (Walker DA, Punt JAG, Taylor RE, eds). London: Arnold; 107–161.

Jenkin D (1996) The radiation treatment of medulloblastoma. J Neurooncol 29: 45–54.

Jenkinson H, Hawkins M (1999) Secondary brain tumours in children with ALL. Lancet 354: 1126.

Jenney MEM (1998) Theoretical issues pertinent to measurement of quality of life. Med Pediatr Oncol Supplement I: 41–45.

Jennings MT, Freeman ML, Murray MJ (1996) Strategies in the treatment of diffuse pontine gliomas: the therapeutic role of hyperfractionated radiotherapy and chemotherapy. J Neurooncol 28: 207–222.

Judkins AR, Mauger J, Ht A, Rorke LB, Biegel JA (2004) Immunohistochemical analysis of hSNF5/INI1 in pediatric CNS neoplasms. Am J Surg Pathol 28: 644–650.

Kaplan AM, Albright AL, Zimmerman RA, Rorke LB, Li H, Boyett JM, et al. (1996) Brainstem gliomas in children. A Children's Cancer Group review of 119 cases. Pediatr Neurosurg 24: 185–192.

Kedar A (1997) Chemotherapy for pediatric brain tumors. Semin Pediatr Neurol 4: 320–332.

Kilday JP, Rahman R, Dyer S, Ridley L, Lowe J, Coyle B, Grundy R (2009) Pediatric ependymoma: biological perspectives. Mol Cancer Res 7: 765–786.

Kim JY, Sutton ME, Lu DJ, Cho TA, Goumnerova LC, Goritchenko L, et al. (1999) Activation of neurotrophin-3 receptor TrkC induces apoptosis in medulloblastomas. Cancer Res 59: 711–719.

Koch R, Scholz M, Nelen MR, Schwechheimer K, Epplen JT, Harders AG (1999) Lhermitte-Duclos disease as a component of Cowden's syndrome. Case report and review of the literature. J Neurosurg 90: 776–779.

Kramer ED, Vezina LG, Packer RJ, Fitz CR, Zimmerman RA, Cohen MD (1994) Staging and surveillance of children with central nervous system neoplasms: recommendations of the Neurology and Tumor Imaging Committees of the Children's Cancer Group. Pediatr Neurosurg 20: 254–262.

Lawrence YR, Li XA, el Naqa I, Hahn CA, Marks LB, Merchant TE, Dicker AP (2010) Radiation dose-volume effects in the brain. Int J Radiat Oncol Biol Phys 76(3 Suppl): S20–27.

Levisohn L, Cronin-Golomb A, Schmahmann JD (2000) Neuropsychological consequences of cerebellar tumour resection in children: cerebellar cognitive affective syndrome in a paediatric population. Brain 123 (Pt 5): 1041–1050.

Lhermitte J, Duclos P (1920) Sur un ganglioneuromed diffus du cortex du cervelet. Bull Assoc Fr Etud Cancer 9: 99–107.

Little MP, de Vathaire F, Shamsaldin A, Oberlin O, Campbell S, Grimaud E, et al. (1998) Risks of brain tumour following treatment for cancer in childhood: modification by genetic factors, radiotherapy and chemotherapy. Int J Cancer 78: 269–275.

Liu GT, Phillips PC, Molloy PT, Balcer LJ, Schut L, Duhaime A-C, Sutton LN (1998) Visual impairment associated with mutism after posterior fossa surgery in children. Neurosurgery 42: 253–257.

Liwnicz BH, Berger TS, Liwnicz RG, Aron BS (1985) Radiation-associated gliomas: a report of four cases and analysis of postradiation tumors of the central nervous system. Neurosurgery 17: 436–445.

Louis DN, Ohgaki H, Wiestler OD, Cavenee WK, Burger PC, Jouvet A, et al. (2007) The 2007 WHO Classification of Tumours of the Central Nervous System. Acta Neuropathol (Berl) 114: 97–109.

Lubin F, Farbstein H, Chetrit A, Farbstein M, Freedman L, Alfandary E, Modan B (2000) The role of nutritional habits during gestation and child life in pediatric brain tumor etiology. Int J Cancer 86: 139–143.

MacDonald SM, Yock TI (2010) Proton beam therapy following resection for childhood ependymoma. Childs Nerv Syst 26: 285–291.

Mandell LR, Kadota R, Freeman C, Douglass EC, Fontanesi J, Cohen ME, et al. (1999) There is no role for hyperfractionated radiotherapy in the management of children with newly diagnosed diffuse intrinsic brainstem tumors: results of a Pediatric Oncology Group phase III trial comparing conventional versus hyperfractionated radiotherapy. Int J Radiat Oncol Biol Phys 43: 959–964.

Mason WP, Goldman S, Yates AJ, Boyett J, Li H, Finlay JL (1998) Survival following intensive chemotherapy with bone marrow reconstitution for children with recurrent intracranial ependymoma. J Neuro-Oncol 37: 135–143.

Merchant TE, Pollack IF, Loeffler JS (2010) Brain tumors across the age spectrum: biology, therapy, and late effects. Semin Radiat Oncol 20: 58–66.

Mulhern R, Hancock J, Fairclough D, Kun L (1992) Neuropsychological status of children treated for brain tumors: a critical review and integrative analysis. Med Pediatr Oncol 20: 181–191.

Mulhern RK, Merchant TE, Gajjar A, Reddick WE, Kun LE (2004) Late neurocognitive sequelae in survivors of brain tumours in childhood. Lancet Oncol 5: 399–408.

Mulhern RK, Palmer SL, Merchant TE, Wallace D, Kocak M, Brouwers P, et al. (2005) Neurocognitive consequences of risk-adapted therapy for childhood medulloblastoma. J Clin Oncol 23: 5511–5519.

Narod SA, Stiller C, Lenoir GM (1991) An estimate of the heritable fraction of childhood cancer. Br J Cancer 63: 993–999.

Needle MN, Goldwein JW, Grass JW, Cnaan A, Bergman I, Molloy P, et al. (1997) Adjuvant chemotherapy for the treatment of intracranial ependymoma of childhood. Cancer 80: 341–347.

Nelen MR, Padberg GW, Peeters EA, Lin AY, van den Helm B, Frants RR, et al. (1996) Localization of the gene for Cowden disease to chromosome 10q22–23. Nat Genet 13: 114–116.

Oberfield SE, Chin D, Uli N, David R, Sklar C (1997) Endocrine late effects of childhood cancers. J Pediatr 131: S37–41.

Packer RJ (1990) Chemotherapy for medulloblastoma/primitive neuroectodermal tumors of the posterior fossa. Ann Neurol 28: 823–828.

Packer RJ (2005) New insights into childhood ependymomas. Curr Neurol Neurosci Rep 5: 107–109.

Packer RJ (2008) Childhood brain tumors: accomplishments and ongoing challenges. J Child Neurol 23: 1122–1127.

Packer RJ, Vezina G (2008) Management of and prognosis with medulloblastoma: therapy at a crossroads. Arch Neurol 65: 1419–1424.

Packer RJ, Sutton LN, Elterman R, Lange B, Goldwein J, Nicholson HS, et al. (1994a) Outcome for children with medulloblastoma treated with radiation and cisplatin, CCNU, and vincristine chemotherapy. J Neurosurg 81: 690–698.

Packer RJ, Boyett JM, Zimmerman RA, Albright AL, Kaplan AM, Rorke LB, et al. (1994b) Outcome of children with brain stem gliomas after treatment with 7800 cGy of hyperfractionated radiotherapy. A Childrens Cancer Group Phase I/II Trial. Cancer 74: 1827–1834.

Perez-Nunez A, Lagares A, Benitez J, Urioste M, Lobato RD, Ricoy JR, et al. (2004) Lhermitte-Duclos disease and Cowden disease: clinical and genetic study in five patients with Lhermitte-Duclos disease and literature review. Acta Neurochir (Wien) 146: 679–690.

Pizer BL, Clifford SC (2009) The potential impact of tumour biology on improved clinical practice for medulloblastoma: progress towards biologically driven clinical trials. Br J Neurosurg 23: 364–375.

Pollack IF (1994) Brain tumors in children. N Engl J Med 331: 1500–1507.

Pollack IF (1997) Posterior fossa syndrome. Int Rev Neurobiol 41: 411–432.

Pollack IF, Hoffman HJ, Humphreys RP, Becker L (1993) The long-term outcome after surgical treatment of dorsally exophytic brain-stem gliomas. J Neurosurg 78: 859–863.

Raisanen JM, Davis RL (1993) Congenital brain tumors. Pathology (Phila) 2(1): 103–116.

Reddick WE, Glass JO, Helton KJ, Langston JW, Xiong X, Wu S, Pui CH (2005) Prevalence of leukoencephalopathy in children treated for acute lymphoblastic leukemia with high-dose methotrexate. AJNR Am J Neuroradiol 26: 1263–1269.

Reddy AT (2005) Atypical teratoid/rhabdoid tumors of the central nervous system. J Neurooncol 75: 309–313.

Relling MV, Rubnitz JE, Rivera GK, Boyett JM, Hancock ML, Felix CA, et al. (1999) High incidence of secondary brain tumours after radiotherapy and antimetabolites. Lancet 354: 34–39.

Ries LAG, Kosary CL, Hankey BF, Miller BA, Harras A, Edwards BK (1998) SEER cancer statistics review, 1973–1995. DHHS Publ No. (NIH) 97–2789.

Riva D, Giorgi C (2000) The cerebellum contributes to higher functions during development: evidence from a series of children surgically treated for posterior fossa tumours. Brain 123 (Pt 5): 1051–1061.

Roach ES, Gomez MR, Northrup H (1998) Tuberous sclerosis complex consensus conference: revised clinical diagnostic criteria. J Child Neurol 13: 624–628.

Robertson PL, Allen JC, Abbott IR, Miller DC, Fidel J, Epstein FJ (1994) Cervicomedullary tumors in children: a distinct subset of brainstem gliomas. Neurology 44: 1798–1803.

Robertson PL, Muraszko KM, Holmes EJ, Sposto R, Packer RJ, Gajjar A, et al. (2006) Incidence and severity of postoperative cerebellar mutism syndrome in children with medulloblastoma: a prospective study by the Children's Oncology Group. J Neurosurg 105(6 Suppl): 444–451.

Rorke LB, Packer RJ, Biegel JA (1996) Central nervous system atypical teratoid/rhabdoid tumors of infancy and childhood: definition of an entity. J Neurosurg 85: 56–65.

Rueckriegel SM, Driever PH, Blankenburg F, Ludemann L, Henze G, Bruhn H (2010) Differences in supratentorial damage of white matter in pediatric survivors of posterior fossa tumors with and without adjuvant treatment as detected by magnetic resonance diffusion tensor imaging. Int J Radiat Oncol Biol Phys 76: 859–866.

Ruggieri M, Pascual Castroviejo I, Di Rocco C (2008) Neurocutaneous Disorders. Vienna and New York: Springer.

Rutkowski S, Cohen B, Finlay J, Luksch R, Ridola V, Valteau-Couanet D, et al. (2010) Medulloblastoma in young children. Pediatr Blood Cancer 54: 635–637.

Rutkowski S, von Bueren A, von Hoff K, Hartmann W, Shalaby T, Deinlein F, et al. (2007) Prognostic relevance of clinical and biological risk factors in childhood medulloblastoma: results of patients treated in the prospective multicenter trial HIT'91. Clin Cancer Res 13: 2651–2657.

Schmahmann JD, Sherman JC (1998) The cerebellar cognitive affective syndrome. Brain 121 (Pt 4): 561–579.

Schmahmann JD, Weilburg JB, Sherman JC (2007) The neuropsychiatry of the cerebellum – insights from the clinic. Cerebellum 6: 254–267.

Schmiegelow M (2006) Endocrinological late effects following radiotherapy and chemotherapy of childhood brain tumours. Dan Med Bull 53: 326–341.

Schmiegelow M, Feldt-Rasmussen U, Rasmussen AK, Poulsen HS, Muller J (2003) A population-based study of thyroid function after radiotherapy and chemotherapy for a childhood brain tumor. J Clin Endocrinol Metab 88: 136–140.

Shapiro S, Mealey JJ, Sartorius C (1989) Radiation-induced intracranial malignant gliomas. J Neurosurg 71: 77–82.

Shih CS, Hale GA, Gronewold L, Tong X, Laningham FH, Gilger EA, et al. (2008) High-dose chemotherapy with autologous stem cell rescue for children with recurrent malignant brain tumors. Cancer 112: 1345–53.

Shore RE, Albert RE, Pasternack BS (1976) Follow-up study of patients treated by X-ray epilation for tinea capitis; resurvey of post-treatment illness and mortality experience. Arch Environmental Health 31: 21–28.

Shu XO, Jin F, Linet MS, Zheng W, Clemens J, Mills J, Gao YT (1994) Diagnostic X-ray and ultrasound exposure and risk of childhood cancer. Br J Cancer 70: 531–537.

Silber JH, Radcliffe J, Peckham V, Perilongo G, Kishnani P, Fridman M, et al. (1992) Whole-brain irradiation and decline in intelligence: the influence of dose and age on IQ score. J Clin Oncol 10: 1390–1396.

Silverman CL, Simpson JR (1982) Cerebellar medulloblastoma: the importance of posterior fossa dose to survival and patterns of failure. Inter J Radiat Oncol Biol Phys 8: 1869–1876.

Sklar CA (1997) Growth and neuroendocrine dysfunction following therapy for childhood cancer. Pediatr Clin North Am 44: 489–503.

Smith MA, Freidlin B, Simon R (1998) Trends in reported incidence of primary malignant brain tumors in children in the United States. J Natl Cancer Inst 90: 1269–1277.

Stark AM, Fritsch MJ, Claviez A, Dorner L, Mehdorn HM (2005) Management of tectal glioma in childhood. Pediatr Neurol 33: 33–38.

Stearns D, Chaudhry A, Abel TW, Burger PC, Dang CV, Eberhart CG (2006) c-myc overexpression causes anaplasia in medulloblastoma. Cancer Res 66: 673–681.

Steinbok P, Hentschel S, Cochrane DD, Kestle JRW (1996) Value of postoperative surveillance imaging in the management of children with some common brain tumors. J Neurosurg 84: 726–732.

Steinlin M, Imfeld S, Zulauf P, Boltshauser E, Lovblad KO, Ridolfi Luthy A, et al. (2003) Neuropsychological long-term sequelae after posterior fossa tumour resection during childhood. Brain 126(Pt 9): 1998–2008.

Stiller CA, Bleyer A (2004) Epidemiology. In: Walker DA, Punt JAG, Taylor RE editor. Brain and Spinal Tumors of Childhood, London: Arnold; 35–49.

Sutton LN, Cnaan A, Klatt L, Zhao H, Zimmerman R, Needle M, et al. (1996) Postoperative surveillance imaging in children with cerebellar astrocytomas. J Neurosurg 84: 721–725.

Tekautz TM, Fuller CE, Blaney S, Fouladi M, Broniscer A, Merchant TE, et al. (2005) Atypical teratoid/rhabdoid tumors (ATRT): improved survival in children 3 years of age and older with radiation therapy and high-dose alkylator-based chemotherapy. J Clin Oncol 23: 1491–1499.

Ternier J, Wray A, Puget S, Bodaert N, Zerah M, Sainte-Rose C (2006) Tectal plate lesions in children. J Neurosurg 104(6 Suppl): 369–376.

Thomas B, Krishnamoorthy T, Radhakrishnan VV, Kesavadas C (2007) Advanced MR imaging in Lhermitte-Duclos disease: moving closer to pathology and pathophysiology. Neuroradiology 49: 733–738.

Varan A, Buyukpamukcu M, Ersoy F, Sanal O, Akyuz C, Kutluk T, Yalcin B (2004) Malignant solid tumors associated with congenital immunodeficiency disorders. Pediatr Hematol Oncol 21: 441–451.

Versteege I, Sevenet N, Lange J, Rousseau-Merck MF, Ambros P, Handgretinger R, et al. (1998) Truncating mutations of hSNF5/INI1 in aggressive paediatric cancer. Nature 394: 203–206.

Vezina LG (1997) Diagnostic imaging in neuro-oncology. Pediatr Clin North Am 44: 701–719.

Walter AW, Mulhern RK, Gajjar A, Heideman RL, Reardon D, Sanford RA, et al. (1999) Survival and neurodevelopmental outcome of young children with medulloblastoma at St. Jude Children's Research Hosptal. J Clin Oncol 17: 3720–3728.

Wirtz CR, Knauth M, Staubert A, Bonsanto MM, Sartor K, Kunze S, Tronnier VM (2000) Clinical evaluation and follow-up results for intraoperative magnetic resonance imaging in neurosurgery. Neurosurgery 46: 1112–1120.

Wisoff JH, Epstein FJ (1984) Pseudobulbar palsy after posterior fossa operation in children. Neurosurgery 15: 707–709.

Yang I, Aghi MK (2009) New advances that enable identification of glioblastoma recurrence. Nat Rev Clin Oncol 6: 648–657.

Zacharoulis S, Moreno L (2009) Ependymoma: an update. J Child Neurol 24: 1431–1438.

Zeltzer PM, Boyett JM, Finlay JL, Albright AL, Rorke LB, Milstein JM, et al. (1999) Metastasis stage, adjuvant treatment, and residual tumor are prognostic factors for medulloblastoma in children: conclusions from the Children's Cancer Group 921 randomized phase III study. J Clin Oncol 17: 832–845.

Zhou XP, Marsh DJ, Morrison CD, Chaudhury AR, Maxwell M, Reifenberger G, Eng C (2003) Germline inactivation of PTEN and dysregulation of the phosphoinositol-3-kinase/Akt pathway cause human Lhermitte-Duclos disease in adults. Am J Hum Genet 73: 1191–1198.

Zuzak TJ, Poretti A, Drexel B, Zehnder D, Boltshauser E, Grotzer MA (2008) Outcome of children with low-grade cerebellar astrocytoma: long-term complications and quality of life. Childs Nerv Syst 24: 1447–1455.

34

Paraneoplastic Cerebellar Syndromes: Neurodegeneration in Langerhans Cell Histiocytosis

Andrea Poretti, Eugen Boltshauser, and Jeremy D. Schmahmann

Paraneoplastic neurological syndromes (PNS) represent remote effects of cancer on the nervous system. PNS can affect any part of the nervous system: in adults the well-known syndromes are peripheral neuropathies (in particular, subacute sensory neuropathies), limbic encephalitis, Lambert-Eaton myasthenic syndrome, neuromyotonia, and so-called paraneoplastic cerebellar degeneration.

PNS in the paediatric age group are exceptionally rare and we focus on three underlying conditions, which are discussed in separate chapters: neurodegeneration in Langerhans histiocytosis (this chapter); paraneoplastic cerebellar degeneration in paediatric Hodgkin disease (Chapter 35); and opsoclonus-myoclonus syndrome (associated with neuroblastoma) (Part 8 Acute Ataxia, Chapter 38).

These paediatric paraneoplastic cerebellar syndromes are quite different regarding pathogenesis, clinical presentation, neuroimaging, treatment, and outcome.

Langerhans cell histiocytosis (LCH) is a granulomatous disorder resulting from clonal proliferation of bone marrow-derived Langerhans cells that reside in the skin and lymph nodes, and in some cases arising from circulating plasmacytoid monocytes. The disorder is rare, occurs mostly in children, with a reported incidence in childhood of 5.4 to 8.9 cases per million children per year (Bernstrand et al. 2005). It also presents in adulthood. The clinical course of LCH is highly variable, ranging from a self-healing solitary bone lesion (single organ system disease affecting skin or bone) to a widely disseminated (multisystem) life-threatening disease involving lungs, liver, spleen, hematopoietic system, and central nervous system (CNS) (Lahey, 1975; Bernstrand et al. 2005). Late sequelae are common and include pulmonary, endocrine, and CNS complications. Neurological symptoms generally appear some years after the diagnosis is established, although they may be the heralding manifestations in some cases. It remains unclear whether LCH is caused by a malignancy or by immune dysregulation. This lack of clear understanding of its pathophysiology renders optimal therapy a challenge. While beyond the scope of this chapter, available treatments include corticosteroids, a range of chemotherapeutic agents, immune modulation with intravenous immunoglobulin, and irradiation to focal bony or other lesions (Grois et al. 1998, 2005; Arceci 1999; Nanduri et al. 2003; Abla et al. 2010).

CNS manifestations of LCH vary widely, both with respect to the pathological underpinnings and the clinical presentations. We consider LCH here because it has a particular predilection for the cerebellum, among other regions. The CNS pathology of this disorder was studied in 12 patients by Grois et al. (2005), whose findings were grouped into three types of lesions. First, tumorous lesions in the meninges or choroid plexus on MRI correspond to circumscribed granulomas like those seen in peripheral organs, with variable presence of CD1a-reactive cells and pronounced CD8-positive (+) T-cell infiltration. Second, granulomas within the brain's connective tissue spaces are accompanied by infiltration of the surrounding CNS parenchyma by CD1a-reactive histiocytes, profound T-cell-dominated inflammation, and severe neurodegeneration characterized by a nearly complete loss of neurons and axons, and gliosis. Third, neurodegenerative lesions lacking infiltration of CD1a+ cells, mainly affecting the cerebellum and brainstem, exhibit a profound inflammatory process dominated by CD8-reactive lymphocytes, associated with tissue degeneration, microglial activation, and gliosis.

Central nervous system involvement in LCH may be primary, or a secondary phenomenon – akin to other paraneoplastic, and possibly immune-mediated postinfectious processes.

Primary brain involvement in Langerhans cell histiocytosis

Primary involvement of the brain is likely to occur in patients with multi-organ disease. The most common CNS manifestation is infiltration of the hypothalamic pituitary region by LCH granuloma, frequently leading to diabetes insipidus and anterior pituitary hormone deficiency (Grois et al. 1998, 2005; Barthez et al. 2000). All other parts of the CNS may be involved, extending from adjacent bone lesions or arising from the meninges, pineal gland or choroid plexus. Additional isolated or multifocal intracerebral space-occupying histiocytic granulomatous lesions cause symptoms dependent on their location (Grois et al. 1998; Prayer et al. 2004). Neuroimaging may show a partially empty sella, lack of the bright signal of the posterior pituitary on T1-weighted images, and granulomatous lesions in the suprasellar region (Prayer et al. 2004).

Neurodegeneration in Langerhans cell histiocytosis

After focal lesions of the pituitary-hypothalamic axis, neurodegenerative changes are the second most frequent pattern of CNS pathology in LCH. These manifest mostly as bilateral symmetric lesions in the cerebellum and basal ganglia of variable signal intensity on MRI, depending on site and stage of the lesion (Prosch et al. 2007; van der Knaap et al. 2008; Wnorowski et al. 2008). The cerebellar pathology is characterized by a T-cell-dominated inflammatory process leading to neuronal and axonal destruction with secondary demyelination (Grois et al. 2005). The prevalence of the neurodegenerative processes on radiological imaging in children with LCH is uncertain and ranges between 4% and 57% in different studies (Prosch et al. 2007; Wnorowski et al. 2008; Laurencikas et al. 2011). In the study of van't Hooft et al. (2008) abnormalities on the MRI were used as a diagnostic criterion for neurodegenerative LCH (ND-LCH). The risk of developing neurodegeneration in LCH has been reported to be greater in patients with craniofacial lesions involving the orbital, temporal, sphenoid, ethmoid, or mastoid bones, and the paranasal sinuses and anterior or middle cranial fossa (Grois et al. 2010), and also in patients with pituitary involvement and diabetes insipidus (Donadieu et al. 2004; Grois et al. 2006).

Neuroimaging findings

In the setting of a history of known LCH, the neuroimaging pattern is quite typical and distinct. Symmetric, non-enhancing, signal hyperintensities are seen in the cerebellum on T2-weighted images, and variable signal hypointensities on T1-weighted images in the hilus of the dentate nuclei and less frequently in the cerebellar white matter (Fig. 34.1a) (Prosch et al. 2007; van der Knaap et al. 2008; Wnorowski et al. 2008). In some cases the dentate nuclei have a hyperintense signal on T1- and hypointense signal on T2-weighted images, representing calcifications (van der Knaap et al. 2008). Homogenous, symmetric T2-hyperintense signal abnormalities have been described in the superior (Fig. 34.1b) and middle cerebellar peduncles, and in the brainstem involving the pontine tegmentum and less frequently the pyramidal tracts (Fig. 34.1a) (Martin-Duverneuil et al. 2006).

Generalized cerebellar atrophy has been reported in several patients (Martin-Duverneuil et al. 2006; Prosch et al. 2007; van der Knaap et al. 2008; Wnorowski et al. 2008). Cerebellar atrophy may not be present on neuroimaging at the commencement of the clinical symptoms of ND-LCH but only on follow-up (Wnorowski et al. 2008), most likely representing the end stage of the pathogical process. This temporal progresssion of the imaging findings in ND-LCH is captured through the sequential neuroimaging findings (Figs 34.2, 34.3) over 17 years in one of our patients whom we first met at the age of 22 years (Case 1, below; Case 8 in Schmahmann et al. 2007). His diagnosis of LCH was established at age 3 by skin biopsy. He developed ND-LCH initially as cerebellar motor signs at the age of 6 years, which progressed through adolescence from subtle to moderate disability, along with neurocognitive and neuropsychiatric problems, discussed below. This case illustrates that during the course of the disease the initial cerebellar white matter neuroimaging signal abnormalities attenuate, giving way to leukoencephalopathy, gliosis of the deep nuclei, and pancerebellar atrophy. We are not aware of another case in the literature to date with longitudinal MRI follow-up extending over such a protracted period of time.

Associated supratentorial findings in some cases include bilateral, mostly symmetric, non-enhancing T2 hypertense areas involving the cerebral white matter, predominantly in the posterior periventricular regions and, less frequently, supratentorial atrophy that may be diffuse, bifrontal predominant, or affecting the corpus callosum (Martin-Duverneuil et al. 2006; Prosch et al. 2007; van der Knaap et al. 2008). Neuroimaging abnormalities do not resolve during the course of the disease, but remain stable, progress, or (as shown in Figs 34.2 and 34.3) evolve to a different pattern of abnormalities (dependent on the study, in 60–100% of patients) (Prosch et al. 2007; van der Knaap et al. 2008). It should be noted that the precise relationship between the progression of neuroimaging abnormalities and the clinical manifestations remains unclear (Prosch et al. 2007).

Signal abnormalities bilaterally in the basal ganglia (particularly the globus pallidus and less often the caudate nucleus) represent the second most common neuroimaging finding in ND-LCH after cerebellar lesions. The globus pallidus typically appears hyperintense on T1-weighted images and, rarely, hyperintense on T2-weighted images (Martin-Duverneuil et al. 2006). Hypointensity of the globus pallidus on susceptibility-weighted images (SWI) representing calcifications has also been reported

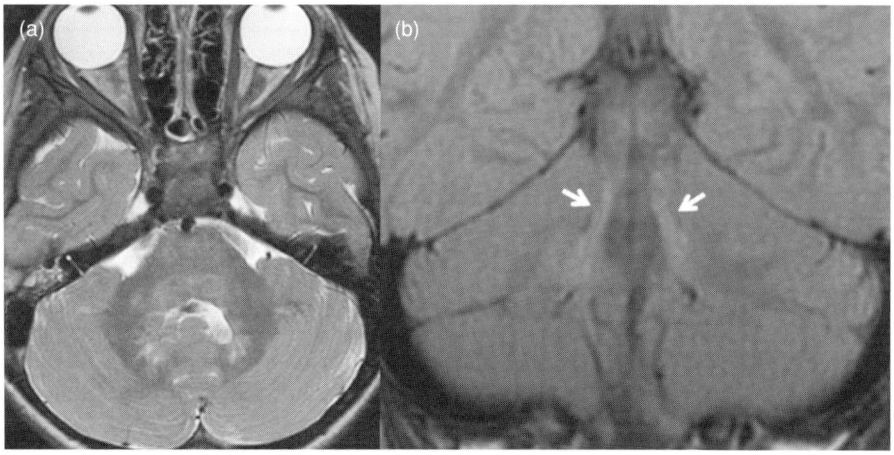

Fig. 34.1. 6-year-old child with inactive Langerhans cell histiocytosis with previous skin and bone involvement. He presented with isolated cognitive impairment. **(a)** Axial T2-weighted MRI showing abnormally high signal in the cerebellar white matter, hilus of the dentate nuclei, and brainstem; **(b)** coronal FLAIR-weighted MRI showing involvement of the superior cerebellar peduncles (white arrows). MRI also revealed multifocal punctuate signal abnormalities in the corpus callosum and supratentorial white matter (not shown).

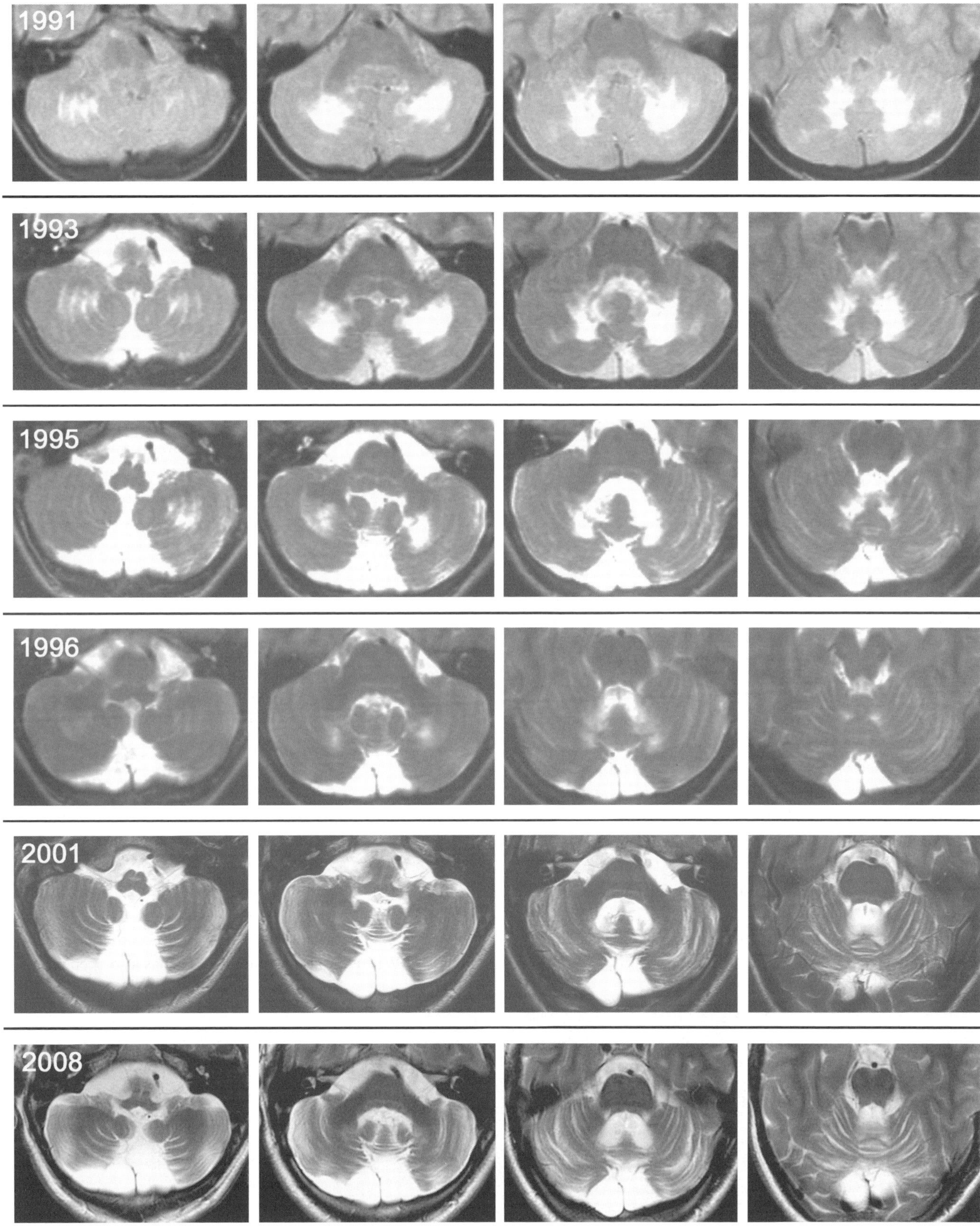

Fig. 34.2. Axial T2-weighted MR images through the cerebellum in Case 1 over 17 years from the age of 8 years (1991) to the age of 25 years (2008). The first sequence of images (1991) was acquired using fluid-attenuated inversion recovery. The images reveal high signal throughout the cerebellar white matter early in the course (1991–1995), with more recent images (2001 and 2008) demonstrating pancerebellar atrophy and attenuated white matter.

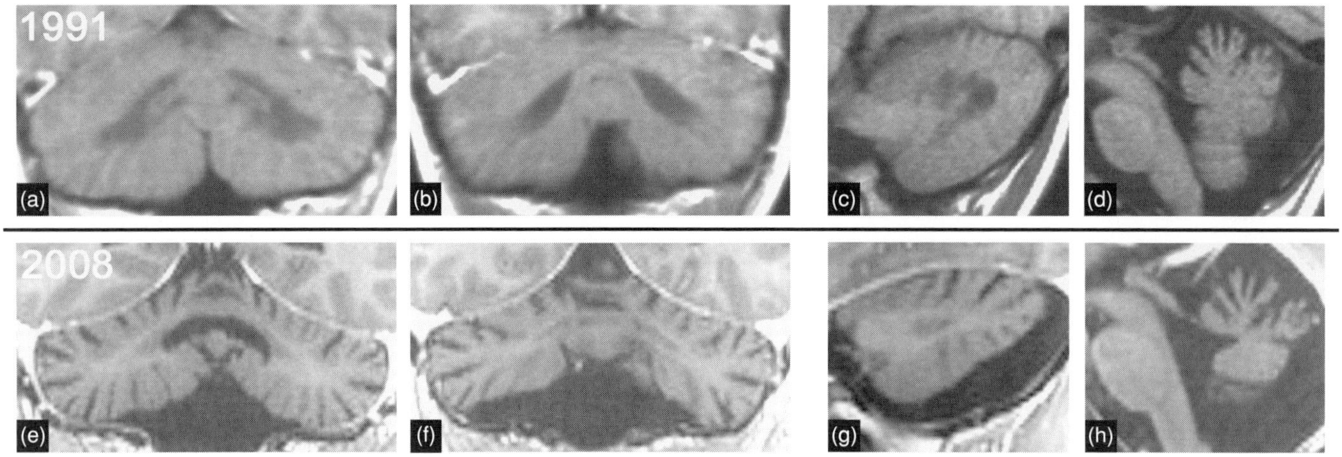

Fig. 34.3. Coronal and sagittal T1-weighted MR images compared over time in Case 1. Hypointensity within the cerebellum in 1991 is seen in the coronal plane **(a, b)**, compared with similar coronal sections in 2008 **(e, f)** showing cerebellar volume loss both in the cerebellar cortex and white matter. The sagittal images in 1991 show hypointensity in the white matter and deep nuclear region **(c)** and only mild superior vermian volume loss in the midsagittal plane **(d)**, compared to the smaller area of hypointensity in 2008 **(g)** and marked volume loss in midsagittal section **(h)**.

(Ertan and Huisman 2010). SWI revealed calcifications in the substantia nigra (Ertan and Huisman 2010).

Clinical manifestations

The clinical presentation of focal lesions in primary CNS LCH is determined by the location of the pathology, whether intra-axial (mostly in the pituitary-hypothalamic axis with diabetes insipidus and hypothalamic endocrine and neurobehavioural disturbances), or meningeal/choroidal disease. In approximately 25% of cases, ND-LCH leads to clinically relevant neurocognitive symptoms at a median of 6 years after initial diagnosis of LCH (Prosch et al. 2007; Wnorowski et al. 2008). However, onset of neurodegeneration may precede other manifestations of LCH by up to 20 years (Prosch et al. 2007; van der Knaap et al. 2008). The clinical picture is heterogeneous, including a spectrum of signs ranging from a subtle cerebellar motor syndrome of tremor, gait disturbance, dysarthria, and dysphagia, together with spasticity and hyperreflexia, to a syndrome of pronounced ataxia, with neurobehavioural problems including cognitive impairment and psychopathology such as obsessive-compulsive disorder (Grois et al. 1998; Shuper et al. 2000; Grois et al. 2010; Mimouni-Bloch et al. 2010). In a long-term follow-up study, ataxia, dysarthria, spasticity, hydrocephalus, and neuropsychiatric disabilities were identified in 4 of 40 of the patients examined by Bernstrand et al. (2005), corresponding to 3 of 16 of the surviving patients with multisystem disease at onset (with or without single bone involvement).

Of the 28 children with LCH studied by Nanduri et al. (2003), 14 had no CNS or hypothalamo-pituitary involvement, 6 had isolated diabetes insipidus, and 7 had lesions in the hypothalamus and/or cerebellum, often with cerebral atrophy. Behavioural abnormalities in the patients with hypothalamic damage included rage attacks and abnormal eating patterns – binge eating, anorexia, or bulimia, as well as claustrophobia, agoraphobia, depression, and aggression. Four patients had signal change in the cerebellar hemispheres and deep nuclei on MRI, while seven had varying degrees of cerebellar ataxia as measured by the International Cooperative Ataxia Rating Scale (Trouillas et al. 1997). The children with lesions in the CNS (hypothalamic and/or cerebellar) had impaired intellectual function (lower full scale, performance, and verbal intellectual quotient), with other domains affected including memory (particularly immediate verbal memory, and immediate and delayed visual memory), attentional systems (interference with learning), linguistic skills (receptive vocabulary and reading comprehension), and mathematical skills (reasoning and numerical operations). Severe psychological disability was noted in some.

Cognitive and behavioural deficits were reported in two children with LCH studied by Whitsett et al. (1999). One with pituitary and hypothalamic involvement developed diabetes insipidus, hyperphagia, obesity and subsequent diabetes mellitus, and on neuropsychological testing showed impairments in full-scale IQ, verbal memory and mental flexibility as well as freedom from distractibility. The child with the characteristic cerebellar lesion (white matter signal abnormality on MRI) was shown at age 15 to have experienced a decline in global intellectual functioning over time, as well as mildly impaired memory (visual more than verbal), mental flexibility, freedom from distractibility, and processing speeds. He was described as immature, impulsive, and socially inept. He would act in a way that ostracized him from others, but seemed bewildered by the consequences of his actions. Although attempts were made to provide him with social skills training, he was unable to apply the basic skills he had been taught.

All nine patients with LCH studied by van't Hooft et al. (2008) had lesions in the cerebellum and basal ganglia, and six in the hypothalamo-pituitary axis. Cognitive deficits were noted in eight cases, particularly involving perceptual tasks, demanding visual-spatial processing skills, and working memory in both the verbal and visual-spatial domains. Subtle deficits in short-term auditory memory were also noted in 14 of the 25 patients studied for long term consequences of LCH by Mittheisz et al. (2007), although overt neurological symptoms were not noted in this cohort.

Whereas the association between infratentorial signal abnormalities and neurological symptoms is not always readily apparent (Prosch et al. 2007; Grois et al. 2010), available evidence suggests that all patients with cerebellar atrophy are clinically symptomatic. Neurological symptoms in ND-LCH have been linked by some investigators to the presence of cerebellar atrophy rather than the nuclear and white matter signal abnormalities (Martin-Duverneuil et al. 2006). Others have identified ND-LCH symptoms with cerebellar gray and/or white matter signal abnormalities without cerebellar atrophy (Wnorowski et al. 2008), a scenario consistent with the history of motor and neuropsychiatric and cognitive impairments in our own patients.

Representative case reports

The following cases illustrate the nature of the cerebellar motor syndrome as well as the cerebellar cognitive affective syndrome that results from cerebellar predominant ND-LCH.

Case 1

(See Fig 34.2 and 34.3; patient included as Case 8 in Schmahmann et al. 2007).

A 22-year-old man was referred to us for his ND-LCH because of major and ongoing problems of behavioural dyscontrol. At 3 months of age he developed a persistent skin rash, which was shown to be LCH when it was biopsied at age 3 years. The disease involved his lungs, skull and skin, and he was treated with vinblastine, vinorelbine, corticosteroids and 750 rad to the right side of the skull. At age 6 he developed problems with balance and running, together with impairments of gross and fine motor coordination. Motor impairments continued to worsen slowly; by age 12 he was diagnosed with cerebellar dysfunction, with abnormal gait and inability to run. He required special education assistance at school, because of decreased IQ measures, performance skills more affected than verbal skills. Hand writing and typing were slow. At age 22 he was described as being 'almost entirely in denial' with multiple emotional problems. He was impetuous, impulsive, self-absorbed, immature, unreliable and demonstrated poor judgment. He took unnecessary risks and was inappropriate in interactions. He perseverated over the loss of a previous job. He was not social, had no friends, and had become socially isolated. He was mildly paranoid, and could be intermittently agitated and aggressive. He refused help, and was 'his own worst enemy'.

Examination at age 22 revealed that he was intermittently cooperative and engaged, but disinhibited and impulsive. He learned four words on the first attempt; at 5 minutes he recalled two spontaneously, one with a clue and one with multiple choice. His semantic fluency was limited to 13 animals in one minute; phonemic fluency was 13 F words and 9 A words in a minute. He had a moderately severe cerebellar motor syndrome, with a score of 51/120 points on the Modified version of the International Cooperative Ataxia Rating Scale (11/34 for posture and gait, 30/68 for kinetic function, 3/10 for speech disorders, and 7/8 for oculomotor disorders) and 13/30 on the Brief Ataxia Rating Scale (3/8 for gait, 2/4 for each of the upper and lower extremities, 1/4 for speech, and $^1/_2$ for eye movements; Schmahmann et al. 2009). He walked independently but there was considerable difficulty with staggering and with half turn, and the speed was slightly reduced. He could stand with his feet together but not in a tandem position, he swayed with his feet together and eyes open, threatening the upright position with his eyes closed. He had moderate impairment with the heel-to-shin test, and mild decomposition of rapid foot tapping. The upper extremity dysmetria was of moderate degree, slightly worse on the left than the right. There was minimal cerebellar dysarthria. He had square wave jerks and downward bobbing occasionally of the eyes at rest, persistent but moderate gaze-evoked nystagmus, saccadic intrusions into ocular pursuit, overshoot and undershoot of the saccade, and saccadic intrusions into the vestibulo-ocular reflex test (VORC).

At age 30 the cerebellar motor syndrome was unchanged. He required frequent supervision at home. He engaged in self-injurious behaviour, ruminated obsessively, demonstrated poor reality testing, and was unable to maintain a job because of sexually inappropriate comments. He showed impaired insight and judgment, and grappled with anxiety and depression (sadness, despair and despondency, lack of interest, guilt, remorse, poor sleep, and suicidal thoughts). He was intermittently violent, requiring the involvement of law enforcement, a situation exacerbated by his use of alcohol. Neuropsychological testing documented his deficits, which were focused heavily in the domains of executive dysfunction, and the issues of mood and behaviour. He showed decline compared to prior testing, including deficits in visual-perceptual tasks more than verbal performance. He received an axis I diagnosis of cerebellar cognitive affective syndrome with a depressive disorder, and axis II diagnosis of narcissistic dependent and antisocial personality features.

The clinical presentation of the patient reported by Shuper et al. (2000) bears an uncanny resemblance to our case 1. Their patient was diagnosed with LCH at age 3 years 6 months. He had been a gifted student in his early years, but at age 16 he developed a cerebellar motor syndrome with marked behavioural features. This included poor attention span, memory impairment, and anomia. The authors report that the patient 'showed very poor insight into reality, with distorted, unorganized, and often aggressive thought content, and bouts of inappropriate laughing. Severe obsessive-compulsive disorder became manifest. The obsessions included persistent ideas, religious rituals, and thought content and phrases that continuously occupied him, leading him to perform intentional repetitive and stereotypical behaviours . . . [that] significantly interfered with his normal personal, occupational, and social activity.' These neuropsychiatric features recapitulate many aspects of the domains of impairment that comprise the neuropsychiatry of the cerebellum (Schmahmann et al. 2007).

Case 2

A highly functioning professional known for meticulous attention to detail developed fatigue and diabetes insipidus in his early 40s. Recalcitrant groin rashes led to biopsy at age 48 that established the diagnosis of LCH. Treatments ensued with multiple chemotherapeutic agents and focal irradiation of the jaw. Cerebellar MRI lesions were first noted at age 51 (T2 hyperintensities in the middle cerebellar peduncles, cerebellar white matter, and perinuclear region of the cerebellum bilaterally). The following year the patient's wife noted that he could not think things through adequately, or complete negotiations, and because of this he was no longer able to work. Judgment became impaired. He would open car doors close to others without paying attention, use sharp knives in an irresponsible manner, and deliver off-color jokes in inappropriate contexts, exhibiting no self-monitoring. Over the next 2 years he developed prominent dysarthria and gait impairment. Hematopoietic stem cell transplant produced marked improvement in systemic symptoms and the cerebellar motor syndrome, but behavioural changes persisted. He began using the internet irresponsibly and was taken in by scams. He became unable to multitask, and had difficulty recognizing the consequence of his own actions. He was inattentive, while at the same time compulsive, ruminative, and perseverative. He had difficulty shifting focus, or engaging in a flow of conversation. He developed occasional spontaneous laughing, and features of passivity, immaturity, and childishness. He was overly gullible and trusting, and oblivious to social boundaries.

His neurological examination revealed a mild to moderate cerebellar motor syndrome (MICARS score 40/120; BARS score 12/30), with minimal saccadic intrusions into pursuit eye movements and the VORC, transient horizontal nystagmus and saccadic hypermetria; prominent cerebellar dysarthria; irregular cadence to his gait and mild widening of stance; jerking in-plane dysmetria with heel-to-shin testing bilaterally; and left more than right upper extremity dysmetria. He was alert and oriented, learned four words on the first attempt, and 5 minutes later recalled three spontaneously and the fourth from multiple choice. Language and praxis were normal. Semantic fluency was reduced to twelve animals in a minute; phonemic fluency reduced to eight F words. Fist-palm-side graphomotor sequencing showed impulsivity and inadequate sequence alternation, and he perseverated when drawing the Luria diagram. His drawings were preserved (clock, three-dimensional cube). Visuospatial functioning had shown deficits on neuropsychological testing 5 years previously, but on re-evaluation at age 57 he was now in the solidly average range. He also exhibited deficits in attention and executive functions (working memory, cognitive flexibility, impulsivity, verbal fluency, processing speed, judgment, and problem solving). He had difficulty learning unstructured linguistic material, partly due to poor learning strategies and his sensitivity to interference from material he had just previously been asked to learn. Learning and recall were stronger when he was provided with structured (contextual) material. Language was normal.

At age 57 the focal cerebellar lesions had subsided, replaced by cerebellar atrophy and mild prominence of the cerebral sulci. Brain positron emission tomographic (PET) scan at this time showed hypometabolism bilaterally in the cerebellum hemispheres, left > right, cerebellar nuclei, and dorsal portion of the mid-pons and midbrain. The cerebral hemispheres were normal.

These cases are consistent with the conclusions of the larger studies of ND-LCH cases cited above that report motor and neurobehavioural phenomena, and they convey some of the difficulties faced by these patients as well as by their families and healthcare providers. The deficits in executive and visual-spatial cognition as well as changes in linguistic function that include limited verbal fluency are consistent with the cognitive impairments of the cerebellar cognitive affective syndrome (Schmahmann and Sherman 1998), and the range and pattern of psychological and behavioural features conform to the five domains postulated to characterize the neuropsychiatry of the cerebellum (Schmahmann et al. 2007), considered in more detail in Chapter 4. It is possible that selected aspects of the cognitive and neurobehavioural impairments arise from non-cerebellar lesions, and in cases where the neuroimaging features are not confined to the cerebellum, caution is warranted in drawing this conclusion. This is particularly true if anterograde amnesia is a major component of the cognitive profile, as that would not be expected from pure cerebellar lesions, but may result from damage to cortical and subcortical areas engaged in memory including the hypothalamus, anterior and/or dorsal thalamic nuclei, and hippocampal formation, or the fibre tracts that link these areas.

Therapeutic strategies

The management of neurodegeneration in LCH has not yet been established. Three therapeutic options have been reported. Transretinoic acid (administered orally at a dose of $45mg/m^2$ daily for 6 weeks and then 2 weeks every month for 1 year) stabilized the neurological signs and symptoms in 10 patients after 1-year follow-up (Idbaih et al. 2004). A combination of intravenous immunoglobulin (monthly or twice-monthly at a dosage of 250–400mg/kg/dose) and chemotherapy (steroid ± vinblastine ± 6-mercaptopurine ± methotrexate) led to stabilization of the neurological deficits and neuroimaging findings in 4 patients administered more than 23 doses of intravenous immunoglobulin and chemotherapy (Imashuku et al. 2008). A regimen of vincristine 1.5mg/m^2 on day 1 and cytosine arabinoside (ARA-C) 100mg/m^2 daily for 5 days or ARA-C alone monthly for 4–19 months decreased the ataxia severity grade and/or the neuroimaging findings in five of seven patients (Allen et al. 2010). A number of other treatments for LCH, mostly in the earlier stages, include chemotherapeutic agents such as vinorelbine, fludarabine, and busulfan; immune modulating agents used in certain forms of cancer – cladribine, imatinib, thalidomide, etanercept, alemtuzumab, retuximab, and lymphocyte immune globulin; and, as noted in Case 2, hematopoietic stem cell transplant. These interventions are best administered in specialized centres.

Principles of management of the motor, cognitive, and affective symptoms in patients at all stages of CNS LCH are similar to those discussed in the general chapters dealing with these manifestations. Both our cases described above showed clinically relevant improvements in comportment and mood with judicious use of antidepressant and/or atypical antipsychotic medications.

Acknowledgments

The authors are grateful to Dr Jeffrey Weilburg, Massachusetts General Hospital Department of Psychiatry, and Dr Jan Drappatz, Dana Farber Cancer Center, Boston, MA, for patient referrals. This work is supported in part by RO1 MH067980, the Birmingham and MINDlink Foundations (JDS). The assistance of Jason MacMore is greatly appreciated.

REFERENCES

Abla O, Egeler RM, Weitzman S (2010) Langerhans cell histiocytosis: Current concepts and treatments. Cancer Treat Rev 36: 354–359.

Allen CE, Flores R, Rauch R, Dauser R, Murray JC, Puccetti D, et al. (2010) Neurodegenerative central nervous system Langerhans cell histiocytosis and coincident hydrocephalus treated with vincristine/cytosine arabinoside. Pediatr Blood Cancer 54: 416–423.

Arceci RJ (1999) The histiocytoses: the fall of the Tower of Babel. Eur J Cancer 35: 747–767.

Barthez MA, Araujo E, Donadieu J (2000) Langerhans cell histiocytosis and the central nervous system in childhood: evolution and prognostic factors. Results of a collaborative study. J Child Neurol 15: 150–156.

Bernstrand C, Sandstedt B, Ahström L, Henter JI (2005) Long-term follow-up of Langerhans cell histiocytosis: 39 years' experience at a single centre. Acta Paediatr 94: 1073–1084.

Donadieu J, Rolon MA, Thomas C, Brugieres L, Plantaz D, Emile JF, et al.; French LCH Study Group (2004) Endocrine involvement in pediatric-onset Langerhans' cell histiocytosis: a population-based study. J Pediatr 144: 344–350.

Ertan G, Huisman TA (2010) Susceptibility-weighted imaging in neurodegeneration in Langerhans cell histiocytosis. J Pediatr 156: 1032.

Grois N, Fahrner B, Arceci RJ, Henter JI, McClain K, Lassmann H, et al. (2010) Central nervous system disease in Langerhans cell histiocytosis. J Pediatr 156: 873–881.

Grois N, Pötschger U, Prosch H, Minkov M, Arico M, Braier J, et al.; DALHX- and LCH I and II Study Committee (2006) Risk factors for diabetes insipidus in Langerhans cell histiocytosis. Pediatr Blood Cancer 42: 438–444.

Grois N, Prayer D, Prosch H, Lassmann H and the CNS LCH Co-operative Group (2005) Neuropathology of CNS disease in Langerhans cell histiocytosis. Brain 128: 829–838.

Grois NG, Favara BE, Mostbeck GH, Prayer D (1998) Central nervous system disease in Langerhans cell histiocytosis. Neuroradiology 41: 443–446.

Idbaih A, Donadieu J, Barthez MA, Geissmann F, Bertrand Y, Hermine O, et al. (2004) Retinoic acid therapy in 'degenerative-like' neuro-Langerhans cell histiocytosis: a prospective pilot study. Pediatr Blood Cancer 43: 55–58.

Imashuku S, Okazaki NA, Nakayama M, Fujita N, Fukuyama T, Koike K, et al., and Japan LCH Study Group (2008) Treatment of neurodegenerative CNS disease in Langerhans cell histiocytosis with a combination of intravenous immunoglobulin and chemotherapy. Pediatr Blood Cancer 50: 308–311.

Lahey E (1975) Histiocytosis x – an analysis of prognostic factors. J Pediatr 87: 184–189.

Laurencikas E, Gavhed D, Stalemark H, van't Hooft I, Prayer D, Grois N, Henter JI (2011) Incidence and pattern of radiological central nervous system Langerhans cell histiocytosis in children: a population based study. Pediatr Blood Cancer 56: 250–257.

Martin-Duverneuil N, Idbaih A, Hoang-Xuan K, Donadieu J, Genereau T, Guillevin R, Chiras J, French Langerhans Cell Histiocytosis Study Group (2006) MRI feaures of neurodegenerative Langerhans cell histiocytosis. Eur Radiol 16: 2074–2082.

Mimouni-Bloch A, Schneider C, Politi KE, Konen O, Gothelf D, Stark B, et al. (2010) Neuropsychiatric manifestations in Langerhans' cell histiocytosis disease: a case report and review of the literature. J Child Neurol 25: 884–887.

Mittheisz E, Seidl R, Prayer D, Waldenmair M, Neophytou B, Pötschger U, et al. (2007) Central nervous system-related permanent consequences in patients with Langerhans cell histiocytosis. Pediatr Blood Cancer 48: 50–56.

Nanduri VR, Lillywhite L, Chapman C, Parry L, Pritchard J, Vargha-Khadem F (2003) Cognitive outcome of long-term survivors of multisystem Langerhans cell histiocytosis: a single-institution, cross-sectional study. J Clin Oncol 21: 2961–2967.

Prayer D, Grois N, Prosch H, Gadner H, Barkovich AJ (2004) MR imaging presentation of intracranial disease associated with Langerhans cell histiocytosis. AJNR Am J Neuroradiol 25: 880–891.

Prosch H, Grois N, Wnorowski M, Steiner M, Prayer D (2007) Long-term MR imaging course of neurodegenerative Langerhans cell histiocytosis. AJNR Am J Neuroradiol 28: 1022–1028.

Schmahmann JD, Sherman JC (1998) The cerebellar cognitive affective syndrome Brain 121: 561–579.

Schmahmann JD, Gardner RC, MacMore J, Vangel M (2009) Development of a brief ataxia rating scale (BARS) based on a modified form of the ICARS. Movement Disorders 24: 1820–1828.

Schmahmann JD, Weilburg JB, Sherman JC (2007) The neuropsychiatry of the cerebellum – insights from the clinic. Cerebellum 6: 254–267.

Shuper A, Stark B, Yaniv Y, Zaizov R, Carel C, Sadeh M, Steinmetz A (2000) Cerebellar involvement in Langerhans' cell histiocytosis: a progressive neuropsychiatric disease. J Child Neurol 15: 824–826.

Trouillas P, Takayanagi T, Hallett M, Currier RD, Subramony SH, Wessel K, et al. (1997) International Cooperative Ataxia Rating Scale for pharmacological assessment of the cerebellar syndrome. The Ataxia Neuropharmacology Committee of the World Federation of Neurology. J Neurol Sci 145: 205–211.

van der Knaap MS, Arts WF, Garbern JY, Hedlund G, Winkler F, Barbosa C, et al. (2008) Cerebellar leukoencephalopathy: most likely histiocytosis-related. Neurology 71: 1361–1367.

Van't Hooft I, Gavhed D, Laurencikas E, Henter JI (2008) Neuropsychological sequelae in patients with neurodegenerative Langerhans cell histiocytosis. Pediatr Blood Cancer 51: 669–674.

Whitsett SF, Kneppers K, Coppes MJ, Egeler RM (1999) Neuropsychologic deficits in children with Langerhans cell histiocytosis. Med Pediatr Oncol 33: 486–492.

Wnorowski M, Prosch H, Prayer D, Janssen G, Gadner H, Grois N (2008) Pattern and course of neurodegeneration in Langerhans cell histiocytosis. J Pediatr 153: 127–132.

35 Paraneoplastic Cerebellar Degeneration in Pediatric Hodgkin Disease

Eugen Boltshauser and Andrea Poretti

Paraneoplastic cerebellar degeneration (PCD) is one presentation within the spectrum of paraneoplastic neurological syndromes (Vedeler et al. 2006; Giometto et al. 2010). In PCD antineuronal antibodies are mainly directed against Purkinje cells (Graus et al. 2010). Yo antibodies are most frequently associated with PCD. In adults almost every type of tumor has been reported in association with PCD. Most frequently associated are tumors of the lung, ovary, breast, and lymphoma. In about 60% of such patients, the neurological symptoms precede the diagnosis of the cancer. Characteristically, the onset of PCD is subacute leading to moderate or severe ataxia with truncal or limb involvement; dysarthria and nystagmus are less commonly observed.

PCD is a well-known rare complication in adults with Hodgkin disease. Hammack et al. (1992) reported a series of 21 patients. In the majority, Hodgkin disease preceded neurological symptoms by 1–54 months. The clinical findings were usually only cerebellar, but some patients had long tract signs and sensory neuropathy. PCD was more common in males (18/21) and in a younger age group. Six of 21 patients had antibodies against Purkinje cells.

Only very few single observations of PCD in pediatric Hodgkin disease are on record. In an 8-year-old boy cerebellar signs including truncal and limb ataxia, dysarthria, and bilateral horizontal nystagmus of acute onset associated with nausea and vomiting were evident 4 years before Hodgkin disease (mass in the anterior mediastinum) was diagnosed. Following treatment neurological signs regressed (Topcu et al. 1992). Hahn et al. (2000) described a 13-year-old boy with truncal ataxia, intention tremor, dysarthria, downbeat nystagmus, diplopia, and progressive cerebellar atrophy observed before Hodgkin disease was diagnosed. Antibodies against Purkinje cells were detected. Despite successful lymphoma treatment, cerebellar symptoms only partially resolved. An 11-year-old boy was observed by Emir et al. (2000), presenting with a cervical mass and severe cerebellar ataxia. MRI revealed cerebellar atrophy. Under chemotherapy neurological symptoms improved markedly.

Hodgkin disease should be considered in the differential diagnosis of (rapidly) evolving cerebellar signs, often associated with neuroimaging evidence of cerebellar atrophy, but initial MRI may be normal. Indeed, the signs of paraneoplastic syndromes commonly precede those of the associated neoplasm. The diagnostic yield of antibodies against Purkinje cells in pediatric Hodgkin disease is not known.

REFERENCES

Emir S, Kutluk MT, Goguş S, Buyukpamukçu M (2000) Paraneoplastic cerebellar degeneration and Horner syndrome: association of two uncommon findings in a child with Hodgkin disease. J Pediatr Hematol Oncol 22: 158–161.

Giometto B, Grisold W, Vitaliani R, Graus F, Honnorat J, Bertolini G (2010) Paraneoplastic neurologic syndrome in the PNS Euronetwork database: a European study from 20 centers. Arch Neurol 67: 330–335.

Graus F, Saiz A, Dalmau J (2010) Antibodies and neuronal autoimmune disorders of the CNS. J Neurol 257: 509–517.

Hahn A, Claviez A, Brinkmann G, Altermatt HJ, Schneppenheim R, Stephani U (2000) Paraneoplastic cerebellar degeneration in pediatric Hodgkin disease. Neuropediatrics 31: 42–44.

Hammack J, Kotanides H, Rosenblum MK, Posner JB (1992) Paraneoplastic cerebellar degeneration. II. Clinical and immunologic findings in 21 patients with Hodgkin's disease. Neurology 42: 1938–1943.

Topcu M, Gucuyener K, Topaloglu H, Renda Y, Akyuz C, Kale G (1992) Paraneoplastic syndrome manifesting as chronic cerebellar ataxia in a child with Hodgkin disease. J Pediatr 120: 275–277.

Vedeler CA, Antoine JC, Giometto B, Graus F, Grisold W, Hart IK, Honnorat J, Sillevis Smitt PA, Verschuuren JJ, Voltz R (2006) Management of paraneoplastic neurological syndromes: report of an EFNS Task Force. Eur J Neurol 13: 682–690.

Part 8
Acute Ataxia

Introductory comments

The four chapters in this section provide a detailed overview of the causes and management of acute ataxia. Individually they cover (1) the definition, epidemiology, differential diagnosis, and suggested clinical approach, (2) acute inflammatory disorders, (3) the opsoclonus-myoclonus syndrome, and (4) all other causes.

36
Acute Ataxia: Epidemiology and Differential Diagnosis

Peter Baxter

Acute ataxia in a child is a neurological emergency requiring immediate assessment and intervention. Although well recognized, there is no formal definition. Working definitions and early case series describe the new onset of clinical ataxia either suddenly, sometimes on waking, or rapidly over a period of a few hours or days (Table 36.1). Ryan and Engle (2003) propose an 'unsteadiness of walking, or of fine motor movement, of less than 72 hours duration, in a previously well child'. While most affected children are previously healthy, some can have pre-existing problems such as epilepsy, while others can have a prodromal event such as a febrile illness or immunization as described below. It might be preferable to define acute ataxia as acute unsteadiness developing over 72 hours or less in a previously unaffected child.

Epidemiology

There is no epidemiological data for acute ataxia as a whole. A Dutch population-based study of acute cerebellar ataxia found an annual incidence of 0.7 per 100 000 hospitalized children under 15 years (van der Maas et al. 2009). This is an underestimate as it excluded non-hospitalized childen and causes other than infection or inflammation. Davis and Marino (2003) estimated an incidence of 1 per 100 000–500 000 children a year. Connolly et al. (1994) reported that acute ataxia accounted for 0.4% of children seen for neurological problems over a 23-year period at one North American children's hospital, but this also excluded non-inflammatory causes. Martínez-González et al. (2006) reported acute ataxia in 0.024% of acute referrals to their hospital's paediatric emergency department.

The age and sex distribution vary with the cause, but it is most prevalent in young children. Data from published series (Table 36.1) show that inflammatory causes including acute demyelination are the most frequent, followed by intoxication and neuropathy. The differential is wide (Table 36.2) and not mutually exclusive: Connolly et al. (1994) describe a child with apparently typical varicella-associated ataxia who

TABLE 36.1
Reported series, excluding case reports

First author/year	Number of children	Period (years)	Inflammatory	Intoxication	Neuropathic	Other
Van der Maas 2009	45	2	36	excluded	excluded	
Martínez-González 2006	39	3	20	10	1	8: trauma (2), paroxysmal vertigo (2), ADEM, paravertebral tumour, intermittent, psychogenic.
Nussinovitch 2003	39	12	29	excluded		excluded metabolic causes
Gieron-Korthals 1994	40	10	14	13	5 (2 Miller Fisher)	8: cerebellar infarction, hyperventilation syndrome, myositis, conversion reaction, Reye syndrome, benign paroxysmal vertigo, meningitis, encephalitis
Connolly 1994	73	23	73	excluded	excluded	excluded
Weiss and Carter 1959	18	20	9			opsomyoclonus (2)
Blaw 1958	8	10	7			1 subacute
King 1958	9	13				all uncertain
Cottom 1957	7				1	
Berglund 1955	6	1	5		1	
Shanks 1950	22	20				
Klingman 1944	7	3	5?			1 opsomyoclonus due to neuroblastoma; 1 uncertain
Griffith 1921	31	–	24			1 post-traumatic (porsanal/published cases)

Blank spaces indicate that information is either unavailable or not reported.

TABLE 36.2
List of possible differential causes

1. Acute encephalopathies and cerebellopathies:
   - infectious
   - parainfectious
   - inflammatory
   - autoimmune/paraneoplastic
   - demyelination
   - intoxication
   - metabolic (see Chapter 27)
   - vascular (see Chapter 32)
   - trauma
   - raised intracranial pressure/acute hydrocephalus
2. Neuropathic (acute-onset sensory ataxia)
3. Space-occupying and structural lesions
4. Epilepsy (especially nonconvulsive status)
6. Acute vertigo
7. Psychogenic
8. Acute presentation of intermittent ataxias

TABLE 36.3
Important features in the history

Time course including any fluctuation

Precipitating events, e.g. infection, trauma

Associated neurological symptoms: alertness, behaviour change, headache, vomiting, visual symptoms, weakness, sensory symptoms; epileptic phenomena

Other associated symptoms, e.g. fever, rash

Recent immunization

Contacts with infection such as chickenpox; recent travel

Medication and recreational drugs including alcohol

Previous health including previous episodes and other neurological problems, e.g. epilepsy

Family history, especially of similar symptoms and drug therapies

Psychosocial history

later re-presented with ataxia due to a cerebellar astrocytoma. Acute ataxia can be the first presentation of an intermittent ataxia, but not usually of a chronic ataxia such as Friedreich ataxia. Individual causes are discussed in detail below or in other relevant sections of this book. In the older series these different pathologies were not always distinguished, so, for example, Klingman and Hodges (1944) include a classic case of neuroblastoma-associated opsomyoclonus-myoclonus, while Berglund et al. (1955) include a case strongly suggestive of acute inflammatory polyneuropathy with an ascending paralysis and raised protein in the cerebrospinal fluid (Table 36.1).

Differential diagnosis and clinical approach

The clinical approach is based on the differential diagnosis, outlined in Table 36.2. Inflammatory causes can be suggested by a history of recent febrile illness, exanthem, contacts (especially varicella zoster), or immunization. Prescribed and over-the-counter medication use as well as recreational drug use, including alcohol, both of the child and of close family members, may point to intoxication. A history suggestive of possible epilepsy is important, both as a possible cause and as an associated symptom in some conditions. Psychological factors may be relevant, especially in older children. While less common, symptoms of possible raised intracranial pressure and meningitis always need to be looked for. These and other suggested standard details of the history are listed in Table 36.3 and discussed in chapters 37 to 39.

Investigations

Many investigations could be considered relevant, but as always should be tailored to the clinical situation and kept as few and as non-invasive as possible. Appropriate tests are suggested in Table 36.4, but in general, for non-neuropathic ataxias and encephalopathies, neuroimaging is often the first step, although it will be normal in many cases. Some authorities state that in cases of typical cerebellar ataxia without additional features

TABLE 36.4
Possible investigations

Acute central ataxia without encephalopathy:
- Neuro-imaging: CT or MRI (preferably) of brain +/– spine
- Blood: serology (viral, mycoplasma)
- Viral cultures (throat swab, urine, stool)
- EEG

Acute central ataxia with encephalopathy:
- Neuro-imaging: CT or MRI (preferably) of brain +/– spine
- Blood: serology (viral, mycoplasma); culture; toxicology; heavy metals; metabolic (liver function tests, ammonia, amino acids, blood gas, lactate, pyruvate, glucose, biotinidase); antithyroid antibodies
- Urine: viral culture; toxicology; amino acids; organic acids
- CSF: pressure; cell count, glucose, protein; viral and bacterial studies (culture including TB, serology, PCR); oligoclonal bands, Ig index; lactate and pyruvate
- Throat swab, and faeces (or rectal swab): viral and bacterial culture
- Mantoux test
- EEG

Sensory ataxia:
- Nerve conduction studies and electromyography
- Cerebrospinal fluid protein
- Blood: anti-GM1 and anti-GQ1b antibodies
- Viral cultures (throat swab, urine, stool)
- Viral and mycoplasma serology
- Stool culture or rectal swab (esp. *C. jejuni*)

Opsoclonus-myoclonus (see Chapter 38):
- Neuro-imaging: CT or MRI (preferably) of brain +/– spine
- Neuroblastoma (see Chapter 38; consult oncologist):
- Chest X-ray
- Ultrasound scan of neck, abdomen and pelvis
- ^{123}I-meta-iodobenzylguanidine (MIBG) scintigraphy scan
- Urine catecholamine metabolites
- If negative: MR imaging neck, chest and abdomen

neuroimaging is unnecessary, but this decision should only be made by a practitioner with adequate experience. Subsequent investigations will be guided by the clinical and imaging findings, taking account of the prevalences in Table 36.1. As well as looking for evidence of infection or inflammation, at presentation it is often useful to save blood and urine samples for later toxicological or metabolic analyses.

REFERENCES

Berglund G, Mossberg H-O, Rydenstam B (1955) Acute cerebellar ataxia in children. Acta Paed Scand 44: 254–262.

Blaw ME, Sheehan JC (1958) Acute cerebellar syndrome of childhood. Neurology 8: 538–542.

Connolly AM, Dodson WE, Prensky AL, Rust RS (1994) Course and outcome of acute cerebellar ataxia. Ann Neurol 35: 673–679.

Cottom DG (1957) Acute cerebellar ataxia. Arch Dis Child 32: 181–188.

Davis DP, Marino A (2003) Acute cerebellar ataxia in a toddler: case report and literature review. J Emerg Med 24: 281–284.

Gieron-Korthals MA, Westberry KR, Emmanuel PJ (1994) Acute childhood ataxia: 10-year experience. J Child Neurol 1994; 9: 381–384.

Griffith JPC (1921) Acute cerebellar encephalitis (acute cerebellar ataxia). Am J Med Sci 1921; 162: 781–789.

King G, Schwarz GA, Slade HW (1958) Acute cerebellar ataxia of childhood; report of nine cases. Pediatrics 21: 731–745.

Klingman WO, Hodges RG (1944) Acute ataxia of unknown origin in children. J Pediatr 24: 536–543.

Martínez-González MJ, Martínez-González S, García-Ribes A, Mintegi-Raso S, Benito-Fernández J, Prats-Viñas JM (2006) Acute onset ataxia in infancy: its aetiology, treatment and follow-up. Rev Neurol 42: 321–324.

Nussinovitch M, Prais D, Volovitz B, Shapiro R, Amir J (2003) Post-infectious acute cerebellar ataxia in children. Clin Pediatr (Phila) 42: 581–584.

Ryan MM, Engle EC (2003) Acute ataxia in childhood. J Child Neurol 18: 309–316.

Shanks RA (1950) Notes on cerebellar ataxia in childhood. Arch Dis Child 25(124): 389–391.

van der Maas NAT, Vermeer-de Bondt PE, de Melker H, Kemmeren JM (2009) Acute cerebellar ataxia in the Netherlands: a study on the association with vaccinations and varicella zoster infection. Vaccine 27: 1970–1973.

Weiss S, Carter S (1959) Course and prognosis of acute cerebellar ataxia in children. Neurology (Minneap) 9: 711–721.

37
Acute Inflammatory Diseases of the Cerebellum

Marc Tardieu

Acute ataxia may be the consequence of an inflammatory reaction within the central nervous system (CNS). The inflammation that leads to ataxia may have various anatomical locations, including the cerebellum, the brainstem, parts of the basal ganglia or even the peripheral nerves. A clinical evaluation carefully looking for associated symptoms, brain magnetic resonance imaging (MRI) performed within days of onset for the most severely affected children or for those with associated symptoms, and a CSF study where there are no signs of raised intracranial pressure, may direct the diagnosis towards an inflammatory disease and help in the anatomical localization of the process. This initial analysis is of the utmost importance because early treatment, which may be urgent, varies according to the target of the inflammatory reaction. Moreover, the long-term outcomes and the risk of later relapses vastly differ between the different conditions and can now be evaluated on initial clinical and radiological findings.

In this chapter, after a short overview on neuro-immunological aspects, the most classic benign acute inflammatory cerebellar ataxia will be reviewed, followed by a discussion of more severe forms. Acute cerebellar ataxia is sometimes differentiated, in reviews and chapters, from acute cerebellitis, the latter being more severe (Gill 2010). In this chapter the two terms are considered as equivalent with benign and severe forms, acute cerebellar ataxia being a clinical description and acute cerebellitis referring to the pathophysiology. In the later section, the autoimmune diseases, which may start as an acute inflammatory cerebellar ataxia but are usually relapsing, will be reviewed, followed by a discussion of differential diagnosis.

Neuro-immunological aspects of acute inflammatory diseases of the cerebellum

Inflammatory diseases of the brain have in common the detection of lymphocytes and monocytes in the brain parenchyma (and therefore their crossing of the blood–brain barrier), the induction of an inflammatory reaction related to the innate immunity and, in some conditions, adaptive immune responses of antigen-specific T- and B-lymphocytes (Ballabh et al. 2004; Bechmann et al. 2006).

The innate immune response is not antigen-specific and it induces the secretion of soluble mediators of the inflammation including cytokines, free radicals and eicosanoids, after ligation of Toll-like receptors. Toll-like receptors (TLR) are a family of receptors that recognize conformational patterns of bacterial products or nucleic acids. TLR-recognizing bacteria (mostly lipopolysaccharides) are usually on the cell surface while TLR-recognizing nucleic acids are expressed in endosomes that have previously internalized viral products. These receptors are specialized and are different for single- or double-stranded nucleic acids and for DNA and RNA. They are also not expressed identically on all types of cells. The innate immunity induced by a virus will then depend on the virus, on the cells being able to recognize its nucleic acids, as well as on the specificity of the TLR–nucleic acid interaction that may change over time. TLRs are highly expressed on microglia, as expected for these mesoderm-derived macrophages, but also on neuroectoderm-derived astrocytes and even neurons. After TLR ligation, cellular activation occurs that is also under the control of paracrine cytokines secreted by blood-derived leukocytes (Levy 2007).

Acute ataxia is thought to be an inflammatory disease because it is frequently associated with a recent viral illness. The CSF is frequently abnormal with a meningitic pattern and there are frequent abnormalities of MRI signal suggesting acute inflammation in one or different parts of the cerebellar pathways. Very few neuropathological studies are available, however, and they are restricted to patients who died after very severe inflammation and posterior fossa oedema (Roulet Perez et al. 1993). Their pathophysiology might not be representative of that in more benign disorders. Acute cerebellar ataxia and the associated cerebellitis probably depend in most cases on an innate immunity reaction with perivascular leukocyte infiltration. The initial trigger is unknown but is most probably the consequence, within the cerebellum or brainstem, of TLR-viral nucleic acid ligation. Although likely to be the most frequent mechanism in acute inflammatory cerebellitis, the induction of the TLR pathways is probably not the only one. The first alternative mechanism is a direct viral replication within resident cells of the cerebellum with a subsequent cytopathogenic effect. This has been demonstrated in experimental infections in mice and may occur in children especially after varicella zoster infection. The second alternative mechanism is an antigen-specific immune response that by definition will occur several days after the initial antigen stimulation. The causal antigen could be a viral protein or even a myelin product and the presence of anti-MOG (myelin oligodendrocyte glycoprotein) antibody has been demonstrated in acute inflammatory demyelination. This first demyelinating event might, finally, turn out to be the initial episode of one of a variety of relapsing autoimmune diseases or of a genetically linked immune deficiency.

Acute benign cerebellitis with acute cerebellar ataxia

Acute cerebella ataxia is characterized by a sudden onset of ataxia following, or in association with, a viral illness. It is a familiar entity to every paediatrician and was described over 140 years ago. Its frequency and its usually benign outcome precluded the constitution of large prospective population-based cohorts. Most of the reported series are hospital-based and probably skewed toward more severe cases. Acute cerebellar ataxia can be observed in children of all ages although, in a combined series of 112 cases, half the cases occurred before 4 years of age (Connolly et al. 1994). The onset of ataxia is usually acute, with a marked gait ataxia and dysmetria. The child adopts a wide-based stance or may avoid standing altogether. Even in the sitting position a young child may look very uncomfortable and unsteady. On attempting to walk, if successful, he sways and staggers. Hypotonia, tremor of the extremities, head and trunk, are usually obvious and in older children, speech is often affected. The speech is slow, without the usual intonations, and syllables are uttered in an explosive manner.

At the onset of the disease, clinical evaluation should carefully explore associated symptoms relating to three areas. The first is related to eye movement: nystagmus is frequently observed (although no precise frequency can be established due to large variations between series) whereas sudden random movements of eyes either spontaneously or during voluntary movement are less frequent (but raise other possible diagnoses). The second are findings which suggest either meningitis or raised intracranial pressure (headache, depressed level of consciousness, vomiting) while neck stiffness is unusual. Any symptom suggesting raised intracranial pressure should prompt further steps detailed below. Finally, myoclonic movement of the arms and any brainstem-related symptoms may be present and tend to be associated with a more severe phenotype.

A history of either fever or a viral infection, in the 2 weeks preceding onset of neurological symptoms, is common. The causative viral infection is sometimes obvious due to a recent or ongoing exanthematous disease (mostly varicella) but is frequently nonspecific. The respective frequency of different viral infections varies according to country and vaccination recommendations. The clinical experience and a few systematic studies suggest that varicella, mumps and Epstein-Barr virus infections are more frequently associated with acute benign cerebellitis than other common viral infections (Connolly et al. 1994; Amlie-Lefond and Jubelt 2009).

The CSF is abnormal in about half of such patients with a mild pleocytosis, mostly lymphocytic, and a moderately elevated protein content. In most benign cases of acute ataxia, the brain MRI is normal.

The disease is self-limiting in benign acute inflammatory ataxia, by definition. Prognostic factors of benign evolution have not been formally evaluated but are generally believed to include mild initial symptomatology, the absence of symptoms or signs of raised intracranial pressure, the absence of abnormal eye movements or brainstem symptoms as well as a normal MRI. The prognostic value of age at onset is unclear. The ataxia resolves completely with an average duration of cerebellar signs of 2 months although mildly affected children can recover completely within a week. Benign cases do not require any treatment, but in more affected or very uncomfortable children, a good symptomatic response has been seen with the use of a short course of steroids (usually 1mg/kg for 7 days, although no formal study has been conducted).

Severe and unusual forms of cerebellitis with acute cerebellar ataxia

Acute cerebellar ataxia with raised intracranial pressure

Acute cerebellitis can induce very severe symptoms usually related to an intense inflammatory reaction with leukocyte infiltration of brain parenchyma and the opening of the blood–brain barrier to soluble factors and water. This leads to posterior fossa or brainstem swelling and should be regarded as a medical and sometimes neurosurgical emergency (Roulet Perez et al. 1993; Kamate et al. 2009).

In contrast to benign forms which consist in relatively pure cerebellar symptoms, severe forms have more global neurological features and an altered mental state in addition to the acute cerebellar symptoms. The altered mental state is one of the most difficult symptoms to evaluate in a young child usually very resistant to clinical evaluation. It could be the consequence of the cerebellar swelling but it may also be part of a polysymptomatic inflammatory disease of the CNS, most frequently acute disseminated enceph-alomyelitis (ADEM), as discussed later. Other associated neurological symptoms usually suggest raised posterior fossa pressure. These include nausea, repetitive yawns, vomiting as well as sixth cranial nerve palsies (due to compression at the brainstem), reduced consciousness level and frequently papilloedema. Symptoms that are more directly related to brainstem involvement are altered respiratory pattern, blood pressure changes or other cranial nerve palsy. These may reflect a life-threatening situation, associated with herniation either upward through the tentorium or downwards through the foramen magnum (Shkalim et al. 2009).

If the situation is not immediately life-threatening, MRI should be performed and may be illuminating. The MRI sequences to be performed are T1, T2, FLAIR and diffusion-weighted sequences in axial, coronal and sagittal planes and should also evaluate the spinal cord. Various aspects of early brain imaging in acute and severe cerebellar ataxia have been described (Horowitz et al. 1991; Shoji et al. 1991; Iester et al. 1995; Sawaishi et al. 1999; Soussan et al. 2003; De Bruecker et al. 2004; Matsukuma et al. 2008). The first is a global swelling of the cerebellum and brainstem with a compressed fourth ventricles and occasionally signs of herniation either upward transtentorially or of the cerebellar tonsils into the foramen magnum. In less acute cases, two other abnormalities are observed, which are usually mutually exclusive: an increased

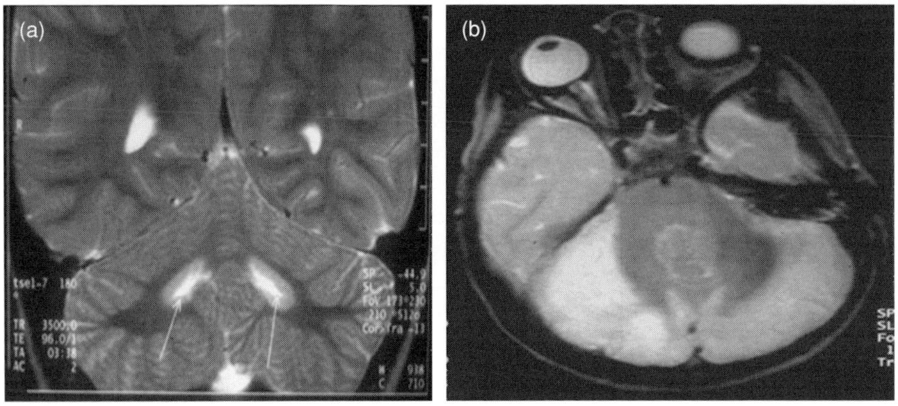

Fig. 37.1. MRI brain imaging in two cases of severe acute cerebellitis. **(a)** An increased signal on a T2-weighted sequence is observed around the dentate nuclei (arrows) and in the cerebellar white matter while cerebellar cortex appears normal. **(b)** On a similar MRI sequence the cerebellar cortex has an increased signal with swelling of the whole cerebellum.

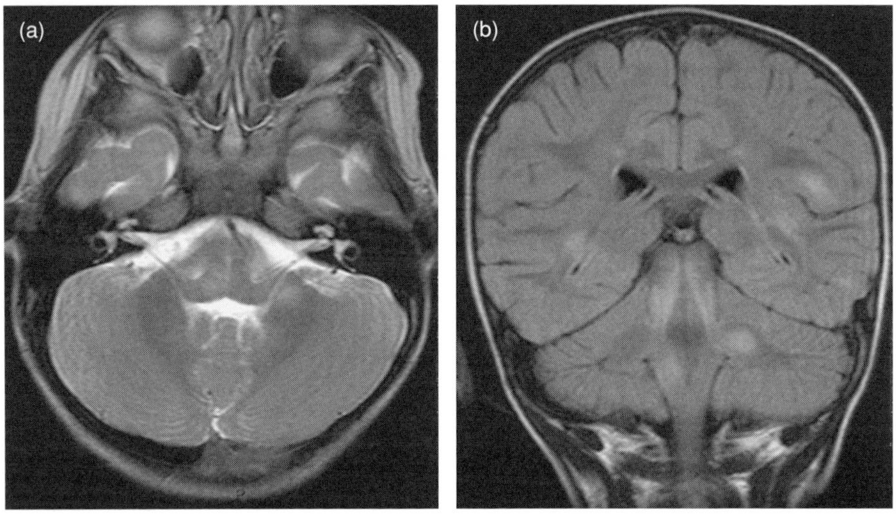

Fig. 37.2. Acute disseminated encephalomyelitis (ADEM) in a 5-year-old child: brainstem, cerebellum and supratentorial multiple white matter lesions are observed on **(a)** T2 and **(b)** FLAIR sequences. The lesions are in poorly demarcated areas.

signal on T2 and FLAIR at the level of the cerebellar cortex that can be either uni- or bilateral, or increased signal around the dentate nucleus and of the cerebellar white matter (Fig. 37.1). Finally, MRI may demonstrate supratentorial lesions in association with infratentorial lesions and, therefore, suggest a multifocal inflammatory process (Fig. 37.2).

Acute swelling of the cerebellum is an emergency which requires medical and sometimes neurosurgical measures and usually intensive care. High-dose pulses of methylprednisolone, as administered in ADEM, are probably the best medical treatment (methylprednisolone, 30mg/kg/day for 3 days with a maximum of 1g/day injected intravenously over 2 hours with careful monitoring of the blood pressure and of the level of consciousness). This may help to reduce the swelling and obviate the need for surgical intervention. However, surgical decompression of the posterior fossa may be life-saving when there are signs of brainstem compression or tonsillar herniation.

The outcome is highly variable. Several cases of rapid deterioration and death have been reported. Thereafter, while complete recovery is observed in the majority, with disappearance of MRI lesions on subsequent imaging, severe cerebellar destruction and atrophy have also been described (Hayakawa and Katoh 1995; Tabarki et al. 1998). If this occurs, the clinical consequences are a combination of predominantly cerebellar motor dysfunction with predominantly cerebellar disorders and an accompanying cognitive deficit.

Persistent cerebellar ataxia and relapsing cerebellar ataxia

Persistent cerebellar ataxia incorporates ataxia of both trunk and limbs, dysarthria and a variety of behavioural problems which persist over time. No strict definition has been proposed but if a cut-off for persistent symptoms is set at 2 months from onset, a third of affected children would be included. Symptoms can be relieved by steroids (usually prednisone 1mg/kg for 10 days and in more severe cases by intravenous high dose of methylprednisolone). However, if cerebellar ataxia persists, the diagnosis should be carefully re-evaluated: from clinical experience, cases of ospsoclonus-myoclonus syndrome and of other inflammatory and non-inflammatory conditions may initially be misdiagnosed as persistent acute cerebellar ataxia. Persistence of marked cerebellar ataxia is associated with mental retardation (UK: learning disability) and behavioural abnormalities that are more frequent if cerebellar atrophy or patchy necrosis are observed on MRI performed 3 months after onset (although no optimal date to evaluate prognosis has been defined).

Relapsing acute cerebellar ataxia is unusual and should be differentiated both from the transient exacerbation of a known pre-existing ataxia during an intercurrent febrile episode and also from acute disseminated relapsing inflammatory diseases of the CNS such as vasculitis or multiple sclerosis. It is best characterized by purely acute cerebellar episodes with signs of inflammation either in the CSF or on cerebellar MRI. No minimum interval between episodes has been defined but 3 months may be accepted by analogy with ADEM. A re-evaluation of the diagnosis is also mandatory, especially if the CSF remains persistently normal. Possible explanations include mitochondrial diseases and episodic ataxia due to ion-channel proteins mutations, as discussed in the final section of this chapter.

Acute inflammatory ataxia as initial presentation in acute disseminated encephalomyelitis or chronic autoimmune, autoinflammatory or infectious disease

Acute inflammatory cerebellar ataxia can be a symptom of a more diffuse inflammatory disease of the nervous system or even of an autoimmune disease that will relapse in the future. The clinical picture is that of a child with acute ataxia, abnormal CSF, with meningitic picture and an elevated protein content, and an abnormal MRI. A very rigorous evaluation is required because of the broad spectrum of possible diagnoses, some of them requiring urgent treatment. The clinical clues are: the patient's age, level of fever, associated clinical symptoms, MRI pattern and, as main biological data, level of the CSF protein and of inflammatory markers in blood. The main possible clinical entities are discussed below.

Tuberculous meningitis

This diagnosis should be considered first although it is now very unusual in Western countries. A combination of acute cerebellar and brainstem symptoms in a persistently febrile child with some degree of mental status alteration, irritability, headache and nuchal rigidity is a frequent presentation. The two main symptoms leading to diagnosis are a very elevated CSF protein content (frequently over 1g/l) and MRI evidence of arachnoiditis (basilar enhancement and meningeal inflammation) and abnormal signal in the parenchyma due to infarcts or enhancing lesions (tuberculoma: ring-enhancing lesions with low intensity on T2-weighted images and intermediate intensity on T1-weighted images). This requires prompt treatment with usually four antituberculous agents.

Acute disseminated encephalomyelitis, clinically isolated syndrome, multiple sclerosis and vasculitis

Acute disseminated encephalomyelitis cannot be confused, by definition, with acute inflammatory ataxia because it must be multifocal, polysymptomatic and associated with some degree of altered mental state, as well as white matter abnormalities on MRI (although this is not part of the definition). The typical white matter lesions are in large poorly demarcated areas both supra- and infratentorially and, in 50% of cases, associated with basal ganglia involvement and in 10% with cortical lesions. However, acute ataxia can be the major initial symptom of more anatomically localized acute inflammatory lesions ('clinically isolated syndrome') leading to the diagnosis of brainstem encephalitis or acute inflammatory lesions of the basal ganglia. Frequently in these children, acute ataxia is not the only neurological symptom, with others occurring either initially or within a few days of onset. The most frequent associated symptoms are cranial nerves palsies, raised intracranial pressure or, in the case of basal ganglia involvement, drooling and buccofacial paresis or severe dyspraxia. MRI usually demonstrates increased signal on T2-weighted sequences in the brainstem or the basal ganglia, frequently associated with localized white matter lesions (Fig. 37.2). These conditions are related to ADEM and will benefit from intravenous methylprednisolone at the same doses as described above. In about 15–20% of cases, a relapse will occur that will raise the diagnosis of multiple sclerosis. Several clinical and radiological factors, observed at onset, are predictive of further relapses and multiple sclerosis: an associated symptom, especially optic neuritis, a high protein content in the CSF with oligoclonal bands on electrophoresis, multiple well-limited lesions of the white matter on T2-weighted and FLAIR sequences of MRI, some of the lesions being perpendicular to the corpus callosum ('Dawson fingers') (Mikaeloff et al. 2004, 2007). Finally, in young adolescents, acute ataxia is among the frequent initial symptoms of multiple sclerosis, while sensory symptoms are less frequent than later, in older individuals. If both the clinical and radiological aspects are very typical of multiple sclerosis with a high risk of further relapses, an immunomodulary treatment with beta-interferon or cop-1 is to be considered after the first event, although a second clinical event is frequently trigger for such treatment.

Vasculitis is a large group of diseases either primary (isolated angiitis of the CNS) or secondary (to systemic conditions), that differ according to the size of the targeted vessel (large, medium or small vessels involvement). Most have a polysymptomatic expression including headache, mental status change and psychiatric conditions, as well as seizures. The most frequent vasculitis is systemic lupus erythematosus, but ataxia is a very unusual sign during its evolution (Bader-Meunier et al. 2005; Appenzeller et al. 2008). Conversely, Behcet disease deserves a special emphasis. One of its two main presentations is the occurrence of small infarcts that are frequently localized in the brainstem and can be expressed as acute ataxia (the second presentation being deep cerebral venous thrombosis and raised intracranial pressure) (Kone-Paut et al. 1998; Atkinson et al. 2008). In the case of arterial vasculitis, MRI demonstrates the typical small ischemic lesions (Fig. 37.3) and the CSF is characterized by inflammatory changes and a high protein content. The diagnosis is further suggested by the Mediterranean origin, the higher frequency of HLA B51 and sometimes the typical aphthous and cutaneous lesions. A course of immunosuppressive treatment is often required, mostly using azathioprine and colchicine.

Haemophagocytic lymphohistiocytosis

Several diseases, the most frequent being familial haemophagocytic lymphohistiocytosis, have in common the occurrence during the course of the disease of acute phases, known as 'haemophagocytic syndrome', 'haemophagocytic lymphohistiocytosis' (HLH) or 'macrophage activation syndrome' (MAS)

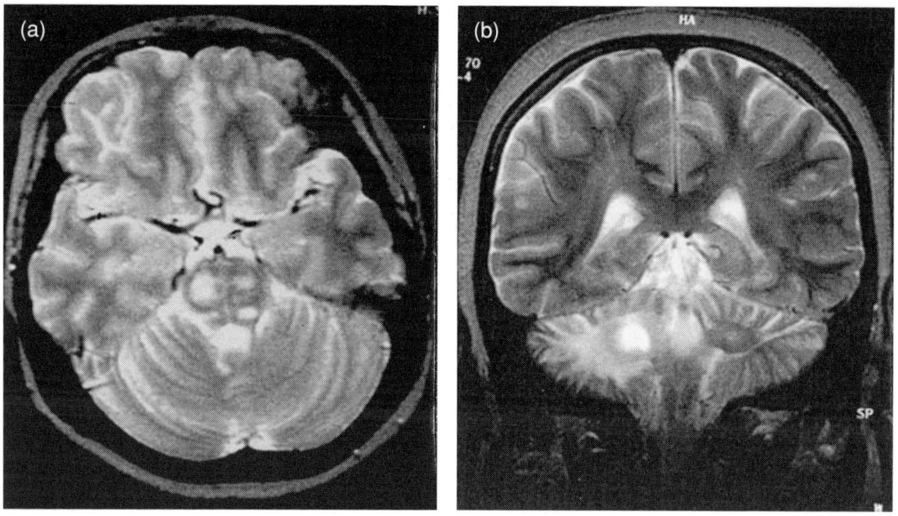

Fig. 37.3. **(a, b)** Isolated vasculitis with brainstem and cerebellar white matter hyperintensity in T2-weighted sequence.

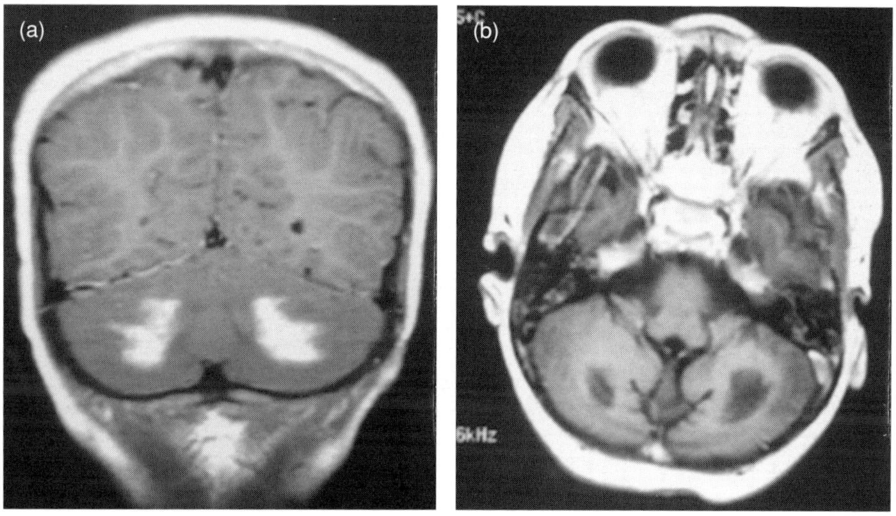

Fig. 37.4. Haemophagocytic lymphohistiocytosis a 5-year-old child with acute onset of lymphohistiocytosis and acute necrotic area in cerebellar white matter on **(a)** FLAIR and **(b)** T1-weighted sequences MRI.

(Haddad et al. 1997; Tardieu and Mahlaoui 2010). MAS is typically a multisystem illness with symptoms of meningitis and encephalitis associated with hepatomegaly, splenomegaly, adenopathy, high fever and signs of intravascular coagulation, but neurological symptoms may be the first and only symptoms of the disease. It occurs most often within the first 18 months of life. However, in older children its initial clinical expression can be acute ataxia (Astigarraga et al. 2004). The MRI will typically demonstrate necrotic lesions of the cerebellar white matter associated with areas of supratentorial white matter high signal (Fig. 37.4).

Miller Fisher syndrome and Guillain-Barré syndrome

An acute inflammatory disease of peripheral nerves (acute poyradiculoneuritis or Guillain-Barré syndrome) can lead to a reduction of muscle power, a sensory loss and a hesitant pattern of movement which can be misdiagnosed as ataxic. The absence of reflexes, the isolated hyperproteinorachia and the electrophysiological studies will lead to the right diagnosis and the appropriate treatment. Miller Fisher syndrome may be more difficult to recognize, although it is infrequent in children. It consists of a combination of acute ataxia, external ophthalmoplegia and areflexia without peripheral weakness. Ophthalmoplegia and sometimes bilateral facial palsy are usually the first symptom and an isolated ataxia is very unusual at onset.

Other diseases mimicking acute inflammatory cerebellar ataxia

Several conditions can mimic acute inflammatory cerebellar ataxia but most of them are usually associated with other symptoms or have a chronic progressive evolution. The range of possibilities is very broad, ranging from cerebellar tumours to genetic cerebellar or spinocerebellar degenerative diseases. A long list of different diseases would not be of practical help. From personal clinical experience, the differential diagnosis at onset of acute cerebellar ataxia in a previously healthy child should focus on five possibilities, listed below.

1. Intoxications: They are usually an easy diagnosis and should be systematically evaluated by appropriate investigation, mostly specific dosages in urine or blood. The spectrum

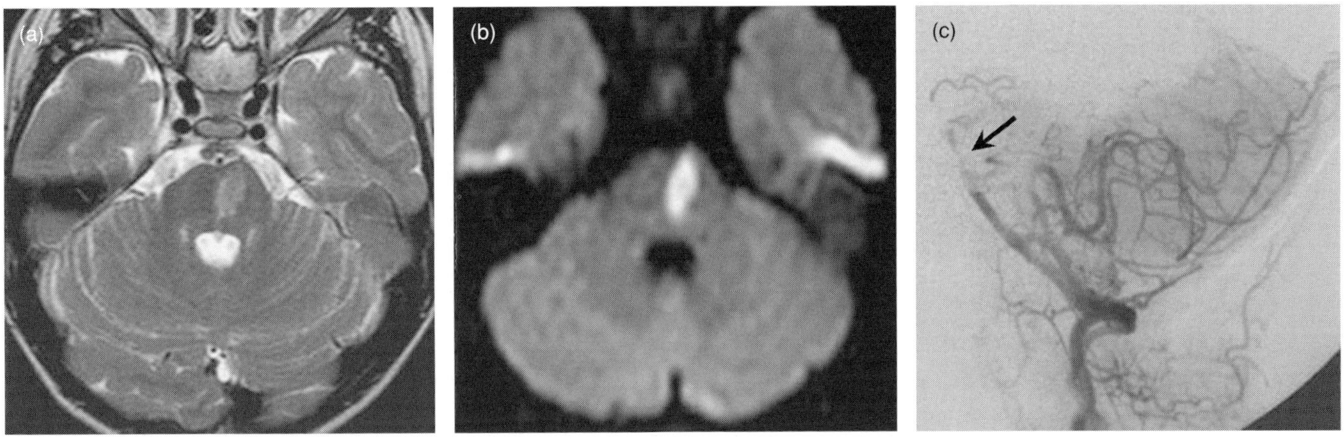

Fig. 37.5. Acute ischaemic lesion in the brainstem: on **(a)** FLAIR and **(b)** diffusion-weighted sequences a lesion is demonstrated in the brainstem with a sharp demarcation at the midline. **(c)** Arteriography demonstrates occlusion of the basilar artery (arrow). (Courtesy of Dr B. Husson.)

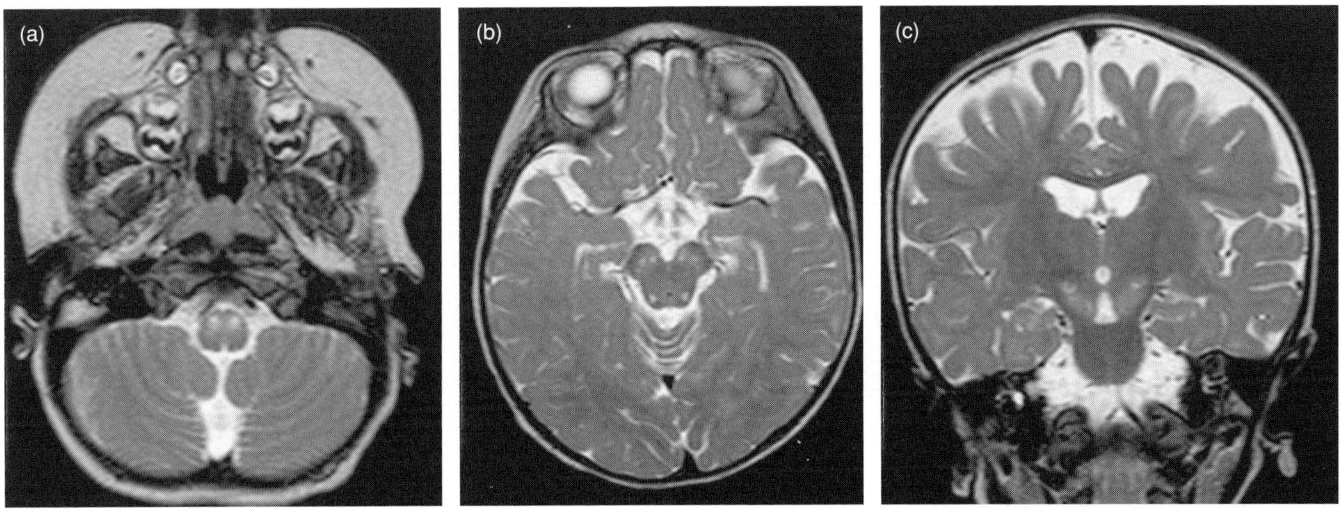

Fig. 37.6. Mitochondrial disease in a child aged 2 years 6 months with acute brainstem and cerebellar symptoms. **(a, b, c)** MRI T2-weighted sequences reveal high signal intensity in the brainstem and the subthalamic area. A quantitative defect in mitochondrial respiratory chain complex I and IV was observed but known mtDNA mutation could not be demonstrated.

of responsible agents varies between countries and cultures. The most frequent ones in Western countries are alcohol, benzodiazepines, and neuroleptic and antiepileptic drugs.

2. Ischaemic strokes: An ataxia of very sudden onset (or observed at awakening) can be the only or the main symptom of an ischaemic stroke. It is usually associated with some degree of hemiparesis, somnolence or cranial nerve palsy. The MRI will provide the main clue, showing on FLAIR and diffusion-weighted sequences a small lesion either in the brainstem (and sometimes lateralized with a sharp demarcation at the midline), the cerebellum or the basal ganglia (Fig. 37.5). A frequent aetiology is an arterial wall dissection frequently at the level of one of the vertebral arteries or and less frequently of the basilar artery producing a thrombus and small downstream embolus.
3. Channelopathy and other inherited familial episodic ataxia: These are very rare conditions. The diagnosis depends on the family history because the disease is transmitted as an autosomal dominant trait. There are several types caused by a missense mutation in the potassium channel gene *KCNA1* or by missense or nonsense mutation in the calcium channel gene *CACNA1A*. In absence of a family history, the diagnosis is more difficult and will be suggested by repetitive bouts of acute ataxia; ion measurements during symptomatic episodes may give a lead to the relevant genetic test (see Chapter 28).
4. Leigh disease and other mitochondrial disorders: Repetitive episodes of ataxia with either brainstem, basal ganglia or cerebellar lesions on MRI should raise the possibility of mitochondrial disorders especially Leigh disease in a young child (Fig. 37.6). Clues to the diagnosis, apart from the MRI features, are the lactate level in CSF (usually higher than 2mmol/L) and the lactate/pyruvate ratio in serum (>20). This syndrome may be the consequence of a variety of causal genetic mutations in both mtDNA or nuclear DNA (see Chapter 27).

5. Opsoclonus-myoclonus syndrome: This syndrome is described in Chapter 38. A misdiagnosis of acute inflammatory cerebellar ataxia is frequent at onset, especially if the pathological eye movements are missed. The diagnosis should be carefully considered if the ataxia is persistent

Two further conditions should also be evaluated.

6. Cerebellar tumours: An acute onset with ataxia is unusual but possible. Neck stiffness, vomiting and associated neurological signs will prompt an MRI.
7. Acute labyrinthitis: This is in fact unusual but nausea and vertigo are clues to diagnosis. Benign paroxysmal vertigo in toddlers is characterized by a sudden, unsteady gait in a child who holds on to a parent for stability. The very short duration and sometimes migraine in one or both parents will suggest the diagnosis.

Conclusion

Acute cerebellar ataxia is a relatively frequent symptom that raises a variety of possible diagnosis with a spectrum of different treatment implications. A very careful clinical evaluation associated with early brain imaging is pivotal in distinguishing the frequent and benign cerebellitis from other inflammatory or non-inflammatory conditions.

REFERENCES

Amlie-Lefond C, Jubelt B (2009) Neurologic manifestations of varicella zoster virus infections. Curr Neurol Neurosci Rep 9:430–434.

Astigarraga I, Prats JM, Navajas A, Fernandez-Teijeiros A, Urberuaga A (2004) Near fatal cerebellar swelling in familial hemophagocytic lymphohistiocytosis. Pediatr Neurol 30:361–364.

Appenzeller S, Cendes F, Costallat LT (2008) Cerebellar ataxia in systemic lupus erythematosus. Lupus 17:1122–1126.

Atkinson M, Moore E, Altinok D, Acsadi G (2008) Cerebral infarct in pediatric neuro-Behcet's disease. J Child Neurol 23:1331–1335.

Bader-Meunier B, Armengaud J-B, Haddad E, Salomon R, Deschênes G, Kone-Paut I, et al. (2005) Initial presentation of childhood-onset systemic lupus erythematosus: a French multicenter study. J Pediatr 146:648–653.

Ballabh P, Braun A, Nedergaard M (2004) The blood-brain barrier: an overview: structure, regulation and clinical implications. Neurobiol Dis 16:1–13.

Bechmann I, Galea I, Perry VH (2006) What is the blood-brain-barrier (not)? Trends in Immunology 28:5–11.

Connolly AM, Dodson WE, Prensky AL, Rust RS (1994) Course and outcome of acute cerebellar ataxia Ann Neurol 35:673–679.

De Bruecker Y, Claus F, Demaerel P, Ballaux F, Sciot R, Lagae L, et al. (2004) MRI findings in acute cerebellitis Eur Radiol 14:1478–1483.

Gill D (2010) Postinfectious ataxia and cerebellitis. In: Inflammatory and Autoimmune Disorders of the Nervous System in Children (Dale RC, Vincent A, eds). London: Mac Keith Press; 190–206.

Haddad E, Salis ML, Jabado N, Blanche S, Fischer A, Tardieu M (1997) Frequency and severity of central nervous system lesions in familial hemophagocytic lymphohistiocytosis. Blood 89:794–800.

Hayakawa H, Katoh T (1995) Severe cerebellar atrophy following acute cerebellitis. Pediatr Neurol 12:159–161.

Horowitz MB, Pang D, Hirsch W (1991) Acute cerebellitis: case report and review. Pediatr Neurosurg 17:142–145.

Iester A, Alpigiani MG, Franzone G, Cohen A, Puleo MG, Tortori-Donati P (1995) Magnetic resonance imaging in right hemisphere cerebellitis associated with homolateral hemiparesis. Child's Nerv Syst 11:118–120.

Kamate M, Chetal V, Hattiholi V (2009) Fulminant cerebellitis: a fatal clinically isolated syndrome. Pediatr Neurol 41:220–222.

Kone-Paut I, Yurdakul S, Bahabri SA, Shafae N, Ozen S, Ozdogan H, Bernard JL (1998) Clinical features of Behcet's disease in children: an international collaborative study of 86 cases. J Pediatr 132:721–725.

Levy O (2007) Innate immunity of the newborn: basic mechanisms and clinical correlates. Nature Rev Immunol 7:379–390.

Matsukuma E, Kato Z, Orii K, Asano T, Orii K, Matsui E, et al. (2008) Acute mumps cerebellitis with abnormal findings in MRI diffusion-weighted images. Eur J Pediatr 16:829–830.

Mikaeloff Y, Adamsbaum C, Husson B, Vallée L, Ponsot G, Confavreux C, et al. (2004) MRI prognostic factors for relapse after acute CNS inflammatory demyelination in childhood. Brain 127:1942–1947.

Mikaeloff Y, Caridade G, Husson B, Suissa S, Tardieu M (2007) Acute disseminated encephalomyelitis cohort study in children: prognostic factors for relapse. Eur J Pediatr Neurol 11:90–95.

Roulet Perez E, Maeder P, Cotting J, Eskenazy-Cottier AC, Deonna T (1993) Acute fatal cerebellar swelling in two children. A rare or an overlooked situation? Neuropediatrics 24:346–351.

Sawaishi Y, Takahashi I, Hirayama Y, Abe T, Mitzutani M, Hirai K, Takada G (1999) Acute cerebellitis caused by Coxiella burnetii. Ann Neurol 45:124–127.

Shkalim V, Amir J, Kornreich L, Scheuerman O, Straussberg R (2009) Acute cerebellitis presenting as tonsillar herniation and hydrocephalus. Pediatr Neurol 41:200–203.

Shoji H, Hirai S, Ishikawa K, Aramaki M, Sato Y, Abe T, Kojima K (1991) CT and MRI imaging of acute cerebellar ataxia. Neuroradiology 33:360–361.

Soussan V, Husson B, Tardieu M (2003) Description and prognostic value of cerebellar MRI lesions in children with severe acute ataxia [in French] Arch Pediatr 10:604–607.

Tabarki B, Husson B, Landrieu P (1998) Acute cerebellar atrophy in encephalitis. J Child Neurol 13:192–195.

Tardieu M, Mahlaoui N (2010) Macrophage activation syndromes. In: Inflammatory and Autoimmune Disorders of the Nervous System in Children (Dale RC, Vincent A, eds). London: Mac Keith Press; 266–274.

38
Opsoclonus-Myoclonus Syndrome

Michael Pike

Opsoclonus-myoclonus syndrome (OMS), also known as dancing eye syndrome, opsoclonus-myoclonus ataxia and Kinsbourne syndrome, was first described by Kinsbourne (Kinsbourne 1962). It is extremely rare, with an incidence in the United Kingdom of 1 per 5 million total population per year, an equal sex ratio and a mean age at onset of 18 months (Pang et al. 2010a). Adult OMS is probably a different entity with overlap – typically associated with small cell lung cancer or breast cancer (the latter often associated with anti-Ri antibodies), though sometimes idiopathic in younger adults (Bataller et al. 2001). Paediatric OMS is associated in many cases (probably about 50%) with neuroblastoma, for which a systematic investigation protocol is required at presentation. The oncological outcome in children with neuroblastoma and OMS is good. Outcome for OMS, with or without neuroblastoma, is diverse but a high proportion will suffer significant long-term cognitive, behavioural and motor sequelae. Treatment for OMS is primarily with steroids and other immunomodulatory therapies but, because of its rarity and the consequent difficulties in conducting therapeutic trials, there is not currently compelling evidence that a particular intervention alters long-term outcome.

Clinical presentation and natural history

Typical presentation

Opsoclonus-myoclonus syndrome presents subacutely, usually over a matter of days. The typical scenario is a toddler of between 12 months and 3 years with a jerky unsteadiness, marked irritability, sleep disturbance and intermittent opsoclonus, in whom a neuroblastoma (usually abdominal or thoracic) may be identified. Opsoclonus consists of rapid, conjugate, multidirectional, back-to-back saccadic eye movements without an intersaccadic interval; ocular flutter, which may rarely be present in OMS, also consists of rapid, conjugate, back-to-back saccadic eye movements but in a single plane. For those unfamiliar with opsoclonus, an example can be viewed on the internet (www.dancingeyes.org.uk).

Diagnostic criteria

The prime features are a movement disorder involving to varying degrees both myoclonus and ataxia, along with opsoclonus and irritability with sleep disturbance. In a proportion of children, probably about 50%, there is an accompanying neuroblastoma. Atypical and incomplete variants have been described (Pang et al. 2010a) and diagnostic criteria have been proposed which require three out of the following four features: (1) opsoclonus or ocular flutter; (2) neuroblastoma; (3) myoclonus and/or ataxia; (4) behavioural disturbance and/or sleep disturbance (often with marked irritability); and the absence of evidence of active CNS infection (Matthay et al. 2005), to which should be added the absence of demyelination on brain MRI, as brainstem demyelination may produce overlapping clinical features (Tsutada et al. 1996).

Delayed diagnosis

Diagnosis is often delayed for a number of reasons. Because of its rarity, a United Kingdom paediatric neurologist who serves a population of, on average, 700 000 will care for a case of OMS perhaps six or seven times in a professional lifetime – clinical familiarity is therefore limited. Second, the opsoclonus is usually intermittent and fleeting, may require close clinical observation over a period of time before it is identified and may be misdiagnosed as another eye movement disorder such as nystagmus or as an epileptic seizure (Haden et al. 2009). Occasionally, opsoclonus may only follow other features of the condition by a period of weeks or months (Pang et al. 2010a) (although this may in fact reflect a delay in recognition of an intermittent and fleeting phenomenon rather than a true delay in onset). Two techniques which may elicit opsoclonus if it is suspected but not readily seen are (1) fixation from far to near and vice versa and (2) eyelid elevation against resistance (Mitchell WG, personal communication). Third, the investigation protocol for identifying an underlying neuroblastoma, assuming that it is initiated, is variable and may be inadequate (Pang et al. 2010a). Fourth, the importance of the behavioural change and sleep disturbance is often underestimated; this is a striking distinguishing feature from the most frequent misdiagnosis which is of the much more common condition, acute cerebellar ataxia. Finally, a small number of children present with atypical OMS accompanied, for example, by dysphagia (Pang et al. 2010a) or early spontaneous improvement (Pang et al. 2010b).

Natural history and outcome

OMS may be monophasic or chronic relapsing. Differences in the underlying pathophysiology of the two patterns of disease remain unclear and do not seem to be influenced by the presence or absence of neuroblastoma. A very occasional child may recover spontaneously, with improvement becoming apparent within a week of onset (Pang et al. 2010b), but the vast majority require treatment. Data on outcome are derived from reports usually of small numbers, often retrospective, referral centre-based (including variously neurological and oncological centres) and probably therefore subject to referral bias. However, outcome does not appear to be affected by the presence or absence of an accompanying neuroblastoma (Catsman-Berrevoets et al. 2009; Krug et al. 2010). In outcome reviews to date a substantial majority (60–100%) are identified as experiencing significant neurological, behavioural and/or cognitive sequelae (Boltshauser et al. 1979; Koh et al. 1994; Hammer et al. 1995; Papero et al. 1995; Pohl et al. 1996; Russo et al. 1997; Plantaz et al. 2000; Hayward et al. 2001; Rudnick et al. 2001; Mitchell et al. 2002; Tate et al. 2005; Klein et al. 2007; De Grandis et al. 2009; Krug et al. 2010). The degree of disability is often not fixed and may fluctuate, perhaps influenced by intercurrent infection. Some authors have identified an association between poor neurological outcome and delayed treatment, young age at onset, severity at onset and relapsing (as opposed to monophasic) course; others have failed to confirm these observations. It may be that some children, perhaps particularly those with chronic relapsing symptoms, experience cumulative neurological damage and therefore a progressive encephalopathy (Mitchell et al. 2002). It seems clear that any evaluation of outcome requires an assessment of both the early symptomatic response and a detailed examination of late motor, cognitive and behavioural function, as the two may not be correlated. Long-term difficulties identified in children with OMS include ataxia, incoordination, attentional, language and visuomotor difficulties, as well as a variety of neuropsychiatric disorders. The language impairment is more expressive than receptive; speech intelligibility as well as output may be reduced; neuropsychiatric disorders include oppositional behaviour, rage attacks, impulsivity, irritability and, sometimes, obsessional-compulsive traits (Mitchell et al. 2002; Turkel et al. 2006).

Genetics and autoimmunity

There are no reports of familial OMS. Hero et al. (2005) identified an association with HLA-DRB1 and an increased prevalence of autoimmune disorders in families of children with OMS has been described (Krasenbrink et al. 2007).

Neuroimaging

Brain imaging, whether CT or MRI, is almost always normal in the acute phase of OMS. Indeed, the presence of an acute imaging abnormality should prompt a re-evaluation of the diagnosis, raising the possibility that this is an active CNS infection or a demyelinating episode. Having said this, the neuroradiological findings in patients with other conditions but with opsoclonus-myoclonus as part of the presenting phenotype may be relevant to the localization of the neuropathological process in OMS. There has also been interest in the use of other neuroimaging modalities in both the acute and the chronic phase in order to localize the pathophysiological process. Single photon emission computed tomography (SPECT) in one child in the acute phase of an illness described as encephalitis, albeit with both opsoclonus and myoclonus, showed increased tracer uptake in the cerebellar vermis; in another child in the chronic phase of OMS there was hypoperfusion on SPECT in the cerebellum diffusely with a midline emphasis (Oguro et al. 1997). Hayward et al. showed cerebellar atrophy in all five children who consented to MRI imaging at long-term follow-up (Hayward et al. 2001); in the more recent Italian study 36% had cerebellar atrophy on long-term follow-up (De Grandis et al. 2009); in neither of these two studies was there a clear association between late cerebellar atrophy and neurological outcome. Voxel-based morphometry (VBM) has shown decreased vermis volume in a group of children in the chronic phase (Bluml et al. 2006). Magnetic resonance spectroscopy (MRS) has not shown consistent abnormalities to date (Kuhn et al. 2002; Bluml et al. 2006).

Electroencephalography

The EEG is either normal or non-specifically slow in acute OMS. It is not usually indicated but may be helpful in the occasional child in whom a diagnosis of epilepsy (including status epilepticus) is under consideration (Haden et al. 2009).

Association with neuroblastoma

Of those children with neuroblastoma, 2–3% have OMS (Rudnick et al. 2001). There remains uncertainty as to the proportion of children with OMS who have neuroblastoma; series range from 7.5% (Pohl et al. 1996) to 100% (Mitchell et al. 2002) and are likely to be subject to (1) selection bias and (2) the effects of very variable investigation protocols for neuroblastoma in children presenting with OMS (Pang et al. 2010a). Even in those children in whom no neuroblastoma has been identified after an exhaustive and sophisticated investigation protocol, the possibility has been raised that neuroblastoma may have been present and spontaneously regressed, as is recognized to be part of the natural history in certain neuroblastoma tumours (Nishihara et al. 2000). The current consensus is that probably approximately 50% of children with OMS have an underlying neuroblastoma but this figure may be subject to change on the basis of the forthcoming prospective and systematic European protocol (see under **The future**, below).

A thorough and systematic approach to the exclusion of neuroblastoma is mandatory in all children presenting with OMS and the following appproach is recommended. A first-line protocol should include chest radiograph and ultrasonography of the neck, abdomen and pelvis with special attention directed at the para-carotid, adrenal and para-vertebral regions along with a spot urine test for adrenal metabolites. If a neuroblastoma is identified, further imaging will be determined by the relevant national or international oncology protocol at the time. If, however, the above investigations are negative, detailed MRI in 4mm sections is required of all areas typically affected by neuroblastoma to include the neck, chest and abdomen with particular focus on the para-vertebral regions (full-length spine from cervical to sacral), the adrenals and the mediastinum. If a tumour is identified it should be further examined with T1-weighted contrast enhancement. An MIBG scintigraphy scan will be required in all children whether or not a neuroblastoma is identified on other imaging modalities in view of its role both in tumour identification and staging.

An under-recognized point to emphasize is that, because OMS-associated neuroblastoma is often low-grade and metabolically inactive, investigations such as urinary adrenal metabolites and MIBG scans which are metabolism-dependent, although a necessary part of neuroblastoma assessment, are not sufficient as investigative tools in isolation as they may produce false-negative results.

Children with neuroblastoma and OMS tend to have good prognosis tumours with lower staging, low-grade histology – often ganglioneuroblastoma, lymphoid infiltrates and absence of N-myc amplification (Koh et al. 1994; Cooper et al. 2001; Gambini et al. 2003) and a markedly better oncological outcome than children with neuroblastoma without the neurological condition (Altman and Baehner 1976; Rudnick et al. 2001), although this is not invariably the case (Hiyama et al. 1994). Rudnick et al. (2001) also reported that the presence of OMS conferred an improved oncological outcome even when disease staging was matched. The neurological outcome, however, seems to be independent of the presence or absence of a neuroblastoma and, where present, of the successful treatment of the underlying neuroblastoma (Boltshauser et al. 1979; Hammer et al. 1995; Plantaz et al. 2000; Klein et al. 2007) although, in one series, an association of worse neurological outcome with lower neuroblastoma stage at presentation was identified (Rudnick et al. 2001).

Atypical presentation of neuroblastoma

There are occasional reports of later presentation of a neuroblastoma not identified at the initial presentation of OMS. The possibility has been raised that immunosuppressive treatment for OMS may facilitate the growth of a previously unidentified neuroblastoma (Chang et al. 2006). Many would favour the natural history of some neuroblastomas and the variation in neuroblastoma investigation protocols as more likely explanations for later neuroblastoma diagnosis in occasional children. The presence or absence of neuroblastoma does not alter the indication for immunosuppressive treatment. Where neuroblastoma is excluded on initial investigation, but the OMS remains intractable, it is wise to repeat the neuroblastoma investigation protocol after 6 months; some clinicians repeat neuroblastoma investigation in all children with initially negative results irrespective of the progress of their OMS.

Other neoplastic and infectious disorders associated with OMS

Occasionally paediatric OMS has been described with neoplastic disorders other than neuroblastoma – for example, acute lymphoblastic leukaemia (Pohl et al. 1996) and hepatoblastoma in Beckwith-Wiedemann syndrome (Wilfong et al. 1992) – also on a presumptively paraneoplastic basis. However, case reports of OMS in association with various infectious agents include both individuals with postinfectious OMS, for example, following streptococcal infection (Candler et al. 2006), *Mycoplasma* (Chemli et al. 2007) and varicella zoster (Pang et al. 2010b), and those who do not have OMS but in whom direct CNS infection produces the clinical features of opsoclonus and myoclonus, presumably because of involvement of the relevant vermian and/or related structures in the infectious process – for example, in mumps (Ichiba et al. 1988), human herpesvirus 6 (Crawford et al. 2007), parainfluenza virus type 3 (McCarthy et al. 1990) and Lyme disease in an adult (Peter et al. 2006). The salutary paper by Cardesa-Salzmann et al. (2006) describes OMS in a child with both evidence of a recent Epstein-Barr virus infection and an underlying neuroblastoma, emphasizing the importance of a systematic search for neuroblastoma in every child.

Neuropathology

Neuropathological data are scarce and not entirely consistent. In the adult form, the only identified abnormality in the autopsies of three patients in one report was a widespread perivascular lymphocyte infiltration (Young et al. 1993). In another autopsy case (Ohara et al. 2007) only the cerebellum was affected and the prominent finding was of diffuse Purkinje cell and dentate neuron loss. One biopsy in a child (who was atypical in having a vermian lesion visible on MRI) reported the lesion as showing Purkinje and granular cell loss with gliosis (Tuchman et al. 1989). In an autopsy of a 6-year-old child with OMS and a neuroblastoma, the abnormalities were restricted to the cerebellum and consisted of demyelination, gliosis and Purkinje cell loss (Ziter et al. 1979). Clerico et al. (1993) described a very unusual child who died with Cushing syndrome said to be secondary to an adrenocorticotropic hormone (ACTH)-secreting ganglioneuroblastoma, and who also had opsoclonus and myoclonus with a mass lesion involving the vermis and left cerebellar hemisphere; the cerebellar lesion was said to be degenerative rather than neoplastic and to show regenerative gliosis with no T- or B-cell infiltration.

Pathophysiology

The presumption is that this is an immune-mediated condition caused by cross-reacting antibodies to a component of neuroblastoma. In those children in whom a neuroblastoma is not identified the condition is ascribed to a previously present but spontaneously regressed neuroblastoma, to a neuroblastoma remaining unidentified because of an insufficiently rigorous investigation protocol or to an alternative immune mechanism, perhaps postinfectious in origin, with a variety of putative and variably characterized infections being responsible (see above).

Although there is as yet no consistent and specific immune marker in OMS, support for the immune-mediated hypothesis derives from a variety of sources. These include the analogous, and more consistently paraneoplastic, adult syndrome which may be associated with anti-Hu or anti-Ri antibodies and the response to immunomodulatory treatments including steroids, intravenous immunoglobulin (IVIG), cyclophosphamide and rituximab (see Treatment section, below). Krasenbrink et al. (2007) identified a substantially increased prevalence of autoimmune disease in first-degree relatives of children with OMS, with autoimmune thyroid and rheumatoid disease being particularly evident.

Neuroblastoma pathological studies indicate that OMS-associated neuroblastomas are characterized by striking lymphocytic infiltration and secondary perivascular lymphoid follicle formation (Cooper et al. 2001; Gambini et al. 2003; Raffaghello et al. 2009), although of note is the lack of evidence for neurological benefit in most cases where neuroblastoma is successfully treated. Children with neuroblastoma and OMS are more likely to have antineuronal antibodies than children with neuroblastoma alone (Antunes et al. 2000). Sera from children with OMS and neuroblastoma have been demonstrated to have increased IgG binding to the surface of a neuroblastoma cell line (SKN-SH cells) compared to sera from children with neuroblastoma alone and healthy controls (Blaes et al. 2005). Autoantibodies to the surface of a neuroblastoma cell line were identified in neuroblastoma-associated OMS sera but were absent in sera from children with neuroblastoma without accompanying OMS and, in one neuroblastoma-negative child whose OMS resolved rapidly and spontaneously, there was an accompanying decrease in serum auto-antibodies (Blaes et al. 2008).

While CSF cell counts are usually normal in OMS, there are characteristic patterns of cell phenotypes including an increased proportion of B-cells, particularly CD5+, CD5-, these findings correlating with disease severity and declining with time from illness onset (Pranzatelli et al. 2004a); an increased proportion also of CD19+ B-cells and of gammadelta T-cells with a relative reduction in CD4+ T-cells and a reduced CD4/CD8 ratio has also been demonstrated by the same group (Pranzatelli et al. 2004b), again correlating with disease severity and unaffected by the presence or absence of an underlying neuroblastoma; peripheral blood in neuroblastoma-associated OMS children reflects a similarly reduced CD4+ T-cell subset and CD4/CD8 ratio but is not otherwise in keeping with CSF findings (Pranzatelli et al. 2004c). More indirect evidence for T-cell involvement comes from the identification of elevated CSF neopterin with normal tetrahydrobiopterin in children with OMS/DES (Pranzatelli et al. 2004d). CSF B-cell activating factor (BAFF) is higher in children with untreated OMS than in treated children and neurological controls (Pranzatelli et al. 2008); the CSF BAFF has been confirmed to be of intrathecal origin in children with OMS, to be elevated in comparison with other inflammatory neurological disorders, to correlate with anti-cerebellar granular neuron antibodies and not to be associated with elevated CSF APRIL, another B-cell activating factor (Fuhlhuber et al. 2009).

A number of individual case reports indicate that the clinical phenotype may occasionally be associated with a variety of other immune-mediated conditions – diabetes mellitus with anti-GAD antibodies possibly cross-reacting with both pancreatic beta-cells and Purkinje cells (Lenti et al. 1999), coeliac disease (Deconinck et al. 2006) and, most recently, anti-N-methyl-D-aspartate receptor encephalitis in a young adult without an underlying tumour (Kurian et al. 2010).

Treatment

Evidence to underpin therapeutic decision-making in OMS is sparse because of the difficulties contingent on therapeutic trials in a disease of such rarity which is also diverse in a variety of respects – paraneoplastic or postinfectious in aetiology, monophasic or chronic relapsing in natural history, outcomes which range from complete recovery in a few to severe chronic neurological disability, along with the need for long-term follow-up and the systematic measurement of neurological morbidity in terms not only of motor function but also of cognition, behaviour and quality of life as outcome measures.

However, treatments which have been used and identified as beneficial in some children can be divided into immunomodulatory, based on the probable immunophysiological basis of the condition, and symptomatic.

Immunomodulatory treatment

Steroids have been used with symptomatic benefit from the time of Kinsbourne (Kinsbourne 1962), but it is not clear that early response correlates with later outcome (Boltshauser et al. 1979). Commonly a dose of prednisolone 1–2mg/kg/day is used for a period of weeks to months until the most prominent symptoms are modified. At that point prednisolone dose is very slowly tapered over a period of weeks to months depending on symptom control. In many cases persistent or fluctuating symptomatology results in prolonged steroid therapy for months to years, with the concomitant side-effects of such a regimen. A number of clinicians have commented on the benefits of corticotrophin (ACTH) as opposed to prednisone or prednisolone and there are anecdotal reports of a therapeutic response when a child unresponsive to prednisone or prednisolone is switched to ACTH, and some evidence is available suggesting that CSF cortisol levels are higher in children treated with ACTH than in those on oral steroid (Pranzatelli et al. 2005a). However, it has not been possible to verify a therapeutic advantage on a systematic basis (Mitchell et al. 2002). High-dose dexamethasone pulses have been shown in small and uncontrolled case series to have produced striking benefit used either alone (Rostásy et al. 2006; Ertle et al. 2008), or with cyclophosphamide (Wilken et al. 2008), in children previously resistant to daily prednisolone monotherapy.

Intravenous immunoglobulin (IVIG) has been reported to improve symptoms in some cases and has been used either on its own (Petruzzi and de Alarcon 1995; Glatz et al. 2003) or in combination with steroid therapy or rituximab (Leen et al. 2008). Currently the US Child Oncology Group is running a randomized trial of IVIG in neuroblastoma-associated OMS with results expected in 2012.

Rituximab, a monoclonal anti-CD20 B-cell antibody, has shown benefit in a number of studies (Bell et al. 2008; Burke and Cohn 2008; Corapcioglu et al. 2008; Leen et al. 2008) with accompanying depletion in presumptively pathogenic CSF B-cells where measured (Pranzatelli et al. 2005b; Pranzatelli et al. 2006; Pranzatelli et al. 2010).

There is some evidence of a therapeutic advantage in neuroblastoma-associated OMS treated with chemotherapy as against those not so treated (Russo et al. 1997; Rudnick et al. 2001). Cyclophosphamide, used for its immunosuppressive rather than its anti-neoplastic effect, has been of benefit in association with pulsed dexamethasone in a small group of previously steroid-resistant children (Wilken et al. 2008).

Plasma exchange may benefit occasional cases (Armstrong et al. 2005) but is frequently ineffective (Blaes 2002).

Mycophenolate mofetil, a lymphocyte proliferation inhibitor, produced some benefits in CSF immune factors, particularly CSF HLA-DR+ activated T-cells, but little sustained clinical benefit (Pranzatelli et al. 2009).

Azathioprine, used as an adjunct to other immunomodulatory treatments, has been helpful in individual cases but requires sustained administration over many months to produce a useful immunosuppressive effect (John Newsom-Davis, personal communication).

Theoretical concern that the paraneoplastic immune response may have a role in controlling the neuroblastoma has been raised. Blaes et al. (2008) identified an inhibitory effect on the proliferation of a neuroblastoma cell line (SKN-SH) in sera from children with both neuroblastoma-positive and -negative OMS. Inhibition of neuroblastoma cell proliferation and apoptosis had also been reported by Korfei et al. (2005). This does not appear to be a significant clinical problem however and, although there is, for example, a single clinical case report of a neuroblastoma identified in a child with OMS 4 months after starting rituximab therapy (Chang et al. 2006), the late identification of neuroblastoma in an occasional child on treatment for OMS is most likely to be because of a more rigorous second investigation protocol.

Symptomatic treatment

A single case report indicated a benefit from gabapentin to both opsoclonus and myoclonus in an adult with OMS (Moretti et al. 2000). A small but well-designed study of piracetam failed to demonstrate a therapeutic effect on the myoclonus associated with OMS (Pranzatelli et al. 2001). There are case reports also of benefit from clonazepam, often in high dosage, in both children and adults with OMS (Garg et al. 1996; Bartos 2006; Paliwal et al. 2010).

In children with chronic OMS, prominent sleep disturbance and aggressive behaviour, trazodone, a hypnotic serotonergic agent not currently readily available in the United Kingdom, was shown to improve both sleep and, perhaps in consequence, behaviour (Pranzatelli et al. 2005c).

As with other rare neurological disorders, professionals should not be inhibited by the rarity of the condition from empirical use of relevant therapy including hypnotics, other symptom-targeted pharmacotherapy, behaviour management techniques, educational support, occupational therapy, physiotherapy, and speech and language therapy.

The future

The Pranzatelli group continues to advance our knowledge of the immunopathological substrate to this condition particularly in the CSF, and to examine the effects of rational customized treatment interventions designed to address these processes.

Two national or multinational trials have opened. The Children's Oncology Group (COG) Trial (Chief Investigator, Pedro de Alarcon) is an oncology-led US trial of children with neuroblastoma-associated OMS in which all children receive steroids and cyclophosphamide with half randomized to receive intravenous immunoglobulin (IVIG); results are expected in early 2012. There is currently a Societe Internationale d'Oncologie Pediatrique en Europe Neuroblastome (SIOPEN)-led European Trial that opened in France in 2011 recruiting children both with and without neuroblastoma. This involved a detailed, systematic and uniform approach to the exclusion of neuroblastoma in children presenting with OMS, partnership between paediatric neurologists and oncologists in participating countries, the use of the same OMS severity scores as the US COG Trial, a Europe-wide combined specialist centre approach to immunological and pathological assessment and an emphasis on longer-term cognitive and behavioural outcomes in the setting of a single-arm trial with treatment progression depending on response, starting with monthly pulsed dexamethasone, escalating where this has been ineffective after 3 months to add pulsed cyclophosphamide and then, again where the child remains significantly symptomatic, to replace cyclophosphamide with rituximab. It is anticipated that US paediatric oncologists will recruit to the European Trial once the COG Trial is complete.

Both of these large-scale trials allowed for the systematic prospective evaluation of treatment response and outcome on a scale which is unprecedented in this rare disorder. Their shared severity scoring system will allow for useful comparison between the trial groups; the European SIOPEN OMS Network of paediatric oncologists, neurologists, pathologists and immunologists will be available to generate further trials, probably randomized and on a transatlantic basis.

REFERENCES

Altman AJ, Baehner RL (1976) Favorable prognosis for survival in children with coincident opso-myoclonus and neuroblastoma. Cancer 37: 846–852.

Antunes NL, Khakoo Y, Matthay KK, Seeger RC, Stram DO, Gerstner E, et al. (2000) Antineuronal antibodies in patients with neuroblastoma and paraneoplastic opsoclonus-myoclonus. J Pediatr Hematol Oncol 22: 315–320.

Armstrong MB, Robertson PL, Castle VP (2005) Delayed, recurrent opsoclonus-myoclonus syndrome responding to plasmapheresis. Pediatr Neurol 33: 365–367.

Bartos A (2006) Effective high-dose clonazepam treatment in two patients with opsoclonus and myoclonus: GABAergic hypothesis. Eur Neurol 564: 240–242.

Bataller L, Graus F, Saiz A, Vilchez JJ, Spanish Opsoclonus-Myoclonus Study Group (2001) Clinical outcome in adult onset idiopathic or paraneoplastic opsoclonus-myoclonus. Brain 124: 437–443.

Bell J, Moran C, Blatt J (2008) Response to rituximab in a child with neuroblastoma and opsoclonus-myoclonus. Pediatr Blood Cancer 502: 370–371.

Blaes F (2002) Immunotherapeutic approaches to paraneoplastic disorders. Expert Opin Biol Ther 2, 4: 419–430.

Blaes F, Fuhlhuber V, Korfei M, Tschernatsch M, Behnisch W, Rostásy K, et al. (2005) Surface-binding autoantibodies to cerebellar neurons in opsoclonus syndrome. Ann Neurol 58: 313–317.

Blaes F, Pike MG, Lang B (2008) Autoantibodies in childhood Opsoclonus-Myoclonus Syndrome. J Neuroimmunol 201–202: 221–226.

Bluml S, Chen V, Panigraphy A (2006) Neuro-imaging of opsoclonus-ataxia sequelae: MRS and voxel-based morphometry. Ann Neurol 60(supp 3): S156.

Boltshauser E, Deonna T, Hirt HR (1979) Myoclonic encephalopathy of infants or 'dancing eyes syndrome'. Report of 7 cases with long-term follow-up and review of the literature (cases with and without neuroblastoma). Helv Paediatr Acta 34: 119–133.

Burke MJ, Cohn SL (2008) Rituximab for treatment of opsoclonus-myoclonus syndrome in neuroblastoma. Pediatr Blood Cancer 50: 679–680.

Candler PM, Dale RC, Griffin S, Church AJ, Wait R, Chapman MD, et al. (2006) Post-streptococcal opsoclonus-myoclonus syndrome associated with anti-neuroleukin antibodies. J Neurol Neurosurg Psychiatry 77: 507–512.

Cardesa-Salzmann TM, Mora J, Garcia Cazorla MA, Cruz O, Munoz C, Campistol J (2006) Epstein-Barr virus related opsoclonus-myoclonus-ataxia does not rule out the presence of occult neuroblastic tumors. Pediatr Blood Cancer 47: 964–967.

Catsman-Berrevoets CE, Aarson FK, van Hemsbergen ML, van Noesel MM, Hakvoort-Cammel FG, van den Heuvel-Eibrink MM (2009) Improvement of neurological status and quality of life in children with opsoclonus myoclonus syndrome at long-term follow-up. Pediatr Blood Cancer 53: 1048–1053.

Chang BH, Koch T, Hopkins K, Malempati S (2006) Neuroblastoma found in a 4-year old after rituximab therapy for Opsoclonus-Myoclonus. Pediatric Neurology 35: 213–215.

Chemli J, Ketata S, Dalhoumi A, Ajmi H, Hassayoun S, Fodha I, Boujafar N, Harbi A (2007) Opsoclonus-myoclonus syndrome associated with Mycoplasma pneumoniae infection. Arch Pediatr 14: 1003–1006. (in French)

Clerico A, Tenore A, Bartolozzi S, Remotti D, Ruco L, Dominici C, Properzi E, Castello MA (1993) Adrenocorticotropic hormone-secreting ganglioneuroblastoma associated with opsomyoclonic encephalopathy: a case report with immunohistochemical study. Med Pediatr Oncol 219: 690–694.

Cooper R, Khakoo Y, Matthay KK, Lukens JN, Seeger RC, Stram DO, et al. (2001) Opsoclonus-myoclonus-ataxia syndrome in neuroblastoma: Histopathologic features – a report from the Children's Cancer Group. Med Pediatr Oncol 36: 623–629.

Corapcioglu F, Mutlu H, Kara B, Inan N, Akansel G, Gurbuz Y, Topcu S (2008) Response to rituximab and prednisolone for opsoclonus-myoclonus-ataxia syndrome in a child with ganglioneuroblastoma. Pediatr Hematol Oncol 258: 756–761.

Crawford JR, Kadom N, Santi MR, Mariani B, Lavenstein BL (2007) Human herpesvirus 6 rhombencephalitis in immunocompetent children. J Child Neurol 22: 1260–1268.

Deconinck N, Scaillon M, Segers V, Groswasser JJ, Dan B (2006) Opsoclonus-myoclonus associated with celiac disease. Pediatr Neurol 344: 312–314.

De Grandis E, Parodi S, Conte M, Angelini P, Battaglia F, Gandolfo C, et al. (2009) Long-term follow-up of neuroblastoma-associated opsoclonus-myoclonus-ataxia syndrome. Neuropediatrics 40: 103–111.

Ertle F, Behnisch W, Al Mulla NA, Bessisso M, Rating D, Mechtersheimer G, et al. (2008) Treatment of neuroblastoma-related opsoclonus-myoclonus-ataxia syndrome with high-dose dexamethasone pulses. Pediatr Blood Cancer 50: 683–687.

Fuhlhuber V, Bick S, Kirsten A, Hahn A, Gerriets T, Tschnernatsch M, et al. (2009) Elevated B-cell activating factor BAFF, but not APRIL, correlates with CSF cerebellar autoantibodies in pediatric opsoclonus-, yoclonus syndrome. J Neuroimmunol 210: 87–91.

Gambini C, Conte M, Bernini G, Angelini P, Pession A, Paolucci P, et al. (2003) Neuroblastic tumors associated with opsoclonus-myoclonus syndrome: histological, immunohistochemical and molecular features of 15 Italian cases. Virchows Arch. 4426: 555–562.

Garg RK, Kar AM, Dixit V (1996) Opsoclonus-myoclonus syndrome in an adult: a case report and response to clonazepam. Indian J Opthalmol 44: 101–102.

Glatz K, Meinck H-M, Wildemann B (2003) Para-infectious opsoclonus-myoclonus syndrome: high dose intravenous immonoglobulins are effective. J Neurol Neurosurg Psychiatry 74: 279–280.

Haden SV, McShane MA, Holt CM (2009) Opsoclonus myoclonus: a non-epileptic movement disorder that may present as status epilepticus. Arch Dis Child 94: 897–899.

Hammer MS, Larsen MB, Stack CV (1995) Outcome of children with opsoclonus-myoclonus regardless of etiology. Pediatr Neurol 13: 21–24.

Hayward K, Jeremy RJ, Jenkins S, Barkovich AJ, Gultekin SH, Kramer J, et al. (2001) Long-term neurobehavioural outcomes in children with neuroblastoma and opsoclonus-myoclonus-ataxia syndrome: relationship to MRI findings and anti-neuronal antibodies. J Pediatr 139: 552–559.

Hero B, Radojska S, Gathof B (2005) Opsomyoclonus syndrome in infancy with or without neuroblastoma is associated with HLA-DRB1. Pediatr Blood Cancer 45: 480.

Hiyama E, Yokoyama T, Ichikawa T, Hiyama K, Kobayashi M, Tanaka Y, et al. (1994) Poor outcome in patients with advanced stage neuroblastoma and coincident opsomyoclous syndrome. Cancer 74: 1821–1826.

Ichiba N, Miyake Y, Sato K, Oda M, Kimoto H (1988) Mumps-induced opsoclonus-myoclonus and ataxia. Pediatr Neurol 4: 224–227.

Kinsbourne M (1962) Myoclonic encephalopathy of infants. J Neurol Neurosurg Psychiatry 25: 271–276.

Klein A, Schmitt B, Boltshauser E (2007) Long-term outcome of ten children with opsoclonus-myoclonus syndrome. Eur J Pediatr 166: 359–363.

Koh PS, Raffensperger JG, Berry S, Larsen MB, Johnstone HS, Chou P, et al. (1994) Long-term outcome in children with opsoclonus-myoclonus and ataxia and coincident neuroblastoma. J Pediatr 125: 712–716.

Korfei M, Fuhlhuber V, Scmidt-Woll T, Kaps M, Preissner KT, Blaes F (2005) Functional characterisation of autoantibodies from patients with pediatric opsoclonus-myoclonus-syndrome. J Neuroimmunol 170: 150–157.

Krasenbrink I, Fuhlhuber V, Juhasz-Boess I, Stolz E, Hahn A, Kaps M, et al. (2007) Increased prevalence of autoimmune disorders and autoantibodies in parents of children with opsoclonus-myoclonus syndrome (OMS). Neuropediatrics 38: 114–116.

Krug P, Schleiermacher G, Michon J, Valteau-Couanet D, Brisse H, Peuchmaur M, et al. (2010) Opsoclonus-myoclonus in children associated or not with neuroblastoma. Eur J Paediatr Neurol 14: 400–409.

Kuhn MJ, Pranzatelli MR, Langheim JM (2002) MR Spectroscopy in children with opsoclonus-myoclonus syndrome. Proceedings of the 40th Annual Meeting of the American Society of Neuroradiology, Vancouver, Canada; 233.

Kurian M, Lalive PH, Dalmau JO, Horvath J (2010) Opsoclonus-myoclonus syndrome in anti-N-methyl-D-aspartate receptor encephalitis. Arch Neurol 67: 118–121.

Leen WG, Weemaes CM, Verbeek MM, Willemsen MA, Rotteveel JJ (2008) Rituximab and intravenous immunoglobulins for relapsing post-infectious opsoclonus-myoclonus syndrome. Pediatr Neurol 39: 213–217.

Lenti C, Bognetti E, Bonfanti R, Bonifacio E, Meschi F (1999) Myoclonic encephalopathy and diabetes mellitus in a boy. Dev Med Child Neurol 41: 489–490.

Matthay KK, Blaes F, Hero B, Plantaz D, De Alarcon P, Mitchell WG, et al. (2005) Opsoclonus myoclonus syndrome in neuroblastoma: a report from a workshop on the dancing eyes syndrome at the advances in neuroblastoma meeting in Genoa, Italy, 2004. Cancer Lett 228: 275–282.

McCarthy VP, Zimmerman AW, Miller CA (1990) Central nervous system manifestations of parainfluenza virus type 3 infections in childhood. Pediatr Neurol 6: 197–201.

Mitchell WG, Davalos-Gonzalez Y, Brumm VL, Aller SK, Burger E, Turkel SB, et al. (2002) Opsoclonus-ataxia caused by childhood neuroblastoma: developmental and neurological sequelae. Pediatrics 109: 86–98.

Moretti R, Torre P, Antonello RM, Nasuelli D, Cazzato G (2000) Opsoclonus-myoclonus syndrome: Gabapentin as a new therapeutic proposal. Eur J Neurol 7: 455–456. (Letter)

Nishihara H, Toyoda Y, Tanaka Y, Ijiri R, Aida N, Takeuchi M, et al. (2000) Natural course of neuroblastoma detected by mass screening: a 5-year prospective study at a single institution. J Clin Oncol 18: 3012–3017.

Oguro K, Kobayashi J, Aiba H, Hojo H (1997) Opsoclonus-myoclonus syndrome with abnormal single photon emission computed tomography imaging. Pediatr Neurol 16: 334–336.

Ohara S, Iijima N, Hayashida K, Oide T, Katai S (2007) Autopsy case of opsoclonus-myoclonus-ataxia and cerebellar cognitive affective syndrome associated with small cell lung carcinoma of the lung. Mov Disord 22: 1320–1324.

Paliwal VK, Chandra S, Verma R, Kalita J, Misra UK (2010) Clonazepam responsive opsoclonus myoclonus syndrome: additional evidence in favour of fastigial nucleus disinhibition hypothesis? J Neural Transm 117: 613–615.

Pang K, de Sousa C, Lang B, Pike MG (2010a) A prospective study of the presentation and management of Dancing Eye Syndrome/Opsoclonus-Myoclonus Syndrome in the United Kingdom. Eur J Paediatr Neurol 14: 156–161.

Pang K, Lynch B, Osborne J, Pike MG (2010b) Dancing eye syndrome with spontaneous recovery and normal neurodevelopment. Eur J Paediatr Neurol 14: 178–181.

Papero PH, Pranzatelli MR, Margolis LJ, Tate E, Wilson LA, Glass P (1995) Neurobehavioral and psychosocial functioning of children with opsoclonus-myoclonus syndrome. Dev Med Child Neurol 37: 915–932.

Peter L, Jung J, Tilikete C, Ryvlin P, Mauguiere F (2006) Opsoclonus-myoclonus as a manifestation of Lyme disease. J Neurol Neurosurg Psychiatry 77: 1090–1091.

Petruzzi MJ, de Alarcon PA (1995) Neuroblastoma-associated opsoclonus-myoclonus treated with intravenously administered immune globulin G. J Pediatr 127: 328–329.

Plantaz D, Michon J, Valteau-Couanet D, Coze C, Chastagner P, Bergeron C, et al. (2000) Opsoclonus-myoclonus syndrome associated with non-metastatic neuroblastoma. Long-term survival. Study of the French Society of Pediatric Oncologists. Arch Pediatr 7: 621–628. (in French)

Pohl KR, Pritchard J, Wilson J (1996) Neurological sequelae of the dancing eye syndrome. Eur J Pediatr 155: 237–244.

Pranzatelli MR, Tate ED, Galvan I, Wheeler A (2001) Controlled pilot study of piracetam for pediatric opsoclonus-myoclonus. Clin Neuropharmacol 24: 352–357.

Pranzatelli MR, Travelstead AL, Tate ED, Allison TJ, Verhulst SJ (2004a) CSF B-cell expansion in opsoclonus-myoclonus syndrome: a bio-marker of disease activity. Mov Dis 19: 770–777.

Pranzatelli MR, Travelstead AL, Tate ED, Allison TJ, Moticka EJ, Franz DN, et al. (2004b) B- and T-cell markers in opsoclonus-myoclonus syndrome: immunophenotyping of CSF lymphocytes. Neurology 62: 1526–1532.

Pranzatelli MR, Travelstead AL, Tate ED, Allison TJ, Lee ND, Fisher J, Jasty R. (2004c) Immunophenotype of blood lymphocytes in neuroblastoma-associated opsoclonus-myoclonus. J Pediatr Hematol Oncol 26: 718–723.

Pranzatelli MR, Hyland K, Tate ED, Arnold LA, Allison TJ, Soori GS (2004d) Evidence of cellular immune activation in children with opsoclonus-myoclonus: cerebrospinal fluid neopterin. J Child Neurol 19: 919–924.

Pranzatelli MR, Chun KY, Moxness M, Tate ED, Allison TJ (2005a) Cerebrospinal fluid ACTH and cortisol in Opsoclonus-Myoclonus: Effect of therapy. Pediatr Neurol 33: 121–126.

Pranzatelli MR, Tate ED, Travelstead AL, Longee D (2005b) Immunologic and clinical responses to Rituximab in a child with Opsoclonus-Myoclonus Syndrome. Pediatrics 115: 115–119.

Pranzatelli MR, Tate ED, Dukart WS, Flint MJ, Hoffman MT, Oksa AE (2005c) Sleep disturbance and rage attacks in opsoclonus-myoclonus syndrome: response to trazodone. J Pediatr 1473: 372–378.

Pranzatelli MR, Tate ED, Travelstead AL, Barbosa J, Bergamini RA, Civitello L, et al. (2006) Rituximab (anti-CD20) adjunctive therapy for Opsoclonus-Myoclonus Syndrome. J Pediatr Hematol Oncol 28: 585–593.

Pranzatelli MR, Tate ED, Hoefgen ER, Swan JA, Colliver JA (2008) Therapeutic down-regulation of central and peripheral B-cell-activating factor (BAFF) production in pediatric opsoclonus-myoclonus syndrome. Cytokine 44: 26–32.

Pranzatelli MR, Tate ED, Travelstead AL, Baumgardenr CA, Gowda NV, Halthore SN, et al. (2009) Insights on chronic relapsing opsoclonus-myoclonus from a pilot study of mycophenolate mofetil. J Child Neurol 24: 316–322.

Pranzatelli MR, Tate ED, Swan JA, Travelstead AL, Colliver JA, Verhulst SJ, et al. (2010) B cell depletion therapy for new-onset opsoclonus-myoclonus. Mov Disord 25: 238–242.

Raffaghello L, Conte M, De Grandis E, Pistoia V (2009) Immunological mechanisms in opsoclonus-myoclonus associated neuroblastoma. Eur J Paediatr Neurol 13: 219–223.

Rostásy K, Wilke B, Baumann M, Müller-Deile K, Bieber I, Gärtner J, et al. (2006) High dose pulsatile dexamethasone therapy in children with opsoclonus-myoclonus syndrome. Neuropediatrics 37: 291–295.

Rudnick E, Khakoo Y, Antunes NL, Seeger RC, Brodeur GM, Shimada H, et al. (2001) Opsoclonus-myoclonus-ataxia syndrome in neuroblastoma: clinical outcome and antineuronal antibodies – a report from the Children's Cancer Group Study. Med Pediatr Oncol 36: 612–622.

Russo C, Cohn SL, Petruzzi MJ, de Alarcon PA (1997) Long-term neurologic outcome in children with opsoclonus-myoclonus associated with neuroblastoma: a report from the Pediatric Oncology Group. Med Pediatr Oncol 28: 284–288.

Tate ED, Allison TJ, Pranzatelli MR, Verhulst SJ (2005) Neuroepidemiologic trends in 105 US cases of pediatric opsoclonus-myoclonus syndrome. J Pediatr Oncol Nurs 22: 8–19.

Tsutada T, Izumi T, Murakami T (1996) Correlation of clinical improvement with pontine lesions in opsoclonus-myoclonus. Osaka City Med J 42: 53–60.

Tuchman RF, Alvarez LA, Kantrowitz AB, Moser FG, Liena J, Moshe SL (1989) Opsoclonus-myoclonus syndrome: Correlation of radiographic and pathological observations. Neuroradiology 31, 3: 250–2.

Turkel SB, Brumm VL, Mitchell WG, Tavare CJ (2006) Mood and behavioral dysfunction with opsoclonus-myoclonus ataxia. J Neuropsychiatry Clin Neurosci 18, 2: 239–241.

Wilfong AA, Parke JT, McCrary JA 3rd (1992) Opsoclonus-myoclonus with Beckwith-Wiedemann syndrome and hepatoblastoma. Pediatr Neurol 8: 77–79.

Wilken B, Baumann M, Bien CG, Hero B, Rostásy K, Hanefeld F (2008) Chronic relapsing opsoclonus-myoclonus syndrome: Combination of cyclophosphamide and dexamethasone pulses. Eur J Paediatr Neurol 12: 51–55.

Young CA, MacKenzie JM, Chadwick DW, Williams IR (1993) Opsoclonus-Myoclonus Syndrome: An autopsy study of three cases. Eur J Med 2: 239–241.

Ziter FA, Bray PF, Cancilla PA (1979) Neuropathologic findings in a patient with neuroblastoma and myoclonic encephalopathy. Arch Neurol 36: 51.

39
Acute Ataxia: Other Causes

Peter Baxter

Intoxication

As shown earlier in Chapter 36 (Table 36.1), intoxication is the second most common cause of acute ataxia in hospital practice. Like inflammatory causes it predominates in younger children, when most ingestion is accidental, but there is also a second peak of incidence in adolescence, when it is usually deliberate (Gieron-Korthals et al. 1994). Martínez-González et al. (2006) describe an ataxic presentation in 1.8% of all children seen for acute ingestion, with a mean age of approximately 40 months and a predominance of boys. Just as the organisms associated with inflammatory ataxias vary according to region and public health measures, the specific toxins associated with ataxia also depend on availability. In both Gieron-Korthals' and Martínez-González' series benzodiazepines were the most frequent agents. Both series include phenytoin and phenobarbital, with in addition carbamazepine and phenothiazines featuring in the former and dextromethorphan and alcohol in the latter. A large number of individual case reports and series describe acute ataxia due to toxic doses of therapeutic drugs such as anticonvulsants, anti-neoplastic agents, and piperazine (worm wobble); inadvertent or deliberate ingestion/inhalation, including Munchausen by proxy, of medical or recreational drugs, such as alcohol; or exposure to environmental toxins such as heavy metals (Lifshitz et al. 2000; Shroff and Houston 2002; Bonkowsky et al. 2005; Lin and Lawrence 2006; Daana et al. 2007; Kohli et al. 2008; O'Brien et al. 2010).

In the first iatrogenic group the likely cause is obvious from the medication history. In the second, inadvertent administration usually occurs in young children who have found agents such as their grandparent's medication or their parent's recreational substances. In the United States in 2008 in terms of intoxication 'the top five most common exposures in children age 5 or less were cosmetics/personal care products (13.5%), analgesics (9.7%), household cleaning substances (9.7%), foreign bodies/toys/miscellaneous (7.5%), and topical preparations (6.9%)' (Bronstein et al. 2009), but most of these will not cause ataxia. In an Indian centre between 2004 and 2006 three of 111 children presented with ataxia, and kerosine (27.9%), medications (19.8%, most often anticonvulsants) or insecticides (11.7%) were the most common substances (Kohli et al. 2008). Deliberate ingestion is a feature of adolescents, either as a suicide or para-suicide attempt or when the dose of recreational agents has been misjudged. More rarely, carers might deliberately administer agents to provoke symptoms, in the Münchhausen by proxy syndrome, or for other reasons. Environmental toxins such as heavy metals are the least common causes of intoxication in most studies. Chronic ataxia can also follow acute or chronic toxicity from lead or drugs such as phenytoin.

Acute ataxia due to intoxication is usually associated with a reduced level of consciousness of variable severity. Seizures and vomiting can be additional features of an acute encephalopathy. The diagnosis is confirmed by blood or urine analysis. If a drug is being administered for medical reasons, blood levels will indicate possible toxicity although there is not always a direct link with the level of intoxication, which in some susceptible individuals can occur within the recommended therapeutic range. This is particularly so where active metabolites might contribute, as with the epoxy metabolite of carbamazepine. Many hospitals carry out a restricted routine analysis of urine samples to look for common toxins, with diagnostic results if they are unexpectedly present. If this screen is negative a full forensic toxicology screen is essential to pursue less frequent substances. Other investigations are less useful. EEGs may be normal or show diffuse slow-wave activity as in any encephalopathy, but can show specific features such as fast activity with benzodiazepine intoxication.

Treatment and outcome depends on the individual toxin, if necessary with advice from national poisoning advisory agencies. Prevention of future ingestion is also important, using physical, psychological and social interventions as appropriate.

Neuropathic ataxia

The most common of this group of causes is an acute inflammatory motor and sensory polyradiculoneuropathy (Guillain-Barré syndrome), which can occur in any age group (Rabie and Nevo 2009). Sensory ataxia, which worsens in the dark or with the eyes closed, has been described as the presenting symptom in 15% but is less common as a presentation than pain and ascending weakness (Jones 1996; Delanoe et al. 1998; Ryan 2005). The level of consciousness is usually normal and cerebellar signs such as nystagmus or dysarthria are absent. Typical findings can include distal weakness, areflexia, a positive Romberg sign, and sensory changes, but in the early stages some of these may not be obvious. Characteristically the onset is preceded by an infection, especially *Campylobacter jejuni* enteritis, but cases can also be associated with many other agents, follow immunization, or have no obvious precipitant (Jones 1996; Rabie and Nevo 2009). In some patients raised blood levels of anti-GM1 antibodies are detectable.

In the most frequent demyelinating type, nerve conduction studies typically show slowing of motor conduction velocity. In the less frequent axonal type of acute neuropathy the neurophysiological findings characteristically show low amplitude compound muscle action potentials on nerve conduction studies and features of denervation on needle electromyography. Nerve conduction studies may not show any abnormalities until several days to a week after onset, by which stage 90% will be diagnostic. The cerebrospinal fluid protein level may not increase for a similar period, when the classic cyto-albuminaemic dissociation occurs. Typical spinal MRI findings include thickening and contrast enhancement of the nerve roots and cauda equina, but the diagnostic and prognostic value of this investigation has yet to be established (Yikilmaz et al. 2010).

The Miller Fisher syndrome is a rare variant, characterized by sensory ataxia, areflexia and external ophthalmoplegia, which has been described in children as young as 2 years of age (Ryan 2005; Torrent et al. 2009). The ophthalmoplegia can be complete or affect only vertical or horizontal movement. Anti-GQ1b antibodies are usually present. Recent series have shown an overlap with Bickerstaff rhombencephalitis, another rare condition mostly described in adults where ataxia and ophthalmoplegia can be associated with a reduced level of consciousness, pupillary abnormalities, facial weakness, bulbar palsy and/or extensor plantar responses. Brainstem involvement has been confirmed in one autopsy study. Up to 60% can have antibodies to GQ1b (Odaka et al. 2003; Steer et al. 2006; Ito et al. 2008; Tsapis et al. 2010). Some adult patients have also been described with acute mydriasis associated with anti-GQ1b (Fleury et al. 2010). Intracranial hypertension has also been described (Pulitanò et al. 2005).

Treatment relies on general support and immune-modulation therapy. If there is autonomic instability or respiratory compromise, intensive care is indicated, but otherwise general nursing care is sufficient. Feeding intervention may be needed. Physiotherapy is important, partly to maintain joint ranges. Pain can be significant and may not respond to agents such as gabapentin, so opiates can be needed (Ryan 2005). If infection has been the underlying trigger it may need treatment, but usually this is not required. Intravenous immunoglobulin accelerates recovery and is usually given as 400mg/kg bodyweight over several hours for 5 successive days. Shorter courses are as effective, but may have a higher relapse rate (Hughes et al. 2006; Rabie and Nevo 2009). In rare patients a repeat course a week or more later has been reported to give additional benefit. Steroids alone are ineffective. The outcome is generally good in young children, although some may require a prolonged convalescence.

Although inflammation is the most common cause, other causes of acute neuropathy also need to be considered. Ataxia has been described as a presenting feature of tick paralysis (Li and Turner 2004; Vedanarayanan et al. 2004), thiamine deficiency (Darcel et al. 2009) and germanium toxicity (Kamijo et al. 1991).

In theory, acute dorsal column impairment can present with ataxia, as in acute tabetic ataxia, but this has not been described in children.

Chronic inflammatory demyelinating polyneuropathy (CIDP) also presents with ataxia which can be relatively acute or subacute in its time course. Distal and proximal weakness and sensory symptoms are usually prominent as well. The course is very variable, with acute, progressive and relapsing-remitting patterns. Immunomodulatory treatment with intravenous immunoglobulin, steroids or plasma exchange form the first line of treatment while agents such as cytotoxic drugs, interferon, or anti-B-cell monoclonal antibodies have been used in resistant cases (Rabie and Nevo 2009).

Space-occupying lesions and structural causes

While the posterior fossa is the most common site for paediatric brain tumours, acute ataxia is not a typical or common presenting feature. Acute ataxia can occur if there is an acute haemorrhage into the tumour (Mesiwala et al. 2001), as discussed in Chapter 33, but is not otherwise a described association. More typically subacute ataxia is seen, usually in association with other signs such as headache, nausea, seizures, squint, personality change, head tilt, and/or cranial nerve palsies (Berglund et al. 1955; Wilne et al. 2007). Nonetheless most authorities recommend early neuroimaging in acute ataxia to exclude space-occupying lesions and other structural causes (Brunberg et al. 2008). The treatment and outcome vary according to the type and stage of the tumour.

Other space-occupying lesions that can rarely present with acute ataxia include tuberculomas (Rolinck-Werninghaus et al. 2001) and cysticercosis (Singh et al. 1996). In addition, acutely raised intracranial pressure due to haemorrhage into other space occupying lesions such as arachnoid cysts elsewhere in the brain can present with ataxia (De et al. 2002). Finally chronic hindbrain herniation due to an Arnold-Chiari malformation may cause ataxia and intermittent giddiness (Williams 1981).

Epilepsy (including nonconvulsive status)

Acute ataxia can occasionally be the initial and sole presentation of epilepsy in a child (Fig. 39.1; Bennett et al. 1982). The diagnosis relies on EEG recording during the symptomatic phase, as interictal EEGs may be normal. Other symptoms of epilepsy may be present but not volunteered until specifically sought in the history. More typically ataxia, usually fluctuant, is a well-recognized feature of nonconvulsive status epilepticus, which can be prominent in children with epileptic syndromes and encephalopathies such as Lennox-Gastaut, Dravet or Angelman syndrome. In addition intermittent or chronic ataxia can be associated with epilepsy through other mechanisms in degenerative conditions such as neuronal ceroid lipofuscinosis, dentatorubropallidoluysian atrophy, or infantile-onset spinocerebellar ataxia, as well as in some metabolic disorders (see Part 5) and Glut-1 deficiency. Iatrogenic or accidental anticonvulsant intoxication can also be a cause.

(a)

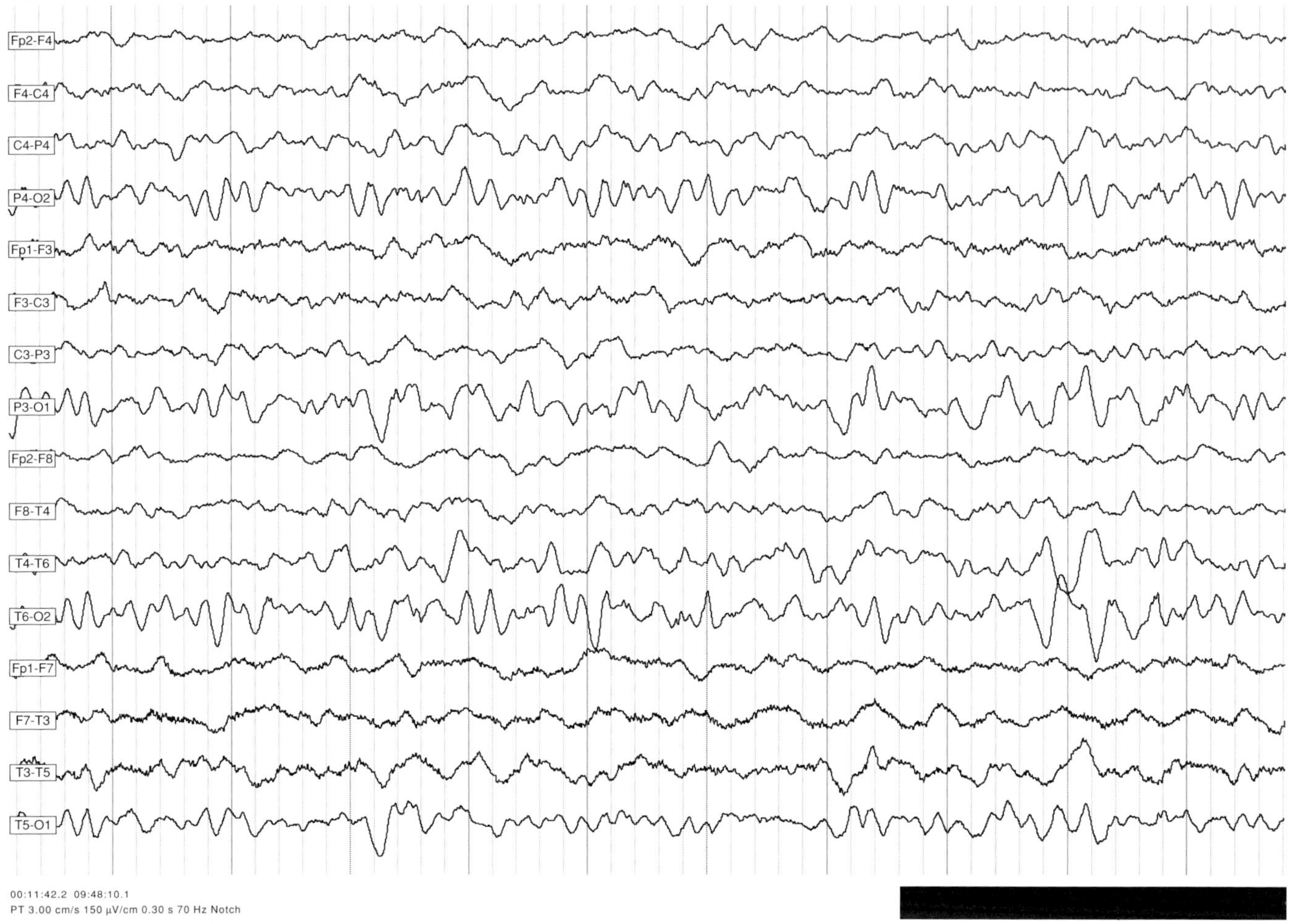

Fig. 39.1. Epileptic ataxia. EEGs: **(a)** interictal and **(b)** during an episode of acute ataxia 10 days apart in a 3-year-old child without any history of epilepsy, showing association with epileptic discharges.

The management is of the underlying epileptic disorder and, if appropriate, or possible, the underlying cause. These will also determine the outcome.

Traumatic

In major brain injury the clinical picture is dominated by the resulting encephalopathy. Minor brain and head trauma can be associated with acute ataxia through several mechanisms:

1. In children with some leukodystrophies, especially eIF2B (vanishing white matter disease), minor injuries can provoke an acute deterioration with ataxia (van der Knaap et al. 1997).
2. In other children ataxia has at times been reported to follow trauma, typically a minor closed head injury. The mechanism is unclear but may be similar to that in the other forms of transient cerebral dysfunction such as visual loss, hemiparesis or reduced level of consciousness that can follow similar mild injuries (Snoek et al. 1984; Yeoh et al. 2006). Stuttering can be associated (Yeoh et al. 2006). More prolonged ataxia is also described (Gohil and Munshi 2006). In some adults there can be signal change in the cerebellar peduncles on MR imaging (Fumeya and Hideshima 1994).
3. In children with dominant episodic ataxia type 2 due to *CACNA1A* mutations, attacks may be triggered by mild head trauma. Children with different mutations in the same gene can develop much more severe reactions such as seizures and oedema after minor head injuries, but they do not usually have prior episodic ataxia (Stam et al. 2009).
4. Minor head trauma can cause vertebral dissection leading to an infarct affecting the cerebellum or its connections (see Chapters 32 and 40).
5. Acutely raised pressure following trauma can also present with ataxia and headache, for example following minor injury causing haemorrhage into an arachnoid cyst (De et al. 2002).
6. Trauma can also cause vertigo through various mechanisms including traumatic perilymphatic fistulae (Kim et al. 2001; Choung et al. 2003).
7. Acute ataxia is also common following posterior fossa surgery, especially tumor resection involving the deep nuclei. It can occur in up to 25% of cases and is typically associated with hypotonia and cerebellar mutism (Wells et al. 2010).

(b)

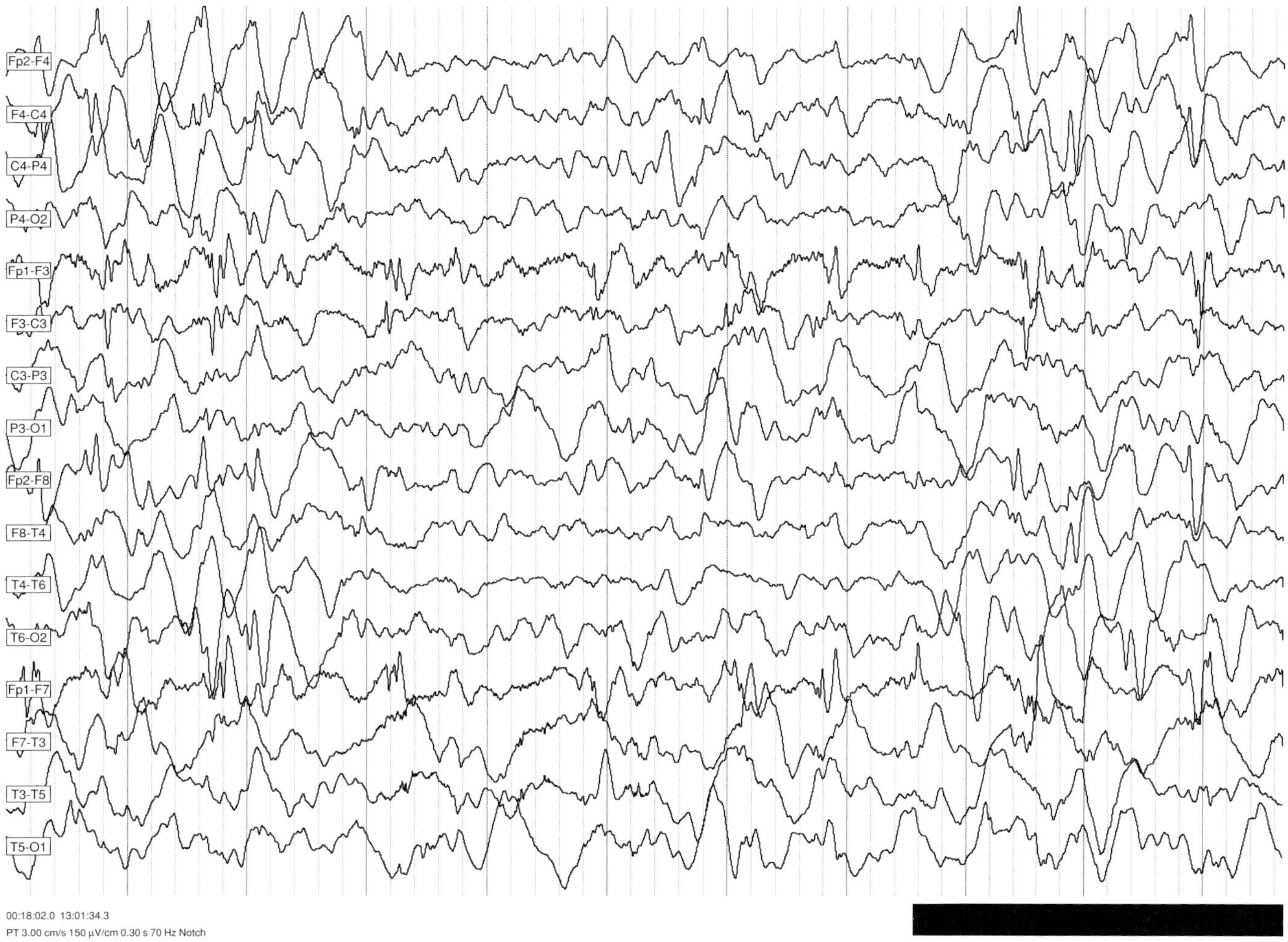

Fig. 39.1. (*continued*)

In all of these the underlying cause determines the management and outcome.

Acute vertigo

In young or nonverbal children it can be difficult to distinguish unsteadiness due to vertigo from other types of ataxia. The most common causes of acute vertigo are acute viral labyrinthitis and benign paroxysmal vertigo. Additional causes include trauma (see above), otitis media, vestibular neuronitis (which can be associated with *Borrelia* infection), benign paroxysmal positional vertigo, Meniere disease and tumors (Choung et al. 2003; Balatsouras et al. 2007). Vertigo, which may be positional, is the most obvious distinguishing feature, while other associated symptoms and signs can include nausea, vomiting, auditory symptoms and nystagmus. The nystagmus is classically spontaneous or positional, independent of gaze direction, and never vertical. The effects of position on vertigo and nystagmus can be tested by the Dix-Hallpike and supine roll manouevres (Bhattacharyya et al. 2008). Otoscopy, audiometry and vestibular function testing can contribute to the diagnosis. Treatment depends on the underlying cause.

Psychogenic ataxia

Acute movement disorders can have a psychogenic origin. Psychogenic ataxia is rarely described in children but may be more common in daily practice (Bisht et al. 2008). It is well described in adults (Baik and Lang 2007). In paediatric reports tremor is a common symptom (Ahmed et al. 2008; Ferrara and Jankovic 2008; Schwingenschuh et al. 2008). When gait is affected, buckling at the knees and/or ataxia are the most common features. As with other somatoform disorders, management relies on the exclusion of organic causes, identification of the likely psychological cause, and psychiatric intervention. The outcome is variable with some children developing significant and prolonged disability (Ahmed et al. 2008; Ferrara and Jankovic 2008; Schwingenschuh et al. 2008).

Rarely psychogenic triggers can provoke acute symptoms in organic disorders. This is best described in the eIF2B leukodystrophy, where fright has been associated with the onset of symptoms (Kaczorowska et al. 2006).

Metabolic and vascular causes

Metabolic and vascular causes of acute ataxia are discussed in Parts 5 and 7, respectively. Wernicke's encephalopathy can be difficult to diagnose, as most children do not show the classical triad of ataxia, diminished consciousness level, and ophthalmoplegia or nystagmus. Most cases are associated with malignancy or with dietary insufficiency (Vasconcelos et al. 1999; Fattal-Valevski et al. 2005). Late-onset biotinidase deficiency can present with ataxia, as well as pyramidal signs and visual impairment (Rahman et al. 1997).

Acute presentation of intermittent ataxias

These are mostly covered in Part 5, or above. The differential diagnosis includes the episodic ataxias types 1 to 4; metabolic disorders such as Leigh syndrome or maple syrup urine disease, Glut-1 deficiency, intoxication and epilepsy. Migraine also enters the differential diagnosis although some cases could be due to *CACNA1A* mutations. Arnold-Chiari malformations have also been associated with intermittent symptoms.

Conclusion

Acute ataxia is a relatively uncommon disorder in children but has a well-characterized list of possible causes, many of which show spontaneous improvement and a good outcome. Most cases are relatively easy to diagnose using the clinical approach and investigations described above.

REFERENCES

Ahmed MAS, Martinez A, Yee A, Cahill D, Besag FMC (2008) Psychogenic and organic movement disorders in children. Dev Med Child Neurol 2008; 50: 300–304.

Baik JS, Lang AE (2007) Gait abnormalities in psychogenic movement disorders. Mov Disord 22: 395–399.

Balatsouras DG, Kaberos A, Assimakopoulos D, Katotomichelakis M, Economou NC, Korres SG (2007) Etiology of vertigo in children. Int J Pediatr Otorhinolaryngol 71: 487–494.

Bennett HS, Selman JE, Rapin I, Rose A (1982) Nonconvulsive epileptiform activity appearing as ataxia. Am J Dis Child 136: 30–32.

Berglund G, Mossberg H-O, Rydenstam B (1955) Acute cerebellar ataxia in children. Acta Paed Scand 44: 254–262.

Bhattacharyya N, Baugh RF, Orvidas L, Barrs D, Bronston LJ, Cass S, et al.; American Academy of Otolaryngology-Head and Neck Surgery Foundation (2008) Clinical practice guideline: benign paroxysmal positional vertigo. Otolaryngol Head Neck Surg 139 (Suppl 4): S47–81.

Bisht J, Sankhyan N, Kaushal RK, Sharma RC, Grover N (2008) Clinical profile of pediatric somatoform disorders. Indian Pediatr 45: 111–115.

Brunberg JA; Expert Panel on Neurologic Imaging (2008) Ataxia. AJNR Am J Neuroradiol 29: 1420–1422.

Bonkowsky JL, Sarco D, Pomeroy SL (2005) Ataxia and shaking in a 2-year-old girl: acute marijuana intoxication presenting as seizure. Pediatr Emerg Care 21: 527–528.

Bronstein AC, Spyker DA, Cantilena LR Jr, Green JL, Rumack BH, Giffin SL (2009) 2008 Annual Report of the American Association of Poison Control Centers' National Poison Data System (NPDS): 26th Annual Report. Clin Toxicol (Phila) 47: 911–1084.

Choung Y-H, Park K, Moon S-K, Kim C-H, Ryu SJ (2003) Various causes and clinical characteristics in vertigo in children with normal eardrums. Int J Pediatr Otorhinolaryngol 67: 889–894.

Daana M, Nevo Y, Tenenbaum A, Taustein I, Berger I (2007) Lamotrigine overdose in a child. J Child Neurol 22: 642–644.

Darcel F, Roussin C, Vallat JM, Charlin C, Tournebize P, Doussiet E (2009) Polyneuropathies in vitamin B1 deficiency in Reunion and Mayotte islands in 70 patients of Maori and Comorian descent. Bull Soc Pathol Exot 102: 167–172.

De K, Berry K, Denniston S (2002) Haemorrhage into an arachnoid cyst: a serious complication of minor head trauma. Emerg Med J 19: 365–366.

Delanoe C, Sebire G, Landrieu P, Huault G, Metral S (1998) Acute inflammatory demyelinating polyradiculopathy in children: clinical and electrodiagnostic studies. Ann Neurol 44: 350–356.

Fattal-Valevski A, Kesler A, Sela BA, Nitzan-Kaluski D, Rotstein M, Mesterman R, et al. (2005) Outbreak of life-threatening thiamine deficiency in infants in Israel caused by a defective soy-based formula. Pediatrics 115: e233–238.

Ferrara J, Jankovic J (2008) Psychogenic movement disorders in children. Mov Disord 23: 1875–1881.

Fleury V, Aqallal A, Lagrange E, Besson G, Caudie C (2010) Acute bilateral mydriasis associated with anti-GQ1b antibody. J Clin Neurosci 17: 514–515.

Fumeya H, Hideshima H (1994) Cerebellar concussion – three case reports. Neurol Med Chir (Tokyo) 34: 612–615.

Gieron-Korthals MA, Westberry KR, Emmanuel PJ (1994) Acute childhood ataxia: 10-year experience. J Child Neurol 9: 381–384.

Gohil JR, Munshi SS (2006) Post concussion ataxia following minor head injury. Indian Pediatr 43: 829.

Hughes RA, Raphael JC, Swan AV, van Doorn PA (2006). Intravenous immunoglobulin for Guillain-Barré syndrome. Cochrane Database Syst Rev (1): CD002063.

Ito M, Kuwabara S, Odaka M, Misawa S, Koga M, Hirata K, Yuki N (2008) Bickerstaff's brainstem encephalitis and Fisher syndrome form a continuous spectrum: clinical analysis of 581 cases. J Neurol 255: 674–682.

Jones HR (1996) Childhood Guillain-Barré syndrome: clinical presentation, diagnosis and therapy. J Child Neurol 11: 4–12.

Kaczorowska M, Kuczynski D, Jurkiewicz E, Scheper GC, van der Knaap MS, Jozwiak S (2006) Acute fright induces onset of symptoms in vanishing white matter disease-case report. Eur J Paediatr Neurol 10: 192–193.

Kamijo M, Yagihashi S, Kida K, Narita S, Nakata F (1991) An autopsy case of chronic germanium intoxication presenting peripheral neuropathy, spinal ataxia, and chronic renal failure. Rinsho Shinkeigaku 31: 191–196.

Kim SH, Kazahaya K, Handler SD (2001) Traumatic perilymphatic fistulas in children: etiology, diagnosis and management. Int J Pediatr Otorhinolaryngol 60: 147–153.

Kohli U, Kuttiat VS, Lodha R, Kabra SK (2008) Profile of childhood poisoning at a tertiary care centre in North India. Indian J Pediatr 75: 791–794.

Li Z, Turner RP (2004) Pediatric tick paralysis: discussion of two cases and literature review. Pediatr Neurol 31: 304–307.

Lifshitz M, Gavrilov V, Sofer S (2000) Signs and symptoms of carbamazepine overdose in young children. Pediatr Emerg Care 16: 26–27.

Lin G, Lawrence R (2006) Pediatric case report of topiramate toxicity. Clin Toxicol (Phila) 44: 67–69.

Martínez-González MJ, Martínez-González S, García-Ribes A, Mintegi-Raso S, Benito-Fernández J, Prats-Viñas JM (2006) Acute onset ataxia in infancy: its aetiology, treatment and follow-up. Rev Neurol 42: 321–324.

Mesiwala AH, Avellino AM, Roberts TS, Ellenbogen RG (2001) Spontaneous cerebellar hemorrhage due to a juvenile pilocytic astrocytoma: case report and review of the literature. Pediatr Neurosurg 34: 235–238.

O'Brien MM, Lacayo NJ, Lum BL, Kshirsagar S, Buck S, Ravindranath Y, et al. (2010) Phase I study of valspodar (PSC-833) with mitoxantrone and etoposide in refractory and relapsed pediatric acute leukemia: a report from the Children's Oncology Group. Pediatr Blood Cancer 54: 694–702.

Odaka M, Yuki N, Yamada M, Koga M, Takemi T, Hirata K, Kuwabara S (2003) Bickerstaff's brainstem encephalitis: clinical features of 62 cases and a subgroup associated with Guillain-Barré syndrome. Brain 126: 2279–2290.

Pulitanò S, Viola L, Genovese O, Chiaretti A, Piastra M, Mariotti P, et al. (2005) Miller-Fisher syndrome mimicking intracranial hypertension following head trauma. Childs Nerv Syst 21: 473–476.

Rabie M, Nevo Y (2009) Childhood acute and chronic immune-mediated polyradiculoneuropathies. Eur J Paediatr Neurol 13: 209–218.

Rahman S, Standing S, Dalton RN, Pike MG (1997) Late presentation of biotinidase deficiency with acute visual loss and gait disturbance. Dev Med Child Neurol 39: 830–831.

Rolinck-Werninghaus C, Kötz K, Magdorf K, Bunikowski R, Staab D, Wahn U (2001) Late clinical manifestation of cerebral tuberculomas in two children with tuberculous meningoencephalitis. Eur J Pediatr 160: 645–648.

Ryan MM (2005) Guillain-Barré syndrome in childhood. J Paediatr Child Health 41: 237–241.

Schwingenschuh P, Pont-Sunyer C, Surtees R, Edwards MJ, Bhatia KP (2008) Psychogenic movement disorders in children: a report of 15 cases and a review of the literature. Mov Disord 23: 1882–1888.

Shroff R, Houston B (2002) Unusual cerebellar ataxia: 'worm wobble' revisited. Arch Dis Child 87: 333–334.

Singh UK, Sinha R, Suman S (1996) An unsteady 12-year-old. Lancet 347: 1158.

Snoek JW, Minderhoud JM, Wilmink JT (1984) Delayed deterioration following mild head injury in children. Brain 107: 15–36.

Stam AH, Luijckx GJ, Poll-Thé BT, Ginjaar IB, Frants RR, Haan J, et al. (2009) Early seizures and cerebral oedema after trivial head trauma associated with the CACNA1A S218L mutation. J Neurol Neurosurg Psychiatry 80: 1125–1129.

Steer AC, Starr M, Kornberg AJ (2006) Bickerstaff brainstem encephalitis associated with Mycoplasma pneumoniae infection. J Child Neurol 21: 533–534.

Torrent LS, Julian AN, Dueñas BP, Osorio AN, Oferil JC (2009) Miller Fisher syndrome in paediatrics: A description of 3 cases. An Pediatr (Barc) 71: 377–378.

Tsapis M, Laugel V, Koob M, de Saint Martin A, Fischbach M (2010) A pediatric case of Fisher-Bickerstaff spectrum. Pediatr Neurol 42: 147–150.

van der Knaap MS, Barth PG, Gabreels FJM, Franzoni E, Begeer JH, Stroink H, et al. (1997) A new leukoencephalopathy with vanishing white matter. Neurology 48: 845–855.

Vasconcelos MM, Silva KP, Vidal G, Silva AF, Domingues RC, Berditchevsky CR (1999) Early diagnosis of pediatric Wernicke's encephalopathy. Pediatr Neurol 20: 289–294.

Vedanarayanan V, Sorey WH, Subramony SH (2004) Tick paralysis. Semin Neurol 24: 181–184.

Wells EM, Khademian ZP, Walsh KS, Vezina G, Sposto R, Keating RF, Packer RJ (2010) Postoperative cerebellar mutism syndrome following treatment of medulloblastoma: neuroradiographic features and origin. J Neurosurg Pediatr 5: 329–334.

Williams B (1981) Chronic herniation of the hindbrain. Ann R Coll Surg Engl 63: 9–17.

Wilne S, Collier J, Kennedy C, Koller K, Grundy R, Walker D (2007) Presentation of childhood CNS tumours: a systematic review and meta-analysis. Lancet Oncol 8: 685–695.

Yeoh HK, Lind CRP, Law AJ (2006) Acute transient cerebellar dysfunction and stuttering following mild closed head injury. Childs Nerv Syst 22: 310–313.

Yikilmaz A, Doganay S, Gumus H, Per H, Kumandas S, Coskun A (2010) Magnetic resonance imaging of childhood Guillain-Barre syndrome. Childs Nerv Syst 26: 103–1108.

Part 9
Extrinsic Insults

40
Trauma to the Posterior Fossa

Daune L. MacGregor

Cerebellar traumatic injury is uncommon and is usually associated with injury to other structures of the head and neck and parenchymal cerebral injury. Isolated cerebellar injury is rare; however, neuroimaging techniques now allow for assessment and treatment approaches.

Traumatic hematomas

Epidural hematomas

Posterior fossa traumatic epidural hematomas (Fig. 40.1) are considered rare, with the incidence being approximately 1% of all head injuries (Dirim et al. 2005) representing 1–3% of all extradural hematomas (Berker et al. 2003). Most published series report both adult and pediatric patients. It is considered that there is a high mortality associated with an epidural hematoma in the posterior fossa and this relates, in part, to nonspecific presenting symptoms. In one series more than half of the patients had associated intradural lesions (Balik et al. 2010).

The causal incidents are usually accidental falls, motor vehicle or bicycle accidents or direct blows to the occipit (accidental or by assault). The presentation after injury can be clinically silent or may include occipital (scalp) swelling, headache, and vomiting. Some patients have brief or transient alterations in consciousness with cerebellar signs. The classic lucid interval associated with epidural hematomas is rarely seen in children with posterior fossa epidural hemorrhages (Berker et al. 2003). The occurrence, however, of a symptom-free initially silent period is reported (Dirim et al. 2005; Karasu et al. 2008). It is recognized that, in children, there is a high rate of occurrence of an epidural hemorrhage without a fracture.

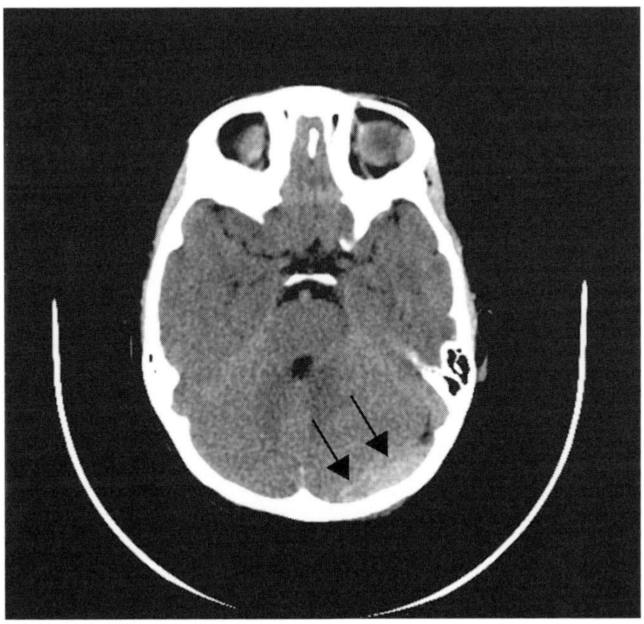

Fig. 40.1. Traumatic head injury in a 4-year-old girl with unenhanced CT image showing an acute hyperdense left posterior fossa epidural haematoma with some compression of the left cerebellar hemisphere. (Courtesy of Dr Manohar Shroff.)

Diagnosis is generally by CT or MR imaging. The management can be conservative with observation only; however, there can be sudden clinical deterioration which is difficult to predict. It is generally felt that surgical management is required if there is mass effect.

Risk factors for morbidity and mortality in children (Karasu et al. 2008) are considered to include the presence of supratentorial extension of the hematoma or other intracranial pathology. Other risk factors include a tear of one of the major sinuses or hemodynamic instability and low initial Glasgow coma score.

The mechanism of epidural hematoma of the posterior fossa is considered nonarterial in 30–40% of cases with an even greater rate occurring in children without associated skull fractures. One series (Dirim et al. 2005) reported that 85% of cases were venous and were as a result of injury to the transverse or sigmoid sinuses (although these cases were associated with occipital skull fracture). The origin of the hemorrhaging is the separation of the periosteal dura from the skull bone and rupture of vessels due to trauma (Dirim et al. 2005). Most hemorrhages will thus expand slowly, being of venous origin, and there is a delay to development of clinical symptomatology. At surgery, there has been an operative confirmation of the venous origin reported (Yilmazlar et al. 2005) which has included tearing of the venous dural sinuses, emissary veins and venous lakes or arachnoid granulation rupture.

In some series (Pillay and Peter 1995) there has been good outcome reported after surgical management – this is felt to be a result of a combination of factors including the subacute evolution of the hemorrhage and an association with minor occipital trauma. This is a common presentation in the 5- to 10-year-old child.

Subdural hematomas

It is reported (d'Avella et al. 2003) that acute subdural hematomas of the posterior fossa are very rare (0.2% of all intracranial traumatic injuries). Case series published include some pediatric patients. The causes are high-velocity motor vehicle accidents as well as low-energy falls. The CT findings are of an extra or retrocerebellar hemorrhage in a concave-convex shape within the posterior fossa.

In one case series (d'Avella et al. 2003), 19 of 24 patients were managed with decompressive suboccipital craniectomy. Surgical evacuation was indicated for hemorrhage thickness greater than 1cm. Better outcome was observed with patients who had admission Glasgow Coma Scores greater than 8 and associated with moderate to mild head injuries. Overall, subdural hematomas in the posterior fossa are felt to have poor prognostic outcome and to be life threatening.

There are a limited number of case reports discussing chronic subdural hematoma and effusions in the posterior fossa (Suzuki et al. 2007), indicated as being more common in children and newborn infants. The mechanisms are as a result of traumatic damage to the posterior fossa and tearing of bridging veins – if chronic, the origin may be due to the transformation of an acute hemorrhage. Traumatic subdural effusions may be acute (with compressive symptoms developing within 3 days of injury) or subacute/chronic (Mori et al. 2007) associated with progressive hydrocephalus. Other causal mechanisms can include anticoagulation therapy or a rupture of an aneurysm or arteriovenous malformation. Chronic posterior fossa subdural effusions usually require surgical management.

One case report of a 6-month-old infant (Tu et al. 2006) describes a unilateral traumatic posterior fossa subdural effusion with secondary hydrocephalus presenting with lethargy, poor appetite, and vomiting 2 weeks after a head injury. The presumed mechanism was an arachnoid membrane tear due to the trauma with CSF efflux (ball valve-like mechanism).

Intracerebellar contusions

Traumatic intraparenchymal cerebellar contusions are similarly rare. The pathophysiological mechanism (d'Avella et al. 2001) of cerebral contusions is the impact of the brain against the hard bony surfaces of the anterior or middle fossa (acceleration-deceleration injury) or falx cerebri (rotational injury). The posterior fossa represents a more confined space than the cerebral calvarium. There are thus different contusional injury mechanisms in the posterior fossa which may include direct occipital injury with local parenchymal displacement or deformation. Rarely, a contrecoup injury can occur associated with frontal bone direct trauma (noting however the protective role of the strap muscles attached from under the inion).

Diffuse axonal injury due to severe rotational trauma can also affect the cerebellum with contusions in the superior vermis, tonsils, and inferior aspects of the cerebellar hemispheres (d'Avella et al. 2002).

There can be delayed progression of involvement with hemorrhaging into contused areas. In a series of ten patients (d'Avella et al. 2002), there was an evolution of the clinical radiological findings and course in all patients – five of whom were children aged 9 to 16 years.

A conservative approach can be used for noncomatose patients with intraparenchymal clots less than 3cm in diameter (d'Avella et al. 2001), otherwise surgical management is recommended.

Traumatic arterial dissection and aneurysm formation

Vertebral artery dissection (Fig. 40.2) presents with occipital headache or posterior neck pain (Arnold and Bousser 2005) and associated symptoms of posterior circulation ischemia (vertigo, vomiting, diplopia, and motor signs). The dissection can occur following traumatic head and neck injury. A relationship to trivial trauma and chiropractic manipulation is described. The initial imaging findings (Jao et al. 2008) are of cerebellar or brainstem infarction or subarachnoid hemorrhage (Schuster et al. 1999).

Extra- and intracranial vertebral artery dissection is described. Intracranial dissection can be isolated or associated with an extracranial extension and basilar artery involvement. Dissection of the posteroinferior cerebellar artery (PICA) may be the result of extension from the intracranial vertebral artery or can be isolated.

Investigations to establish the diagnosis (Jao et al. 2008) include diffusion-weighted magnetic resonance studies, wall imaging (T1-fat suppression technique), CT and MR angiography. Conventional (cervical four-vessel) angiography will show focal stenosis with fusiform aneurymal dilatation. Prominent fusiform dilatation (which may be associated with a saccular pouch) is considered as a pseudoaneurysm. Three-dimensional reconstruction angiography demonstrates the dissection site.

The pathophysiology which may explain vertebral artery and PICA dissection relates to a number of factors (Jao et al. 2008). The PICA has considerable anatomic variability (Schuster et al. 1999). There is a higher incidence of internal elastic lamina defects near the origin of the PICA. The intradural portion is more susceptible to rupture as there is lack of an external elastic lamina with fewer elastic fibers in the media.

Intracranial traumatic aneurysms can be caused by penetrating wounds with related skull fractures (Sure et al. 1999). Traumatic impact on other arterial structures and the tentorium are considered causal and there is one case report of rotatory trauma resulting in a form of tear-out injury of a perforating artery. In this case, there was a delayed diagnosis with subarachnoid hemorrhage and the finding of a PICA aneurysm.

Initial treatment is usually with anticoagulation to prevent artery-to-artery emboli, and long-term treatment involves the use of antiplatelet agents. Surgical management or embolization (Jao et al. 2008) is necessary in ruptured dissecting aneurysms.

Special considerations

Posterior fossa syndrome and cerebellar mutism

Transient cerebellar mutism is rare but recognized as being associated with midline cerebellar lesions, most commonly related to posterior fossa tumor resection (Koh et al. 1997). There are cases reported following severe head trauma with cerebellar hemisphere and peduncle contusion and hemorrhage.

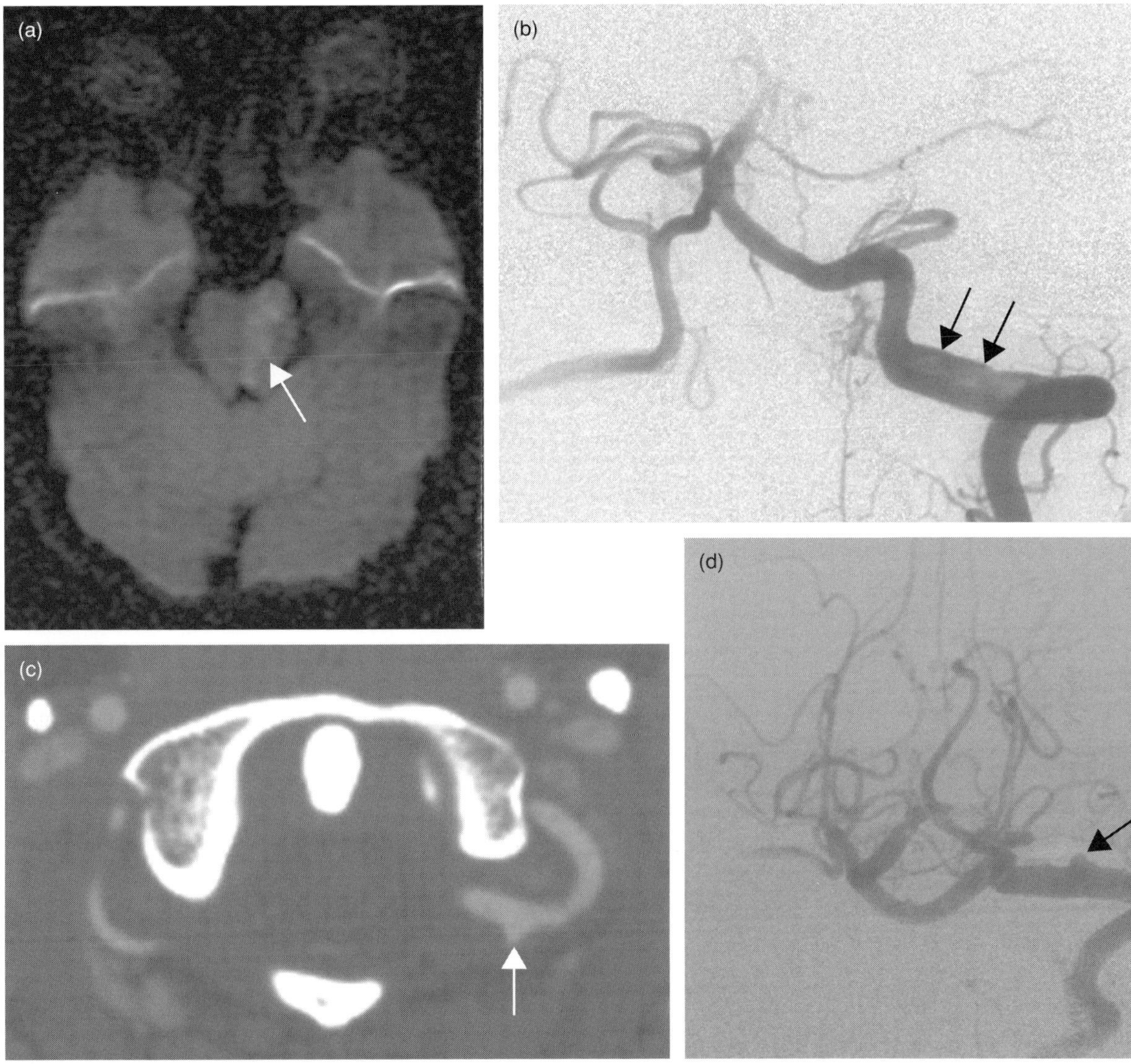

Fig. 40.2. Vertebral artery dissection in a 12-year-old boy with acute infarction in the left midbrain (with diffusion restriction) **(a)** and angiographic filling defect in left vertebral artery. **(b)** Note the small pseudoneurysm at this site on the follow up CT **(c)** and follow up angiography **(d)**. (Courtesy of Dr. Manohar Shroff.)

The mutism occurs in the setting of intact cranial nerve function. As the mutism resolves, articulation is characterized by impaired fluency and modulation of speech.

Posterior fossa syndrome with mutism, cerebellar signs, oromotor and oculomotor apraxia with emotional lability (Morris et al. 2009) can be seen with infratentorial injury. Similarly, this is most commonly reported after posterior fossa neurosurgical procedures.

A recent study using postoperative MRI and diffusion tensor imaging (Morris et al. 2009) suggests that posterior fossa syndrome may be related to multiple bilateral injuries to the proximal dentatothalamo-cortical pathways.

Birth-related cerebellar injury

Preterm infants

Cerebellar injury is seen in 2.3–3% of preterm infants with birthweight less than 1500 grams and 19% of those weighing less than 750 grams (Steggerda et al. 2009). It is thus considered to occur frequently in very preterm infants.

Improved detection of cerebellar injury is achieved by serial ultrasonographic imaging with additional views of the posterior fossa structures using the mastoid and posterior fontanels. Magnetic resonance imaging is required for detection of smaller punctate cerebellar hemorrhages.

It is felt that the developing cerebellum is highly vulnerable to injury (Steggerda et al. 2009) with the risk of destruction of immature cerebellar structures and effect on long-term neurodevelopmental outcome.

A recent report (Bednarek et al. 2008), which included six very low birthweight preterm infants, demonstrated cerebellar injury using mastoid fontanel ultrasonographic studies. The hemorrhagic lesions detected were acquired – and found at approximately 7 days of life. These can be associated with intraventricular hemorrhage and germinal matrix haemorrhage, but isolated cerebellar injuries and hemorrhages can occur.

An outcome study of cerebellar infarction in preterm infants showed neurodevelopmental disabilities with cognitive impairment, hypotonia, and microcephaly (Bednarek et al. 2008).

Term infants

Cerebellar injury and hemorrhage in term infants is no longer considered rare, given the improved resolution of newer imaging techniques (Limperopoulos et al. 2009). The causal factors are frequently traumatic delivery, forceps or vacuum assisted delivery, and prolonged labor (with cranial molding). With traumatic delivery, there is distortion and disruption of the venous structures in the skull and there can be direct cerebellar vermal laceration (Limperopoulos et al. 2009). The pathogenesis of injury, however, is likely to be multifactorial.

In a case series of 23 term infants (Limperopoulos et al. 2009), those with larger cerebellar lesions had long-term outcome assessment showing hemispheral and vermis atrophy with motor, cognitive, language, and behavioral deficits. A concerning association with autism was reported in children with atrophy of the superior cerebellar vermis.

In term infants, posterior fossa hemorrhage presentation is usually at several days of life (Usul et al. 2005) with lethargy and irritability. Brainstem and cranial nerve signs may follow with respiratory distress.

Diagnosis is by CT or MRI. Treatment can be by surgical evacuation or conservative observational management assessing for acute deterioration.

FRACTURES OF THE CLIVUS AND RETROCLIVAL EPIDURAL HEMATOMA

Pediatric patients are included in a series of patients (Ochalski et al. 2009) with central cranial base fractures and craniocervical junction injuries – there are thus clival fractures which may be oblique, transverse or longitudinal. The mechanisms of injury are predominantly motor vehicle accident-related, with other causes including falls, assaults and crush injuries. These injuries are associated with high-energy trauma (Paterakis et al. 2005).

Associated complications include cerebral spinal fluid leak (rhinorrhea or otorrhea), cranial nerve injuries, and hemorrhage.

Retroclival fractures with epidural hematoma are very rare and in some cases there is atlanto-axial or atlanto-occipital dislocations with ligament disruption (Kwon et al. 2008) and venous rupture. In these cases, the mechanism is cervical hyperextension or hyperflexion. These patients have multiple cranial nerve pareses.

Fractures of the clivus were considered to be fatal because of brainstem trauma or vertebrobasilar arterial injury and occlusion (Menkü et al. 2004). More recently, hospitalized patients managed by multidisciplinary surgical teams have had a lower mortality rate but there remains a high incidence of poor long-term outcome (Ochalski et al. 2009).

Outcome of traumatic cerebellar injury

The cerebellum has important functions for motor learning and coordination (Steinlin 2008). There is evidence to support cerebellar contributions to attention, language sequencing, memory, and visual spatial skills (Frank et al. 2007). It is suggested that childhood cerebellar injury or dysfunction can result in neurocognitive problems.

Focal cerebellar infarction (Steinlin 2008) results in impairment of cognition, attention, and short-term memory. There is concern, however, that studies to assess post-injury cognitive function (Frank et al. 2007) may misinterpret or overinterpret the role of the cerebellum. Well-controlled lesional studies are needed.

A small case series (Schmahmann et al. 2007) described neuropsychiatric problems in patients with congenital and acquired cerebellar lesions including traumatic injury. Abnormal behavior included distractability, hyperactivity, anxiety, stereotypic behaviors, and aggression. The 'cerebellar cognitive affective syndrome' is felt to represent dysregulation of affect with lesions of the limbic cerebellum (vermis and fastigial nucleus).

Interesting animal studies using the neonatal rat (Willson et al. 2007) showed that unilateral transection of the olivocerebellar pathway (by pedunculotomy) at different ages resulted in transcommissural reinnervation which was associated with spatial learning (using locomotor tests and a water maze). Another animal model used to assess post-traumatic brain injury pathophysiological changes (Park et al. 2007) suggested that there is susceptibility to selective Purkinje cell loss and white matter involvement (Matschke et al. 2007). Cerebellar atrophy after mild (Matschke et al. 2007) and moderate to severe traumatic brain injury (Spanos et al. 2007) is the result of reduced cerebellar white matter volume.

Damage to the cerebellum may be structure specific and related to projection areas which are at risk for fiber degeneration. Disruption of the frontal cerebellar system may contribute to cognitive and behavioral sequelae. The cerebellum may affect striatal activity (Centonze et al. 2008). Plasticity in the striatum may function in mediating motor symptoms after cerebellar injury. In a series of children with severe head trauma (Soto-Ares et al. 2001) six patients had cerebellar atrophy associated with frontal or temporal lesions. It is thought that there may be interruption of the afferent input from the corticopontocerebellar pathways with resultant fiber degeneration.

Comment

As traumatic injury to the cerebellum in isolation has been uncommon, there has been little study of the outcome and sequelae of such injuries. The availability of neurodiagnostic imaging and an array of new treatment approaches has allowed for a greater understanding of the nature of cerebellar traumatic injury and improved outcomes.

While the motor and coordination aspects of the cerebellar function have been well understood, there is growing appreciation of the role of the cerebellum in cognition and behavior.

Lesional studies will now allow a greater understanding of the neuropsychological aspects of cerebellar injury and the effects on functioning. The very complex interplay of the connections between the cerebrum and cerebellum require continued study and assessment. The availability of diffusion tensor imaging will assist in studies of post-injury cerebellar functioning.

REFERENCES

Arnold M, Bousser MG (2005) Clinical manifestations of vertebral artery dissection. Handbook on cerebral artery dissection. Front Neurol Neurosci 20: 77–86.

Balik V, Lehto H, Hoza D, Sulla J, Hernesniemi J (2010) Posterior fossa extradural haematomas. Cen Eur Neurosurg 71: 167–172.

Bednarek N, Akhavi A, Pietrement C, Mesmin F, Loron G, Morville P (2008) Outcome of cerebellar injury in very low birth-weight Infants: 6 case reports. J Child Neurol 23: 906–911.

Berker M, Cataltepe O, Özcan OE (2003) Traumatic epidural haematoma of the posterior fossa in childhood: 16 new cases. Br J Neurosurg 17: 226–229.

Centonze D, Rossi S, De Bartolo P, De Chiara V, Foti F, Musella A, et al. (2008) Adaptations of glutamatergic synapses in the striatum contribute to recovery from cerebellar damage. Eur J Neurosci 27: 2188–2196.

d'Avella D, Cacciola F, Angileri S, Cardali S, La Rosa G, Germanò A, Tomasello F (2001) Traumatic intracerebellar hemorrhagic contusions and hematomas. J Neurosurg Sci 45: 29–37.

d'Avella D, Servadei F, Scerrati M, Tomei G, Brambilla G, Angileri FF, et al. (2002) Traumatic intracerebellar hemorrhage: Clinicoradiological analysis of 81 patients. Neurosurgery 50: 16–27.

d'Avella D, Servadei F, Scerrati M, Tomei G, Brambilla G, Massaro F, et al. (2003) Traumatic acute subdural haematomas of the posterior fossa: clinicoradiological analysis of 24 patients. Acta Neurochirurgica (Wien) 145: 1037–1044.

Dirim BV, Örük C, Erdoğan N, Gelal F, Uluç E (2005) Traumatic posterior fossa hematomas. Diagn Interv Radiol 11: 14–18.

Frank B, Schoch B, Richter S, Frings M, Karnath HO, Timmann D (2007) Cerebellar lesion studies of cognitive function in children and adolescents – limitations and negative findings. Cerebellum 6: 242–253.

Jao T, Liu HM, Tang SC, Jeng JS (2008) Dissection of the posterior inferior cerebellar artery in a young adult with cerebellar infarct. Acta Neurol Taiwan 17: 243–247.

Karasu A, Sabanci PA, Izgi N, Imer M, Sencer A, Cansever T, Canbolat A (2008) Traumatic epidural hematomas of the posterior cranial fossa. Surg Neurol 69: 247–252.

Koh S, Turkel SB, Baram TZ (1997) Cerebellar mutism in children: report of six cases and potential mechanisms. Pediatr Neurol 16: 218–219.

Kwon TH, Joy H, Park YK, Chung HS (2008) Traumatic retroclival epidural hematoma in a child. Neurol Med Chir (Toyko) 48: 347–350.

Limperopoulos C, Robertson RL, Sullivan NR, Bassan H, Plessis AJ (2009) Cerebellar injury in term infants: clinical characteristics, magnetic resonance imaging findings, and outcome. Pediatr Neurol 41: 1–8.

Matschke J, Laas R, Schulz F (2007) Cerebellar atrophy following mild head injury in a 4-year-old girl. Pediatr Neurosurg 43: 330–333.

Menkü A, Koc RK, Tucer B, Durak AC, Akdemir H (2004) Clivus fractures: clinical presentations and courses. Neurosurg Rev 27: 194–198.

Mori H, Ohashi H, Nonaka Y, Oi S (2007) Traumatic subacute subdural effusion in the posterior fossa associated with secondary acute hydrocephalus in a neonate. J Neurosurg 107: 159–162.

Morris EB, Phillips NS, Laningham FH, Patay Z, Gajjar A, Wallace D, et al. (2009) Proximal dentatothalamocortical tract involvement in posterior fossa syndrome. Brain 132: 3087–3095.

Ochalski PG, Spiro RM, Fabio A, Kassam AB, Okonkwo DO (2009) Fractures of the clivus: A contemporary series in the computed tomography era. Neurosurgery 65: 1063–1069.

Park E, Ai J, Baker AJ (2007) Cerebellar injury: clinical relevance and potential in traumatic brain injury research. Progr Brain Res 161: 327–338.

Paterakis KN, Karantanas AH, Hadjigeorgiou GM, Anagnostopoulos V, Karavelis A (2005) Retroclival epidural hematoma secondary to a longitudinal clivus fracture. Clin Neurol Neurosurg 108: 67–72.

Pillay R, Peter JC (1995) Extradural haematomas in children. S Afr J Med J 85: 672–674.

Schmahmann JD, Weilburg JB, Sherman JC (2007) The neuropsychiatry of the cerebellum – insights from the clinic. Cerebellum 6: 254–267.

Schuster JM, Santiago P, Elliott JP, Grady MS, Newell DW, Winn HR (1999) Acute traumatic posteroinferior cerebellar artery aneurysms: report of three cases. Neurosurgery 45: 1465–1468.

Soto-Ares G, Vinchon M, Delmaire C, Abecidan E, Dhellemes P, Pruvo JP (2001) Cerebellar atrophy after severe traumatic head injury in children. Child's Nerv Syst 17: 263–269.

Spanos GK, Wilde EA, Bigler ED, Cleavinger HB, Fearing MA, Levin HS, et al. (2007) Cerebellar atrophy after moderate-to-severe pediatric traumatic brain Injury. Am J Neuroradiol 28: 537–542.

Steggerda SJ, Leijser LM, Wiggers-de Bruïne FT, van der Grond J, Walther FJ, van Wezel-Meijler G (2009) Cerebellar injury in preterm infants: Incidence and findings on US and MR images. Radiology 252: 190–199.

Steinlin M (2008) Cerebellar disorders in childhood: cognitive problems. Cerebellum 7: 607–610.

Sure U, Becker R, Petermeyer M, Bertalanffy H (1999) Aneurysm of the posterior inferior cerebellar artery caused by a traumatic perforating artery tear-out mechanism in a child. Child's Nerv System 15: 354–356.

Suzuki C, Maeda M, Matsushima N, Takamura M, Matsubara T, Taki W, Takeda K (2007) Spontaneous chronic subdural hematoma of the posterior fossa. J Neuroradiol 34: 213–215.

Tu PH, Lui TN, Hsu HH, Lee ST (2006) Unilateral traumatic posterior fossa subdural effusion in an infant. J Clin Neurosci 13: 128–130.

Usul H, Karaasian G, Cakir E, Kuzeyl K, Mungan I, Baykal S (2005) Conservative management of spontaneous posterior fossa subdural hematoma in a neonate. J Clin Neurosci 12: 196–198.

Willson ML, Bower AJ, Sherrard RM (2007) Developmental neural plasticity and its cognitive benefits: olivocerebellar reinnervation compensates for spatial function in the cerebellum. Eur J Neurosci 25: 1475–1483.

Yilmazlar S, Kocaeli H, Dogan S, Abas F, Aksoy K, Kofali E, Doygun M (2005) Traumatic epidural haematomas of nonarterial origin: analysis of 30 consecutive cases. Acta Neurochir (Wien) 147: 1241–1248.

41
Toxic Agents

Andrea Poretti and Eugen Boltshauser

Experience in adults

It is well known from clinical observations in adults that the cerebellum is vulnerable to a large range of toxic agents (Timmann and Diener 2000; Manto 2010).

Purkinje cells (particularly sensitive to alcohol and phenytoin) and granule cells are the most important target for toxic substances (Fonnum and Lock 2000, 2004).

The most relevant toxic agents are alcohol, several drugs such as phenytoin, antineoplastic drugs, and lithium, heavy metals (mercury, lead, and thallium), several 'industrial' organic solvents, insecticides, herbicides, heroin, and cocaine.

Chronic intoxication (overuse) may lead to a permanent ataxic syndrome, often with evident cerebellar atrophy on neuroimaging (e.g., alcohol consumption and chronic phenytoin treatment). Although phenytoin is no longer recommended as a first-line treatment in epilepsy, it is remarkable that up to the present case reports of recognized and missed intoxications are still being published (Brostoff et al. 2008). Acute exposure may prompt acute reversible signs, but may also result in permanent cerebellar damage, as in phenytoin intoxication (Kuruvilla and Bharucha 1997; Alioglu et al. 2000) and drug abuse. Heroin-induced leukencephalopathy typically involves the cerebellar white matter (with sparing of the dentate nuclei), but sparing of the cerebellum has been observed as well (Wolters et al. 1982; Ryan et al. 2005; Offiah and Hall 2008). Cocain-dependent individuals were found to have reduced cerebellar gray matter compared to controls (Sim et al. 2007). Cocaine consumption seems to pose an increased risk for developing cerebellar infarctions. Overdose of metronidazole can prompt reversible changes within the dentate nuclei (Heaney et al. 2003; Bonkowsky et al. 2007).

Drugs which may trigger cerebellar ataxia are lithium salts, phenytoin, valproate, amiodarone, metronidazole, procainamide, and isoniazid (Marmolino and Manto 2010).

Experience in children and adolescents

Because of different potential exposure and consumption of toxic agents, the problem of cerebellotoxic agents is fortunately small in the pediatric age.

Phenytoin is almost out of use for chronic antiepileptic treatment in developed countries, but is still used occasionally in status epilepticus. Cerebellar atrophy has been repeatedly documented in chronic phenytoin treatment (Baier et al. 1984; personal observation).

Valproate is a widely used anticonvulsant drug and tremor (reversible) is a known side-effect. Truncal ataxia and cerebellar atrophy have been reported in a 10-year-old child with Lennox Gastaut syndrome and valproate toxicity (Ghosh et al. 2011).

Vigabatrin is first-line treatment in patients with infantile spasms and tuberous sclerosis. Reversible T2-hyperintensities in thalami, globi pallidi, dentate nuclei, brainstem, and corpus callosum have been reported (Pearl et al. 2009).

Antineoplastic chemotherapy: In clinical practice cerebellotoxicity is not recognised as a relevant complication. Cerebral leukencephalopathy, often demonstrable by neuroimaging, is a known side-effect of systemic and intrathecal/intraventricular application of drugs such as methotrexate as well as cytarabine. The cerebellum is not a primary target as judged from neurological examination and imaging.

Drug abuse (heroin, cocaine, methadone)

We have encountered accidental drug intoxication by heroin in a toddler leading to severe cerebellar and cerebral leukencephalopathy with permanent sequelae (Fig. 41.1). Cerebellar infarctions were reported in adolescent males associated with acute marijuana use (Geller et al. 2004). Mills et al. reported acute cerebellitis representing a toxic encephalopathy with supra- and infratentorial leukoencephalopathy and swelling of the cerebellum causing hydrocephalus following accidental ingestion of methadone by a 3-year-old girl (Mills et al. 2008). The follow-up MRI 2 months later revealed tissue loss with atrophy of the cerebellar hemispheres. Zanin et al. reported a 30-month-old girl, who developed ataxia, dysarthria, and abnormal movements 5 days after methadone intoxication. Despite a normal MRI in the acute state, 19 days and 4 weeks after the intoxication MRI showed signal abnormalities in the temporomesial regions, basal ganglia, substantia nigra, and subtle changes involving the cerebellar cortex (Zanin et al. 2010).

Poisoning

Inhaled elemental mercury toxicity has been reported in three siblings with history of fever, increasing irritability, fatigue, malaise, insomnia, headache, anorexia, and ataxia (Florentine and Sanfilippo 1991). Carbon monoxide intoxication typically affect the deep gray matter, but cerebral cortex and cerebral white matter can be also involved. Damage of the cerebellum (particularly sparing the cerebrum) is rare (Mascalchi et al. 1996; Yang and Jeon 2011). In cyanide intoxication cerebellar and cerebral gray matter are particularly affected (Barkovich 2005).

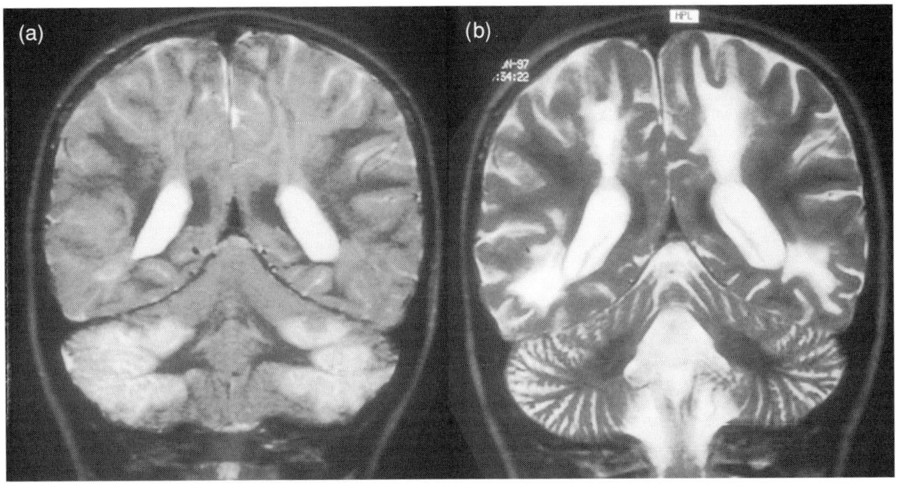

Fig. 41.1. Serial coronal T2-weighted MR imaging of a child with accidental heroin intoxication: **(a)** at 3 years in the acute phase showing hyperintensity of the cerebellar cortex as well as widespread signal changes in the cerebral white matter; **(b)** 3 months later demonstrating symmetric atrophy of the cerebellar hemispheres and supratentorial leukoencephalopathy. (Reprinted with permission from Poretti A et al. Eur J Paediatr Neurol. 2008; 12: 155–167.)

REFERENCES

Alioglu Z, Sari A, Velioglu SK, Özmenoglu M (2000) Cerebellar atrophy following acute phenytoin intoxication. J Neuroradiol 27: 52–55.

Baier WK, Bck U, Doose H, Klinge H, Hirsch W (1984) Cerebellar atrophy following diphenylhydantoin intoxication. Neuropediatrics 15: 76–81.

Barkovich AJ (2005) Toxic and metabolic brain disorders. In: Barkovich AJ, editor. Pediatric Neuroimaging. Philadelphia: Lippincott Williams & Wilkins; 130–131.

Bonkowsky JL, Sondrup C, Benedict SL (2007) Acute reversible cerebellar lesions associated with metronidazole therapy. Neurology 68: 180.

Brostoff JM, Birns J, McCrea D (2008) Phenytoin toxicity: an easily missed cause of cerebellar syndrome. J Clin Pharm Ther 33: 211–214.

Florentine MJ, Sanfilippo DJ (1991) Elemental mercury poisoning. Clin Pharm 10: 213–221.

Fonnum F, Lock EA (2000) Cerebellum as a target for toxic substances. Toxicol Lett 112–113: 9–16.

Fonnum F, Lock EA (2004) The contributions of excitotoxicity, glutathione depletion and DNA repair in chemically induced injury to neurones: exemplified with toxic effects on cerebellar granule cells. J Neurochem 88: 513–531.

Geller T, Loftis L, Brink DS (2004) Cerebellar infarction in adolescent males associated with acute marijuana use. Pediatrics 113: e365–370.

Ghosh VB, Kapoor S, Prakash A, Bhatt S (2011) Cerebellar atrophy in a child with valproate toxicity. Indian J Pediatr. 78: 999–1001.

Heaney CJ, Campeau NG, Lindell EP (2003) MR imaging and diffusion-weighted imaging changes in metronidazole (flagyl)-induced cerebellar toxicity. AJNR Am J Neuroradiol 24: 1615–1617.

Kuruvilla T, Bharucha NE (1997) Cerebellar atrophy after acute phenytoin intoxication. Epilepsia 38: 500–502.

Manto MU (2010) Toxic agents. In: Cerebellar Disorders (Manto MU, ed.). New York: Cambridge University Press; 157–170.

Marmolino D, Manto M (2010) Past, present and future therapeutics for cerebellar ataxias. Curr Neuropharmacol 8: 41–61.

Mascalchi M, Petruzzi P, Zampa V (1996) MRI of cerebellar white matter damage due to carbon monoxide poising: case report. Neuroradiology 38: S73–S74.

Mills F, MacLennan SC, Devile CJ, Saunders DE (2008) Severe cerebellitis following methadone poisoning. Pediatr Radiol 38: 227–229.

Offiah C, Hall E (2008) Heroin-induced leukoencephalopathy. Characterization using MRI, diffusion-weighted imaging, and MR spectroscopy. Clin Radiol 63: 146–152.

Pearl PL, Vezina LG, Saneto RP, McCarter R, Molloy-Wells E, Heffron A, et al. (2009) Cerebral MRI abnormalities associated with vigabatrin therapy. Epilepsia 50: 184–194.

Ryan A, Molloy FM, Farrell MA, Hutchinson M (2005) Fatal toxic leukoencephalopathy: clinical, radiological, and necropsy findings in two patients. J Neurol Neurosurg Psychiatry 76: 1014–1016.

Sim ME, Lyoo IK, Streeter CC, Covell J, Sarid-Segal O, Ciraulo DA, et al. (2007) Cerebellar gray matter volume correlates with duration of cocaine use in cocaine-dependent subjects. Neuropsychopharmacology 32: 2229–2237.

Timmann D, Diener HC (2000) Alcoholic cerebellar degeneration (including ataxias that are due to other toxic causes). In: Handbook of Ataxia Disorders (Klockgether T, ed.). New York: Marcel Dekker; 571–605.

Wolters EC, van Wijngaarden GK, Stam FC, Rengelink H, Lousberg RJ, Schipper ME, Verbeeten B (1982) Leucoencephalopathy after inhaling 'heroin' pyrolysate. Lancet 2: 1233–1237.

Yang HJ, Jeon BS (2011) Selective cerebellar degeneration following carbon monoxide poisoning. AJNR Am J Neuroradiol 32: E39.

Zanin A, Masiero S, Severino MS, Calderone M, Da Dalt L, Laverda AM (2010) A delayed methadone encephalopathy: clinical and neuroradiological findings. J Child Neurol 25: 748–751.

42
Gluten Ataxia

Andrea Poretti and Eugen Boltshauser

Coeliac disease or gluten sensitivity is a chronic, immune-mediated, inflammatory disorder of the small intestine triggered by the ingestion of gluten (Barker and Liu 2008; Zawahir et al. 2009). Its overall prevalence varies between 0.4% and 1.3% in the childhood population (Rewers 2005). Coeliac disease involves both the innate and adaptive immune system with three main features: presence of the human leukocyte antigen (HLA) type II molecules DQ2 or DQ8, specific antibodies to transglutaminase-2, and dependence on exposure to gluten, that is, full remission following the implementation of a strict gluten-free diet (Zawahir et al. 2009). The response to gluten results in characteristic damage to the villi, resulting in malabsorption. Therefore, toddlers and young children classically present with failure to thrive, diarrhea, and abdominal distension some time after the introduction of gluten in the diet, but more often they present with subtle gastrointestinal symptoms such as constipation (Barker and Liu 2008; Zawahir et al. 2009). The standard diagnostic criterion remains the duodenal biopsy. However, a stepwise approach is needed, starting with a high degree of clinical suspicion and serological tests. These include antigliadin IgA and IgG (nonspecific), antideamidated gliadin (highly sensitive and specific, but not widely used and validated), antiendomysial IgA (highly sensitive and specific, but expensive and operator dependent), and antitransglutaminase-2 IgA and IgG (highly sensitive and specific, and not operator dependent) (Zawahir et al. 2009).

Particularly in older children, the clinical presentation can be dominated by extraintestinal symptoms ('atypical manifestation') causing a significant delay in the diagnosis. Dermatitis herpetiformis, unexplained short stature, delayed puberty, vitamin deficiencies, iron deficiency anaemia unresponsive to therapy, recurrent aphthous stomatitis, elevated transaminases, dental enamel hypoplasia, autoimmune thyroiditis, arthritis, arthralgias, and neuropsychiatric symptoms are the most common extraintestinal symptoms associated with coeliac disease (Barker and Liu 2008; Zawahir et al. 2009).

In adults, the prevalence of neurological dysfunction in patients with coeliac disease has been estimated to be between 10% and 25% (Hadjivassiliou et al. 2010). Peripheral neuropathy, cerebellar ataxia, encephalopathy, headaches, epileptic seizures, myopathy, myelopathy, stiff-man syndrome, and myoclonic ataxia are possible neurological manifestations of coeliac disease (Hadjivassiliou et al. 2003, 2010). In adults, gluten ataxia presents at a mean age of 53 years, affects both trunk and limbs, is always associated with positive IgG and/or IgA antigliadin antibodies, and brain MRI can show various degrees of cerebellar atrophy (Hadjivassiliou et al. 2010).

Current evidence suggests that neurological symptoms in coeliac disease are immune mediated, while deficiency of vitamins and trace elements rarely plays a part (Hadjivassiliou et al. 2010). Postmortem studies showed patchy loss of Purkinje cells in the cerebellar cortex as well as diffuse infiltration mainly of T-lymphocytes within the cerebellar white matter and marked perivascular cuffing with inflammatory cells (Hadjivassiliou et al. 2010). Experimental studies suggest an antibody cross-reactivity between antigenic epitopes on Purkinje cells and gluten peptides (Hadjivassiliou et al. 2010). The concept of gluten ataxia is not accepted by all authors and is highly controversial. Some authors find antigliadin antibodies in patients with sporadic and genetically confirmed spinocerebellar ataxia. Abele et al. determined antigliadin antibodies in 95 patients with ataxia and 73 controls (Abele et al. 2003). Antibodies were positive in 8% of the controls, 19% of patients with sporadic ataxia, 8% of patients with recessive ataxia, and 15% of patients with dominant ataxia (Abele et al. 2003). The authors concluded that positivity for antigliadin antibodies may be a consequence, not the cause, of cerebellar degeneration, raising some controversy about the entity of gluten ataxia (Abele et al. 2003; Bushara and Hallett 2004).

Children with coeliac disease have an increased risk of developing neurological complications during childhood, but the overall prevalence of neurological involvement in children is lower than in adults (Lionetti et al. 2010). Explanations for this difference may include the following: the relatively short duration of gluten exposure in children (insufficient to cause involvement of the nervous system), the early elimination of gluten from the diet, a strict adherence to a gluten-free diet (both may be preventive for the development of neurological symptoms), and a different susceptibility to immune-mediated disorders (Lionetti et al. 2010).

Neurological manifestations of coeliac disease in children are headache and neuropathy (Lionetti et al. 2010). Lionetti et al. found that children with coeliac disease at diagnosis had a significantly higher prevalence of headaches than healthy controls (24.8% versus 8%) (Lionetti et al. 2009). A similar prevalence has been reported by Zelnik et al. (2004). Adherence to a gluten-free diet led to an amelioration of headache in about three-quarters of the children (Lionetti et al. 2009). Cakir et al. and Ruggieri et al. reported mixed patterns of axonal motor and sensory polyneuropathy, pure sensory polyneuropathy, and acute predominantly motor demyelinating neuropathy in children with coeliac disease (Cakir et al. 2007; Ruggieri et al. 2008).

Cerebellar ataxia in children with coeliac disease has been explored in just a few studies (Lionetti et al. 2010). Kieslich et al. reported mild ataxia in two children (2.7%), whereas Zelnick et al. found ataxia (gait and limb ataxia as well as nystagmus) in six patients with coeliac disease (5.4%) (Kieslich et al. 2001; Zelnik et al. 2004). However, in a prospective study including 835 children with coeliac disease, Ruggieri et al. did not find children with cerebellar ataxia (Ruggieri et al. 2008). Therefore, a possible association between coeliac disease and cerebellar ataxia in children remains unclear. An explanation for the difference between the apparently high prevalence of ataxia in adults with coeliac disease and the low or null prevalence in children could be the age-related effect of coeliac disease on the cerebellum and/or the possible preventive action of the early gluten-free diet.

REFERENCES

Abele M, Schols L, Schwartz S, Klockgether T (2003) Prevalence of antigliadin antibodies in ataxia patients. Neurology 60: 1674–1675.

Barker JM, Liu E (2008) Celiac disease: pathophysiology, clinical manifestations, and associated autoimmune conditions. Adv Pediatr 55: 349–365.

Bushara K, Hallett M (2004) Prevalence of antigliadin antibodies in ataxia patients. Neurology 62: 1237–1238.

Cakir D, Tosun A, Polat M, Celebisoy N, Gokben S, Aydogdu S, et al. (2007) Subclinical neurological abnormalities in children with celiac disease receiving a gluten-free diet. J Pediatr Gastroenterol Nutr 45: 366–369.

Hadjivassiliou M, Grunewald R, Sharrack B, Sanders D, Lobo A, Williamson C, et al. (2003) Gluten ataxia in perspective: epidemiology, genetic susceptibility and clinical characteristics. Brain 126: 685–691.

Hadjivassiliou M, Sanders DS, Grunewald RA, Woodroofe N, Boscolo S, Aeschlimann D (2010) Gluten sensitivity: from gut to brain. Lancet Neurol 9: 318–330.

Kieslich M, Errazuriz G, Posselt HG, Moeller-Hartmann W, Zanella F, Boehles H (2001) Brain white-matter lesions in celiac disease: a prospective study of 75 diet-treated patients. Pediatrics 108: E21.

Lionetti E, Francavilla R, Maiuri L, Ruggieri M, Spina M, Pavone P, et al. (2009) Headache in pediatric patients with celiac disease and its prevalence as a diagnostic clue. J Pediatr Gastroenterol Nutr 49: 202–207.

Lionetti E, Francavilla R, Pavone P, Pavone L, Francavilla T, Pulvirenti A, et al. (2010) The neurology of coeliac disease in childhood: what is the evidence? A systematic review and meta-analysis. Dev Med Child Neurol 52: 700–707.

Rewers M (2005) Epidemiology of celiac disease: what are the prevalence, incidence, and progression of celiac disease? Gastroenterology 128: S47–S51.

Ruggieri M, Incorpora G, Polizzi A, Parano E, Spina M, Pavone P (2008) Low prevalence of neurologic and psychiatric manifestations in children with gluten sensitivity. J Pediatr 152: 244–249.

Zawahir S, Safta A, Fasano A (2009) Pediatric celiac disease. Curr Opin Pediatr 21: 655–660.

Zelnik N, Pacht A, Obeid R, Lerner A (2004) Range of neurologic disorders in patients with celiac disease. Pediatrics 113: 1672–1676.

Checklists

Andrea Poretti and Eugen Boltshauser

In this chapter we provide checklists for selected clinical and neuroimaging aspects. These lists can be used as 'memo lists'; they are not meant to be complete. The conditions listed are in random order. Note that for a given condition a range of findings may occur, which do not all have to be present (spectrum) to make a diagnosis. For the listed items we provide significant clinical or neuroimaging references.

TABLE 1
Congenital ataxia

Comment: This table lists conditions which (according to the literature and own experience) may present as congenital ataxia. Neuroimaging is important in this category. The final diagnosis often rests on additional disease-specific (clinical, ophthalmological, and neuroimaging) findings.

Disease		Comments	References
Nonprogressive congenital ataxia (often familial occurrence, mostly with autosomal recessive inheritance)		Early evidence of cerebellar ataxia, without progression on follow-up, cognitive impairment common; variable neuroimaging (normal, small cerebellum, small cerebellum with widened interfolial spaces)	Chapter 9; Steinlin et al. 1998; Steinlin et al. 1999
Cerebellar malformations	Dandy-Walker malformation (DWM)	At birth mostly asymptomatic, as infant macrocephaly and hydrocephalus, as child ataxia (50%) and cognitive impairment in about 50% of the cases; MRI diagnostic	Chapter 10; Bolduc and Limperopoulos 2009
	Joubert syndrome and related disorders (JSRD)	Ataxia, hypotonia, cognitive impairment, retinal dystrophy (not consistent), nephronophthisis (not consistent), postaxial polydactyly (not consistent), hypoplasia/dysplasia of the vermis, molar tooth sign	Chapter 11; Doherty 2009
	Rhombencephalosynapsis (RS)	Ataxia often mild, head nodding possible, often cognitive impairment; MRI diagnostic	Chapter 16; Poretti et al. 2009a
	Cerebellar agenesis	Only minute remnants of cerebellar tissue; flat pons; all patients symptomatic, mostly severe motor (ataxia) and cognitive impairment; remarkably all patients older than 2 years achieved independent walking	Chapter 7
	Cerebellar hypoplasia (CH)	Occurring in a wide range of genetic and acquired conditions (see checklist about CH), which can be associated with a spectrum of neuroimaging anomalies and clinical findings	Chapter 8; Wassmer et al. 2003
Congenital oculomotor apraxia type Cogan		Ocular motor apraxia, ataxia, mostly normal cognition, vermis hypoplasia (inconsistent)	Kondo et al. 2007; Orssaud et al. 2009
Cerebellar disruptions	Unilateral cerebellar hypoplasia (UCH)	Variable outcome ranging from almost normal development to marked developmental impairment; ataxia frequent but not a leading sign; involvement of the vermis often associated with a poorer cognitive outcome	Chapter 30; Poretti et al. 2010a
	Extreme preterm birth	Cerebellar hemispheres predominantly affected, vermis small, flat pons; significantly poorer motor and cognitive development as in similar preterms with normal cerebellum	Chapter 31; Messerschmidt et al. 2008
Metabolic disorders occasionally presenting as congenital ataxia	L-2-Hydroxyglutaric aciduria	Ataxia, macrocephaly, seizures, pyramidal signs, regression; distinct neuroimaging pattern with T2W-hyperintensity of subcortical cerebral white matter and dentate nuclei	Steenweg et al. 2010
	Glutaric aciduria type 1	Unusual as congenital ataxia; usual manifestation as acute encephalopathic crise with striatal injury and subsequently dystonia; various symptoms including tremor, dyskinesias, and ataxia in escaping the acute encephalopathic crise	Kölker et al. 2007; Korman et al. 2007
	Congenital disorders of glycosylation Ia	Ataxia, hypotonia, mental retardation (UK: learning disability), visceromegaly, retinitis pigmentosa, inverted nipples, ascites, pericardial effusion	Eklund and Freeze 2006
	Congenital disorders of glycosylation Iq	Ataxia, hypotonia, mental retardation (UK: learning disability), nystagmus, optic nerve atrophy, visual impairment, coloboma	Morava et al. 2010
	Pyruvate dehydrogenase (PDH) deficiency	Four phenotypic groups possible: neonatal encephalopathy with lactic acidosis, nonprogressive infantile encephalopathy, Leigh syndrome, and relapsing episodes of ataxia with axonal neuropathy	Barnerias et al. 2010
	Glucose transporter type 1 (GLUT1) deficiency	Motor and mental developmental delay, seizures with infantile onset, acquired microcephaly, dystonia, spasticity	Brockmann 2009; Leen et al. 2010
Early stage of infantile onset progressive ataxia	Ataxia teleangiectasia (Louis Bar syndrome)	Progressive ataxia, acquired ocular motor apraxia, ocular and cutaneous telangiectasia, choreoathetoid movements	Crawford et al. 2000

TABLE 1
(*continued*)

Disease		Comments	References
	Infantile-onset spinocerebellar ataxia (IOSCA)	After 1 year of age ataxia, muscle hypotonia, loss of deep-tendon reflexes, and athetosis; at school age ophthalmoplegia and sensorineural deafness; at adolescence sensory axonal neuropathy, optic atrophy, and in females hypergonadotrophic hypogonadism; myoclonic jerks or focal clonic seizures	Koskinen et al. 1994
	Mitochondrial disorders	Variable clinical manifestation	Hanna et al. 1995; Barnerias et al. 2010
	Marinesco-Sjögren syndrome	Early-onset (not necessarily congenital) cataracts, mild to severe cognitive impairment, hypotonia, muscle weakness, short stature, various skeletal abnormalities	Slavotinek et al. 2005
White matter disorders	Vanishing white matter disease (early childhood-onset form)	Onset of ataxia at the age of 1–2 years, subsequently generally progressive deterioration resulting in increasing difficulty in walking, tremor, spasticity, dysarthria, and seizures, later dysphagia and optic atrophy; acute encephalopathic crises following mild head trauma or febrile illness	van der Knaap et al. 2006
	Hypomyelination and congenital cataract	Congenital cataract, developmental delay, slowly progressive neurological impairment with spasticity, cerebellar ataxia, and mild-to-moderate mental retardation beginning at the age of 12–16 months	Biancheri et al. 2007
	Hypomyelination, hypogonadotropic hypogonadism and hypodontia (4H)	Early-onset ataxia, delayed dentition, hypomyelination and cerebellar atrophy	Wolf et al. 2007
Syndromes	Rett syndrome	Ataxia, dementia, autism, acquired microcephaly, hand stereotypies, epilepsy	Naidu et al. 2001
	Angelman syndrome	Ataxia, cognitive impairment, abnormal behaviour, epilepsy, microcephaly, absent speech	Williams 2005
KCNJ10 mutations		Multisystem channelopathy disorder consisting of early-onset epilepsy, ataxia, sensorineural deafness, and tubulopathy	Bockenbauer et al. 2009
NEUROD1 mutations (2q31)		Neonatal diabetes mellitus, ataxia, deafness, myopia, cerebellar hypoplasia	Rubio-Cabezas et al. 2010
CACNA1A mutation		Ataxia, mental retardation, dyskinesia, recurrent episodes of coma	Blumkin et al. 2010
Benign hereditary chorea (mutations in the *NKX2*-1 gene)		Early-onset chorea and ataxia, delayed motor development; tendency to improve	Fernandez et al. 2001; Kleiner-Fisman et al. 2003
Sensory ataxia in severe forms of hereditary hypomyelinating neuropathy		Nonprogressive weakness, areflexia, hypotonia, very slow nerve-conduction	Phillips et al. 1999
Midline tumours in the posterior fossa		Rarely midline tumours of the posterior fossa can present as congenital ataxia	Dobrovoljac et al. 2002

A new form of congenital cerebellar ataxia associated with epilepsy and cognitive impairment has been recently described in patients with mutations in the *KIAA0226* gene and called Salih ataxia (Assoum et al. 2010).

TABLE 2
Acute ataxia

Comment: In acute ataxia the onset of the symptoms is within hours, 'overnight', or within a few days. Bacterial meningitis and cerebellar tumours do not present as acute ataxia. At the first episode a disorder causing intermittent ataxia can present as acute ataxia.

Disease		Comments	References
Intoxication		Several drugs (such as benzodiazepines, phenytoin, carbamazepine, antihistamines, tricyclic antidepressants), alcohol, solvents, mercury; possible manifestation of Münchhausen syndrome by proxy	Manto 2010
Infection	Acute cerebellar ataxia	Commonly affects children aged 1 to 4 years, mostly 1 to 3 weeks after viral infection (mostly varicella, mumps, parvovirus, Epstein-Barr virus), self-limiting	Sawaishi and Takada 2002
Inflammation	Acute disseminating encephalomyelitis (ADEM)	Diagnosis made on the basis of neuroimaging and CSF examination; depending on the overall situation, steroid medication may be considered	Tenembaum et al. 2007
	Miller-Fisher syndrome	Diagnosis based on the presence of the clinical triad: ophthalmoplegia, areflexia, and ataxia (sensory rather than cerebellar); mydriasis and poor pupillary reaction possible	Garrett and Ryan 2002; Lo 2007
	Multiple sclerosis (MS) (rare)	Ataxia is the presenting feature in about 5–15% of the patients with MS and is particularly common (about 50%) in children younger than 10 years	Banwell et al. 2007
Paraneoplastic	Opsoclonus-myoclonus syndrome	May be associated with an occult neuroblastoma or ganglioneuroma; the course is often protracted and fluctuating; steroid therapy is usually efficient; variant without opsoclonus reported	Klein et al. 2007
Vascular	Posterior circulation stroke (rare)	Presenting symptoms can be nonspecific (nausea, vomiting, headache, gait ataxia); life-threatening complications possible (brainstem compression, hydrocephalus), peak on the third day	Ganesan 2002; Edlow et al. 2008
	Vertebral artery dissection (rare)	Often spontaneous (or due to minimal trauma), pain in the back of the neck, face, or head as presenting symptom	Bacigaluppi et al. 2006; Lin et al. 2007
	Cerebellar haemorrhages (rare)	Most commonly associated with arteriovenous malformations	Stapf et al. 2003
Trauma	Cerebellar haemorrhage or contusion, postconsussion syndrome	History is mandatory; in postconcussive syndrome gait ataxia is more marked than nystagmus or limb ataxia; associated headache and dizziness are possible	D'Avella et al. 2002
Benign paroxysmal torticollis of childhood		Episodic attacks lasting minutes to days with tilt of the head to one side, pallor, irritability, malaise, vomiting, or ataxia, and remitting spontaneously	Cuveillier and Lepine 2010
Basilar migraine		Can be associated with vertigo, cranial nerve dysfunction, nausea, and vomiting	Lapkin and Golden 1978; Evans and Linder 2002
Pseudoataxia due to nonconvulsive epileptic status		Ataxia with or without alteration of consciousness; absence of clonic movements, but minor myoclonus and atonic episodes possible	Bennett et al. 1982
Functional or psychogenic		Patients appear to stagger, gait often not wide-based, falls are rare; clinical signs are inconsistent and often fail to conform to neuroanatomic distributions	Hinson and Haren 2006

Modified from Ryan MM, Engle EC (2003) Acute ataxia in childhood. J Child Neurol 18: 309–316.

TABLE 3
Intermittent ataxia

Comment: 'Intermittent ataxia' refers to intermittent ataxia in patients who are symptom-free in the interval. The first sign may be presenting as an 'acute ataxia'. 'Episodic ataxias' refer to dominantly inherited channelopathies. Intermittent ataxias of metabolic origin are mostly caused by decompensation of disorders of 'intermediary metabolism'.

Disease			Comments	References
Intoxication			Several drugs (such as benzodiazepines, phenytoin, carbamazepine, antihistamines, tricyclic antidepressants), alcohol, solvents, mercury; possible as Münchhausen syndrome by proxy	Manto 2010
Infection	Recurrence of acute cerebellar ataxia		Commonly affect children aged 1 to 4 years, mostly 1 to 3 weeks after viral infection (mostly varicella, mumps, parvovirus, Epstein-Barr virus), self-limiting	Sawaishi and Takada 2002
Inflammation	Multiple sclerosis (MS) (rare)		Ataxia is the presenting feature in about 5–15% of the patients with MS and is particularly common (about 50%) in children younger than 10 years	Banwell et al. 2007
Paraneoplastic	Opsoclonus-myoclonus syndrome		May be associated with an occult neuroblastoma; the course is often protracted and fluctuating; steroid therapy is usually efficient	Klein et al. 2007
Metabolic	Mitochondrial disorders	Pyruvate dehydrogenase deficiency	Four phenotypic groups possible: neonatal encephalopathy with lactic acidosis, nonprogressive infantile encephalopathy, Leigh syndrome, and relapsing episodes of ataxia with axonal neuropathy, first attack (duration of more than 1 week) can be misdiagnosed as cerebellitis or Guillain-Barré syndrome	Barnerias et al. 2010
		Pyruvate decarboxylase deficiency	There are 2 major presentations: metabolic and neurologic; the metabolic form presents as severe lactic acidosis in the newborn period, usually leading to death, the neurologic form shows hypotonia, lethargy, seizures, cognitive impairment, and spasticity; between these 2 forms there are intermediate forms with intermittent episodes of lactic acidosis and cerebellar ataxia	Livingstone et al. 1984
		Leigh syndrome (rare as intermittent ataxia)	Leigh syndrome is a progressive neurodegenerative disorder; decompensation often with lactic acidosis occurring during an intercurrent illness is typically associated with regression; a period of recovery may follow the initial decompensation, but, if recovery occurs, it is usually incomplete	Finsterer 2008
	Amino acidopathies	Maple syrup urine disease (intermittent variant)	Normal early growth and development with episodic intermittent decompensations mimicking the classic phenotype (poor feeding, irritability, lethargy, opisthotonus, focal dystonia, "fencing", "bicycling")	Simon et al. 2006
		Hartnup disease	Light-sensitive dermatitis, emotional instability, psychotic manifestations, seizures, dystonia	Cheon et al. 2010
	Urea cycle disorders (deficiency of ornithine transcarbamylase, arginase, carbamoylphosphate synthetase, arginosuccinate synthetase, or arginosuccinase)		Intermittent mental status changes such as lethargy or somnolence, agitation or disorientation, and significant personality changes associated with intercurrent illness, recurrent seizures or other movement disorders such as ataxia	Smith et al. 2005
	Organic acidopathies	Untreated partial biotinidase deficiency	Ataxia, seizures, hypotonia, hearing loss, vision problems, alopecia, eczematous skin rash, conjunctivitis, candidiasis; in children with untreated partial biotinidase deficiency (10–30% of mean normal serum biotinidase activity) the symptoms are usually mild and occur only in stress situations such as a prolonged infection	Swango et al. 1998
		Isovaleric acidaemia	Approximately 50% of cases are acute, severe neonatal illness often with rapid death and 50% are chronic episodic (metabolic acidosis, seizures, ataxia, coma) with asymptomatic intervals	Tanaka 1990
		Methylmalonic and propionic acidaemia	Repeated relapses with acute encephalopathy, lethargy, seizure, ataxia, and dystonia, precipitated by excessive protein intake, intercurrent infection, or constipation	Deodato et al. 2006
	Carnitine acetyltransferase deficiency (very rare)		Intermittent ataxia, oculomotor palsy, hypotonia, mental confusion, and disturbances of consciousness	DiDonato et al. 1979
	Glucose transporter type 1 (GLUT1) deficiency		Motor and mental developmental delay, seizures with infantile onset, acquired microcephaly, ataxia, dystonia, spasticity	Brockmann 2009

TABLE 3
(*continued*)

Disease		Comments	References
Basilar migraine		Can be associated with vertigo, cranial nerve dysfunction, nausea, and vomiting	Lapkin and Golden 1978; Evans and Linder 2002
Vascular	Transient ischaemic attacks	Can be caused by sickle cell disease, vasculitis, arterial dissection, arterial hypoplasia, subclavian steal syndrome	Bojinova et al. 2000
Benign paroxysmal vertigo		Episodic attacks with severe vertigo, occurring without warning and resolving spontaneously after minutes to hours	Cuveillier and Lepine 2010
Benign paroxysmal torticollis of childhood		Episodic attacks lasting minutes to days with tilt of the head to one side, pallor, irritability, malaise, vomiting, or ataxia, and remitting spontaneously	Cuveillier and Lepine 2010
Paroxysmal tonic upgaze of childhood		Episodes of variably sustained conjugate upward deviation of the eyes, with neck flexion and downbeating saccades in attempted downgaze; exacerbation with febrile illnesses; ataxia can be confined to episodes or can persist	Ouvrier and Billson 2005
Pseudoataxia due to non-convulsive epileptic activity (rare)			Bennett et al. 1982

Modified from Ryan MM, Engle EC (2003) Acute ataxia in childhood. J Child Neurol 18: 309–316.

TABLE 4
Episodic ataxias

Comment: 'Episodic ataxias' (EA) refer to dominantly inherited channelopathies characterized by intermittent episodes of cerebellar dysfunction with or without interictal neurologic dysfunction. See Chapter 28.

	EA1	EA2	EA3	EA4	EA5	EA6*	EA7**
OMIM	160120	108500	606554	606552	601949	600111	611907
Gene locus	12q13	19p13	1q42	unknown	2q22–q23	5p	19q13
Gene	*KCNA1*	*CACNA1A*	unknown	unknown	*CACNB4*	*SLC1A3*	unknown
Age at onset (years)	2–20	2–20	1–42	23–60	<20	5	<20
Attack duration	seconds–minutes	hours	1 minute–6 hours	brief	hours	hours–days	hours–days
Tinnitus (intraictal)	infrequent	no	usual	occasional	no	no	no
Myokymia (interictal)	usual	no	usual	no	no	no	no
Nystagmus (interictal)	no	usual, downbeat	occasional	usual	usual	no	no
Epilepsy (associated)	occasional	infrequent	occasional	occasional	usual	yes	no
Response to acetazolamide	occasional	usual	usual	no	transient	no	no

In EA2 there is also slowly progressive cerebellar dysfunction and atrophy and in 50% migraines; * 1 case; ** 1 family.
Modified from Jen JC, et al. (2007) Primary episodic ataxias: diagnosis, pathogenesis and treatment. Brain 130: 2484–2493.

TABLE 5
Progressive ataxias

Comment: The context of history and findings, particularly 'ataxia plus' symptoms, often allow targeted diagnostic investigations. However, despite extensive work-up the final diagnosis remains unknown in a considerable proportion of progressive ataxias. It is particularly important not to miss the rare treatable causes.

Disease		Comments	References
Sphingolipidoses	Late-onset GM2 gangliosidosis	Onset of ataxia between 2 and 10 years, followed by regression	Maegawa et al. 2006
	Niemann Pick type C	Classically truncal and limb ataxia and vertical supranuclear gaze palsy (manifesting as increased latency in initiation of vertical saccades) in middle-late childhood, progressive cognitive impairment, behavioural disturbances; seizures (40%), cataplexy (20%), visceromegaly	Wraith et al. 2009
	Late-infantile metachromatic leukodystrophy*	Onset between 1 and 2 years with weakness, hypotonia, slurred speech, and clumsiness; later ataxia, dysarthria, regression, spasticity, epileptic seizures, peripheral neuropathy; in the final stage decerebrate posturing	Lugowska et al. 2005
	Krabbe disease* (late infantile and juvenile)	Onset after 1 year of age with ataxia, vision loss, regression, irritability, later spasticity	Barone et al. 1996
Neuronal ceroid lipofuscinosis (NCL) (late infantile and juvenile)		Late infantile: onset at the age of 1–4 years, starting with epilepsy followed by regression, ataxia, extrapyramidal and pyramidal signs, rapidly progressive visual impairment since about 4–6 years; juvenile: onset at the age 4–10 years, starting with rapidly progressive visual impairment, followed by ataxia, myoclonic seizures, and regression	Kohlschütter and Schulz 2009
Giant axonal neuropathy*		Severe early onset peripheral sensorimotor neuropathy, cognitive impairment, ataxia, and characteristic tightly curled hair	Koop et al. 2007
Abnormalities of DNA repair	Ataxia teleangiectasia (Louis Bar syndrome)	Progressive cerebellar ataxia beginning between ages 1 and 4, acquired ocular motor apraxia, choreoathetosis; ocular telangiectasias later; increased risk for malignancy, immunodeficiency, marked elevated α-fetoprotein	Crawford et al. 2000
	Cockayne syndrome (type 1)	Progressive impairment of vision, hearing, and central and peripheral nervous system function beginning in the first year; ataxia, spasticity, pigmentary retinopathy, cataract, and optic atrophy as not consistent additional symptoms	Cleaver et al. 2009
Mitochondrial	Kearns-Sayre syndrome	Multisystemic disorder with onset before age 20 years, pigmentary retinopathy, progressive external ophthalmoplegia, cerebellar ataxia, and cardiac conduction block	DiMauro and Schon 2003
	Myoclonic epilepsy with ragged red fibres (MERRF)	Onset in childhood with myoclonus (often the first symptom) followed by epilepsy, ataxia, weakness, and dementia; additionally often hearing loss, short stature, optic atrophy, and cardiomyopathy	DiMauro and Schon 2003
	Neurogenic muscle weakness, ataxia, and retinitis pigmentosa (NARP)	Proximal neurogenic muscle weakness with sensory neuropathy, ataxia, and pigmentary retinopathy, onset in early childhood	DiMauro and Schon 2003
Peroxisomal	Adrenoleukodystrophy (ALD)	Isolated progressive ataxia is a rare manifestation of ALD; onset typically between 4 and 8 years of age with behavioural changes and progressive impairment of cognition, vision, hearing, and motor function	Moser et al. 2007
	Refsum disease	Anosmia and early-onset retinitis pigmentosa, neuropathy, deafness, ataxia, and ichthyosis	Wills et al. 2001
Other metabolic	Abetalipoproteinaemia	Sensory neuropathy, diarrhoea, very low cholesterol, acanthocytosis	Zamel et al. 2008
	Vitamin E deficiency	Onset typically at puberty with progressive ataxia, loss of proprioception, areflexia, and retinitis pigmentosa	Di Donato et al. 2010
	Cerebrotendinous xanthomatosis	Infantile-onset diarrhea, childhood-onset cataract, adolescent- to young adult-onset tendon xanthomas, and adult-onset (rarely in the childhood) progressive neurologic dysfunction (dementia, psychiatric disturbances, pyramidal and/or cerebellar signs, and seizures)	Keren and Falik-Zaccai 2009
	Mevalonic aciduria	Impaired motor and cognitive development, failure to thrive, progressive cerebellar ataxia, dysmorphic features, progressive visual impairment, and recurrent febrile, lymphadenopathy, arthralgia, and skin rashes	Haas and Hoffmann 2006
	L-2-hydroxyglutaric aciduria	Ataxia, macrocephaly, seizures, pyramidal signs, regression	Steenweg et al. 2010

TABLE 5
(*continued*)

Disease		Comments	References
Leukodystrophies	Pelizaeus-Merzbacher disease	Typical manifestation in infancy or early childhood with nystagmus, hypotonia, and cognitive impairment; later progressive spasticity and ataxia	Golomb et al. 2004
	Vanishing white matter disease	Early childhood or late childhood/juvenile onset of spasticity, optic atrophy, and ataxia with progressive course, which can be exacerbated by rapid deterioration during febrile illnesses or following head trauma	van der Knaap et al. 2006; Labauge et al. 2009
	Megalencephalic leukoencephalopathy with subcortical cysts (MLC)	Progressive ataxia and spastic quadriplegia, dysarthria, dysphagia, and epileptic seizures	Blattner et al. 2003
	Salla disease	Ataxia, hypotonia, nystagmus, regression	Varho et al. 2002
Spinocerebellar degenerations	Friedreich ataxia	Slowly progressive ataxia, onset usually 5–15 years, associated with absent lower limb reflexes, loss of position and vibration sense, and spasticity in the lower limbs; about 2/3 have cardiomyopathy and 1/3 diabetes mellitus	Pandolfo 2009
	Ataxia-oculomotor apraxia type 1 (AOA1)	Ataxia, ocular motor apraxia, dystonia, chorea, peripheral neuropathy, cerebellar atrophy, hypoalbuminaemia	Le Ber et al. 2003
	Ataxia-oculomotor apraxia type 2 (AOA2)*	Ataxia, ocular motor apraxia (not consistent), dystonia, chorea, peripheral neuropathy, cerebellar atrophy, elevated α-fetoprotein (about 2–4×)	Anheim et al. 2009
	Spinocerebellar ataxias (SCA), particularly type 7 (SCA7)**	Ataxia, retinal degeneration (macular degeneration, optic atrophy, pigmentary renitopathy), slow saccades	Miller et al. 2009
Midline tumours in the posterior fossa		Progressive ataxia; signs of high intracranial pressure due to obstructive hydrocephalus common, but not constant	Dörner et al. 2007

* Ataxia is not the leading sign; ** recently renamed as SCAR-1 (spinocerebellar ataxia, recessive, non-Friedreich type 1) because of nonconsistent ocular motor apraxia; progressive cerebellar ataxia has been reported in mutations in PEX10 gene (Régal et al. 2010).

TABLE 6
Treatable causes of inherited ataxia

Comment: In this context 'treatable' implies improvement, not necessarily cure by the intervention.

Disease	Treatment	References
Abetalipoproteinaemia	Vitamin E supplementation	Zamel et al. 2008
Vitamin E deficiency (autosomal recessive inherited or due to chronic cholestasis or short-bowel syndrome)	Vitamin E supplementation	Mariotti et al. 2004; Zamel et al. 2008
Biotinidase deficiency	Biotin supplementation	Wolf 2010
Cerebrotendinous xanthomatosis	Chenodeoxycholic acid	Pierre et al. 2008
Coenzyme Q10 deficiency	Coenzyme Q10 supplementation	Montini et al. 2008
Glucose transporter type 1 (GLUT1) deficiency	Frequent snacks rich in carbohydrates, ketogenic diet	Baranano and Hartman 2008
Maple syrup urine disease	Diet (restriction in leucine, isoleucine, and valine), thiamine	Strauss et al. 2010
Pyruvate dehydrogenase deficiency	Ketogenic diet	Baranano and Hartman 2008
Refsum disease	Phytanic acid free diet	Wills et al. 2001
Urea cycle defects	Diet, sodium benzoate	Walker 2009
Friedreich ataxia*	Idebenone	Pineda et al. 2008
Niemann-Pick disease type C*	Miglustat	Pineda et al. 2010

* Controversial, if treatment or intervention is effective; gluten ataxia is not listed as it is not inherited (see Chapter 42 and Hadjivassiliou et al. 2010).

TABLE 7
Ataxia and ocular motor apraxia

Comment: Ocular motor apraxia (OMA) implies impaired generation of voluntary saccades and is associated with head 'thrusts' during attempted shifts of gaze. The terminology is controversial and both terms "oculomotor" as well as "ocular motor" are commonly used. The oculomotor nerve is not involved. Therefore, we prefer "ocular motor" apraxia.

Disease	Additional findings	References
Congenital OMA type Cogan*	Ataxia, mostly normal cognition, vermis hypoplasia (inconsistent)ß	Kondo et al. 2007; Orssaud et al. 2009
Joubert syndrome and related disorders*	Ataxia, hypotonia, cognitive impairment, retinal dystrophy (not consistent), nephronophthisis (not consistent), postaxial polydactyly (not consistent), hypoplasia/dysplasia of the vermis, molar tooth sign	Weiss et al. 2009; Sturm et al. 2010
Gaucher disease type 3*	Cognitive regression, myoclonic seizures, squint, splenomegaly, fever, growth retardation, aseptic bone necrosis, storage cells in bone marrow	Accardo et al. 2005
Abnormal brain anatomy (corpus callosum agenesis, brainstem dysgenesis)*	Variable, depending on the disease	Sargent et al. 1997
Ataxia-teleangiectasia (Louis-Bar syndrome)**	Progressive ataxia, choreoathetoid movements, ocular and cutaneous teleangiectasia, immunodeficiency, endocrine abnormalities, cerebellar atrophy, marked elevated α-fetoprotein	Lewis et al. 1999; Shaikh et al. 2009
Ataxia oculomotor apraxia type 1 (AOA1)**	Ataxia, dystonia, chorea, peripheral neuropathy, cerebellar atrophy, hypoalbuminaemia	Le Ber et al. 2003
Ataxia oculomotor apraxia type 2 (AOA2)**, ***	OMA not consistent, ataxia, dystonia, chorea, peripheral neuropathy, cerebellar atrophy, elevated α-fetoprotein (about 2–4×)	Anheim et al. 2009
Mitochondrial disorders (rare)**	Variable, depending on the mitochondrial disorder	Punal et al. 1998

* Congenital onset of OMA; ** noncongenital onset of OMA (acquired in Louis-Bar syndrome and mitochondrial disorders); *** recently renamed as SCAR-1 (spinocerebellar ataxia, recessive, non-Friedreich type 1) because of nonconsistent ocular motor apraxia.

TABLE 8
Ataxia and progressive external ophthalmoplegia

Disease	Additional findings	References
Kearns Sayre syndrome	Retinopathy, myopathy, cognitive impairment, heart block, diabetes mellitus	Gronlund et al. 2010
POLG mutation	Epilepsy, nystagmus, extrapyramidal movement disorders, peripheral neuropathy, liver involvement in Alpers disease	Wong et al. 2008
TWINKLE mutation	Axonal neuropathy, deafness, cataracts, depression, levodopa responsive parkinsonism	Lewis et al. 2002
Infantile-onset spinocerebellar ataxia (IOSCA)	After 1 year of age ataxia, muscle hypotonia, and athetosis; at school age ophthalmoplegia and sensorineural deafness; at adolescence neuropathy, optic atrophy, and in females hypergonadotrophic hypogonadism; later seizures	Koskinen et al. 1994

TABLE 9
Ataxia and retinopathy

Disease		Additional findings	References
Syndromic	Joubert syndrome and related disorders (particularly JBTS3 and JBTS5)	Ocular motor apraxia, hypotonia, cognitive impairment, nephronophthisis (not consistent), postaxial polydactyly (not consistent), vermian hypoplasia/dysplasia, molar tooth sign	Doherty et al. 2009; Sturm et al. 2010
	Bardet-Biedl syndrome	Speech disorder, developmental delay, anosmia, behavioural abnormalities, truncal obesity, postaxial poyldactyly, hypogonadism, renal anomalies	Tobin and Beales 2007
Metabolic	Kearns Sayre syndrome	External ophthalmoplegia, myopathy, cognitive impairment, heart block, diabetes mellitus	Isashiki et al. 1998
	MELAS*	Stroke-like episodes, focal seizures, cognitive regression, short stature, diabetes mellitus, heart block	Gronlund et al. 2010
	Neuropathy, ataxia, and retinitis pigmentosa (NARP)	Peripheral neuropathy, epilepsy, cognitive regression	Kerrison et al. 2000

TABLE 9
(*continued*)

Disease		Additional findings	References
	Coenzyme Q10 deficiency	Encephalomyopathy with recurrent myoglobinuria, brain involvement and ragged red fibres; severe infantile multisystemic disease; ataxia; Leigh syndrome with growth retardation, ataxia, and deafness; isolated myopathy	Quinzii et al. 2007
	Refsum disease	Demyelinating neuropathy, cataract, anosmia, elevated phytanic acid	Fogel and Perlman 2007
	Vitamin E deficiency	Sensory neuropathy, low serum vitamin E	Fogel and Perlman 2007
	Abetalipoproteinaemia	Sensory neuropathy, diarrhoea, very low cholesterol, acanthocytosis	Fogel and Perlman 2007
	Early-onset methylmalonic aciduria	Acute neurological deterioration with ataxia, extrapyramidal symptoms, cognitive regression, and psychiatric disturbances, pancytopenia, megaloblastic anaemia	Gerth et al. 2008
	Congenital disorders of glycosylation (CDG)	Retinitis pigmentosa (not consistent), hypotonia, mental retardation, visceromegaly, inverted nipples, ascites, pericardial effusion	Morava et al. 2009
Neuro-degenerative	Neuronal ceroid lipofuscinoses	Epileptic seizures, myoclonia, dystonia, cognitive regression, microcephaly	Birch 1999
	Autosomal dominant spinocerebellar ataxia type 7 (SCA7)	Ataxia, retinal degeneration (macular degeneration, optic atrophy, pigmentary retinopathy), slow saccades	Miller et al. 2009
	Wolfram syndrome (DIDMOAD, MIM #598500)	Diabetes mellitus, optic atrophy, diabetes insipidus, deafness, renal tract abnormalities, psychiatric disorders, gonadal disorders, ataxia, peripheral neuropathy, cognitive impairment	Ganie and Bhat 2009
	Posterior column ataxia and retinitis pigmentosa (PCARP, MIM #609033)	Retinitis pigmentosa, areflexia, nycalopia, peripheral visual loss, sensory ataxia, peripheral neuropathy, scoliosis, camptodactyly, achalasia	Rajadhyaksha et al. 2010

* MELAS, mitochondrial encephalomyopathy, lactic acidosis, and stroke-like episodes. Retinopathy has also been reported in *PEX10* mutations (Regal et al. 2010).

TABLE 10
Ataxia and cataract

Disease	Additional findings	References
Marinesco-Sjögren syndrome	Ataxia, mild to severe cognitive impairment, hypotonia, muscle weakness, short stature, various skeletal abnormalities	Slavotinek et al. 2005
Refsum disease	Demyelinating neuropathy, retinitis pigmentosa, anosmia, elevated phytanic acid	Wills et al. 2001
Cerebrotendinous xanthomatosis	Cognitive impairment, peripheral neuropathy, spasticity, infantile-onset diarrhea, tendon xanthomas	Keren and Falik-Zaccai 2009
Hypomyelination and congenital cataract	Congenital cataract, developmental delay, slowly progressive neurological impairment with spasticity, cerebellar ataxia, and mild-to-moderate cognitive impairment beginning at the age of 12–16 months	Biancheri et al. 2007
Portneuf ataxia	Ataxia, spasticity, hyperreflexia, urinary urgency, scoliosis, dystonia, cognitive impairment, optic atrophy, cataract, hearing impairment	Thiffault et al. 2006
TWINKLE mutation	Axonal neuropathy, deafness, cataracts, depression, levodopa responsive parkinsonism	Lewis et al. 2002
VLDLR-associated cerebellar hypoplasia	Cognitive impairment, ataxia, occasionally seizures, short stature	Boycott et al. 2009
CDG type Iq	Congenital ataxia, severe visual impairment, variable eye malformations, variable degree of cerebellar hypoplasia	Morava et al. 2010

TABLE 11
Ataxia and polyneuropathy

Comment: Neuropathies may be mild particularly in the early stage and may not be clinically obvious. Nerve conduction studies are recommended.

Disease	Characteristics of neuropathy	References
Abetalipoproteinaemia	Sensory, axonal	Zouari et al. 1998
Ataxia oculomotor apraxia type 1 (AOA1)	Sensorimotor, axonal	Le Ber et al. 2003
Ataxia oculomotor apraxia type 2 (AOA2)*	Sensori(motor), axonal	Anheim et al. 2009
Ataxia teleangiectasia (Louis-Bar syndrome)	Sensory, axonal	Crawford et al. 2000
Autosomal recessive spastic ataxia of Charlevoix-Saguenay (ARSACS)	Sensori(motor), axonal	Vermeer et al. 2008
Cerebrotendinous xanthomatosis	Sensorimotor, axonal	Verrips et al. 2000
Congenital ataxia and neuropathy (due to mutations in the *TDP1* gene)	Sensorimotor, axonal	Takashima et al. 2002
Friedreich ataxia	Sensori(motor), axonal	Zouari et al. 1998
Infantile-onset spinocerebellar ataxia (IOSCA)	Sensori(motor), axonal	Koskinen et al. 1994
Late-onset GM2 gangliosidosis	Neuropathy is a very rare symptoms – if present, is sensorimotor and axonal	Shapiro et al. 2008
Neuropathy, ataxia, and retinitis pigmentosa (NARP)	Sensori(motor), axonal	Kerrison et al. 2000
Posteror column ataxia and retinitis pigmentosa (PCARP)	Sensory plus posterior column	Rajadhyaksha et al. 2010
Refsum disease	Sensorimotor, demyelinating	Wills et al. 2001
Sensory ataxic neuropathy, dysarthria and ophthalmoparesis (POLG-related)	Sensory, axonal	van Goethem et al. 2003
Vitamin E deficiency	Sensory, axonal	Zouari et al. 1998

* Recently renamed as SCAR-1 (spinocerebellar ataxia, recessive, non-Friedreich type 1) because of non-consistent oculomotor apraxia; an axonal motor neuropathy has been recently reported in two patients with progressive ataxia and marked cerebellar atrophy due to mutations in the *PEX10* gene (Regal et al. 2010).

TABLE 12
Ataxia and spasticity

Disease	Comments	References
Autosomal recessive spastic ataxia of Charlevoix-Saguenay (ARSACS)	Ataxia, dysarthria, spasticity, extensor plantar reflexes, distal muscle wasting, distal sensorimotor neuropathy predominant in the legs, and horizontal gaze nystagmus	Vermeer et al. 2008
Hypomyelination and congenital cataract	Congenital cataract, developmental delay, slowly progressive neurological impairment with spasticity, cerebellar ataxia, and mild-to-moderate cognitive impairment; onset at the age of 12–16 months	Biancheri et al. 2007
Krabbe disease (late infantile and juvenile)	Onset after 1 year of age with ataxia, visual loss, regression, irritability, later spasticity	Barone et al. 1996
Late-onset GM2 gangliosidosis	Onset of ataxia between 2 and 10 years, followed by regression	Maegawa et al. 2006
Megalencephalic leukoencephalopathy with subcortical cysts (MLC)	Progressive ataxia and spastic quadriplegia, dysarthria, dysphagia, and epileptic seizures	Blattner et al. 2003
Pelizaeus-Merzbacher disease	Typical manifestation in infancy or early childhood with nystagmus, hypotonia, and cognitive impairment; later spasticity and ataxia; increased prevalence of congenital stridor	Golomb et al. 2004
Portneuf ataxia	Ataxia, spasticity, hyperreflexia, urinary urgency, scoliosis, dystonia, cognitive impairment, optic atrophy, cataract, hearing impairment	Thiffault et al. 2006
Spinocerebellar ataxias (SCA), particularly type 7 (SCA7)	Ataxia, retinal degeneration (macular degeneration, optic atrophy, pigmentary renitopathy), slow saccades	Miller et al. 2009
Vanishing white matter disease	Early childhood or late childhood/juvenile onset of spasticity, optic atrophy, and ataxia with progressive course; exacerbations often prompted by febrile illnesses or head trauma	van der Knaap et al. 2006

Additionally: Klebe et al. reported spastic paraparesis with mild ataxia and sensory neuropathy in an Algerian family and mapped the gene locus on chromosome 2q37.3 (SPG30) (Klebe et al. 2006); Bouslam et al. reported autosomal recessive spastic ataxia with gene locus on chromosome 17p13 in a consanguineous Moroccan family (Bouslam et al. 2007).

TABLE 13
Ataxia 'plus' (additional suggestive signs or symptoms in selected ataxias)

Specific sign or symptom	Disease
Aniridia	Gillespie syndrome
Anosmia	Refsum disease
Cardiomyopathy	Congenital disorders of glycosylation (CDG)
	Friedreich ataxia
	Mitochondrial disorders (e.g. Kearns-Sayre syndrome, MELAS, POLG mutation)
Chorea	Ataxia oculomotor apraxia type 1 and 2 (AOA1 and AOA2)
	Ataxia teleangiectasia (Louis-Bar syndrome)
	Benign hereditary chorea (mutations in the *NKX2-1* gene)
	Dentatorubropallidoluysian atrophy (DRPLA)
	Late-onset GM2 gangliosidosis
	L-2-hydroxyglutaric aciduria (choreodystonia)
Eye malformations	CDG Iq
Ichthyosis	Refsum disease
	Trichothiodystrophy (ichthyosiform erythroderma)
Hearing impairment	Infantile-onset spinocerebellar ataxia (IOSCA)
	Mitochondrial disorders (e.g. KSS, MELAS, POLG mutations, SANDO)
	Coenzyme Q10 deficiency
	Refsum disease
	Wolfram syndrome (DIDMOAD, MIM #598500)
	KCNJ10 mutations (epilepsy, ataxia, sensorineural deafness, and tubulopathy)
	NEUROD1 mutations (neonatal diabetes, ataxia, deafness, myopia)
Hypodontia	Hypomyelination, hypogonadotropic hypogonadism and hypodontia (4H)
Myoclonus	Ataxia oculomotor apraxia type 2 (AOA2)
	Ataxia telangiectasia (Louis-Bar syndrome)
	Cerebrotendinous xanthomatosis
	Dentatorubropallidoluysian atrophy (DRPLA)
	Glucose transport type 1 (GLUT1) deficiency
	Late-onset GM2 gangliosidosis
	Mitochondrial disorders, particularly MERRF
	Neuronal ceroid lipofuscinosis (particularly late-infantile and juvenile forms)
	Niemann-Pick disease type C
Telangiectasias	Ataxia teleangiectasia (Louis Bar syndrome)
Tightly curled hair	Giant axonal neuropathy

TABLE 14
Cerebellar hypoplasia in childhood

Comments: Cerebellar hypoplasia (CH) (defined as volume reduction) occurs in a wide range of genetic and acquired conditions. A given (e.g. genetic) condition may be associated with a spectrum of neuroimaging anomalies, i.e. not all affected patients have CH. For example, *FOXC1* mutations may be associated with Dandy-Walker malformation, cerebellar hypoplasia, or even mega cisterna magna. Many patients with nonprogressive cerebellar ataxia, a static condition, may have a smaller cerebellum with enlarged interfolial spaces, mimicking atrophy. We consider this finding to be cerebellar hypoplasia. The nomenclature in the literature is not consistent.

Type	Disease	Additional features	References
Prenatal infection	Cytomegalovirus (CMV)	Lissencephaly, polymicrogyria, white matter abnormalities, ventriculomegaly, periventricular calcification	Poretti et al. 2009c, Fink et al. 2010
Teratogen	Anticonvulsant drugs, retinoic acid		Squier et al. 1990
	Cocaine		Bellini et al. 2000
Chromosomal defects	Trisomy 13	Holoprosencephaly, microcephaly, micro/anophthalmia, neural tube defects, corpus callosum agenesis	Rosati and Gauriglia 1999
	Trisomy 18	Holoprosencephaly, hydrocephalus, corpus callosum agenesis, choroid plexus cysts	Lin et al. 2006
	Partial trisomy 12q and monosomy 21q	Microcephaly, ventriculomegaly	Chen et al. 2006
	Trisomy 17 mosaicism	Cognitive impairment, peripheral motor and sensory neuropathy, zonular cataract, short stature, body asymmetry	Terhal et al. 2004
Metabolic	Adenylosuccinase deficiency	Early isolated CH, late cerebellar atrophy with periventricular white matter abnormalities	Edery et al. 2003
	Some mitochondrial disorders	Enlarged ventricles, basal ganglia and brainstem abnormalities	Saneto et al. 2008
	Zellweger syndrome (rare)	Abnormal gyration (polymicrogyria, pachygyria), heterotopia, leukencephalopathy, germinolytic cysts	Weller S et al. 2008
	Nonketotic hyperglycinaemia (rare)	Delayed myelination, corpus callosum agenesis	Shah et al. 2005
	Mucopolysaccharidosis type I (rare)	Enlarged perivascular and subarachnoid spaces, cerebral atrophy, white matter abnormalities, ventriculomegaly	Matheus et al. 2004
	Congenital disorders of glycosylation Ia	Brainstem hypoplasia, white matter atrophy or hypoplasia	Sparks 2006
	Congenital disorder of glycosylation Iq	Cerebellar vermis hypoplasia	Morava et al. 2010
	Smith-Lemli-Opitz syndrome	Callosal abnormalities, arachnoid cyst	Caruso et al. 2004
	Sulfite oxidase deficiency	Generalized brain edema, subsequently white matter cystic encephalomalacia	Hoffmann et al. 2007
Migrational disorders	*LIS1* lissencephaly	Lissencephaly with posterior gradient	Uyanik et al. 2007
	RELN lissencephaly	Lissencephaly with anterior gradient, pontine hypoplasia	Hong et al. 2000
	TUBA1A lissencephaly	Lissencephaly with centro-posterior gradient, agenesis of corpus callosum, brainstem hypoplasia	Kumar et al. 2010
	DCX lissencephaly	Lissencephaly with anterior gradient in males, subcortical band heterotopia in females	Jissendi-Tchofo et al. 2009
	ARX lissencephaly	Lissencephaly with temporo-posterior gradient, corpus callosum agenesis	Jissendi-Tchofo et al. 2009
	VLDLR migration disorder	Pontine hypoplasia, reduced gyral pattern, afolial cerebellum, short stature	Boycott et al. 2009
	TUBB2B polymicrogyria	Bilateral asymmetrical polymicrogyria (anterior gradient), fusion of caudate, putamen, and internal capsule, corpus callosum dysgenesis, small pons	Jaglin et al. 2009
	TUBB3 polymicrogyria	Perisylvian polymicrogyria/frontoparietal gyral disorganization, corpus callosum hypoplasia, fusion or hypertrophy of the caudate nucleus and putamen, brainstem hypoplasia	Poirier et al. 2010
	FLNA-associated heterotopia	Bilateral periventricular nodular heterotopias, hippocampal malformations (inconsistent), macrocephaly (inconsistent)	Parrini et al. 2006
Congenital muscular dystrophies (CMD)	Primary merosin-deficient CMD	White matter abnormalities with frontotemporal predominance, bilateral occipital cortical dysplasia, brainstem hypoplasia	Leite et al. 2005
	Walker-Warburg syndrome	Congenital hydrocephalus, cobblestone lissencephaly, thin corpus callosum, absent septum pellucidum, hypoplastic pons, cerebellar cysts, kinking of the brainstem	Clement et al. 2008
	Fukuyama CMD	Polymicrogyria frontotemporal, pachygyria occipital, white matter abnormalities, pons hypoplastic, cerebellar cysts	Clement et al. 2008
	Muscle-eye-brain disease	Polymicrogyria with fronto-occipital gradient, abnormal white matter, thin corpus callosum, cerebellar cysts, brainstem cleft, hypoplastic pons	Clement et al. 2008

TABLE 14
(*continued*)

Type	Disease	Additional features	References
	GPR56 mutations	Bilateral frontoparietal polymicrogyria, pontine hypoplasia, cerebellar dysplasia, cerebellar cysts, thin corpus callosum, abnormal white matter	Bahi-Buisson et al. 2010
Genetic	Cayman Ataxia	Marked developmental delay	Bomar et al. 2003
	OPHN1 mutation	Frontotemporal atrophy, enlargement of the lateral ventricles	Zanni et al. 2005
	CASK-associated CH	Brainstem hypoplasia, reduced gyral pattern, microcephaly	Takanashi et al. 2010
	FOXC1 mutation	Dandy-Walker malformation, mega cisterna magna	Aldinger et al. 2009
	X-linked congenital ataxia (Xq11.21-q21.3)	Isolated global CH, normal cognition	Illarioshkin et al. 1996
	X-linked congenital ataxia (Xq25-q27.1)	Isolated global CH, normal cognition	Zanni et al. 2008
	Autosomal recessive ataxia (9q34-qter)	Cognitive impairment, short stature, albinism (inconsistent)	Delague et al. 2001
	Cerebellar Ataxia with Mental retardation, Optic atrophy, and Skin abnormalities (CAMOS) (*ZNF592* mutation)	Cognitive impairment, spasticity, speech disorder, microcephaly, short stature, optic atrophy, osmophilic skin vessels	Delague et al. 2002; Nicolas et al. 2010
	Autosomal recessive ataxia (20q11-q13)	Normal cognition, mild spasticity, short stature	Tranebjaerg et al. 2003
	Autosomal recessive ataxia (17p)	Cognitive impairment (may be severe), speech impairment (dysarthria-absent speech), short stature, hirsutism, coarse face	Turkmen et al. 2006
	Autosomal recessive ataxia (16q21-q23)	Epilepsy, cognitive impairment, reduced tendon reflexes	Gribaa et al. 2007
	Gene locus unknown (due to familial history autosomal recessive inheritance)	Muscular hypotonia as first symptom, ataxia, cognitive impairment	Personal observation
	NEUROD1 mutation (2q31)	Neonatal diabetes mellitus, ataxia, deafness, myopia	Rubio-Cabezas et al. 2010
Syndromic	Ritscher-Schinzel syndrome (3C)	Dandy-Walker malformation, hydrocephalus	Leonardi et al. 2001
	Hoyeraal-Hreidarsson syndrome	Delayed myelination of cerebral white matter, hypoplastic corpus callosum	Kuwashima 2009
	Gillespie syndrome	Partial aniridia, cerebellar ataxia, and cognitive impairment	Marien et al. 2008
	CHARGE syndrome	Arrhinencephaly/hypoplastic olfactory bulbs, holoprosencephaly, septum pellucidum agenesis, nodular heterotopia, Dandy-Walker malformation	Sanlaville and Verloes 2007
	Velocardiofacial syndrome	Septum pellucidum abnormalities, polymicrogyria, corpus callosum hypoplasia, white matter abnormalities, ventriculomegaly	Campbell et al. 2006
	PHACE(S) association	Dandy-Walker malformation, vermis hypoplasia, cortical dysplasia, subcortical and subependymal gray matter heterotopia, agenesis of the corpus callosum, cerebral vascular anomalies	Metry et al. 2009
	Oculocerebrocutaneous syndrome	Giant dysplastic tectum rotated upward, large posterior fossa, frontal predominant polymicrogyria, periventricular nodular heterotopia, corpus callosum agenesis, interhemispheric cysts, ventriculomegaly, occipital meningocele (inconsistent)	Moog et al. 2005
	Endosteal sclerosis	Delayed myelination	Ozgen et al. 2005
	Oculodentodigital dysplasia	Midbrain hypoplasia, thin cervical spinal cord	Amador et al. 2008
	Nonprogressive ataxia with iris heterochromia	Iris heterochromia, non progressive congenital ataxia, cognitive impairment	Lamonica et al. 2010
	Joubert-like syndromes (vermis hypoplasia)	Morning glory disc anomaly, dysplastic kidneys, no molar tooth sign	Janecke et al. 2004
		Hypotonia, cognitive impairment, impaired vision, colobomas; ventriculomegaly, no molar tooth sign	Kroes et al. 2005
	Neurofibromatosis type 1 (not consistent)	Optic pathway and other gliomas, T2-weighted hyperintensities in basal ganglia, brainstem and cerebellum	Personal observations

CH has also been reported, not consistently, in acrocallosal syndrome (Fernandez et al. 2008), pseudo-TORCH syndrome (Abdel-Salam and Zaki 2009), cri-du-chat syndrome or distal 5p deletion (Chen et al. 2004), Pallister-Killian syndrome (Saito et al. 2006), Galloway-Mowat syndrome (Steiss et al. 2005), Sengers syndrome (Perry and Sladky 2008), Cohen syndrome (Waite et al. 2010), and in 2 patients with additionally postnatal growth failure, microcephaly, mental retardation, cataracts, large joint contractures, osteoporosis, and cortical dysplasia (Shotelersuk et al. 2003).

TABLE 15
Unilateral cerebellar hypoplasia

Comment: In this context hypoplasia refers to a smaller volume, irrespective of its pathogenetic mechanism.

Disease		Additional neuroimaging findings	References
PHACE(S) association (inconsistent)		Dandy-Walker malformation, cerebellar/vermis hypoplasia, cortical dysplasia, subcortical and subependymal gray matter heterotopia, agenesis of the corpus callosum, cerebral vascular anomalies	Metry et al. 2009
Prenatal cerebellar disruptions	Cerebellar cleft	Uni- or bilateral cleft in one/both cerebellar hemispheres, vermis spared, malorientation of the cerebellar foliation, irregular gray/white matter junction, lack of the normal architecture of the white matter confined to the region adjacent to the cleft	Poretti et al. 2009b
	Unilateral cerebellar hypoplasia (UCH)	Inconsistent involvement of the vermis, variable volume of the posterior fossa, brainstem asymmetry	Poretti et al. 2010a

TABLE 16
Cerebellar atrophy in childhood: a pattern-recognition approach

Comments: In a single MRI study, progressive cerebellar atrophy (CA) cannot be distinguished from static (residual) atrophy (Poretti et al. 2008). In many patients with nonprogressive cerebellar ataxia, MRI demonstrates enlarged interfolial spaces mimicking CA. In view of the static course we consider this to be cerebellar hypoplasia (CH). Postnatal-onset metabolic or genetic CAs do not result in pontine atrophy.

Pattern	Disease	References
Pure CA	Ataxia-telangiectasia	Tavani et al. 2003
	Ataxia-telangiectasia-like disorder (ATLD)	Delia et al. 2004
	Late-onset GM2 gangliosidosis	Maegawa et al. 2006
	Ataxia-oculomotor apraxia type 1	Le Ber et al. 2003
	Ataxia-oculomotor apraxia type 2*	Le Ber et al. 2004
	Progressive encephalopathy with edema, hypsarrhythmia and optic atrophy (PEHO)	Klein et al. 2004
	Autosomal recessive spastic ataxia of Charlevoix-Saguenay (ARSACS)	Richter et al. 1993
	CACNA1A mutation (including episodic ataxia type 2, SCA6, familial hemiplegic migraine type 1)	Wada et al. 2002
	Mevalonate kinase deficiency	Simon et al. 2004
	Predominant dystonia with CA	Le Ber et al. 2006
	Familial adult myoclonic epilepsy type 3	Carr et al. 2007
	Some mitochondrial disorders	Lamperti et al. 2003
CA and hypomyelination	Pelizaeus-Merzbacher disease	Plecko et al. 2003
	Pelizaeus-Merzbacher-like disease	Henneke et al. 2008
	Salla disease	Sonninen et al. 1999
	Hypomyelination, hypogonadotropic hypogonadism and hypodontia (4H)	Wolf et al. 2007
	Hypomyelination with atrophy of basal ganglia and cerebellum (HABC)	van der Knaap et al. 2007
	Trichothiodystrophy (Tay syndrome)	Yoon et al. 2005
	Galactosemia	Nelson et al. 1992
	Cerebellar ataxia with elevated cerebrospinal free sialic acid (CAFSA)	Mochel et al. 2009

TABLE 16
(*continued*)

Pattern		Disease	References
CA and progressive white matter abnormalities	Frontal predominance	Infantile neuroaxonal dystrophy (INAD)	Farina et al. 1999
	Periventricular predominance	Neuronal ceroid lipofuscinoses (particularly late-infantile type)	Seitz et al. 1998
		Niemann-Pick disease type C	Palmieri et al. 1994
		Adenylosuccinase deficiency	Edery et al. 2003
	Occiptial predominance	Early-onset peroxisomal disorders	Bams-Mengerink et al. 2006
	Subcortical predominance	L-2-hydroxyglutaric aciduria	Moroni et al. 2000
		Kearns-Sayre syndrome	Chu et al. 1999
	Diffuse cerebral	Vanishing white matter disease	van der Knaap et al. 2006
		Some mitochondrial disorders	Saneto et al. 2008
	Cerebellar predominance	Peroxisomal disorders	Weller et al. 2008
		Cerebrotendinous xanthomatosis	Vanrietvelde et al. 2000
	Brainstem predominance	Wilson disease	Taly et al. 2007
		Peroxisomal disorders	Kurihara et al. 1993
		Leigh syndrome	Lee et al. 2009
		Dentato-rubral-pallido-luysian atrophy (DRPLA)	Brunetti-Pierri et al. 2006
	Multifocal	Some mitochondrial disorders	Diogo et al. 2010
		Galactosemia	Nelson et al. 1992
		Infantile neuroaxonal dystrophy (INAD)	Farina et al. 1999
		L-2-Hydroxyglutaric aciduria	Moroni et al. 2000
CA and signal change of the dentate nucleus		L-2-Hydroxyglutaric aciduria	Moroni et al. 2000
		Wilson disease	Taly et al. 2007
		Cerebrotendinous xanthomatosis	Vanrietvelde et al. 2000
CA and cerebellar cortex T2-hyperintensity		Infantile neuroaxonal dystrophy (INAD)	Farina et al. 1999
		Marinesco-Sjögren syndrome (MSS)	Georgy et al. 1998
		Some mitochondrial disorders	Valanne et al. 1998
		Congenital disorders of glycosylation 1a (CDG)	Sparks 2006
CA and basal ganglia involvement	Calcifications	Kearns-Sayre syndrome	Chu et al. 1999
		Other mitochondrial disorders	Dinopoulos et al. 2005
		Cockayne syndrome	Koop et al. 2010
		Aicardi-Goutières syndrome	Uggetti et al. 2009
	Atrophy	Hypomyelination with atrophy of basal ganglia and cerebellum (HABC)	van der Knaap et al. 2007
		Wilson disease (late)	Taly et al. 2007
		Huntington chorea (inconsistent)	Fennema-Notestine et al. 2004
	Signal changes	Mitochondrial disorders	Haas and Dietrich 2004
		Wilson disease	Taly et al. 2007
		3-Methylglutaconic aciduria	Arbelaez et al. 1999

* Recently renamed as SCAR-1 (spinocerebellar ataxia, recessive, non-Friedreich type 1) because of nonconsistent ocular motor apraxia.
CA has also been reported in hereditary spastic paraplegias (particularly types 7, 11, and 32) (Dreha-Kulaczewski et al. 2006; Depienne et al. 2007), giant axonal neuropathy (Koop et al. 2007), succinic semialdehyde dehydrogenase deficiency (Acosta et al. 2010), methemoglobinemia type II (Fusco et al. 2010), *PEX10* mutations (Régal et al. 2010), progressive cerebello-cerebral atrophy due to disruptions of the selenocysteine formation (Agamy et al. 2010), fatty acid 2-hydroxylase gene mutations (Edvardson et al. 2008), *MED17* mutations (Kaufmann et al. 2010), SLC9A6 mutations (Gilfillan et al. 2008), *MECP2* duplication (Reardon et al. 2010), and autosomal recessive spastic ataxia with frequent white matter changes mapping to 2q33-34 (Thiffault et al. 2006).
Modified from Poretti A. et al. (2008b) Differential diagnosis of cerebellar atrophy in childhood. Eur J Paediatr Neurol 12: 155–167.

TABLE 17
Acquired cerebellar atrophy in childhood

Condition		Comments	References
Extreme preterm		Risk factors: gestational age <30 weeks, intraventricular haemorrhages	Messerschmidt et al. 2005
Neonatal hypoxic-ischemic encephalopathy		Term, superior vermis atrophy	Sargent et al. 2004
Postinflammatory (= post 'cerebellitis')		Exceptional observations, often clinically 'silent'	De Bruecker et al. 2004
Multiple sclerosis		Brainstem also affected, possible in adolescents	Edwards et al. 1999
Post-traumatic brain injury		Moderate-severe trauma, global atrophy	Spanos et al. 2007
Paraneoplastic	Paediatric Hodgkin disease	Rare, diffuse cerebellar dysfunction	Hahn et al. 2000
	Langerhans cell histiocytosis	Global atrophy, abnormalities of cerebellar white matter, brainstem, nuclei dentate, and basal ganglia	Prosch et al. 2007
	Opsoclonus-myoclonus syndrome		Klein et al. 2007
Chronic epilepsy		Not due to intoxication with antiepileptic drugs	Hermann et al. 2005
Radiation therapy			Personal observation
Posterior fossa surgery			Szathmari et al. 2010
Malnutrition	Vitamin B12 deficiency	Related to breastfeeding in vegan mothers and mothers with subclinical pernicious anaemia, cerebral > cerebellar atrophy	von Schenck et al. 1997
Toxic	Phenytoin and other antiepileptic drugs	Children, adolescents	Manto 2010
	Tacrolimus	Children, adolescents	Kaleyias et al. 2006
	Incidental intoxications	Children, adolescents	Personal observation
	Alcohol, solvents, heavy metals, drugs (heroin, cocaine)	Adolescents	Timmann and Diener 2000; Manto 2010

Modified from Poretti A, et al. (2008b) Differential diagnosis of cerebellar atrophy in childhood. Eur J Paediatr Neurol 12: 155–167.

TABLE 18
Unilateral cerebellar atrophy in childhood

Disease	Comments	References
Sequelae after unilateral cerebellitis	Cerebellitis usually has bilateral involvement, rarely unilateral	Melek et al. 2006
Sequelae after unilateral ischaemic infarction	Rarely isolated, different aetiologies possible (embolic, traumatic, toxic)	Geller et al. 2004
Sequelae after unilateral traumatic brain injury		Personal observation
Following posterior fossa surgery		Personal observation
Rasmussen encephalitis	Unilateral CA ipsilateral to the supratentorial involvement	Takeoka et al. 2003
Crossed cerebro-cerebellar diaschisis	Unilateral CA contralateral to a supratentorial lesion of different aetiology	Kozic and Kostic 2001
Unexplained origin	Child with epilepsy	Poretti et al. 2008b

Modified from Poretti A, et al. (2008b) Differential diagnosis of cerebellar atrophy in childhood. Eur J Paediatr Neurol 12: 155–167.

TABLE 19
Ataxia without cerebellar atrophy in childhood

Disease	Typical findings	References
Friedreich ataxia	Ataxia, sensory neuropathy, areflexia, hypertrophic cardiomyopathy, cervical cord atrophy	Fogel and Perlman 2007
Vitamin E deficiency	Ataxia, sensory neuropathy, low serum vitamin E	Fogel and Perlman 2007
Abetalipoproteinaemia	Ataxia, sensory neuropathy, diarrhoea, very low cholesterol, acanthocytosis	Fogel and Perlman 2007
Refsum disease	Ataxia, retinitis pigmentosa, cataract, anosmia, demyelinating polyneuropathy, elevated phytanic acid	Fogel and Perlman 2007
Glucose transporter type 1 deficiency	Ataxia, infantile epilepsy, delayed development, acquired microcephaly, hypoglycorrhachia	Klepper et al. 2005
Angelman syndrome	Ataxia, cognitive impairment, abnormal behaviour, epilepsy, macrocephaly, absent speech	Williams 2005
Rett syndrome	Ataxia, dementia, autism, acquired microcephaly, hand stereotypies, epilepsy	Naidu et al. 2001

Modified from Poretti A, et al. (2008b) Differential diagnosis of cerebellar atrophy in childhood. Eur J Paediatr Neurol 12: 155–167.

TABLE 20
Cerebellar cortex hyperintensity

Comment: Cerebellar cortex hyperintensity is best seen in FLAIR sequences, but may be missed in T2-weighted MRI. It is an inconsistent finding in a given disorder and may not be consistent in a follow-up MRI in the same patient. A diagnosis has not been reached in all patients.

Disease	Additional neuroimaging findings	References
Infantile neuroaxonal dystrophy (INAD)	Cerebellar atrophy, pallidum T2 hypointensity	Farina et al. 1999
Marinesco-Sjögren syndrome (MSS)	Cerebellar atrophy; cerebellar cortex T2-weighted hyperintensity not consistent	Harting et al. 2004
Congenital disorders of glycosylation 1a (CDG)	Cerebellar and brainstem atrophy, white matter atrophy or hypoplasia	Sparks 2006
Mitochondrial disorder	Cerebellar and cerebral atrophy, involvement of basal ganglia and white matter	Scaglia et al. 2005
Coenzyme Q10 deficiency	Cerebellar atrophy	Susan Blaser 2011 (pers. comm.)
DOOR syndrome	Cerebellar and pontine hypoplasia, delayed myelination	Nomura et al. 2009
Congenital ataxia	Cerebellar hypoplasia (inconsistent)	Personal observation

Cerebellar cortex hyperintensity has been reported in cyanide intoxication (Barkovich 2005). DOOR, Deafness, Onychdystrophy, Osteodystrophy, and Mental Retardation).

TABLE 21
Abnormalities of the dentate nuclei

Disease		Dentate nucleus	Additional neuroimaging findings	References
Metabolic	Leigh syndrome	T2W↑	T2W-hyperintensity of putamen, caudate nuclei, thalamus, red nuclei, tegmentum, and periaquiductal gray matter, diffuse white matter abnormalities supratentorially, cerebral atrophy	Lee et al. 2009
	Glutaric aciduria type 1	T2W↑	T2W-hyperintensity of putamen and caudate nuclei, atrophy fronto-temporally and dilatation of the sylvian fissures, temporal arachnoid cysts	Twomey et al. 2003
	L-2 hydroxyglutaric aciduria	T2W↑	Global atrophy, T2W-hyperintensity of the superficial cerebral white matter and subcortical U-fibres, deep white matter relatively spared	Steenweg et al. 2009
	Mucopolysaccharidoses	FLAIR↓ mixed T2W-signal	Dilatation of the Virchow-Robin spaces, cribriform appearance of white matter, corpus callosum, and basal ganglia, craniocervical junction compression, occasionally arachnoid cysts	Matheus et al. 2004
	Infantile Refsum disease	T2W↑	Symmetrical signal change involving corticospinal tracts and corpus callosum	Cakirer and Savas 2005
	Maple syrup urine disease (MSUD)	T2W↑	T2W-hyperintensity and restricted diffusion involving brainstem, corticospinal tracts, cerebellar white matter, thalami, globi pallidi, and posterior limb of internal capsule	Di Rocco et al. 2004
	Wilson disease	T1W↑	T2W-hyperintensity of putamen and cortical white matter, cerebellar and cerebral atrophy, Panda sign	Taly et al. 2007
	Cerebrotendinous xanthomatosis	T2W↑	Cerebellar atrophy, inhomogeneous white matter	Vanrietvelde et al. 2000
White matter diseases	Adrenoleukodystrophy	T2W↑	T2W-hyperintensity of the white matter, affecting splenium of corpus callosum and parieto-occipital white matter (80%) or frontal white matter, rostrum, and genu of the corpus callosum (20%)	Loes et al. 2003
	Canavan disease	T2W↑	Diffuse symmetric T2W-hyperintensity of subcortical (early) and deep (late) white matter, thalami, and globi pallidi	Brismar et al. 1990
	Krabbe disease	T2W↑	T2W-hyperintensity of the deep cerebral and cerebellar white matter, basal ganglia, and thalami	Provenzale et al. 2009
	Megalencephalic leukoencephalopathy with cysts (MLC)	T2W↑	T2W-hyperintensity of the white matter with sub-cortical cysts especially in the anterior, temporal, and fronto-parietal regions	van der Knaap and Scheper 2008
Merosin-negative muscular dystrophy		T2W↑	T2W-hyperintensity of the white matter with fronto-temporal predominance, cortical dysplasia	Leite et al. 2005
Aicardi-Goutières syndrome		Calcifications	Cerebral atrophy, white matter abnormality, cerebral calcification	Uggetti et al. 2009

Abnormalities of the dentate nuclei have also been reported in Langerhans cell histiocytosis (Prosch et al. 2007), neurofibromatosis type 1 (Mentzel et al. 2005), varicella infections (Baskin and Hedlund 2007), periventricular leukomalacia (Baker et al. 1988), cerebellar ischaemia (Fulham et al. 1992), and transiently associated with vigabatrin therapy (Pearl et al. 2009). For an excellent review of nucleus dentatus in neuropediatric diseases see McErlean et al. (2010).

TABLE 22
Cerebellar calcifications

Disease	Additional neuroimaging findings	References
Aicardi-Goutières syndrome	Cerebral atrophy, white matter abnormality, cerebral calcification	Rice et al. 2009
Cockayne syndrome	Cerebral and cerebellar atrophy, basal ganglia calcifications	Koop et al. 2010
Histiocytosis related	Abnormalities of cerebellar white matter, brainstem, basal ganglia, and cerebral white matter, spinal cord lesions (inconsistent)	Prosch et al. 2007
Kearns-Sayre syndrome	Cerebellar and cerebral atrophy, T2-weighted hyperintensity of white matter, thalami, and basal ganglia, basal ganglia calcifications	Chu et al. 1999
MELAS	Severe cortical atrophy, cerebellar atrophy, stroke-like lesions (mostly occipital)	Saneto et al. 2008

Cerebellar calcifications have been reported in neurofibromatosis type 2 (Mayfrank et al., Neuroradiology, 1990, 32: 33–37; personal observation).

TABLE 23
Abnormalities of the cerebellar white matter in metabolic and genetic diseases

Disease		Additional neuroimaging findings	References
Metabolic	Maple syrup urine disease (MSUD)	T2W-hyperintensity and restricted diffusion involving brain stem, corticospinal tracts, dentate nuclei, thalami, globi pallidi, and posterior limb of internal capsule	Di Rocco et al. 2004
	Kearns-Sayre syndrome	Cerebellar and cerebral atrophy, T2W-hyperintensity of thalami, globi pallidi, substantia nigra, pons, and medulla oblongata, basal ganglia calcifications	Chu et al. 1999
	MELAS	Cerebellar atrophy, severe cortical atrophy, stroke-like lesions (mostly occipital)	Valanne et al. 1998
	Navajo neuropathy	Comma-shaped T2W-hyperintensity of the cerebellar white matter, patchy T2W-hyperintensity of the frontal and parietal white matter	Williams et al. 1990
White matter diseases	Zellweger syndrome	Abnormal gyration (polymicrogyria, pachygyria), heterotopia, leukencephalopathy, germinolytic cysts, cerebellar hypoplasia	Weller S et al. 2008
	D-bifunctional protein deficiency	Perisylvian polymicrogyria, frontoparietal pachygyria, cerebral leukencephalopathy	Gronborg et al. 2010
	Krabbe disease	T2W-hyperintensity of the deep cerebral white matter, basal ganglia, dentate nuclei, and thalami	Provenzale et al. 2009
	Pelizaeus-Merzbacher disease	Global hypomyelination, cerebral and cerebellar atrophy	Plecko et al. 2003
	Pelizaeus-Merzbacher-like disease	Global hypomyelination, cerebral and cerebellar atrophy	Henneke et al. 2008
	Adrenoleukodystrophy	T2W-hyperintensity of the white matter, affecting splenium of corpus callosum and parieto-occipital white matter (80%) or frontal white matter, rostrum, and genu of the corpus callosum (20%)	Loes et al. 2003
	Metachromatic leukodystrophy	Diffuse symmetric white matter T2W-hyperintensity, subcortical U-fibres initially spared	Eichler et al. 2009

Additionally, Yalcinkaya et al. reported a girl with diabetes insipidus, ataxia, and pyramidal signs and progressive white matter abnormalities starting in the cerebellum (Yalcinkaya et al. 2002). For a general review of white matter diseases see the excellent review by Schiffmann and van der Knaap (2009).

Acquired abnormalities: T2-weighted hyperintensities of the cerebellar white matter have been described in varicella infections (Baskin and Hedlund 2007), Langerhans cell histiocytosis (Prosch et al. 2007), haemophagocytic lymphohistiocytosis (Van Egmond et al. 2011, personal communication), carbon monoxide poisoning (Mascalchi et al. 1996), and heroin intoxication (Offiah and Hall 2008).

White matter abnormalities in neurofibromatosis type 1 (Chapter 29; Mentzel et al. 2005).

TABLE 24
Small pons

Comment: Note that genetic and metabolic disorders with postnatal onset do *not* result in pontine atrophy.

Disease		Additional neuroimaging findings	References
Cerebellar disruptions	Cerebellar agenesis	Only minute remnants of cerebellar tissue corresponding to the middle cerebellar peduncles, anterior vermis, and flocculi, variable volume of the posterior fossa, extensive cerebral white matter loss reminiscent of periventricular leukomalacia (not consistent)	Poretti et al. 2009c
	Vanishing cerebellum in Chiari type II	Typical findings of Chiari type II malformation, marked destruction (hypoplasia) of one cerebellar hemisphere	Boltshauser et al. 2002
	Extreme preterm birth	Cerebellar hemispheres predominantly affected, vermis small and with variably preserved shape, fourth ventricle of variable size	Messerschmidt et al. 2005
Lissencephalies	*RELN* lissencephaly	Lissencephaly with anterior gradient, severe cerebellar hypoplasia	Hong et al. 2000
	VLDLR migration disorders	Pontine hypoplasia, simplified gyral pattern, afolial cerebellum	Boycott et al. 2009
	TUBA1A lissencephaly	Lissencephaly with centro-posterior gradient, cerebellar hypoplasia, agenesis of corpus callosum, ventriculomegaly	Kumar et al. 2010
Congenital muscular dystrophies (CMD)	Walker-Warburg syndrome	Congenital hydrocephalus, cobblestone lissencephaly, thin corpus callosum, absent septum pellucidum, cerebellar hypoplasia, cerebellar cysts, brainstem kinking	Clement et al. 2008
	Muscle-eye-brain disease	Polymicrogyria with fronto-occipital gradient, abnormal white matter, thin corpus callosum, cerebellar hypoplasia, cerebellar cysts	Clement et al. 2008
	Fukuyama CMD	Polymicrogyria with fronto-occipital gradient, pachygyria occipital, white matter abnormalities, cerebellar hypoplasia, cerebellar cysts	Clement et al. 2008
	GPR56 mutations	Bilateral frontoparietal polymicrogyria, cerebellar hypoplasia and dysplasia, cerebellar cysts, thin corpus callosum, abnormal white matter	Bahi-Buisson et al. 2010
	CMD with merosin deficiency	White matter abnormalities with fronto-temporal predominance, bilateral occipital cortical dysplasia, cerebellar hypoplasia	Leite et al. 2005
Metabolic	Congenital disorders of glycosylation	Cerebellar and white matter hypoplasia and/or atrophy	Sparks 2006
	Deafness, Onychodystrophy, Osteodystrophy, and mental Retardation syndrome (DOOR)	Cerebellar hypoplasia, T2-weighted hyperintensity of the cerebellar cortex, delayed myelination	James et al. 2007
Other genetic	*CASK* mutation	Severe cerebellar hypoplasia, simplified gyral pattern, thin and unmyelinated corpus callosum	Takanashi et al. 2010
	PTF1A mutation	Cerebellar agenesis	Sellick et al. 2004
	Pontine tegmental cap dysplasia (PTCD)	Vaulted pontine tegmentum, hypoplasia and dysplasia of the vermis, atypical molar tooth sign, absence of the middle cerebellar peduncles	Barth et al. 2007
	Pontocerebellar hypoplasias (PCH)	Cerebellar hypoplasia, mild cerebral atrophy and delayed myelination (all PCH forms)	Steinlin et al. 2007; Navamar et al. 2009
	CHARGE syndrome	Arrhinencephaly/hypoplastic olfactory bulbs, holoprosencephaly, septum pellucidum agenesis, nodular heterotopia, Dandy-Walker malformation	Sanlaville and Verloes 2007
	Cri-du-chat syndrome	Mild isolated pontine hypoplasia	Ninchoji and Takanshi 2010
Anencephaly		Anencephaly, primordium of cerebellum resembling cerebellar atrophy	Poretti et al. 2010b
Möbius syndrome (inconsistent)		Hypoplasia of the VIth, VIIth, XIIth nuclei	Pedraza et al. 2000

TABLE 25
Macrocerebellum

Disease	Additional neuroimaging findings	References
Sotos syndrome	Ventricular abnormalities, increased extracerebral fluid spaces, midline abnormalities, and migration anomalies	Schaefer et al. 1997
Costello syndrome	Macrocerebellum progressive causing cerebellar tonsillar herniation and hydrocephalus, Chiari type I, syrinx formation	Gripp et al. 2010
Williams syndrome	'Small cerebrum'	Jones et al. 2002
Macrocephaly–capillary malformation	Hydrocephalus, asymmetric lateral ventricle, white matter defects, hemimegalencephaly, Chiari type I, polymicrogyria, cortical dysplasia	Conway et al. 2007
Alexander disease	Symmetric cerebral white matter abnormalities with a frontal preponderance, periventricular rim of decreased signal intensity on T2-weighted images, abnormalities of the basal ganglia, thalami, and brainstem, contrast enhancement involving several brain structures	van der Knaap et al. 2005
Fucosidosis	Hypomyelination and T1-weighted hyperintensity of putamina and globi pallidi	Kau et al. 2011
Lhermitte-Duclos syndrome	Non-enhancing gyriform pattern, hypointensity on T1-weighted images, striated pattern with isointense bands in the area of hyperintensity on T2-weighted images	Nowak and Trost 2002
Nonsyndromal macrocerebellum	Deficient or delayed myelination of the cerebral white matter, subcortical band heterotopia	Bodensteiner et al. 1997

TABLE 26
Hemicerebellar megalencephaly

Comment: Cerebellar enlargement is ipsilateral to hemimegalencephaly.

Disease	Additional neuroimaging findings	References
Isolated hemicerebellar megalencephaly	Hemimegalencephaly	Flores-Sarnat 2008
Epidermal naevus syndrome	Hemimegalencephaly, patchy macrogyria, microgyria, heterotopia, vascular malformations, brain tumours, intracranial/intraspinal lipomas, gliomatosis	Sugarman 2007
Klippel-Trenaunay syndrome	Hemimegalencephaly, arteriovenous malformations and aneurysms	Oduber et al. 2008
Neurofibromatosis type 1	Optic pathway and other gliomas, T2-weighted hyperintensities in brainstem, cerebellar white matter, basal ganglia, hemimegalencepahly	Payne et al. 2010
Proteus syndrome	Hemimegalencephaly, subependymal calcified nodules, periventricular cysts	Dietrich et al. 1998
Tuberous sclerosis	Cortical tuber, subependymal nodule, giant cell astrocytoma, white matter radial migration lines, hemimegalencephaly	Galluzzi et al. 2002
Hypomelanosis of Ito	Hemimegalencephaly, heterotopia, polymicrogyria, white matter signal abnormalities, enlarged perivascular spaces	Chapman and Cardenas 2008
Macrocephaly–capillary malformation	Hemimegalencephaly, hydrocephalus, asymmetric lateral ventricle, white matter defects, Chiari type I, hemimegalencephaly, cavum septum pellucidum, polymicrogyria, cortical dysplasia	Conway et al. 2007

TABLE 27
Molar tooth sign

Comment: The typical molar tooth sign (MTS) is characterized by thickened and elongated superior cerebellar peduncles with parallel course, and an abnormally deep interpeduncular fossa. In the 'atypical' MTS the superior cerebellar peduncles are not thickened and elongated, but show an almost horizontal orientation and a convergent course, and the depth of the interpeduncular fossa is only mild.

Disease	MTS	Additional findings	References
Pure Joubert syndrome	Typical	Hypoplasia/dysplasia of the vermis, ataxia, OMA, hypotonia, cognitive impairment, postaxial polydactyly	Doherty 2009
Joubert syndrome and retinal dystrophy	Typical	Hypoplasia/dysplasia of the vermis, ataxia, OMA, hypotonia, cognitive impairment, retinal dystrophy, postaxial polydactyly	Gleeson et al. 2004
Senior-Löken syndrome	Typical	Hypoplasia/dysplasia of the vermis, ataxia, OMA, hypotonia, cognitive impairment, cystic dysplastic kidneys, nephronophthisis, retinal dystrophy	Gleeson et al. 2004
Dekaban-Arima syndrome	Typical	Hypoplasia/dysplasia of the vermis, ataxia, OMA, hypotonia, cognitive impairment, cystic dysplastic kidneys, retinal dystrophy	Gleeson et al. 2004
COACH syndrome	Typical	Hypoplasia/dysplasia of the vermis, ataxia, OMA, hypotonia, cognitive impairment, coloboma, hepatic fibrosis, postaxial polydactyly	Brancati et al. 2009
Oral-facial-digital syndrome type VI (OFD VI)	Typical	Hypoplasia/dysplasia of the vermis, abnormalities of the tectum, enlarged posterior fossa and prepontine cisterna, ataxia, OMA, hypotonia, cognitive impairment, tongue hamartoma, mesaxial polydactyly, additional frenula, hypothalamic hamartoma	Poretti et al. 2008a
Malta syndrome	Typical	Hypoplasia/dysplasia of the vermis, ataxia, OMA, hypotonia, cognitive impairment, cystic dysplastic kidneys, retinal dystrophy	Gleeson et al. 2004
Meckel-Gruber syndrome	Typical	Hypoplasia/dysplasia of the vermis, ataxia, OMA, hypotonia, cognitive impairment, cystic dysplastic kidneys, occipital encephalocele, dysplasia of the bile ducts, postaxial polydactyly	Frank et al. 2008
Pontine tegmental cap dysplasia (PTCD)	Atypical	Flat profile of the ventral pons, vaulted pontine tegmentum, hypoplasia and dysplasia of the vermis, absence of the middle cerebellar peduncles, hearing impairment, facial, palsy, bilateral sensory trigeminal nerve involvement, ataxia	Barth et al. 2007

COACH, cerebellar vermis hypoplasia, oligophrenia, ataxia, coloboma, and hepatic fibrosis; OMA, ocular motor apraxia.

TABLE 28
Abnormal tectum

Tectal finding	Disease	Additional neuroimaging findings	References
Enlarged	Walker-Warburg phenotype	Congenital hydrocephalus, cobblestone lissencephaly, thin corpus callosum, absent septum pellucidum, cerebellar and pontine hypoplasia, cerebellar cysts, brainstem kinking	Clement et al. 2008
	Postsegmentation malformations (dorsal and ventral clefts)	Dorsal and ventral clefts, elongation of midbrain and medulla, small pons and vermis, absent corpus callosum	Barkovich et al. 2007
Enlarged and rotated	Oculocerebrocutaneous syndrome	Cerebellar hypoplasia with absent vermis, large posterior fossa, frontal predominant polymicrogyria, periventricular nodular heterotopia, corpus callosum agenesis, ventriculomegaly, interhemispheric cysts, occipital meningocele (inconsistent)	Moog et al. 2005
Long and thick	Abnormal brainstem segmentation (short pons)	Short pons, long medulla, thin midbrain tegmentum, dorsal and ventral clefts in the pons	Barkovich et al. 2007
	L1 syndrome	Severe hydrocephalus, rippled ventricular wall after shunt placement, hypoplasia of the corpus callosum, large massa intermedia, hypoplasia of the cerebellar vermis	Kanemura et al. 2006
Short and thin	Abnormal brainstem segmentation (short midbrain/long pons)	Short midbrain, long pons, large superior vermis	Barkovich et al. 2007
Short and thick	Oral-facial-digital syndrome type VI (OFD VI)	Hypoplasia/dysplasia of the vermis, molar tooth sign, enlarged posterior fossa and prepontine cisterna, hypothalamic hamartoma	Poretti et al. 2008a
Thick and rounded	Muscle-eye-brain disease phenotype	Polymicrogyria with fronto-occipital gradient, abnormal white matter, thin corpus callosum, cerebellar hypoplasia, cerebellar cysts, brainstem cleft	Clement et al. 2008
Beaking	Chiari 2 malformation	Small posterior fossa and cerebellar volume, vermian herniation below foramen magnum, upward herniation of the superior vermis, wrapping of the cerebellar hemispheres around the brainstem, dysplastic tentorium cerebelli, inferior displacement of the lower brainstem, medullary-cervical kink, aqueduct stenosis	Juranek and Salman 2010
Dysplastic	Some cases of Joubert syndrome	Hypoplasia/dysplasia of the vermis, molar tooth sign, absence of pyramidal and superior cerebellar peduncles, decussation, encephalocele (inconsistent)	Doherty 2009

TABLE 29
Brainstem clefts

Comments: The most common clefts are ventral longitudinal and midline, involving the pons. Dorsal midline clefts are localized in the region of the median longitudinal fasciculus; therefore, these patients have abnormal horizontal gaze. Ventral clefts are associated with cerebellar malformations, small middle cerebellar peduncles, and diminished or absent anterior transverse pontine axons (probably due to absence of the decussation of the middle cerebellar peduncles). Transverse clefts are situated where the transverse axonal bundles normally connect between the ventral and dorsal longitudinal fascicles.

Cleft localization		Disease	Cleft characteristics	Neuroimaging findings	References
Midbrain	Dorsal	Midbrain dysgenesis (in a patient with trisomy 14)	Longitudinal	Longitudinal cleft, midbrain dysgenesis	Barkovich et al. 2009
Pons	Dorsal	Walker-Warburg phenotype	Small longitudinal cleft in the region of the brainstem kinking	Congenital hydrocephalus, cobblestone lissencephaly, thin corpus callosum, absent septum pellucidum, cerebellar and pontine hypoplasia, cerebellar cysts	Barkovich et al. 2007
		Postsegmentation malformations (dorsal and ventral clefts)	Deep, longitudinal, in the midline	Dorsal pontine concavity, cerebellar hypoplasia (not consistent)	Barkovich et al. 2007
	Ventral	Muscle-eye-brain disease phenotype	Small, longitudinal, midline	Polymicrogyria with fronto-occipital gradient, abnormal white matter, thin corpus callosum, cerebellar hypoplasia, small middle cerebellar peduncles, cerebellar cysts	Barkovich et al. 2007
		Horizontal clefts (reported in 2 cases of Godenhar syndrome)	Horizontal (left to right), in the middle of the pons with small band of tissues ventral to the cleft	Short and extremely narrow pons, small middle cerebellar peduncles	Barkovich et al. 2007; Pane et al. 2004
		Postsegmentation malformations (dorsal and ventral clefts)	Deep, longitudinal, midline, can be asymmetric	Small pons and cerebellum, elongated medulla, absent corpus callosum, mildly enlarged midbrain tectum	Barkovich et al. 2007
	Dorso-ventral	Abnormal brainstem segmentation (short pons)	Deep, longitudinal, midline	Short pons, long medulla, thin midbrain tegmentum	Barkovich et al. 2007
		Postsegmentation malformations (dorsal and ventral clefts)	Deep, longitudinal, in the midline	Short pons, long medulla, variable midbrain (normal, small, long) and corpus callosum (absent, thick), tectum long and thick	Barkovich et al. 2007
		Horizontal gaze palsy and progressive scoliosis due to *ROBO3* mutation	Prominent, longitudinal, in the midline	Hypoplastic pons and medulla, flat pons, butterfly-shaped medulla	Bosley et al. 2005

In postsegmentation malformation with midbrain enlargement and dorsoventral midline hyperintensity, dorsoventral midline stripes of hyperintensity in the midbrain have been reported (Barkovich et al. 2007).

REFERENCES

Abdel-Salam GM, Zaki MS, Saleem SN, Gaber KR (2008) Microcephaly, malformation of brain development and intracranial calcification in sibs: pseudo-TORCH or a new syndrome. Am J Med Genet A 146A: 2929–2936.

Accardo AP, Pensiero S, Perissutti P (2005) Saccadic analysis for early identification of neurological involvement in Gaucher disease. Ann N Y Acad Sci 1039: 503–507.

Acosta MT, Munasinghe J, Pearl PL, Gupta M, Finegersh A, Gibson KM, Theodore WH (2010) Cerebellar atrophy in human and murine succinic semialdehyde dehydrogenase deficiency. J Child Neurol 25: 1457–1461.

Agamy O, Ben Zeev B, Lev D, Marcus B, Fine D, Su D, et al. (2010) Mutations disrupting selenocysteine formation cause progressive cerebello-cerebral atrophy. Am J Hum Genet 87: 538–544.

Aldinger KA, Lehmann OJ, Hudgins L, Chizhikov VV, Bassuk AG, Ades LC, et al. (2009) FOXC1 is required for normal cerebellar development and is a major contributor to chromosome 6p25.3 Dandy-Walker malformation. Nat Genet 41: 1037–1042.

Amador C, Mathews AM, Del Carmen Montoya M, Laughridge ME, Everman DB, Holden KR (2008) Expanding the neurologic phenotype of oculodentodigital dysplasia in a 4-generation Hispanic family. J Child Neurol 23: 901–905.

Anheim M, Monga B, Fleury M, Charles P, Barbot C, Salih M, et al. (2009) Ataxia with oculomotor apraxia type 2: clinical, biological and genotype/phenotype correlation study of a cohort of 90 patients. Brain 132: 2688–2698.

Arbelaez A, Castillo M, Stone J (1999) MRI in 3-methylglutaconic aciduria type 1. Neuroradiology 41: 941–942.

Assoum M, Salih MA, Drouot N, H'Mida-Ben Brahim D, Lagier-Tourenne C, AlDrees A, et al. (2010) Rundataxin, a novel protein with RUN and diacylglycerol binding domains, is mutant in a new recessive ataxia. Brain 133: 2439–2447.

Bacigaluppi S, Rusconi R, Rampini P, Annoni F, Zavanone ML, Carnelli V, Gaini SM (2006) Vertebral artery dissection in a child. Is 'spontaneous' still an appropriate definition? Neurol Sci 27: 364–368.

Bahi-Buisson N, Poirier K, Boddaert N, Fallet-Bianco C, Specchio N, Bertini E, et al. (2010) GPR56-related bilateral frontoparietal polymicrogyria: further evidence for an overlap with the cobblestone complex. Brain 133: 3194–3209.

Baker LL, Stevenson DK, Enzmann DR (1988) End-stage periventricular leukomalacia: MR evaluation. Radiology 168: 809–815.

Bams-Mengerink AM, Majoie CB, Duran M, Wanders RJ, Van Hove J, Scheurer CD, et al. (2006) MRI of the brain and cervical spinal cord in rhizomelic chondrodysplasia punctata. Neurology 66: 798–803.

Banwell B, Ghezzi A, Bar-Or A, Mikaeloff Y, Tardieu M (2007) Multiple sclerosis in children: clinical diagnosis, therapeutic strategies, and future directions. Lancet Neurol 6: 887–902.

Baranano KW, Hartman AL (2008) The ketogenic diet: uses in epilepsy and other neurologic illnesses. Curr Treat Options Neurol 10: 410–419.

Barkovich AJ (2005) Toxic and metabolic brain disorders. In: Barkovich AJ, editor. Pediatric Neuroimaging. Philadelphia: Lippincott Williams & Wilkins; pp. 130–131.

Barkovich AJ, Millen KJ, Dobyns WB (2007) A developmental classification of malformations of the brainstem. Ann Neurol 62: 625–639.

Barkovich AJ, Millen KJ, Dobyns WB (2009) A developmental and genetic classification for midbrain-hindbrain malformations. Brain 132: 3199–3230.

Barnerias C, Saudubray JM, Touati G, De Lonlay P, Dulac O, Ponsot G, et al. (2010) Pyruvate dehydrogenase complex deficiency: four neurological phenotypes with differing pathogenesis. Dev Med Child Neurol 52: e1–9.

Barone R, Bruhl K, Stoeter P, Fiumara A, Pavone L, Beck M (1996) Clinical and neuroradiological findings in classic infantile and late-onset globoid-cell leukodystrophy (Krabbe disease). Am J Med Genet 63: 209–217.

Barth PG, Majoie CB, Caan MW, Weterman MA, Kyllerman M, Smit LM, et al. (2007) Pontine tegmental cap dysplasia: a novel brain malformation with a defect in axonal guidance. Brain 130: 2258–2266.

Baskin HJ, Hedlund G (2007) Neuroimaging of herpesvirus infections in children. Pediatr Radiol 37: 949–963.

Bellini C, Massocco D, Serra G (2000) Prenatal cocaine exposure and the expanding spectrum of brain malformations. Arch Intern Med 160: 2393.

Bennett HS, Selman JE, Rapin I, Rose A (1982) Nonconvulsive epileptiform activity appearing as ataxia. Am J Dis Child 136: 30–32.

Bernard G, Shevell M (2008) The wobbly child: an approach to inherited ataxias. Semin Pediatr Neurol 15: 194–208.

Biancheri R, Zara F, Bruno C, Rossi A, Bordo L, Gazzerro E, et al. (2007) Phenotypic characterization of hypomyelination and congenital cataract. Ann Neurol 62: 121–127.

Birch DG (1999) Retinal degeneration in retinitis pigmentosa and neuronal ceroid lipofuscinosis: An overview. Mol Genet Metab 66: 356–366.

Blattner R, Von Moers A, Leegwater PA, Hanefeld FA, Van Der Knaap MS, Kohler W (2003) Clinical and genetic heterogeneity in megalencephalic leukoencephalopathy with subcortical cysts (MLC). Neuropediatrics 34: 215–218.

Blumkin L, Michelson M, Leshinsky-Silver E, Kivity S, Lev D, Lerman-Sagie T (2010) Congenital ataxia, mental retardation, and dyskinesia associated with a novel CACNA1A mutation. J Child Neurol 25: 892–897.

Bockenhauer D, Feather S, Stanescu HC, Bandulik S, Zdebik AA, Reichold M, et al. (2009) Epilepsy, ataxia, sensorineural deafness, tubulopathy, and KCNJ10 mutations. N Engl J Med 360: 1960–1970.

Bodensteiner JB, Schaefer GB, Keller GM, Thompson JN, Bowen MK (1997) Macrocerebellum: neuroimaging and clinical features of a newly recognized condition. J Child Neurol 12: 365–368.

Bojinova V, Dimova P, Belopitova L (2000) Clinical manifestations of cerebrovascular hypoplasias in childhood. J Child Neurol 15: 166–171.

Bolduc ME, Limperopoulos C (2009) Neurodevelopmental outcomes in children with cerebellar malformations: a systematic review. Dev Med Child Neurol 51: 256–267.

Boltshauser E, Schneider J, Kollias S, Waibel P, Weissert M (2002) Vanishing cerebellum in myelomeningocoele. Eur J Paediatr Neurol 6: 109–113.

Bomar JM, Benke PJ, Slattery EL, Puttagunta R, Taylor LP, Seong E, et al. (2003) Mutations in a novel gene encoding a CRAL-TRIO domain cause human Cayman ataxia and ataxia/dystonia in the jittery mouse. Nat Genet 35: 264–269.

Bosley TM, Salih MA, Jen JC, Lin DD, Oystreck D, Abu-Amero KK, et al. (2005) Neurologic features of horizontal gaze palsy and progressive scoliosis with mutations in ROBO3. Neurology 64: 1196–1203.

Bouslam N, Bouhouche A, Benomar A, Hanein S, Klebe S, Azzedine H, et al. (2007) A novel locus for autosomal recessive spastic ataxia on chromosome 17p. Hum Genet 121: 413–420.

Boycott KM, Bonnemann C, Herz J, Neuert S, Beaulieu C, Scott JN, et al. (2009) Mutations in VLDLR as a cause for autosomal recessive cerebellar ataxia with mental retardation (dysequilibrium syndrome). J Child Neurol 24: 1310–1315.

Brancati F, Iannicelli M, Travaglini L, Mazzotta A, Bertini E, Boltshauser E, et al. (2009) MKS3/TMEM67 mutations are a major cause of COACH syndrome, a Joubert syndrome related disorder with liver involvement. Hum Mutat 30: E432–442.

Brismar J, Brismar G, Gascon G, Ozand P (1990) Canavan disease: CT and MR imaging of the brain. AJNR Am J Neuroradiol 11: 805–810.

Brockmann K (2009) The expanding phenotype of GLUT1-deficiency syndrome. Brain Dev 31: 545–552.

Brunetti-Pierri N, Wilfong AA, Hunter JV, Craigen WJ (2006) A severe case of dentatorubro-pallidoluysian atrophy (DRPLA) with microcephaly, very early onset of seizures, and cerebral white matter involvement. Neuropediatrics 37: 308–311.

Cakirer S, Savas MR (2005) Infantile Refsum disease: serial evaluation with MRI. Pediatr Radiol 35: 212–215.

Campbell LE, Daly E, Toal F, Stevens A, Azuma R, Catani M, et al. (2006) Brain and behaviour in children with 22q11.2 deletion syndrome: a volumetric and voxel-based morphometry MRI study. Brain 129: 1218–1228.

Carr JA, van der Walt PE, Nakayama J, Fu YH, Corfield V, Brink P, Ptacek L (2007) FAME 3: a novel form of progressive myoclonus and epilepsy. Neurology 68: 1382–1389.

Caruso PA, Poussaint TY, Tzika AA, Zurakowski D, Astrakas LG, Elias ER, et al. (2004) MRI and 1H MRS findings in Smith-Lemli-Opitz syndrome. Neuroradiology 46: 3–14.

Chapman K, Cardenas JF (2008) Hemimegalencephaly in a patient with a neurocutaneous syndrome. Semin Pediatr Neurol 15: 190–193.

Chen CP, Lee CC, Chang TY, Town DD, Wang W (2004) Prenatal diagnosis of mosaic distal 5p deletion and review of the literature. Prenat Diagn 24: 50–57.

Chen CP, Chern SR, Lin CC, Wang TH, Li YC, Hsieh LJ, et al. (2006) Prenatal findings and molecular cytogenetic analyses of partial trisomy 12q (12q24.32 – >qter) and partial monosomy 21q (21q22.2 – >qter). Prenat Diagn 26: 313–320.

Cheon CK, Lee BH, Ko JM, Kim HJ, Yoo HW (2010) Novel mutation in SLC6A19 causing late-onset seizures in Hartnup disorder. Pediatr Neurol 42: 369–371.

Chu BC, Terae S, Takahashi C, Kikuchi Y, Miyasaka K, Abe S, et al. (1999) MRI of the brain in the Kearns-Sayre syndrome: report of four cases and a review. Neuroradiology 41: 759–764.

Cleaver JE, Lam ET, Revet I (2009) Disorders of nucleotide excision repair: the genetic and molecular basis of heterogeneity. Nat Rev Genet 10: 756–768.

Clement E, Mercuri E, Godfrey C, Smith J, Robb S, Kinali M, et al. (2008) Brain involvement in muscular dystrophies with defective dystroglycan glycosylation. Ann Neurol 64: 573–582.

Conway RL, Pressman BD, Dobyns WB, Danielpour M, Lee J, Sanchez-Lara PA, et al. (2007) Neuroimaging findings in macrocephaly-capillary malformation: a longitudinal study of 17 patients. Am J Med Genet A 143A: 2981–3008.

Crawford TO, Mandir AS, Lefton-Greif MA, Goodman SN, Goodman BK, Sengul H, Lederman HM (2000) Quantitative neurologic assessment of ataxia-telangiectasia. Neurology 54: 1505–1509.

Cuvellier JC, Lepine A (2010) Childhood periodic syndromes. Pediatr Neurol 42: 1–11.

D'Avella D, Servadei F, Scerrati M, Tomei G, Brambilla G, Angileri FF, et al. (2002) Traumatic intracerebellar hemorrhage: clinicoradiological analysis of 81 patients. Neurosurgery 50: 16–25.

De Bruecker Y, Claus F, Demaerel P, Ballaux F, Sciot R, Lagae L, et al. (2004) MRI findings in acute cerebellitis. Eur Radiol 14: 1478–1483.

Delague V, Bareil C, Bouvagnet P, Salem N, Chouery E, Loiselet J, Megarbane A, Claustres M (2001) Nonprogressive autosomal recessive ataxia maps to chromosome 9q34–9qter in a large consanguineous Lebanese family. Ann Neurol 50: 250–253.

Delague V, Bareil C, Bouvagnet P, Salem N, Chouery E, Loiselet J, Megarbane A, Claustres M (2002) A new autosomal recessive non-progressive congenital cerebellar ataxia associated with mental retardation, optic atrophy, and skin abnormalities (CAMOS) maps to chromosome 15q24-q26 in a large consanguineous Lebanese Druze Family. Neurogenetics 4: 23–27.

Delia D, Piane M, Buscemi G, Savio C, Palmeri S, Lulli P, Carlessi L, Fontanella E, Chessa L (2004) MRE11 mutations and impaired ATM-dependent responses in an Italian family with ataxia-telangiectasia-like disorder. Hum Mol Genet 13: 2155–2163.

Deodato F, Boenzi S, Santorelli FM, Dionisi-Vici C (2006) Methylmalonic and propionic aciduria. Am J Med Genet C Semin Med Genet 142C: 104–112.

Depienne C, Stevanin G, Brice A, Durr A (2007) Hereditary spastic paraplegias: an update. Curr Opin Neurol 20: 674–680.

Di Donato I, Bianchi S, Federico A (2010) Ataxia with vitamin E deficiency: update of molecular diagnosis. Neurol Sci 31: 511–515.

Di Rocco M, Biancheri R, Rossi A, Allegri AE, Vecchi V, Tortori-Donati P (2004) MRI in acute intermittent maple syrup urine disease. Neurology 63: 1078.

DiDonato S, Rimoldi M, Moise A, Bertagnoglio B, Uziel G (1979) Fatal ataxic encephalopathy and carnitine acetyltransferase deficiency: a functional defect of pyruvate oxidation? Neurology 29: 1578–1583.

Dietrich RB, Glidden DE, Roth GM, Martin RA, Demo DS (1998) The Proteus syndrome: CNS manifestations. AJNR Am J Neuroradiol 19: 987–990.

DiMauro S, Schon EA (2003) Mitochondrial respiratory-chain diseases. N Engl J Med 348: 2656–2668.

Dinopoulos A, Cecil KM, Schapiro MB, Papadimitriou A, Hadjigeorgiou GM, Wong B, et al. (2005) Brain MRI and proton MRS findings in infants and children with respiratory chain defects. Neuropediatrics 36: 290–301.

Diogo L, Cordeiro M, Garcia P, Fineza I, Moura C, Oliveira CR, et al. (2010) Value of brain magnetic resonance imaging in mitochondrial respiratory chain disorders. Pediatr Neurol 42: 196–200.

Dobrovoljac M, Hengartner H, Boltshauser E, Grotzer MA (2002) Delay in the diagnosis of paediatric brain tumours. Eur J Pediatr 161: 663–667.

Doherty D (2009) Joubert syndrome: insights into brain development, cilium biology, and complex disease. Semin Pediatr Neurol 16: 143–154.

Dorner L, Fritsch MJ, Stark AM, Mehdorn HM (2007) Posterior fossa tumors in children: how long does it take to establish the diagnosis? Childs Nerv Syst 23: 887–890.

Dreha-Kulaczewski S, Dechent P, Helms G, Frahm J, Gartner J, Brockmann K (2006) Cerebral metabolic and structural alterations in hereditary spastic paraplegia with thin corpus callosum assessed by MRS and DTI. Neuroradiology 48: 893–898.

Edery P, Chabrier S, Ceballos-Picot I, Marie S, Vincent MF, Tardieu M (2003) Intrafamilial variability in the phenotypic expression of adenylosuccinate lyase deficiency: a report on three patients. Am J Med Genet A 120A: 185–190.

Edlow JA, Newman-Toker DE, Savitz SI (2008) Diagnosis and initial management of cerebellar infarction. Lancet Neurol 7: 951–964.

Edvardson S, Hama H, Shaag A, Gomori JM, Berger I, Soffer D, et al. (2008) Mutations in the fatty acid 2-hydroxylase gene are associated with leukodystrophy with spastic paraparesis and dystonia. Am J Hum Genet 83: 643–648.

Edwards SG, Gong QY, Liu C, Zvartau ME, Jaspan T, Roberts N, Blumhardt LD (1999) Infratentorial atrophy on magnetic resonance imaging and disability in multiple sclerosis. Brain 122: 291–301.

Eichler F, Grodd W, Grant E, Sessa M, Biffi A, Bley A, et al. (2009) Metachromatic leukodystrophy: a scoring system for brain MR imaging observations. AJNR Am J Neuroradiol 30: 1893–1897.

Eklund EA, Freeze HH (2006) The congenital disorders of glycosylation: a multifaceted group of syndromes. NeuroRx 3: 254–263.

Evans RW, Linder SL (2002) Management of basilar migraine. Headache 42: 383–384.

Farina L, Nardocci N, Bruzzone MG, D'Incerti L, Zorzi G, Verga L, et al. (1999) Infantile neuroaxonal dystrophy: neuroradiological studies in 11 patients. Neuroradiology 41: 376–380.

Fennema-Notestine C, Archibald SL, Jacobson MW, Corey-Bloom J, Paulsen JS, Peavy GM, et al. (2004) In vivo evidence of cerebellar atrophy and cerebral white matter loss in Huntington disease. Neurology 63: 898–995.

Fernandez C, Soulier M, Coulibaly B, Liprandi A, Benoit B, Giuliano F, et al. (2008) Acrocallosal syndrome in fetus: focus on additional brain abnormalities. Acta Neuropathol 115: 151–156.

Fernandez M, Raskind W, Matsushita M, Wolff J, Lipe H, Bird T (2001) Hereditary benign chorea: clinical and genetic features of a distinct disease. Neurology 57: 106–110.

Fink R, Thapa MM, Ishak GE, Pruthi S (2010) Neuroimaging of pediatric central nervous system cytomegalovirus infection. Radiographics 30: 1779–1796.

Finsterer J (2008) Leigh and Leigh-like syndrome in children and adults. Pediatr Neurol 39: 223–235.

Flores-Sarnat L (2008) Hemimegalencephaly syndrome. In: Malformations of the Nervous System (Sarnat HB, Curatolo P, eds). New York: Elsevier; 153–176.

Fogel BL, Perlman S (2007) Clinical features and molecular genetics of autosomal recessive cerebellar ataxias. Lancet Neurol 6: 245–257.

Frank V, den Hollander AI, Bruchle NO, Zonneveld MN, Nurnberg G, Becker C, et al. (2008) Mutations of the CEP290 gene encoding a centrosomal protein cause Meckel-Gruber syndrome. Hum Mutat 29: 45–52.

Fulham MJ, Brooks RA, Hallett M, Di Chiro G (1992) Cerebellar diaschisis revisited: pontine hypometabolism and dentate sparing. Neurology 42: 2267–2273.

Fusco C, Soncini G, Frattini D, Della Giustina E, Vercellati C, Fermo E, Bianchi P (2011) Cerebellar atrophy in a child with hereditary methemoglobinemia type II. Brain Dev 33: 357–360.

Galluzzi P, Cerase A, Strambi M, Buoni S, Fois A, Venturi C (2002) Hemimegalencephaly in tuberous sclerosis complex. J Child Neurol 17: 677–680.

Ganesan V, Chong WK, Cox TC, Chawda SJ, Prengler M, Krikham FJ (2002) Posterior circulation stroke in childhood: risk factors and recurrence. Neurology 59: 1552–1556.

Ganie MA, Bhat D (2009) Current developments in Wolfram syndrome. J Pediatr Endocrinol Metab 22: 3–10.

Garrett J, Ryan P (2002) A child with Miller Fisher syndrome. J Paediatr Child Health 38: 414–416.

Geller T, Loftis L, Brink DS (2004) Cerebellar infarction in adolescent males associated with acute marijuana use. Pediatrics 113: e365–370.

Georgy BA, Snow RD, Brogdon BG, Wertelecki W (1998) Neuroradiologic findings in Marinesco-Sjogren syndrome. AJNR Am J Neuroradiol 19: 281–283.

Gerth C, Morel CF, Feigenbaum A, Levin AV (2008) Ocular phenotype in patients with methylmalonic aciduria and homocystinuria, cobalamin C type. J AAPOS 12: 591–596.

Gilfillan GD, Selmer KK, Roxrud I, Smith R, Kyllerman M, Eiklid K, et al. (2008) SLC9A6 mutations cause X-linked mental retardation, microcephaly, epilepsy, and ataxia, a phenotype mimicking Angelman syndrome. Am J Hum Genet 82: 1003–1010.

Gleeson JG, Keeler LC, Parisi MA, Marsh SE, Chance PF, Glass IA, et al. (2004) Molar tooth sign of the midbrain-hindbrain junction: occurrence in multiple distinct syndromes. Am J Med Genet A 125A: 125–134.

Golomb MR, Walsh LE, Carvalho KS, Christensen CK, DeMyer WE (2004) Clinical findings in Pelizaeus-Merzbacher disease. J Child Neurol 19: 328–331.

Gribaa M, Salih M, Anheim M, Lagier-Tourenne C, H'Mida D, Drouot N, et al. (2007) A new form of childhood onset, autosomal recessive spinocerebellar ataxia and epilepsy is localized at 16q21-q23. Brain 130: 1921–1928.

Gripp KW, Hopkins E, Doyle D, Dobyns WB (2010) High incidence of progressive postnatal cerebellar enlargement in Costello syndrome: brain overgrowth associated with HRAS mutations as the likely cause of structural brain and spinal cord abnormalities. Am J Med Genet A 152A: 1161–1168.

Gronborg S, Krätzner R, Spiegler J, Ferdinandusse S, Wanders RJ, Waterham HR, Gärtner J (2010) Typical cMRI pattern as diagnostic clue fro D-bifunctional protein deficiency without apparent biochemical abnormalities in plasma. Am J Genet A 152A: 2845–2849.

Gronlund MA, Honarvar AK, Andersson S, Moslemi AR, Oldfors A, Holme E, et al. (2010) Ophthalmological findings in children and young adults with genetically verified mitochondrial disease. Br J Ophthalmol 94: 121–127.

Haas D, Hoffmann GF (2006) Mevalonate kinase deficiencies: from mevalonic aciduria to hyperimmunoglobulinemia D syndrome. Orphanet J Rare Dis 1: 13.

Haas R, Dietrich R (2004) Neuroimaging of mitochondrial disorders. Mitochondrion 4: 471–490.

Hadjivassiliou M, Sanders DS, Grunewald RA, Woodroofe N, Boscolo S, Aeschlimann D (2010) Gluten sensitivity: from gut to brain. Lancet Neurol 9: 318–330.

Hahn A, Claviez A, Brinkmann G, Altermatt HJ, Schneppenheim R, Stephani U (2000) Paraneoplastic cerebellar degeneration in pediatric Hodgkin disease. Neuropediatrics 31: 42–44.

Hanna MG, Nelson I, Sweeney MG, Cooper JM, Watkins PJ, Morgan-Hughes JA, Harding AE (1995) Congenital encephalomyopathy and adult-onset myopathy and diabetes mellitus: different phenotypic associations of a new heteroplasmic mtDNA tRNA glutamic acid mutation. Am J Hum Genet 56: 1026–1033.

Harting I, Blaschek A, Wolf NI, Seitz A, Haupt M, Goebel HH, et al. (2004) T2-hyperintense cerebellar cortex in Marinesco-Sjogren syndrome. Neurology 63: 2448–2449.

Henneke M, Combes P, Diekmann S, Bertini E, Brockmann K, Burlina AP, et al. (2008) GJA12 mutations are a rare cause of Pelizaeus-Merzbacher-like disease. Neurology 70: 748–754.

Hermann BP, Bayless K, Hansen R, Parrish J, Seidenberg M (2005) Cerebellar atrophy in temporal lobe epilepsy. Epilepsy Behav 7: 279–287.

Hinson VK, Haren WB (2006) Psychogenic movement disorders. Lancet Neurol 5: 695–700.

Hoffmann C, Ben-Zeev B, Anikster Y, Nissenkorn A, Brand N, Kuint J, Kushnir T (2007) Magnetic resonance imaging and magnetic resonance spectroscopy in isolated sulfite oxidase deficiency. J Child Neurol 22: 1214–1221.

Hong SE, Shugart YY, Huang DT, Shahwan SA, Grant PE, Hourihane JO, et al. (2000) Autosomal recessive lissencephaly with cerebellar hypoplasia is associated with human RELN mutations. Nat Genet 26: 93–96.

Illarioshkin SN, Tanaka H, Markova ED, Nikolskaya NN, Ivanova-Smolenskaya IA, Tsuji S (1996) X-linked nonprogressive congenital cerebellar hypoplasia: clinical description and mapping to chromosome Xq. Ann Neurol 40: 75–83.

Isashiki Y, Nakagawa M, Ohba N, Kamimura K, Sakoda Y, Higuchi I, et al. (1998) Retinal manifestations in mitochondrial diseases associated with mitochondrial DNA mutation. Acta Ophthalmol Scand 76: 6–13.

Jaglin XH, Poirier K, Saillour Y, Buhler E, Tian G, Bahi-Buisson N, et al. (2009) Mutations in the beta-tubulin gene TUBB2B result in asymmetrical polymicrogyria. Nat Genet 41: 746–752.

James AW, Miranda SG, Culver K, Hall BD, Golabi M (2007) DOOR syndrome: clinical report, literature review and discussion of natural history. Am J Med Genet A 143A: 2821–2831.

Janecke AR, Muller T, Gassner I, Kreczy A, Schmid E, Kronenberg F, et al. (2004) Joubert-like syndrome unlinked to known candidate loci. J Pediatr 144: 264–269.

Jen JC, Graves TD, Hess EJ, Hanna MG, Griggs RC, Baloh RW (2007) Primary episodic ataxias: diagnosis, pathogenesis and treatment. Brain 130: 2484–2493.

Jissendi-Tchofo P, Kara S, Barkovich AJ (2009) Midbrain-hindbrain involvement in lissencephalies. Neurology 72: 410–418.

Jones W, Hesselink J, Courchesne E, Duncan T, Matsuda K, Bellugi U (2002) Cerebellar abnormalities in infants and toddlers with Williams syndrome. Dev Med Child Neurol 44: 688–694.

Juranek J, Salman MS (2010) Anomalous development of brain structure and function in spina bifida myelomeningocele. Dev Disabil Res Rev 16: 23–30.

Kaleyias J, Faerber E, Kothare SV (2006) Tacrolimus induced subacute cerebellar ataxia. Eur J Paediatr Neurol 10: 86–89.

Kanemura Y, Okamoto N, Sakamoto H, Shofuda T, Kamiguchi H, Yamasaki M (2006) Molecular mechanisms and neuroimaging criteria for severe L1 syndrome with X-linked hydrocephalus. J Neurosurg (5 Suppl Pediatrics) 105: 403–412.

Kau T, Karlo C, Güngor T, Prietsch V, Kellenberger CJ, Scheer I, Boltshauser E (2011) Increased cerebellar volume in the early stage of fucosidosis: a case control study. Neuroradiology 53: 509–516.

Kaufmann R, Straussberg R, Mandel H, Fattal-Valevski A, Ben-Zeev B, Naamati A, et al. (2010) Infantile cerebral and cerebellar atrophy is assocaited with a mutation in the MED17 subunit of the transcription preinitiaion mediator complex. Am J Hum Genet 87: 667–670.

Keren Z, Falik-Zaccai TC (2009) Cerebrotendinous xanthomatosis (CTX): a treatable lipid storage disease. Pediatr Endocrinol Rev 7: 6–11.

Kerrison JB, Biousse V, Newman NJ (2000) Retinopathy of NARP syndrome. Arch Ophthalmol 118: 298–299.

Klebe S, Azzedine H, Durr A, Bastien P, Bouslam N, Elleuch N, et al. (2006) Autosomal recessive spastic paraplegia (SPG30) with mild ataxia and sensory neuropathy maps to chromosome 2q37.3. Brain 129: 1456–1462.

Klein A, Schmitt B, Boltshauser E (2004) Progressive encephalopathy with edema, hypsarrhythmia and optic atrophy (PEHO) syndrome in a Swiss child. Eur J Paediatr Neurol 8: 317–321.

Klein A, Schmitt B, Boltshauser E (2007) Long-term outcome of ten children with opsoclonus-myoclonus syndrome. Eur J Pediatr 166: 359–363.

Kleiner-Fisman G, Rogaeva E, Halliday W, Houle S, Kawarai T, Sato C, et al. (2003) Benign hereditary chorea: clinical, genetic, and pathological findings. Ann Neurol 54: 244–247.

Klepper J, Scheffer H, Leiendecker B, Gertsen E, Binder S, Leferink M, et al. (2005) Seizure control and acceptance of the ketogenic diet in GLUT1 deficiency syndrome: a 2- to 5-year follow-up of 15 children enrolled prospectively. Neuropediatrics 36: 302–308.

Kohlschutter A, Schulz A (2009) Towards understanding the neuronal ceroid lipofuscinoses. Brain Dev 31: 499–502.

Kolker S, Christensen E, Leonard JV, Greenberg CR, Burlina AB, Burlina AP, et al. (2007) Guideline for the diagnosis and management of glutaryl-CoA dehydrogenase deficiency (glutaric aciduria type I). J Inherit Metab Dis 30: 5–22.

Kondo A, Saito Y, Floricel F, Maegaki Y, Ohno K (2007) Congenital ocular motor apraxia: clinical and neuroradiological findings, and long-term intellectual prognosis. Brain Dev 29: 431–438.

Koop M, Laugel V, Durand M, Fothergill H, Dalloz C, Sauvanaud F, et al. (2010) Neuroimaging in Cockayne syndrome. AJNR Am J Neroradiol 31: 1623–1630.

Koop O, Schirmacher A, Nelis E, Timmerman V, De Jonghe P, Ringelstein B, et al. (2007) Genotype-phenotype analysis in patients with giant axonal neuropathy (GAN). Neuromuscul Disord 17: 624–630.

Korman SH, Jakobs C, Darmin PS, Gutman A, van der Knaap MS, Ben-Neriah Z, et al. (2007) Glutaric aciduria type 1: clinical, biochemical and molecular findings in patients from Israel. Eur J Paediatr Neurol 11: 81–89.

Koskinen T, Santavuori P, Sainio K, Lappi M, Kallio AK, Pihko H (1994) Infantile onset spinocerebellar ataxia with sensory neuropathy: a new inherited disease. J Neurol Sci 121: 50–56.

Kozic D, Kostic VS (2001) Crossed cerebrocerebellar atrophy. Arch Neurol 58: 1929–1930.

Kroes HY, Nievelstein RJ, Barth PG, Nikkels PG, Bergmann C, Gooskens RH, et al. (2005) Cerebral, cerebellar, and colobomatous anomalies in three related males: Sex-linked inheritance in a newly recognized syndrome with features overlapping with Joubert syndrome. Am J Med Genet A 135: 297–301.

Kumar RA, Pilz DT, Babatz TD, Cushion TD, Harvey K, Topf M, et al. (2010) TUBA1A mutations cause wide spectrum lissencephaly (smooth brain) and suggest that multiple neuronal migration pathways converge on alpha tubulins. Hum Mol Genet 19: 2817–2827.

Kurihara M, Kumagai K, Yagishita S, Imai M, Watanabe M, Suzuki Y, Orii T (1993) Adrenoleukomyeloneuropathy presenting as cerebellar ataxia in a young child: a probable variant of adrenoleukodystrophy. Brain Dev 15: 377–380.

Kuwashima S (2009) Hoyeraal-Hreidarsson syndrome: magnetic resonance imaging findings. Jpn J Radiol 27: 324–327.

Labauge P, Horzinski L, Ayrignac X, Blanc P, Vukusic S, Rodriguez D, et al. (2009) Natural history of adult-onset eIF2B-related disorders: a multi-centric survey of 16 cases. Brain 132: 2161–2169.

Lamonica DA, Maximino LP, Abramides DV, Souza DH, Richieri-Costa A (2010) Nonprogressive congenital cerebellar ataxia, iris heterochromia, mental retardation and language impairment in two brothers. Clin Dysmorphol 19: 76–78.

Lamperti C, Naini A, Hirano M, De Vivo DC, Bertini E, Servidei S, et al. (2003) Cerebellar ataxia and coenzyme Q10 deficiency. Neurology 60: 1206–1208.

Lapkin ML, Golden GS (1978) Basilar artery migraine. A review of 30 cases. Am J Dis Child 132: 278–281.

Le Ber I, Moreira MC, Rivaud-Pechoux S, Chamayou C, Ochsner F, Kuntzer T, et al. (2003) Cerebellar ataxia with oculomotor apraxia type 1: clinical and genetic studies. Brain 126: 2761–2772.

Le Ber I, Bouslam N, Rivaud-Pechoux S, Guimaraes J, Benomar A, Chamayou C, et al. (2004) Frequency and phenotypic spectrum of ataxia with oculomotor apraxia 2: a clinical and genetic study in 18 patients. Brain 127: 759–767.

Le Ber I, Clot F, Vercueil L, Camuzat A, Viemont M, Benamar N, et al. (2006) Predominant dystonia with marked cerebellar atrophy: a rare phenotype in familial dystonia. Neurology 67: 1769–1773.

Lee HF, Tsai CR, Chi CS, Lee HJ, Chen CC (2009) Leigh syndrome: clinical and neuroimaging follow-up. Pediatr Neurol 40: 88–93.

Leen WG, Klepper J, Verbeek MM, Leferink M, Hofste T, van Engelen BG, et al. (2010) Glucose transporter-1 deficiency syndrome: the expanding clinical and genetic spectrum of a treatable disorder. Brain 133: 655–670.

Leite CC, Lucato LT, Martin MG, Ferreira LG, Resende MB, Carvalho MS, et al. (2005) Merosin-deficient congenital muscular dystrophy (CMD): a study of 25 Brazilian patients using MRI. Pediatr Radiol 35: 572–579.

Leonardi ML, Pai GS, Wilkes B, Lebel RR (2001) Ritscher-Schinzel cranio-cerebello-cardiac (3C) syndrome: report of four new cases and review. Am J Med Genet 102: 237–242.

Lewis RF, Lederman HM, Crawford TO (1999) Ocular motor abnormalities in ataxia telangiectasia. Ann Neurol 46: 287–295.

Lewis S, Hutchison W, Thyagarajan D, Dahl HH (2002) Clinical and molecular features of adPEO due to mutations in the Twinkle gene. J Neurol Sci 201: 39–44.

Lin HY, Lin SP, Chen YJ, Hung HY, Kao HA, Hsu CH, et al. (2006) Clinical characteristics and survival of trisomy 18 in a medical center in Taipei, 1988–2004. Am J Med Genet A 140: 945–951.

Lin JJ, Lin KL, Chou ML, Wong AM, Wang HS (2007) Cerebellar infarction in the territory of the superior cerebellar artery in children. Pediatr Neurol 37: 435–437.

Livingstone IR, Gardner-Medwin D, Pennington RJ (1984) Familial intermittent ataxia with possible X-linked recessive inheritance. Two patients with abnormal pyruvate metabolism and a response to acetazolamide. J Neurol Sci 64: 89–97.

Lo YL (2007) Clinical and immunological spectrum of the Miller Fisher syndrome. Muscle Nerve 36: 615–627.

Loes DJ, Fatemi A, Melhem ER, Gupte N, Bezman L, Moser HW, Raymond GV (2003) Analysis of MRI patterns aids prediction of progression in X-linked adrenoleukodystrophy. Neurology 61: 369–374.

Lugowska A, Berger J, Tylki-Szymanska A, Loschl B, Molzer B, Zobel M, Czartoryska B (2005) Molecular and phenotypic characteristics of metachromatic leukodystrophy patients from Poland. Clin Genet 68: 48–54.

Maegawa GH, Stockley T, Tropak M, Banwell B, Blaser S, Kok F, et al. (2006) The natural history of juvenile or subacute GM2 gangliosidosis: 21 new cases and literature review of 134 previously reported. Pediatrics 118: e1550–1562.

Manto MU (2010) Toxic agents. In: Manto MU, editor. Cerebellar disorders. New York: Cambridge University Press; pp. 157–70.

Marien P, Brouns R, Engelborghs S, Wackenier P, Verhoeven J, Ceulemans B, De Deyn PP (2008) Cerebellar cognitive affective syndrome without global mental retardation in two relatives with Gillespie syndrome. Cortex 44: 54–67.

Mariotti C, Gellera C, Rimoldi M, Mineri R, Uziel G, Zorzi G, et al. (2004) Ataxia with isolated vitamin E deficiency: neurological phenotype, clinical follow-up and novel mutations in TTPA gene in Italian families. Neurol Sci 25: 130–137.

Mascalchi M, Petruzzi P, Zampa V (1996) MRI of cerebellar white amtter damage due to carbon monoxide poising: case report. Neuroradiology 38: S73–S74.

Matheus MG, Castillo M, Smith JK, Armao D, Towle D, Muenzer J (2004) Brain MRI findings in patients with mucopolysaccharidosis types I and II and mild clinical presentation. Neuroradiology 46: 666–672.

McErlean A, Abdalla K, Donoghue V, Ryan S (2010) The dentate nucleus in children: normal development and patterns of disease. Pediatr Radiol 40: 326–339.

Melek E, Ozyer U, Erol I, Alehan F, Muhtesem Agildere A (2006) +H-proton-magnetic resonance spectroscopic findings in a patient with acute hemicerebellitis presenting without localized signs: a case report. Eur J Paediatr Neurol 10: 202–206.

Mentzel HJ, Seidel J, Fitzek C, Eichhorn A, Vogt S, Reichenbach JR, et al. (2005) Pediatric brain MRI in neurofibromatosis type I. Eur Radiol 15: 814–822.

Messerschmidt A, Brugger PC, Boltshauser E, Zoder G, Sterniste W, Birnbacher R, Prayer D (2005) Disruption of cerebellar development: potential complication of extreme prematurity. AJNR Am J Neuroradiol 26: 1659–1667.

Messerschmidt A, Fuiko R, Prayer D, Brugger PC, Boltshauser E, Zoder G, et al. (2008) Disrupted cerebellar development in preterm infants is associated with impaired neurodevelopmental outcome. Eur J Pediatr 167: 1141–1147.

Metry D, Heyer G, Hess C, Garzon M, Haggstrom A, Frommelt P, et al. (2009) Consensus statement on diagnostic criteria for PHACE syndrome. Pediatrics 124: 1447–1456.

Miller RC, Tewari A, Miller JA, Garbern J, Van Stavern GP (2009) Neuro-ophthalmologic features of spinocerebellar ataxia type 7. J Neuroophthalmol 29: 180–186.

Mochel F, Sedel F, Vanderver A, Engelke UF, Barritault J, Yang BZ, et al. (2009) Cerebellar ataxia with elevated cerebrospinal free sialic acid. Brain 132: 801–809.

Montini G, Malaventura C, Salviati L (2008) Early coenzyme Q10 supplementation in primary coenzyme Q10 deficiency. N Engl J Med 358: 2849–2850.

Moog U, Jones MC, Bird LM, Dobyns WB (2005) Oculocerebrocutaneous syndrome: the brain malformation defines a core phenotype. J Med Genet 42: 913–921.

Morava E, Wosik HN, Sykut-Cegielska J, Adamowicz M, Guillard M, Wevers RA, et al. (2009) Ophthalmological abnormalities in children with congenital disorders of glycosylation type I. Br J Ophthalmol 93: 350–354.

Morava E, Wevers RA, Cantagrel V, Hoefsloot LH, Al-Gazali L, Schoots J, et al. (2010) A novel cerebello-ocular syndrome with abnormal glycosylation due to abnormalities in dolichol metabolism. Brain 133: 3210–3220.

Moroni I, D'Incerti L, Farina L, Rimoldi M, Uziel G (2000) Clinical, biochemical and neuroradiological findings in L-2-hydroxyglutaric aciduria. Neurol Sci 21: 103–108.

Moser HW, Mahmood A, Raymond GV (2007) X-linked adrenoleukodystrophy. Nat Clin Pract Neurol 3: 140–151.

Naidu S, Kaufmann WE, Abrams MT, Pearlson GD, Lanham DC, Fredericksen KA, et al. (2001) Neuroimaging studies in Rett syndrome. Brain Dev 23: S62–71.

Namavar Y, Barth PG, Kasher PR, van Ruissen F, Brockmann K, Bernert G, et al. (2009) Clinical, neuroradiological and genetic findings in pontocerebellar hypoplasia. Brain 134: 143–156.

Nelson MD, Jr., Wolff JA, Cross CA, Donnell GN, Kaufman FR (1992) Galactosemia: evaluation with MR imaging. Radiology 184: 255–261.

Nicolas E, Poitelon Y, Chouery E, Salem N, Levy N, Megarbane A, Delague V (2010) CAMOS, a nonprogressive, autosomal recessive, congenital cerebellar ataxia, is caused by a mutant zinc-finger protein, ZNF592. Eur J Hum Genet 18: 1107–1113.

Ninchoji T, Takanashi J (2010) Pontine hypoplasia in 5p-syndrome: a key MRI finding for a diagnosis. Brain Dev 32: 571–573.

Nomura T, Koyama N, Yokoyama M, Awaya A, Yokochi K (2009) DOOR syndrome concomitant with non-convulsive status epilepticus and hyperintense cerebellar cortex on T2-weighted imaging. Brain Dev 31: 75–78.

Nowak DA, Trost HA (2002) Lhermitte-Duclos disease (dysplastic cerebellar gangliocytoma): a malformation, hamartoma or neoplasm? Acta Neurol Scand 105: 137–145.

Oduber CE, van der Horst CM, Hennekam RC (2008) Klippel-Trenaunay syndrome: diagnostic criteria and hypothesis on etiology. Ann Plast Surg 60: 217–223.

Offiah C, Hall E (2008) Heroin-induced leukoencephalopathy. Characterization using MRI, diffusion-weighted imaging, and MR spectroscopy. Clin Radiol 63: 146–152.

Orssaud C, Ingster-Moati I, Roche O, Bui Quoc E, Dufier JL (2009) Familial congenital oculomotor apraxia: clinical and electro-oculographic features. Eur J Paediatr Neurol 13: 370–372.

Ouvrier R, Billson F (2005) Paroxysmal tonic upgaze of childhood – a review. Brain Dev 27: 185–188.

Ozgen HM, Overweg-Plandsoen WC, Blees-Pelk J, Besselaar PP, Hennekam RC (2005) Cerebellar hypoplasia-endosteal sclerosis: a long term follow-up. Am J Med Genet A 134A: 215–219.

Palmeri S, Battisti C, Federico A, Guazzi GC (1994) Hypoplasia of the corpus callosum in Niemann-Pick type C disease. Neuroradiology 36: 20–22.

Pandolfo M (2009) Friedreich ataxia: the clinical picture. J Neurol 256 Suppl 1: 3–8.

Pane M, Baranello G, Battaglia D, Donvito V, Carnevale F, Stefanini MC, et al. (2004) Severe abnormalities of the pons in two infants with Goldenhar syndrome. Neuropediatrics 35: 234–238.

Parrini E, Ramazzotti A, Dobyns WB, Mei D, Moro F, Veggiotti P, et al. (2006) Periventricular heterotopia: phenotypic heterogeneity and correlation with Filamin A mutations. Brain 129: 1892–1906.

Payne JM, Moharir MD, Webster R, North KN (2010) Brain structure and function in neurofibromatosis type 1: current concepts and future directions. J Neurol Neurosurg Psychiatry 81: 304–309.

Pearl PL, Vezina LG, Saneto RP, McCarter R, Molloy-Wells E, Heffron A, et al. (2009) Cerebral MRI abnormalities associated with vigabatrin therapy. Epilepsia 50: 184–194.

Pedraza S, Gamez J, Rovira A, Zamora A, Grive E, Raguer N, Ruscalleda J (2000) MRI findings in Mobius syndrome: correlation with clinical features. Neurology 55: 1058–1060.

Perry MS, Sladky JT (2008) Neuroradiologic findings in Sengers syndrome. Pediatr Neurol 39: 113–115.

Phillips JP, Warner LE, Lupski JR, Garg BP (1999) Congenital hypomyelinating neuropathy: two patients with long-term follow-up. Pediatr Neurol 20: 226–232.

Pierre G, Setchell K, Blyth J, Preece MA, Chakrapani A, McKiernan P (2008) Prospective treatment of cerebrotendinous xanthomatosis with cholic acid therapy. J Inherit Metab Dis. 2008 epub Dec 27.

Pineda M, Arpa J, Montero R, Aracil A, Domínguez F, Galván M, et al. (2008) Idebenone treatment in paediatric and adult patients with Friedreich ataxia: long-term follow-up. Eur J Paediatr Neurol 12: 470–475.

Pineda M, Perez-Poyato MS, O'Callaghan M, Vilaseca MA, Pocovi M, Domingo R, et al. (2010) Clinical experience with miglustat therapy in pediatric patients with Niemann-Pick disease type C: a case series. Mol Genet Metab 99: 358–366.

Plecko B, Stockler-Ipsiroglu S, Gruber S, Mlynarik V, Moser E, Simbrunner J, et al. (2003) Degree of hypomyelination and magnetic resonance spectroscopy findings in patients with Pelizaeus Merzbacher phenotype. Neuropediatrics 34: 127–136.

Poirier KJ (2010) Mutations in the neuronal ß-tubulin subunit TUBB3 result in malformation of cortical development and neuronal migration defects. Hum Mol Genet 19: 4462–4473.

Poretti A, Brehmer U, Scheer I, Bernet V, Boltshauser E (2008a) Prenatal and neonatal MR imaging findings in oral-facial-digital syndrome type VI. AJNR Am J Neuroradiol 29: 1090–1091.

Poretti A, Wolf NI, Boltshauser E (2008b) Differential diagnosis of cerebellar atrophy in childhood. Eur J Paediatr Neurol 12: 155–167.

Poretti A, Alber FD, Burki S, Toelle SP, Boltshauser E (2009a) Cognitive outcome in children with rhombencephalosynapsis. Eur J Paediatr Neurol 13: 28–33.

Poretti A, Huisman TA, Cowan FM, Del Giudice E, Jeannet PY, Prayer D, et al. (2009b) Cerebellar cleft: confirmation of the neuroimaging pattern. Neuropediatrics 40: 228–233.

Poretti A, Prayer D, Boltshauser E (2009c) Morphological spectrum of prenatal cerebellar disruptions. Eur J Paediatr Neurol 13: 397–407.

Poretti A, Limperopoulos C, Roulet-Perez E, Wolf NI, Rauscher C, Prayer D, et al. (2010a) Outcome of severe unilateral cerebellar hypoplasia. Dev Med Child Neurol 52: 718–724.

Poretti A, Meoded A, Ceritoglu E, Huisman TA, Boltshauser E (2010b) Postnatal in-vivo MRI findings in anencephaly. Neuropediatrics 41: 264–266.

Prosch H, Grois N, Wnorowski M, Steiner M, Prayer D (2007) Long-term MR imaging course of neurodegenerative Langerhans cell histiocytosis. AJNR Am J Neuroradiol 28: 1022–1028.

Provenzale JM, Peddi S, Kurtzberg J, Poe MD, Mukundan S, Escolar M (2009) Correlation of neurodevelopmental features and MRI findings in infantile Krabbe's disease. AJR Am J Roentgenol 192: 59–65.

Punal JE, Rodríguez E, Pintos E, Campos Y, Castro-Gago M (1998) Congenital ocular motor apraxia associated with myopathy, external hydrocephalus and NADH dehydrogenase deficiency. Brain Dev 20: 175–178.

Quinzii CM, DiMauro S, Hirano M (2007) Human coenzyme Q10 deficiency. Neurochem Res 32: 723–727.

Rajadhyaksha AM, Elemento O, Puffenberger EG, Schierberl KC, Xiang JZ, Putorti ML, et al. (2010) Mutations in FLVCR1 cause posterior column ataxia and retinitis pigmentosa. Am J Hum Genet 87: 643–654.

Reardon W, Donoghue V, Murphy AM, King MD, Mayne PD, Horn N, Birk Moller L (2010) Progressive cerebellar degeneration changes in the severe mental retardation syndrome caused by duplication of MECP2 and adjacent loci on Xq28. Eur J Pediatr 169: 941–949.

Régal L, Ebberink MS, Goemans N, Wanders RJA, De Meirleir L, Jaeken J, Schrooten M, Van Coster R, Waterham HR (2010) Mutations in PEX10 are cause of autosomal recessive ataxia. Ann Neurol 68: 259–263.

Rice GI, Bond J, Asipu A, Brunette RL, Manfield IW, Carr IM, et al. (2009) Mutations involved in Aicardi-Goutieres syndrome implicate SAMHD1 as regulator of the innate immune response. Nat Genet 41: 829–832.

Richter A, Morgan K, Bouchard JP, Poirier J, Mercier J, Gosselin F, Melançon SB (1993) Clinical and molecular genetic studies on autosomal recessive spastic ataxia of Charlevoix-Saguenay (ARSACS). Adv Neurol 61: 97–103.

Rosati P, Guariglia L (1999) Cerebellar hypoplasia: could it be a sonographic finding of abnormal fetal karyotype in early pregnancy? Fetal Diagn Ther 14: 365–367.

Rubio-Cabezas O, Minton JA, Kantor I, Williams D, Ellard S, Hattersley AT (2010) Homozygous mutations in NEUROD1 are responsible for a novel syndrome of permanent neonatal diabetes and neurological abnormalities. Diabetes 59: 2326–2331.

Ryan MM, Engle EC (2003) Acute ataxia in childhood. J Child Neurol 18: 309–316.

Saito Y, Masuko K, Kaneko K, Chikumaru Y, Saito K, Iwamoto H, et al. (2006) Brain MRI findings of older patients with Pallister-Killian syndrome. Brain Dev 28: 34–38.

Saneto RP, Friedman SD, Shaw DW (2008) Neuroimaging of mitochondrial disease. Mitochondrion 8: 396–413.

Sanlaville D, Verloes A (2007) CHARGE syndrome: an update. Eur J Hum Genet 15: 389–399.

Sargent MA, Poskitt KJ, Jan JE (1997) Congenital ocular motor apraxia: imaging findings. AJNR Am J Neuroradiol 18: 1915–1922.

Sargent MA, Poskitt KJ, Roland EH, Hill A, Hendson G (2004) Cerebellar vermian atrophy after neonatal hypoxic-ischemic encephalopathy. AJNR Am J Neuroradiol 25: 1008–1015.

Sawaishi Y, Takada G (2002) Acute cerebellitis. Cerebellum 1: 223–228.

Scaglia F, Wong LJ, Vladutiu GD, Hunter JV (2005) Predominant cerebellar volume loss as a neuroradiologic feature of pediatric respiratory chain defects. AJNR Am J Neuroradiol 26: 1675–1680.

Schaefer GB, Bodensteiner JB, Buehler BA, Lin A, Cole TR (1997) The neuroimaging findings in Sotos syndrome. Am J Med Genet 68: 462–465.

Schiffmann R, van der Knaap MS (2009) Invited article: an MRI-based approach to the diagnosis of white matter disorders. Neurology 72: 750–759.

Seitz D, Grodd W, Schwab A, Seeger U, Klose U, Nagele T (1998) MR imaging and localized proton MR spectroscopy in late infantile neuronal ceroid lipofuscinosis. AJNR Am J Neuroradiol 19: 1373–1377.

Sellick GS, Barker KT, Stolte-Dijkstra I, Fleischmann C, Coleman RJ, Garrett C, et al. (2004) Mutations in PTF1A cause pancreatic and cerebellar agenesis. Nat Genet 36: 1301–1305.

Shah DK, Tingay DG, Fink AM, Hunt RW, Dargaville PA (2005) Magnetic resonance imaging in neonatal nonketotic hyperglycinemia. Pediatr Neurol 33: 50–52.

Shaikh AG, Marti S, Tarnutzer AA, Palla A, Crawford TO, Straumann D, et al. (2009) Gaze fixation deficits and their implication in ataxia-telangiectasia. J Neurol Neurosurg Psychiatry 80: 858–864.

Shapiro BE, Logigian EL, Kolodny EH, Pastores GM (2008) Late-onset Tay-Sachs disease: the spectrum of peripheral neuropathy in 30 affected patients. Muscle Nerve 38: 1012–1015.

Shotelersuk V, Desudchit T, Suwanwela N (2003) Postnatal growth failure, microcephaly, mental retardation, cataracts, large joint contractures, osteoporosis, cortical dysplasia, and cerebellar atrophy. Am J Med Genet A 116A: 164–169.

Simon A, Kremer HP, Wevers RA, Scheffer H, De Jong JG, Van Der Meer JW, Drenth JP (2004) Mevalonate kinase deficiency: Evidence for a phenotypic continuum. Neurology 62: 994–997.

Simon E, Flaschker N, Schadewaldt P, Langenbeck U, Wendel U (2006) Variant maple syrup urine disease (MSUD) – the entire spectrum. J Inherit Metab Dis 29: 716–724.

Slavotinek A, Goldman J, Weisiger K, Kostiner D, Golabi M, Packman S, et al. (2005) Marinesco-Sjogren syndrome in a male with mild dysmorphism. Am J Med Genet A 133A: 197–201.

Smith W, Kishnani PS, Lee B, Singh RH, Rhead WJ, Sniderman King L, et al. (2005) Urea cycle disorders: clinical presentation outside the newborn period. Crit Care Clin 21: S9–17.

Sonninen P, Autti T, Varho T, Hamalainen M, Raininko R (1999) Brain involvement in Salla disease. AJNR Am J Neuroradiol 20: 433–443.

Spanos GK, Wilde EA, Bigler ED, Cleavinger HB, Fearing MA, Levin HS, et al. (2007) Cerebellar atrophy after moderate-to-severe pediatric traumatic brain injury. AJNR Am J Neuroradiol 28: 537–542.

Sparks SE (2006) Inherited disorders of glycosylation. Mol Genet Metab 87: 1–7.

Squier W, Hope PL, Lindenbaum RH (1990) Neocerebellar hypoplasia in a neonate following intra-uterine exposure to anticonvulsants. Dev Med Child Neurol 32: 737–742.

Stapf C, Khaw AV, Sciacca RR, Hofmeister C, Schumacher HC, Pile-Spellman J, et al. (2003) Effect of age on clinical and morphological characteristics in patients with brain arteriovenous malformation. Stroke 34: 2664–2669.

Steenweg ME, Salomons GS, Yapici Z, Uziel G, Scalais E, Zafeiriou DI, et al. (2009) L-2-Hydroxyglutaric aciduria: pattern of MR imaging abnormalities in 56 patients. Radiology 251: 856–865.

Steenweg ME, Jakobs C, Errami A, van Dooren SJ, Adeva Bartolome MT, Aerssens P, et al. (2010) An overview of L-2-hydroxyglutarate dehydrogenase gene (L2HGDH) variants: a genotype-phenotype study. Hum Mutat 31: 380–390.

Steinlin M, Zangger B, Boltshauser E (1998) Non-progressive congenital ataxia with or without cerebellar hypoplasia: a review of 34 subjects. Dev Med Child Neurol 40: 148–154.

Steinlin M, Styger M, Boltshauser E (1999) Cognitive impairments in patients with congenital nonprogressive cerebellar ataxia. Neurology 53: 966–973.

Steinlin M, Klein A, Haas-Lude K, Zafeiriou D, Strozzi S, Muller T, et al. (2007) Pontocerebellar hypoplasia type 2: variability in clinical and imaging findings. Eur J Paediatr Neurol 11: 146–152.

Steiss JO, Gross S, Neubauer BA, Hahn A (2005) Late-onset nephrotic syndrome and severe cerebellar atrophy in Galloway-Mowat syndrome. Neuropediatrics 36: 332–335.

Strauss KA, Wardley B, Robinson D, Hendrickson C, Rider NL, Puffenberger EG, et al. (2010) Classical maple syrup urine disease and brain development: principles of management and formula design. Mol Genet Metab 99: 333–345.

Sturm V, Leiba H, Menke MN, Valente EM, Poretti A, Landau K, Boltshauser E (2010) Ophthalmological findings in Joubert syndrome. Eye (Lond) 24: 222–225.

Sugarman JL (2007) Epidermal nevus syndromes. Semin Cutan Med Surg 26: 221–230.

Swango KL, Demirkol M, Huner G, Pronicka E, Sykut-Cegielska J, Schulze A, et al. (1998) Partial biotinidase deficiency is usually due to the D444H mutation in the biotinidase gene. Hum Genet 102: 571–575.

Szathmari A, Thiesse P, Galand-Desmé S, Mottolese C, Bret P, Jouanneau E, et al. (2010) Correlation between pre- or postoperative MRI findings and cerebellar sequelae in patients with medulloblastomas. Pediatr Blood Cancer 15: 1310–1316.

Takanashi J, Arai H, Nabatame S, Hirai S, Hayashi S, Inazawa J, et al. (2010) Neuroradiologic features of CASK mutations. AJNR Am J Neuroradiol 31: 1619–1622.

Takashima H, Boerkoel CF, John J, Saifi GM, Salih MA, Armstrong D, et al. (2002) Mutation of TDP1, encoding a topoisomerase I-dependent DNA damage repair enzyme, in spinocerebellar ataxia with axonal neuropathy. Nat Genet 32: 267–72.

Takeoka M, Kim F, Caviness VS, Jr., Kennedy DN, Makris N, Holmes GL (2003) MRI volumetric analysis in Rasmussen encephalitis: a longitudinal study. Epilepsia 44: 247–251.

Taly AB, Meenakshi-Sundaram S, Sinha S, Swamy HS, Arunodaya GR (2007) Wilson disease: description of 282 patients evaluated over 3 decades. Medicine (Baltimore) 86: 112–121.

Tanaka K (1990) Isovaleric acidemia: personal history, clinical survey and study of the molecular basis. Prog Clin Biol Res 321: 273–290.

Tavani F, Zimmerman RA, Berry GT, Sullivan K, Gatti R, Bingham P (2003) Ataxia-telangiectasia: the pattern of cerebellar atrophy on MRI. Neuroradiology 45: 315–319.

Tenembaum S, Chitnis T, Ness J, Hahn JS (2007) Acute disseminated encephalomyelitis. Neurology 68: S23–S36.

Terhal P, Sakkers R, Hochstenbach R, Madan K, Rabelink G, Sinke R, Giltay J (2004) Cerebellar hypoplasia, zonular cataract, and peripheral neuropathy in trisomy 17 mosaicism. Am J Med Genet A 130A: 410–414.

Thiffault I, Rioux MF, Tetreault M, Jarry J, Loiselle L, Poirier J, et al. (2006) A new autosomal recessive spastic ataxia associated with frequent white matter changes maps to 2q33–34. Brain 129: 2332–2340.

Timmann D, Diener HC (2000) Alcoholic cerebellar degeneration (including ataxias that are due to other toxic causes). In: Klockgether T, editor. Handbook of ataxia disorders. New York: Marcel Dekker, Inc.; pp. 571–605.

Tobin JL, Beales PL (2007) Bardet-Biedl syndrome: beyond the cilium. Pediatr Nephrol 22: 926–936.

Tranebjaerg L, Teslovich TM, Jones M, Barmada MM, Fagerheim T, Dahl A, et al. (2003) Genome-wide homozygosity mapping localizes a gene for autosomal recessive non-progressive infantile ataxia to 20q11-q13. Hum Genet 113: 293–295.

Turkmen S, Demirhan O, Hoffmann K, Diers A, Zimmer C, Sperling K, Mundlos S (2006) Cerebellar hypoplasia and quadrupedal locomotion in humans as a recessive trait mapping to chromosome 17p. J Med Genet 43: 461–464.

Turkmen S, Guo G, Garshasbi M, Hoffmann K, Alshalah AJ, Mischung C, et al. (2009) CA8 mutations cause a novel syndrome characterized by ataxia and mild mental retardation with predisposition to quadrupedal gait. PLoS Genet 5: e1000487.

Twomey EL, Naughten ER, Donoghue VB, Ryan S (2003) Neuroimaging findings in glutaric aciduria type 1. Pediatr Radiol 33: 823–830.

Uggetti C, La Piana R, Orcesi S, Egitto MG, Crow YJ, Fazzi E (2009) Aicardi-Goutieres syndrome: neuroradiologic findings and follow-up. AJNR Am J Neuroradiol 30: 1971–1976.

Uyanik G, Morris-Rosendahl DJ, Stiegler J, Klapecki J, Gross C, Berman Y, et al. (2007) Location and type of mutation in the LIS1 gene do not predict phenotypic severity. Neurology 69: 442–447.

Valanne L, Ketonen L, Majander A, Suomalainen A, Pihko H (1998) Neuroradiologic findings in children with mitochondrial disorders. AJNR Am J Neuroradiol 19: 369–377.

van der Knaap MS, Salomons GS, Li R, Franzoni E, Gutierrez-Solana LG, Smit LM, et al. (2005) Unusual variants of Alexander's disease. Ann Neurol 57: 327–338.

van der Knaap MS, Pronk JC, Scheper GC (2006) Vanishing white matter disease. Lancet Neurol 5: 413–423.

van der Knaap MS, Linnankivi T, Paetau A, Feigenbaum A, Wakusawa K, Haginoya K, et al. (2007) Hypomyelination with atrophy of the basal ganglia and cerebellum: follow-up and pathology. Neurology 69: 166–171.

van der Knaap MS, Scheper GC (2008) Megalencephalic leukoencephalopathy with subcortical cysts. In: Pagon RA, Bird TC, Dolan CR, Stephens K, editors. GeneReviews. Seattle: University of Washington.

Van Goethem G, Martin JJ, Dermaut B, Lofgren A, Wibail A, Ververken D, et al. (2003) Recessive POLG mutations presenting with sensory and ataxic neuropathy in compound heterozygote patients with progressive external ophthalmoplegia. Neuromuscul Disord 13: 133–142.

Vanrietvelde F, Lemmerling M, Mespreuve M, Crevits L, De Reuck J, Kunnen M (2000) MRI of the brain in cerebrotendinous xanthomatosis (van Bogaert-Scherer-Epstein disease). Eur Radiol 10: 576–578.

Varho TT, Alajoki LE, Posti KM, Korhonen TT, Renlund MG, Nyman SR, et al. (2002) Phenotypic spectrum of Salla disease, a free sialic acid storage disorder. Pediatr Neurol 26: 267–273.

Vermeer S, Meijer RP, Pijl BJ, Timmermans J, Cruysberg JR, Bos MM, et al. (2008) ARSACS in the Dutch population: a frequent cause of early-onset cerebellar ataxia. Neurogenetics 9: 207–214.

Verrips A, van Engelen BG, ter Laak H, Gabreels-Festen A, Janssen A, Zwarts M, et al. (2000) Cerebrotendinous xanthomatosis. Controversies about nerve and muscle: observations in ten patients. Neuromuscul Disord 10: 407–414.

von Schenck U, Bender-Gotze C, Koletzko B (1997) Persistence of neurological damage induced by dietary vitamin B-12 deficiency in infancy. Arch Dis Child 77: 137–139.

Wada T, Kobayashi N, Takahashi Y, Aoki T, Watanabe T, Saitoh S (2002) Wide clinical variability in a family with a CACNA1A T666m mutation: hemiplegic migraine, coma, and progressive ataxia. Pediatr Neurol 26: 47–50.

Waite A, Somer M, O'Driscoll M, Millen K, Manson FD, Chandler KE (2010) Cerebellar hypoplasia and Cohen syndrome: a confirmed association. Am J Med Genet A 152A: 2390–2393.

Walker V (2009) Ammonia toxicity and its prevention in inherited defects of the urea cycle. Diabetes Obes Metab 11: 823–835.

Wassmer E, Davies P, Whitehouse WP, Green SH (2003) Clinical spectrum associated with cerebellar hypoplasia. Pediatr Neurol 28: 347–351.

Weiss AH, Doherty D, Parisi M, Shaw D, Glass I, Phillips JO (2009) Eye movement abnormalities in Joubert syndrome. Invest Ophthalmol Vis Sci 50: 4669–4677.

Weller S, Rosewich H, Gartner J (2008) Cerebral MRI as a valuable diagnostic tool in Zellweger spectrum patients. J Inherit Metab Dis epub Apr 14.

Williams CA (2005) Neurological aspects of the Angelman syndrome. Brain Dev 27: 88–94.

Williams KD, Drayer BP, Johnsen SD, Johnson PC (1990) MR imaging of leukoencephalopathy associated with Navajo neuropathy. AJNR Am J Neuroradiol 11: 400–402.

Wills AJ, Manning NJ, Reilly MM (2001) Refsum's disease. QJM 94: 403–406.

Wolf B (2010) Clinical issues and frequent questions about biotinidase deficiency. Mol Genet Metab 100: 6–13.

Wolf NI, Harting I, Innes AM, Patzer S, Zeitler P, Schneider A, et al. (2007) Ataxia, delayed dentition and hypomyelination: a novel leukoencephalopathy. Neuropediatrics 38: 64–70.

Wong LJ, Naviaux RK, Brunetti-Pierri N, Zhang Q, Schmitt ES, Truong C, et al. (2008) Molecular and clinical genetics of mitochondrial diseases due to POLG mutations. Hum Mutat 29: E150–E172.

Wraith JE, Baumgartner MR, Bembi B, Covanis A, Levade T, Mengel E, et al. (2009) Recommendations on the diagnosis and management of Niemann-Pick disease type C. Mol Genet Metab 98: 152–165.

Yalcinkaya C, Arslanoglu I, Islak C, Aydin A, Boltshauser E (2002) Progressive white-matter disease with primary cerebellar involvement: a separate entity? Neuroradiology 44: 775–779.

Yoon HK, Sargent MA, Prendicille JS, Poskitt KJ (2005) Cerebellar and cerebral atrophy in trichothiodystrophy. Pediatr Radiol 35: 1019–1023.

Zamel R, Khan R, Pollex RL, Hegele RA (2008) Abetalipoproteinemia: two case reports and literature review. Orphanet J Rare Dis 3: 19.

Zanni G, Saillour Y, Nagara M, Billuart P, Castelnau L, Moraine C, et al. (2005) Oligophrenin 1 mutations frequently cause X-linked mental retardation with cerebellar hypoplasia. Neurology 65: 1364–1369.

Zanni G, Bertini E, Bellcross C, Nedelec B, Froyen G, Neuhauser G, et al. (2008) X-linked congenital ataxia: a new locus maps to Xq25-q27.1. Am J Med Genet A 146A: 593–600.

Zouari M, Feki M, Ben Hamida C, Larnaout A, Turki I, Belal S, et al. (1998) Electrophysiology and nerve biopsy: comparative study in Friedreich's ataxia and Friedreich's ataxia phenotype with vitamin E deficiency. Neuromuscul Disord 8: 416–425.

Index

Note: page numbers in *italics* refer to figures and tables

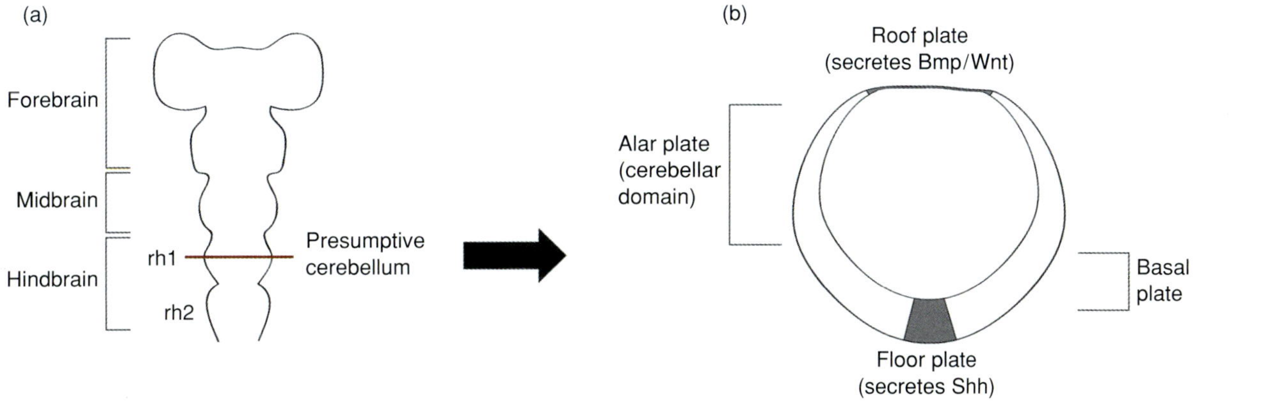

Plate 1. (Figure 1.1) Early neural tube development. **(a)** The early neural tube forms three primary vesicles that will form the forebrain, midbrain, and hindbrain, respectively, from anterior to posterior. The hindbrain is further subdivided into seven rhombomeres. The first two rhombomeres are illustrated (rh1 and rh2). The cerebellum is derived from rhombomere 1. **(b)** In cross-section at the level of rhombomere 1 [red line in (a)] the roof, alar, basal, and floor plates are evident. The cerebellum arises from the alar plate of rhombomere 1. The roof plate is a source of Bmp and Wnt signaling molecules, while the floor plate is a source of Shh.

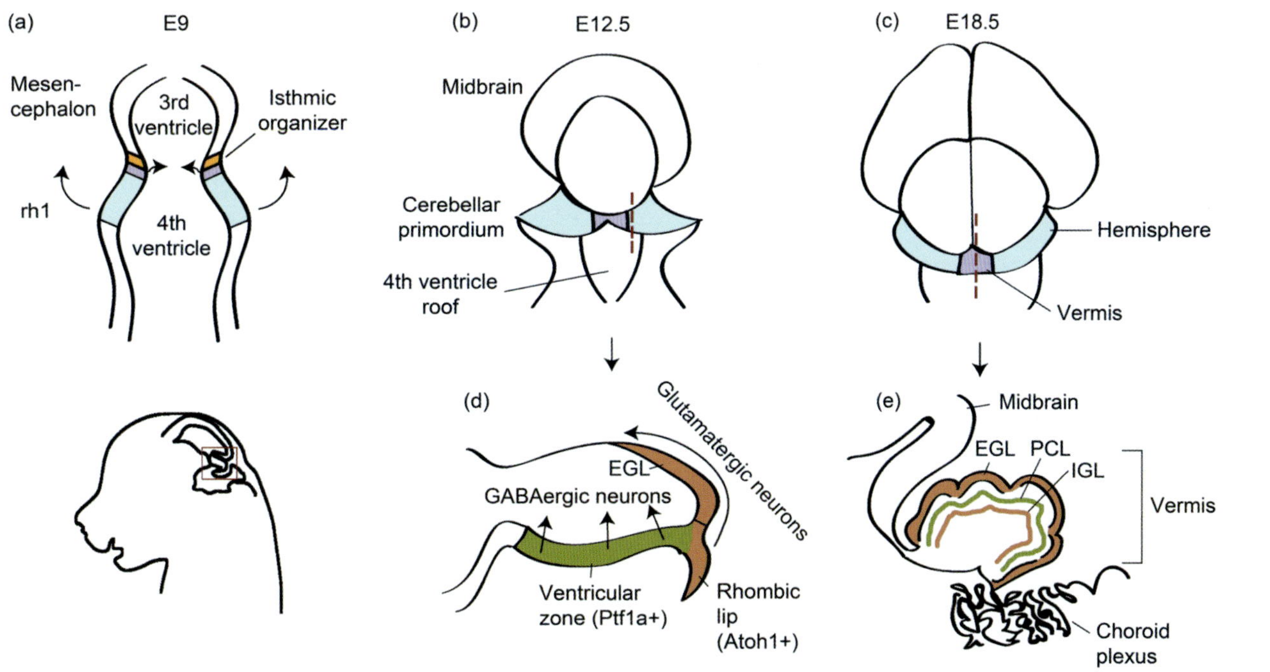

Plate 2. (Figure 1.2) The developing morphology of the embryonic mouse cerebellum at three stages of development. **(a–c)** Schematic dorsal views of the developing cerebellum from embryonic day 9 (E9) through E18.5. **(a)** At E9, the cerebellar territory is defined with anterior regions of rhombomere 1 (rh1) fated to become the cerebellar vermis and more posterior regions fated to become hemispheres, **(b)** after medial/lateral rotation of the bilateral cerebellar anlage wings by E12.5 **(c)** which eventually fuse on the midline to form a contiguous cerebellar anlage by E18.5. **(d)** At E12.5, the ventricular zone and rhombic lip regions of neurogenesis are evident in parasagittal view [indicated by red dotted line in (b)]. The ventricular zone gives rise to all GABAergic cerebellar neurons and the rhombic lip gives rise to glutamatergic neurons. The nascent EGL is also indicated. **(e)** At E18.5, following cell division and migration, a parasagittal schematic section reveals the locations of EGL, PCL (Purkinje cell layer), and IGL (internal granule cell layer). The fourth ventricle roof plate has also differentiated into the choroid plexus epithelium. The lower left panel shows the position of the developing cerebellum (inside red square) relative to the rest of the brain and is relevant to panels (d) and (e).

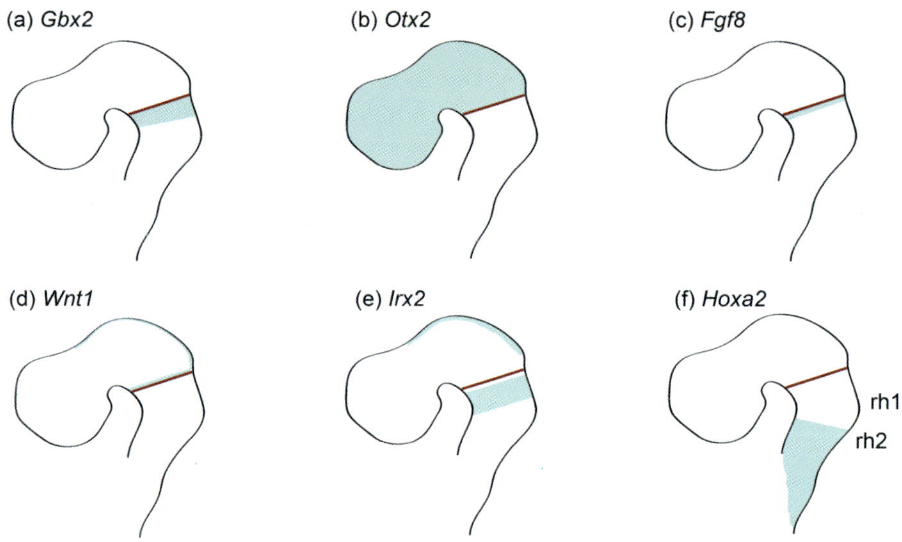

Plate 3. (Figure 1.3) Schematic side views of E9.5 mouse embryos illustrating the expression patterns of multiple genes (blue shading) around the mid-hindbrain boundary (red line). Each gene has been shown to be essential in establishment of the cerebellar territory along the anterior/ posterior axis of the neural tube and influence positioning of the isthmic organizer. **(a, b)** The interface of *Gbx2* and *Otx2* transcription factor encoding genes at the mid-hindbrain boundary determines the expression of the secreted factor **(c)** Fgf8, a critical effector of isthmic organizer function, which in turn regulates the expression domain of **(d)** Wnt1, another essential isthmic organizer secreted factor. **(e)** The transcription factor Irx2 is required for Fgf8 function to define the cerebellar territory and **(f)** Hoxa2, yet another transcription factor, is expressed posteriorly from the rhombomere (rh) 1/2 boundary and defines the posterior limit of the cerebellar territory.

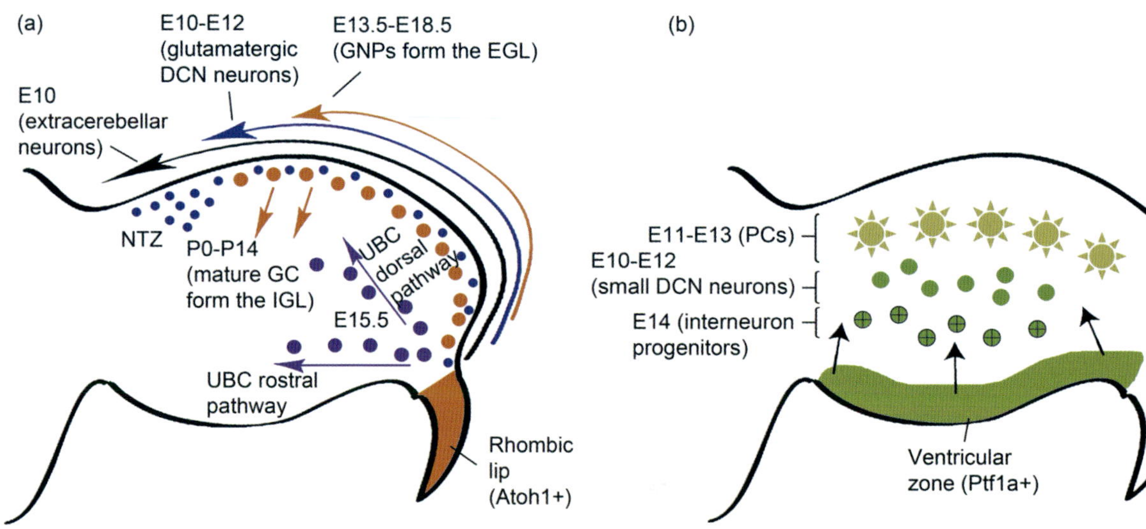

Plate 4. (Figure 1.4) Sagittal sections through the E16.5 cerebellum showing the migratory paths followed by various cerebellar neurons superimposed from a variety of developmental stages. **(a)** The rhombic lip produces glutamatergic neurons and traditionally has been defined by expression of the transcription factor Atoh1. Granule neuron progenitors (GNPs, orange), unipolar brush cells (UBCs, pink), and interneurons of deep cerebellar nuclei (DCN, purple) exit the rhombic lip in overlapping waves of neurogenesis, with the earliest neurons to exit the rhombic lip end up contributing to extracerebellar nuclei. Approximate exit times are indicated with arrows showing the direction of migration for these cells. The GNPs travel along a subpial tangential route to form the external granule layer (EGL) where they proliferate extensively, and eventually migrate inwards as mature granule cells along the Bergmann glial fibers (not shown in figure) through a radial route to form the internal granule layer (IGL) (see text). The UBCs migrate along two pathways – the dorsal pathway leading into the cerebellar white matter and a rostral pathway leading towards the ventricular zone and eventually the brainstem (Englund et al. 2006). The glutamatergic interneurons of the DCN follow a rostral subpial migratory path beginning from the rhombic lip and migrating to a transitory region called the nuclear transitory zone (NTZ) (Fink et al. 2006) from where they then migrate through the white matter via a poorly understood migration patter to settle deep inside the cerebellar base. **(b)** The ventricular zone, defined by expression of the transcription factor Ptf1a, gives rise to all GABAergic neurons of the cerebellum, also in overlapping waves of neurogenesis with timing indicated. The Purkinje cells (green stars) travel radially from the ventricular zone towards the surface along the fibers of radial glial cells and settle just underneath the IGL (see text). The interneuron progenitors (green with black outlines and crosses) and small neurons of the DCN (green) also travel radially away from the ventricular zone towards the prospective white matter remaining in the prospective white matter for several days before migrating to their final destinations in the cerebellar cortex and becoming committed to their final fates.

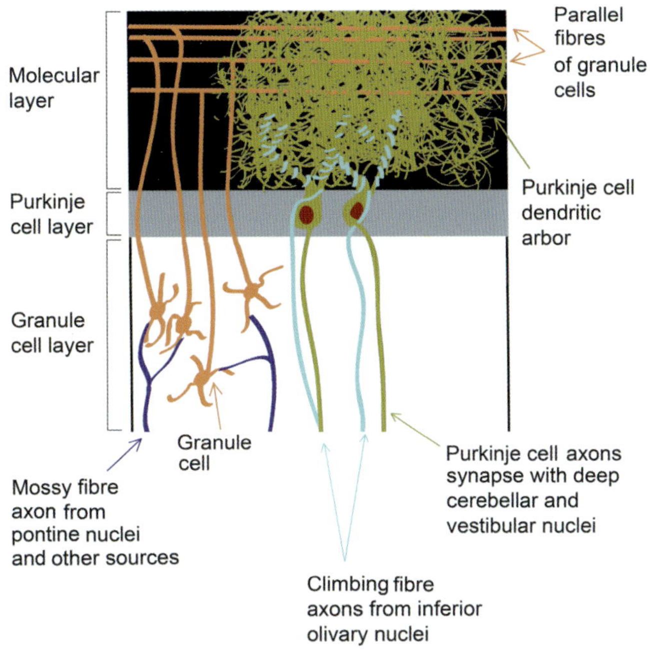

Plate 5. (Figure 1.5) Mature circuitry of the cerebellar cortex. Afferent input to the cerebellum is from two sources: mossy fibers (purple) and climbing fibers (blue). Granule cells (orange) receive mossy fiber (purple) inputs from multiple sources and project their extensive T-shaped axons (parallel fibers, yellow) to synapse onto the branches of dendritic arbor of Purkinje cells (green) within the upper segment of the molecular layer. Purkinje cell dendrites also receive inputs from the climbing fibers of the inferior olive (blue) within the lower segment of the molecular layer. All afferent output of the cerebellar cortex is from the axons of the Purkinje cells (green) which project to either the deep cerebellar nuclei within the base of the cerebellar cortex or the vestibular nuclei adjacent to the cerebellum.

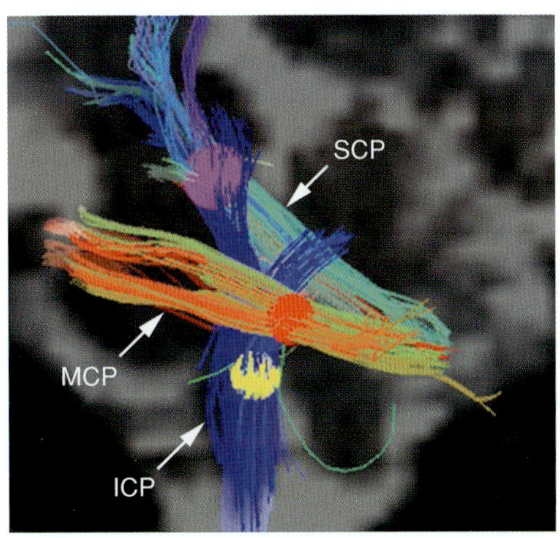

Plate 7. (Figure 2.3) Superior (SCP), middle (MCP) and inferior (ICP) cerebellar peduncles in human identified with diffusion spectrum magnetic resonance imaging, overlaid on a diffusion weighted image of cerebellum and brainstem. (From Granziera et al. 2009.)

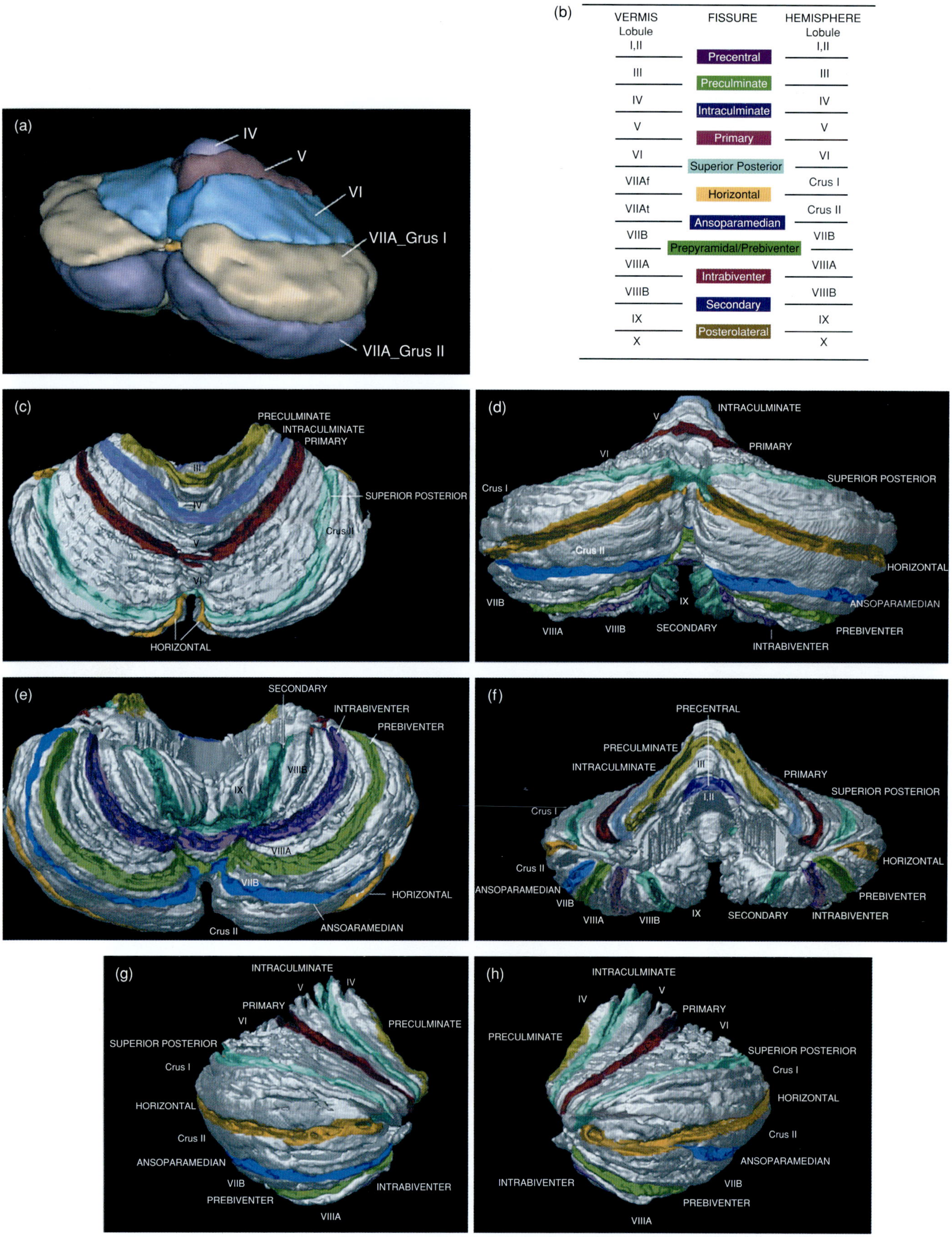

Plate 6. (Figure 2.2) Surface reconstructions of the human cerebellum derived from magnetic resonance images. **(a)** The cerebellum is viewed from the right posterior superior aspect, showing lobules IV through crus II as labeled. **(b)** Diagram illustrating the relationship of the named cerebellar fissures to the lobules in the vermis and hemispheres. The named fissures are demarcated in color according to the convention in (b), and the fissures and lobules are identified. The cerebellum is viewed from **(c)** superior, **(d)** posterior, **(e)** inferior, **(f)** anterior, **(g)** right lateral, and **(h)** left lateral aspects. ((a) from Makris et al. 2005; (b–h) from Schmahmann et al. 1999, 2000.)

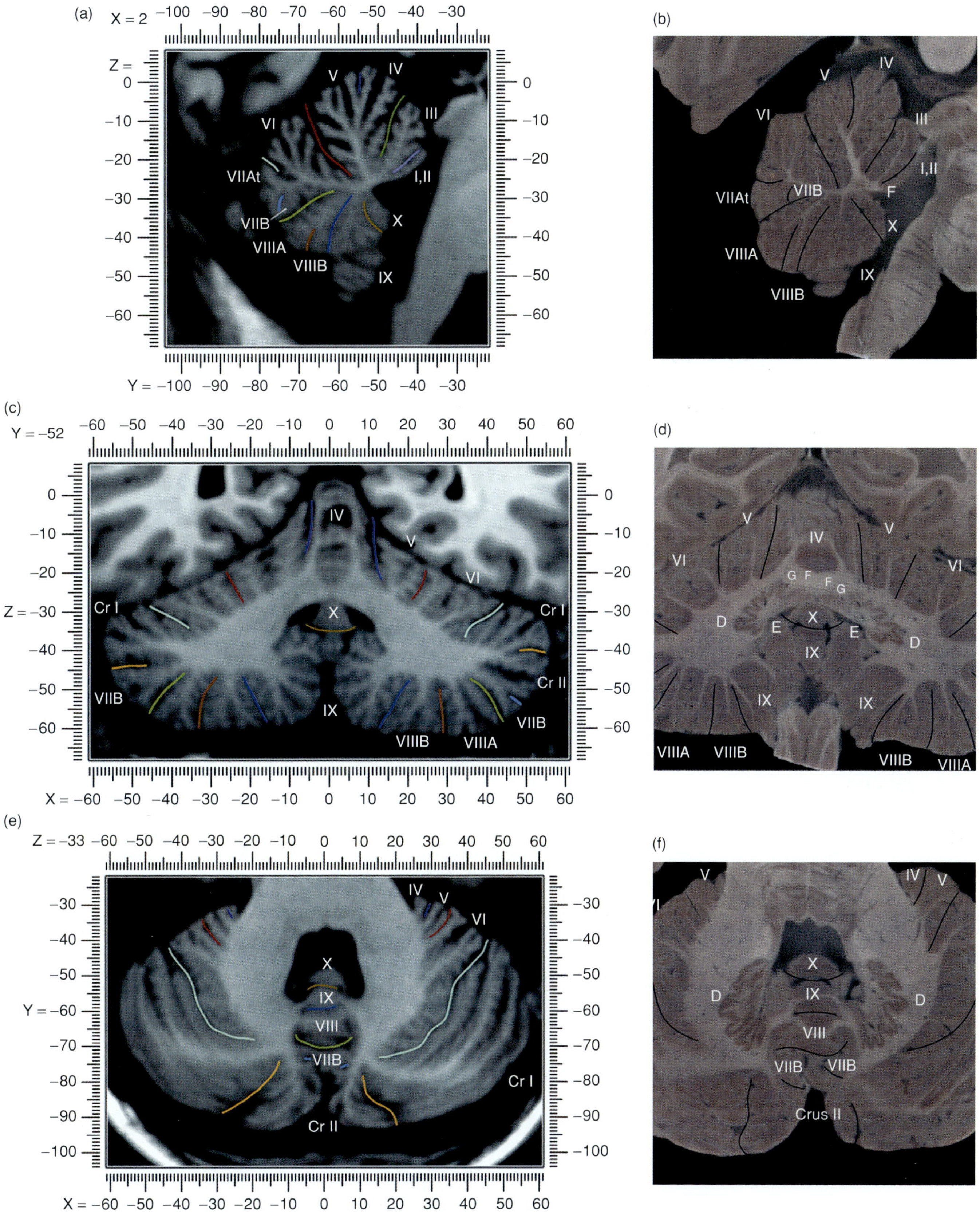

Plate 8. (Figure 2.4) Images of the human cerebellum on MRI (left panel) and postmortem cryosection (right panel). The cerebellum is sectioned in the sagittal plane 2mm to the right of midline in **(a)** and **(b)**; in the coronal plane 52mm behind the anterior commissure–posterior commissure (AC-PC) line in **(c)** and **(d)**; and in the transverse plane 33mm below the AC-PC line in **(e)** and **(f)**. Fissures are color coded according to the convention used in Fig. 2.2(b–h), and the lobules are designated. Deep cerebellar nuclei are identified in the cryosection brain: E, emboliform nucleus; F, fastigial nucleus; G, globose nucleus; D, dentate nucleus. (From Schmahmann et al. 2000.)

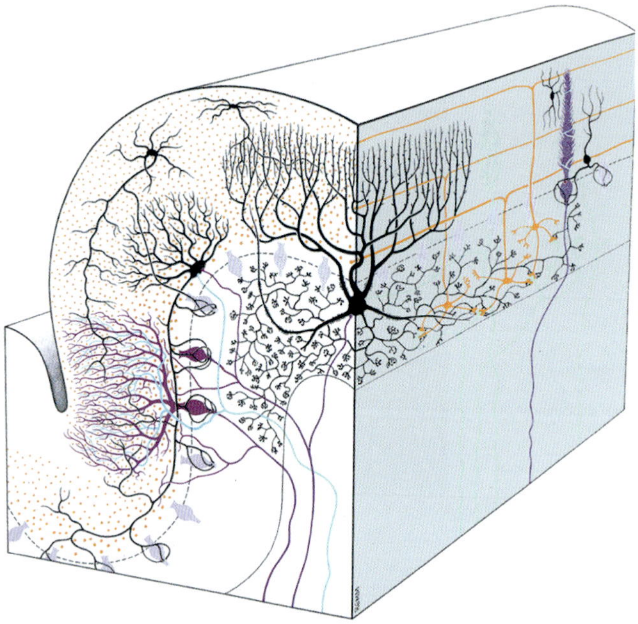

Plate 9. (Figure 2.5) Organization of the cerebellar cortex. A single cerebellar folium is shown sectioned in its longitudinal axis (diagram right) and transversely (left). Purkinje cells are red; superficial and deep stellate, basket and Golgi cells are black; granule cells and ascending axons and parallel fibers are yellow; mossy and climbing fibers are blue. Also shown are the glomeruli with mossy fiber rosettes, claw-like dendrites of granule cells, and Golgi axons. Lugaro and unipolar brush cells are not shown. (Diagram of Eccles, Ito, Szengothai 1967, as redrawn in Gray's Anatomy 1995.)

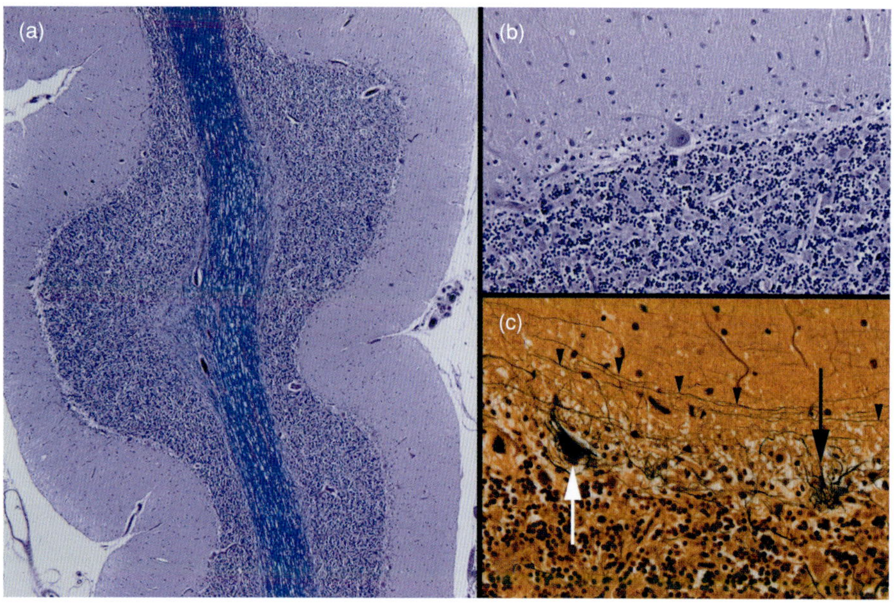

Plate 10. (Figure 2.6) Photomicrographs of the human cerebellar cortex. **(a)** Low power view of a cerebellar folium showing white matter (stained blue) coursing between the apposed leaves of the cerebellar cortex: granular layer innermost, Purkinje cell (Purkinje cell) monolayer intermediate, and molecular layer outermost. 4× magnification, stained with hematoxylin and eosin (H&E). **(b)** The Purkinje cell layer is seen between the molecular layer (above) and the granule cell layer (below). Note the eosinophilic (pink stained) glomeruli throughout the granular layer. 20× magnification, H&E. **(c)** Cerebellar cortex derived from a patient with spinocerebellar ataxia type 7 to show axons of basket cells (arrowheads) coursing horizontally in the Purkinje cell layer, enveloping a Purkinje cell in the basket of axon terminal ramifications (white arrow) and forming an 'empty basket' around a degenerated Purkinje cell (black arrow). 40× magnification, silver stain. (Photographs courtesy of Dr. Matthew Frosch, C.S. Kubik Laboratory for Neuropathology, Massachusetts General Hospital.)

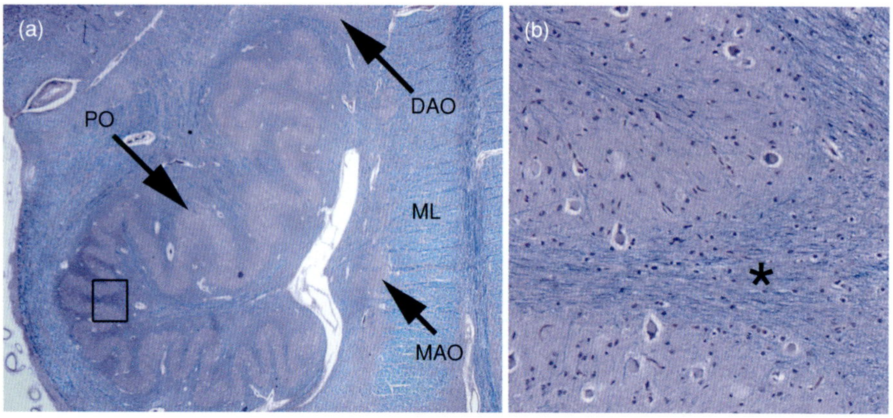

Plate 11. (Figure 2.7) Photomicrographs of human inferior olivary complex. **(a)** Low power view of the ventral part of the right medulla sectioned in a slightly oblique plane. 4× magnification, H&E. The principal olivary nucleus (PO), and dorsal (DAO) and medial accessory olivary nuclei (MAO) are labeled, laterally adjacent to the medial lemniscus (ML). **(b)** Higher magnification view shows neurons in the principal olive, and the hilum of the olive (asterisk) through which the olivocerebellar fibers (stained blue) course to the contralateral cerebellum. 10× magnification, H&E. (Photographs courtesy of Dr. Matthew Frosch, C.S. Kubik Laboratory for Neuropathology, Massachusetts General Hospital.)

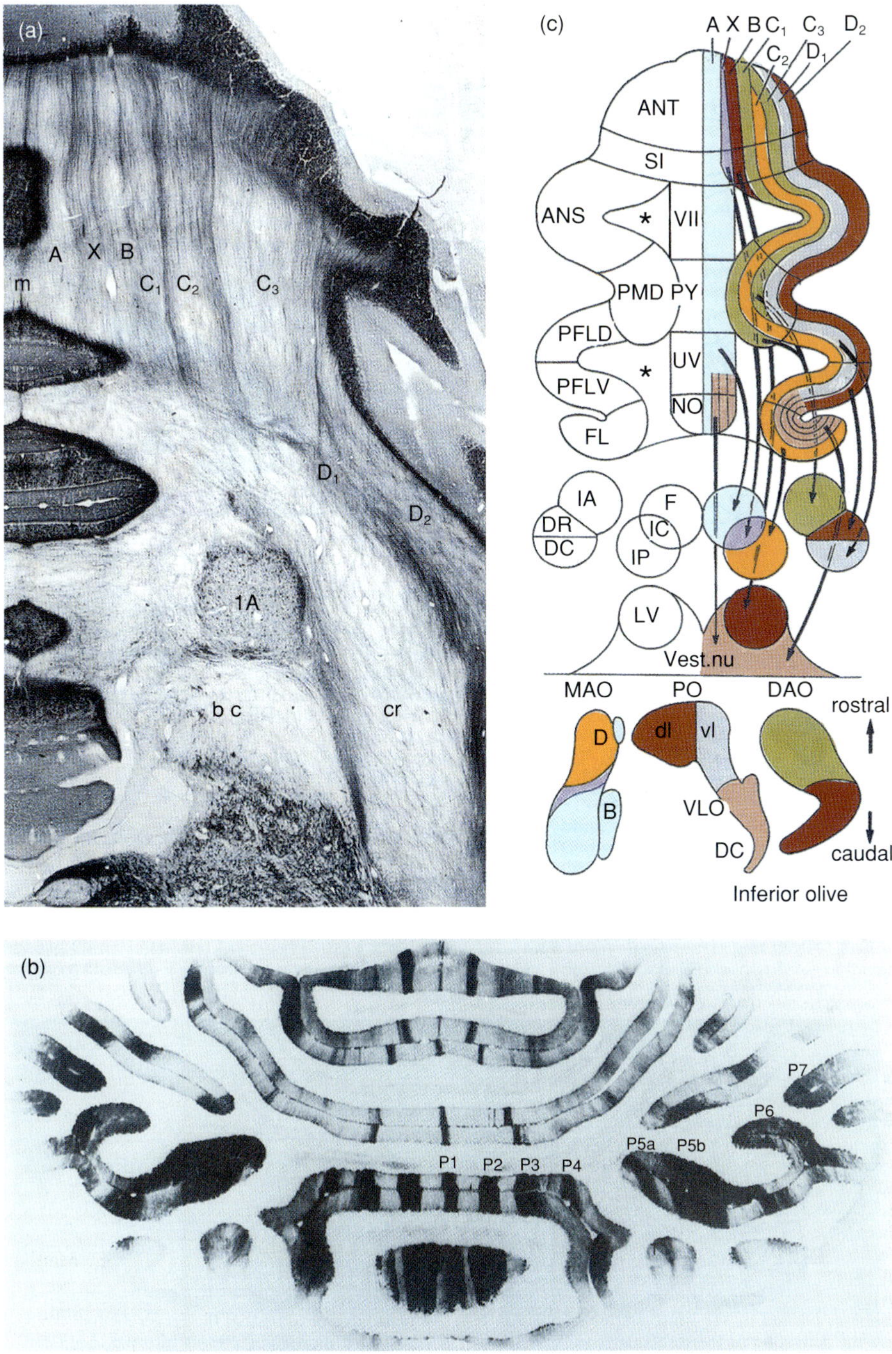

Plate 12. (Figure 2.8) Diagrams depicting parasagittal zones and connections in the cerebellum. **(a)** Transverse section through the anterior lobe of monkey cerebellum stained for acetylcholinesterase, showing white matter compartments. **(b)** Frontal section through the cerebellum of an adult rat to show Purkinje cells stained with immunoperoxidase for zebrin I. The immunoreactive Purkinje cells align to form parasagittal bands in the vermis and hemispheres. **(c)** Color-coded diagram showing the zonal arrangement of cerebellar corticonuclear (above) and olivocerebellar projections (below) on a flattened cerebellar cortex of the cat. Cerebellum – zones A, X, B, C1, C2, C3, D1, D2; ANS, ansiform lobule; ANT, anterior lobe; FL, flocculus; IA, anterior interposed nucleus; bc, brachium conjunctivum; cr, restiform body; NO, nodulus; P1–7, parasagittal zones in the rat cerebellum; PFL (D/V), (dorsal/ventral) paraflocculus; PMD, paramedian lobule; PY, pyramis; SI, lobulus simplex (lobule VI); UV, uvula. Cerebellar nuclei – DC, ventrocaudal dentate nucleus; DR, rostromedial dentate nucleus; IC, interstitial cell group; IP, posterior interposed nucleus; F, fastigial nucleus. Inferior olivary nucleus – B, ß cell group; D, dorsomedial cell column; DAO, dorsal accessory olive; DC, dorsal cap; dl, dorsal leaf; MAO, medial accessory olive; PO, principal olive; vl, ventral leaf; VLO, ventrolateral outgrowth. Vest. nu, vestibular nuclei; LV, lateral vestibular nucleus. ((a) and (c) from Voogd and Glickstein 1998. (b) from Leclerc et al. 1990.)

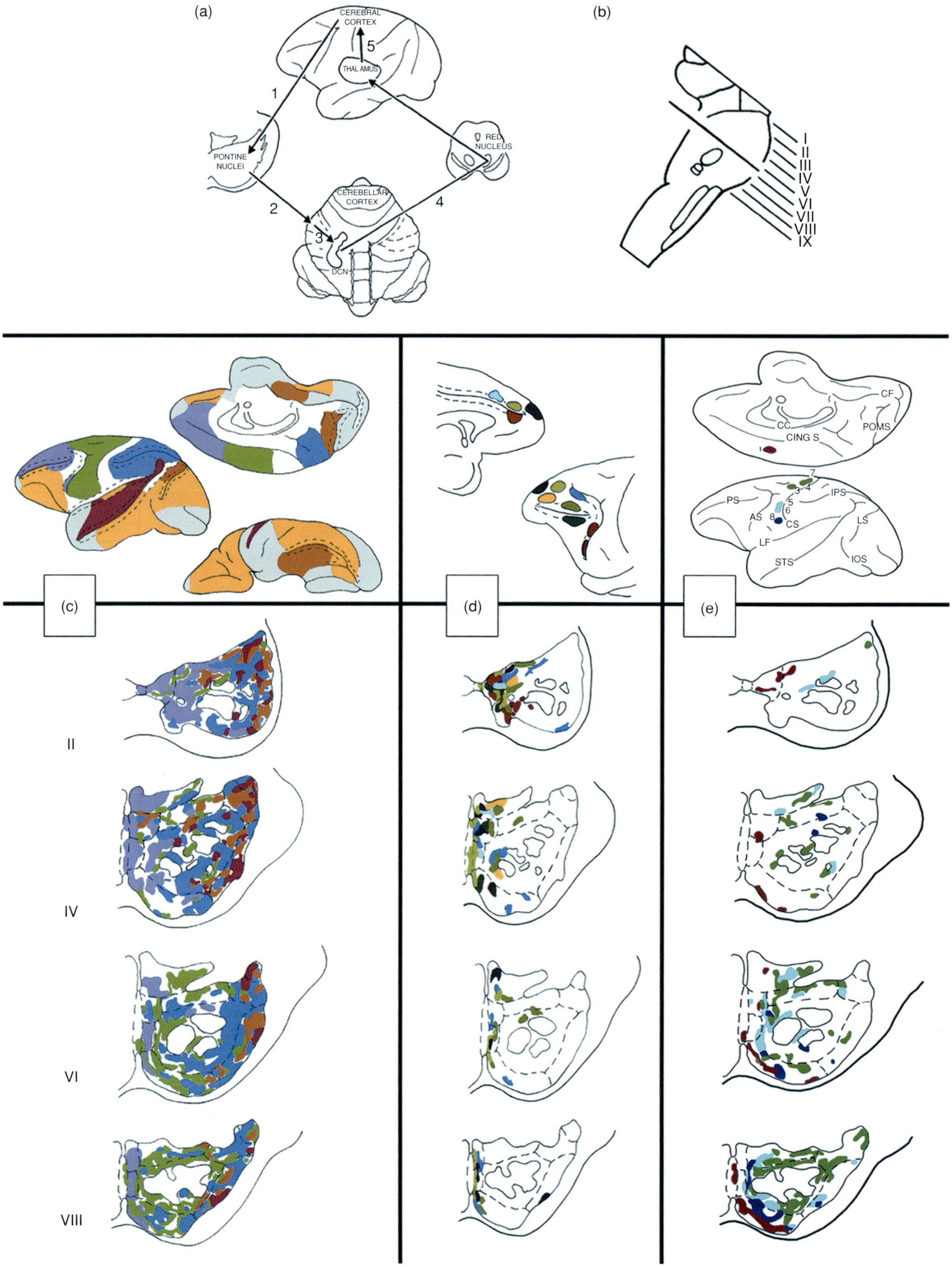
(a)
CEREBRAL CORTEX
5
THALAMUS
1
PONTINE NUCLEI
RED NUCLEUS
2
CEREBELLAR CORTEX
4
3
DCN
(b)
I
II
III
IV
V
VI
VII
VIII
IX
CF
CC
CING S
POMS
7
3
4
IPS
PS
5
6
AS
8
CS
LS
LF
STS
IOS
(c)
(d)
(e)
II
IV
VI
VIII

Plate 13. (Figure 2.10) (*opposite*) Diagrammatic representations of the feedfoward limb of the corticopontine projections in rhesus monkey. **(a)** Schematic of the crossed cerebrocerebellar connections, or cerebrocerebellar loops. 1. Two-stage feedforward limb of cerebral cortex projections to the ipsilateral pontine nuclei. 2. Pontocerebellar projections through the middle cerebellar peduncle to the contralateral cerebellar hemisphere. 3. Cerebellar cortex projections to the deep cerebellar nuclei (DCN) begin the two-stage feedback limb. 4. Projections from the DCN via the contralateral red nucleus to the thalamus. 5. Thalamic projections to the same (or similar) regions of the cerebral cortex from which the corticopontine projection originated. **(b)** Plane of section through the pons from which the rostrocaudal levels II through VIII are taken in the schematics (c–e). **(c)** Composite color-coded summary diagram illustrating the distribution within selected regions of the basis pontis of projections from association and paralimbic areas shown on medial, lateral, and orbital views of the cerebral hemisphere in the prefrontal (purple), posterior parietal (blue), superior temporal (red), and parastriate and parahippocampal regions (orange), and from motor, premotor, and supplementary motor areas (SMA) (green). Other cerebral areas known to project to the pons are depicted in white. Cortical areas with no pontine projections are shown in yellow (from anterograde and retrograde studies) or gray (from retrograde studies). Dashed lines in the hemisphere diagrams represent sulcal cortices. Dashed lines in the pons diagrams represent pontine nuclei; solid lines depict corticofugal fibers. The projections are characterized by a complex mosaic of terminations in the pontine nuclei. Each cerebral cortical region has preferential sites of pontine terminations; there is interdigitation of terminations, but almost no overlap. **(d)** Color-coded summary diagram of distribution within the basis pontis of projections from the medial and lateral convexities of the prefrontal cortex. **(e)** Color-coded summary diagram of projections to the pontine nuclei from motor and supplementary motor cortices. Injection sites in the cerebral cortex in (e) (filled areas) are color-coded: SMA, red; trunk and leg, green; hand, light blue; face-hand overlapping area, dark blue. The terminations are predominantly in the caudal half of the pons; SMA projections are most medial, and the face, hand, and leg projections are progressively more laterally situated. ((a–c) from Schmahmann 1996 and Schmahmann and Pandya 1997b. (d) from Schmahmann and Pandya 1997a. (e) from Schmahmann et al. 2004.)

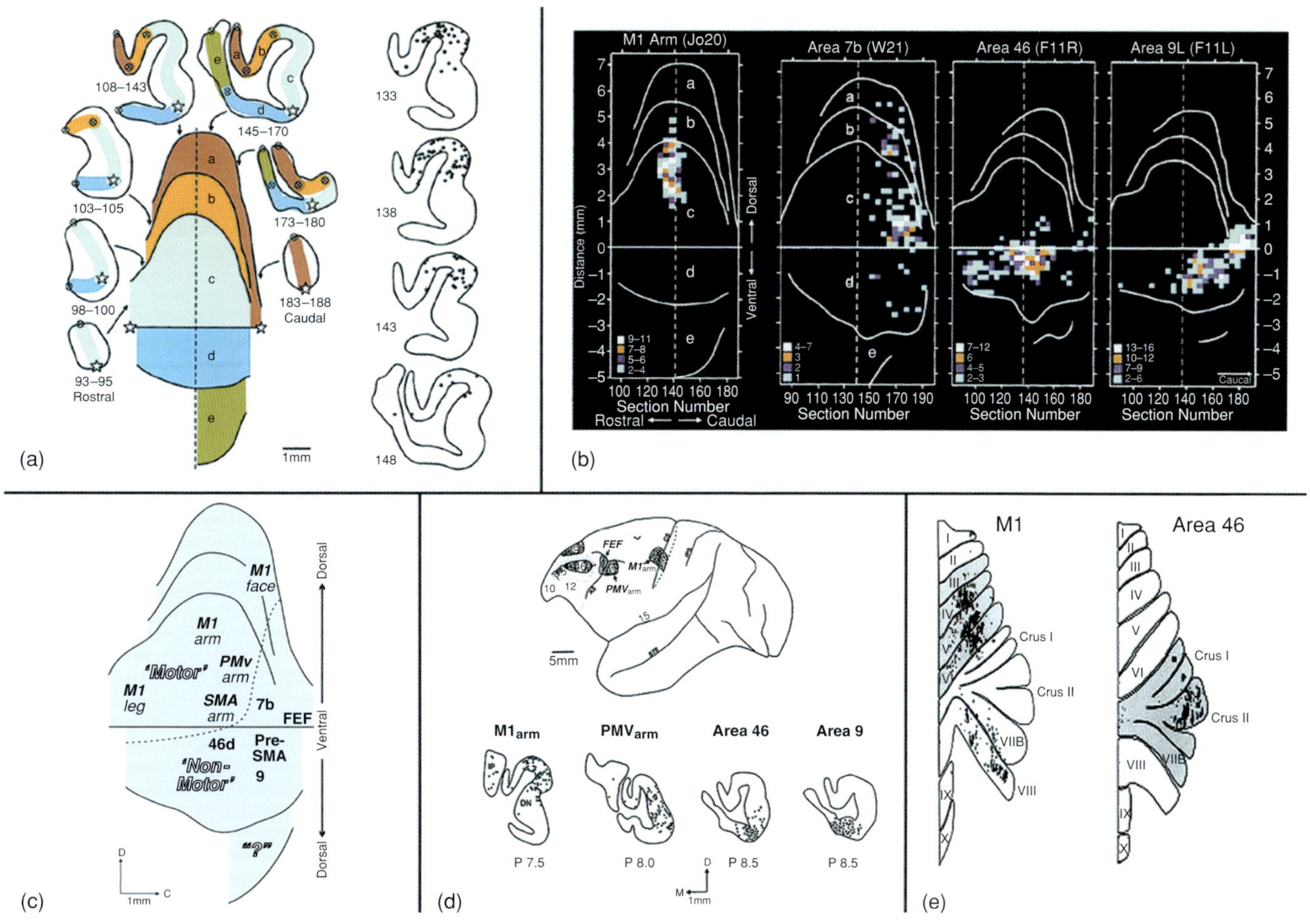

Plate 14. (Figure 2.11) Diagrams depicting cerebellar feedback projections to the cerebral cortex in cebus monkey. **(a)** Unfolded map of the dentate nucleus (in color) created by unfolding serial coronal sections through the nucleus. Each section is aligned to the junction of the c and d segments (open star). Dashed vertical line indicates the rostrocaudal center of the nucleus. Cross-sections of the dentate nucleus on the right show the location of 'second order' neurons (dots) labeled after transport of herpes simplex virus type 1 (HSV1) from the arm representation of M1. **(b)** Unfolded maps of the dentate nucleus illustrate the neurons labeled after virus injections into the arm representation in M1, posterior parietal cortex area 7b, and mid-dorsolateral prefrontal cortex areas 46 and 9-lateral. **(c)** Summary diagram showing the origins of dentate nucleus projections to primary motor cortex (M1) representations of the leg, arm and face; ventral premotor area (PMv); inferior parietal lobule (area 7b); and the mid-dorsolateral prefrontal cortex (areas 46 and 9L). **(d)** Lateral view of monkey brain (top) shows the locations of viral tracer injections in the M1 – arm, PMv – arm, and prefrontal cortex areas 46 and 9. The resulting retrogradely labeled neurons in the cerebellar dentate nucleus (bottom) are indicated by solid dots. **(e)** Flattened representation of cerebellum to show the folia linked with M1 motor cortex (left) and prefrontal cortex area 46 (right) using viral tracers that travel in the anterograde direction (H129 strain of HSV1) and retrograde direction (rabies virus). ((a) and (b) from Dum and Strick 2003; (c) from Strick et al. 2009; (d) from Middleton and Strick 1997; (e) from Kelly and Strick 2003.)

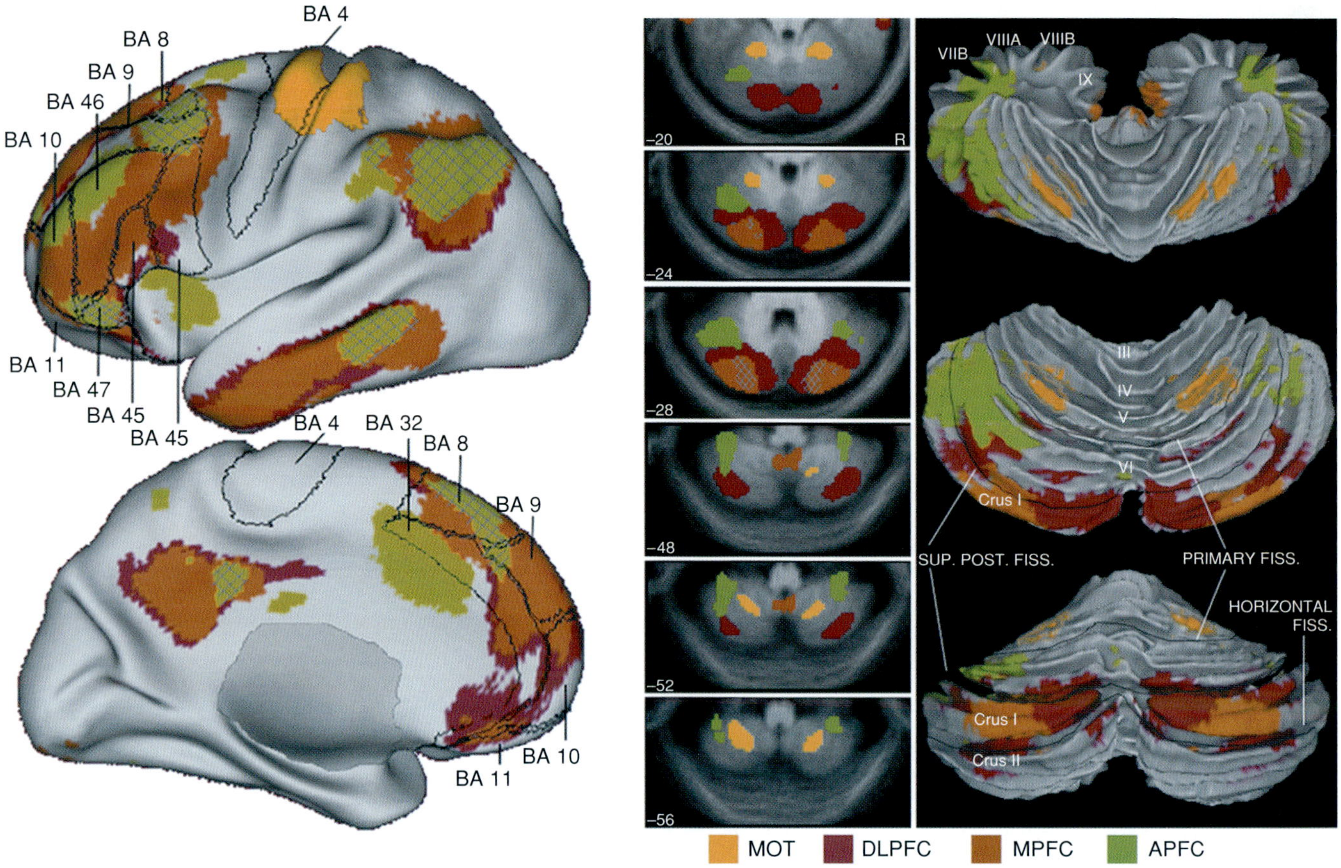

Plate 15. (Figure 2.12) Provisional map of human cerebellar connectivity with the frontal cortex as determined by functional connectivity MRI. Seed regions were placed in the motor cortex (MOT) shown in yellow, dorsolateral prefrontal cortex (DLPFC) in red, medial prefrontal cortex (MPFC) in orange, and anterior prefrontal cortex (APFC) in green. Correlation maps with frontal lobe and other cerebral cortical areas are shown in the cerebral hemisphere diagrams at left (hatched regions represent overlap of two correlation maps; parietal and temporal lobes not labeled); in the cerebellum in rostral-to-caudal axial sections in the middle panel; and in surface reconstructions of the cerebellum in the right panel (inverted anterior view; dorsal view; posterior view). The cerebral cortical motor correlations are in cerebellar lobules IV, V, and VIIIA; the majority of the mapped portion of the posterior cerebellum (lobules VI and crus I and crus II) is associated with prefrontal (cognitive) regions of the neocortex. Approximate borders of relevant labeled Brodmann areas (BA) are shown in the prefrontal and motor cortices. Cerebellar nomenclature as in Schmahmann et al. (1999, 2000). (Images adapted from Krienen and Buckner 2009.)

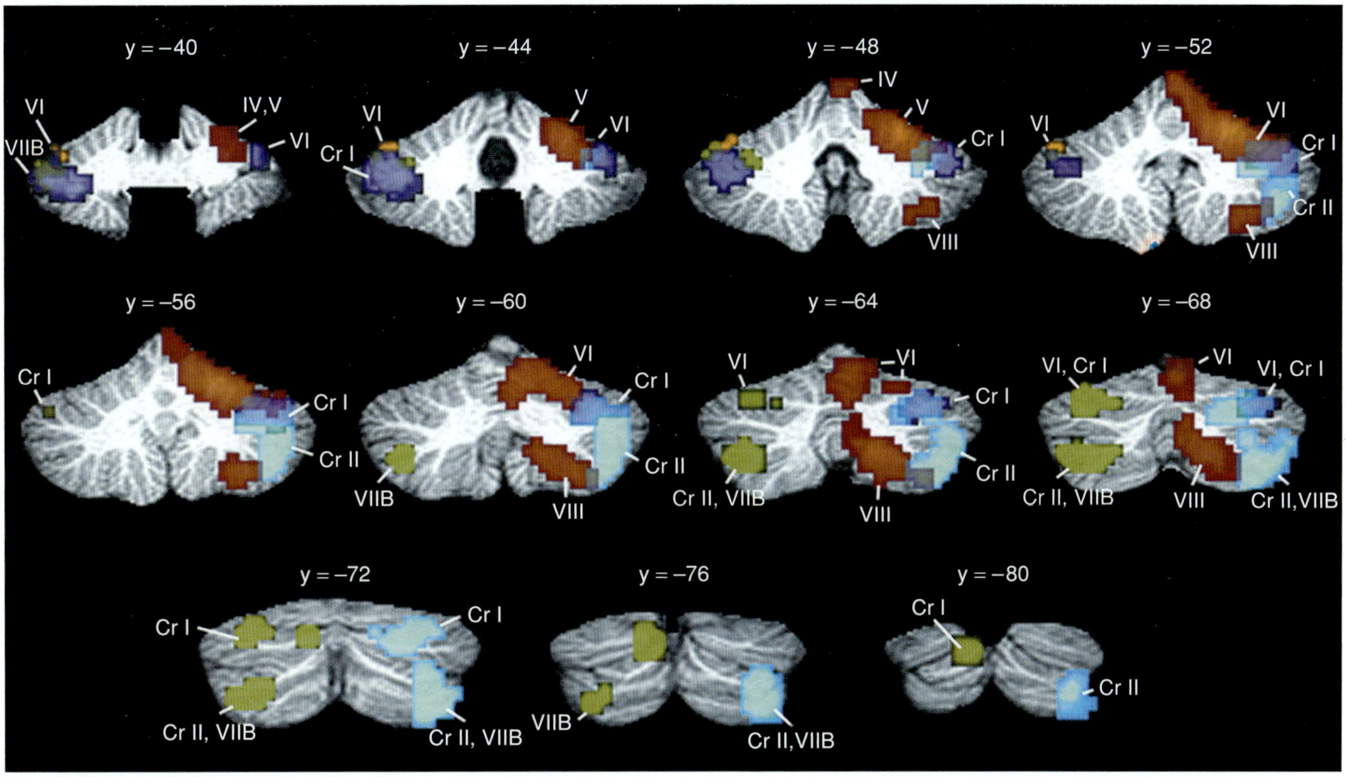

Plate 16. (Figure 2.13) Representative rostral (y = −44) to caudal (y = −80) coronal sections through a human cerebellum showing activation patterns in a functional magnetic resonance imaging experiment in a single individual. Tasks investigated sensorimotor function (finger tapping, shown in red), language (verb generation, blue), spatial cognition (mental rotation, green), working memory (N-back, purple), and emotional processing (viewing images from the International Affective Picture System, yellow). Cerebellar lobules are labeled according to Schmahmann et al. 1999, 2000. The right cerebellar hemisphere is shown on the right. (From Stoodley et al. 2010.)

Plate 17. (Figure 4.1) Copy and 5-minute delayed recall of the Rey-Osterrieth figure by a 15-year-old boy with cerebellar agenesis.

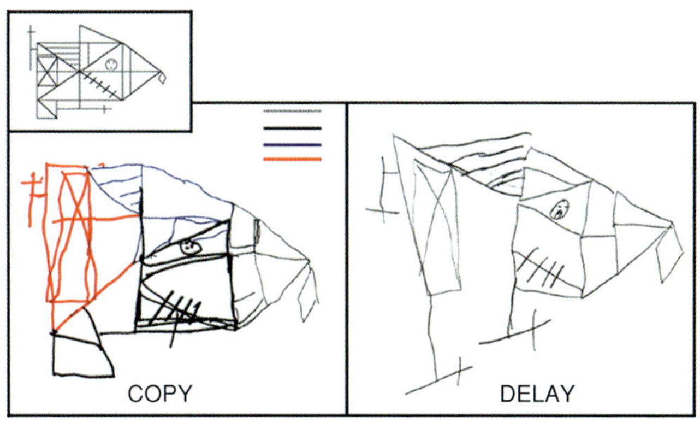

Plate 18. (Figure 6.3(c)) Three-dimensional surface shaded reconstruction of a CT dataset allows detailed study of the skull and skull base as well as the craniocervical junction.

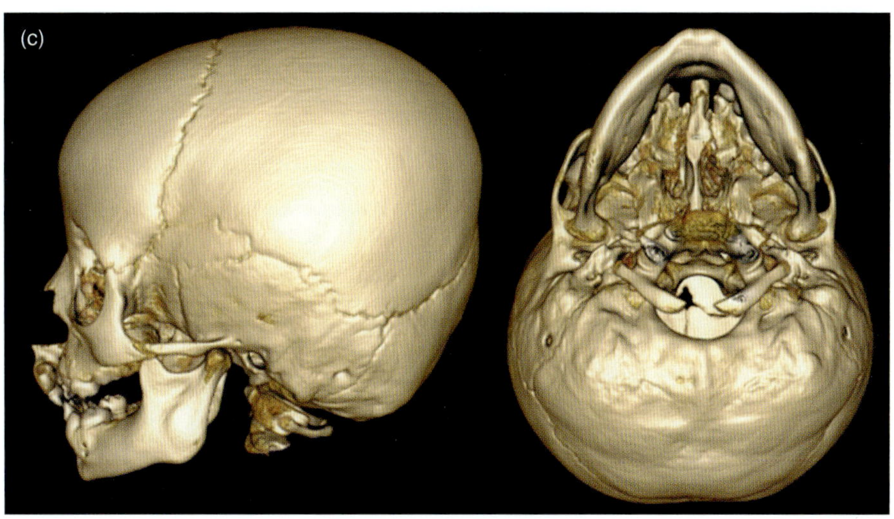

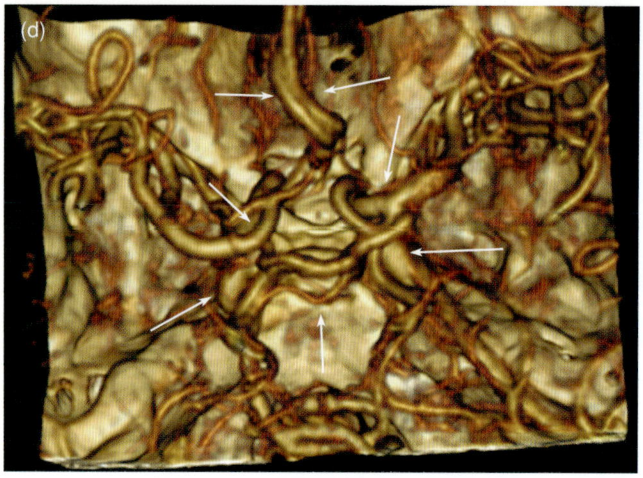

Plate 19. (Figure 6.3(d)) Three-dimensional reconstruction of a contrast-enhanced CT angiography. The circulus arteriosus Willisi is seen from above, projected on the osseous skull base (arrows).

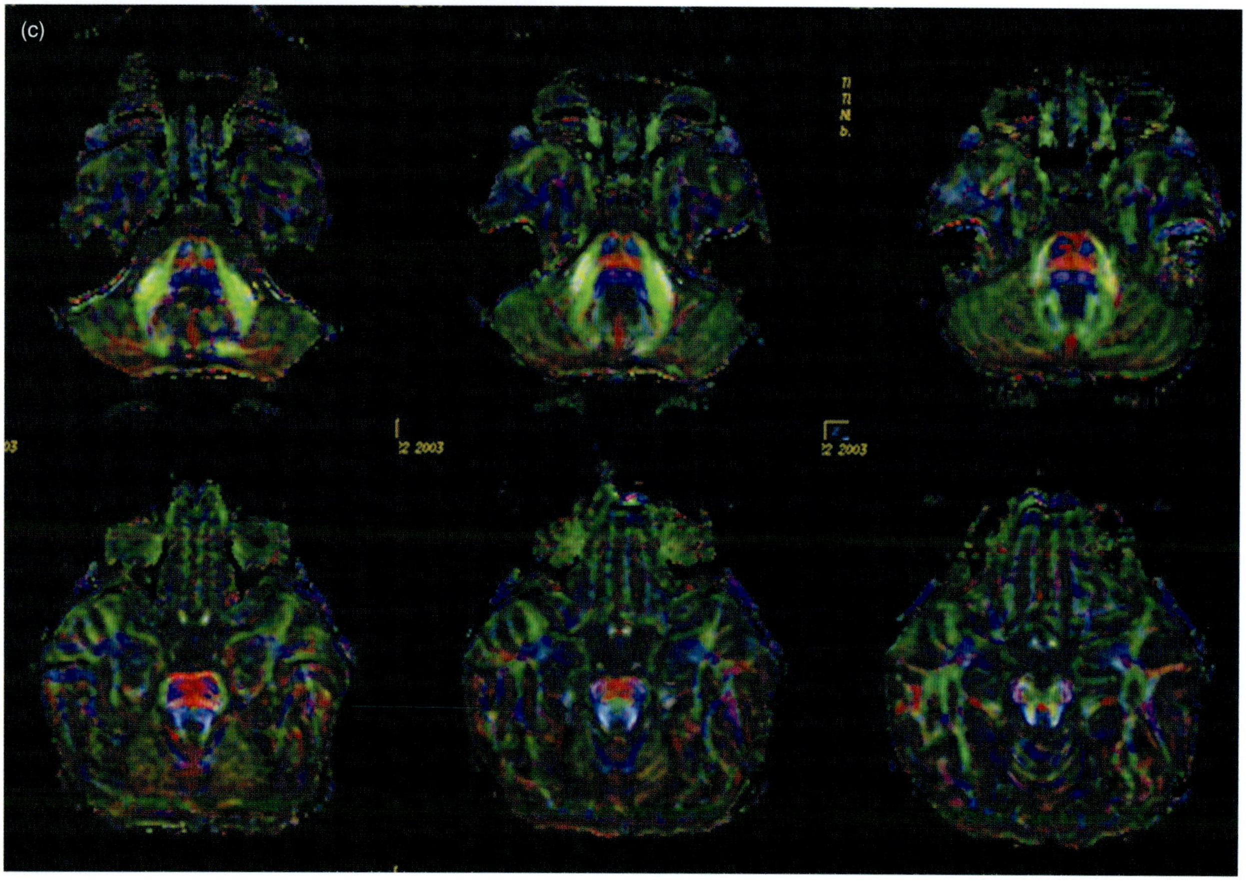

Plate 20. (Figure 6.7(c)) Color-coded FA maps show the predominant diffusion direction, course of the various white matter tracts (green: anterior-posterior; red: left-right; blue: superior-inferior).

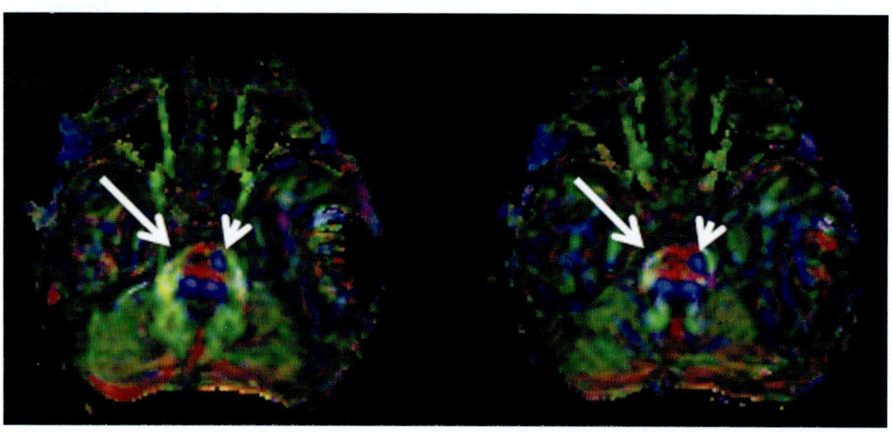

Plate 21. (Figure 6.8) Example of a pathologic color-coded fractional anisotropy (FA) map. The descending corticospinal tract (blue) is absent on the right (large arrow) due to a large supratentorial infarction in the ipsilateral motor cortex. The left corticospinal tract (arrowhead) is preserved and can easily be depicted.

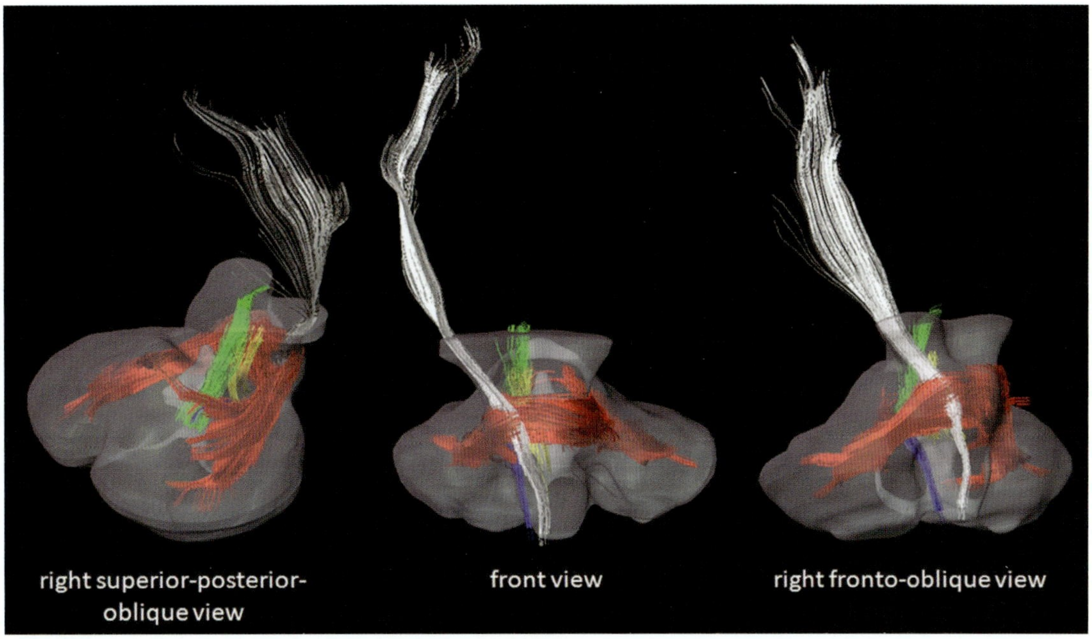

Plate 22. (Figure 6.9) Color-coded multiplanar, three-dimensional reconstruction of various fiber tracts (tractography) within the brainstem and cerebellum from a diffusion tensor dataset. The corticospinal, corticobulbar, and corticopontine tracts, the medial lemniscus, the inferior, middle, and superior cerebellar tract, and transverse pontine fibers are displayed. (Courtesy of Dr Kenichi Oishi, Johns Hopkins Hospital, Baltimore, USA.)

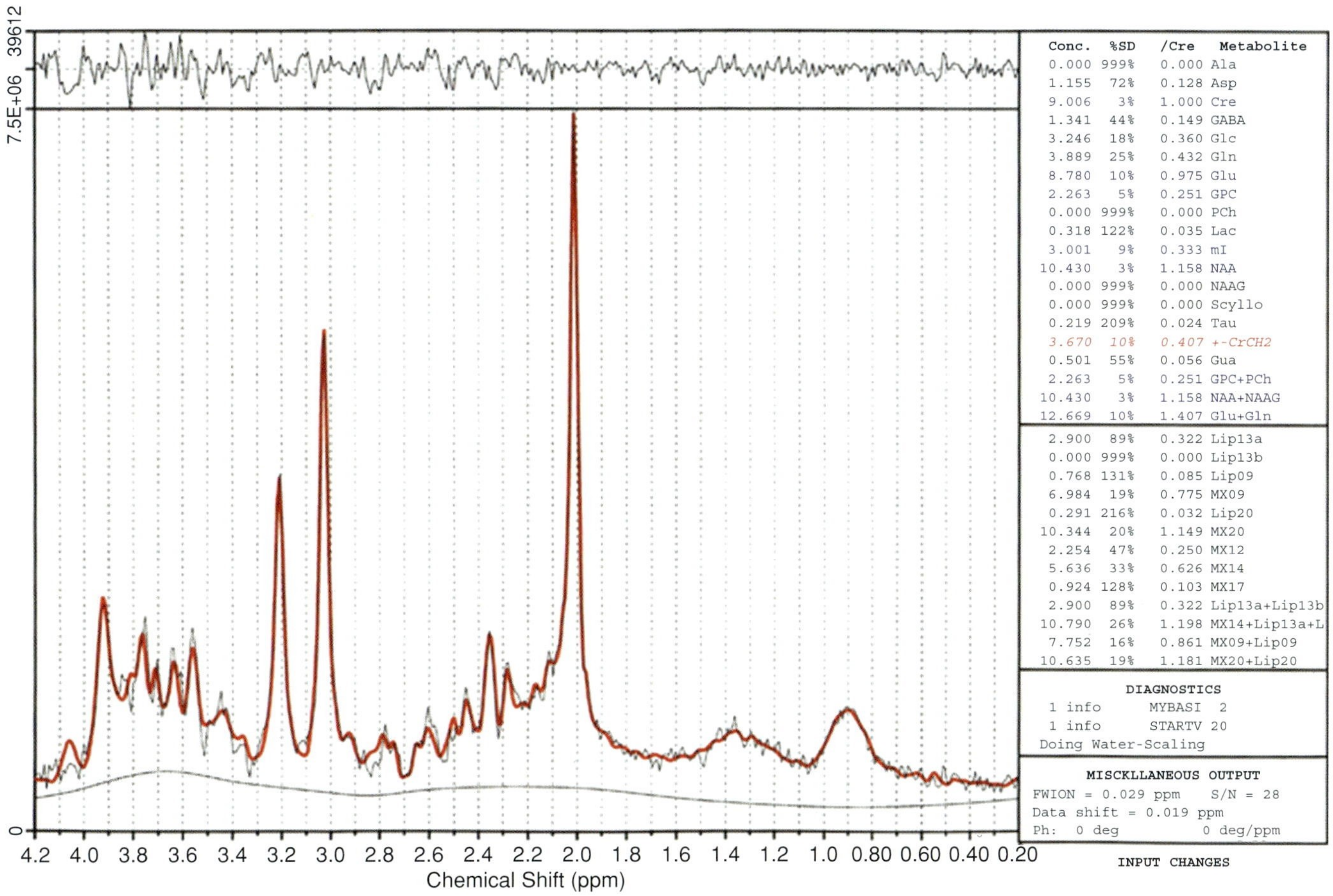

Plate 23. (Figure 6.13) [1]H Magnetic resonance spectroscopy of the cerebellar white matter. The dominant peak is *N*-acetylaspartate (at 2ppm). Additional peaks are creatine and choline. The metabolite concentration is calculated from the normalized surface area underneath the peak.

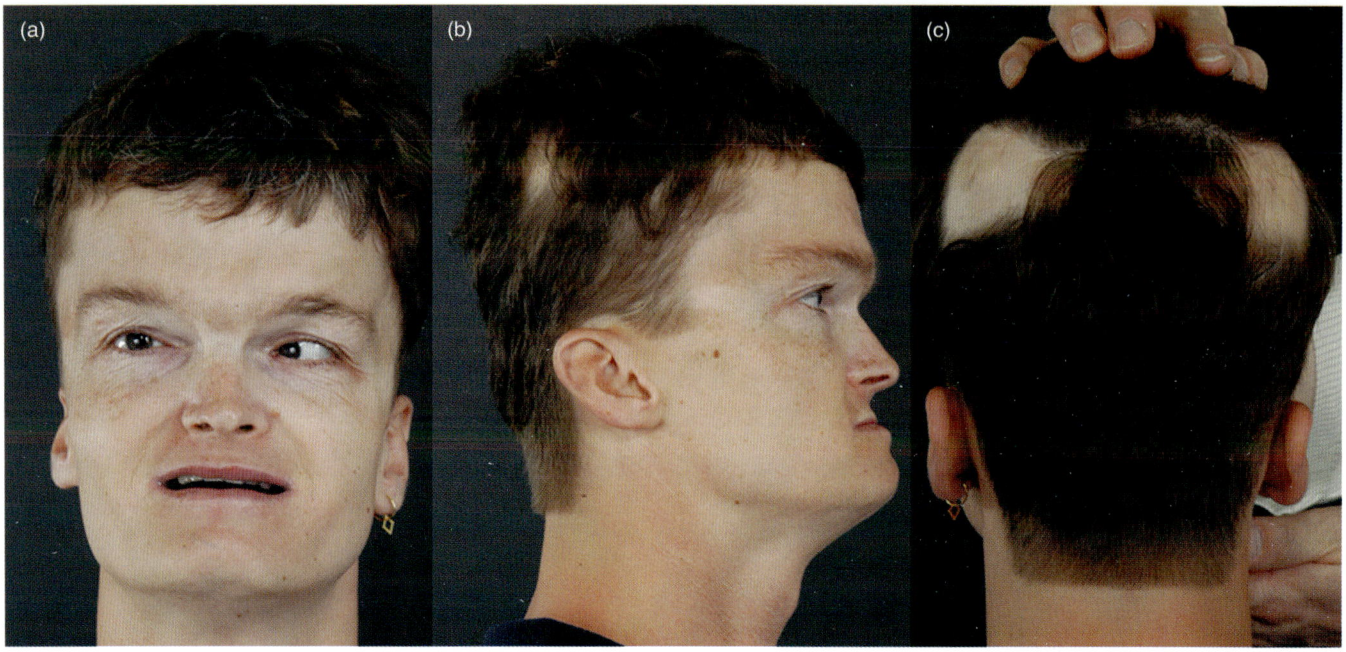

Plate 24. (Figure 16.1) Gómez-López-Hernández syndrome in a 34-year-old patient. **(a)** Front view showing broad, high forehead, hypertelorism, strabismus, small nose, and short and flat philtrum. Note the premature aging and scars on the forehead. **(b)** Right side view demonstrating pronounced brachyturricephaly, low-set, posteriorly rotated ears, prognathism, midface hypoplasia, and parietal alopecia. **(c)** Posterior view revealing bilateral parietal alopecia. (Reprinted with permission from Poretti A et al. Eur J Med Genet 2008; 51(3): 197–208.)

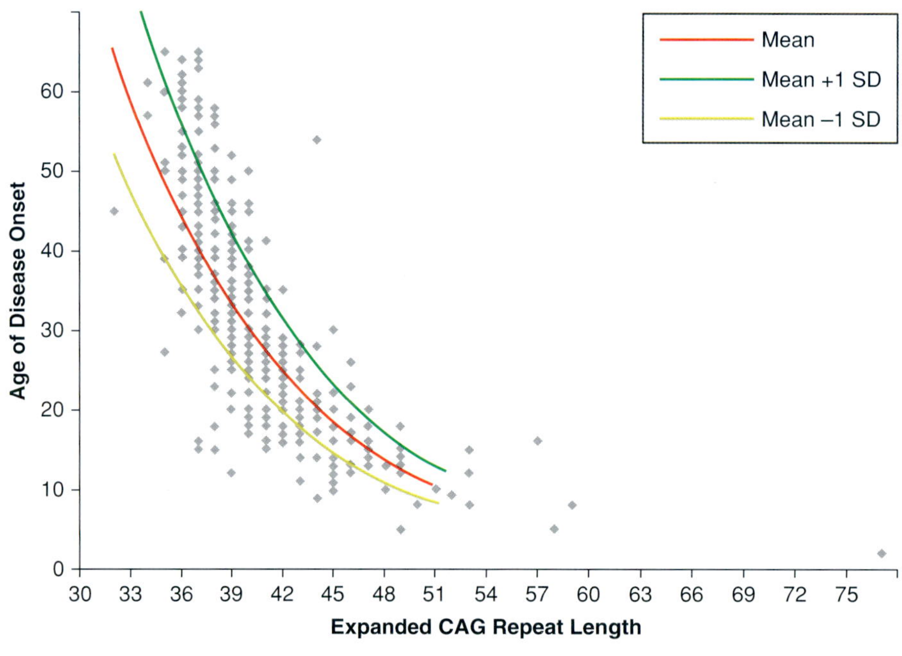

Plate 25. (Figure 24.2) Scatterplot of SCA2 CAG repeat length and age at onset in Cuban SCA2 patients: dashed and dotted red and yellow lines denote one standard deviation boundaries for age at onset. (Reproduced with permission from Pulst S et al. Brain 2005; 128: 2297–2303.)

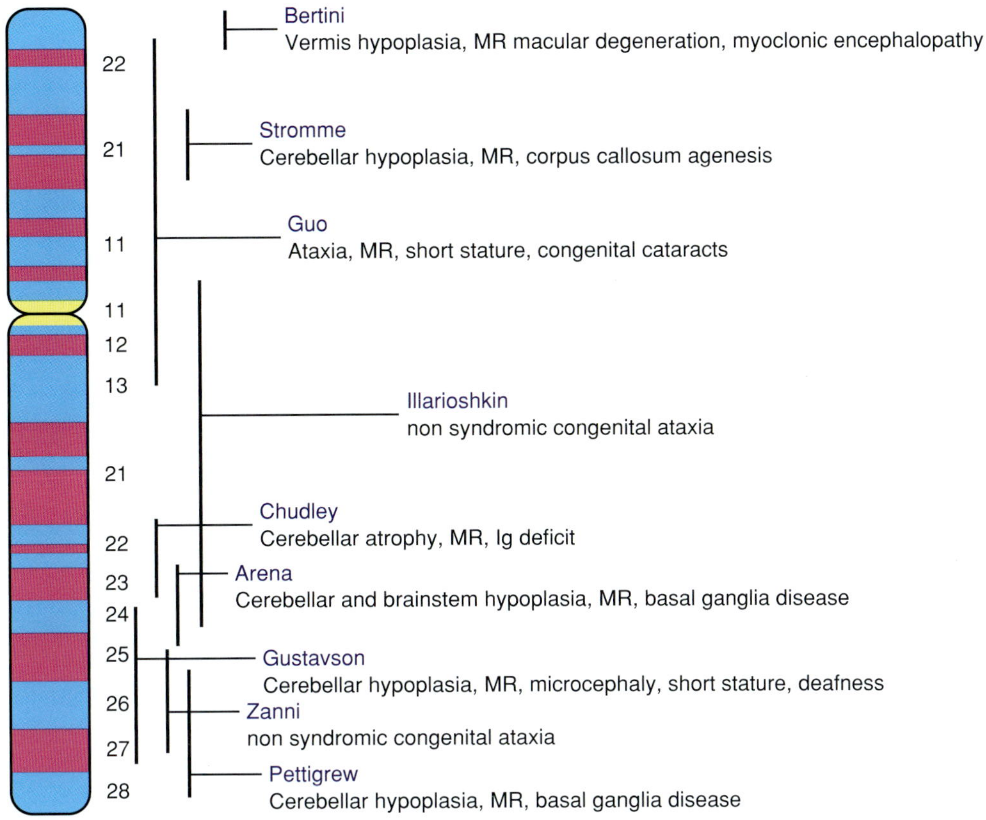

Plate 26. (Figure 25.3) Ideogram of the X-chromosome with linkage mapping limits of families with X-linked cerebellar disorders.

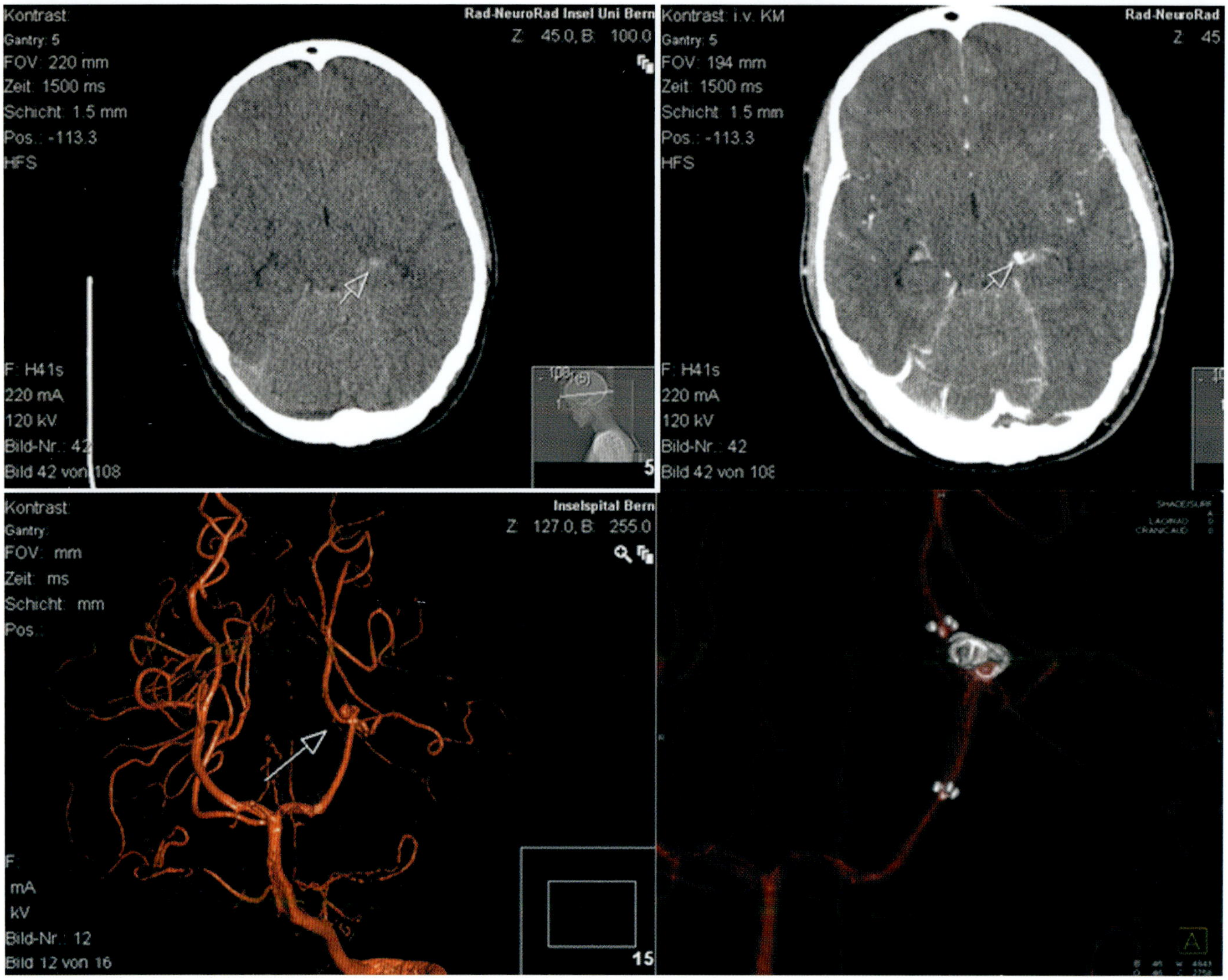

Plate 27. (Figure 32.8) Non-contrast-CT (upper left image) indicates subtle subarachnoid haemorrhage (SAH) in the perimesencephal cistern (Fisher I). Angio-CT (upper right image) indicates an aneurysm in the ambient cistern as source of the SAH. Three-dimensional rotation angiography (lower row) confirms a bilobulated aneurysm of the left posterior cerebral artery arising with a broad neck from the branching into the calcarine and occipitotemporal arteries. Three-dimensional digital abstraction angiography after endovascular treatment shows the electrolytically detachable coils in the aneurysm and normal flow through the adjacent posterior cerebral artery protected by a neuroform stent, which bridges the wide neck of the aneurysm and keeps the coils inside the aneurysm.

Materialwirtschaft mit SAP S/4HANA®

SAP PRESS

SAP PRESS ist eine gemeinschaftliche Initiative von SAP SE und der Rheinwerk Verlag GmbH. Unser Ziel ist es, Ihnen als Anwendern qualifiziertes SAP-Wissen zur Verfügung zu stellen. SAP PRESS vereint das Know-how der SAP und die verlegerische Kompetenz von Rheinwerk. Die Bücher bieten Ihnen Expertenwissen zu technischen wie auch zu betriebswirtschaftlichen SAP-Themen.

Damit Sie nach weiteren Titeln Ihres Interessengebiets nicht lange suchen müssen, haben wir eine kleine Auswahl zusammengestellt.

Maximilian Münkel
Materialwirtschaft mit SAP S/4HANA – Customizing
649 Seiten, 2021, gebunden
ISBN 978-3-8362-8346-5
www.sap-press.de/5303

Yvonne Lorenz, Birgit Kleinebekel, Uwe Schedl, Matthias Schlaubitz
Qualitätsmanagement mit SAP S/4HANA
827 Seiten, 2021, gebunden
ISBN 978-3-8362-7990-1
www.sap-press.de/5220

Alexander Wolf, Christoph Sting
Produktionsplanung und -steuerung mit SAP S/4HANA. Das Praxishandbuch
692 Seiten, 2021, gebunden
ISBN 978-3-8362-7873-7
www.sap-press.de/5182

André Käber
Warehouse Management mit SAP. Effektive Lagerverwaltung mit WM.
Inkl. Stock Room Management.
666 Seiten, 4., aktualisierte und erweiterte Auflage 2021, gebunden
ISBN 978-3-8362-8437-0
www.sap-press.de/5333